Craniomaxillofacial Trauma

In memory of

Harold Delf Gillies (1882–1960)
Born Dunedin, New Zealand

and

Hugh Bell Cairns (1896–1952)
Born Port Pirie, Australia

two great surgeons whose work remains fundamental in the management of craniomaxillofacial injuries.

For Churchill Livingstone

Commissioning Editor: Miranda Bromage
Copy Editor: Robin Watson
Indexer: Laurence Errington
Design Direction: Erik Bigland
Project Manager: Mark Sanderson
Sales Promotion Executive: Caroline Boyd

Craniomaxillofacial Trauma

A System of Multidisciplinary Management by Members of the Australian Craniofacial Unit

EDITED BY

D. J. David

Head of Department of Plastic and Reconstructive Surgery and Australian Craniofacial Unit, Women's and Children's Hospital and Royal Adelaide Hospital, Adelaide, South Australia

D. A. Simpson

Clinical Professor of Neurosurgery, University of Adelaide; Honorary Neuropathologist, Institute of Medical and Veterinary Science; Senior Research Associate, National Health and Medical Research Council Road Accident Research Unit, University of Adelaide, Adelaide, South Australia

ILLUSTRATIONS BY
Deirdre Cain

Director of the Medical Illustration Unit, Royal Adelaide Hospital, Adelaide, South Australia

CHURCHILL LIVINGSTONE

EDINBURGH   HONG KONG   LONDON   MADRID   MELBOURNE   NEW YORK
AND   TOKYO   1995

CHURCHILL LIVINGSTONE

Medical Division of Pearson Professional Limited

Distributed in the United State of America by Churchill Livingstone Inc., 650 Avenue of the Americas, New York N.Y. 10011, and by associated companies, branches and representatives throughout the world.

© Pearson Professional Limited 1995

First published 1995

ISBN 0 443 04414 7

British Library Cataloguing in Publication Data
A catalogue record for this book is available from the British Library.

Library of Congress Cataloging in Publication Data
A catalog record for this book is available from the Library of Congress.

The publisher's policy is to use **paper manufactured from sustainable forests**

Printed in Great Britain by BPC Wheatons Ltd, Exeter

Contents

Contributors

This book was written by members of the Australian Craniofacial Unit, with assistance from members of the NH & MRC Road Accident Research Unit, University of Adelaide.

Each chapter was prepared by a group of authors whose names appear at the head of the relevant chapter as well as in this list. An asterisk (*) identifies those who have contributed to chapters prepared by other authors.

Amanda H. Abbott BDS BScDent (Hons) PhD
Senior Research Scientist, Australian Craniofacial Unit, Women's and Children's Hospital, Adelaide, South Australia
(*Chapter 7, Appendix II*)

John R. Abbott BScDent (Hons) MDS PhD FADM
Deputy Director, Craniofacial Research, Women's and Children's Hospital, Adelaide; Senior Visiting Dental Consultant, Plastic and Reconstructive Surgery, Royal Adelaide Hospital, Adelaide, South Australia
(*Chapters 5, 10*, 12, 21, 22**)

J. A. Barritt OAM DipSocSci
Senior Social Worker, Plastic and Reconstructive Surgery Unit, Australian Craniofacial Unit, Royal Adelaide Hospital and Women's and Children's Hospital, Adelaide, South Australia
(*Chapters 10, 22**)

Tasman Brown AM MDS DDSc FRACDS FICD
Emeritus Professor, Department of Dentistry, University of Adelaide; Consultant Research Director, Australian Craniofacial Unit, Women's and Children's Hospital, Adelaide, South Australia
(*Chapters 2, 12, 19*, 22*, 23*)

Stephen B. Cantrell DDS MD
Craniofacial Surgery Fellow, Australian Craniofacial Unit; Affiliate Registrar, Plastic and Reconstructive Surgery, Royal Adelaide Hospital, Adelaide, South Australia
(*Chapter 21**)

B. Clark BDS MB BS FRCR
Consultant Radiologist, Women's and Children's Hospital, Adelaide, South Australia
(*Chapter 7, Appendix II*)

Rodney D. Cooter MB BS MD (Adel) FRACS
Senior Lecturer in Plastic and Reconstructive Surgery, University of Adelaide; Consultant Plastic and Reconstructive Surgeon, The Queen Elizabeth Hospital, Woodville, South Australia
(*Chapters 2* and 6*)

John L. Crompton MB BS FRACO FRACS
Clinical Lecturer, Department of Surgery, University of Adelaide; Head of Neuro-ophthalmology Unit, Royal Adelaide Hospital, Adelaide; Consultant Ophthalmologist to the Surgeon-General, Australian Defence Forces, Canberra, Australia
(*Chapters 2*, 6*, 14, 18, 22*, Appendix IV*)

Lachlan L. Daenke BDS DipAppPsych FRACDS
Private Endodontic Practice, Adelaide; Endodontic Consultant to Australian Craniofacial Unit, Adelaide, South Australia
(*Chapter 12*)

David J. David AC FRCS FRCS (Ed)
Head, Department of Plastic and Reconstructive Surgery and Australian Craniofacial Unit, Women's and Children's Hospital and Royal Adelaide Hospital; Chief of Surgery, Women's and Children's Hospital, Adelaide, South Australia
(*Chapters 1, 2, 5*, 8, 9, 11, 16, 21, 23*)

Robert M. Edwards MB MS BS FFARACS FANZCA
Anaesthetist, Australian Craniofacial Unit, Royal Adelaide Hospital; Director of Anaesthesia and Intensive Care, Modbury Hospital; Commissioner, Operations Branch, St John Ambulance Service, South Australia
(*Chapters 8, 9*, 10, 20*)

Michael E. Hammerton MB BS FRACO FRACS
Senior Consultant Ophthalmologist, Women's and Children's Hospital, Adelaide, South Australia
(*Chapters 2*, 5*, 9*, 14, 18*, 19*, 22*)

Ahmad Hanieh MB ChB FRCS (Glas) FRACS
Director, Department of Neurosurgery, Adelaide Women's and Children's Hospital; Lecturer, University of Adelaide, Adelaide, South Australia
(*Chapters 13*, 19*)

M. M. Jay MB FRCS FRACS
Senior Visiting Specialist in
Otorhinolaryngology, Royal Adelaide
Hospital; Consultant Otorhinolaryngologist
to Australian Craniofacial Unit, Adelaide,
South Australia
(*Chapters 11*, 21, 22**)

I. O. W. Leitch MB BS FRACS
Senior Visiting Plastic Surgeon and Surgeon-
in-Charge of Burns Unit, Royal Adelaide
Hospital; Colonel, Royal Australian Army
Medical Corps
(*Chapters 3*, 4*, 5*, 17*)

A. J. McLean ScD
Director, NH & MRC Road Accident
Research Unit, University of Adelaide,
Adelaide, South Australia
(*Chapters 3, 4, Appendix I*)

Mark H. Moore MB ChB FRACS
Craniofacial Surgeon, Australian
Craniofacial Unit; Senior Visiting Plastic
Surgeon, Royal Adelaide and Women's and
Children's Hospitals; Clinical Senior
Lecturer, University of Adelaide, Adelaide,
South Australia
(*Chapters 8*, 11, 19*)

Michael A. C. Nugent BD ScQLD DOrth RCS
MS FRACDS FRCS MS FSDRACS
Senior Visiting Consultant in Orthodontics,
Women's and Children's Hospital, Adelaide,
South Australia
(*Chapter 21*)

Peter L. Reilly MD BS BMedSc (Hons) FRACS
Director of Research and Development,
Department of Neurosurgery, Royal
Adelaide Hospital; Neurosurgeon, Women's
and Children's Hospital; Clinical Senior
Lecturer, University of Adelaide, Adelaide,
South Australia
(*Chapters 2, 13*)

Donald A. Simpson AM DUniv MS FRCS
FRACS
Clinical Professor of Neurosurgery,
University of Adelaide; Honorary
Neuropathologist, Institute of Medical and
Veterinary Science; Senior Research
Associate, NH & MRC Road Accident
Research Unit, University of Adelaide,
Adelaide, South Australia
(*Chapters 1, 3, 4, 5, 9*, 13, 18*, 19*, 20,
22*, 23*, Apprndix I*)

E. Tan MB BS FRACS MMed
Senior Visiting Plastic Surgeon, Royal
Adelaide and Women's and Children's
Hospitals, Adelaide, South Australia
(*Chapters 14*, 15, 16, 17*, 18*)

John Tomich MB BS FRACS
Consultant Otolaryngologist, Australian
Craniofacial Unit, Women's and Children's
Hospital, Adelaide, South Australia
(*Chapters 2*, 6*, 8*, 15**)

James Trott MB BS FRCS(Glasg) FRACS
Deputy Head, Australian Craniofacial Unit;
Senior Visiting Plastic Surgeon, Royal
Adelaide Hospital and Women's and
Children's Hospital, Adelaide, South
Australia
(*Chapters 6, 9, 10*, 11, 20**)

Ruth V. Walter BS BSocAdmin
Senior Social Worker, Psychiatric Unit,
The Queen Elizabeth Hospital, Adelaide,
South Australia
(*Chapters 10, 17**)

Andrew Murray Whyte BDS(Hons) MB ChB
FFDRSCI DDRRCR FRCR FRACR
Visiting Specialist in Radiology, Flinders
Medical Centre, Bedford Park; Radiologist
to the Joint Consultative Clinic for Head
and Neck Cancer, Royal Adelaide Hospital,
Adelaide, South Australia
(*Chapter 7*)

M. M. Wood BSc(Hons) PhD FBPSS
Associate Professor, Academic Mental
Health Unit, University of New South
Wales; Deputy Director, Rehabilitation and
Community Services, Kenmore Hospital,
Goulburn, New South Wales, Australia
(*Chapter 22, Appendix III*)

P. Woodroffe BA(Hons)
Senior Clinical Psychologist, Department of
Neurosurgery, Women's and Children's
Hospital, Adelaide, South Australia
(*Appendix III*)

Preamble

The craniomaxillofacial (CMF) region has central importance in almost every aspect of human life. If we define this region in anatomical terms, it corresponds to the norma frontalis of cranial osteology: the skull from the coronal suture to the symphysis menti. Here are located the end organs of the special senses of vision, smell and taste: only hearing lies just outside the CMF zone. Here are the upper visceral components of the respiratory and alimentary tracts; behind the frontal bone are the frontal lobes of the brain, of critical importance in intellect, communication and personality. The CMF region is innervated by the cranial nerves, and it receives most of the blood supply of the common carotid arteries. Most importantly, it is the face. The bone of the CMF region and the associated soft tissues, the eyes, and the facial mimetic movements are together the basis of facial aesthetics, and they underlie many aspects of human self-esteem. In preparing this book, we have tried to consider the CMF region from all these viewpoints and, if we have extended somewhat beyond the anatomical confines of the norma frontalis, it is because trauma in the CMF region affects the head as a whole. Blunt impacts and penetrating wounds in the facial area may produce dramatic local injuries, but they may also cause damage in remote parts of the brain of far greater significance in the quantum of long-term disability.

CMF trauma is common in peace and in war; it traverses the conventional boundaries of the surgical specialties and may engage plastic, ENT, and oral surgeons, neurosurgeons and ophthalmic surgeons. Long-term sequelae include functional impairments in many activities: there may be disturbances in mastication, respiration, sight, smell, hearing, lacrimation and salivation and, not least, there may be impairments in the functions of the brain. Aesthetic impairments are common. Psychosocial sequelae include the effects of all these impairments, interacting with the personality of the victim. All the surgical specialists concerned in primary care of CMF trauma have to deal with these sequelae; so do social workers, psychiatrists and specialists in rehabilitation medicine.

CMF trauma presents a seemingly infinite diversity of injury patterns, challenging both in diagnosis, management and biophysical analysis. All the skills of surgeons with specialist commitments in the CMF region are demanded in repair of CMF injuries. Supplementary skills may be needed, notably in microvascular repair and prosthetic reconstruction. Great experience is often necessary to evaluate priorities and timing, even when the overall needs of the patient are clear. Such experience comes only from study of a large number of cases.

The pioneering work of the French plastic surgeon Paul Tessier established craniofacial surgery as a discipline in its own right. His achievement was based chiefly in responses to the challenges seen in congenital deformities, and his work has led to the development of craniofacial units throughout the world. The structure of the modern craniofacial unit makes it ideally fitted to undertake the holistic care of the victims of CMF trauma, and to bring to their manifold problems the wide intellectual perspectives and technical skills evolved in the surgery of CMF diseases of other types. However, many cases of CMF trauma must be managed in less specialized units, often by surgeons with little experience of these very complex injuries.

This book has been written with two main aims. The first is to present the system of specialized CMF trauma management evolved in the Australian Craniofacial Unit (ACFU) since its foundation in 1975. This multidisciplinary unit, which is based on two long-established teaching hospitals, now treats some 400 Australian victims of CMF injury annually; it also acts as a referral centre for the management of complex problems arising from injuries sustained elsewhere in the world, notably in South East Asia and in the Middle East. Our experience has generated studies into patterns of CMF fractures and cerebral injuries, with implications both in management and injury prevention. These researches have drawn on the experience of the ACFU in three-dimensional imaging, and on the work of the National Health and Medical Research Council (NH & MRC) Road Accident Research Unit in analyzing the craniocerebral injuries caused by traffic crashes.

Our second aim has been to show the relevance of this specialized system in general trauma practice. The work of the ACFU is integrated in a trauma management service that has been developed in the state of South Australia in response to the challenges of distance and demography: this state is large (approximately 984 000 km^2) and thinly populated (approximately 1.4 million), and many cases of acute trauma must necessarily be managed in remote places, at least in the first instance. We believe that we have learned, often from our own errors, some lessons that may be helpful to any medical practitioner confronted with injuries in the CMF region.

Adelaide   D.J.D.
1995   D.A.S.

Acknowledgements

The authors of this book acknowledge with much gratitude the help given by colleagues in the Royal Adelaide and Women's and Children's Hospitals, the Institute of Medical and Veterinary Science and the Child Health Research Institute; they are too numerous to list, but we wish to thank especially Professor B. Vernon-Roberts, Dr D. Hansman and Dr L. Reade, without whom our chapter on the pathology of injury and repair would have been wholly inadequate, and Dr A. T. Davis for his valuable comments on post-traumatic stress. Mr Kingsley Coulthard (Pharmacist at the Women's and Children's Hospital, Adelaide) and Ms Jill Lenton (Dietician at the Royal Adelaide Hospital) advised us in their fields of special expertise, as did Dr J. LaBrooy, Dr M. Gaughwin and Dr P. Harding (Physicians at the Royal Adelaide Hospital) and Dr K. Cheney (Haematologist, Australian Red Cross). Dr J. Barker contributed valuably with respect to the orthodontic correction of deformities. Dr O. Holubowycz (NH & MRC Road Accident Research Unit) gave us much advice and unpublished statistics on the epidemiology of alcohol and road crashes. Mrs Andrea Simpson and other legal friends assisted us in the sections on medicolegal issues. Ms Julie Baker gave much help in the preparation of chapters dealing with various aspects of ophthalmology.

Vice-Admiral Sir James Watt, Dr J. Knott (Australian National University), Mr D. J. Penn (Imperial War Museum) and Dr G. A. Ryan helped us most generously in our consideration of the history of cranio-maxillofacial trauma. Professor Sir William Manchester of the University of Auckland (NZ) shared with us some of his unique experience in mandibular reconstruction and Professors S. A. Shapiro (North Indiana University, USA), A. Sahar (Tel-Aviv University, Israel) and Nguyen Thuong Xuan (Viet-Duc Hospital, Hanoi, Vietnam) gave us, with equal generosity, some of their experience in the management of cranio-cerebral injuries.

Illustrations were kindly contributed by Mr R. Cooter from his unpublished MD thesis, Dr Prema Iyer, Dr V. Luks, Dr L. C. Richards, Dr A. Sandhu and Professor G. C. Townsend, and from overseas by Dr Carleton Gajdusek of the National Institute for Neurological Diseases and Stroke, Bethesda, Maryland, USA; other acknowledgements are made in appropriate legends. Most of the photographic illustrations were prepared in the Foundation Studios, Women's and Children's Hospital, whose staff we thank for their skill and patience. We thank Mr Colin Smith (Archivist of the Royal Australasian College of Surgeons) for access to wartime illustrations by Sir Daryl Lindsay.

Dr G. Guzman-Stein and Dr L. H. Lim were instrumental in preparing case audits and helped us in many other ways. Dr S. B. Cantrell was particularly helpful in the preparation of Chapter 21 with his many modern suggestions. Mrs Louise Netherway undertook the final preparation of the typescript and assisted us in other tedious labours, all done with great efficiency.

D.J.D.
D.A.S.

CHAPTER 1

Historical perspectives

D. A. Simpson   D. J. David

CAUSES OF INJURY IN THE CRANIOMAXILLOFACIAL REGION

THE HEAD AS A TARGET IN WAR AND CRIME

Primate evolution has made the human head very vulnerable to frontal impacts. In other species, the face is more protective: birds have beaks, reptiles have armoured snouts and most mammals have prognathous jaws, evolved to house large olfactory organs or for predatory mastication, but also serving to absorb impact energy. In the evolution of *Homo sapiens*, the sense of smell has become less important and mastication less aggressive. Concurrently, the nose and jaws have receded (Fig. 1.1A), and the cerebral hemispheres — enormous when compared with other primates — bulge forward in the frontal region, an attractive target for blows and missiles (Fig. 1.1B). The frontal skull is thick and has considerable defensive value, both for the brain and for the eyes recessed in the bony orbits, but this skeletal protection has limits and often fails when challenged by blunt or sharp objects.

The vulnerability of the human head would have fewer consequences if we were less pugnacious and less inventive. But *Homo sapiens* is both aggressive and ingenious: wars and murderous assaults are older than recorded history and in these conflicts the face and head have always been a favoured target. Hand-held clubs, spears and swords have been in military use since remote antiquity and so have missiles. Slingshots and arrows were not new when Troy fell, about 1250 BC; Homer's *Iliad* (c. 800 BC) has many very precise references to missile wounds of the brain and face, penetrating wounds from arrows and bronze-pointed javelins, and blunt impacts

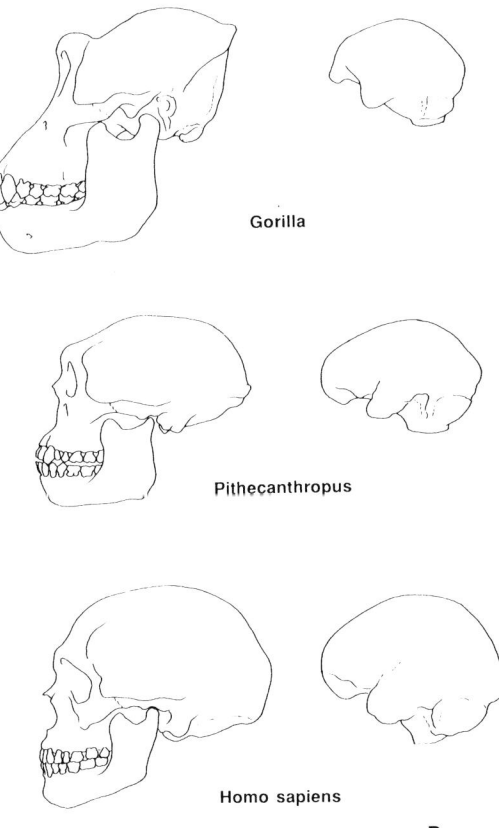

Gorilla

Pithecanthropus

Homo sapiens

A   B

Fig. 1.1 The face in primates: a changing target. Craniofacial evolution in the gorilla, a primitive hominid (*Pithecanthropus*), and man (*Homo sapiens*). Reproduced by permission from W. E. LeGros Clark, *The Antecedents of Man*. 2nd edn, 1962, Edinburgh University Press. **A** The facial skeleton shows recession of the jaws and increasing prominence of the frontal bone. **B** Endocranial casts show increase in the bulk and prominence of the frontal and temporal lobes of the brain.

by stones that could shatter a soldier's helmet; Adamson (1977) found mention of 59 head or neck wounds in Homer's Iliad, of which 45 were lethal.

Weapons driven by human muscles have limited killing power. Muscular energy can be stored in a stretched bow or a tensed catapult and released to propel an arrow or a bolt; the long history of human violence records many facial and cerebral wounds from these weapons. Perhaps the most famous is the death of Harold, king of the Saxons, supposedly from an orbitocranial arrow wound, sustained in 1066, a year renowned as one of the only two 'memorable' dates in English history (Sellars & Yeatman 1930). Asian history records a similar arrow wound, equally dramatic and better authenticated: the second battle of Panipat (1556) was won, and the future of India was decided, when a Mughal arrow blinded the brilliant Hindu general Hemu at a tactical crisis in the battle. Missiles propelled by chemical energy have far greater power. Gunpowder — a mixture of saltpetre, charcoal and sulphur — came into use c. AD 1300, and by the sixteenth century was employed by all civilized armies. Cannon, mines and the matchlock muskets of Spanish, Turkish and Japanese professional soldiers made this century the age of the gunpowder empires, and inflicted appalling wounds that were so often septic that they seemed to be poisoned.

Advances in the design of offensive weapons were paralleled by improved systems of defence, and the obvious vulnerability of the face and head inspired the helmet (Gurdjian 1973). Awareness of the need for brain protection is evident in the leather and metal helmets worn by soldiers in Mediterranean and Middle East armies well before 1200 BC. Greek soldiers also saw a need for facial protection: Greek heavy infantry used well-designed helmets that covered the whole face, with a nasal bar to ward off sword slashes (Fig. 1.2). These full-face helmets restricted vision, and Greek warriors are often shown with their helmets pushed up; the introduction of hinged visors in the European Middle Ages gave the option of an open-faced helmet, and important persons used visored helmets well into the seventeenth century (Fig. 1.3). As late as 1641, a French army commander is said to have inadvertently blown out his brains by pushing up his visor with a loaded pistol. But these visors also reduced the user's field of vision, and some soldiers preferred to take their chances without facial protection. Francois de Guise (1519–1563) got a lance through his face in this way at the attack on Boulogne in 1545: the iron point went in below the eye and out behind the ear, lodging so firmly that it had to be extracted with blacksmith's pincers (Paré 1649, Hamby 1967).

Advances in musketry and military organization exposed the soldier to increasing numbers of missiles, with increasing accuracy and hitting power (Parker 1988). In

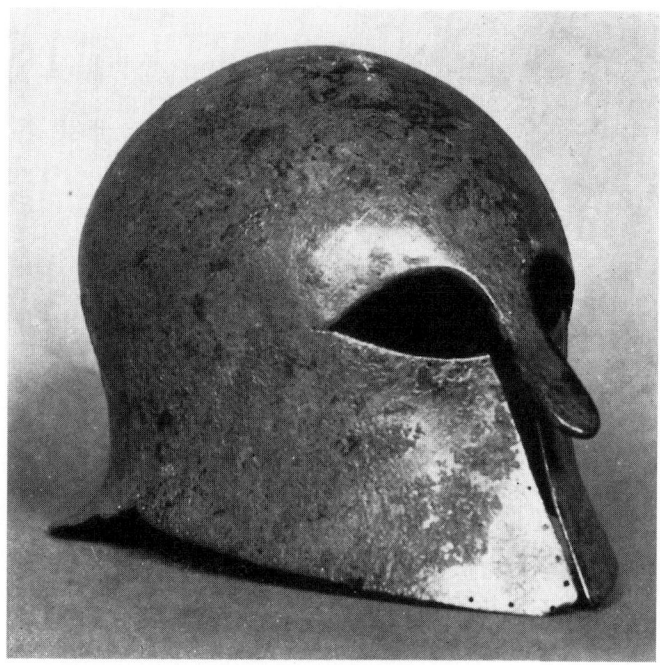

Fig. 1.2 The Corinthian helmet. Bronze helmet, used by Greek heavy infantry (hoplites) in the fifth century BC. Reproduced by permission from E. S. Gurdjian, *Head Injury from Antiquity to the Present with Special Reference to Penetrating Head Wounds*, 1973, Charles C. Thomas, Springfield, Illinois.

the seventeenth century, what would now be called the military–industrial complex, led by arms magnates in Liège, Holland and Sweden, organized mass production of standardized firearms in great quantities. The smooth-bored musket increasingly dominated the battlefield (Figs 1.4 and 1.5A); it was soon supplemented by the rifle, more accurate and with greater muzzle velocity. Snipers were armed with rifles as early as the Thirty Years War (1618–1648); rifles were used by guerillas on both sides of the War of American Independence (1775–1781), and by British light infantry in 1800. Breechloaders gave faster rates of fire, but the early designs were unreliable, and in the fierce battles of the American Civil War (1861–1865) both sides chiefly relied on muzzle-loading 0.58 in. rifled muskets firing 'minny balls', the cylindroconical lead bullets designed by C. E. Minié, a French officer of Chasseurs (Fig. 1.5B). The international armament industry became very competitive: designs were rapidly improved and in the Franco-Prussian War (1870–1871), single-shot breech-loading rifles were in service in both armies. Magazine rifles were introduced in the chief European armies by 1890, and also machine guns. These weapons fired smaller bullets, approximately 0.3 in. in diameter (Fig. 1.5C), driven by new propellants more powerful than gunpowder, giving greater range and impact force. Cordite, a smokeless mixture of nitrocellulose and nitroglycerine, gave the British .303 in. service rifles of

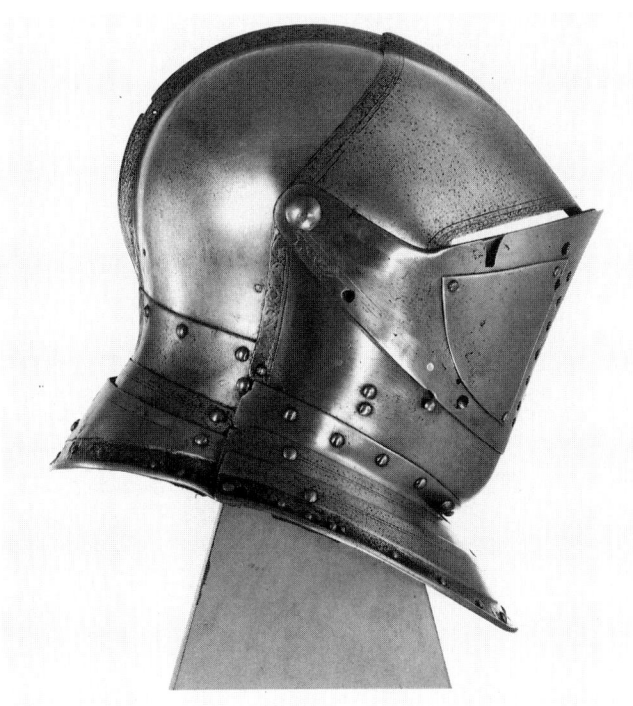

A

1900 a muzzle velocity in the range 600–800 m/s, whereas smoothbore muskets fired with black powder seldom bettered 300 m/s. The first Hague Convention (1899) outlawed expanding bullets, but to offset this humane aspiration, new bullet designs produced high velocity missiles able to cause still more massive tissue destruction. The effects of higher muzzle velocities on the face and brain are discussed in Chapter 4. Automatic rifles and hand-held submachine guns came into general military use during World War II (1939–1945), at first for close combat, but later as standard equipment; today, the Russian Kalashnikov 7.62 mm assault rifle is the characteristic weapon of the terrorist/freedom fighter throughout the world.

Naval cannon appeared very early, and became the decisive weapon at sea, where the impact of roundshot was multiplied by splinters struck from the ship's timbers. Cannon firing musket balls in bags or in a tin case inflicted appalling wounds at close range. Richard Wiseman (c. 1622–1676), then a young surgeon serving on the king's side in the English Civil War (1642–1646), noted this at the siege of Taunton.

One of Colonel John Arundell's men, in storming the Works, was shot in the Face by Case-shot. He . . . was carried off among the dead and laid in an empty house.

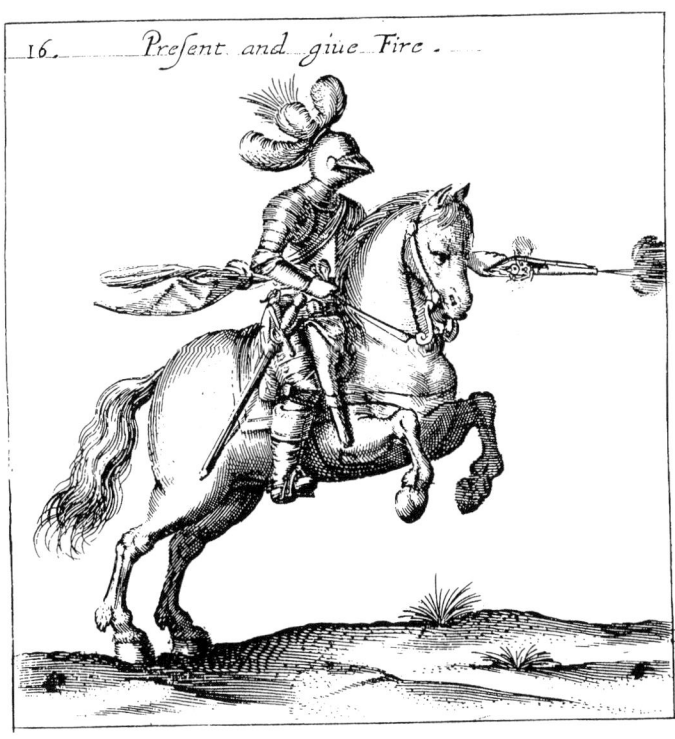

B

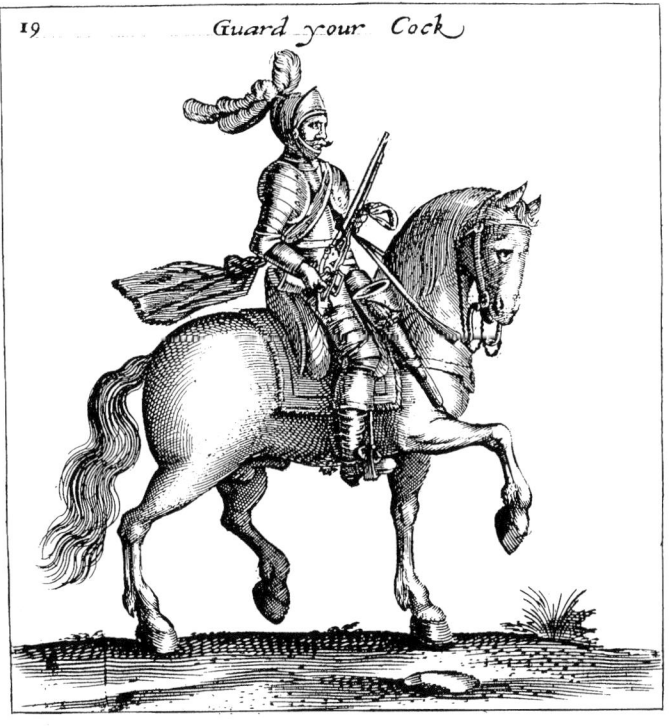

C

Fig. 1.3 Full head protection in the sixteenth and seventeenth centuries. A Tournament helmet, made for King Henry VIII of England in 1540. The hinged visor gave facial protection but limited vision. By courtesy of the Board of Trustees of the Royal Armouries, UK. **B** Cavalry trooper of the Thirty Years War, charging with his visor down. **C** After he has fired, he reloads with his visor up. From John Cruso, *Militarie Instructions for the Cavallerie*, 1632.

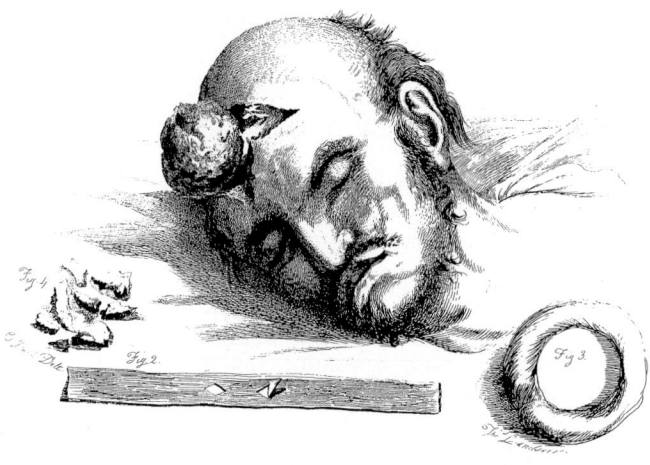

Fig. 1.4 Frontal missile wounds in the Napoleonic wars. Cerebral fungus or herniation resulting from a musket ball wound, presumably sustained at Waterloo 18th June, 1815. Herniations of this type have been a common sequel of battlefield wounds as late as World War II. From C. Bell, *Illustrations of the Great Operations of Surgery*, 1821.

In the morning early, the Colonel marching by that house heard a knocking within against the Door. Some of the Officers desiring to know what it was, lookt in, and saw this man standing by the Door without Eye, Face, Nose, or Mouth . . . . His Face, with his Eyes, Nose, Mouth, and forepart of the Jaws, with the Chin, was shot away, and the remaining parts of them driven in. One part of the Jaw hung down by his Throat, and the other part pasht into it. I saw the Brain working out underneath the lacerated Scalp on both sides between his Ears and Brows. (Wiseman 1977)

The man lived at least 6 days, being able to drink by holding down the root of his tongue.

Concurrently, advances were made in killing by fragmentation missiles. Hand-thrown grenades and bombs shot from mortars were used in the sixteenth and seventeenth centuries; shells fired from howitzers came somewhat later. Difficulties in devising accurate fuses were slowly overcome; in the siege of Gibraltar (1781) Henry Shrapnel, a young English officer, saw the benefits of fusing shells so that they would burst in the air and by the time of the American Civil War, explosive shells accounted for a sizeable minority of head wounds (Otis, 1870). In the great wars of the twentieth century, more soldiers were killed or wounded by shells than by bullets (Reister, 1975). In World War I (1914–1918), shrapnel shells charged with high explosives such as trinitrotoluene caused so many head wounds that steel helmets came back to give head protection especially against relatively low velocity fragmentation missiles (p. 115). Such helmets remain a military necessity, and are now fitted with polycarbonate visors for eye protection; steel has been replaced by laminated composites of aramid fibres (Kevlar®), giving 35% greater protection without increased weight.

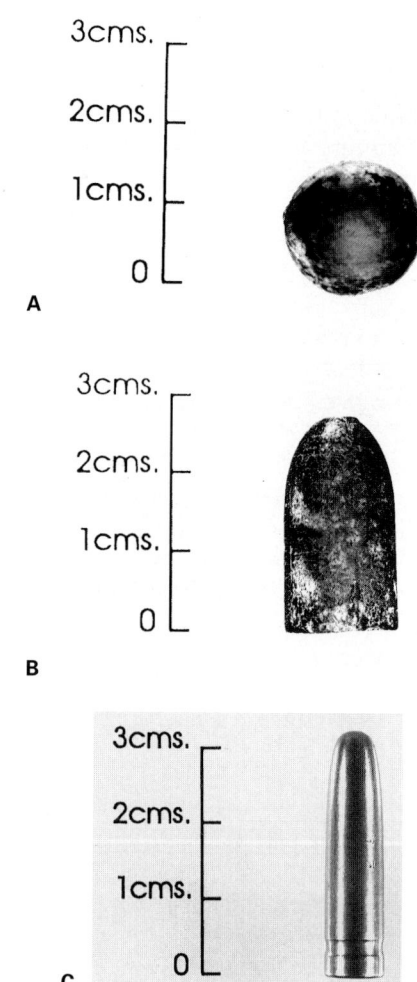

Fig. 1.5 A century of military missiles. A British service musket ball, diameter 0.693 in., as used at Waterloo. By courtesy of the Trustees of the Imperial War Museum, London. **B** British Enfield 1853 rifle bullet, diameter 0.550 in., with a hollow base to engage in the rifling of the barrel when fired. Such bullets were used by both sides in the American Civil War, though lacking the grooving of the United States Army pattern Minié bullet. By courtesy of the Trustees of the Imperial War Museum, London. **C** British Army Service rifle bullet, diameter 0.303 in., as used in the First and Second World Wars: probably a Mark VI bullet, approved in 1904.

The brothers Wright, and also Graf Zeppelin, made it possible to drop bombs from the air. This was also outlawed by the Hague convention, but ten years after the Wrights' first flight in 1903, the potential of air attacks was being eagerly touted by science-fiction writers like H. G. Wells and by the nascent aerospace industry (Grahame-White & Harper 1914). High explosive bombs were used early in World War I, and also incendiary bombs, containing phosphorus and other combustibles.

Fire is a very ancient weapon and wartime facial burns have a long history. Byzantine warships carried 'Greek fire', an inflammable liquid containing bitumen, naphtha or pitch, which was sprayed by bellows through copper nozzles (Watt 1980); this was used in sea fights with the Arabs as early as the seventh century AD. In 1915, burning oils propelled by compressed nitrogen were used in trench warfare, initially with terrifying effect. Since the first use of gunfire in naval war, burns have been a dreaded feature of sea fights; even modern warships burn furiously, as was seen in the Falklands War. Fire is a horrible concomitant of air warfare, both for aircrew and for the victims of bombing; napalm (a mixture of petroleum and palm oil derivatives) has often been dropped from aircraft, with varying degrees of discrimination, and white phosphorus has also been used. These agents are capable of inflicting very severe facial burns (Fig. 17.11).

As might be expected, firearms were early used in crime as well as in war: muskets and pistols were used in several sixteenth-century political assassinations, and private ambushes are mentioned by surgical writers of the period. As military firearms evolved and diversified, the criminal classes were quick to see the utility of the smaller handguns. Pistols, originally used chiefly as a cavalry weapon, were easily hidden in pockets or under cloaks; in violent societies, pistols came to replace the sword for 'self-protection' and as a part of the male image. British duellists took to pistols rather than swords in the eighteenth century, and became even more dangerous. It seems that the usual target was the trunk, but head wounds were not unknown. The Irish surgeon Sylvester O'Halloran (1728–1807), in his racy account (1793) of the high incidence of head injuries in Munster ('our people, invincibly brave, ... and highly irritable, soon catch fire ... to this add the frequent abuse of spirituous liquors, particularly whiskey...') reported one such duel: the gallant 0'C., an excellent shot, was himself struck by a ball in the temple and died of what reads like cerebritis. These duels were usually fought with single-shot pistols. There was felt to be a need for pistols capable of more than one shot and in 1835, Samuel Colt patented his famous revolver: it was not a new idea, but Colt's reliable weapons became popular throughout the world, and their descendants are still very much with us. While rifles can be used in hunting animals, pistols are primarily intended to kill people, and as soon as they became cheap enough to be purchased by the lower classes, governments began to try to restrict possession of these dangerous weapons to those considered to be socially responsible. In 1602, the viceroy of Catalonia prohibited pistols less than 90 cm long, 'in an attempt to reduce the death rate in the principality' (Elliott, 1963); the spirited Catalans greatly resented this early gun law and it had little effect. Later gun laws have had varied success, but no government has succeeded in the logical measure of total abolition, except the Tokugawa administration in Japan. Ieyasu, the first and greatest Tokugawa shogun, took control of the firearms industry in 1609, and his successors cut back

production until the nation was virtually without guns (Parker 1988).

THE HEAD IN TRAFFIC ACCIDENTS

War is of course not the only historic cause of injuries of the face and head. Traffic accidents are today the leading cause of serious head injuries in most parts of the world, and these also have a long history. The horse has been domesticated for more than four millennia. In Iraq, the Sumerians used horses to pull chariots around 2000 BC and somewhat later horses were ridden, with control by bridles and bits. Nobody who has ridden or driven horses will doubt that this great technical achievement must have led almost immediately to accidents and head injuries. There is an account of a Chinese chariot accident in the oracular archives of the Shang dynasty (c. 1600–1000 BC): one of King Wuding's courtiers was thrown out of his chariot when it hit an obstacle at high speed. (Gao Jian-Guo, personal communication.) A few hundred years later there is a literary reference to a chariot accident causing craniofacial injury in Homer's *Iliad*. Eumelus is thrown in the course of a very dirty chariot race, when his vehicle is sabotaged by the goddess Athene: he suffers facial abrasions and is temporarily speechless, but recovers. No doubt there were many such accidents; a galloping horse can reach a speed of 50 km/h, and at this speed fatal head injuries can easily result from falls, impacts against trees or other overhanging objects, or collisions with pedestrians. In imperial Rome, better roads and a very self-indulgent aristocracy gave rise to complaints about bad driving (Ammanius Marcellinus quoted by Gibbon 1854). Juvenal (c. AD 60–140) also listed heavy road transport as one of the lethal hazards of Roman traffic.

In the Renaissance, there are several case reports of facial and cranial injuries from riding accidents. Giovanni da Vigo (?1460–1520) mentions a gentleman in the service of the duke of Urbino who fell from his horse onto a rock surface: his whole face swelled, and he was mute for 20 days, but recovered with a permanent speech defect that sounds like a dysphasia. Transport accidents were common in the seventeenth century. In the civilian practice of Richard Wiseman, such accidents apparently accounted for a fifth of all the reported injuries; a typical example is the Lady who was wounded 'down the whole length of the Forehead to the Nose, also transverse the left Eye-brow...; her Eye and Face were also much bruised. It happened to her travelling in a Hackney-Coach [i.e. a taxi], upon the jetting [jolting] whereof she was thrown out of the hinder Seat against a Bar of Iron in the forepart of the Coach' (Wiseman 1977). In the eighteenth century, Percivall Pott (1714–1788) described 43 cases of head injury, of which 12 (27.9%) were riding or carriage

Table 1.1 Head injuries in eighteenth century London (from Pott 1779)

		No. of cases	%
Industry	Scaffolding	5	
	Cranes	2	
	Other	4	
	Total	11	25.6
Roads	Carriages and carts	6	
	Riding horses	5	
	Hitting horses	1	
	Total	12	27.9
Assault etc.	By relatives or neighbours	4	
	By rioters	2	
	By school masters	1	
	By the French (naval war)	1	
	Suicides	1	
	Total	9	20.9
Sport	Cricket	2	
	Quoits	1	
	Cudgels	1	
	Total	4	9.3
Miscellaneous	(including falls)	7	16.3
Total		43	100.00

accidents, some of them alcohol-related: the series gives a picture very familiar to modern accident surgeons (Table 1.1).

In the nineteenth century, the horse was supplemented by steam power. Passenger-carrying steam trains came in England in 1825, and as early as 1839 the Great Western Railway provided a fine museum specimen of a skull base fracture for the Royal College of Surgeons. Steam road carriages followed, but were restrained by a speed limit of 4 miles/h, enforced by an act of parliament that required a man holding a red flag to precede the steam car.

The modern motor car was born in 1884–1886, when Gottlieb Daimler (1834–1900) invented an effective internal combustion engine powered by petrol, and installed it in a four-wheeled vehicle; the horseless carriage then became a practicable means of road transport (Overy 1992, Lay 1993). At first the killing power of the motor car was underestimated, and complaints centred on its effects on the emotional balance of horses. The first automobile crash is said to have occurred in France, in 1893, when a vehicle driven by Baron de Zuylen struck a motor brake belonging to the Comte de Dion; happily these noblemen escaped serious injury (Ryan 1965). Lay (1993) gives 1896 as the year of the first motor martyrs; a London pedestrian, Ms Bridget Driscoll, was killed despite warning cries from the driver of a car, and in the same year Emile Levassor was killed in a motor race from Paris to Marseilles. In 1899, one of Daimler's fine wagonettes demonstrated its killing power near Harrow (UK). A wheel broke — it was made of inferior (non-British) oak — at perhaps 14 miles/h (Fig. 1.6). The

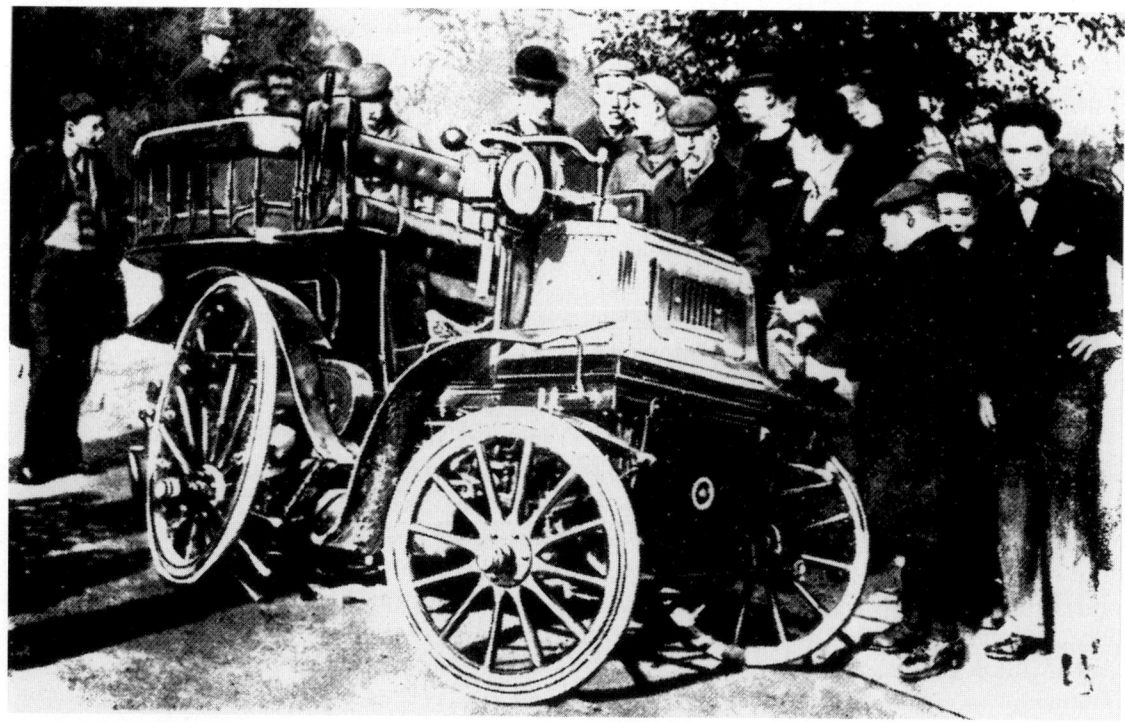

Fig. 1.6 'Sad fatality at Harrow'. Accident to a Daimler waggonette driven by Engineer E. A. Sewell when carrying five gentlemen on 25 February 1899. The right rear wheel collapsed at an estimated speed of 15 miles/h: Sewell and his front seat passenger were ejected and killed. By courtesy of Dr G. A. Ryan.

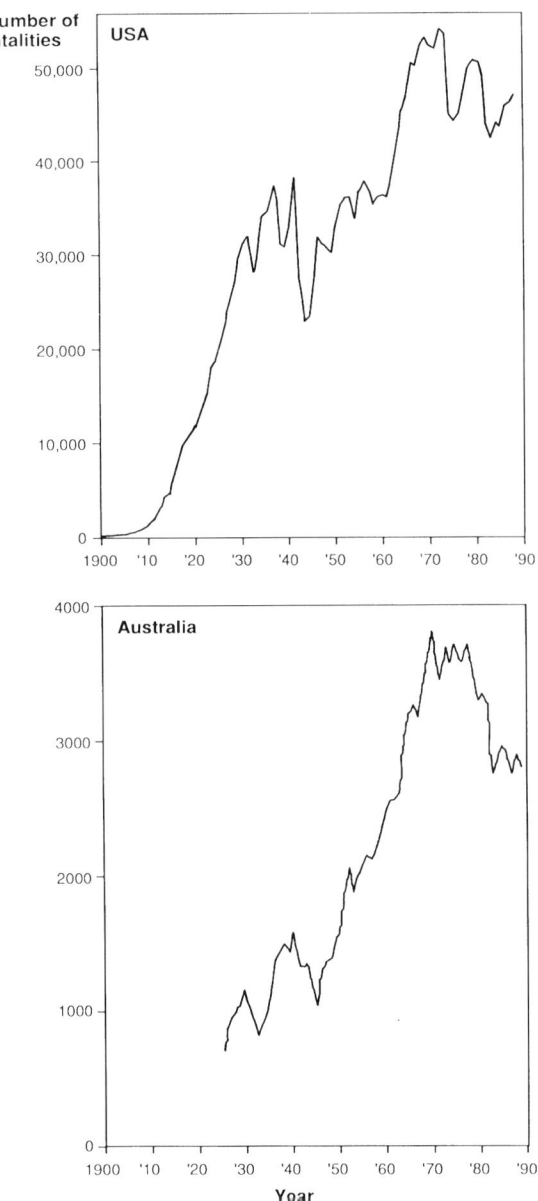

Fig. 1.7 Road deaths in the USA and Australia, 1900–1990. The graphs show simultaneously a fall after 1970, presumably as a result of safety measures. By courtesy of J. W. Knott (in press) and L. Evans (1991).

driver (Engineer E. A. Sewell) was killed instantly, and a passenger, Major J. S. Richer, died a few days later in coma (Anonymous 1899). After the World War I the rising mortality rate from car crashes caused great public concern in the USA and other motorized societies, and this has mounted ever since, until at last concern has been implemented in legislation and the road toll has in most countries begun to fall (Fig. 1.7).

THE HEAD AS A TARGET IN SPORT

Boxing is an ancient sport. Greek and Roman boxers fought wearing the cestus, a leather knuckleduster, and there are literary accounts of well-placed blows damaging the face and brain. In Vergil's *Aeneid* (written 30–19 BC) a champion boxer wears gloves loaded with lead and iron, and stained with blood and brains from previous sporting contests. In nineteenth-century England, boxing was made more humane by padded gloves and by the rules associated with the 8th Marquis of Queensberry, Oscar Wilde's adversary, described by him as the screaming scarlet marquis. Boxing persists today, as the only sport in which brain injury, real or token, is the chief aim.

In the past, there were other sports in which the head and face were targets. Roman gladiators suffered head wounds; the great Galen (c. AD 131–199) spent some years as surgeon to the gladiators of his native town Pergamon, and mentions their depressed skull fractures. Medieval tournaments often ended with head injuries; even the formalized contests of Renaissance elites could have unhappy consequences. Both Henry VIII of England (1491–1547) and Henri II of France (1519–1559) suffered head impacts when jousting in full armour. Henry VIII survived this head injury, and also another sustained in pole vaulting: his apologists have attributed his later behaviour to traumatic or anoxic brain damage. Henri II died of an accidental orbitocranial wound complicated by a chronic subdural haematoma or empyema. For the lower classes there were other martial sports, such as cudgels. Percivall Pott (1779) mentions a young player who received a blow on the forehead: 'it did not seem to himself or to the spectators a severe one, but as it produced blood, it was deemed by the laws of the game a broken head', and he lost the match, as well as developing what sounds like an extradural abscess.

Sports played with balls, or bats and balls, are not intended to cause craniofacial injuries, but have often done so. Again, Pott provides a typical eighteenth-century example: a boy struck in the forehead by a cricket bat, who later developed a frontal extradural abscess, cured by trephining. Cricket ball injuries of the head or face became quite common in the twentieth century, with the rise of fast bowling aimed at the body of the batsman; in the 1977/8 World Cup Cricket Series, a leading batsman first appeared wearing a helmet, and since then serious players of cricket usually wear helmets with visors. Baseball batsmen also use helmets. Football might be thought less likely to lead to head injuries, but the vigour of the game and its opportunities for head contacts make this, in all its forms, a common cause of craniofacial injury, in the past as now. Sir Thomas Elyot (c. 1495–1546) saw the Tudor form of football as 'nothyng but beastely fury and extreme violence, whereof proceedeth hurte and consequently rancour and malice do remayne with thym that be wounded.' However, football is not usually thought to demand protective headgear, except in the USA where fullface helmets have long been considered necessary for serious players. Richard Schneider (1966), an authority on the American form of this robust game, collected 225 cases of serious or fatal injury from football over a 5-year period: of these, 75% were craniocerebral injuries.

CRANIOFACIAL INJURY IN FALLS AND INDUSTRIAL ACCIDENTS

Falls must always have been responsible for such injuries. Industrial head injuries are doubtless as old as building scaffolds and underground mines; in Pott's (1779) series of head injuries, industrial accidents were almost as numerous as road accidents. Steam engines, introduced into the mining industry in England as early as 1712, presumably increased the risks. In the nineteenth century, concern over industrial accidents was widespread; Hudson (1877) described head injuries among Cornish miners, and mentioned the routine use of protective hard hats. Facial burns and scalds were also a frequent concomitant of the industrial revolution.

FACIAL MUTILATION

In the ancient world, punitive facial mutilation was a favoured way of humiliating and tormenting one's enemies (Adamson, 1990). Later, such mutilations were reserved for criminals, especially those of low social rating; in 1637, the King of England's judges removed the ears of a barrister, a clergyman and a doctor of medicine, and this was meant as an especially humiliating punishment for persons of upper middle class status, who would not ordinarily be penalized in this way. In India, nasal mutilation was used on a large scale and for a long time. Thus, Tipu Sultan (1750–1799) the brilliant ruler of Mysore, when at war with the British, offered a pagoda (gold coin weighing about 3.4 g) for each nose removed from a supporter of the English East India Company (McDowell, 1977); modern plastic surgery has been dated from the successful treatment of a victim of this campaign (p. 16). Still more recently, similar mutilations were reported in Africa, during wars of liberation: persons caught smoking enemy cigarettes were likely to lose their lips.

Apart from these punitive disfigurements of the face, many ancient and recent cultural practices involve mutilations of the face and orofacial soft tissues, whether as rituals or for aesthetic reasons. Examples of decorative mutilation include chipping and filing tooth crowns, tooth adornment with inlays or overlays of various materials, evulsion of teeth, facial tattooing, septal perforation, piercing and plugging of the lips, removal of the uvula and facial scarring (Wilson et al 1992).

In most parts of the world today, judicial and political penalties do not include facial mutilation; it is perhaps the only historic cause of facial injury that has been largely eliminated. Decorative mutilations are also less prevalent, though it is possible to find parallels with these in some aspects of modern aesthetic surgery.

THE EVOLUTION OF SURGICAL CONCEPTS AND TECHNIQUES

CRANIOMAXILLOFACIAL SURGERY IN ANTIQUITY

The record of craniomaxillofacial (CMF) trauma over the last 4000 years is paralleled by the history of endeavours to heal the wounds, mend the fractures and restore an acceptable appearance, undertaken by men and women who can be called surgeons, whether they were seen by their contemporaries as priests, wizards, physicians or skilled craftsmen. The Edwin Smith Papyrus, written about 1600 BC but conveying much older thinking (Breasted 1930), gives in didactic form the practice of an Egyptian surgeon. Cases are described, with treatment policies: nasal fractures and dislocated mandibles are to be treated, but skull fractures with neurological signs such as a squint or gait disorder, or infected jaw fractures, are illnesses not to be treated (Hoffmann-Axthelm, 1982). Whereas much Egyptian medicine is concerned with drugs and incantations, the surgeon behind this papyrus seems rational and objective. Majno (1991) notes that Egyptian wound treatment included skin closure by adhesive tapes and possibly by sutures; he has tested the bactericidal action of the favourite Egyptian wound salve, honey and grease, and found it effective against staphylococci and coliform bacilli.

In ancient Iraq, medical literature surviving in cuneiform inscriptions stresses the therapeutic role of magic. Excavations from Nineveh are said to have discovered scalpels, a saw and a bronze trephine, but there is apparently no literary evidence of surgical treatment, beyond the famous malpractice laws of Hammurabi enacting amputation for unsuccessful operations on persons of noble rank, and lesser penalties for accidents in operations on slaves.

Information on Indian medicine stems from the Sanskrit Vedas; these include the Susruta Samhita, supposedly written around 600 BC, which describes surgical procedures including restoration of a mutilated nose by swinging down a pedicled flap from the forehead. This procedure is the Indian rhinoplasty, practised by members of a specific caste over the next 2000 years and still in general use (Fig. 17.18).

The surviving memorials of trauma management in antiquity portray the responses of thoughtful surgeons confronted with the challenge of facial wounds and skull fractures. Doubtless there were many such surgeons who left no written memorials, yet transmitted their skills and experience verbally to enrich surgical thinking in India, the Middle East and the eastern Mediterranean.

GRAECO-ROMAN AND ARABIC SURGERY OF THE HEAD AND FACE

In the fifth century BC, Kos, a small Greek island state, produced the towering but shadowy personality of Hippocrates (c. 470–400 BC). The Hippocratic collection, the body of writings attributed to him but now thought to have been written somewhat later, inaugurated a succession of surgical texts that were extended through the Hellenistic and Roman periods, to live on for more than a thousand years in Byzantine compilations. In the field of CMF surgery, the most interesting works in the Hippocratic collection are the treatises 'On Wounds in the Head' and 'On Joints' (Hippocrates, 1927). The first describes trephining for head wounds. It is clear that the operator was careful and thoughtful, with a proper regard for the dangers of penetrating the intact dura mater, and had plenty of experience of wound infection. It is much less obvious why he operated. It appears that depressed fractures of the skull were left to suppurate, in the expectation that the bone fragments would sequestrate and be discharged; fissured fractures were, however, explored aggressively. De Moulin (1988) states that the operator was looking for intracranial bleeding; Majno (1991) sees the operation as intended to let out blood that would otherwise turn to pus. The management of various types of fractures of the mandible is more comprehensible. The fracture was immobilized by interdental wiring, using gold wire or thread, and splinted externally with leather glued to the skin and tied behind the head. Union was expected in only 20 days. Hippocratic surgery also included primary suture of some wounds, especially in the face: the wound was stitched up after being washed out with wine, and dressed with an ointment containing copper oxide and honey. Majno (1991) has tested the antibacterial effect of wine and found it quite potent: it appears that this is due to polyphenols in the wine, not to ethyl alcohol.

The Roman conquest of Greece widened the influence Greek culture; Roman medicine was a partnership based on Italian organizational skills and Greek science. The teachings of Hippocrates and the discoveries of his successors in Alexandria were studied and elaborated by Roman writers such as Cornelius Celsus (c. AD 30). Celsus has been disparaged as a popularizer of current medical knowledge, not an original thinker, yet his very readable work is representative of the best state of the art in imperial Rome. Celsus (1938) gave a good account of plastic closure of areas of facial tissue loss, by two quadrangular advancement flaps sutured together to close the defect; he used thread sutures. Nasal injuries were seen as causes of deformity and airway obstruction: nasal displacements were reduced with the fingers or with a probe or a quill in the nostril(s), and immobilized by internal and external splints. Fractures and dislocations of the mandible were described; interdental horsehair ligatures were used. His account of the surgery of head injury gives some idea of the indications for trephining the skull. He enquired first about neurological symptoms, such as vomiting, loss of speech, and obscured vision. These symptoms might point to a skull fracture in need of treatment. More serious symptoms, such as coma ('torpor'), suggested that the dura mater was violated, and operation might be ineffective. Irritation of the meninges was seen as a cause of harm — a concept that was to have a long life. Celsus recognized the danger of bleeding under the intact skull, presumably extradural, and advised operation for cranial osteomyelitis. His tools included the modiolus, an iron cylindrical trephine, and the terebra, ancestor of the modern perforator: large areas of bone were excised by making a ring of holes with the terebra and joining the holes with chisel cuts. All in all, it appears that the operative craniofacial surgery of Celsus went to the limits of what was then possible, given the absence of anaesthesia and the consequent need for speed and dexterity: Celsus noted that the surgeon must be compassionate, yet unmoved by his patient's screams.

Galen (c. AD 130–199) is a greater figure in medical biology than in the history of surgery. It is even suggested that he had no practical surgical experience, but this is nonsense. In his work as physician to the gladiators of Pergamon, he certainly had to treat the less fortunate sportsmen, and he wrote confidently of operations on the skull (Galen, 1976). His animal experiments suggest remarkable manual dexterity, and he was a fine anatomist, though he had to study monkeys and other animals, being debarred from using human cadavers. (Human anatomy had been studied in the cadaver in Hellenistic Egypt, but this invaluable aid to good surgery had been abandoned.) His experiments included making brain lesions in conscious animals: he was able to demonstrate the serious effects of damage to the cerebral ventricles, especially the fourth ventricle, and he noted similar effects from accidents in trephining the human head. The awareness of the lethal effects of cerebral compression, both from clinical observation and from animal experiment, foreshadows a central concept in modern neurosurgical thinking. But Galen's main surgical legacy was a very complete system of pathophysiology; his concepts of cardiorespiratory and neurological function were profoundly wrong, but they were very convincing and had enormous influence. Whatever its scientific demerits, Galen's system gave surgeons a set of working dogmas that were doubtless just as helpful as more correct knowledge would have been, given the limitations of what was possible. The Catalan Joseph Trueta (1897–1977), in our times a most influential military surgical writer and a great surgical biologist, blames Galen for many things, and particularly for a fundamental error that prevented progress for fourteen centuries — the belief that suppuration is a benign and indeed essential process in wound healing. In this, he is contrasted with Hippocrates (Trueta 1944). This seems rather unfair. There were writers before Galen who saw suppuration as a favourable event, while Galen himself clearly regarded healing by first intention, i.e. without suppuration, as the most desirable outcome (De Moulin 1988).

Graeco-Roman medicine gave very serviceable rules for the management of facial injuries; for craniocerebral injuries, the Hippocratic legacy was less helpful but at least the basic surgical armamentarium was defined. Galen's concepts of humoral pathology and his emphasis on venesection were certainly unhappy; he bears much responsibility for the 'therapeutic' bleeding of wounded persons over the next 1700 years. After Galen's death, there were no great speculative or experimental medical biologists in the declining Roman world, but his ideas, and those of his predecessors, were kept alive by surgeons in the Byzantine cities, and by them transmitted to the Arab world.

The great surge of Islam established a brilliant and tolerant cultural unity from Delhi to Cordoba. In the intellectual centres of the Eastern and Western Caliphates, Graeco-Roman medicine was studied and advanced. But surgery received relatively less attention, and most of the great figures of Arab medical science were primarily concerned with internal medicine. The chief exception was Albucasis, in Arabic Abu'l-Qasim (936–1013). His surgical textbook was translated into Latin in Toledo, and widely read in western Europe; he reiterated Hippocratic teaching on the treatment of fractures of the mandible by dental ligatures and external splints. It is also relevant that Albucasis is credited with the belief that atmospheric air will infect wounds. This concept, not an unreasonable deduction from everyday experience, was to have wide currency, and especially in the misunderstanding of brain infections.

MEDIEVAL SURGERY OF THE SKULL AND FACE

Some ten centuries separate the political and social disintegration of the Western Roman Empire from the dawn of the Renaissance in Italy. In that long period, Western Europe produced few surgical writers of distinction or originality, and little of what was written is relevant to the theme of this book. To a considerable extent, learning was confined to the ecclesiastical establishment, and as clerics were prohibited by the Church from shedding blood, there was a cleavage between the learned physician who did not operate and the surgical craftsman who did not study. Nevertheless the picture of medieval scientific sterility and clerical obscurantism has been much exaggerated. In Italy especially, there were priests who did

operate, even after this was banned by the Fourth Lateran Council in 1215. In Salerno, a multicultural seaport south of Naples, a lay medical school emerged around 900, and flourished for some 300 years: the surgeons of Salerno studied anatomy, performed autopsies, and reported many cases of cranial and facial wounds, including a fatal extradural haematoma from a slingshot impact (De Moulin 1988). Before operating on the brain, the Salernitan surgeon washed his hands, a practice that had to be rediscovered in the nineteenth century, and also abstained from sexual intercourse and eating garlic. Universities, perhaps the greatest intellectual achievement of the Middle Ages, established medical faculties, first in Bologna (1156) but soon elsewhere, and in Italy these universities taught surgery and anatomy, with cadaver dissections from the early fourteenth century at latest. De Moulin (1988) has reviewed the surgical practice of French writers such as Henri de Mondeville (c. 1260–1320) and Guy de Chauliac (c. 1298–1368): both gave attention to head injury management, and had sensible things to say on wound healing.

THE SIXTEENTH CENTURY

Seen in retrospect, this century appears as a time of exhilarating intellectual adventure. The religious revolution in Europe shattered old beliefs and assumptions. The oceanic voyages of discovery expanded the world enormously, and brought back new diseases and new drugs. Humanist scholars rediscovered or renovated Greek and Latin texts, and the printing press spread their findings in an enlarged intellectual community that extended from Poland to Portugal and beyond to the Americas. Medical texts were studied more widely: Celsus was printed in 1478, and much of Galen's work was published in Latin translation in 1490. An increased interest in human anatomy followed. Surgery, stimulated by the effects of the terrifying new firearms, shared in the expansion of medical science. The northern Italian universities, already old as centres of learning, were in the vanguard of the advance of surgical thinking. Padua, the university of the powerful republic of Venice, was pre-eminent, and its professorial chairs were held by a number of outstanding physician-surgeons, one of whom was Andreas Vesalius (1514–1564) of Brussels.

1543 is often given as the landmark year of Renaissance science, when Vesalius brought out his great textbook of anatomy, *De Humani Corporis Fabrica*. Vesalius was at once a learned Galenist — there are more than 200 citations of Galen in the index of his book — and an iconoclastic revolutionary, correcting Galen's anatomical errors on the basis of his own meticulous dissections. His book gave surgeons a superbly illustrated textbook that emphasized function as well as structure. In particular, it gave a fine description of the skull and facial skeleton, and of the external morphology of the brain and cranial nerves. Vesalius was himself a daring surgeon, not least in the field of CMF trauma, as is evident in a famous case report from his practice after he left Padua. In 1562, Don Carlos, the young and very unsatisfactory crown prince of Spain, fell down a flight of steps 'in hasty following of a wench', and suffered a contused wound of the scalp, which became infected. His conscious level worsened, and Vesalius, who was then one of the royal physicians, evidently diagnosed intracranial suppuration. 'Dr. Vesalius was of the opinion that the lesion was inside and that there was no other remedy but to penetrate the skull to the membranes'. This was not done, but the later course of the illness makes it clear that Vesalius was right in his diagnosis (Simpson 1987).

The sixteenth century saw many notable surgical authors who wrote on the management of CMF trauma. Berengario da Carpi (c. 1460–1530) wrote a book, De Fractura Cranei, dealing specifically with head injuries, and remarkable for its emphasis on their symptomatology. This work also figures the instruments of the time; it is interesting to see that the modiolus has guards to prevent overpenetration, and the terebra or perforator is supplemented by a burr (Fig. 1.8) of modern design. Other influential writers were the Italian Giovanni da Vigo (c. 1460–1520), an enthusiast for the cautery, and the German Hieronymus Braunschweig (1450–1533). Also from the Germanic world was the great Paracelsus (Philipp Bumbastus von Hohenheim, c. 1494–1541). Paracelsus exemplifies the Renaissance, in his flamboyant iconoclasm — he ceremoniously burned one of the chief traditional textbooks — and his readiness to explore new fields; even in his interests in magic and the occult, to us less admirable, there is a gusto that still fascinates. In surgery, his *Grosse Wundarznei* and his *Spitalbuch* have much to say about wound treatment, but they are even more remarkable for the author's total rejection of the traditional separation of medicine and surgery: 'there can be no surgeon who is not also a physician' (Pagel 1982). But the best known, best loved and most typical Renaissance surgeon is Ambroise Paré (c. 1510–1590), and his writings have much that is relevant in an evaluation of the evolution of the surgery of CMF trauma.

Paré was born in Bourg-Hersent, a small village in Mayenne, but went early to Paris. It appears that he learned his profession as apprentice to a barber-surgeon, and also in the Hôtel-Dieu, the chief public hospital in Paris. He had no university education: in France, unlike Italy, universities did not teach academic surgery. Paré went to Italy in 1537 as personal surgeon to a commander in the French royal army; thereafter, he served in many campaigns in the wars with the German emperor Charles V and his allies. In 1559, he attended his king Henri II

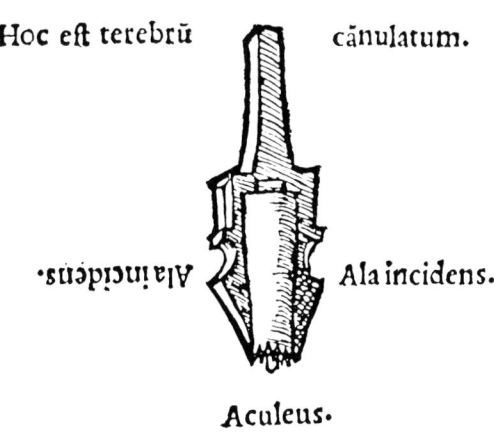

A

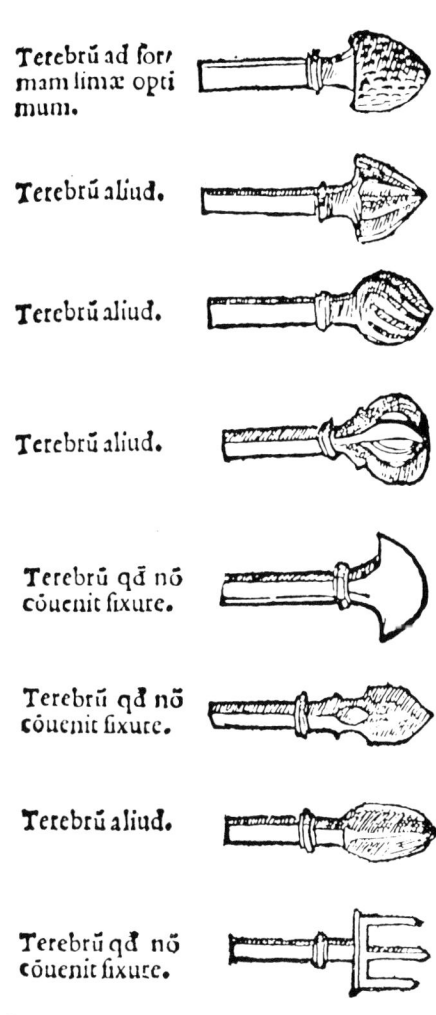

B

Fig. 1.8 Cranial surgery in the Renaissance. Craniotomy instruments used by Berengario da Carpia, 1518. **A** Modiolus or trephine, with adjustable guard against overpenetration. **B** Range of perforators and burrs.

after the fatal tourney accident described above, together with Vesalius, who was sent to Paris by the concerned king of Spain, Philip II. Paré also attended many leading figures in the religious wars that broke out after the death of Henri II. He became immensely experienced, he designed many surgical instruments and prostheses and he wrote many books — in vigorous French because he was a poor Latinist. His management of head injuries is described in the tenth book of his 'Complete Works' (Paré, 1649). His chief indication for operation on the head appears to have been a compound depressed fracture, to relieve pressure on the meninges and to allow the escape of 'corrupt and putrid blood'. It is not always clear whether this meant evacuation of pus or blood clot. He used a trephine on a brace, a gimlet perforator, and also a compass saw for larger bone resections. Great care was taken to preserve the dura mater; bone fragments were removed with elevators and forceps. Bone still attached to the pericranium was not removed. Simple scalp wounds were pulled together with a few sutures, or otherwise closed; deeper wounds were often left open to granulate.

Paré described his management of injuries of the face and jaws, and of the eyes, in the same book. Facial wounds were carefully sutured with waxed thread, or closed with strips of sticking plaster sutured together (Fig. 1.9). Fractures of the mandible were treated as advised by Hippocrates, with interdental wiring using gold or silver wire and an external leather restraint sewn to the patient's night-cap. Union of the fracture was expected in 20 days, unless 'inflammation' should supervene. Presumably the figure of 20 days is derived from Hippocrates: Paré qualified it by noting that patients vary in the time needed for union. Paré had little to say about midfacial fractures, though he quoted the gratifying case of a soldier who suffered a disfiguring compound wound of the upper jaw, which became infested with worms because of delay in getting surgical aid, and stank. With appropriate local medication and delayed suture, the wound eventually healed very well. Nasal wounds and fractures were discussed in more detail. Paré noted that an amputated nose could not be replaced, but if there was any adherence to the rest of the adjacent flesh, 'from whence it may receive life and nourishment', then it should be sewn back. His ability to treat eye injuries was limited, but he removed corneal foreign bodies, using a speculum, and was aware that penetrating eye wounds could heal well if the pupil was not injured. Human milk was an excellent irrigating fluid for injured eyes, especially if the donor was suckling a girl. Paré's contemporary Georg Bartisch (1535–1605), court oculist in Dresden, was more adventurous as an eye surgeon: he described the operation of enucleation, and is said to have been the first to note sympathetic ophthalmia as a sequel of eye injury (Albert & Diaz-Rohena, 1989).

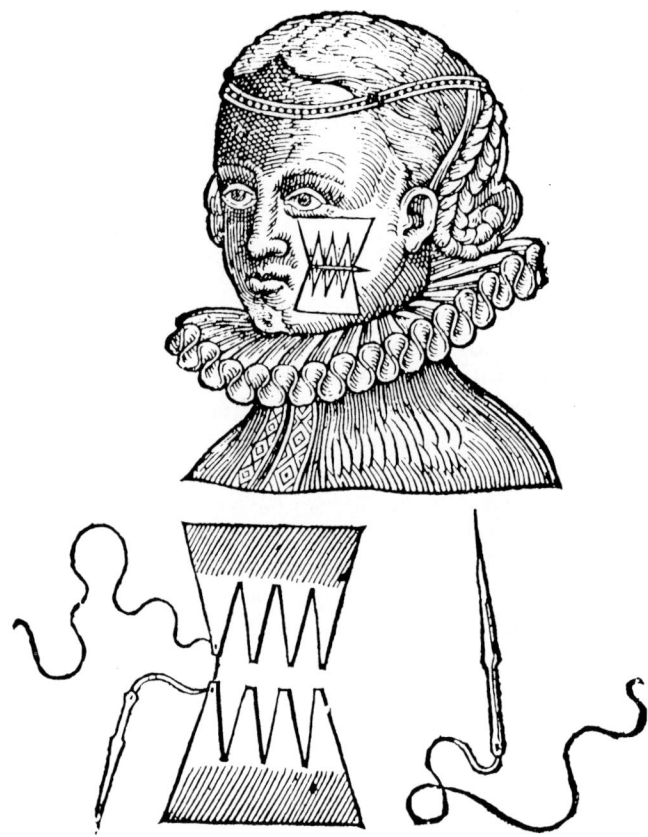

Fig. 1.9 Skin closure in the Renaissance. Pare's 'dry suture' for wounds of the cheek: pieces of cloth are gummed to the skin and sutured together with thread.

Paré described in much detail his various wound dressings; distilled spirits were often used, and may have had some antimicrobial effect, though of course he could not know this. He used frequent venesections for head injuries, in line with traditional Galenic practice, bleeding from the cephalic vein 'according to the strength of the patient.'

One procedure not in Paré's repertoire was repair of facial tissue loss by a pedicle graft. However, his remarkable contemporary Gaspare Tagliacozzi (1545–1599) was active in this field. Tagliacozzi held a professorial chair in the university of Bologna, and was a very gifted surgeon. To repair noses slashed off in civil or military clashes, he used a pedicle skin graft taken from the inner surface of the arm, sutured to the freshened nasal defect (Fig. 1.10). The arm was bandaged to the head and trunk until union was established. Tagliacozzi's rhinoplasty was a staged procedure, and might take up to five months. He used a similar flap to restore defects in the lips and ears, noting that restoration of a whole ear was not possible. Done without anaesthesia, these operations must have needed great skill in the surgeon and great fortitude in the patient. Tagliacozzi's well-illustrated book is a classic in the history of plastic surgery, but the operation was not

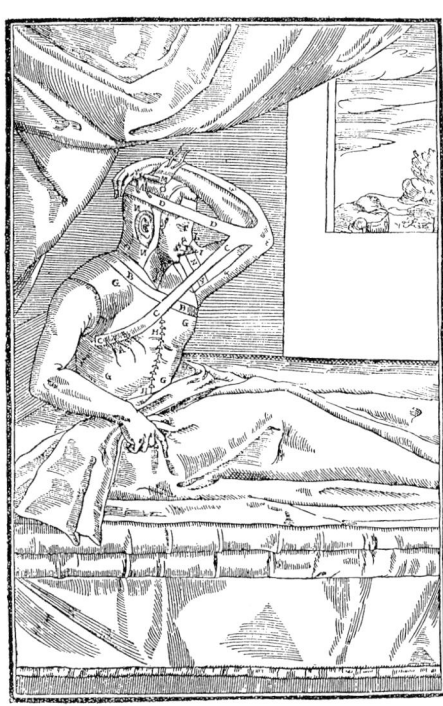

Fig. 1.10 Tagliacozzi's rhinoplasty. A pedicled graft from the forearm has been sutured to the mutilated nose, and the arm is immobilized. From G. Tagliacozzi, *De Curtorum Chirugia per Insitionem*, 1597.

The form of a nofe artificially made, both alone by it felf, and alfo with the upper-lip covered as it were with the hair of the beard,

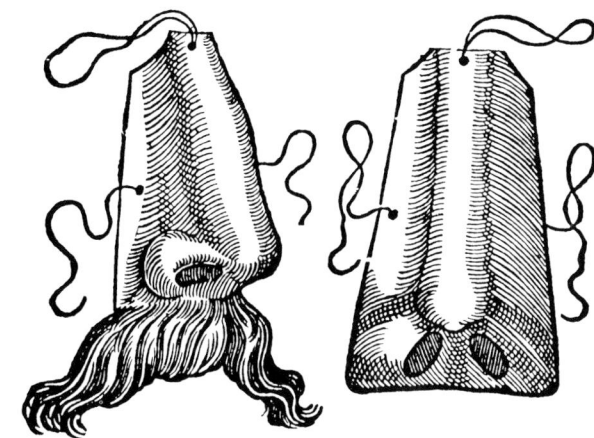

Fig. 1.11 Pare's prosthesis for a mutilated nose. The prosthesis was made from gold, silver, paper, or glued cloth, and was coloured appropriately; it was secured to the head or to the hat.

widely performed, and the principle of the autogenous pedicle graft was obscured by more or less fantastic tales of homografted noses taken from the rumps of proletarian donors (Gnudi & Webster, 1989).

It is always dangerous to read modern concepts into the minds of the scientists of the past. Renaissance science included much thaumaturgy and belief in astrology and alchemy was widespread; surgeons were not immune to these seductive aberrations. But one can see in the writings of the elite surgeons of the sixteenth century three themes of enduring importance: themes that had indeed been evident in Graeco Roman surgical practice, but had not previously come so clearly into focus.

First, wound healing and tissue repair were seen as natural if still mysterious processes, and were studied objectively. Early in the century, it had been thought that gunshot wounds were poisoned, and should be purified by the cautery or by irrigation with boiling oil. As is well known, Paré rejected this doctrine on the basis of clinical observation. Paré gave attention to the putrefying effect of the air and the depraved humours of the victim, but suppuration was seen in natural terms as the effect of tissue damage by the force of the missile — 'the vehemency of the contusion, dilaceration and fracture, caused by the bullets too violent entry' — and to the effects of indriven fragments of cloth, missiles, splinters of bone and bruised flesh (Paré 1649). His contemporary Leonardo Botallo (1530–?) showed that gunpowder is not poisonous, and also attributed the septic complications

of gunshot wounds to indriven foreign matter (Trueta, 1944).

Second, there was general concern to protect the brain from the secondary effects of trauma. It is not always clear whether operations on the head were done to evacuate pus or blood clot, or indeed whether they were done prophylactically. But it does appear that there was awareness of the danger of intracranial collections. The distinction between pus and blood may not have seemed so fundamental as it does now, since it was believed that blood was transformed into pus as a natural process.

Lastly, there was full awareness of the aesthetic importance of facial wounds. Here again, Paré speaks for the period, when he warns that bad management of facial wounds will 'leave deformed scars in the most specious (precious) and beautifull part of the body' (Paré 1649). This awareness, in that beauty-loving age, doubtless inspired Tagliacozzi's amazing operations and Paré's elaborate designs for facial prostheses (Fig. 1.11). The impact of facial disfigurement is a main theme in this book.

THE SEVENTEENTH AND EIGHTEENTH CENTURIES

In these centuries, the philosophy of experimental science became generally accepted, and Galen's physiology was slowly discarded. Wound healing became better understood, especially after the work of John Hunter (1728–1793). He established that healing by primary union, without suppuration, must be the surgical ideal, and should be promoted by wound closure. Like Paré, he favoured closure by adherent plasters because sutures induced ulceration, perhaps from the use of contaminated thread. He studied pus with the primitive microscopes of the time and saw white blood cells; he could not establish their significance, but he came as close to understanding the nature of infection as was possible before Pasteur's work. Most importantly, he denied that air, in itself, could induce suppuration.

Bone healing was also studied: De Moulin (1988) cites the experimental work of the Dutch physician Anton De Heide (1646–169?) on long bone and cranial fractures in dogs. The anatomy of the facial structures, especially the air sinuses, the salivary glands and their ducts, was clarified: the Danish anatomist/bishop Niels Stensen (1638–1686) and the Cromwellian physician Thomas Wharton (c. 1616–1673) are commemorated by the parotid and submandibular ducts respectively. Thomas Willis (1621–1675) published a fine neuroanatomical textbook, illustrated by the young Christopher Wren, which was especially important in defining the anatomy of the cerebral circulation. Understanding of the pathophysiology of head injuries made slower progress. As late as 1752, John Hunter's learned brother William (1718–1783) could say 'as to the uses of the different parts of the brain, we are quite ignorant' (Dowd 1972). However, at the end of the period, one concept of fundamental importance was enunciated: the Monro-Kelly doctrine (Lundberg 1983). The Scottish anatomist Alexander Monro II (1733–1817) stated that the skull is 'a case of bone' whose contents are incompressible and of constant volume; with some important modifications, this observation underlies the modern concept of raised intracranial pressure (p. 36).

The wars of the seventeenth century produced some fine surgeons, notably the German Johann Schultes (1595–1645), better known as Scultetus, a graduate of Padua who practised in Ulm during the Thirty Years War. His management of head injuries has been perceptively studied by Louis Bakay (1971), himself a distinguished neurosurgeon and a competent Latinist. Bakay has shown that Scultetus's procedures were little different from those of Paré and his predecessors, both in technique and in rationale. His surgical armamentarium included the hand trephine, various nibblers and two more complex tools that doubtless express the ingenuity of German craftsmen: a rotary saw and a screw on a tripod to elevate depressed fractures (Fig. 1.12). His medical treatment was traditional: his patients were given enemas and bled vigorously to reduce fever and inflammation. Faith in therapeutic venesection was to persist well into the nineteenth century, despite the intelligent scepticism of the British naval surgeon James Yonge (1646–1721), a pioneer in the study of haemostasis (Watt 1975). In the eighteenth century, Henri-François Le Dran (1685–1770) of Paris and Percivall Pott (see p. 5) of London recognized the clinical importance of the lucid interval before worsening in conscious level, as an indication of extradural haemor-

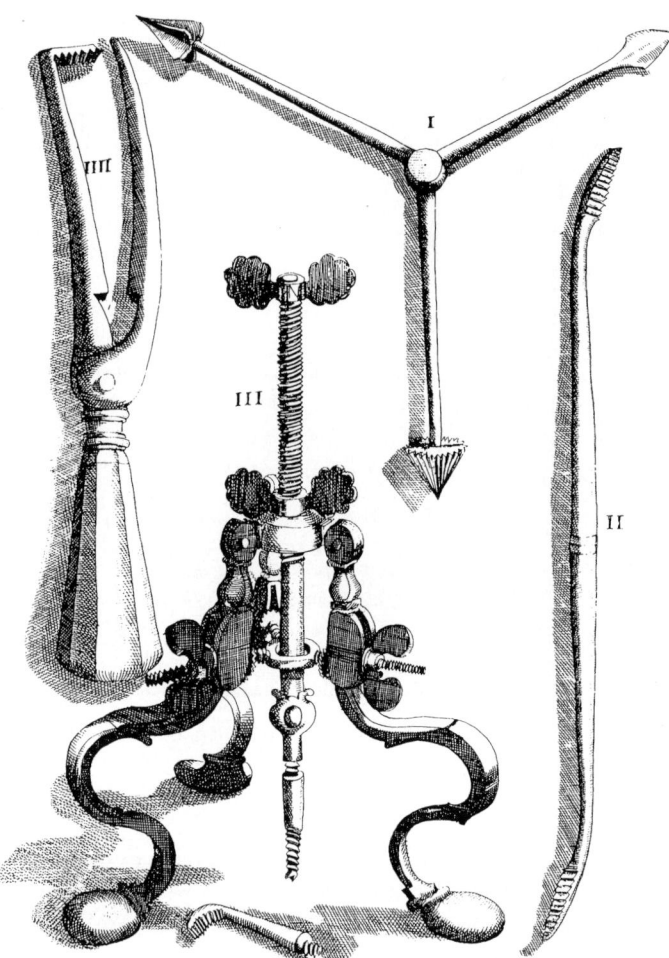

Fig. 1.12 Cranial surgery in the Thirty Years War. A perforator with three points, a simple elevator, an adjustable screw elevator, and a pair of bone forceps. From J. Scultetus, *Armamentarium Chirurgicum*, 1655.

rhage, and one must see this as a very notable conceptual advance. Several eighteenth-century writers show awareness of the crucial distinction between the primary effects of head injury and the secondary — often remediable — complications. An article on trephination in the famous French *Encyclopedie* (Anonymous 1765) quoted the royal surgeon F. R. Quesnay (1694–1774) on the indications for operation: these stressed late-onset ('consecutif') symptoms, in contrast to the primary ('primitif') effects of injury. Both Quesnay and Pott (better known for his puffy tumour of the scalp, associated with cranial osteomyelitis) were also very ready to trephine linear fractures on suspicion of underlying mischief, or even prophylactically (Fig. 1.13). By the end of the eighteenth century, there was general agreement on the detrimental effects of cerebral compression and readiness to relieve it immediately by operation at the site of impact: 'when a Blow upon the Head is attended with considerable Symptoms, you cannot enquire too soon into the State of the Cranium by making a large Incision upon that Part which

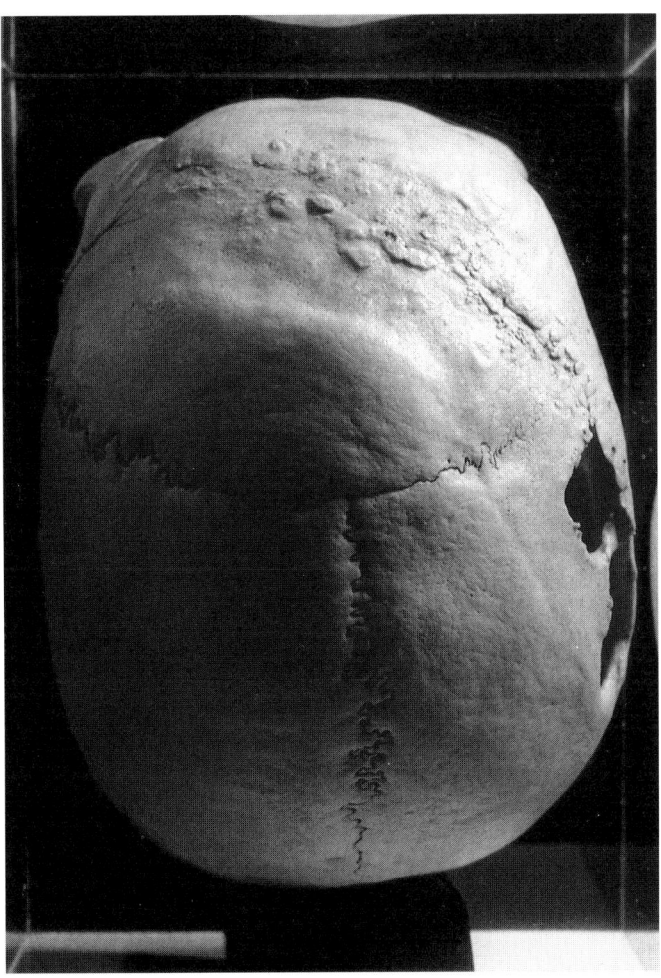

Fig. 1.13 Cranial surgery in the Age of Reason. Skull trephined, possibly by John Hunter. On the right there are two healed trephine holes. Extending across the frontal region, is a healed fracture, with many bony nodules, suggesting chronic inflammation. Reproduced by courtesy of Trustees of the Hunterian Collection, Royal College of Surgeons, England: Catalogue of the pathological series P459.

has received the Blow; and it is far more preferable to make a useless Incision, than to neglect it in a dubious Case' (Le Dran 1740). The surgeons of this period were keen observers, and one comment by Pott deserves record, because of its relevance to CMF trauma: 'I think that I have seen more patients get well, whose injuries have been in or under the frontal bone, than any other bones of the cranium. If this should be found to be generally true, may not the reason be worth enquiring into?' In Chapter 4, this prophetic observation is related to modern research on frontal impacts.

One can see in this period increasing skill in dealing with facial fractures. Richard Wiseman (p. 3) described the reduction of mandibular dislocations along what were then orthodox lines, but also described innovative approaches to fractures of the midfacial skeleton. In one case, a child aged 8 years, he reduced such a fracture with a hook behind the hard palate: the dislocation

recurred, and the only recourse available was for members of the family and the child himself to take turns in holding the maxillary segment forward until it became fixed in the proper position. This was done with a good result. Wiseman also described several cases of bullet wounds in the face: he was at pains to extract the slug or ball, especially if it was of iron or brass, as being more likely to 'rust' than lead (p. 153), and he emphasized the danger of indriven rags. In one case, a pistol ball lodged in the nose: it caused chronic discharge — 'a fretting ichor' — and had to be removed through the palate. The palatal defect was closed with a plate.

In dental surgery, there is also evidence of conceptual and technical progress, with use of dental methods in the management of facial fractures. Jean-Francois Capperon (?–1763), Louis XV's dentist, collaborated with the surgeon Henri-Francois Le Dran in a way that anticipated modern craniofacial practice. In 1729 Le Dran treated a man injured in a road traffic accident; he had been run over and both the mandible and the maxilla were fractured. Le Dran immobilized both fractures by dental ligation. 'Being little acquainted with this Method, I thought proper, for the Benefit of the Patient, to desire Mr. Capron, Operator for the Teeth to his Majesty, to go to the Hospital and perform this Operation' — perhaps the first record of interdisciplinary collaboration in the management of CMF trauma. Interdental ligation was not an innovative procedure, but later in the century a new means of immobilization was designed for mandibular fractures: a kind of G-clamp, with iron plates fitting on the teeth above and under the chin below (Rowe & Killey 1955).

THE NINETEENTH CENTURY

Napoleonic surgery

The savage battles of the Napoleonic wars produced some great surgeons, but it cannot be said that the theory and practice of the surgery of CMF injuries changed very much in the first half of the nineteenth century. Robert Liston (1794–1847), a Scot who became Professor of Surgery in the new North London (later University College) Hospital, gave a good, succinct account of his treatment of fractures of the nose, maxilla and 'inferior maxilla' (mandible). He used interdental wiring, or 'a machine with blunt hooks and screws, to be had of the instrument-makers', but in general his treatment was little in advance of eighteenth-century practice. However, it is noteworthy that he used metal cap splints fitted to the teeth of the upper and lower jaws and soldered together to immobilize the mandible before excision of a tumour: a device which was to have much application in fracture management (Liston, 1846). He gave credit for this to 'my friend Mr. Nasmyth of Edinburgh', presumably the Scottish dentist Alexander Nasmyth (1789–1848). The cranial surgery of the period is well exemplified by the writings of George Guthrie (1785–1856), who served as an army surgeon from the unusually young age of 16. In 1847, he published a vivid treatise on head injuries, in which the indications for trephining are somewhat more precise than in earlier publications. He operated urgently to elevate compound depressed fractures, to prevent what he called cerebral irritation: his case reports suggest that this was bacterial infection. He also operated for cerebral compression; his cases include five extradural haematomas, trephined on the battlefield, with three recoveries. Guthrie was convinced of the value of bleeding: one of his patients was bled some 4 litres in 3 days, and also purged (Guthrie 1847).

Facial repair was little advanced from Renaissance times. The Indian rhinoplasty became known outside India after 1793, when one of the victims of Tipu Sultan's terror mutilations (p. 8) underwent successful rhinoplasty by an Indian surgeon (McDowell, 1977), and this operation was performed by several European surgeons thereafter. Carl Ferdinand von Gräfe (1787–1840) of Berlin used both the Indian and the Tagliacotian rhinoplasties. Carl Reiche (1796–1860), one of his pupils, reported an apparatus (Fig. 1.14) for fixing a fractured maxilla to a steel head band (Hoffmann-Axthelm 1991). But if Paré and Tagliacozzi had returned to the surgical world of 1845, they would have seen little to surprise

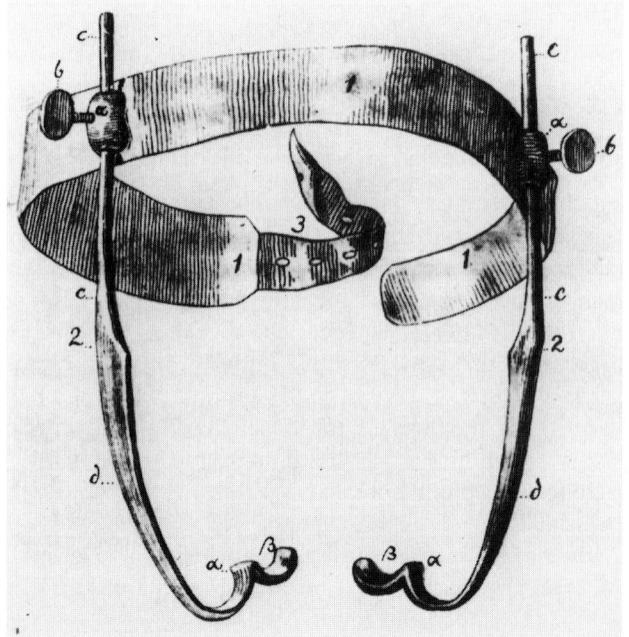

Fig. 1.14 Prussian maxillofacial surgery in the Age of Biedermeier. Apparatus for splinting fractured maxilla from a headband, devised by C. C. F. Reiche of Berlin, and reported in 1822. By courtesy of Professor W. Hoffmann-Axthelm.

them. Over the next 50 years, the theory and practice of surgery changed beyond recognition.

Anaesthesia and the Listerian revolution

In 1846, ether was first given, in Boston, to permit painless surgery; Liston performed the first operation under ether in Europe in the same year. In 1865, Joseph Lister (1827–1912) first used carbolic acid to prevent microbial wound infection. These landmark events inaugurated modern surgery, yet much had to be done before these revolutionary discoveries became relevant in the routine management of CMF injuries.

John Snow (1813–1858), pioneer of scientific anaesthesiology, noted as early as 1848 that the risk of inhalation of blood made anaesthesia in the surgery of the jaws especially hazardous, and this problem remained unsolved until the advent of endotracheal anaesthesia some 60 years later. Major operations on the facial skeleton were done under chloroform or ether, usually given with a face mask. This entailed very real risks, and for some time, jaw injuries were often managed without anaesthesia. Likewise, the advent of antiseptic surgery was not at first of much significance in the management of jaw injuries: fear of infection continued and it was many decades before internal fixation of mandibular fractures by wiring was considered an acceptable procedure, though the procedure had been described as early as 1846 by M. Fouchard in France and around the same time by Gurdon Buck (1807–1877: see below) in the USA (Rowe & Killey 1955). Indeed, the chief nineteenth-century advances in the management of jaw fractures came from the use of new dental technologies for external fixation. Organized training in dentistry began around 1840, in several countries, but most notably in the USA, producing a generation of capable dentists some of whom made important contributions in the fixation of jaw fractures. In many instances, they utilized new dental techniques and materials, such as vulcanized rubber; metal casting, swaged splints and wire fixation were also used in new ways. In the USA, four dentists were particularly innovative in the treatment of jaw fractures: Thomas Bryan Gunning (1813–1889), James Baxter Bean (1834–1870), Thomas Lewis Gilmer (1849–1931), and Edward Hartley Angle (1850–1930).

In 1861 Gunning, a New York dentist, immobilized mandibular fractures with hard vulcanized rubber splints, made from dental impressions in wax and fixed to the teeth by gold screws; where necessary, the splint was also fixed to the intact maxilla, nutrition being maintained through a hole in the vulcanite splint. Gunning also used his splints in edentulous patients, and for this purpose 'Gunning-type' splints are still in use (p. 522). His papers make fascinating reading (Gunning 1866–7): his cases of mandibular fractures included himself and an unnamed 'distinguished statesman in Washington', who was in fact Lincoln's secretary of state and rival W. H. Seward (1801–1872). Seward had suffered a bilateral compound mandibular fracture in a road accident; nine days later, an inept assassin tried to cut his throat and inflicted an extensive facial wound. Gunning's polite record of his successful treatment of these injuries is a maxillofacial classic.

This attempted assassination took place at the end of the American Civil War, which has been described as the first modern war. It is certainly the first large war to be documented in great detail. G. A. Otis (1870) wrote a magnificent surgical history of the war, giving statistics relating to 3312 hospitalized gunshot wounds of the face (mortality 11.4%), 4350 gunshot wounds of the skull (mortality 59.2%), and 1190 gunshot wounds of the eye, with loss of sight of at least one eye in some 75%. The victims are identified by name or initials, and range in military magnitude from Jefferson Coates of the 7th Wisconsin Volunteeers, aged 20, wounded at Gettysburg by a conoidal ball through both orbits, surviving blind and anosmic but 'in good spirits', to 'AL, aged 56 years', who is clearly the commander-in-chief Abraham Lincoln (1809–1865) himself, assassinated by a Derringer pistol shot in the brain (p. 140).

Head injuries of all types were often complicated by intracranial infection; it cannot be said that the war produced real advances in the management of cranial wounds (Table 1.2). The Northern armies were served by a special eye hospital, but the management of eye wounds does not appear to have gone beyond excision of irreparably damaged eyes and the provision of glass eyes. Ophthalmoscopy had been introduced in clinical practice in 1851 by Hermann von Helmholtz (1821–1894) and had inaugurated the development of ophthalmology as a clinical science. But ophthalmoscopy was rarely used in the diagnosis of eye injuries in this war and Otis saw it as a superfluous refinement. Among the documented cases of eye injury, there were 40 cases of so-called sympathetic ophthalmitis, though only four went on to blindness. William McKenzie (1791–1868) had given a brilliant description of six cases of this condition in 1830, but it seems likely that its natural history (p. 412) was not yet understood. Secondary haemorrhage from injuries of the face were often fatal, despite heroic operations to ligate major arteries. The treatment of mandibular injuries does appear to have made progress. Gunning's vulcanite splints and prostheses received admiring comment from Otis, who also referred to interdental splints devised for Confederate wounded by Bean of Atlanta, Georgia. Bean's splints were also of vulcanite; like Gunning, he took plaster casts of the fractured mandible, put the pieces into occlusion with the intact maxilla, and then made a vulcanite splint to maintain the apposition (Hoffmann-Axthelm, 1982). Plastic surgical repairs of residual facial deformity were recorded in only 32 cases; some of these were seen as successful, notably three by the pioneer plastic surgeon Gurdon Buck, but Otis was pessimistic about the utility of such procedures in the vast majority of facial injuries.

Oral and maxillofacial surgery

After the Civil War, American dental surgery advanced rapidly. Gilmer, co-founder of the Dental School of North Western University, is credited with the introduction of the practice of immobilizing the fractured mandible to the intact maxilla by interdental wiring to preserve a correct occlusal position; he also tried open fixation of a mandibular fracture with platinum wire (McDowell 1977). Edward Angle, the father of orthodontics, pioneered the study of post-traumatic malocclusion and its treatment by devising the comprehensive classification of occlusion that bears his name (p. 347). He also laid the foundations for the use of bands and arch wires to immobilize the teeth in correcting malocclusion, and advocated a similar system for fixation of mandibular fractures (Fairbank 1936, Hoffmann-Axthelm 1982). The evolution of oral surgery from dentistry was well established by the end of the nineteenth century, and in several American centres, jaw fractures were seen as problems for the oral surgeon rather than for the general surgeon, who was otherwise responsible for trauma management (Johnson 1936). Nevertheless, the most seminal work on maxillofacial fractures at this time came from a French general surgeon, René Le Fort (1869–1951) of Lille. His studies on 35 cadavers subjected to blunt facial impacts (Le Fort 1901) are of enduring importance.

Le Fort's research methodology was robust. Cadaver heads were struck with a block of wood, or thrown against the edge of a marble table, until the skull cracked; the soft

Table 1.2 Mortality from penetrating wounds of the head in wars from 1853 to 1970 (modified from Gurdjian 1973)

	Mortality (%)
Pre-Listerian era	
Crimean War (1853–5)	74
American Civil War (1861–5)	59–72
Antiseptic era	
South African War (1899–1902)	40–50 (Rawling 1915)
World War I (1914–8)	35–50 (29: Cushing 1918)
Antibiotic era	
Second World War (British Army) (1939–45)	14
Korean War (UN Army) (1950–2)	10
Vietnam War (US Army) (1960–75)	10

The range of percentages in earlier wars reflects differences in wound categorization and sources of data.

tissues were then removed and the fracture or fractures inspected. Le Fort considered nine types of impact:

1. Anteroposterior impact on the upper lip: this tended to produce the transverse (horizontal) lower maxillary fracture described by Alphonse Guérin (1817–1895) in 1866.

2. Lateral impact on the lower part of the maxilla: such impacts were likely to injure the mandible and malar bones, but could also separate the whole upper jaw.

3. Impact from below on the upper alveolar margin: this caused a large symmetrical fracture through the nasal notch, the orbit, below the malar bones and the pterygoid processes, detaching the midface as a large fragment, often with other fractures such as a sagittal crack through the hard palate (p. 294).

4. Impact from in front on the midface: this produced similar fractures.

5. Impact from above downwards on the root of the nose: Le Fort did not himself study this impact, but quoted two cases from the literature.

6. Impact from below upwards on the mandible: fractures of the mandible were often seen but the effect was also to impact the upper alveolar arch from below, causing the fracture pattern resulting from impacts 3 and 4.

7. Impacts on the malar bone — four variants: these impacts forced the malar bone into the maxillary sinus, but could also cause other fractures, running across the midface.

8. Simultaneous facial and cranial impacts: impacts over a large area could separate the whole face from the skull base.

9. Impacts at multiple sites/from multiple directions: Le Fort did not study these himself, but noted that they can occur.

From these findings, correlated with reported clinical experience and with the architecture of the facial skeleton, Le Fort identified his well-known lines of weakness (p. 293). One ran between the skull (i.e. the neuro-cranium) and the facial skeleton, and fractures in this plane could result from either frontal or lateral impacts on the maxillary complex. This is now called the Le Fort III fracture, and it is interesting that the discoverer saw it as a fracture along the plane that protects the brain box (le boîte crânienne). He identified a second line of weakness in the midface, not wholly independent of the first line, running from the root of the nose above the nasal canal (sic) into the orbital floor and back to the pterygomaxillary fissure. This is the Le Fort II fracture. His third line of weakness ran from the lower margin of the piriform aperture across the canine fossa, below the malar bone and into the pterygomaxillary fissure. He called this the Guérin fracture, but his description is far clearer than that of Guérin, and the term Le Fort I fracture is now usual.

Neurosurgery

While modern concepts of maxillofacial surgery were thus being formulated, neurosurgery was taking shape under the liberating influences of anaesthesia and antisepsis/asepsis. For long cranial operations, inhalational anaesthesia was an obvious advance, though early techniques often caused brain swelling. The Listerian antiseptic method was of enormous importance in reducing the risk of cerebral infection. Earlier in the nineteenth century, many surgeons had become much more reluctant to operate on the head than their predecessors had been. In the period 1860–1876, four London teaching hospitals recorded mortality rates from trephining in excess of 75%; the mortality for this operation was little lower in the American Civil War. These appalling figures doubtless express not only actual deaths from hospital infection but also deaths after operations delayed because of fear of infection (Hudson 1877). After 1880 surgeons began to operate on the brain with increasing confidence: not only compound skull fractures but also extradural haematomas were treated surgically, and the infective complications of cranial trauma were recognized and treated — sometimes successfully. William Macewen (1848–1924) of Glasgow described cerebral abscesses with great clarity and detail. Of the 64 cases reported in his book (Macewen 1893), 11 had various kinds of post-traumatic intracranial suppuration, and six of these made good recoveries after surgical drainage. Macewen also made important contributions in the prevention of brain infection by proper primary wound cleansing and suture. Greater readiness to operate on the brain also led to more interest in cerebral physiology and especially in the physiology of raised intracranial pressure: this work was summarized by the Swiss surgeon Theodor Kocher (1841–1917) in a remarkable monograph on brain injuries (Kocher 1901), which includes experimental work done in Berne by the brilliant young American surgeon who was to be the founder of modern neurosurgery — Harvey Cushing (1869–1939).

Radiology

Lastly, the nineteenth century saw the advent of in vivo imaging of bone and organs. Conrad Röntgen (1845–1923) described his 'new kind of rays' late in 1895, and radiology entered the field of CMF trauma as early as 1898, as a means of localizing intraocular and intracranial missiles. Thereafter, clinical radiology grew with a speed that seems amazing today, when innovative procedures are delayed by so many safeguards, necessary and unnecessary.

WORLD WAR I, 1914–1918

Carnage

Modern concepts of the specialized management of CMF trauma took shape during this long and dreadful war. In 1914, these concepts were still embryonic. It was still an age of omnicompetent general surgeons. Admittedly, ophthalmology, ENT surgery and oral surgery were recognized disciplines, and although there were very few committed neurosurgeons in the world, it was accepted that the surgery of the brain required special knowledge and skills. Plastic surgical techniques had evolved from rhinoplasty to employ skin flaps in many situations, and split-skin grafts had been known for some 40 years, but plastic procedures were usually performed by general surgeons. The chief surgical textbooks of the period contained chapters on the surgery of the brain and the jaws by men with a special interest in these fields, and from these one can deduce that the common CMF injuries of peacetime were well understood. Nor were missile wounds ignored: indeed, the surgical literature from Wilhelm II's Germany showed an ominous preoccupation with the effects of the new weapons. Yet when war broke out in August 1914, the army medical services of the chief combatants — Germany, Austria–Hungary, France, Russia and Great Britain — were soon overwhelmed by the sheer numbers of wounds of the head. It is said (Zilz, 1917) that in France and Belgium alone, there were 90 000 head injuries in the first 10 months of war. Facial wounds aroused special concern, because of their appalling appearance and because the victims survived in large numbers, often bitterly aware of disfigurement. Brain wounds also received attention, especially when the high incidence of delayed death from brain abscess became tragically apparent. Eye wounds, very numerous from the new fragmentation missiles, made the blinded soldier a familiar figure. It is said that eye wounds required removal of the eye in two cases out of three. Perhaps this high rate of enucleation in part reflected a dread of sympathetic ophthalmitis, which in fact appears to have been a rare complication in this and later wars (Albert & Diaz-Rohena 1989); nevertheless, only 6 months after the outbreak of war, British ophthalmologists were aware that the risks of the demon of ophthalmitis did not justify sacrificing a damaged eye if there was some useful vision (Jessop 1915).

Specialist management: Morestin, Gillies and Cushing

Management plans took different courses in the various combatant countries, yet converged at the end of the war. For France, the war was chiefly fought on French soil, not far from civilian hospitals of great distinction, well equipped to give multidisciplinary care for maxillofacial injuries. In Hippolyte Morestin (1869–1919), Paris had already a plastic surgeon of acknowledged genius, and the dental management of jaw injuries had been well taught by Claude Martin (1843–1911) of the Lyon school of military medicine (Hoffmann-Axthelm 1982). French wartime literature contains many references to the benefits of collaboration between surgeons, stomatologists

and dental technicians in the management of jaw injuries; a short-lived bilingual periodical, *La Restauration Maxillofaciale*, was published to foster this collaboration. German medical authorities also saw the importance of organized multidisciplinary centres for the care of facial injuries: a 225-bed hospital was allotted for this purpose in Düsseldorf as early as August 1914. Brain wounds were given special attention both in France and in Germany: the famous Parisian hospital La Salpêtrière cared for many thousands of brain-injured soldiers, and the University Clinic in Frankfurt am Main played a similar role for Germans wounded on the Western Front: it was here that the neurologist Kurt Goldstein (1878–1965) inaugurated modern neurorehabilitation. For Austria-Hungary, the war was fought on many fronts, often under great logistic handicaps: perhaps for this reason, the pros and cons of early versus late closure of head wounds came into clear focus in Austrian surgical thinking. The Viennese Nobel Laureate Robert Baranyi (1876–1936), during the siege of Przemysl, argued for primary closure. Austrian surgeons on more remote fronts, where wounds were already stinking when first seen, saw this as Utopian and accepted the formation of a brain hernia as the best hope of avoiding a lethal brain infection (Albrecht & Feuchtinger 1916). It seems that the Russian armies, fighting under notorious administrative handicaps, failed to evolve special services for CMF injuries, although fine work was done by individuals, notably V. P. Filatov of Odessa. He is credited with the invention of the tubular pedicle skin graft (McDowell 1977)

For the British army, the position was somewhat different. The chief effort was in France and Belgium: the trench line changed very little during the war, and medical policy dictated that primary surgical treatment should be done within a few miles of the line. British surgeons believed that brain wounds travelled badly after operation, and for this reason definitive treatment was done as soon as possible, often in advanced hospitals. In this there seems to have been a divergence from French policy: the leading French neurosurgeon of the day, Thierry de Martel (1875–1940), believed that brain wounds did not require urgent operation (Chatelin & de Martel 1918). British surgeons also agreed that eye wounds should be treated as soon as possible. But maxillofacial wounds did not seem so urgent, and were sent for definitive treatment in England; there were obvious psychological advantages in this. In 1917, the Queen's Hospital was established at Sidcup in Kent for these injuries, eventually disposing of 1000 beds and treating about 5000 cases. It became the focus of innovative CMF surgery of the highest quality, under the inspiration of the New Zealand surgeon Harold Gillies (1882–1960). Gillies had originally been an ENT surgeon; he had been impressed by French work on facial injuries and inspired British military medical authorities to form a special hospital for such cases. Australian, Canadian, New Zealand and US sections were added; the Australian section was commanded by Henry Newland (1873–1969), a South Australian general surgeon and one of the founders of Australian plastic surgery and neurosurgery (Hughes 1972). Gillies' team included the dental surgeon W. Kelsey Fry (1889–1963), Ivan Magill (1888–1986) the pioneer of endotracheal anaesthesia, and Henry Tonks (1862–1937), a distinguished academic artist whose delicate pastel drawings of facial wounds are haunting reminders of the brutality of war (Bennett 1986). Tonks was joined by the young Australian artist Daryl Lindsay (1889–1976): his water-colours of similar wounds in Australian soldiers are less well known but are equally precise and moving (Fig. 1.15).

US troops did not come to the Western Front in substantial numbers until 1918, but individual US surgeons were associated with French and British units much earlier, and two of these made very important contributions in CMF surgery. V. H. Kazanjian (1879–1974), a Harvard dental specialist, worked at first in prosthetic reconstructions: he later became a leading plastic surgeon (Converse 1977). Harvey Cushing, already the acknowledged leader of American neurosurgery, served with a British frontline medical unit in 1917, and demonstrated the merits of early wound exploration and closure in two classic papers, which are still well worth reading (Cushing 1918a,b). He reported a rigorous analysis of 133 head wounds with dural penetration treated over 3 months during the terrible battles around Passchendaele: in this period, his early mortality fell from 54.5% to 28.8%, an improvement attributed by him to better technique rather than to case selection. Cushing is not remembered as a modest man, but this report is remarkable for its generosity to British colleagues and for a total absence of comment on the fact that the work was done in a casualty clearing station dangerously close to battles which the author vividly described in the diary he kept during his exhausting work (Cushing 1936).

The end of World War I saw the management of CMF trauma well advanced. Gillies and his team had firmly established the value of the multidisciplinary team in the total care of maxillofacial injuries. His remarkable book (Gillies 1920) described the contribution of the dental prosthetist in fixation of jaw fractures (Fig. 1.16); he detailed the various skin flaps evolved to repair regional facial defects, including the tubed pedicle grafts for which he is famous. This procedure was first used by him in a case of burns, a field in which he also made fundamental contributions, in management strategy as well as in techniques; his principles of burn management, still very relevant, are discussed in Chapter 17. The battle of Jutland (31 May/1 June 1916) brought naval casualties to Sidcup, among them Able Seaman Vicarage, one of the few pioneering patients whose name has not been forgotten (Fig. 1.17). Vicarage had suffered appalling facial burns in a cordite fire in the battleship HMS Malaya; Gillies

gave him a new face 18 months later by swinging two tubed pedicle grafts from the chest (Gillies 1920, case 338; Pound 1964).

Gillies also used and extended French techniques (Imbert & Real 1917) of free bone grafting, using iliac or costochondral grafts. Bone grafts had been used with success in long bone injuries; in the later years of the war, several small series of mandibular reconstructions with free grafts were published, but the results were not brilliant (Cole 1918), sepsis being a frequent cause of failure (Fig. 1.18). Gillies has a central place in the history of the management of CMF injuries, and he was a great teacher. Many Sidcup techniques have become standard procedures, but perhaps more fundamental has been the Sidcup emphasis on aesthetic reconstruction as the prerequisite of psychological recovery.

Concurrently, Cushing had shown the merits of early operations, by neurosurgeons, for craniocerebral wounds; X-ray control, gentle debridement by suction and irrigation became routine procedures, and Baranyi's vision of primary wound closure was accepted as standard policy.

Advances in anaesthesia made these surgical achievements possible. Cushing, and some German plastic surgeons (Lexer 1931), favoured local or regional blocks, but Magill's routine use of endotracheal anaesthesia for CMF trauma showed the way to the future (Rowbotham & Magill 1921).

In retrospect, one can see some gaps in this record of achievement. The need for long-term neurorehabilitation was ignored or soon forgotten. Good as interdisciplinary collaboration between dentists and plastic surgeons had been in war, there was in many countries no systematic professional formulation for continuing this collaboration in peacetime. Nor did the need for routine collaboration between plastic surgeons, oral surgeons and neurosurgeons emerge during the war; indeed, increasing specialization may have made this collaboration less likely. Earlier in the war, a military writer on the surgery of the head could discuss brain and jaw wounds together, in the knowledge that the same surgeon might well treat both forms of CMF trauma (Rawling 1915). Later in the war, a definite conceptual separation is evident. Thus, Cushing made reference to the problems of craniocerebrofacial wounds, but did not enlarge on the contribution of the plastic surgeon; his preferred use of triradiate scalp incisions (Fig. 1.19) suggests that he would have benefited from collaboration of this type. These issues remained unresolved and perhaps unrecognized in the post-war years.

WORLD WAR II, 1939–1945

Logistics: Tönnis and Cairns

This war saw important advances in the logistic and organizational aspects of CMF trauma management, both in the field of maxillofacial surgery and in neurosurgical

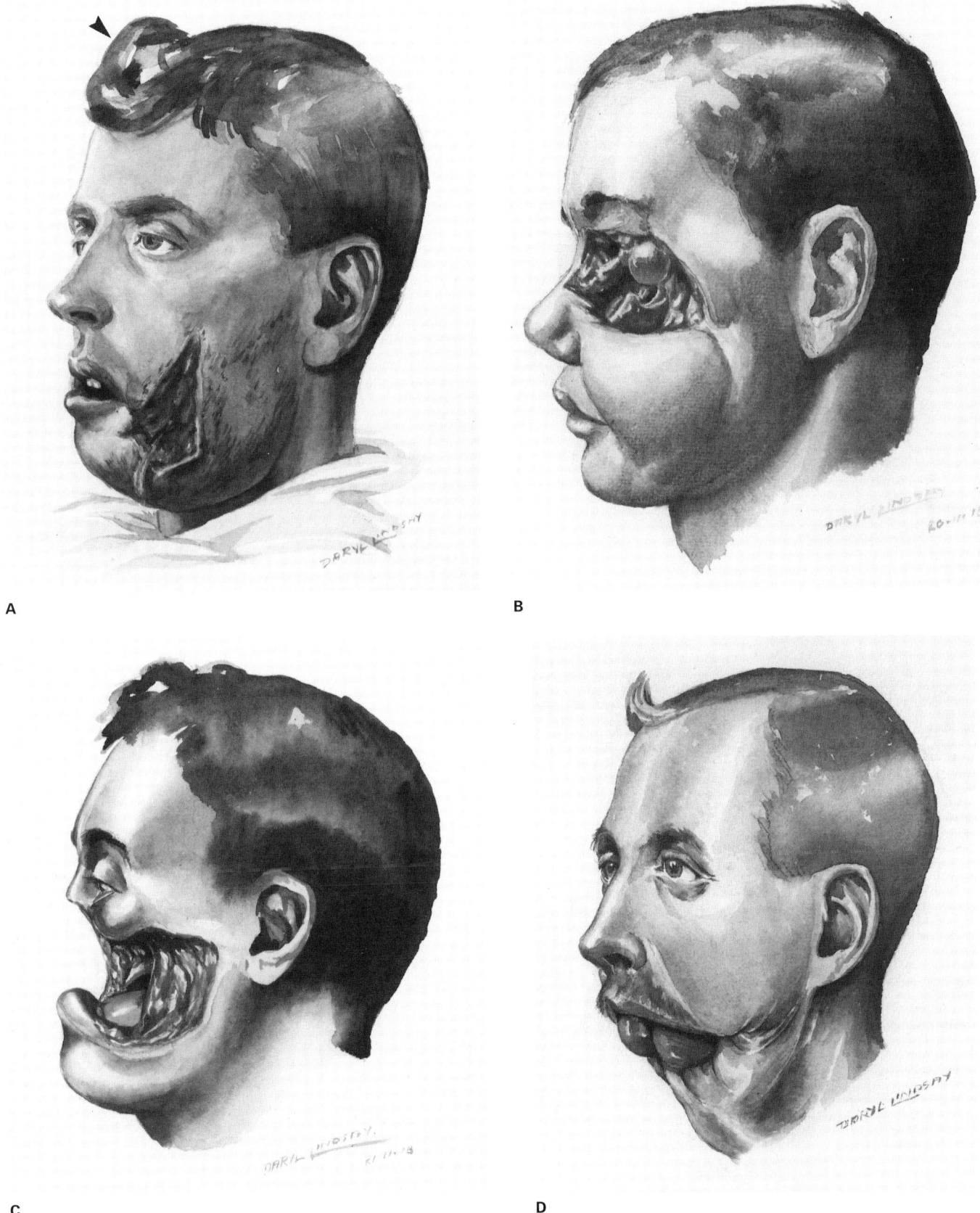

Fig. 1.15 The disasters of war. Four young wounded soldiers, treated in Queen Mary's Hospital, Sidcup, 1918–9. Watercolours by Sir Daryl Lindsay. By courtesy of the Royal Australasian College of Surgeons. **A** Facial and frontal wounds: the frontal swelling appears to be a cerebral hernia. **B** Massive orbital destruction. **C** Massive ablation of upper jaw and nose. **D** Ablation of lower jaw.

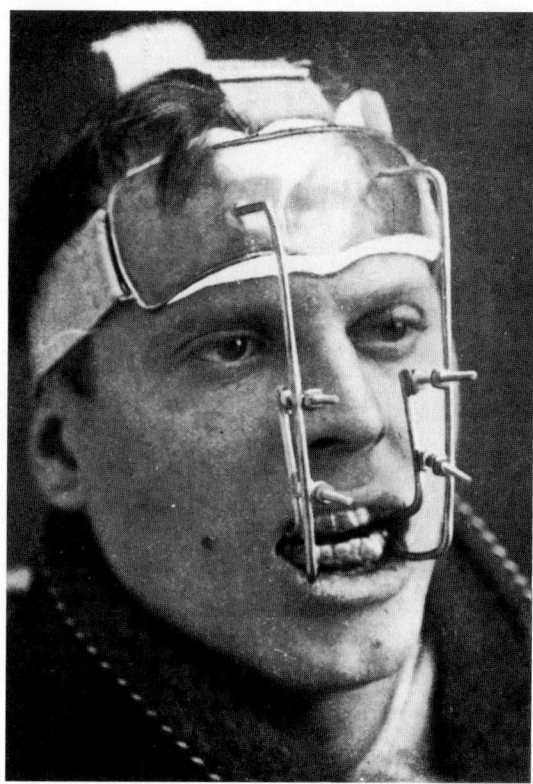

Fig. 1.16 Maxillary fixation in World War I. Apparatus for forward replacement of the maxilla, devised by Major Rischworth, a New Zealand dental surgeon. From H. Gillies (1920), *Plastic Surgery of the Face*, Oxford University Press.

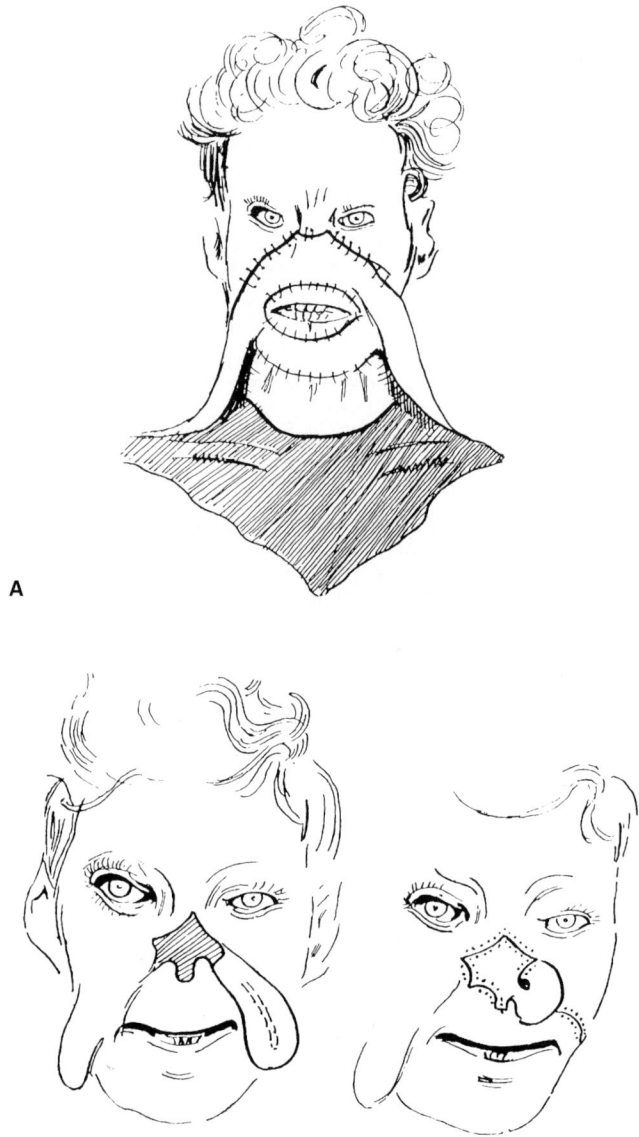

Fig. 1.17 Tubular pedicle grafts for facial deformity after burns: Gillies' first case. The patient had been severely burned some 18 months earlier. Gillies planned to excise the scar tissue and replace it with two flaps of vascularized skin from the thorax. He was inspired to convert these flaps into tubes. **A** Diagram of the plan of operation. The flaps took well, but the skin over the nose became necrotic. **B** When the pedicles were vascularized, the left pedicle was detached and used to cover the nose. Later operations corrected ectropion on both sides, and replaced the eyebrows with scalp grafts. The nose was reconstructed with an allograft of cartilage. The final appearance was considered to be aesthetically successful, and the eyelid functions were much improved.

treatment. These wartime developments have had enduring consequences in peacetime surgery. At the beginning of the war, two great neurosurgeons were in positions of power in their respective countries: Wilhelm Tönnis (1898–1978) as consultant surgeon to the German airforce (Luftwaffe), and Hugh Cairns (1896–1952) as neurosurgical consultant in the British army. Both had served in the World War I, and both saw the need for an integrated service that would give expert neurosurgical care as soon as possible, and would maintain that care until rehabilitation was completed.

Tönnis created, from the outset of the war, a comprehensive service of this type. Great use was made of air transport. When Poland was attacked in 1939, Luftwaffe aircraft, chiefly the famous three-engined Junkers JU52, brought some 2500 casualties back to established neurosurgical units in Berlin, Breslau and Vienna: the average flying time was under three hours. Priority was given to brain, eye and jaw wounds. The Luftwaffe was not the first service to use aircraft in this way; indeed, aircraft had been used for peacetime accident cases in outback Australia for many years. But the Luftwaffe's massive achievement impressed even its enemies, and other combatants soon organized air ambulance services. The small Australian air force pioneered with such a service

in the Middle East theatre of war. In the Pacific theatre, where there was often no alternative means of transport, US medical authorities deployed special air evacuation units, providing trained medical and nursing staff for care of patients in military transport aircraft; these anticipated the modern air medical and paramedical retrieval teams.

Hugh Cairns, a South Australian and the much-loved

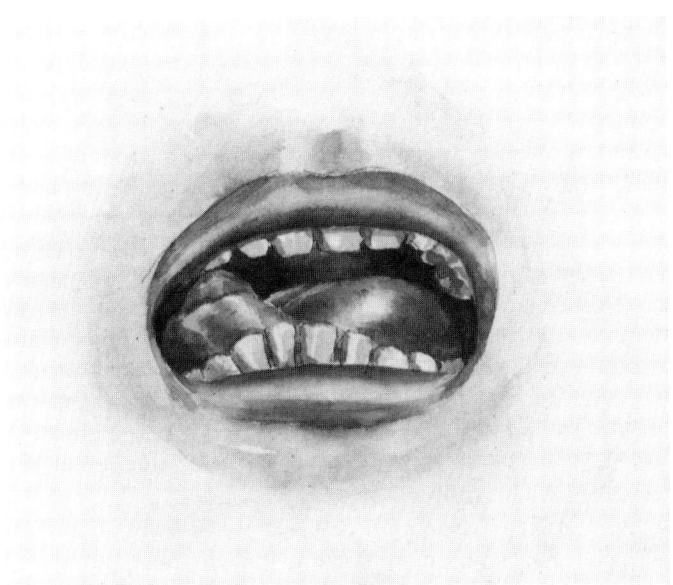

Fig. 1.18 Bone grafting in World War I. Tibial bone graft (arrow) extruding from the mandible: wounded soldier treated September 1917 to February 1919. Watercolour by Sir Daryl Lindsay. By courtesy of Royal Australasian College of Surgeons.

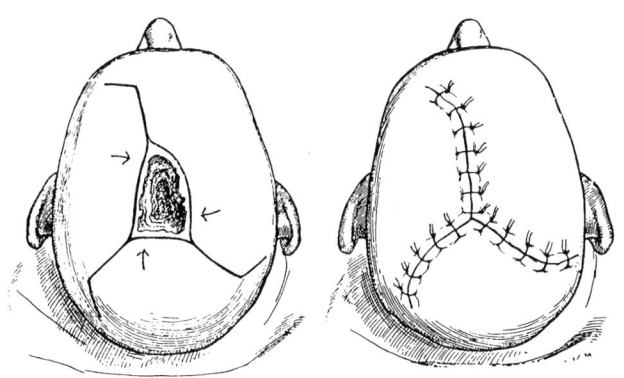

Fig. 1.19 Scalp closure in World War I. Cushing's well known tripod or three-legged incision for wounds of the cranial vault. Personal experience has shown that closure by a rotating flap is usually preferable. From Cushing (1918).

founder of the Oxford neurosurgical school (Fraenkel 1991), approached the logistic challenge of head injuries in a somewhat different way. He established a 300-bed base hospital for head injuries in Oxford, but his most original concept was the 'mobile neurosurgical unit', a small self-contained team that could go anywhere. These very flexible units, staffed by a dozen persons of whom only one was a fully trained neurosurgeon, were equipped to work either close to the battlefield, or in a base hospital; Cairns (1947) has told their story well and for the present purpose it is only necessary to say that these teams both advanced the technical management of brain wounds and pioneered in the multidisciplinary management of complex craniofacial injuries.

The Trinity

Maxillofacial wound management had a parallel evolution. Harold Gillies and Kelsey Fry, with the prestige and experience of their Sidcup achievements, were well qualified to advise on the organization of services in this field. Base units were established in Great Britain, the best known being in Basingstoke under Gillies himself. Rooksdown House in Basingstoke became a great teaching centre during and after the war: from it came the classic textbook *Fractures of the Facial Skeleton*, written by two great oral surgeons, Norman Rowe (1915–1991) and Homer Charles (Paddy) Killey (1915–1976). In addition to the base maxillofacial and plastic units, mobile units analogous to Cairns's mobile neurosurgical units were formed and deployed in various theatres; eventually there were six of these in the British army and two more in India.

There were also in the British army special mobile opthalmological units, deployed as far forward as possible (Goulden 1953). It was common practice to group special neurosurgical, ophthalmological and maxillofacial units closely together: as early as 1943, this grouping was being called 'The Trinity'. This interdisciplinary grouping can be related to the increasing interest in complex craniofacial and cranio-orbital wounds, which constituted up to a quarter of all brain injuries in one large series.

Concern over the treatment of injuries involving the anterior cranial fossa was relatively new. Between the two world wars, neurosurgeons had begun to repair the anterior fossa in cases of post-traumatic cerebrospinal fluid leak: Walter Dandy (1886–1946) had reported a successful case in 1926. Wartime experience of a high incidence of infection after wounds opening the paranasal air sinuses made it logical to carry out such repairs as part of the primary wound closure. However, many wounds of this type showed extensive tissue loss in the fronto-orbital region, and elaborate plastic procedures were needed to close the defects. Thus, interdisciplinary collaboration in CMF trauma management was carried a step further. This is evident in the remarkable *War Surgery Supplement* of the *British Journal of Surgery* which appeared in 1947: it was edited by Cairns, and includes superb illustrations, many of which show craniofacial wounds (Fig. 1.20).

The war saw advances in management of faciomaxillary trauma. Bone grafting of mandibular fractures became increasingly successful. In England, Gillies' pupil Rainsford Mowlem (1902–1988), also a New Zealander, demonstrated the value of cancellous bone (Mowlem 1944). Blocker & Stout (1949) performed what would now be called a meta-analysis of US wartime experience of bone grafts, and found a final success rate of 97%. However, the authors noted that poor follow-up made this imposing achievement somewhat suspect. Fixation of fractures of the mandible by external pins (Fig. 1.21) was also used where other means failed: fear of infection had deterred

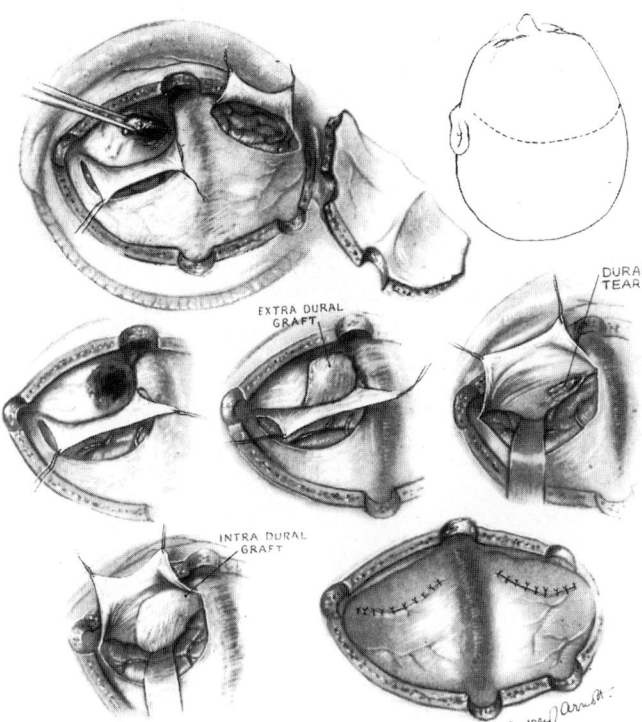

Fig. 1.20 Craniofacial wound in World War II. Repair of an orbitonasofrontal wound, caused by a shell fragment, which had lodged in the ethmoid air cells. Drawn by Audrey Arnot, whose illustrations of operations done by Cairns and his pupils are rightly famous. From Calvert (1947), by courtesy of Messrs Heinemann.

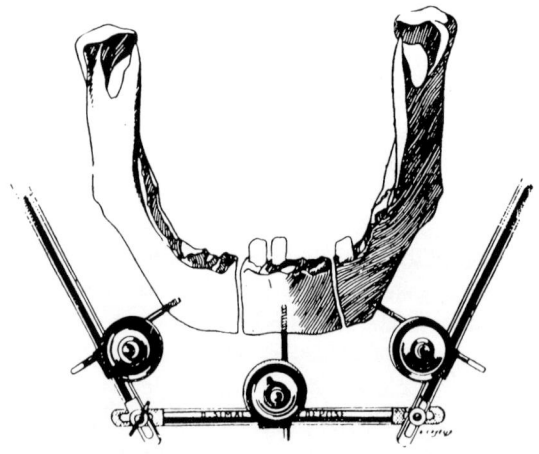

Fig. 1.21 External fixation in World War II. Pin fixation of mandibular fracture, the method employed by Roger Anderson for other fractures, and by G. Maurel in 1940. From Rowe & Killey (1955).

surgeons from much use of open fixation of mandibular fractures, but the advent of chemotherapy opened up this possibility also (Fry 1953). Maxillary fractures received more attention than in the past; fixation to a plaster headcap became a routine procedure (Wallace 1985).

Sulphonamides and penicillin

Chemotherapy was the great innovation of this period. Surgeons dealing with wounds in World War I had tried many external antiseptic agents without success and the need for an antibacterial agent in the circulating blood had been recognized. Antisera had been tried with no effect; urotropine, now a forgotten drug, had been given in the hope that it would generate formaldehyde in the tissues. But until the discovery of the sulphonamides in 1935, there was no chemotherapeutic agent of real worth. Sulphonamides were indeed effective, especially against streptococci, and they were given liberally, sometimes to the neglect of good surgery; Tönnis (1943) wrote critically of 'sulphonamide fanatics' who did not appreciate the primary importance of operative wound closure. However, penicillin was far more potent, and its advent in 1942 was particularly effective in the treatment and prevention of brain infections. Penicillin was brought into surgical use by Cairns, in collaboration with his fellow South Australian Howard Florey (1898–1968); it proved its value in CMF trauma management in the 1943 Italian campaign.

World War II brought the surgery of brain wounds in general, and especially craniofacial wounds, to a stage that is recognizably close to modern practice (Table 1.2): later wars have emphasized the lessons learned then, and have only slightly modified them (p. 373). Head injury rehabilitation was also stimulated by the challenge of so many young men with neurological disabilities. In Russia, Aleksandr Luria (1902–1977) advanced views on the nature of recovery from brain injury that have since inspired many workers in this field; in the USA, the importance of systematic rehabilitation was emphasized by Goldstein, who had emigrated to New York from Nazi Germany.

MULTIDISCIPLINARY MANAGEMENT

Road crashes and trauma management

After 1945, the USA and Western Europe experienced a mounting pandemic of injuries due to road crashes, and within a few years, increasing motorization brought this pandemic to most other parts of the world. Injuries in the CMF region attracted particular attention, and not only as causes of death: with better airway management and nutritional support, prolonged survival in what was later called the vegetative state became a common sequel of severe brain injury.

Surgeons responded to the challenge of these CMF injuries, often with multiple injuries elsewhere, in many ways. These responses are now largely embodied in modern thought and practice. Much of what was innovative in the decade after the World War II is still very relevant, and will be discussed in appropriate parts of this book: in this chapter, only a few major developments are considered.

Accident prevention became, perhaps for the first time in surgical history, a leading consideration. In the USA, the neurosurgeon Elisha Gurdjian (1900–1985) and the engineer Herbert Lissner (1907–1965) made Wayne State University in Detroit a multidisciplinary centre for research in the bioengineering aspects of head impacts, and this has had enormous importance in head and face protection. Colonel John P. Stapp and other volunteers explored the effects of high velocity accidents on themselves and on anaesthetized animals, using a rocket-propelled sled devised by German wartime research workers concerned with aircraft crashes. Stapp saw the relevance of these studies to road accidents and annual Stapp Car Crash Conferences commemorate his initiative and courage. In Oxford, Cairns inspired the physicist A. H. S. Holbourn (1907–1962) to investigate the dynamics of closed head injuries, and this led directly to Sabina Strich's historic discovery of what is now called diffuse axonal injury (p. 139). In Australia, the concern of a number of surgeons did much to give that country priority in the mandatory use of crash helmets and seat belts and in alcohol control.

Trauma management benefited from advances in diagnostic radiology. Brain imaging began in 1918 with air contrast ventriculography and encephalography, but these procedures had little place in the management of acute brain injuries. Cerebral angiography, first reported by the Portuguese neurologist Egas Moniz (1875–1955) in 1927, was used to exclude complications of head injury as early as 1936 (Lohr quoted by Lima 1950). After 1950 percutaneous angiography was increasingly used even in acute cases (Fig. 1.22). However, these invasive procedures were largely superseded by computed tomography (CT), which came into clinical use in 1973. Tomography with a moving X-ray source and conventional silver halide film was used to visualize facial fractures as early as 1940 (Culler 1940); plain tomography was found invaluable in delineating the temporomandibular joint and the cribriform plate. In 1973, the British physicist G. N. Hounsfield's inspired combination of computer analysis with scintillation detection made computed axial tomography the safest and most effective means of imaging the brain, and it still holds this place in trauma management despite the later advent of magnetic resonance imaging (p. 186). The first generation of CT scanners did not provide sufficient definition to visualize facial fractures, but later models could do this, and with software programs allowing three-dimensional reconstruction, the visualization of facial trauma was further advanced.

These increasingly complex methods of imaging the damaged brain and the shattered face brought logistic problems: there was a large capital cost and trained radiological staff had to be available at short notice. The care of the comatose patient was also very demanding. Modern

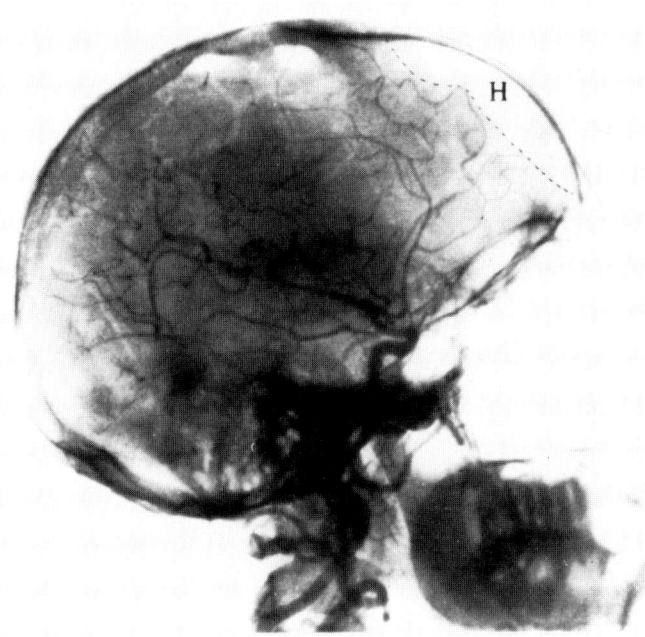

Fig. 1.22 Portuguese contribution: cerebral angiography. Cerebral angiography, introduced by Egas Moniz, has been an important advance in the management of CMF injuries. The Lisbon school pioneered intracarotid injection of thorotrast, which visualized surface clots very well. Unfortunately, the long-term complications of this radioactive contrast agent were often devastating. From Lima (1950), by courtesy of Oxford University Press.

coma care began around 1950 with the general use of tracheotomy, both for the 'stoved-in face' (Nelson 1958), and for the comatose craniocerebral injury where death from respiratory complications would have been inevitable 20 years earlier (Echols et al 1950). The success of tracheotomy encouraged other methods of maintaining normal cerebral physiology, especially oxygenation and intracranial pressure (ICP). Continuous ICP monitoring was introduced in France in 1951 (Guillaume & Janny 1951) and in Sweden a few years later (Lundberg 1983); monitoring has since become a routine part of neurosurgical intensive care, in conjunction with mechanical ventilation. Intensive care was even more demanding in medical and nursing staff and in laboratory services. Only large, well-funded metropolitan hospitals could meet these needs, yet in most countries it became evident that road crashes, unlike the industrial accidents of the nineteenth century, often occurred far from major hospitals.

The concept of the 'trauma centre' was evolved to provide expensive, highly specialized multidisciplinary management for the victims of severe peacetime trauma. This concept had indeed its roots in the experience of World War II, after which Hugh Cairns and his successors had established in Oxford a trauma service that embodied this philosophy. But experience in the long and tragic war in Vietnam brought new insights and techniques. There, one side enjoyed total air superiority: helicopters could be used to transport the wounded to mobile surgical hospitals with unprecedented speed and greatly superior results. In West Germany and somewhat later in the USA, similar rescue services were developed for road and other civilian injuries, and based on metropolitan hospitals. In San Francisco, rapid transport to centralized trauma management was compared favourably with less systematic care in another area, Orange County. Trunkey (1983), in a very influential paper, made a case for regional trauma centres, and these have been widely accepted in the USA and Canada. Today, the concept of the Trauma Centre is implicit in the multidisciplinary management of severe CMF trauma in many parts of the world, not least in Australia, a country which suffers more than most from what has been called the tyranny of distance — the logistic constraints of geography and demography.

Advent of craniofacial surgery

After 1970, a new surgical philosophy began to modify and refine the management of facial injuries. In the preceding decade, Paul Tessier and his colleagues at the Hôpital Foch in Paris had devised innovative surgical procedures to correct congenital facial dysmorphisms, especially those involving severe orbital deformity. In doing this, Tessier created the subspecialty of craniofacial surgery, which in his hands embodied not only a variety of carefully designed anatomical corrections in three dimensions, but also a multidisciplinary, team-based system of assessment and holistic treatment. Tessier's achievements in the surgery of congenital malformations lie outside the scope of this book. But the insights and the methods of craniofacial surgery have greatly enriched the management of CMF trauma.

Tessier was trained in the grand mainstream of French surgical teaching, which has stressed the importance of trauma since the time of Paré, and his formative experiences began during the World War II. He has told how in 1944, only 2 years after his internship, he became an assistant in the Centre of Maxillo-Facial Surgery in the Paris Military Region, which treated many facial wounds in the tough fighting that liberated Paris. In 1946, this army service was transferred to the Hôpital Foch, which for a while housed separate military and civilian units. It will surprise nobody who loves France that these units 'did not appreciate each other'; as an expression of this mood, the senior army surgeon refused to give the young Tessier access to the hospital's prosthodontic department. This forced Tessier to develop that reliance on internal fixation which is so fundamental in modern craniofacial technique (Wolfe & Berkowitz 1989). Paris was not the only place where it proved hard to maintain wartime co-operation, both interdisciplinary and personal, in peace-time surgery, where the isolationism of each specialty becomes stronger as time passes; it is not the smallest of

Tessier's achievements that he institutionalized the multi-disciplinary craniofacial team. Such teams need constant practice; Tessier (1971) emphasized that engagement in a busy trauma service keeps the team's skills sharp and ready to deal with the more complex problems of dysmorphia.

Tessier inspired many young plastic surgeons to form craniofacial units. What is now the Australian Craniofacial Unit began in 1974, when one of us (D.J.D) saw a need for a service of this type in South Australia, and entered into close collaboration with a small group of neuro-surgeons already much engaged in trauma management; several of them also had some acquaintance with missile trauma in less peaceful countries. Similar groups, each with its own mix of specialties and its own personal dynamics, were established at the same time in a number of centres in North America, Europe and elsewhere. The treatment of CMF trauma received great impetus from multidisciplinary groups of this type.

Internal fixation of facial fractures

In 1942, Adams of Memphis (Tennessee) advocated internal suspension and fixation of midface fractures by wiring (Fig. 1.23); he reported a low incidence of infection, and the advent of chemotherapy made surgeons braver in accepting techniques involving open exposure of fractures. Tessier's reconstructive techniques entailed internal fixation of mobilized components of the facial skeleton by wires passed through small drill holes, and the success of these procedures encouraged many surgeons to use similar methods to fix fractures of the mandible and maxilla. Metal plates offered greater stability than wires. Metal plates had been used for fixing long bone fractures since the nineteenth century, but the use of inappropriate types of steel had led to inflammatory complications resulting from metallic corrosion. In the decade preceding World War II, experimental studies had shown the importance of biocompatibility in implanted materials. Venable et al (1937) championed the alloy Vitallium, but chromium – nickel–molybdenum (18/8/Mo) steel was also found to perform well in the tissues, and was easier to forge. With the availability of these biocompatible metals, the Swiss Arbeitsgemeinschaft für Osteosynthese-fragen (AO) reopened in 1958 the question of internal fixation of fractures, and soon European maxillofacial surgeons were successfully plating fractures of the facial skeleton (p. 237). Titanium, originally used in ortho-paedic procedures, was found to be better tolerated than steel or vitallium, and has been used widely for facial fracture fixation and cranioplasty (pp. 270 and 549).

Contemporary management of CMF injuries

From the shared experience of many workers in the

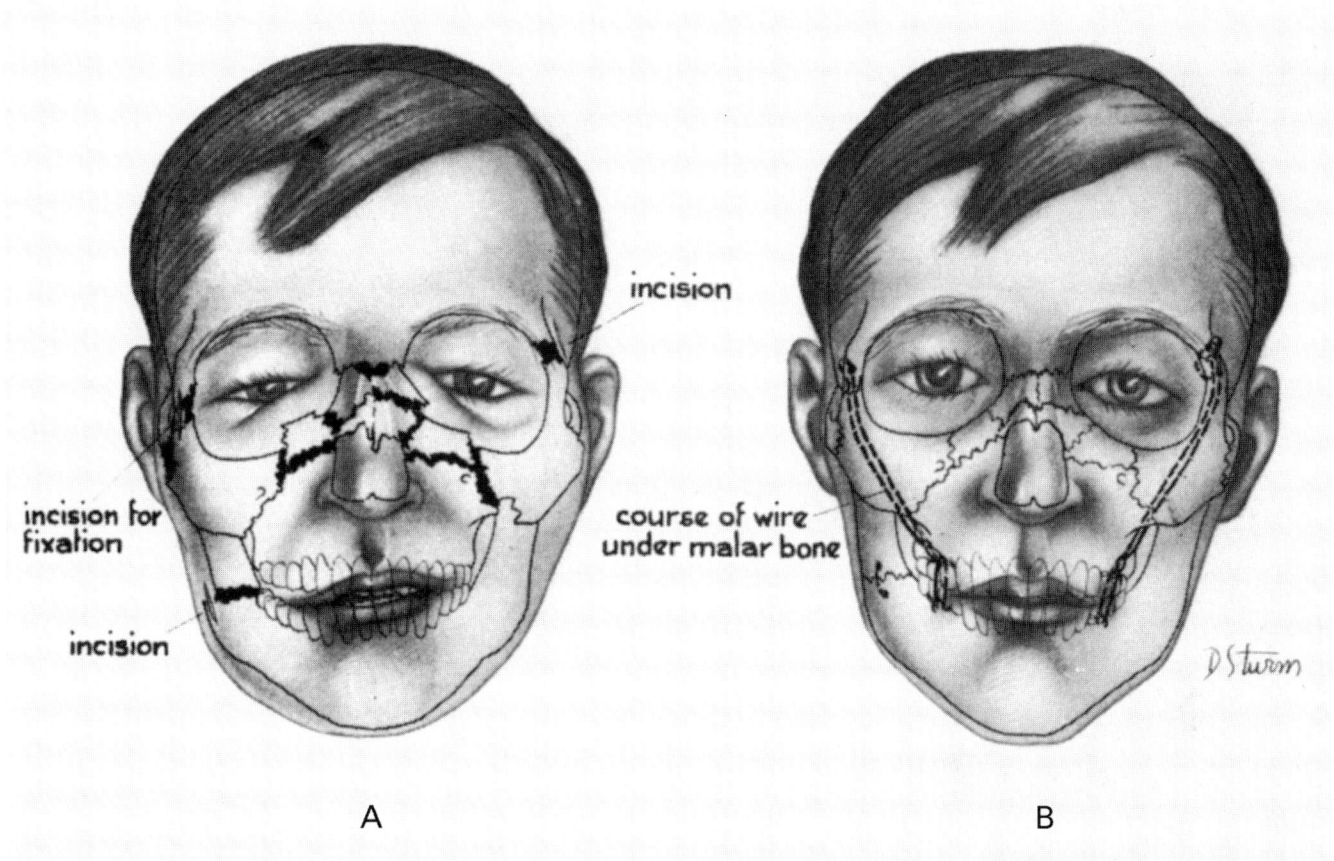

Fig. 1.23 Internal fixation of midfacial fractures. The use of internal fixation of fractures by wiring of the middle third of the face was reported by Adams (1942). His paper is a landmark in the management of CMF injuries. **A** Comminuted fracture of maxilla, presumably Le Fort III type, with fractures of both zygomas; fracture of right mandible. **B** The fractures have been reduced by open operation; the maxillary component was fixed with wires secured to upper teeth and passed to the frontal bone on each side. The left zygoma and the mandible were also fixed by wiring. From Adams (1942).

management of CMF trauma has emerged what can be called the craniofacial perspective:

1. Complex injuries demand a team. Tessier began his work with the orbit as the centrepiece: he deployed there the skills of both the maxillofacial surgeon and the neurosurgeon. Other structures in the CMF region demand other skills, especially in the oral area.

2. Modern methods of imaging show the nature of the damage, and allow decision on the timing of surgical correction: delay is often beneficial, but the neurosurgical and ophthalmological complications of CMF trauma sometimes need urgent action.

3. Wide exposure of the craniofacial skeleton is needed, either through the bicoronal scalp flap, or through one of a choice of periorbital, intraoral and extraoral incisions.

4. Modern craniofacial surgery follows Tessier in aiming to effect internal fixation by primary bone grafts, together with wires, plates and screws. Small plates constructed of biologically acceptable materials have greatly facilitated fixation.

5. Microvascular repair, introduced some 30 years ago (Jacobson & Suarez 1960), has enlarged the scope of grafting with soft tissues and with bone; aspects of the remarkable history of microvascularized bone grafts are given on p. 623.

6. Advances in prosthetic design and materials can supplement surgical correction of traumatic defects by a range of intraoral and extraoral prostheses, including osseo-integrated implants.

7. Advances in conservative dentistry have made it possible to salvage injured teeth that would have been condemned in the past. The science of endodontics has come of age, and the rationale and techniques of endodontic therapy are now integrated in the modern management of maxillofacial trauma.

The surgery of CMF injuries has come a long way in the last four millennia and without doubt it will go further. This book is an endeavour to assess current techniques, and to identify the chief principles of treatment. In the perspective of history, these principles are not new, but their interpretation is constantly changing, and finality remains an unattainable goal.

REFERENCES

Adams W M 1942 Internal wiring fixation of facial fractures. Surgery 12: 523–540

Adamson P B 1977 A comparison of ancient and modern weapons in the effectiveness of producing battle casualties. J R Army Med Corps 123: 93–103

Adamson P B 1990 Medical complications associated with security and control of prisoners of war in the ancient Near East. Med Hist 34: 311–319

Albert D M, Diaz-Rohena R 1989 A historical review of sympathetic ophthalmia and its epidemiology. Surv Ophthalmol 24: 1–14

Albrecht P, Feuchtinger R 1916 Über die offene und geschlossene Wundbehandlung bei Gehirnschüsse. Wien Med Wochenschr 67: 14–22

Angle E H 1890 A new method for the treatment of fractures of the maxillae. Intern Dent J NY 11: 330 (Cited by Rowe & Killey 1955, p 890)

Anonymous 1765 Encyclopedie ou dictionnaire raisonné des sciences, des arts et des métiers. Trépan, trépaner. Faulche, Neufchastel, Vol 16, pp 590–593

Anonymous 1899 Sad fatality at Harrow. The Autocar, pp 174–179

Bakay L 1971 The treatment of head injuries in the Thirty Years' War (1618–1648). Thomas, Springfield, Illinois

Bennett J P 1986 Henry Tonks and his contemporaries. Br J Plast Surg 39: 1–34

Blocker T G, Stout R A 1949 Mandibular reconstruction, World War II. Plast Reconstr Surg 4: 153–156

Breasted J H 1930 The Edwin Smith papyrus. University of Chicago Press, Chicago

Cairns H 1947 Neurosurgery in the British Army, 1939–1945. Br J Surg, War Surgery Suppl I: 9–26

Celsus, A Cornelius 1938 De medicina. Transl W G Spencer, Loeb Classical Library. Heinemann, London

Chatelin C, de Martel T 1918 Wounds of the skull and brain (Military Medical Manuals). University of London Press, London

Cole P P 1918 Ununited fractures of the mandible: their incidence, causation and treatment. Br J Surg 6: 57–72

Converse J M 1977 Introduction to plastic surgery. In: Converse J M, McCarthy J G (eds) Plastic reconstructive surgery, 2nd edn. Saunders, Philadelphia, Vol 1

Culler A U 1940 Fractures of orbit; demonstration of orbit by planigraphy (body section radiography). Trans Am Ophthalmol Soc 28: 348–369

Cushing H 1918a Notes on penetrating wounds of the brain. Br Med J i: 221–226

Cushing H 1918b A study of a series of wounds involving the brain and its enveloping structures. Br J Surg 5: 558–684

Cushing H 1936 From a surgeon's journal, 1915–1918. Little, Brown & Co., Boston

Dandy W 1926 Pneumocephalus (intracranial pneumatocele or aerocele). Arch Surg 12: 949–982

De Moulin D 1988 A history of surgery. Nijhoff, Dordrecht

Dowd N 1972 Hunter's lectures of anatomy (facsimile). Elsevier, Amsterdam

Echols D H, Llewellyn R, Kirgis H D, Rehfeldt F C, García-Bengochea F 1950 Tracheotomy in the management of severe head injuries. Surgery 28: 801–811

Elliott J H 1963 The revolt of the Catalans. A study in the decline of Spain, 1598–1640. Cambridge University Press. Cambridge

Elyott T 1531 Boke named the Governour. From Encyclopedia Britannica, 11th edn: Football. Cambridge University Press, Cambridge, Vol 10, p 617

Evans I 1991 Traffic safety and the driver. Van Nostrand Reinhold, New York

Fairbank L C 1936 A short history of the treatment of maxillary fractures. Milit Surg 78: 95–103

Fraenkel G J 1991 Hugh Cairns, first Nuffield Professor of Surgery, University of Oxford. Oxford University Press, Oxford

Fry W K 1953 Maxillo-facial injuries. In: Cope Z (ed) History of the Second World War. UK Medical Series: Surgery. HMSO, London, Ch 9

Galen 1976 On the affected parts. Translation from the Greek text with explanatory notes. Transl Siegel R E. Karger, Basel

Gibbon E 1854 The history of the decline and fall of the Roman empire. Ed Smith W. Murray, London, Vol 4, pp 77–83

Gillies H D 1920 Plastic surgery of the face. Frowde, Hodder & Stoughton, London

Gnudi M T, Webster J P 1989 The life and times of Gaspare Tagliacozzi. Classics of Medicine Library. H Reichner, New York

Goulden C B 1953 Ophthalmology. In: Cope Z (ed) History of the Second World War. UK Medical Series: Surgery HMSO, London, Ch 15

Grahame-White C, Harper H 1914 The aeroplane. Jack, London

Guérin A 1866 Des fractures des maxillaires superieures. Archives generales de medicin, ser 6, 8: 1–13

Guillaume J, Janny P 1951 Manometrie intracrânienne continué. Intérêt de la méthode et premiers resultats. Rev Neurol (Paris) 84: 131–142

Gunning T B 1866–7 The treatment of fracture of the lower jaw by interdental splints. NY Med J 3: 433–448; 4: 11–29, 274–277

Gurdjian E S 1973 Head Injury from antiquity to the present with special reference to penetrating head wounds. Thomas, Springfield, Illinois

Guthrie G J 1847 On injuries of the head affecting the brain. Churchill & Renshaw, London

Hamby W B 1967 Ambroise Paré, surgeon of the Renaissance. Green, St Louis

Hippocrates 1927 Works. Transl W T Witherinton, Loeb Classical Library. Heinemann, London, Vol 3

Hoffmann-Axthelm W 1982 The treatment of maxillofacial fractures and dislocations in historical perpective. In: Oral and maxillofacial traumatology. Krüger E, Schilli W (eds) Quintessence, Chicago

Hoffmann-Axthelm W 1991 Festvortrag zur 40. Jahrestagung der Deutschen Gesellschaft für Mund-, Kiefer- und Gesichtschirurgie Fortschr Kiefer Gesichtschir 36: 1–5

Hudson 1877 On the use of the trephine in depressed fractures of the skull. Br Med J 2: 75–76

Hughes J E 1972 Henry Simpson Newland. Griffin Press, Adelaide

Imbert L, Real P 1917 La greffe osseuse dans les fractures mandibulaires a large perte de substance. La Restauration Maxillo-faciale 1: 20–32

Jacobson J H, Suarez E L 1960 Microsurgery in anastomosis of small vessels. Surg Forum 11: 243–245

Jessop W H H 1915 Discussion on ophthalmic injuries in warfare. Trans Ophthalmol Soc UK 35: 1–13

Johnson L W 1936 Plastic surgery in relation to the armed forces: past, present and future. Milit Surg 79: 90–120

Knott J W (In press) Road traffic accidents in New South Wales, 1881–1991. Austral Econ Hist Rev 24

Kocher T 1901 Hirnerschütterung, Hirndruck und chirurgische Eingriffe bei Hirnkrankheiten. Hölder, Vienna

Lay M G 1993 Ways of the world. A history of the world's roads and the vehicles that used them. Primavera, Sydney (Also published by Rutgers University Press)

Le Dran H F 1740 Observations in surgery. Transl J S Surgeon, 2nd edn. Hodges, London

Le Fort R 1901 Etude experimentale sur les fractures de la machoire superieure. Revue de chirurgie 23: 208–227, 360–379, 479–507 [See MacDowell (1977) for a translation and commentary by Paul Tessier]

Lexer E 1931 Die gesamte Wiederherstellungschirurgie. Barth, Leipzig

Lima P A 1950 Cerebral angiography. Oxford University Press, Oxford

Liston R 1846 Practical surgery, 4th edn. John Churchill, Soho

Lundberg N 1983 The saga of the Monro-Kellie doctrine. In: Ishii S, Nagai H, Brock M (eds) Intracranial pressure. Springer, Berlin, Vol 5, pp 68–75

Macewen W 1893 Pyogenic infective diseases of the brain and spinal cord. Maclehose, Glasgow

Majno M 1991 The healing hand. Man and wound in the ancient world. Harvard University Press, Cambridge

McDowell F 1977 The sourcebook of plastic surgery. Williams & Wilkins, Baltimore

Mowlem R 1944 Cancellous chip bone graft. Lancet 2: 746–748

Nelson T G 1958 Tracheotomy: a clinical and experimental study. Williams & Wilkins, Baltimore

O'Halloran S 1793 A new treatise on the different disorders arising from external injuries of the head. Robinson, London

Otis G A 1870 The medical and surgical history of the War of the Rebellion (1861–65). Surgeon General, Washington, DC, Part 1, Vol 2

Overy R 1992 The wheels — and wings — of progress. Hist Today 42: 21–27

Pagel W 1982 Paracelsus. Karger, Basel

Paré A 1649 The Workes of that famous Chirurgeon Ambrose Parey. Translated out of Latin and compared with the French by Tho: Johnson. Cotes & Dugard, London

Parker G 1988 The military revolution. Military innovation and the rise of the West, 1500–1800. Cambridge University Press, Cambridge

Pott P 1779 The chirurgicall works of Percivall Pott, FRS. Lowndes, London, Vol 1

Pound R 1964 Gillies — surgeon extraordinary. Michael Joseph, London

Rawling L B 1915 Surgery of the head. Oxford War Primers. Frowde, Hodder & Stoughton, London

Reister F A 1975 Medical statistics in World War II. Office of the Surgeon General, Department of the Army, Washington, DC

Rowbotham E S, Magill I 1921 Anaesthetics in the plastic surgery of the jaw and face. Proc R Soc Med 14, Section of Anaesthetics: 17–27

Rowe N L, Killey H C 1955 Fractures of the facial skeleton. Livingstone, Edinburgh

Ryan G A 1965 Injuries and injury production in traffic accidents in metropolitan Adelaide. Unpublished thesis for the degree of Doctor of Medicine, University of Adelaide

Schneider R C 1966 Serious and fatal neurosurgical football injuries.

Clin Neurosurg 12: 226–236

Sellars W C, Yeatman R J 1930 1066 and all that: a memorable history of England. Methuen, London

Simpson D 1987 Awareness of tragedy. Child's Nerv Syst 3: 135–139

Tessier P 1971 Total osteotomy of the middle third of the face for faciostenosis or for sequelae of Le Fort 3 fractures. Plast Reconstr Surg 48: 533–541

Tönnis W 1943 Grundsätzliche Bemerkungen zur operativen Wundbehandlungen bei Hirnschüssen. Zentralbl Neurochir 8: 1–5

Trueta J 1944 The principles and practice of war surgery, 2nd edn. Hamish Hamilton, London

Trunkey D D 1983 Trauma. Sci Am 249: 20–27

Venable C S, Stuck W G, Beach A 1937 The effects on bone of the presence of metals: based on electrolysis. Ann Surg 105: 917–938

Wallace J 1988 A new frame for craniomaxillary fixation. Br J Oral Maxillofac Surg 23: 304–307

Watt J 1975 The injuries of four centuries of naval warfare. Ann R Coll Surg Engl 57: 3–24

Watt J 1980 The burns of seafarers under oars, sail and steam. Injury 12: 69–81

Wilson D F, Grappin G, Miquel J L 1992 Traditional, cultural and ritual practices involving the teeth and orofacial soft tissues. In: Prabhu S R, Wilson D F, Daftary D K, Johnson N W (eds) Oral diseases in the tropics. Oxford University Press, Oxford, pp 91–120

Wiseman R 1977 Of wounds, of gun-shot wounds, of fractures and luxations. (Facsimile reprint from Severall Chirurgicall Treatises, 1676.) Kingsmead, Bath

Wolfe S A Berkowitz S 1989 Plastic surgery of the facial skeleton. Little, Brown & Co., Boston, ppxiv–xvii

Zilz J 1917 Pathologische Anatomie und Ballistik der Kieferverletzungen. Wien Med Wschr 67: 819–823

CHAPTER 2

Functional anatomy

T. Brown   D. J. David   P. L. Reilly
Contributing authors: J. Crompton   M. Hammerton
J. Tomich

DEFINITION OF THE CRANIOMAXILLOFACIAL REGION

An understanding of trauma in this region presupposes an appreciation of the bony and soft tissue anatomy of the entire head, including the skull and the cranial viscera. The skull comprises three principal structures: the calvaria or vault, the cranial base and the facial skeleton. The calvaria provides mechanical protection for the brain against external violence. The cranial base provides a platform for the brain, with exit foramina for the cranial vessels and nerves. It is the template of the skull: from it is suspended the facial skeleton and above it rises the dome-shaped vault. Base and vault constitute the neurocranium. The facial bones (sometimes called the viscerocranium) enclose the eyes, the upper parts of the airway, and the upper digestive tract; they are coated with muscles and ligaments which give the face much of its form and function. The frontal component of the head, designated the craniomaxillofacial (CMF) region by clinicians, comprises the facial skeleton and the associated viscera and integuments, together with the anterior cranial fossa, the calvaria anterior to the coronal sutures, and the frontal lobes of the brain (Fig. 2.1).

THE BONES AND THEIR ARTICULATIONS

Calvaria

This part of the skull is formed chiefly by the frontal, parietal, temporal and occipital bones. The thick frontal bone forms the forehead and is connected anteriorly with the facial skeleton by the frontonasal, frontomaxillary and frontozygomatic sutures. The thin paired orbital plates

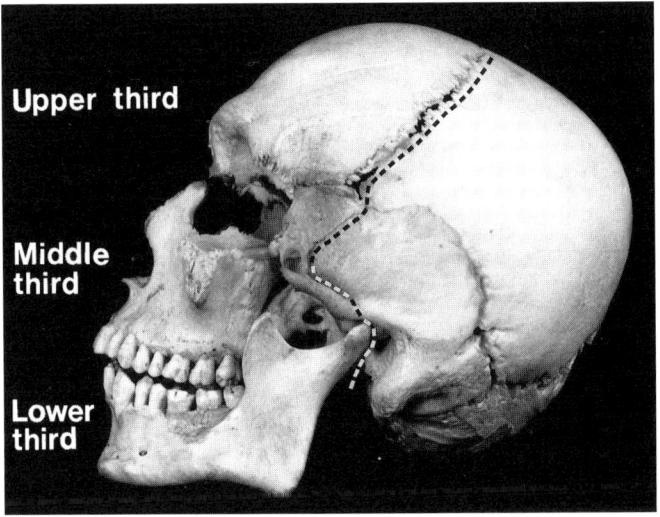

Fig. 2.1 Demarcation of the craniomaxillofacial region. A disjoined view of a normal skull: the dotted line shows the demarcation of the CMF region by the coronal suture, the sphenoid bone and the external auditory meatus. Within this region, it is usual to divide the face into thirds: upper, middle and lower.

curve posteriorly to articulate with other components of the cranial base by the sphenofrontal and fronto-ethmoid sutures. Posteriorly the frontal bone articulates with the parietal bones by the coronal suture. The parietal and occipital bones, which are outside the CMF region as here defined, articulate with each other, with the temporal bones and with the greater wings of the sphenoid laterally. The temporal bone forms part of the cranial base and its squamous part articulates with the mandible by the temporomandibular joint. The calvarial bones are in principle composed of inner and outer plates of cortical bone,

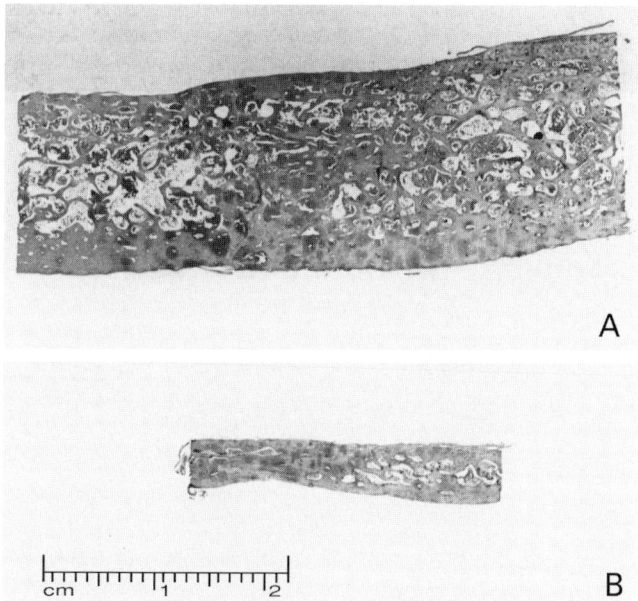

Fig. 2.2 Adult and infant calvarial structure. Sections of parietal bone of adult (**A**) and of 1-year-old infant (**B**). (H & E stain).

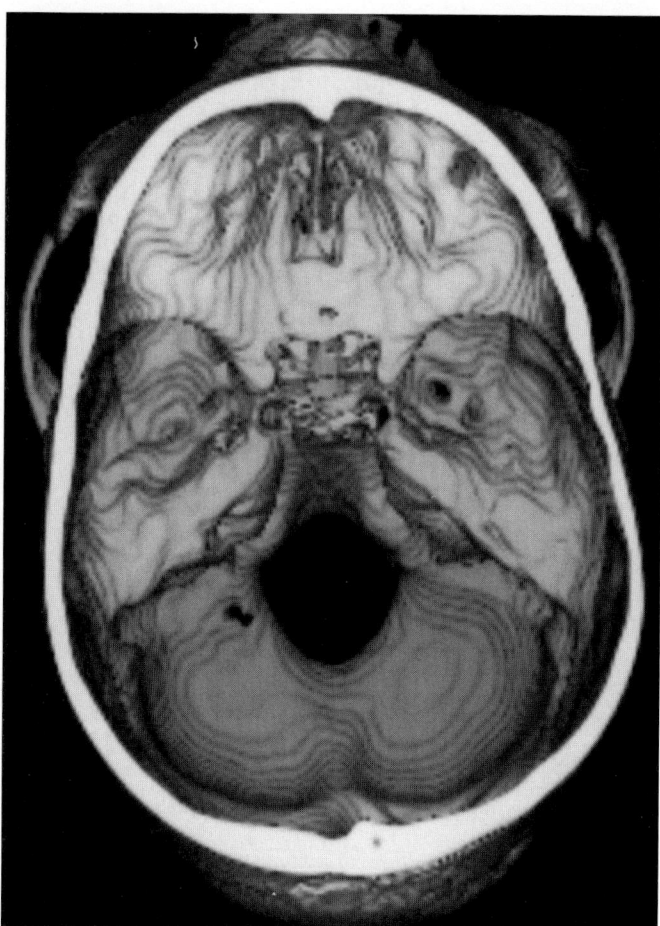

Fig. 2.3 The anterior cranial fossa. Interior of skull, reconstructed from fine cut (1.5 mm) CT scan. The slice lines give a contour map of the anterior and middle cranial fossae, showing bony prominences which correspond with impressions in the frontal and temporal lobes; in closed head injury, contusions are often seen in relation to these. In contrast, the posterior fossa contours are smooth.

separated by cancellous bone which in childhood contains haemopoietic marrow (Fig. 2.2). The layer of cancellous bone constitutes a plane of cleavage, often burst open in comminuted calvarial fractures, and exploited surgically in taking calvarial bone grafts (p. 241).

Cranial base

The cranial base is divided into the anterior, middle and posterior fossae: while only the anterior fossa enters into the CMF region, the anterior part of the middle fossa and the central part of the posterior fossa are important relations (Fig. 2.3).

The anterior cranial fossa

The anterior cranial fossa is bounded anteriorly and laterally by the frontal bone which contains the frontal air sinuses. The largest part of the floor of the anterior cranial fossa is formed by the curved orbital roofs. Medially the floor on each side dips downwards to the cribriform plate, which, with the crista galli, is a part of the ethmoid bone. The cribriform plate is directly related to the roof of the nose; on either side lie the anterior and middle ethmoid air cells. The lesser wing of the sphenoid laterally forms the crescentic posterior borders of the fossa. Centrally the body of the sphenoid roofs over the sphenoid sinuses; the optic canals run lateral to the body, being formed by the two roots of the lesser wing of the sphenoid (p. 57). Fractures of the anterior fossa floor may therefore involve the frontal, ethmoid or sphenoid sinuses or the nasal cavity itself through the cribriform plate; the optic canals

may also be involved when the fracture line runs posteriorly (p. 419). The extent of the frontal sinuses is extremely variable, ranging from almost no pneumatization to extensive pneumatization involving the roof of the orbits. The dura of the cribriform plate is penetrated by the fine olfactory nerves; they are accompanied by arachnoidal sheaths (Lang 1983). Stripping dura from the cribriform plate will lead to anosmia, and possibly to CSF leakage.

In making extradural approaches to the supraorbital region, certain anatomical features need to be borne in mind. The orbital roof may dip steeply down towards the cribriform plate which itself may be quite narrow. On average the cribriform plate is 8 mm below the nasion, the most deeply depressed point on the bridge of the nose (Lang 1983). In frontal craniotomies, access is greatly improved by temporary removal of a bar of bone including the upper margins of the orbits: this entails opening the frontal sinuses.

The middle cranial fossa

This is composed of portions of two bones — the sphenoid and the temporal bone. The sphenoid is surely the most fascinating bone in the craniofacial complex. It sits centrally as the keystone of the skull and has its manifestations in the middle fossa, anterior fossa, infratemporal fossa, pterygomaxillary fossa and orbital cavity. The body of the sphenoid forms the centre of the middle fossa and is in close proximity to the vital neurovascular structures in the cavernous sinuses. Anteriorly, the middle fossa is formed by the greater and lesser wings of the sphenoid, and between these the superior orbital fissure; the wings form part of the lateral wall of the orbit. Laterally the middle fossa is formed by the squamous temporal bones, articulating with the mandibular condyles on their inferior surfaces. Its posterior aspect is buttressed by the strong petrous temporal bones. At the anterior margin of the apex of the petrous temporal bone is a cluster of foramina (lacerum, ovale, spinosum); the bone is penetrated by the ear clefts and traversed by the carotid canal. Although the petrous temporal bones are inherently strong their anterior borders are relatively weakened and the foramina act as areas of stress concentration. The common hinge fracture of the skull base runs along this line of weakness, crossing the midline through the body of the sphenoid. Medially, the middle fossa ascends to join the pituitary fossa (sella turcica).

The floor of the middle fossa is penetrated by branches of the trigeminal nerve — the ophthalmic nerve through the superior orbital fissure, the maxillary nerve through the foramen rotundum and the mandibular nerve through the foramen ovale. The internal carotid artery lies immediately beneath the floor in the carotid canal, which may have no bony roof; this artery ascends into the cavernous sinus. The artery then curves upwards and forwards to pierce the dura medial to the anterior clinoid process. The middle meningeal artery also pierces the floor of the middle fossa, through the foramen spinosum posterolateral to the foramen ovale.

Facial skeleton

Nasal bones

These fragile bones are connected above with the frontal bone by the frontonasal suture and together they separate the frontal processes of the maxillae with which they also articulate. Posteriorly the joined nasal bones are attached to the perpendicular plate of the ethmoid and to the nasal spine of the frontal bone.

Ethmoid bone

The ethmoid bone is delicate and complex. The cribriform plate is perforated by the exit foramina of the olfactory filaments, running from the olfactory bulb to the nasal epithelium. Lang (1983) found on average about 40 osseous perforations on each side; however, there are fewer dural perforations, as the olfactory filaments are grouped into larger bundles as they pass into the dura. The central perpendicular plate of the ethmoid contributes dorsally to the crista galli, and ventrally to the nasal septum; it articulates with the vomer and the septal cartilage. The medial and lateral plates enclose the ethmoid air cells on each side; the lateral plates, suspended from the cribriform plate above, form the medial orbital wall. The lateral wall is paper-thin, hence its alias lamina papyracea, and in some individuals there are bony dehiscences. The ethmoid bone provides the skeletal elements of the superior and middle nasal conchae, also known as turbinate bones. The inferior concha is a separate bone articulating with the maxilla and palatine bone. The ethmoid bone is connected to the frontal bone, the sphenoid bone, the nasal bones and the maxillae.

Zygomatic bones

These form the prominence of each cheek and contribute to the lateral wall and inferior margin of each orbit. The zygomatic bone is interposed between the frontal bone, the sphenoid bone and the maxilla and connects with the zygomatic process of the temporal bone forming the zygomatic arch. It is the length of this arch which determines the forward projection of the cheek bone, and in reconstructing the arch after injury, it is important to maintain its anteroposterior dimension (p. 316).

Maxillae

These paired bones form the keystone of the midface (Fig. 2.4). Anteriorly the maxillae join in the midline, below and behind the anterior nasal spine. They contain the teeth of the upper jaw and together with the palatine bones form the hard palate; they enclose the largest air spaces in the skull, the maxillary air sinuses, which occupy most of their bodies. The terminal branches of the infraorbital nerve and artery exit through the infraorbital foramina below the inferior orbital margins. The paired frontal processes of the maxilla connect with the frontal bone above and the nasal bones medially. Laterally the maxillae flare out to join with the zygomatic bones at the zygomaticomaxillary sutures. The very thin orbital floor components of the maxillae are connected to the ethmoid bone medially. Posteriorly the maxillae articulate with the palatine bones and the pterygoid processes of the sphenoid bone. The keystone position of the maxillae enable them to absorb the forces of mastication. These physiological forces are transmitted from the occluding teeth to the cranial base through the maxillae, which articulate with the frontal and zygomatic bones by the

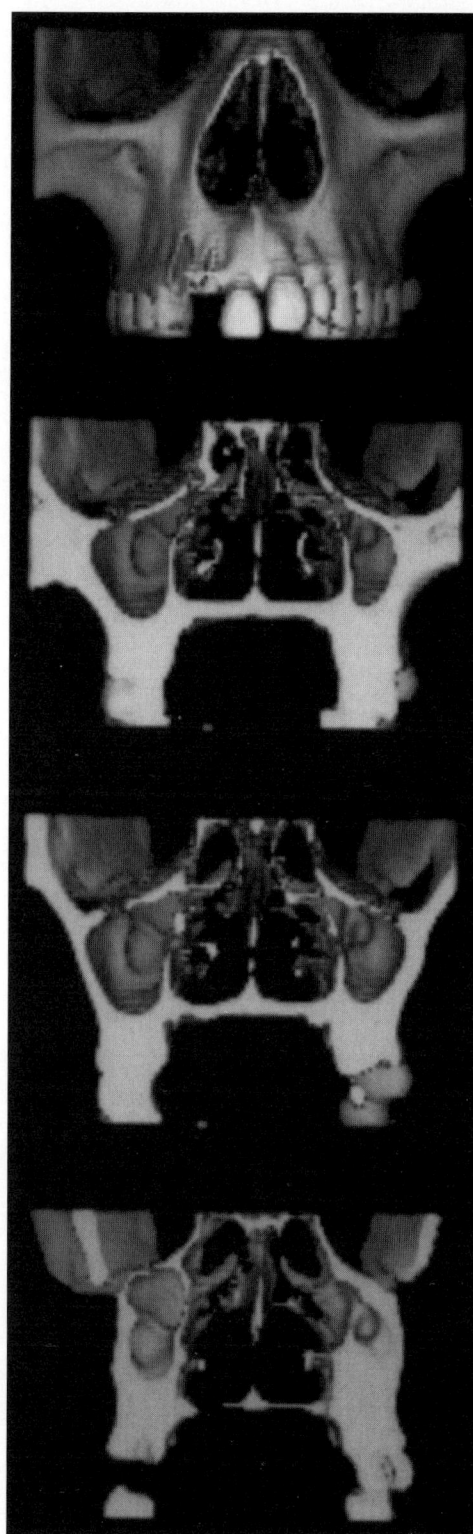

Fig. 2.4 The maxillae. Seen in coronal section, the maxillae comprise dense alveolar bone supporting the teeth, connected transversely by the strong hard palate. The vertical elements of the midface are stronger laterally and behind; centrally the walls of the nasal cavity and the septum are very thin.

frontomaxillary and zygomaticomaxillary sutures. Thus the maxilla is an essential component of the system of vertical pillars or buttresses discussed below, together with the nasal septum, the ethmoid bone, and the strong buttresses provided by the junction of the pyramidal process of the palatine bone and the pterygoid laminae of the sphenoid bone. The maxilla is composed of thin plates of compact bone, which contain little cancellous bone, except in the alveolar region, where the upper teeth and their roots are embedded in bone of this type; nevertheless these thin plates are able to carry heavy loads when stressed in the vertical plane. They are less able to sustain horizontal stresses. The thinness of the maxilla must be remembered when screws are inserted in reconstructing the vertical buttresses of the facial skeleton with miniplates (p. 304); the walls of the maxillary air sinus are often only 0.5 mm thick or even less, but thicker bone is found lateral to the piriform aperture.

Mandible

This robust bone occupies a prominent and exposed position in the facial skeleton. It articulates with the cranial base through its condyles which lie in the glenoid fossae: condyle and glenoid fossa form the temporomandibular joint (TMJ), a synovial joint divided into two cavities by a disc of fibrocartilage (Fig. 2.5). This important joint acts as a hinge, but also allows sliding movement in the anteroposterior plane.

The mandible comprises a number of named components: the condyles, the coronoid processes, the rami, the angles and the two halves of the body, joined anteriorly at the symphysis. The body of the mandible is shaped like a horseshoe, though more open posteriorly; the rami, vertical platelike pillars, project upwards from the free ends of the horseshoe. Viewed from the lateral aspect, the ramus forms an angle of about 120° with the body of the bone in the adult, slightly more in the very young and the elderly. Viewed from the superior aspect there is a slight divergence of the rami. The alveolar portion of the bone supporting the molar teeth does not follow the same line as that formed by the lower border of the mandible.

From a functional viewpoint, the mandible can be regarded as two conjoined L-shaped cantilevers, acting under the influence of the masticatory muscles. The temporalis muscle inserts predominantly into the medial surface of the coronoid process, the masseter to the lateral surface of the ramus and angle. The medial pterygoid muscle inserts on the medial surface of the angle and lower ramus; together with the masseter, it forms a powerful sling acting on the ramus of the mandible. The two heads of the lateral pterygoid muscle unite to insert into the anterior part of the capsule of the TMJ and the pterygoid fovea of the neck of the condyle, with a few

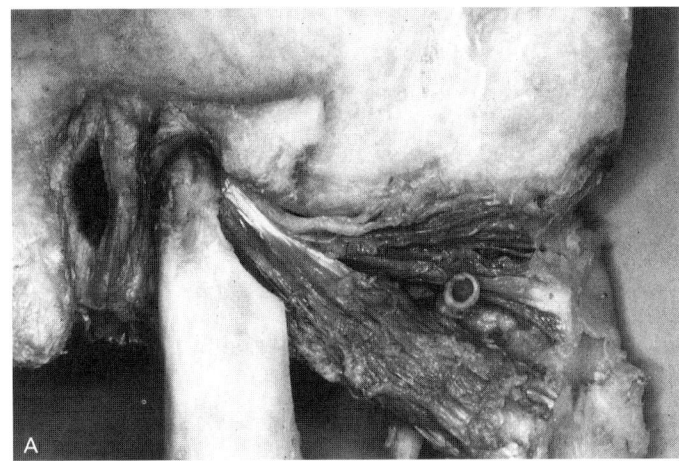

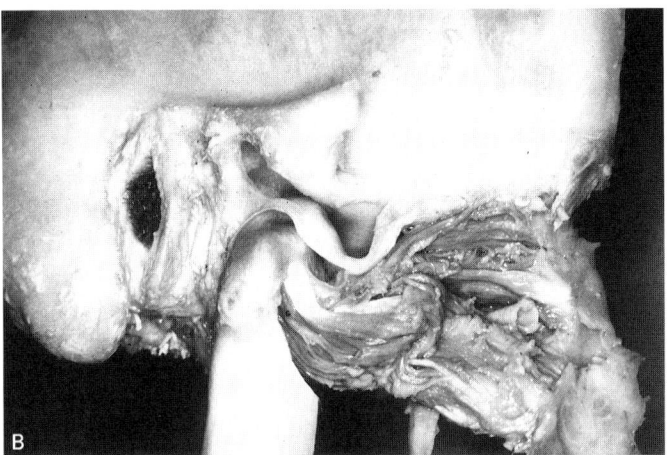

Fig. 2.5 Dissection of the temporomandibular joint and lateral pterygoid muscle. A The condyle of the mandible is in its resting position, located within the articular fossa; the temporomandibular disk is hardly visible. **B** The mandibular condyle is pulled forwards and downwards to simulate the action of the lateral pterygoid muscle during a jaw-opening movement. The fusion of the superior and inferior pterygoid heads and their insertion into the neck of the mandible are shown. The temporomandibular disk with the insertion of a few fibres of the superior head of the lateral pterygoid into its anterior region is clearly visible. Photographs by courtesy of Professor G.C. Townsend, The University of Adelaide.

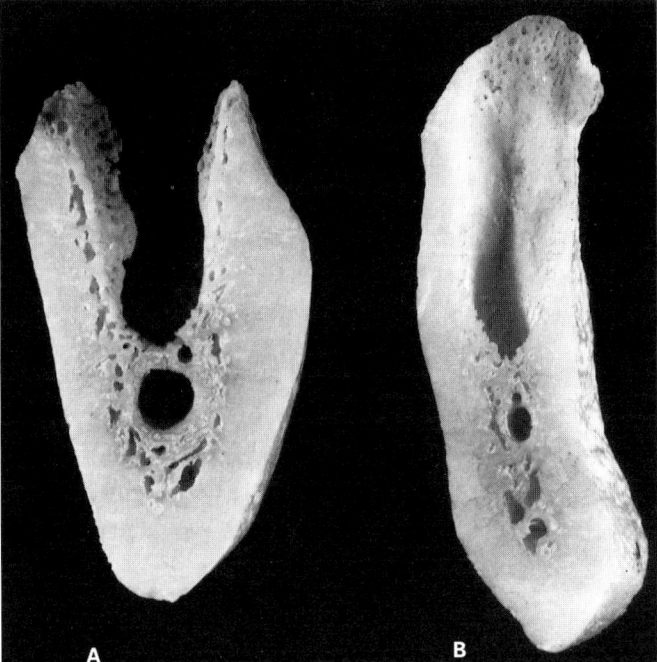

Fig. 2.6 Adult mandible. A The mandible is sectioned through the second molar socket: the mandibular canal is about 3 mm in greatest diameter. On the buccal surface, the cortical plate is 2.7 mm thick at its thinnest point. **B** The mandible is sectioned through the socket of the canine tooth: the canal, now termed the incisive canal, is ~1 mm in diameter. The cortical plates are 2.5–3 mm thick.

fibres passing to the articular disc (Fig. 2.5). The action of this muscle is important in functional recovery after intracapsular fracture of the condyle, and its insertion must be preserved (p. 286).

In cross-section, the body of the mandible is seen as a flattened tube or U, being composed of strong inner and outer cortical plates of bone, between which are inserted the teeth and their roots, embedded in cancellous bone (Fig. 2.6). The plates of compact bone have the typical structure for such a tissue, being built up of haversian systems (osteons) and composed in the outer surface by circumferential lamellae. Between the two plates of cortical bone runs the mandibular or inferior dental canal, containing the inferior dental nerve on its way from the

mandibular foramen to the mental foramen. Knowledge of the location of this nerve is of great importance in siting screws for plate fixation. The mandible is well adapted to withstand the vertical forces generated in mastication; it has areas of weakness, notably at the condylar process, the angle (especially if there is an unerupted third molar), and in the vicinity of the canine tooth (Abbott et al 1992; p. 264).

The morphology of the mandible and the maxilla reflect the state of the dentition. In infancy and childhood, the jaws become progressively more prominent as the tooth buds successively enlarge and erupt. Loss of the teeth, especially in old age, results in regression of the alveoli and muscular processes, with a significant reduction in the strength of the jaws. Alveolar regression is associated with a relative upward migration of the inferior dental nerve — another factor to be remembered when screws are inserted.

Computer coding of CMF bones

Cooter & David (1989) have devised an alphanumeric system of coding fractures of the skull according to their anatomical sites, coded alphabetically, and to their severity, coded by a numerical scale (0–3). The bones of the skull are classed as major zones; the sutures and

Table 2.1 Major and minor zones in the calvaria and skull base, identified alphabetically (Cooter & David 1989)

Major zone	Major code	Minor zone	Minor code
Frontal	F	calvarial	FC
		frontal sinus anterior	FSA
		frontal sinus posterior	FSP
		anterior fossa	FA
		cribriform plate	FCP
		coronal suture	F:P
Parietal	P	Calvarial	PC
		Sagittal suture	P:P
		squamosal suture	P:T
		lambdoid suture	P:OC
Sphenoidal	S	lesser wing	SL
		greater wing	SG
		sph.-frontal suture	S:F
		basal	SB
		sph.-occ. synchond.	S:OC
Temporal	T	calvarial	TC
		basal	TB
		petrous	TP
Occipital	OC	cavarial	OCC
		basal	OCB

Table 2.2 Major and minor zones of the facial skeleton, identified alphabetically (Cooter & David 1989)

Major zone	Major code	Minor zone	Minor code
Naso-ethmoidal	NE	nasal bone	N
		naso-frontal suture	N:F
		maxill. frontal process	NMX
		ant. ethmoid	EA
		post. ethmoid	EP
Zygomatic	Z	arch	ZA
		body	ZB
		zyg.-frontal suture	Z:F
		zyg. maxill. suture	Z:MX
Orbital	O	roof	OR
		medial wall	OM
		lateral wall	OL
		floor	OF
		inferior rim	OI
		superior rim	OS
Maxillary	MX	ant. wall	MXA
		buttress	MXB
		palate	MXP
		dento-alveolar	MXD
		pterygoid	MXT
Mandibular	MD	condyle	MDC
		coronoid process	MDP
		ramus	MDR
		angle	MDA
		body	MDB
		symphyseal	MDS
		dento-alveolar	MDD

Table 2.3 Numerical coding of fracture severity (Cooter & David 1989)

0	=	no fracture
1	=	undisplaced fracture
2	=	obviously displaced fracture
3	=	comminuted and/or compound fracture

various bone parts or regions are classed as minor zones. The code letters for the major and minor zones are set out in Tables 2.1 and 2.2; the severity scale is set out in Table 2.3. The clinical use of this alphanumeric system is considered in Chapter 11.

THE CRANIOMAXILLOFACIAL CAVITIES

Cranial cavity

The cranial cavity is lined by the dura mater, a strong membrane of great surgical importance. It is composed of interlacing collagen fibres, and some elastic fibres, interspersed with fibrocytes and fibroblasts. The dura mater is both the inner periosteum of the skull bones and the outer meningeal investment of the brain, and in keeping with its dual roles, it is composed of two separable layers. The outer layer is osteogenic; it contains the meningeal arteries and veins, and also the meningeal nerves; the dura, unlike the brain and the leptomeninges, is pain-sensitive. The inner layer is separated from the arachnoid by the subdural space, which is lined by flat cells of fibroblastic type. Nabeshima et al (1975) considered that the subdural space is really intradural since electron microscopy shows that the outer layer of the arachnoid is composed of mesothelial cells with tight junctions: in their interpretation, this layer is the true barrier between dura and arachnoid, and the subdural space is a cleft in a fascial plane within the dura. Haines et al (1993) have endorsed this concept. However this may be, the subdural space is very real and very important in the surgical pathology of head injuries, and it is very easily opened up, even by the entry of air into the cranial cavity, if intracranial pressure is low (Fig. 19.14).

Once the cranial sutures have fused and the fontanelles have closed, the walls of the cranial cavity are rigid and the total intracranial volume is fixed. The three major components (brain, spinal fluid and blood) are incompressible: an increase in any one of these three, or the addition of another volume such as a clot or abscess, will cause a rise in intracranial pressure (ICP) unless an equal volume is displaced extracranially. Cerebrospinal fluid (CSF) can be displaced from the cranium, through the foramen magnum to the more distensible spinal subarachnoid space. Venous blood can be displaced via the dural venous sinuses to the extracranial veins. This compensatory capacity is limited both in volume and in rate of displacement. Once the compensatory reserve is exceeded, ICP rises exponentially. In patients with head injuries compensatory reserve may be reduced by brain swelling, which may take several days to subside. Intracranial surgery is then rendered difficult by the inability to retract the brain without excessive force (p. 377) and nursing care and anaesthesia must be conducted in such a way as to prevent any additional rises in ICP. This may be increased inadvertently by overhydration, hypercarbia, hyperpyrexia and the use of volatile anaesthetic agents (p. 252). The clinical measurement of ICP is discussed in Chapter 13: in adults it is normally 5–15 mmHg, being somewhat lower in children and lower still in infants.

Orbital cavity

The orbit is pyramidal in shape (Fig. 2.7). It contains the globe of the eye, the optic nerve, and the external ocular muscles, embedded and sheathed in the orbital fat; the lacrimal gland lies in the upper outer corner of the orbit, in a bony shallow fossa. The orbital cavity is not as high as it is wide and the globe of the eye is therefore nearer to the roof and floor than to the sides (Deuschle 1969). The maxillary component of the orbital floor is very thin as is the medial orbital wall formed by the lateral plate of the ethmoid; these parts of the orbit are often fractured, either as part of a more extensive midfacial fracture, or in isolation as an effect of hydraulic pressure transmitted to the orbital floor through the orbital fat after blunt impact on the globe of the eye (p. 104). The orbital roof is also thin and may be fractured easily; such fractures are often part of a more extensive craniofacial injury, especially an injury resulting from oblique frontal impact. In contrast, the orbital margins are relatively thick, and constitute strong vertical and transverse components of the facial skeleton. Lang (1983), quoting G. Oehmann, gives the following mean lengths of the adult orbit:

roof: 50.5 mm
floor: 48.4 mm
lateral wall: 47.2 mm
medial wall: 40.5 mm

The eye is protected from blunt trauma by the orbital rim, this protection being least effective in the inferolateral area. The optic canal enters the orbit at the apex of the pyramid: Lang (1983) found that the canal is on average 9.8 mm long and 4.6 mm wide at its narrowest point. The optic nerve is often injured within the canal, either by impact forces transmitted through the intact bone of the canal (Jend & Jend-Rossmann 1984) or orbital contents, or when a fracture enters the canal. The nerve is protected from impact by the orbital fat and from stretching by its tortuosity.

Nasal cavity

The irregularly shaped nasal cavity extends from the roof of the mouth to the skull base and communicates with the other pneumatized cavities in the craniofacial region (Fig. 2.8). It is divided in the midline by the nasal septum comprised in part by the crest of the maxilla, the vomer, and the vertical plate of the ethmoid, together with its cartilaginous component. It is further subdivided by the three paired conchae (turbinate bones). The inferior concha demarcates the inferior meatus, into which debouches the nasolacrimal duct. The middle concha demarcates the middle meatus, which is extended anteriorly as the ethmoid infundibulum; into this drain the ostia of the anterior ethmoid air cells, the maxillary air sinus, and in some individuals the frontal sinus. In other individuals, the frontal sinus drains directly into a recess of the middle meatus, the anatomy being dependent on the position of the uncinate process (Stammberger 1991). Many anatomists have described the frontal sinus drainage as an actual duct (frontonasal or nasofrontal duct). Stammberger has shown that this is a rare finding; in most individuals, the ostium of the frontal sinus lies at the junction of two funnel-shaped cavities — the upper leading down from the floor of the sinus and the lower extending up as the frontal recess, which opens into the middle meatus or infundibulum. In this book, the terms frontonasal duct and frontal recess are used interchangeably and with no implication that the drainage system is either a cylindrical duct or a funnel-shaped recess. The superior concha, which is often split into two components, demarcates the superior meatus, into which drain the posterior ethmoid air cells. Above and posterior to the superior concha is the spheno-ethmoid recess, in which the sphenoid air sinuses have their ostia.

The nasal cavity is enclosed by the bony and cartilaginous skeleton of the nose. This comprises an upper immobile bony portion and a lower, mobile cartilaginous portion. Pollock (1992) subdivides the cartilaginous element further, into a middle subregion which equates with the upper lateral nasal cartilages, and a lower area corresponding to the lower lateral or alar cartilages.

The upper osseous portion comprises the paired nasal bones capping a pyramid whose base is formed by the frontal process of the maxilla on each side. Articulating above with the frontal bone, the nasal bone is thick; inferiorly it becomes thin as it meets the upper lateral cartilages. Lying deep to the nasal bones is the perpendicular plate of the ethmoid, and the septal cartilage, and with the vomer at the bone–cartilaginous junction of the septum. In the middle section the upper lateral cartilages overlie the septal cartilage alone, whilst more inferiorly the alar cartilages are tethered to the anterior nasal spine via their medial crura.

The septal cartilage varies in thickness, being strongest and providing most support superiorly at its junction with the vomer. The caudal end and dorsal border are also thickened with a central, relatively thin portion. The cartilage connects to the perpendicular plate of the ethmoid posterosuperiorly, and to the vomerine groove

A   B

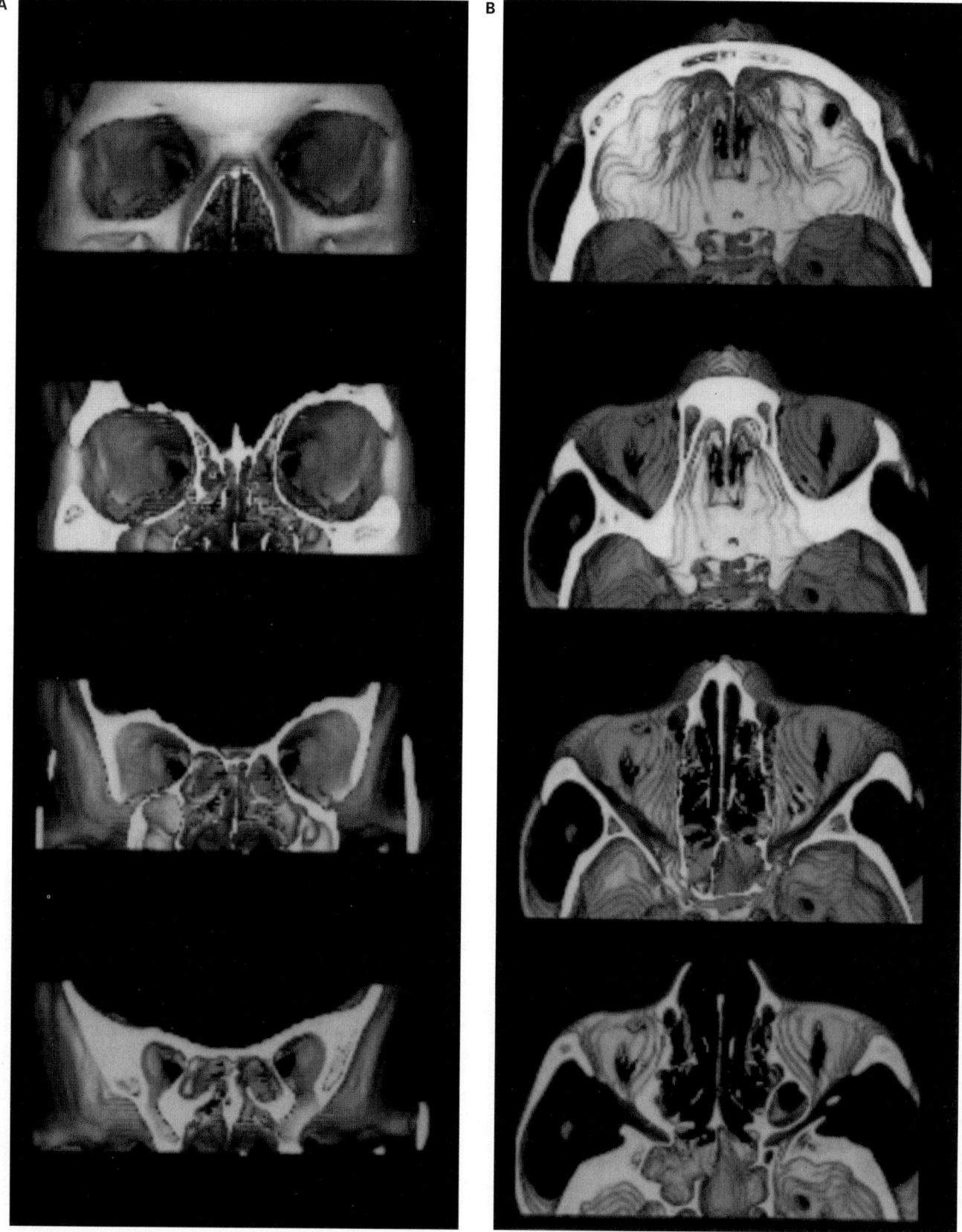

Fig. 2.7 The orbital cavities. A Coronal CT sections show that the lateral wall is relatively thick, the floor and medial wall very thin, the roof variable but sometimes very thin. **B**. Horizontal sections show the pyramidal shape and the close relations with the ethmoid air sinuses.

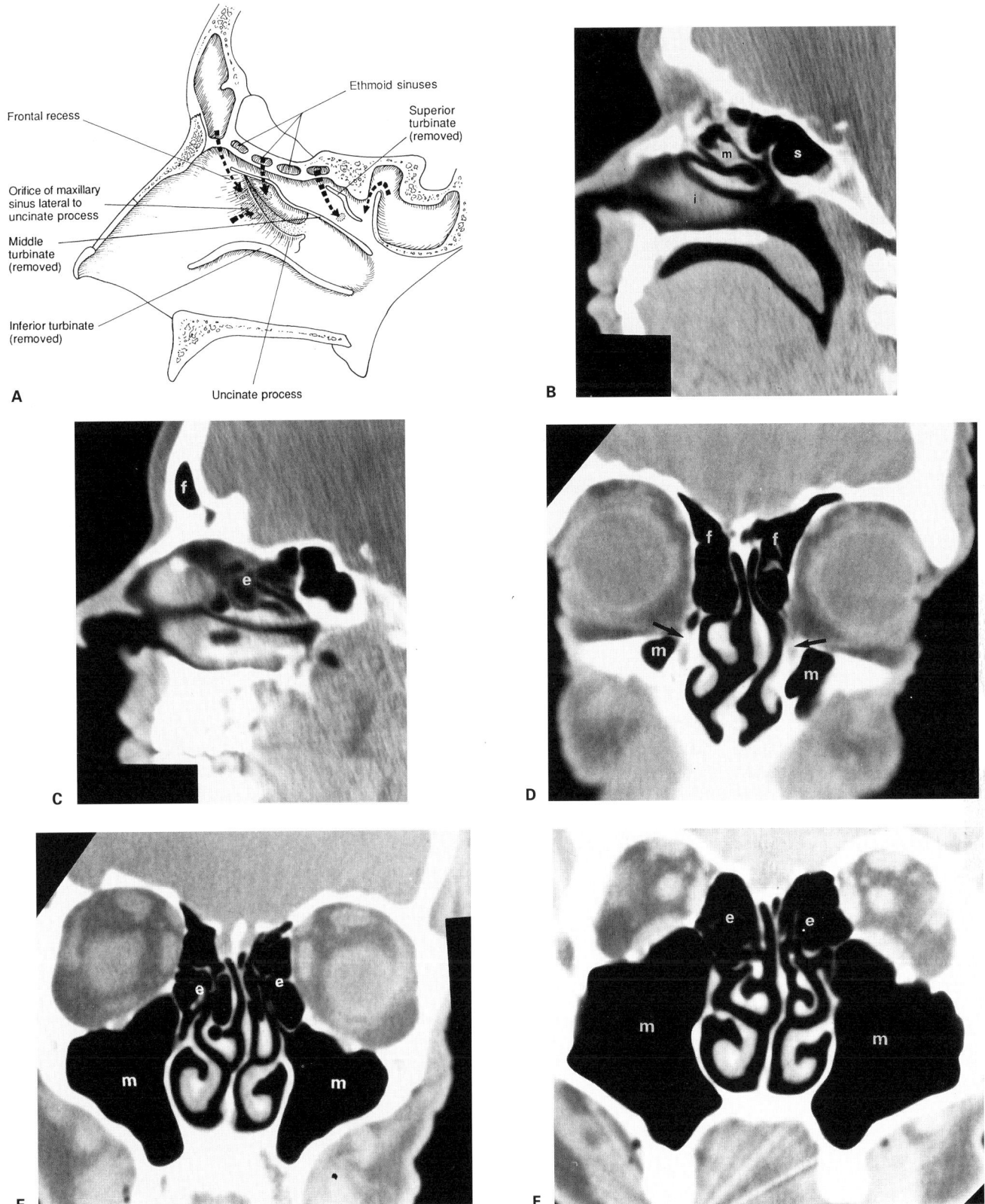

Fig. 2.8 The nasal cavity and paranasal air sinuses. A Diagram shows the lateral wall of the nasal cavity after removal of the turbinate bones. The drainage routes of the paranasal air sinuses are shown (broken arrows). **B** CT scan: a parasagittal cut shows the inferior (i) and middle (m) nasal conchae; the upper part of the bulla ethmoidalis is seen above the attachment of the middle concha. The sphenoid (s) sinus is well seen. **C** CT scan: more laterally, the ethmoid (e) and frontal (f) air sinuses are seen. **D** CT scan: an anterior frontal cut shows the frontal (f) and anterior ethmoid (f) air cells; the maxillary air sinuses (m) are also seen. The lacrimal ducts (arrows) are seen on each side. **E** CT scan: more posteriorly, the maxillary air sinuses (m) are well developed. On the right side, an arrow indicates the site of the drainage of the maxillary air sinuses into the nasal cavity under cover of the uncinate process. The ethmoid air cells (e) are separated from the orbital contents only by the thin lamina papyracea. **F** CT scan: skull more posteriorly, the maxillary (m) and posterior ethmoid (e) air cells are well developed; the ethmoid air cells have a large surface relation to the dura of the anterior cranial fossa.

postero-inferiorly. Septal injury is of great importance in more severe nasal fractures, and if not treated may cause nasal obstruction (p. 333).

The nasal cavity is lined with pseudostratified columnar ciliated epithelium (Moran et al 1991), except in the nasal vestibule and nostrils, where the epithelium is stratified squamous, becoming keratinized as it approaches the skin. The epithelium contains goblet cells, secreting mucus, and ciliated cells. The mucus forms on the surface of the nasal cavity in two layers: a fluid inner layer, termed the sol phase, and a viscous outer layer, the gel phase (Stammberger 1991). The cilia beat continually in the sol layer, slowly moving the overlying gel layer back to the pharynx; foreign material caught on the viscid surface layer is thus moved out of the nasal cavity and swallowed. The nasal epithelium is adherent to the periosteum or perichondrium of the underlying skeletal structures, and contains mucous and serous glands, as well as many blood vessels; the epithelium regenerates well after injury. The nasal conchae have a bony skeleton, covered with a thick mucosa containing venous sinuses with erectile properties. The erectile tissue intermittently dilates and contracts in the normal nasal cycle which regulates air flow through one nostril or the other. In the roof of the nose above the superior concha, the epithelium over an area of about 2 cm² is specialized for olfaction: here are found the ciliated olfactory receptor cells. These are bipolar neurons which send their axons through the olfactory filaments to the olfactory bulb; they have considerable regenerative capacity, being replaced by undifferentiated basal cells, but this capacity is lost if the olfactory bulb is destroyed (Fig. 2.9).

The skin cover of the nasal skeleton and cartilages is of variable thickness. Fascial interconnections exist between the lower cartilaginous structures aiding in the maintenance of shape and structure. These tend to be strong in the region between the alar domes but more lax in the junction between alar and upper lateral cartilages.

Paranasal air sinuses

These sinuses are lined with columnar ciliated epithelium, containing mucus-secreting goblet cells; both cilia and goblet cells are less numerous than in the nasal mucosa. The mucus is transported by ciliary action to the ostia of the sinuses, and then into the nasal cavity; endoscopic studies (Stammberger 1991) have shown that each sinus has its characteristic pattern of transport of mucus secretions.

The anatomy of the paranasal air sinuses is very variable, and these variations are best studied in high-resolution thin-section CT scans (Fig. 2.8B–F). This is especially important when endonasal or transnasal surgery is planned.

Maxillary sinuses

At birth, all the paranasal sinuses are rudimentary. The maxillary sinuses are present as narrow slits or pouches in the wall of the nasal cavity; they expand slowly at first, and more rapidly after the eruption of the permanent dentition. In adult life, the maxillary sinus usually fills the entire body of the maxilla; it may even extend into the zygomatic arch and below the floor of the nose. The maxilla has fragile walls and is easily fractured.

Ethmoid sinuses

The labyrinthine ethmoid air cells are variable in number,

OLFACTORY BULB

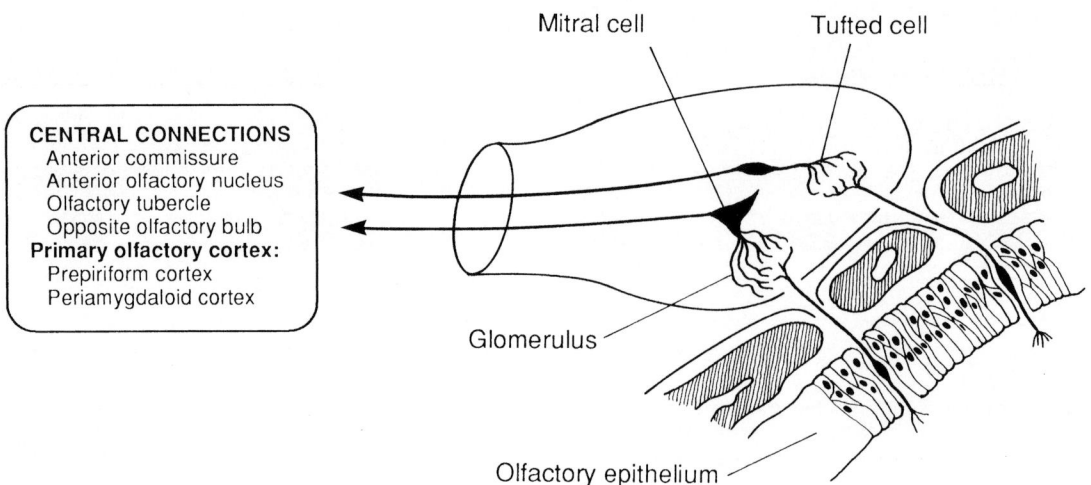

Fig. 2.9 Olfactory pathways. The diagram shows the olfactory bulb in the cribriform fossa, and its connections with the olfactory epithelium; some of the centripetal pathways are shown, with their central connections

shape and size. They are well formed but small at birth, when they have no direct relation with the dura of the anterior cranial fossa; however, they expand rapidly and by the third year of life they are quite capacious, being separated from the dura by only a thin plate of bone, and in relation to the anterior fossa over an area of about 5 cm² (Caldicott et al 1973). In adult life, ethmoid pneumatization may be extensive; the crista galli, and even structures outside the ethmoid bone, may be pneumatized.

Frontal sinuses

The frontal sinus develops between the inner and outer tables of the frontal bone; pneumatization is said to be-

come evident during the third year, but in our experience these air sinuses do not usually develop a relationship with the anterior cranial fossa until the age of 4 years or even later. The anterior and posterior walls of the frontal sinus may be quite thin and easily fractured. The sinuses may be large and then contribute to the fullness and shape of the frontonasal region.

Sphenoid sinuses

These sinuses are evident at birth but enlarge slowly and are the last of the paranasal sinuses to establish a relation to the anterior cranial fossa (Fig. 2.10); much of their development takes place after puberty.

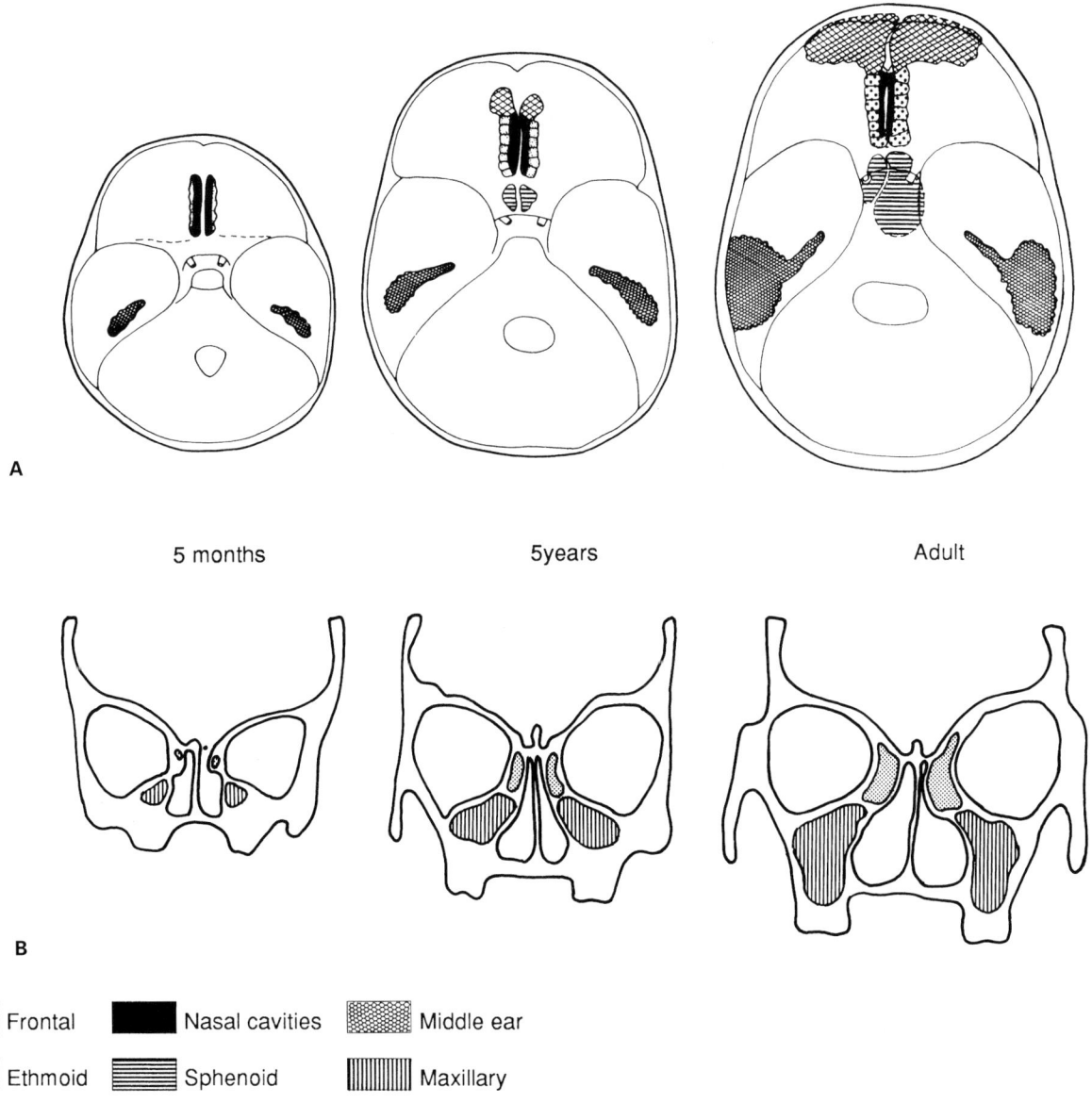

Fig. 2.10 Growth of the paranasal air sinuses. Diagrams, based on dissections or CT scans, show the approximate size of the air sinuses at 5 months, 5 years and in adult life. There is much individual variation. **A** The air sinuses as seen from above, showing areas separated by thin bone from the dura mater. After Caldicott et al (1973), by courtesy of the *Journal of Neurosurgery*. **B** The air sinuses as seen from in front.

Ostia

The orifices of the paranasal sinuses (Fig. 2.8A) have surgical importance. If they are obstructed, the secretions of the sinus are retained and a tension mucocele or chronic sinusitis may result. The frontal sinus ostium and frontal recess are often involved in depressed frontal fractures, and post-traumatic frontal mucoceles are not uncommon; measures to prevent infection or mucocele formation are discussed on page 372. The ethmoid ostia may also be blocked, resulting in local infection or orbital cellulitis. Farmand & Gottsauner (1991) reported on the findings of endoscopy of the maxillary air sinuses after injury; they could visualize the ostium of the sinus in only half their cases, but concluded that it is rarely obstructed except when there is a severe deviation of the nasal septum.

Oral cavity

The oral cavity is incompletely enclosed by the inner surface of the alveolar processes and the lingual surfaces of the teeth: these form lateral anterior walls, the roof being formed by the hard palate. Posteriorly, the mouth is continuous with the oropharynx, the posterior wall of which is formed by the upper two cervical vertebrae. It is lined by stratified non-keratinizing squamous epithelium, which is heaped up in papillae of several types over the surface of the tongue: the filiform and circumvallate papillae contain chemoceptive cells organized in taste buds and responsible for perception of the basic tastes — salt, sweet, sour and bitter. The oral cavity is irrigated by saliva from the sublingual, submandibular and parotid salivary glands and from numerous smaller buccal and labial glands (see below).

Alveoli and teeth

The teeth are supported by the alveolar processes of the maxillae and mandible. The alveolar bone is formed as the teeth develop from tooth germs, emerge and eventually take up their positions within the dental arches. When teeth are lost through disease or trauma, the alveolar processes or parts of them are resorbed; the edentulous jaw may indeed be devoid of all alveolar processes (Fig. 19.11) and is then extremely fragile.

Between about 6 months and 2 years, the primary dentition of eight incisors, four canines and eight molars erupts through the alveolar bone and covering gum tissue (Table 2.4). The permanent teeth, eight incisors, four canines, eight premolars and twelve molars erupt later, between about 6–20 years (Tables 2.5 and 2.6). For a period of time, around 6–14 years, the mixed dentition is present with some teeth from both deciduous and permanent dentitions (Fig. 2.11).

Table 2.4 Emergence times of deciduous teeth (months) in two Caucasian populations studied longitudinally

A Maxilla

Population*	Authors	n	i^1	i^2	c	m^1	m^2
Umea, Sweden	Lysell et al (1962)	171	10.2	11.4	19.2	16.0	29.1
London, England	Leighton (1968)	84	9.2	10.6	18.2	14.7	26.3

B Mandible

Population*	Authors	n	i^1	i^2	c	m^1	m^2
Umea, Sweden	Lysell et al (1962)	171	8.0	13.2	19.7	16.3	27.1
London, England	Leighton (1968)	84	7.3	11.5	18.3	14.8	25.7

* Male and female data combined in absence of significant differences between sexes.

Table 2.5 Emergence times of permanent teeth (years) in South Australian school children*

A Maxilla

		I^1	I^2	C	Pm^1	Pm^2	M^1	M^2
Males	5th Percentile	5.8	6.4	9.5	8.9	9.7	5.1	10.3
	Median	7.4	8.6	11.8	11.3	12.1	6.7	12.7
	95th Percentile	9.1	10.9	14.2	13.6	14.4	8.4	15.1
	Range	3.3	4.5	4.7	4.7	4.8	3.3	4.8
Females	5th Percentile	5.6	6.0	8.8	8.6	9.2	4.8	9.9
	Median	7.2	8.2	11.2	10.8	11.7	6.6	12.3
	95th Percentile	8.7	10.5	13.7	13.0	14.2	8.3	14.7
	Range	3.1	4.5	4.9	4.4	5.0	3.6	4.8

B Mandible

		I_1	I_2	C	Pm_1	Pm_2	M_1	M_2
Males	5th Percentile	5.0	6.0	8.9	9.0	9.7	5.0	9.8
	Median	6.6	7.8	11.0	11.2	12.1	6.6	12.2
	95th Percentile	8.3	9.6	13.1	13.3	14.5	8.3	14.5
	Range	3.3	3.6	4.2	4.3	4.9	3.5	4.7
Females	5th Percentile	4.8	5.7	8.0	8.5	9.1	4.9	9.4
	Median	6.4	7.5	10.1	10.6	11.7	6.4	11.8
	95th Percentile	8.0	9.3	12.2	12.7	14.2	8.0	14.1
	Range	3.2	3.5	4.2	4.3	5.1	3.1	4.7

* Percentiles derived by logistic regression of data from over 37 000 children aged 4–16 years who were examined in 1988 (Diamanti 1991).

Each tooth is held firmly in its socket within the alveolus by the tough periodontal ligament passing between cementum on the tooth root and the cortical lamina dura lining the tooth socket. The periodontal ligament has an important sensory function also as it contains proprioceptive nerve endings that provide information to guide mandibular movements during function. The morphology of a tooth and its supporting structures is

Table 2.6 Emergence times of permanent teeth (years) in four populations

A   Maxilla

Population	Authors		I^1	I^2	C	Pm^1	Pm^2	M^1	M^2
USA (Blacks)	Garn et al (1972)	Males	6.8	8.1	10.9	10.2	10.8	6.5	12.3
		Females	6.8	7.9	10.2	9.7	10.5	6.2	12.0
USA (Whites)	Garn et al (1972)	Males	7.3	8.4	11.5	10.9	11.5	6.2	12.5
		Females	7.1	7.8	10.7	10.4	10.8	6.4	11.7
Hong Kong (Chinese)	Lee et al (1965)	Males	7.4	8.7	11.3	9.8	10.9	6.4	12.6
		Females	7.2	8.3	10.4	9.5	10.4	6.2	12.0
New Guinea (Kaiapit)	Malcolm & Bue (1970)	Males	6.5	7.4	10.7	10.2	11.3	5.7	11.2
		Females	6.7	7.3	9.3	9.5	10.4	5.7	10.3

B   Mandible

Population	Authors		I_1	I_2	C	Pm_1	Pm_2	M_1	M_2
USA (Blacks)	Garn et al (1972)	Males	6.1	7.2	10.2	10.3	11.2	6.2	11.9
		Females	5.8	6.7	9.4	9.7	10.7	5.9	11.3
USA (Whites)	Garn et al (1972)	Males	6.2	7.5	10.9	11.0	11.8	6.2	10.2
		Females	6.4	7.1	9.9	10.5	11.2	6.2	11.5
Hong Kong (Chinese)	Lee et al (1965)	Males	6.2	7.5	10.5	10.4	11.3	6.0	11.9
		females	6.1	7.2	9.6	9.8	10.7	5.9	11.3
New Guinea (Kaiapit)	Malcolm & Bue (1970)	Males	6.2	6.8	10.0	10.4	11.4	5.2	11.3
		Females	6.5	6.9	8.9	10.1	10.4	5.5	10.3

* From data tabulated by Eveleth & Tanner (1976).

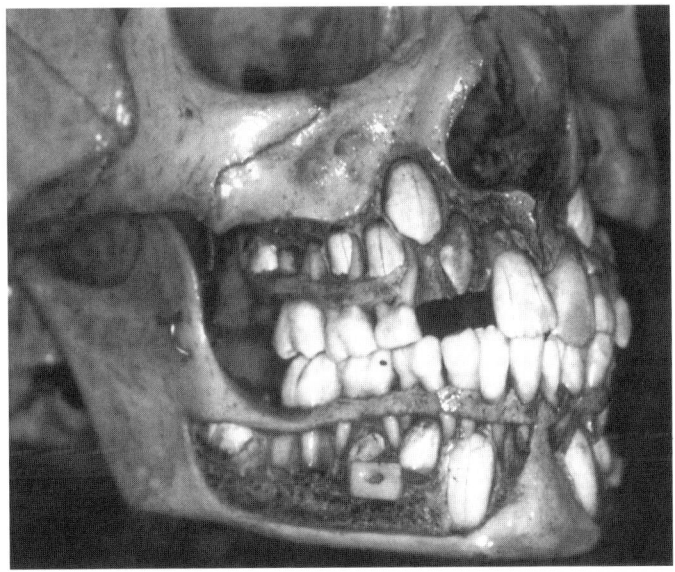

Fig. 2.11 The mixed dentition. Dissection of a young (8–9-year-old) skull showing some permanent incisors and the first permanent molars fully erupted. Also visible are the primary molars and a number of succedaneous permanent teeth developing within their crypts.

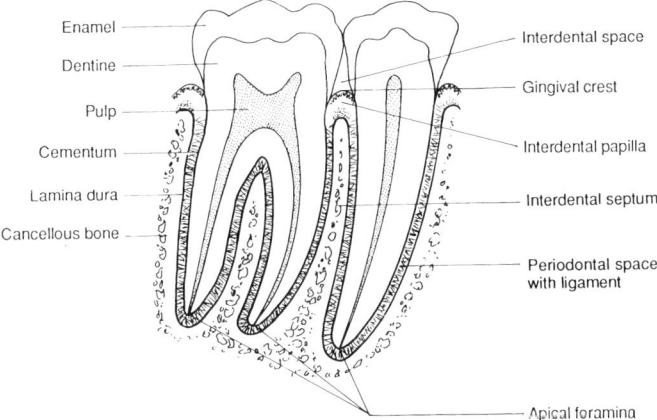

Fig. 2.12 Morphology of teeth and surrounding tissues. Section through a mandibular second premolar and first molar showing internal dental structures and the features of the alveolus and interdental region.

shown in Fig. 2.12. Relations of teeth and alveoli can be visualized in a panoramic radiograph of the jaws (Fig. 2.13).

Normally each tooth contacts a neighbouring tooth at the regions of maximum crown curvature (Fig. 2.12). The adjacent tooth roots, each within their individual sockets, are separated by wedges of alveolar bone which form the interdental septa. These septa are composed of cancellous bone with a thin covering of compact cortical bone termed the lamina dura. A healthy lamina dura appears as a thin radio-opaque line on radiographs. The septa are covered by gingival tissue which extends some distance into the interdental space. This tissue is known as the interdental papilla.

The gingival tissues, which act as cuffs around all the teeth, are composed of tough stratified squamous epithelium and fibrous connective tissue. The gingival crest is the free part of tissue separated from the neck of the tooth by a capillary space, the gingival crevice. Gingivae are attached to the necks of teeth at their gingival attachments and to the periodontal ligaments and septal bone. This region, where the gingival tissues surround the teeth,

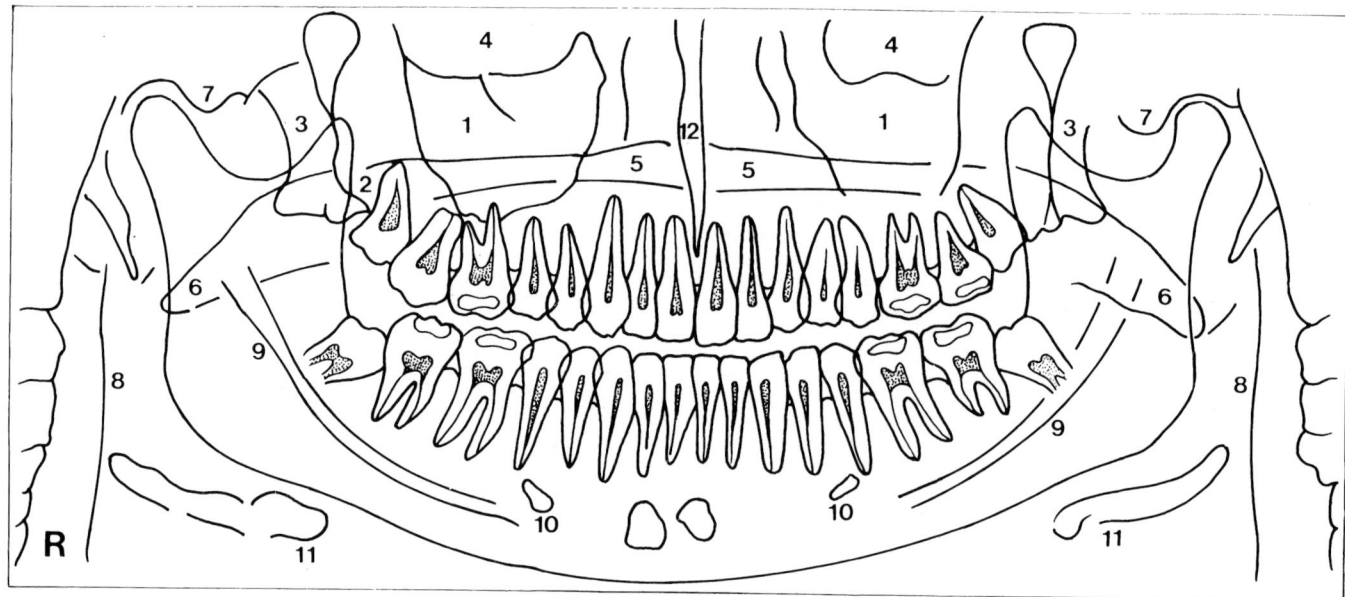

Fig. 2.13 Anatomical relations of the teeth and alveoli. Drawing of an orthopantomogram showing the principal anatomical relations of the teeth and alveoli: (1) maxillary sinus; (2) maxillary tuberosity; (3) lateral pterygoid plate; (4) orbital cavity; (5) hard palate; (6) soft palate; (7) articular eminence; (8) posterior pharyngeal wall; (9) inferior alveolar (mandibular) canal; (10) mental foramen; (11) hyoid bone; (12) nasal septum.

is light pink in colour and tightly bound to the underlying fibrous tissue, giving the characteristic 'orange-peel' appearance of healthy gums. Over the apical part of the alveolus, however, the gingival tissues merge, at the vermilion border, with the alveolar mucosa which is reddish and highly vascular like the epithelium lining the oral cavity.

In the upper jaw, the maxillary sinus is an important superior relation to the premolars and molars, often extending from the region of the first premolar posteriorly as far as the maxillary tuberosity which it often invades, particularly in later life. In radiographs, the maxillary posterior tooth roots sometimes appear to perforate the floor of the sinus but there is a layer of bone, albeit very thin, separating the roots from the lining of the sinus.

Immediately behind the maxillary third molar lies the tuberosity, the hamular notch and the hamular process of the medial pterygoid plate around which the tendon of the tensor palati muscle passes. The hard palate can be seen on orthopantomograms lying above the level of the tooth roots.

In the mandible, the most important relation of the tooth roots and alveoli is the mandibular or inferior alveolar canal (Fig. 2.6) with its enclosed neurovascular bundle. This canal passes very close to the third molar roots and, rarely, it may be encircled by them. The canal passes below the posterior teeth to the mental foramen located in the region of the apex of the second premolar tooth. Here, the canal divides into mental and incisive terminations.

Another important relation of the lower alveolus is the lingual nerve which arises in the infratemporal fossa and

gains access to the oral cavity by passing below a small ridge of bone lingual to the last mandibular tooth, which in the adult is the third molar. In this position the nerve is protected only by this ridge of bone, which has been termed the endalveolar crest, and by the covering mucosa (Volchansky & Makings 1984; Penhall 1992). Figure 2.14 illustrates the relations of the maxillary and mandibular alveoli in the region of the second molar. The mylohyoid muscle, suspended from the mylohyoid lines on each side of the mandible and attached in front to the inside of the symphysis and below to the hyoid bone, forms the interface between the intraoral structures and those lying in the submandibular region. Important structures lie superior to the mylohyoid muscle in the floor of the mouth in close relation to the mandibular alveolus: the sublingual gland, submandibular duct, lingual nerve and at a deeper level the hypoglossal nerve and lingual artery.

GEOMETRIC CONCEPTS OF THE CRANIOFACIAL SKELETON

There have been several attempts to produce geometric models of the craniofacial skeleton. These models present simplified interpretations of the complex anatomy of the bony structural pillars that transmit the forces of mastication, devised to further the understanding of fracture patterns (Fig. 2.15).

The dispersion of masticatory forces through vertical bony columns to the broad areas of the skull base was appreciated by Le Fort himself (p. 17). Rowe & Killey (1955) emphasized the mechanical strength of the alveoli and the transverse palatal arch, on which rest the

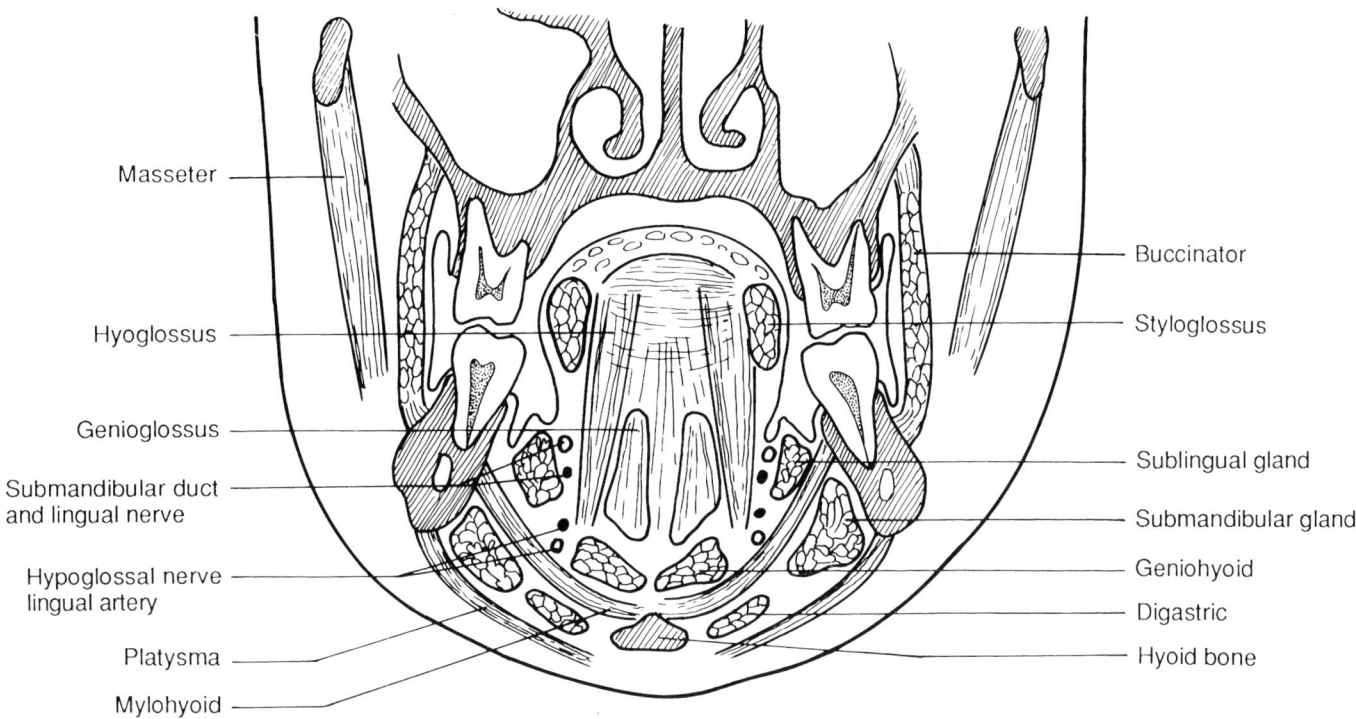

Masseter

Hyoglossus

Genioglossus

Submandibular duct
and lingual nerve

Hypoglossal nerve
lingual artery

Platysma

Mylohyoid

Buccinator

Styloglossus

Sublingual gland

Submandibular gland

Geniohyoid

Digastric

Hyoid bone

Fig. 2.14 Sublingual and submandibular regions. Coronal section in the region of the second molars showing the sublingual and submandibular relations of the teeth and alveoli.

paired buttresses of the maxillae, the palatine-pterygoid buttresses posteriorly and the zygomatic complexes laterally; they saw additional support in the central buttress of the vomer and ethmoid vertical plate (Fig. 2.15A). In a functional analysis of the facial skeleton, Sicher & Du Brul (1975) considered that the facial structures were anchored to the skull base by three pairs of curved vertical pillars: the canine pillar, the zygomatic pillar, and the pterygoid pillar (Fig. 2.15B). Sturla et al (1980) performed cadaver impaction studies, on the basis of which they proposed a lattice-shaped structure whose central and lateral vertical pillars spanned between a superior cranial shelf and an inferior palatal platform (Fig. 2.15C). Their lattice shaped model had a layout resembling the architectural concept of Rowe & Killey (1955): both were essentially anatomical schematizations of the face with the thin laminae of bone removed. The projection of these vertical facial pillars to the main structural zones of the cranial base has been reviewed by Fain (1980) who examined the effects of facial bone trauma on the basal structures. The concept of structural pillars of the facial skeleton has also formed a basis for fracture management whereby the anterior vertical buttresses are reconstituted to preserve the facial height (Manson et al 1980; Gruss & Mackinnon 1986).

In a less anatomical fashion, Gentry et al (1983) conceived the face geometrically as a series of triplanar osseous struts (Fig. 2.15D; Tables 7.1–7.3; p. 183). They identified three major struts in the horizontal plane, five

in the sagittal plane, and two in the coronal plane; also considered were the relationships of the soft tissues to each strut. This analysis was based on high resolution computer tomography of the traumatized face, and was not designed to illustrate mechanical concepts of the facial skeleton. Luce (1984) also proposed a less anatomical format when he illustrated the relationship between the anterior cranial fossa, frontal sinus, orbits and the ethmoid air cells with a diagram in which each region is depicted as a box. This cellular concept of CMF anatomy is of interest in relation to the mechanical role of the paranasal air sinuses. The sinuses form a large aerated honeycomb: from a teleological view, this structure seems designed to absorb the energy of facial impact and so to protect the brain and the sensory organs (Blanton & Biggs 1969). When force is transmitted from below, the pyramidal orientation of these sinuses, with the maxillary sinuses forming the base and the sphenoid sinus as the apex, constitutes an architectural structure that is particularly well suited to a protective, energy-absorbing role (Riu et al 1960).

The forces required to fracture the craniofacial bones are impressively high; in Chapter 4, the data derived from cadaver studies are reviewed. It is necessary to relate the skeletal anatomy of a fracture to the direction of the impacting force as well as to its magnitude. The facial skeleton is well adapted to withstand the vertical forces of mastication, but it is less tolerant of forces in the horizontal plane, which may detach the alveolar complex

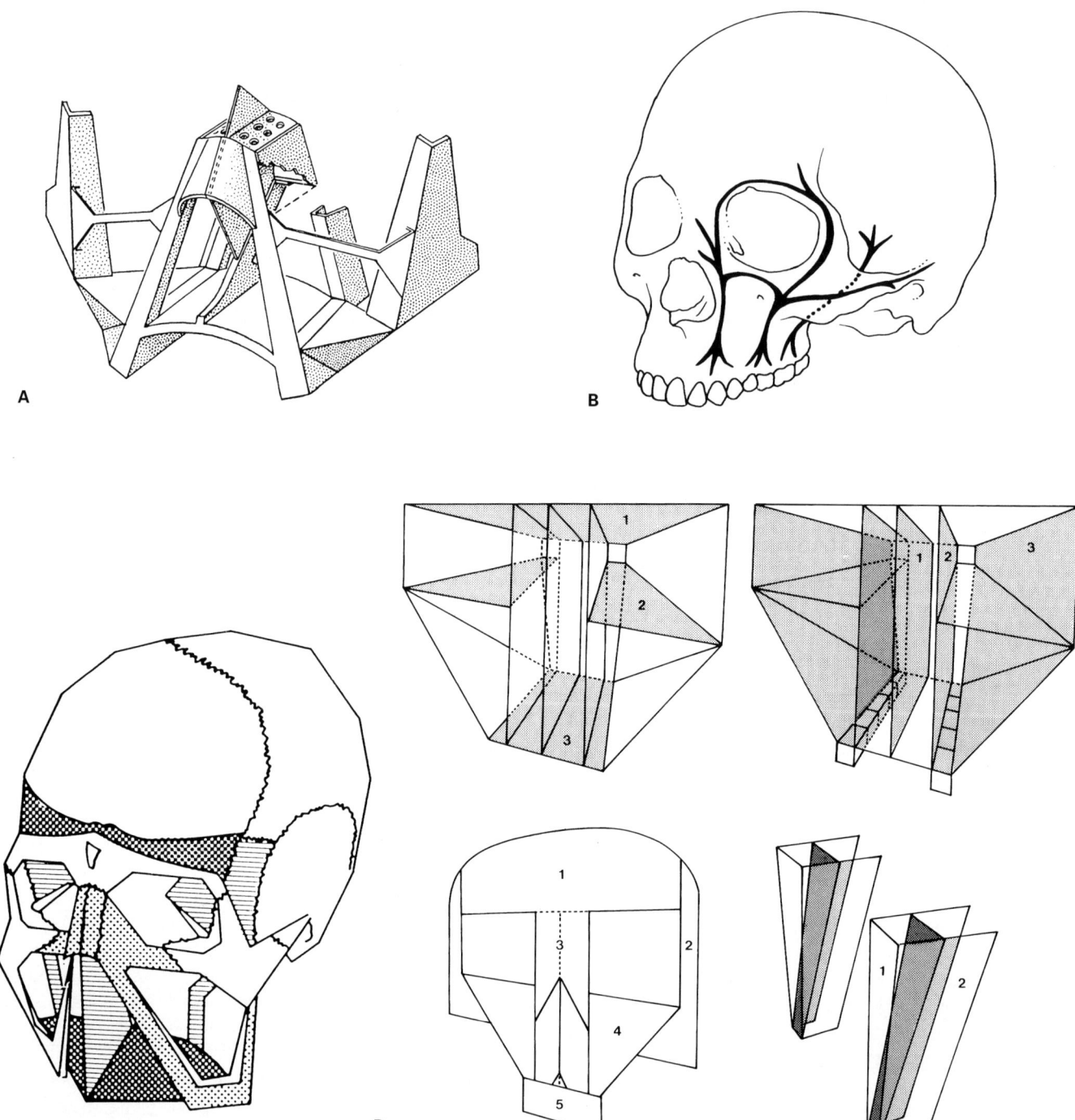

Fig. 2.15 Geometric concepts of the facial skeleton. The complex structure of the facial skeleton has been considered in terms of its capacity to absorb the forces of mastication, and diagrammatic interpretations have been published. **A** Rowe & Killey (1955) saw three paired girders transmitting force evenly to the skull base, with an additional midline strut; in their architectural diagram, the arched palate and the inferior orbital rims join the anterior and lateral girders. **B** Sicher & Du Brul (1975) also recognized the importance of the three paired pillars in transmitting force to the skull base. These authors gave greater prominence to the horizontal pillars connecting the curved vertical pillars, especially the supraorbital bar. Redrawn after Sicher & Du Brul by courtesy of Messrs Mosby, St Louis. **C** Sturla et al (1980) emphasized the importance of the vertical pillars, but also stressed the importance of the transverse platforms — the hard palate below and the frontal and sphenoid bones above. Reproduced by courtesy of *Plastic & Reconstructive Surgery* and the authors. **D** Gentry et al (1983) studied thin-section CT scans of cadavers and identified: (i) three horizontal struts (shaded): superior (1), middle or orbital (2), and inferior or palatal (3); (ii) three sagittal struts (shaded): median or septal (1), parasagittal (2) and lateral (3); (iii) five anterior coronal struts: frontal (1), zygomaticofrontal (2), nasofrontal (3), anterior maxillary (4), and anterior alveolar (5); (iv) two paired posterior coronal struts: posterior maxillary (1) and pterygoid (abutting on 1). This complex schematization can be clearly related to anatomical structures seen in coronal and axial scans. Reproduced by courtesy of *American Journal of Roentgenology* and the authors.

from its supports, or cause complete craniofacial disjunction. The bones of the craniofacial region are intricately linked and the majority of their junctions are immovable sutures. As a result of this configuration there is a high propensity for a stereotyped pattern of fracturing to result from a single blow and the angle of impact may be an important determinant of the final fracture pattern. From a knowledge of the normal spatial relationships of the bones, their major structural components and their impact tolerances, a clear insight can be gained into the dynamic responses to severe impact, the final result of which is the fracture pattern.

BLOOD VESSELS

The blood supply of a region is studied to assess the viability of structures selected for skin flaps and bone flaps, to design surgical approaches and to deal with primary and secondary haemorrhage. Modern concepts of craniofacial surgery have added the need to understand the effects of wide periosteal stripping of the craniofacial skeleton on fracture healing, and to know how to preserve blood vessels and nerves contained in the soft tissues (p. 293). Furthermore, microvascular surgical reconstruction now has a great and increasing role in all aspects of CMF surgery, and this demands knowledge of the vascularity of a region and the potential scope for microvascular anastomosis.

Arterial supply

The arterial blood supply of the CMF structures is derived from branches of the external and internal carotid arteries. There is free anastomosis across the midline (Har-Shai et al 1992) and anastomosis between the internal and external systems in the region of the orbital and nasal cavities (Fig. 2.16).

The common carotid artery divides, usually at the level of the disc between the third and fourth cervical vertebrae, into the internal and external carotid arteries. The internal carotid artery does not branch in the neck and proceeds to enter the base of skull through the carotid canal in the petrous temporal bone. The artery leaves the carotid canal at the foramen lacerum and pierces the dura mater; it then runs forward within the cavernous sinus for about 2 cm before turning upwards and piercing the dura again to enter the subarachnoid space. Within the cavernous sinus, the internal carotid artery gives rise to several small but important arteries. Following Parkinson (1984), most surgical anatomist authors identify the meningohypophyseal trunk, the artery of the inferior cavernous sinus, and McConnell's artery supplying the capsule of the pituitary gland (Stephens & Stilwell, 1969). The meningohypophyseal artery typically gives rise to

three branches: the tentorial artery, the dorsal meningeal artery and the inferior hypophyseal artery, which supplies the posterior lobe of the pituitary gland (see below). Lang (1983) describes two arterial trunks, a superior caroticocavernous trunk supplying the pituitary and the clival region, and a lateral caroticocavernous trunk supplying the trigeminal ganglion and the ocular motor nerves. Avulsion of one of these branches can be a cause of carotid-cavernous fistula (pp. 146 and 392). The internal carotid artery then gives off its important branch the ophthalmic artery. From this arises the anterior ethmoid artery which arises in the orbit, enters the ethmoid in its own canal, traverses the cribriform plate, and enters the nose through the cribro-ethmoid canal to anastomose with branches of the maxillary artery. The ophthalmic artery also gives rise to the central artery of the retina and the supraorbital and supratrochlear arteries, which anastomose with the facial artery (Fig. 2.16). The internal carotid artery then gives off the anterior choroidal, anterior cerebral and middle cerebral arteries and anastomoses with the vertebrobasilar system through the circle of Willis. The details of the vascular supply of the brain lie outside the scope of this book.

The external carotid artery gives off named branches to the pharynx, occiput, thyroid, tongue and face; it then divides into the superficial temporal artery and the maxillary artery.

Together with the ophthalmic and occipital arteries, the superficial temporal artery supplies the scalp, and is therefore the nutrient artery of many useful flaps. It divides into two main branches, anterior (frontal) and posterior (parietal), and there are several variations on this pattern (Marano et al 1985). These main branches (which are usually palpable) divide repeatedly, and as they near their terminations they become more superficial; this can prejudice the survival of galeal flaps dissected away from the scalp (Har-Shai et al 1992). The superficial temporal artery contributes to the temporalis muscle and fascia, though the main supply of the temporalis muscle is the deep temporal artery.

The maxillary artery's relationship to the condylar neck and posterior maxilla is important surgically (p. 293), and its anastomosis with the internal system, in and about the nose, has significance in primary and secondary haemorrhage from this area. The maxillary artery gives rise to the middle meningeal artery, which enters the middle cranial fossa, sending an anterior branch to the region of the pterion, and the inferior dental artery, which enters the mandibular canal.

The middle meningeal artery supplies a wide area of the dura mater; it contributes to the supply of the anterior cranial fossa, anastomosing with branches of the ophthalmic artery, the posterior and anterior ethmoid arteries, and with the small accessory meningeal artery,

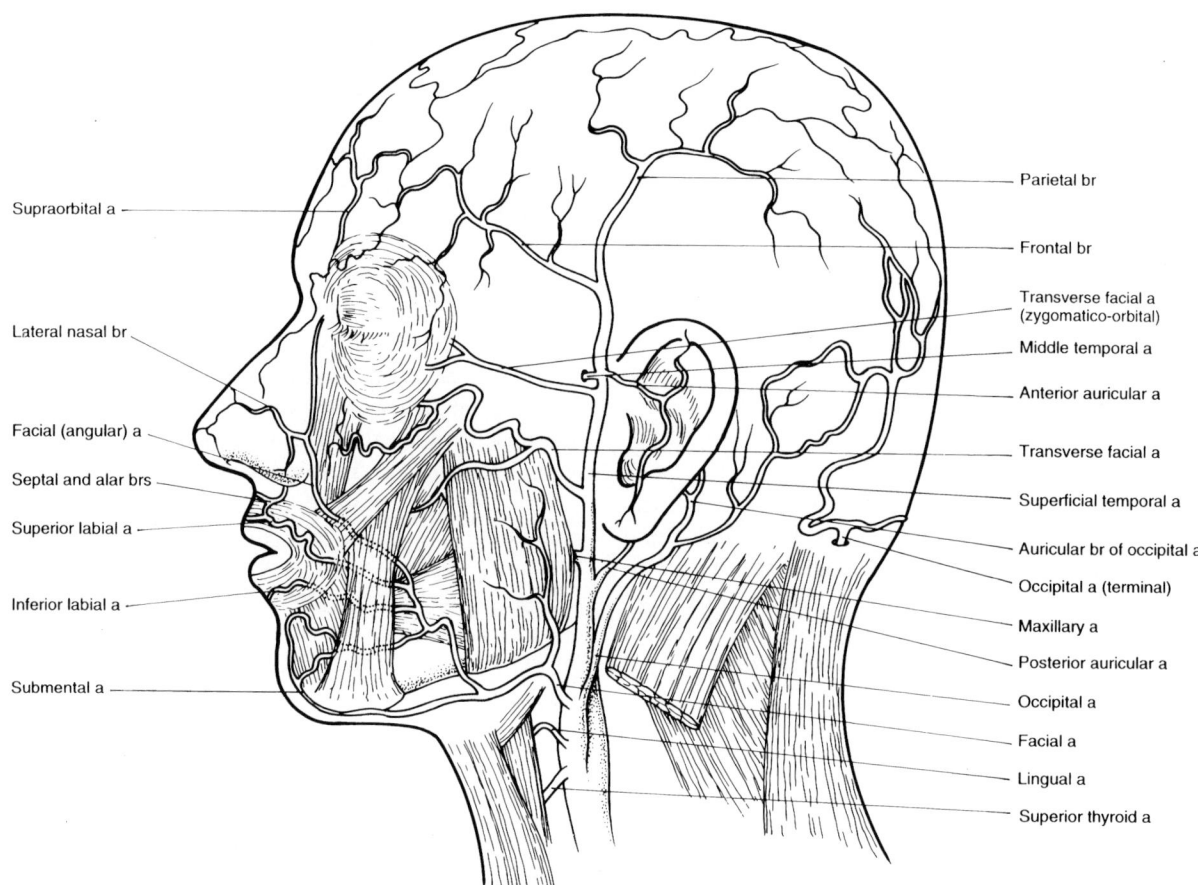

Supraorbital a

Lateral nasal br

Facial (angular) a

Septal and alar brs

Superior labial a

Inferior labial a

Submental a

Parietal br

Frontal br

Transverse facial a (zygomatico-orbital)

Middle temporal a

Anterior auricular a

Transverse facial a

Superficial temporal a

Auricular br of occipital a

Occipital a (terminal)

Maxillary a

Posterior auricular a

Occipital a

Facial a

Lingual a

Superior thyroid a

Fig. 2.16 Arteries of the face and scalp. With the exception of the supraorbital artery (a branch of the ophthalmic artery), all the named arteries in the diagram are derived from the external carotid artery. There are many variations in origin, calibre and anastomoses; these variations often determine the feasibility of microvascular replantations. Redrawn after *Gray's Anatomy* and other sources.

which may arise from it or from the maxillary artery itself. The extradural haemorrhages complicating impacts in the CMF region (p. 385) are usually the result of bleeding from the small meningeal arteries in the anterior fossa rather than from the main trunk of the middle meningeal artery, which is typically lacerated by vertical fractures of the temporal bone. The flat bones of the calvaria receive their blood supply from the pericranium externally, and internally from the dura mater, whose outer layer is functionally equivalent to the pericranium.

Further in its course, the maxillary artery supplies the maxilla and the palate, through the infraorbital artery, the greater palatine artery and the superior dental arteries, and terminates as the sphenopalatine artery. The teeth and their supporting structures are supplied by the inferior and superior dental branches of the maxillary artery but with contributions from the lingual and facial arteries. As the maxillary artery crosses the pterygomaxillary fissure it gives rise to the posterior superior dental artery from which branches enter the maxilla through small foramina above the maxillary tuberosity. These then divide into

smaller branches supplying the upper molar and premolar teeth, the lining of the maxillary sinus and the surrounding alveolus. Other branches run outside the alveolus to supply the alveolar mucosa and other soft tissues in the posterior maxillary region. The maxillary artery passes anteriorly along the infraorbital canal, becoming the infraorbital artery and giving off the anterior, and sometimes middle, superior dental branches to the remaining teeth and supporting tissues. The infraorbital artery provides terminal branches to the upper lip and to the nasal vestibular tissues.

The maxillary artery also gives palatine branches as it crosses the pterygomaxillary fissure. The greater palatine artery enters a canal, passes downwards and emerges through the greater palatine foramen in the posterior region of the palate. From here it passes forwards supplying the palatal mucosa and the gingival tissues on the lingual surfaces of the maxillary teeth. In the region of the incisors it anastomoses with the terminal nasal branches of the maxillary artery emerging through the incisive canal. Lesser palatine arteries also emerge near the posterior border of the hard palate to supply the soft palate where they communicate with branches of the tonsillar and ascending pharyngeal arteries.

The mandibular teeth are supplied by the inferior dental artery. Passing forwards in the mandibular canal the inferior dental artery supplies the posterior mandibular teeth, tooth sockets and cancellous bone of the mandible before dividing into mental and incisive branches in the region of the premolar teeth. The mental branch emerges through the mental foramen to supply lower lip, cheeks and gum tissue as far as the midline where it anastomoses with branches of the facial artery. The incisive branch continues within the mandible to supply anterior teeth and supporting bone.

The buccal mucosa over the mandible is supplied by the buccal branch of the maxillary artery which pierces the buccinator muscle to gain access to the intraoral region. Anastomoses with branches of the facial artery occur in this region also. The lingual mucosa in the mandible is supplied by branches of the lingual artery.

The lingual artery supplies principally the tongue and the floor of the mouth. It arises from the external carotid artery near the tip of the greater cornu of the hyoid bone where it lies on the middle constrictor of the pharynx. The artery then loops above the tip of the hyoid and is crossed by the hypoglossal nerve before descending to enter the floor of the mouth by passing beneath the hyoglossus muscle. Near the anterior border of hyoglossus the lingual artery gives its submental branch to the sublingual gland and floor of the mouth and continues as the deep artery of the tongue which gives many branches to the muscles and mucosa of the tongue.

The facial artery is the main nutrient of the facial musculature and soft tissues. It arises in the neck from the external carotid just superior to the lingual artery. It then passes upwards, grooving the submandibular gland, before passing over the gland and descending between the gland and the ramus of the mandible. While in the neck it gives the ascending palatine and tonsillar branches to the region of the oral fauces. The facial artery crosses the lower border of the mandible at the anterior border of the masseter muscle where the arterial pulse can be felt quite readily. The facial artery takes a tortuous course across the face giving branches to lower and upper lips; it terminates at the side of the nose where it becomes the angular artery, usually passing in its course within the muscles of the region. During its course across the face, the facial artery anastomoses with other arteries in the region, particularly branches of the maxillary, superficial temporal and ophthalmic arteries. The chief superficial facial branches are shown in Fig. 2.16. It is of surgical importance to note that the mandible is unique in the CMF region in the nature of its blood supply. The other facial bones, like the calvarial bones, derive their blood supply from superficial periosteal arteries. The mandible has in addition a central artery, the inferior dental artery, and in this it is comparable with the limb bones. The inferior dental artery is vulnerable in fractures of the body of the mandible. In elderly people, this artery is often obliterated, presumably from atherosclerosis (Bradley 1975; Pogrel et al 1987).

The facial artery is the artery of choice in providing blood supply by microsurgical anastomosis for a free bone graft in restoring a mandibular defect (p. 621). The superficial temporal artery has also been used, or even the occipital artery; the superior thyroid artery is sometimes too small. All the branches of the external carotid artery have relatively thin walls and are apt to go into spasm when microvascular anastomosis is done.

Venous drainage

The posterior part of the superficial facial venous system (Fig. 2.17) drains into the external jugular vein through the retromandibular vein from the upper part of the face and temporal region; the facial vein, arising in the medial canthal region, drains into the internal jugular vein, but has anastomotic connections both with the external jugular vein and the cavernous sinus. There are no valves in the superficial facial veins. There are deep venous systems of surgical significance, the lingual veins, the pharyngeal plexus and the pterygoid plexus, all of which drain into the internal jugular vein. The large pterygoid plexus, lying around the pterygoid muscles, anastomoses with the facial vein and also with the cavernous sinus; it receives venous blood from the meninges and the orbit as well as from the subtemporal region. The venous drainage of the orbit is in communication with both the pterygoid plexus and with the cavernous sinus; these communications become very obvious in the presence of a carotid-cavernous fistula (Fig. 13.14) and are relevant in determining the spread of infection.

The venous drainage of the maxillary and mandibular teeth is through veins that accompany the arteries and pass forward into the anterior facial vein or backward into the pterygoid plexus and so into the cervical jugular system.

The venous blood from the cranial cavity finds its way out through the sagittal transverse and sigmoid sinuses to the jugular veins, and to a much lesser extent through the cavernous sinus system to the facial venous plexuses. The cavernous sinus is an intradural blood space situated adjacent to the pituitary fossa and body of the sphenoid sinus (Fig. 2.18). It is pyramidal, with the apex anteriorly, and lies between two layers of dura. The medial and inferior walls are formed by the periosteal dura of the body of the sphenoid and the dural fold which forms the lateral wall of the pituitary fossa. The superior surface is

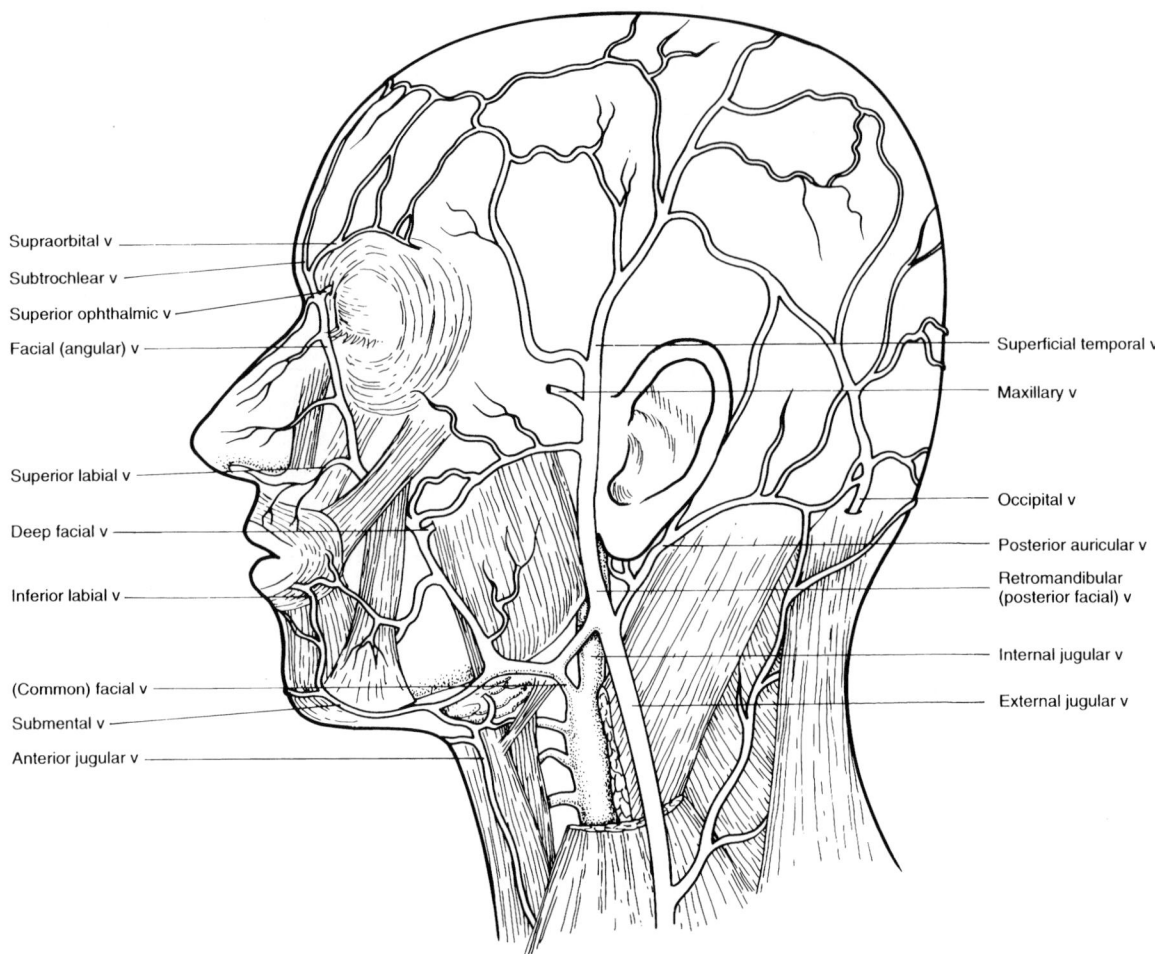

Supraorbital v

Subtrochlear v

Superior ophthalmic v

Facial (angular) v

Superior labial v

Deep facial v

Inferior labial v

(Common) facial v

Submental v

Anterior jugular v

Superficial temporal v

Maxillary v

Occipital v

Posterior auricular v

Retromandibular (posterior facial) v

Internal jugular v

External jugular v

Fig. 2.17 Superficial veins of the face and scalp. These show even more variations in origin, calibre and anastomoses than the arteries, and are also of importance in microvascular replantations. The superficial veins anastomose with the deep venous system at many points: (i) at its origin, the facial (angular) vein connects with the superior ophthalmic vein, and so with the cavernous sinus; (ii) the maxillary vein connects with the pterygoid venous plexus; (iii) the occipital, superficial temporal and supraorbital veins connect through emissary veins (not shown) with dural veins and venous sinuses. These connections may be routes for spread of infection, resulting in cavernous sinus thrombophlebitis or subdural abscess (p. 147). Redrawn after *Gray's Anatomy* and other sources.

triangular and formed by the free and the attached edges of the tentorium and by the interclinoid ligament.

Medially the cavernous sinus is related to the pituitary fossa and the sphenoid air sinus; laterally to the temporal lobe. The posterior wall lies within the posterior fossa and is related to the brain stem. The apex of the cavernous sinus is related to the apex of the orbit and the superior orbital fissure. Inferiorly lies the sphenoid air sinus.

The major venous tributaries of the sinus are: the superior ophthalmic vein which leaves the orbit through the superior orbital fissure to enter the cavernous sinus anteriorly; the sphenoparietal sinus which lies along the edge of the lesser wing of the sphenoid; the superior and inferior petrosal sinuses which connect the cavernous sinus with the sigmoid sinus and jugular bulb respectively; the superficial and deep middle cerebral veins.

The cavernous sinuses on each side are united by a variable pattern of intercavernous sinuses which lie within the dural wall of the pituitary fossa and by a basilar plexus of dural veins which lie between the dura overlying the clivus. Other venous tributaries connect the cavernous sinuses to extracranial venous plexuses such as the pterygoid plexus. The sinus contains the internal carotid artery, and the third, fourth, fifth and sixth cranial nerves. Within the cavernous sinus the internal carotid artery gives rise to the small but important branches described above (p. 47).

Lymphatic drainage

Lymphatic vessels from the scalp and the superficial facial tissues drain into named and unnamed lymph nodes: the chief of these are the submental, submandibular, parotid, retroauricular and occipital nodes. These in turn drain

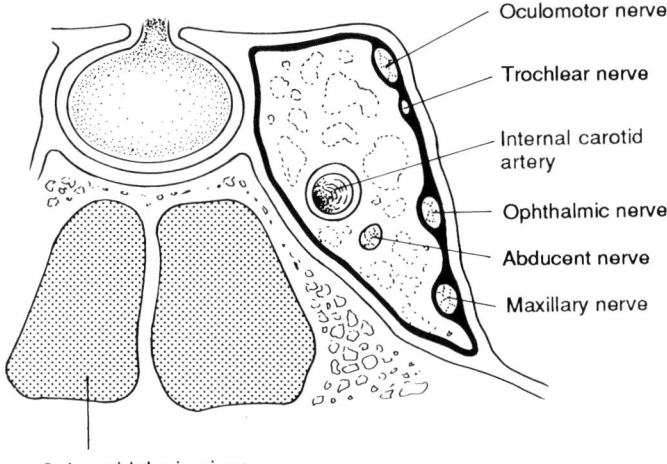

Sphenoidal air sinus

Fig. 2.18 The cavernous sinus. The diagram shows the sinus and its contents in coronal section. The sixth (abducent) cranial nerve is within the lumen of the sinus. The maxillary and ophthalmic branches of the fifth cranial nerve are embedded in the deep dural plate of the lateral wall of the sinus, as are the third (oculomotor) and fourth (trochlear) nerves: Lang (1983) has shown that these nerves are sheathed in arachnoid for short distances after they enter the wall of the sinus.

into deep cervical nodes. Lymphatics from the deeper oral viscera and from the nasal, nasopharyngeal and tympanic cavities also drain into deep cervical nodes. Lymph drainage of the teeth and supporting tissues reaches regional nodes in the sublingual and submandibular region before entering the deep cervical vessels. The dura mater has a rich lymphatic system (Millen & Woollam 1962), but the brain, like the eye, has no lymphatic drainage.

BRAIN

Within the cranial cavity is the brain, lying in the protective bath of CSF provided by the subarachnoid cisterns. Magnetic resonance imaging (MRI) makes it possible to visualize cerebral lesions and anatomical structures as small as 5 mm in diameter, or even smaller. Knowledge of the gross anatomy of the brain has therefore become clinically more relevant than in the past, while functional neuroanatomy remains indispensable in understanding the neurological effects of head injury. However, gross anatomy is best studied in correlative atlases (Lang 1983; Duvernoy 1991), and clinical neuroanatomy is too vast a subject to be reviewed here; for those interested in the anatomy of nuclei and fibre systems, Brodal (1981) and Carpenter & Sutin (1983) provide very detailed textbooks, while Noback et al (1991) give a well-illustrated introductory account. However, it is necessary to consider the clinical and surgical anatomy of those parts of the brain which are in direct relation to the frontal bone and the floor of the anterior fossa, and to consider their functions in the context of CMF trauma.

Frontal lobes

Any part of the brain may be injured by impacts striking the CMF region (p. 138), but the frontal lobes are especially vulnerable. The neuroanatomy of the frontal lobes is therefore clinically very important in understanding post-traumatic cerebral disabilities (p. 653) and their neuropsychological evaluation (Appendix III).

The inferior surface of each frontal lobe conforms closely with the contours of the anterior cranial fossa. Medially, the narrow gyrus rectus extends back from the region of the crista galli to the level of the tuberculum sellae. It is bounded laterally by the olfactory sulcus, in which rests the olfactory tract, and medially by the interhemispheric fissure; it extends back to the medial olfactory stria, one of the terminal components of the olfactory tract. Lateral to the olfactory sulcus are the orbital gyri, overlying the orbital plates and often showing sulci conforming with ridges in the bony surface. Histologically, these gyri are composed of typical six-layered neocortex, and except in the posterior part, the cortex shows numerous granule cells, especially in layer IV. It is usual to identify this granular part of the frontal cortex by the Brodmann numbers 9, 10 and 11, though one may be sceptical of the precise demarcations in the mosaic maps of cortical areas devised by Korbinian Brodmann (1868–1918) and later students of the cytoarchitectonics of the cortex (Fig. 2.19). Posteriorly, the cortex contains fewer granule cells, and indeed the most posterior part is agranular (area 13 in current terminology); there is considerable individual variation in the demarcations of these areas (Beck et al 1950).

The orbital cortex receives a strong projection from

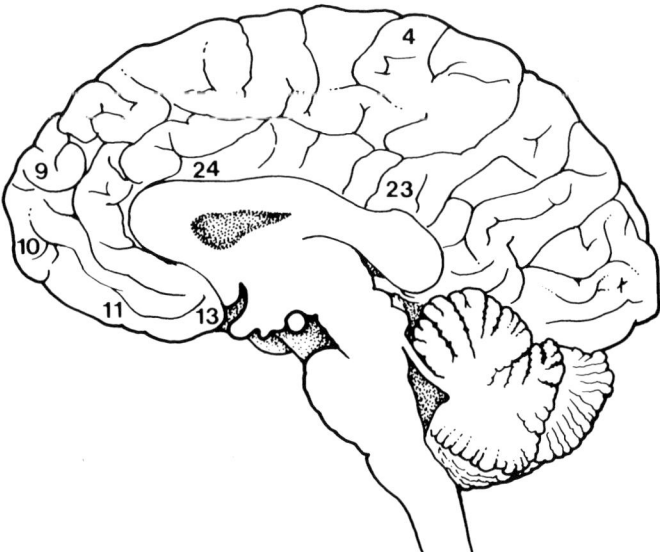

Fig. 2.19 Medial aspect of cerebral hemisphere. Diagram showing the chief cortical areas of the medial frontal lobe; the numerals indicate cortical areas identified by Brodmann.

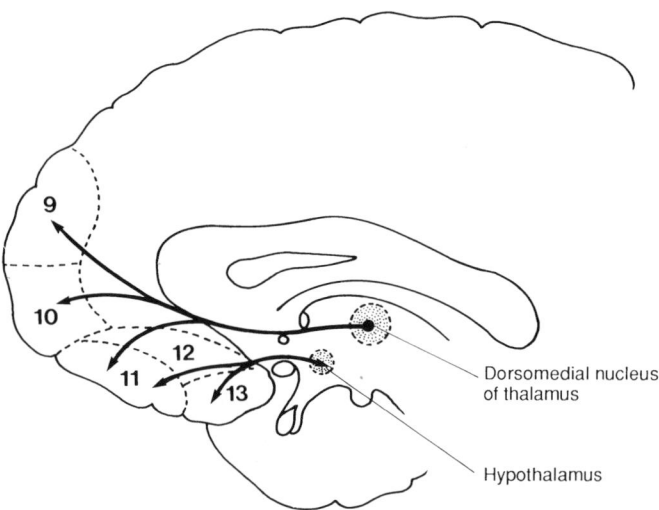

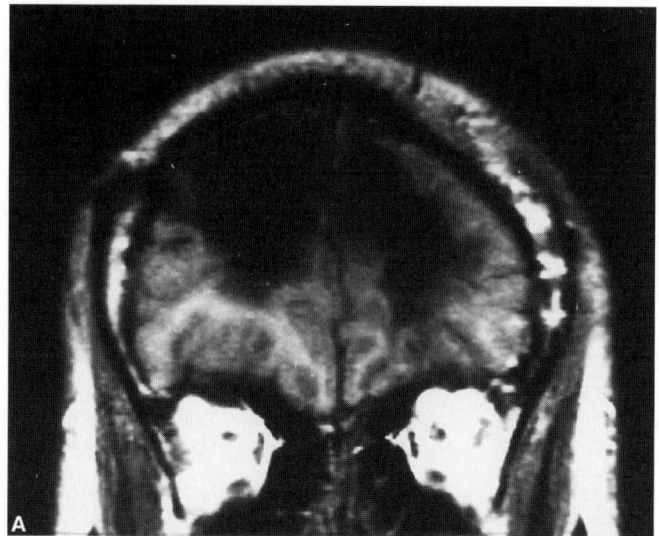

Fig. 2.20 **Fibre connections of prefrontal and orbital cortex.** The granular prefrontal areas have strong two-way connections with the dorsomedial nucleus of the thalamus through the thalamofrontal bundle. The posterior orbital cortex has connections with the hypothalamus through the medial forebrain bundle.

the dorsomedial nucleus of the thalamus through the compact thalamofrontal bundle (Fig. 2.20). There are also numerous fibre connections with the hypothalamus, suggesting autonomic functions. The orbital frontal cortex is often damaged in anterior fossa fractures, especially when the orbital plates are shattered. The clinical effects are striking only when the damage is massive and bilateral (Fig. 2.21). Surgical isolation of the orbital cortex, by cutting through the white matter, was a standard operation in the era of limited psychosurgery. It was found that bilateral lesions of this selective type caused flattening of mood, or sometimes mild euphoria, but without intellectual deficits detectable by the tests then available (Tow & Lewin 1953). More extensive lesions extending back into the posterior orbital cortex, the anterior striatum and the basofrontal nuclei, were sometimes complicated by severe apathy or even stupor, nutritional disturbances and persisting urinary incontinence (Beck et al 1950).

The medial surface of the frontal lobe is related to the medial segment of the falx and to the opposite frontal lobe (Fig. 2.19). Anteriorly and inferiorly, the cortex is granular and is an extension of areas 9–11. Posteriorly is the large cingulate gyrus (areas 23 and 24), curving around the corpus callosum. The cingulate gyrus receives fibres from the anterior nucleus of the thalamus, which is connected with the mammillary body in the hypothalamus (Fig. 2.22) through the mammillothalamic tract. The medial mammillary nucleus in turn receives a tightly organized, point-to-point projection from the hippocampal complex (Simpson 1952) through the fornix. The cingulate gyrus, the mammillary nuclei and the hippocampal complex have been conceptualized as part of the limbic

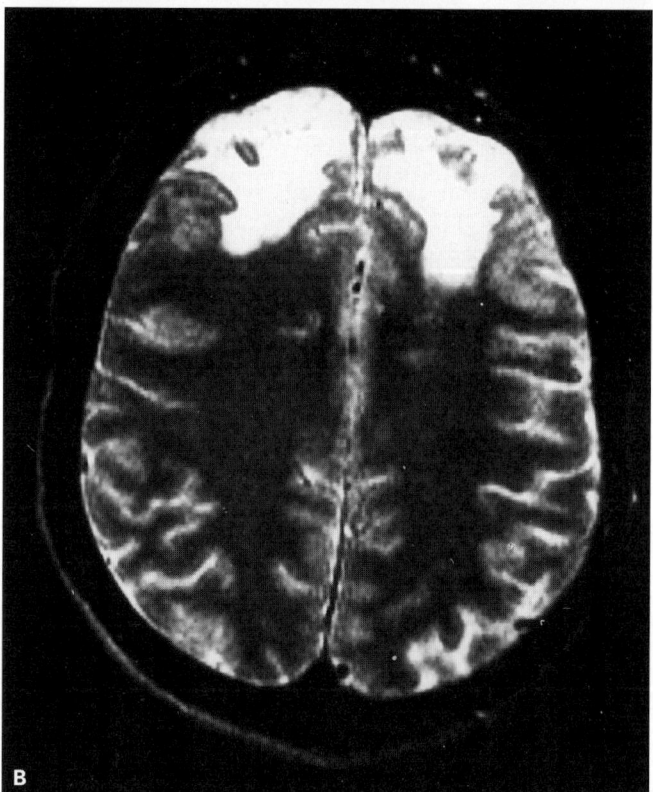

Fig. 2.21 **Bifrontal polar damage.** MRI scan of a young man who had suffered a central frontal impact in a car crash at age 5 years. The victim has a stable personality and intelligence within the normal range. **A** Low signal abnormalities in the T1-weighted coronal image: the white matter is largely destroyed, especially in the dorsomedial quadrants. **B** Bifrontal high signal abnormalities in T2-weighted images.

system, and functionally related both to mood and to memory. The cingulate gyrus is rarely injured in isolation, but psychosurgical cingulate ablation was once much used for obsessive states; the effects of this operation included transient memory impairment (Whitty & Lewin 1960),

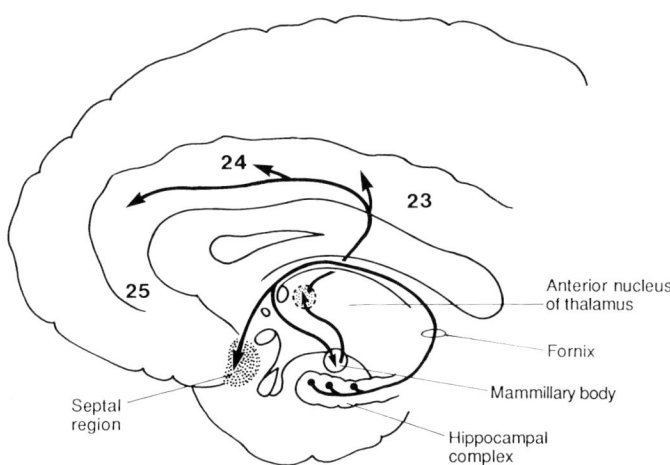

Fig. 2.22 Pathways connecting the mammillary nuclei with the anterior thalamic nucleus and the cingulate gyrus. Neurons in the subiculum (part of the hippocampal complex) project through the fornix to the medial mammillary nucleus and also to the septal nuclei and other basal forebrain structures.

but this did not constitute a permanent disability. Lesions in the mammillary bodies (Dusoir et al 1990), or bilateral destruction of the hippocampal complex, cause gross impairments of memory.

On its convex lateral surface, the frontal lobe is related to the frontal bone, and more posteriorly to the parietal bone (Fig. 2.23), since the precentral gyrus — the poste-

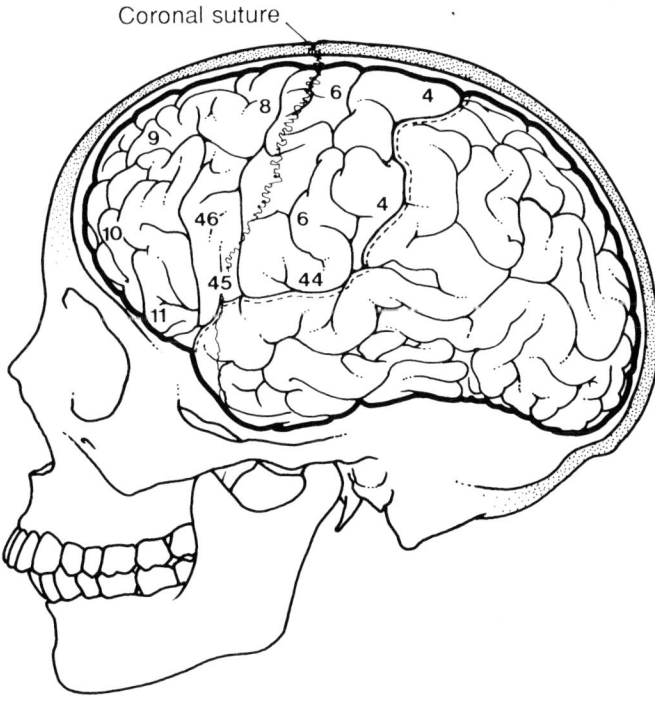

Fig. 2.23 Frontal convexity, in relation to coronal suture. The anatomical frontal lobe is demarcated (dashed lines) by the central sulcus and the sylvian fissure. The chief cortical areas are identified by Brodmann's numbers.

rior limit of the frontal lobe — lies well behind the coronal suture. Anteriorly, the cortex is rich in granule cells and is a part of areas 9–11: thus, these cortical areas are located on all the surfaces of the frontal pole and are often called prefrontal cortex. More posteriorly, the cortex (areas 8, 6, 45 and 46) shows fewer granule cells, and large pyramidal cells become more conspicuous; the precentral gyrus (area 4) is agranular, containing large pyramidal neurons, some of which send axons to synapse directly on spinal motor neurons. The posterior frontal convexity cortex is concerned especially with motor function, including limb movements (areas 4, 6 and 8) and conjugate eye movement (area 8); on the dominant side, the frontal cortex is concerned with expressive speech (supposedly areas 44 and 45). Traumatic lesions posterior to the coronal suture are often associated with contralateral limb or facial weakness, or with non-fluent dysphasia when the dominant hemisphere is injured. But lesions in the prefrontal region, even those causing substantial cortical and subcortical damage, may show no limb signs or speech impairment, and in the past this has given the mistaken impression that this is a 'silent area'. In fact, bilateral prefrontal lesions often cause very disabling changes in intellect and personality.

At present, the evidence does not allow exact correlations between the neuropsychological effects of frontal lobe injury and localized damage to specific cortical areas. But there is general agreement that destruction of the dorsolateral quadrants of the frontal lobes is more disastrous than damage to the inferior and medial quadrants, which may cause little or no obvious clinical impairment (Fig. 2.21). From his large experience of the effects of psychosurgery and of head injury, Walsh (1978, 1985) has made some general correlations between lesion site and neuropsychological sequelae. He associates the dorsolateral cortex with the ideational preparation and execution of actions; patients with lesions in this region may suffer severe intellectual disabilities in planning and learning, despite normal performance in standard IQ tests. There is a characteristic difficulty in integrating data to solve a problem; thinking tends to be rigid or inflexible (Walsh 1978), and this is reflected in the content of speech, though rigid thinking is seen after injuries elsewhere in the brain. The medial frontal cortex, presumably including the anterior cingulate gyrus, is concerned with self-initiated action and sustaining behaviour at an appropriate level. Severe damage in this region may explain the adynamia — lack of drive — so often seen after frontal lobe damage. Walsh (1985) relates the basal (orbitofrontal) and basomedial cortex with 'the flexible control of excitation and inhibition and the emotional control of behaviour': large bilateral lesions in this region may be associated with socially disastrous disinhibition, loss of insight and egotistic behaviour. In practice, the frontal lobe lesions seen after CMF injury are rarely confined exactly to a particular region, and when they are, the effects are not always what one would forecast. But the changes in personality and behaviour described by Walsh and others are very familiar as disastrous sequelae of frontal lobe damage: they are seen in various combinations, which no doubt express differences in anatomical damage as well as different pretraumatic personalities.

Corpus callosum

The genu and the rostrum of the corpus callosum constitute a massive commissural system joining the two frontal lobes. In our experience, surgical lesions in the middle and posterior sections of the corpus callosum may cause mild but detectable impairments of interhemispheric transfer (Jeeves et al 1979), but later writers have not confirmed this, and certainly small surgical transections in the body of the corpus callosum are well tolerated. Surgical transection of the genu does not cause any obvious clinical effects.

The corpus callosum is often injured in closed head injuries. MRI scans visualize callosal lesions well (Fig. 5.16), though it should be remembered that there are numerous variations in the normal structure of the body of the commissure.

Basal forebrain nuclei

The posterior margins of the gyrus rectus and the medial orbital gyri are demarcated by the bifurcation of the olfactory tract. The tract forms a lateral olfactory stria, which goes to the primary olfactory cortex in the medial temporal region (see below), and a medial stria which terminates in the basal forebrain area. Posterior to the termination of the olfactory tract is the anterior perforated substance, so called because it is perforated by the medial striate arteries and more laterally by the recurrent artery of Heubner, a branch of the anterior cerebral artery. Dorsal and posterior to the anterior perforated substance are a number of important basal frontal nuclei, which are linked with the frontal cortex by the medial forebrain bundle (Fig. 2.20) and with the hippocampal complex by the anterior component of the fornix (Fig. 2.22). Of these, the basal nucleus of Meynert, the medial septal nucleus and certain other cell masses are composed of large neurons which send cholinergic axons to the neocortex and also to the limbic system. These magnocellular basal nuclei are thought to be a cholinergic arousal or modulatory system and dysfunction in this system has been seen as part of Alzheimer's dementia; to our knowledge, this has not been postulated in post-traumatic dementia, but as the area is sometimes damaged in closed head injuries, the possibility deserves consideration.

Temporal lobes

These lie postero-inferior to the frontal lobes to which they are linked by several fibre systems. The anatomy of the temporal lobes is too complex to be reviewed here: it is however important to note that the medial parts of the temporal lobes contain the hippocampus and the amygdaloid nucleus, and these are both connected with the basal forebrain nuclei and diencephalon (Fig. 2.22). Of all the structures concerned in the functions of memory, Amaral (1987) concluded 'that the hippocampal formation and the amygdaloid complex are principal candidates for roles in memory processing', and clinical experience has shown that bilateral ablation of these structures can cause very severe and prolonged impairment of memory. Graff-Radford et al (1990) have argued that it is necessary to destroy components of both the hippocampal and amygdaloid systems to produce permanent amnesias, but this is still debatable.

Brief post-traumatic memory impairment is the chief clinical characteristic of minor head injury, and the duration of post-traumatic amnesia is a much used measure of the severity of the injury (p. 384). At present, it cannot be said with confidence what are the anatomical correlates of post-traumatic amnesia, or of the prolonged dysmnesias that sometimes follow head injuries from which in other respects the patient appears to have made a good recovery. But it is noteworthy that bilateral contusions or ischaemic infarctions of the medial and polar temporal lobes are very common results of blunt impact to the head.

Cerebral blood supply

The frontal lobes receive their arterial supply from branches of the anterior cerebral artery, while the middle cerebral artery makes an important contribution to the supply of the frontal convexity. The proximal parts of both arteries send striate branches to the basal frontal nuclei, and, together with the anterior choroidal and posterior cerebral arteries, supply the basal ganglia and the diencephalon.

Two superficial venous systems drain the frontal cortex. Several large veins from the frontal convexity bridge the subarachnoid space to enter the sagittal sinus; laterally, veins run into the superficial middle cerebral vein to drain ultimately into the transverse sinus, with an anastomotic connection to the sagittal sinus. These anastomoses usually prevent venous infarction when cortical veins or even the anterior third of the sagittal sinus are injured; however, it is unwise to presume on this, and even the origin of the sagittal sinus should not be divided unless there is a real need to transect the falx (p. 380). Rupture of the medial bridging veins is one of the causes of subdural bleeding and haematoma formation after head impact.

Hypothalamus

This small but vital area lies posterior to the basal frontal nuclei and the optic chiasm; it forms the ventral walls and floor of the third ventricle. From it the vascular infundibulum or pituitary stalk runs forward and downward to join the posterior lobe of the pituitary gland (neurohypophysis) (Fig. 2.24). The mammillary nuclei constitute the posterior part of the hypothalamus. The hypothalamus has an array of nuclei, which are concerned with the regulation of body temperature, various vegetative and metabolic functions, and certain aspects of behaviour, including aggression. Hypothalamic nuclei also regulate the endocrine activity of the pituitary gland.

The well-defined paraventricular and supraoptic nuclei (Fig. 2.25A) are composed of large neurons which synthesize the peptide hormones vasopressin and oxytocin. These hormones pass by axoplasmic flow to the pituitary stalk and the neurohypophysis, from which they are liberated into the blood stream. Vasopressin is liberated in response to changes in serum osmolality, to which osmoceptive cells in the nuclei respond; vasopressin preserves homeostasis in water balance by regulating diuresis. Damage to the stalk results in diabetes insipidus. The hormonal output of the adenohypophysis (anterior lobe and pars intermedia) is regulated by a different system (Fig. 2.25B). Neurons in the ventral hypophysis, especially the small-celled tuberal nuclei, liberate hypophysiotropic peptides (hormonal releasing or inhibiting factors) into the system of portal vessels running down the infundibulum into the gland, and these induce the release of stored hormones formed by the cells of the adenohypophysis. The hypothalamus is often damaged in severe head injuries (Crompton 1971), and partial or complete lesions of the pituitary stalk are also often seen, especially in cases of anterior fossa fracture (p. 382).

Pituitary gland (hypophysis)

The gland is well protected in the sella turcica. It has its own capsule, separate from the dura-periosteum of the sella. On either side, it is flanked by the cavernous sinuses; ventrally it is separated from the sphenoid air sinus by a variable thickness of bone. It is covered by the diaphragma sellae, which is an extension of the dura of the skull base. The diaphragma has a central foramen through which the infundibulum passes to join the posterior lobe of the pituitary gland, of which it is functionally and histologically a part. There is an arachnoid cistern around the infundibulum, which extends into the sella to spread out over the surface of the anterior lobe (Lang 1983).

Direct injury to the pituitary gland is unusual, at least in surviving cases. Fractures through the body of the

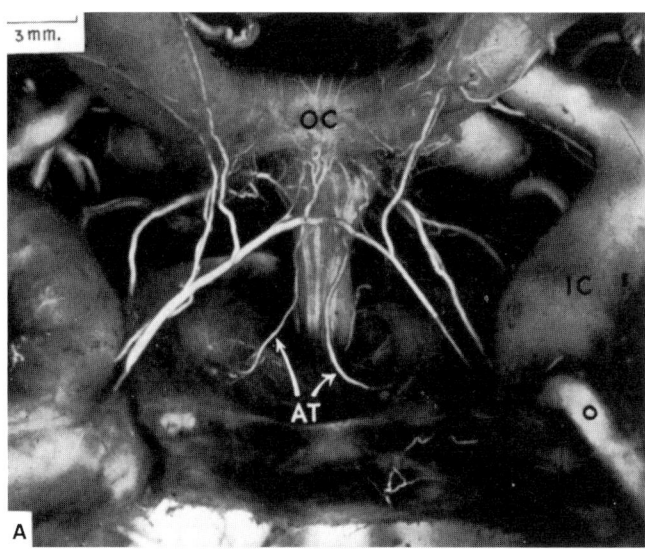

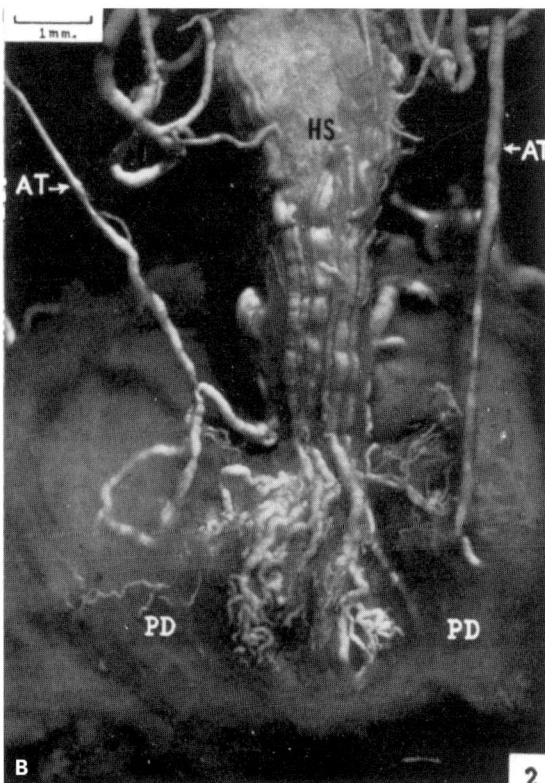

Fig. 2.24 Arterial supply and portal drainage of the hypothalamus and pituitary stalk. A The superior hypophyseal arteries run from the internal carotid arteries (IC) to supply the optic chiasma (OC) and then give descending arteries to the stalk. One of these, the artery of the trabecula (AT), goes directly to the posterior lobe of the pituitary gland. The ophthalmic artery (O) is not normally involved in the blood supply of the pituitary gland. **B** Large portal veins run down along the hypophyseal stalk (HS) to enter the vascular sinusoids of the anterior lobe of the pituitary (pars distalis — PD). Reproduced by permission from Xuereb et al (1954a,b).

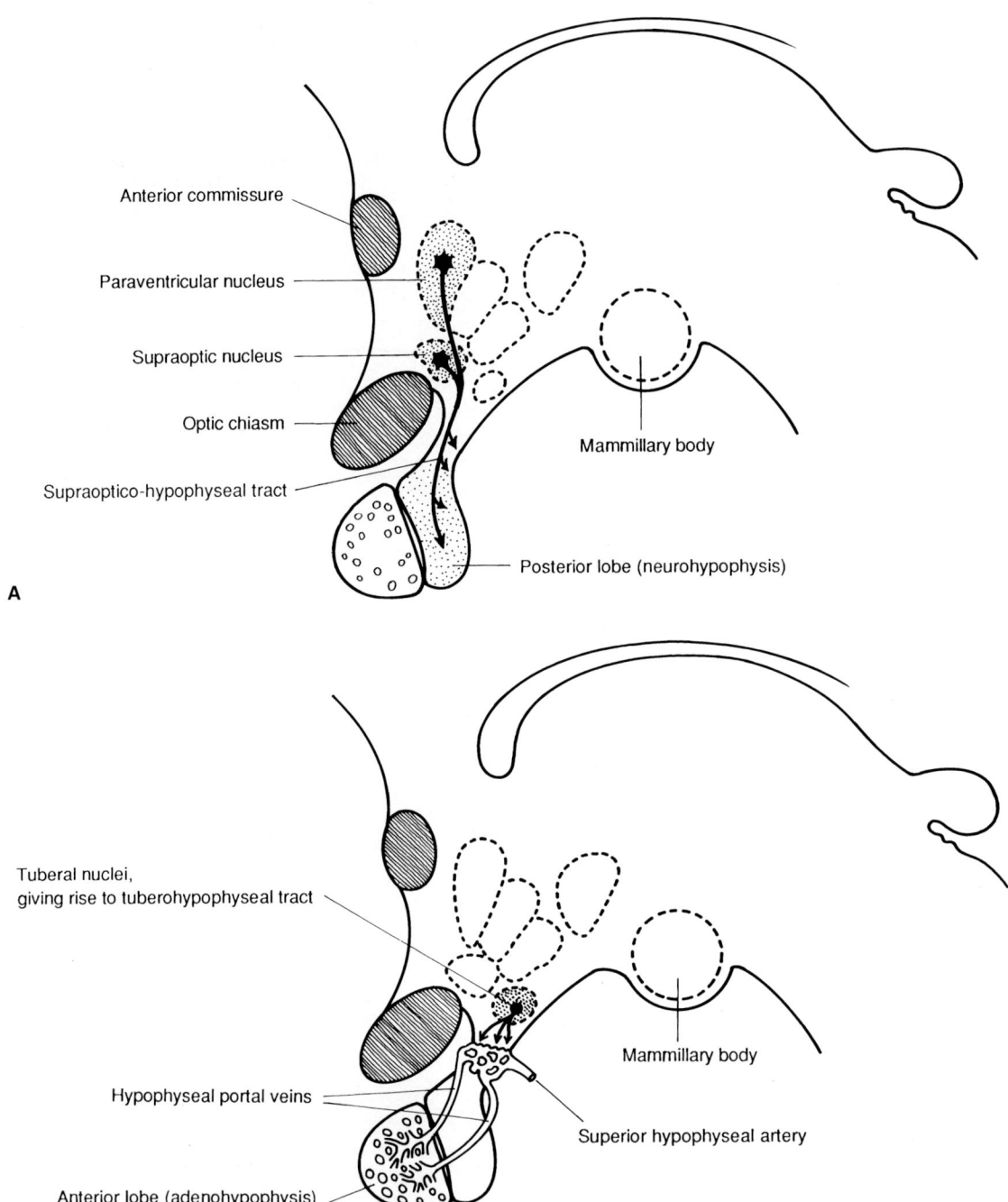

Fig. 2.25 Hypothalamic control of pituitary secretion. A Vasopressin and oxytocin are secreted in the paraventricular and supraoptic nuclei of the hypothalamus and transported in the axons of the supraoptico-hypophyseal tract to the posterior lobe of the pituitary gland: these hormones are then released into the circulation. **B** Hypothalamic releasing hormones are formed in the hypothalamus and transported to a capillary plexus formed by the superior hypophyseal arteries around the median eminence and infundibular stem of the hypothalamus; these hormones there enter into the vascular system and are taken by the portal veins to the adenohypophysis. Here they stimulate, or inhibit, the release of the hormones of the adenohypophysis.

sphenoid may injure the gland, and in theory could open a fistulous communication with the subarachnoid space, but in our experience CSF leakage through the sella turcica is rare. However, the pituitary may be infarcted by trauma to its blood supply.

The gland has a dual blood supply. It receives a direct supply from the inferior hypophyseal artery (p. 47). It is also supplied by the superior hypophyseal artery, arising from the internal carotid artery after it leaves the cavernous sinus (Fig. 2.24A). The superior hypophyseal arteries send branches to capillaries in the hypothalamus and the infundibulum (Xuereb et al 1954a,b); from these capillaries arise portal veins which run down the infundibulum to the sinusoids in the adenohypophysis (Fig. 2.24B). These portal veins convey the hypophysiotropic factors elaborated in the hypothalamus; transection of the pituitary stalk interrupts this pathway, and usually causes infarction of much of the gland. In our experience, the subcapsular glandular tissue may be spared, perhaps because it is supplied by the inferior hypophyseal arteries. Hypopituitarism is occasionally seen after head injury (Winternitz & Dzur 1976), and presumably the basis is an infarction of the adenohypophysis. Daniel et al (1959) showed that autopsy evidence of infarction is quite often seen after severe head injuries of different types; transection of the superior portal vessels seems the likeliest cause.

Disturbed function of the neurohypophysis is a commoner finding in CMF injuries. Damage to the hypothalamus, or traumatic transection of the infundibulum, interrupts the hypothalamohypophyseal tract, causing failure of vasopressin secretion and temporary or permanent diabetes insipidus (p. 382). The converse state of overproduction of vasopressin is common after brain injury as a stress response, and often reaches a level inappropriate to the physiological requirements of the injured person (Fox et al 1971).

CRANIAL NERVES

First (olfactory) nerve

The sensory receptors are in the olfactory epithelium in the roof of the nose. The fine olfactory filaments traverse the cribriform plate in bundles, which are enclosed in an arachnoid sheath, and terminate in the olfactory bulb (Fig. 2.9). The complex central connections of the olfactory tract are described by Carpenter & Sutin (1983) and in more detail by Shipley & Reyes (1991); for present purposes, it is relevant that secondary sensory axons from the olfactory bulb run back in the olfactory tract and the lateral olfactory stria to the primary olfactory cortical areas (prepiriform cortex and periamygdaloid cortex) in the medial temporal lobe. While it is likely that post-traumatic anosmia is usually due to damage to the fragile olfactory filaments, bulb or tract, the possibility that damage to the central connections may be responsible has not been excluded; Sumner (1976) suggested that post-traumatic loss of both taste and smell could be due to central damage, though we have not seen a case that supports this interpretation. Lesions in the primary olfactory cortex may result in epileptic seizures with an olfactory aura, but this type of epilepsy is rare after head injury. The tract and bulb are exposed in intradural subfrontal craniotomies, and the bulb is easily avulsed from the olfactory fossa. However, the bulb can be preserved by freeing it from the overlying gyrus rectus.

Second (optic) nerve

In the orbit, the optic nerve runs back in the centre of the cone of muscles; this segment of the nerve is about 25 mm long. The complex anatomical relations are described and illustrated by Lang (1983) and by Blinkov et al (1986). The nerve then enters the optic canal, between the roots of the lesser wing of the sphenoid bone. Ventral to the nerve runs the ophthalmic artery. This artery has a surgically important relation to the nerve: it arises from the internal carotid artery (see above), usually ventromedial to the nerve, but the point of origin is variable. The final section of the optic nerve is intra cranial: the nerve runs back to the chiasm, a distance ranging from 7 to 16 mm (Lang 1983). The nerve can be injured in any part of its course (p. 418), but clinical interest has centred on the intracanalicular section (Fig. 2.26), since here the possibility of remediable compression arises. Maniscalco & Habal (1978) dissected 83 cadavers, of unspecified ages, and found that the canals were on average 9.22 mm long, ranging from 5.5 to 11.5 mm. The canal is elliptical in cross-section, the widest diameter being horizontal at the intracranial end and vertical at the narrower orbital end. The wall of the canal is thickest at the orbital end of the canal, sometimes called the optic ring, and it is here that the canal is narrowest. On its medial side, the canal has a close relation with the sphenoid air sinus, and indeed there is usually a bulge in the wall of the sinus, representing the canal (p. 420). In some individuals, there is a bony deficiency in the canal, when the optic nerve is covered only by dura mater and the mucosa of the sinus (Renn & Rhoton 1975).

The optic nerve is formed from the axons of the retinal ganglion cells. Fibres from the nasal half of each retina, serving the temporal half of each visual field, run back in the nerve, those from the macula being in the centre; they decussate in the optic chiasm, where they are joined by uncrossed nasal fibres from the opposite eye to form the optic tract (Fig. 2.27). The fibre arrangement explains the field defects seen in cases of CMF trauma. Thus, injuries of the optic nerve, if not complete, may cause central visual loss of scotomatous type when the macular bundle is damaged. When the superior surface of the nerve is damaged — not a rare event — there is an inferior horizontal field defect, sometimes bilateral. Injury of the decussating chiasmal fibres gives a bitemporal hemianopia. Injury at the part of the optic nerve joining the chiasm — the anterior chiasmal angle — may affect the upper temporal field of the opposite eye, because the decussating lower nasal fibres from the opposite retina loop a variable distance into the ipsilateral optic nerve;

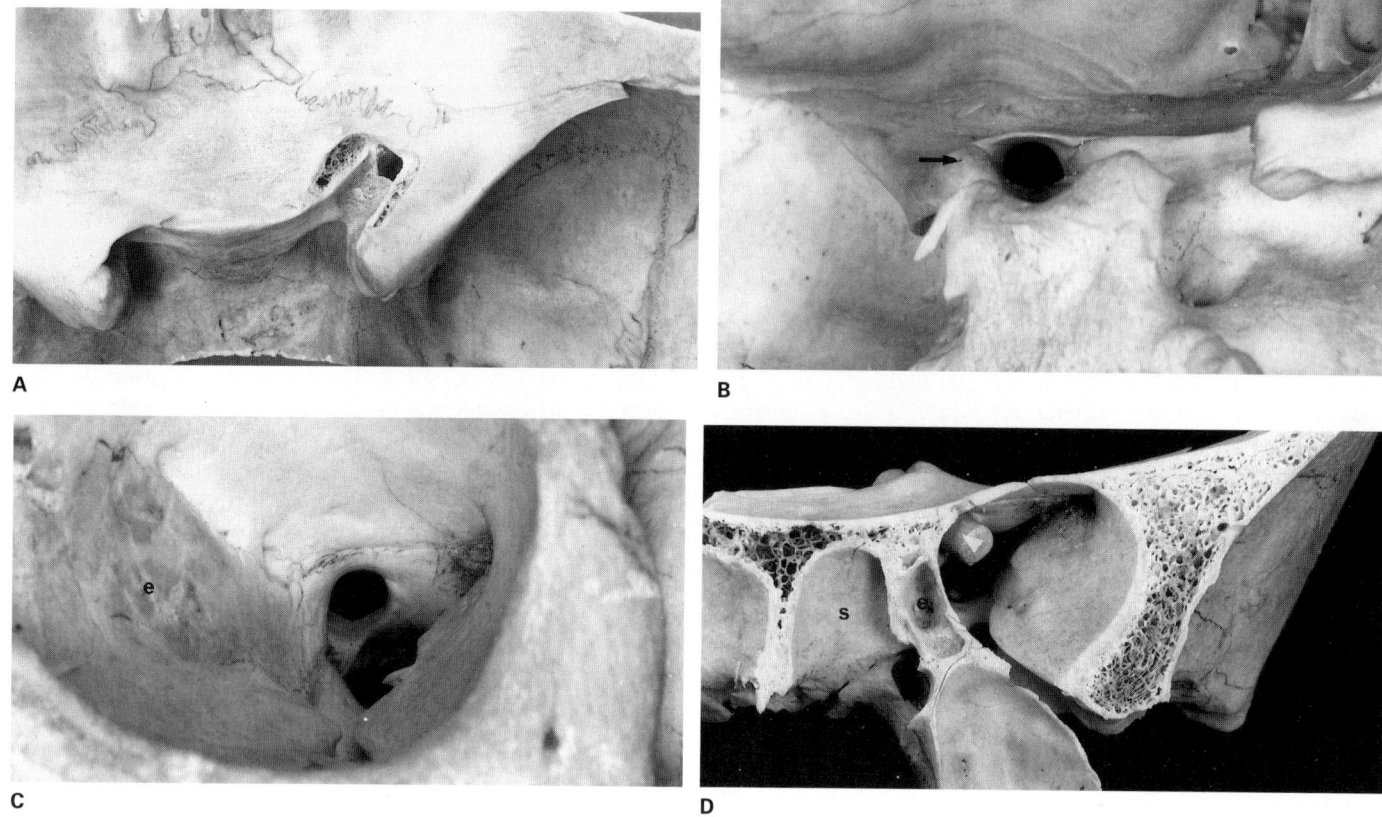

Fig. 2.26 Optic canal. The canal lies between the two roots of the lesser wing of the sphenoid bone. It transmits the optic nerve and the ophthalmic artery. It is in close but variable relation with the sphenoid and ethmoidal air sinuses. **A** The right optic canal is exposed by removal of its thick roof. It is a funnel-shaped canal, narrowing as it enters the orbit. **B** Seen from behind over the dorsum sellae, the optic canal is oval and narrowed in the vertical diameter. In life, the sharp upper margin is prolonged back by a thin fold of dura, the falciform process. The anterior clinoid processes (arrow) lie lateral to the optic nerves. **C** Seen from in front through the orbit, the optic canal is formed by a thick bony ring; it is narrowed in the horizontal diameter. The lamina papyracea of the ethmoid bone (e) lies medially. **D** The canal, containing the optic nerve (simulated: white arrow head), has a medial relationship with the sphenoid (s) and posterior ethmoid (e) air sinuses. In this specimen, there is poor pneumatization and the canal is protected by a relatively thick layer of bone. In many cases, the canal bulges into the sphenoid sinus and the optic nerve may be covered by a very thin layer of bone, or even by mucosa only.

the field defect sometimes takes the form of a junctional scotoma. Posterior to the chiasm, field defects are homonymous.

The optic nerve is surrounded by a sheath of dura mater and an extension of the subarachnoid space; at the inner orifice of the optic foramen, the dural sheath leaves the nerve to merge with the dura of the anterior and middle cranial fossae, while the arachnoid sheath forms part of a cistern around the nerve.

Third (oculomotor) fourth (trochlear) and sixth (abducent) nerves

These nerves arise in the midbrain (third and fourth nerves) and lower pons (sixth nerve). They course through the subarachnoid space to enter the cavernous sinus through separate portals. The third nerve pierces the dura midway between the anterior and posterior clinoid processes and runs in the lateral wall of the sinus. The portal of the fourth nerve is more posterior and lateral;

it also runs in the wall of the sinus. The sixth nerve enters the dura over the clivus and runs through the inferior petrosal sinus to enter the cavernous sinus, where it lies between the internal carotid artery and the dural envelope of the trigeminal ganglion (Fig. 2.18). These nerves are sheathed by sleeves of arachnoid as they enter the dura (Lang 1983). They leave the sinus to enter the orbit through the superior orbital fissure, together with the ophthalmic division of the trigeminal nerve. Before it leaves, the third nerve divides into two divisions. The superior division supplies the superior rectus muscle and the levator palpebrae superioris. The larger inferior division supplies the medial and inferior rectus muscles and the inferior oblique muscle. It also sends parasympathetic fibres to innervate the smooth muscles of the iris and the ciliary body, through the ciliary ganglion and the short ciliary nerves. It is thus the motor component of the light, accommodation and convergence reflexes. The fourth nerve passes above the upper tendinous head of the superior rectus muscle to supply the superior oblique muscle.

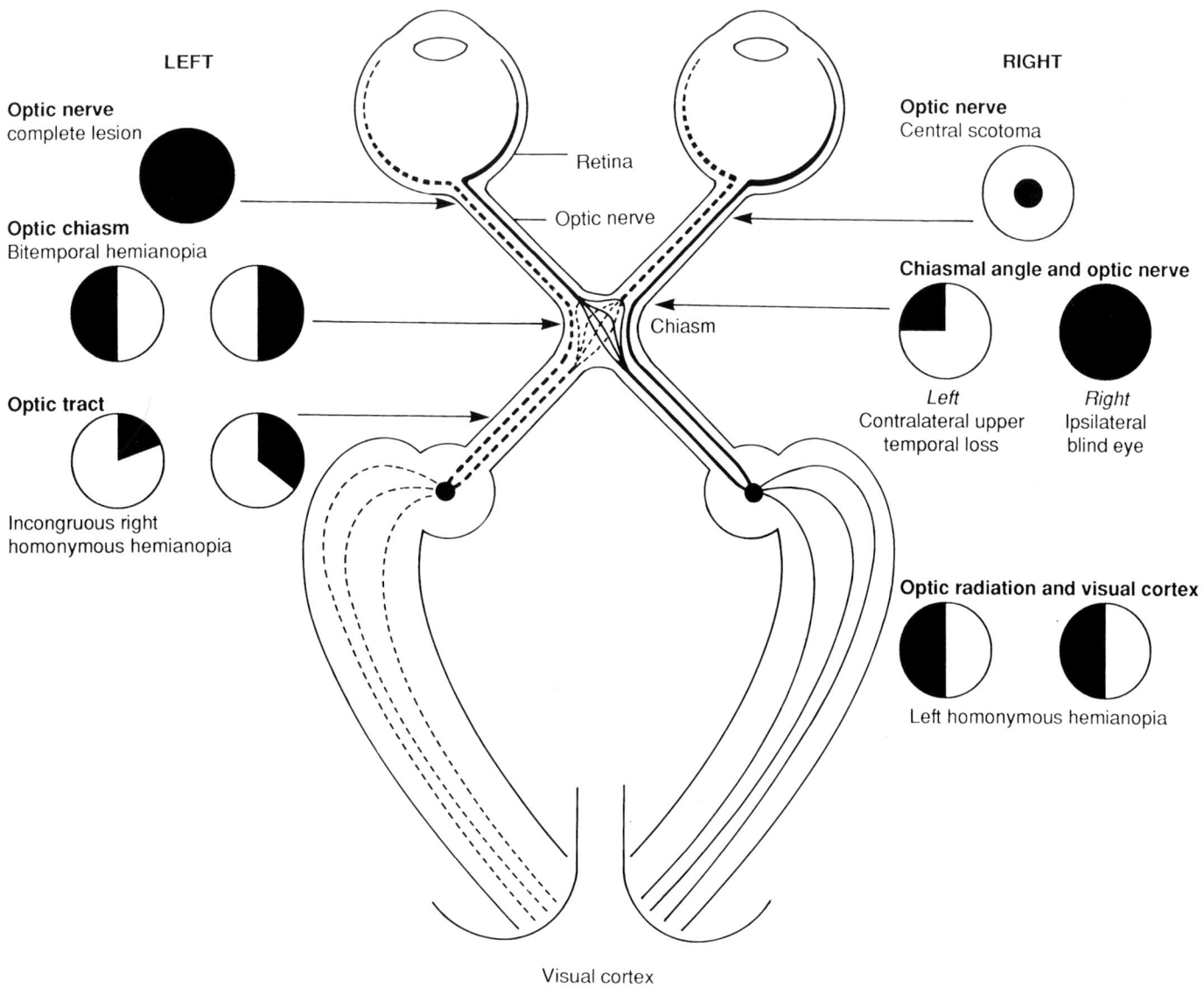

Fig. 2.27 Visual pathways. The diagram shows the nasal and temporal retinal fibres passing through the optic nerve, with the nasal fibres (subserving the temporal hemifield) decussating in the chiasm, synapsing in the lateral geniculate body and then passing in the optic radiation to the visual cortex. Lesions of an optic nerve produce a unilateral visual field defect, except at the anterior chiasmal angle where a junctional scotoma with a contralateral upper temporal field loss is produced, as shown in the diagram. Chiasmal lesions produce bitemporal field defects. Retrochiasmal lesions produce homonymous field defects which become more congruous as the fibres pass back towards the visual cortex.

The sixth nerve passes below the upper tendinous head, together with both divisions of the third nerve, to supply the lateral rectus muscle.

The sympathetic nerves supplying the pupillary dilator muscle usually join and travel with the sixth nerve in the cavernous sinus, though in some individuals they may travel with the third or fourth nerve.

These nerves are often injured. Nuclear or supranuclear damage is seen as a result of severe brainstem damage. The nerves may be contused or avulsed either at their origins from the brainstem (Heinze 1969), or where they pierce the dura; this usually results from a severe impact, though third and fourth nerve paralyses occasionally follow less severe violence. The third nerve

may be compressed in its subarachnoid course by an anterior transtentorial herniation: the parasympathetic fibres are especially sensitive, and pupillary paralysis is therefore the classical sign of transtentorial herniation (Fig. 2.28). Posterior transtentorial herniation may be evident as signs of compression of the midbrain nuclear and supranuclear control of third nerve function — bilateral ptosis and inability to look up. The sixth nerve is often injured in transverse petrous fractures, presumably in its intradural course. All three nerves may be involved in the cavernous sinus, either by the primary injury or from the effects of a carotid-cavernous sinus fistula. Because of the often close relationship of the sixth nerve and the sympathetic pupillodilator fibres,

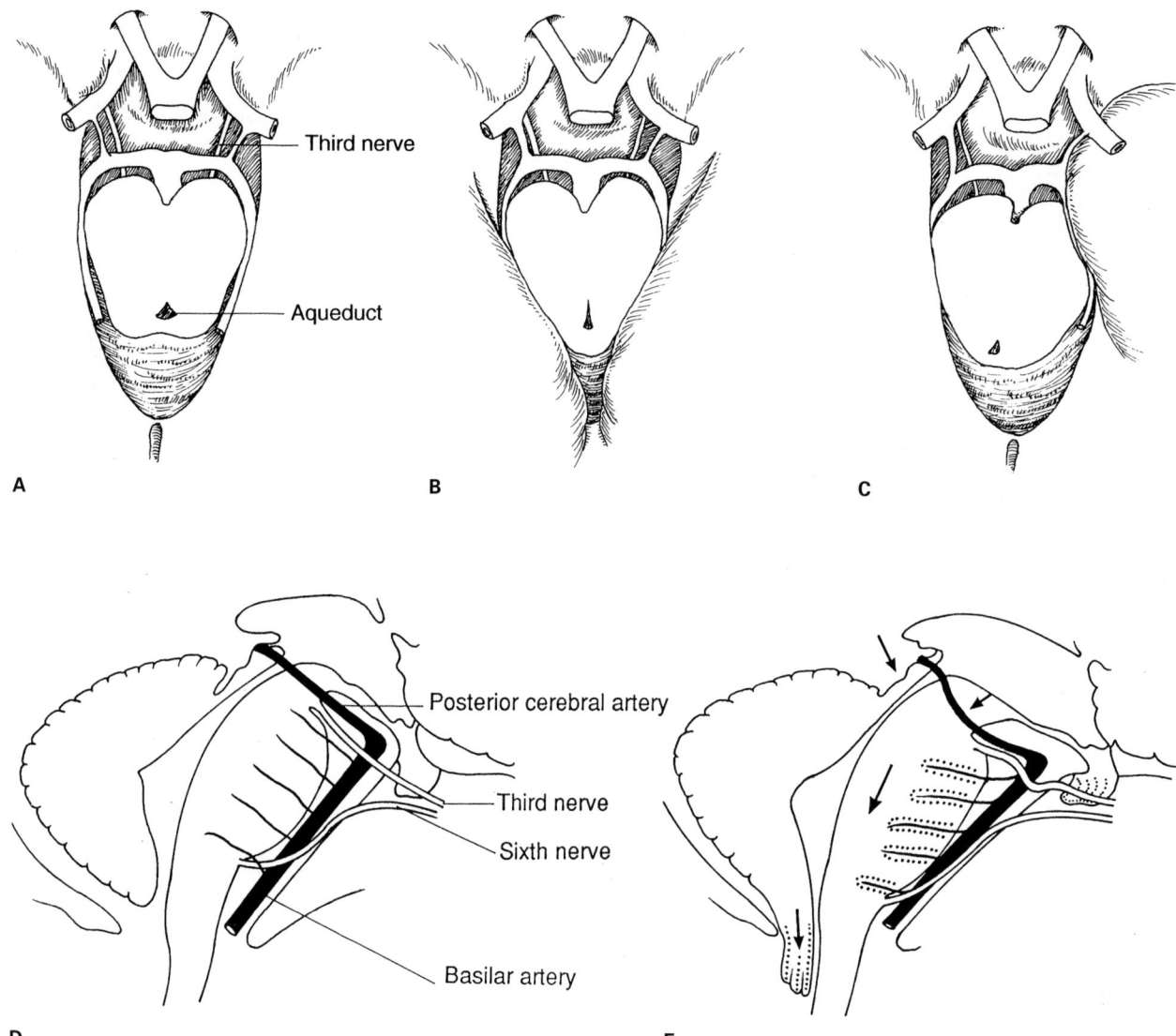

Fig. 2.28 Clinical anatomy of intracranial displacements. An intracranial mass, such as a haematoma, may expand and displace cerebral tissue medially under the falx and downwards through the tentorial hiatus. **A** The normal tentorial hiatus: the midbrain, seen from above in horizontal section, is surrounded by the quadrigeminal and ambiens cisterns (not shown). Anteriorly are the basilar artery and the third nerves running forward to the cavernous sinuses; the posterior cerebral arteries curve around the upper brainstem on their way to supply the occipital visual cortex. **B** Posterior transtentorial herniation: the medial temporal lobes on both sides are forced into the hiatus and compress the dorsal midbrain (*clinical signs: bilateral ptosis, inability to look up and drowsiness*). One or both posterior cerebral arteries may be blocked (*clinical signs: hemianopia or cortical blindness*). The quadrigeminal cisterns are compressed (*CT signs: obliteration of cisterns.* **C** Anterior transtentorial herniation: one medial temporal lobe is displaced by an ipsilateral mass lesion, e.g. a middle meningeal extradural haematoma, into the hiatus, compressing the lateral side of the midbrain and kinking the third nerve (*clinical signs: ipsilateral pupillary dilatation and ptosis, drowsiness*). **D** The normal brainstem in sagittal section: the basilar artery supplies the pons and ventral midbrain. **E** Brainstem displacement and cerebellar herniation: accompanying transtentorial herniation is a downward displacement of the whole brainstem. The blood supply of the pons and midbrain is imperilled; there may be haemorrhages (Duret type) into the ventral brainstem (*clinical signs: deepening coma, decerebration, bradycardia, fixed pupils, respiratory failure*). The cerebellar tonsils are forced into the foramen magnum.

the combination of a Horner's syndrome and a sixth nerve paralysis suggests a lesion in the cavernous sinus. Injury in the superior orbital fissure from skull base fracture may result in simultaneous oculomotor and ophthalmic nerve paralysis. The clinical signs of paralyses of these nerves are set out in Table 2.7, and are further discussed in Chapter 6.

Fifth (trigeminal) nerve

This large nerve takes origin from the upper pons; its brainstem nuclei extend from the midbrain to the second cervical cord segment. Its motor and sensory roots run through the subarachnoid space to the trigeminal sensory ganglion, lying snugly in its dural cave lateral to the

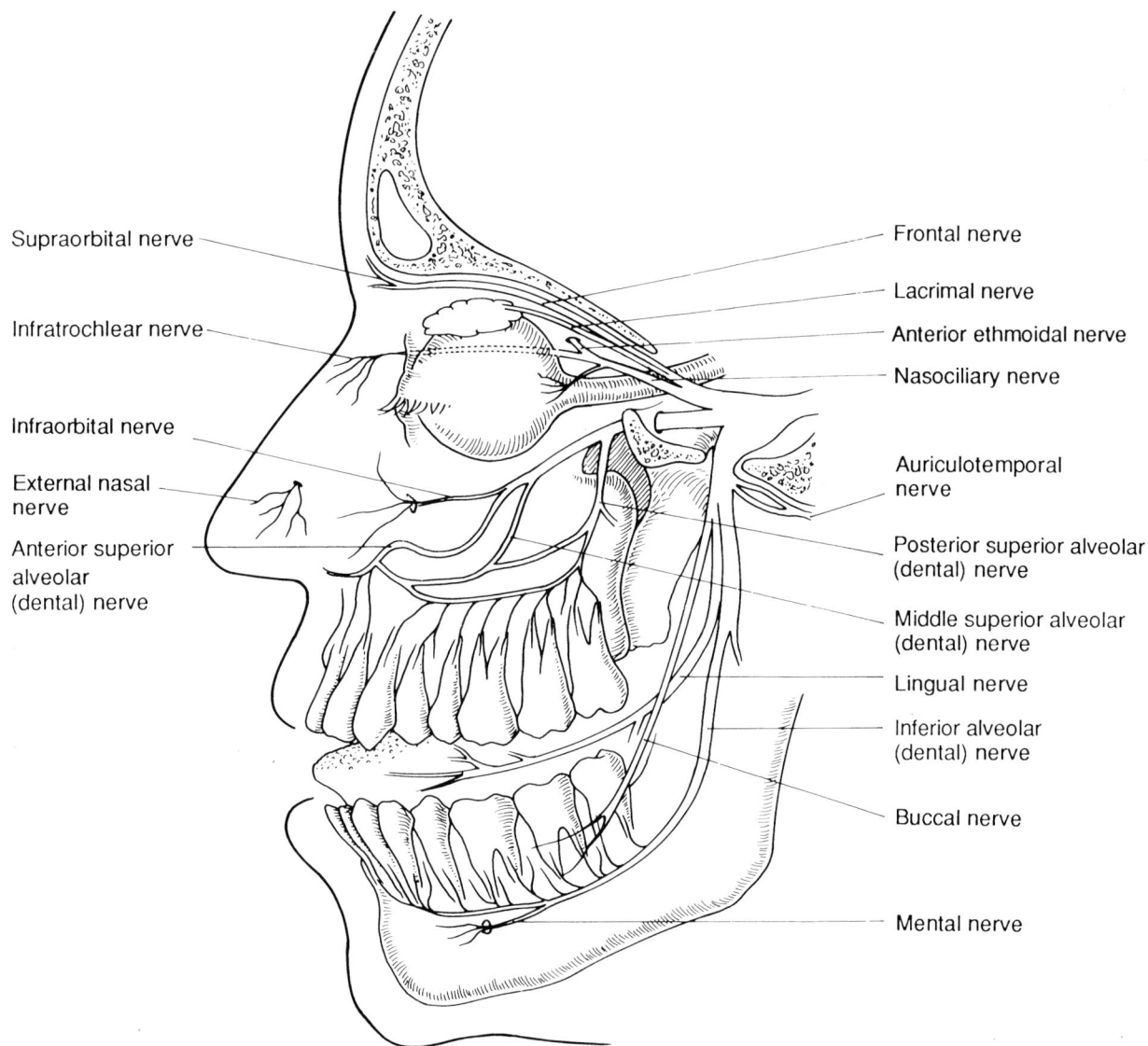

Fig. 2.29 The trigeminal nerve. Diagram of the sensory distribution of the trigeminal nerve. The intracranial course of the anterior ethmoidal nerve is not shown: after entering the ethmoid bone, the nerve passes across the cribriform fossa anterior to the filaments of the olfactory nerve and enters the nasal cavity, which it supplies, to terminate as the external nasal nerve.

cavernous sinus. The motor root passes below the ganglion to enter the mandibular division. Injuries of the roots or the ganglion are rare. Through its three divisions, the trigeminal nerve supplies sensation to almost all the structures in the CMF region (Fig. 2.29): the ophthalmic division provides sensation to the forehead, the maxillary division to the middle third of the face and the mandibular division sensation to the lower face, as well as innervating the muscles of mastication. The supraorbital and supratrochlear nerves emerge from the orbit separately over the supraorbital margin; the supraorbital nerve passes through a notch or foramen, from which it has to be freed by chisel cuts in the standard frontal exposure of the orbits (p. 238). The infraorbital nerve passes through the orbital floor and the infraorbital foramen, supplying

sensation to the lateral side of the nose and upper lip and the maxillary teeth via the superior alveolar nerves. Zygomaticofacial and zygomaticotemporal branches emerge through foramina in the bones, being often damaged during periosteal stripping as well as by trauma. The inferior dental nerve enters the mandibular canal (Fig. 2.6) at the lingula and traverses the body of the mandible to give sensation to the posterior teeth; in this part of its course, the nerve is easily injured (p. 265). The nerve terminates as the mental and incisive nerves to provide sensation to the anterior teeth, chin and lower lip.

Seventh (facial) nerve

This largely motor nerve has its nucleus of origin in the

pons. It runs through the subarachnoid space into the internal auditory meatus and enters the petrous temporal bone, to emerge at the stylomastoid foramen. It then runs into the substance of the parotid gland from which it emerges to supply the muscles of facial expression (Fig. 2.30). Kempe (1980) has shown by stimulation under local anaesthesia that there is functional segregation in the facial nerve even within the stylomastoid canal. He has identified three components, each constituting a fascicle. One innervates the perioral muscular sphincter, the orbicularis oris and a second supplies the ocular sphincter, the orbicularis oculi. The third fascicle, termed by Kempe the mimic fascicle, supplies a crescent of facial muscles including the frontalis muscle, the zygomaticus major, the levator labii superioris, the depressor anguli oris, the mentalis and the platysma (Fig. 2.30A).

Through its chorda tympani branch, the facial nerve transmits sensation from taste buds in the anterior two thirds of the tongue (Fig. 2.31). The facial nerve also contains parasympathetic secretomotor fibres to the lacrimal and the submandilular and sublingual salivary glands, via the chorda tympani and the greater superficial petrosal nerve (Fig. 2.32). These secretomotor fibres have their cells of origin in the superior salivatory nucleus, in the pons.

Injuries of the facial nerve are common, both in its petrous course and in the region of the parotid gland. These injuries are discussed in Chapter 15.

Eighth (vestibular and cochlear) nerves

These nerves are outside the scope of this book; their

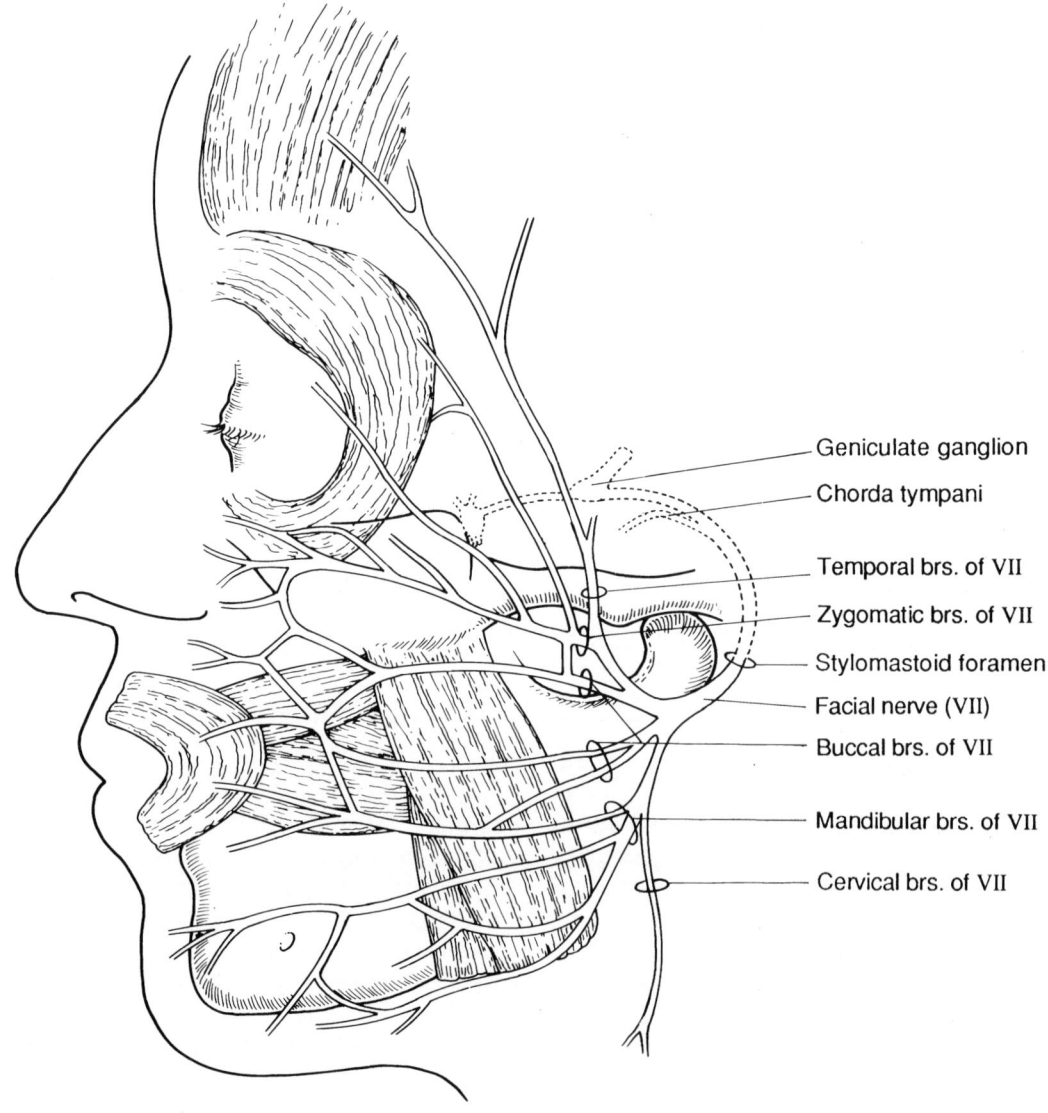

A

Fig. 2.30 The facial nerve. A Within the petrous temporal bone the nerve is already divided into fascicles destined to innervate individual muscles of facial expression. Kempe (1980) has identified three groups innervating: (1) the orbicularis oris sphincter, (2) the orbicularis oculi sphincter, (3) the muscles of facial expression. Reproduced by courtesy of the *Journal of Neurosurgery.*

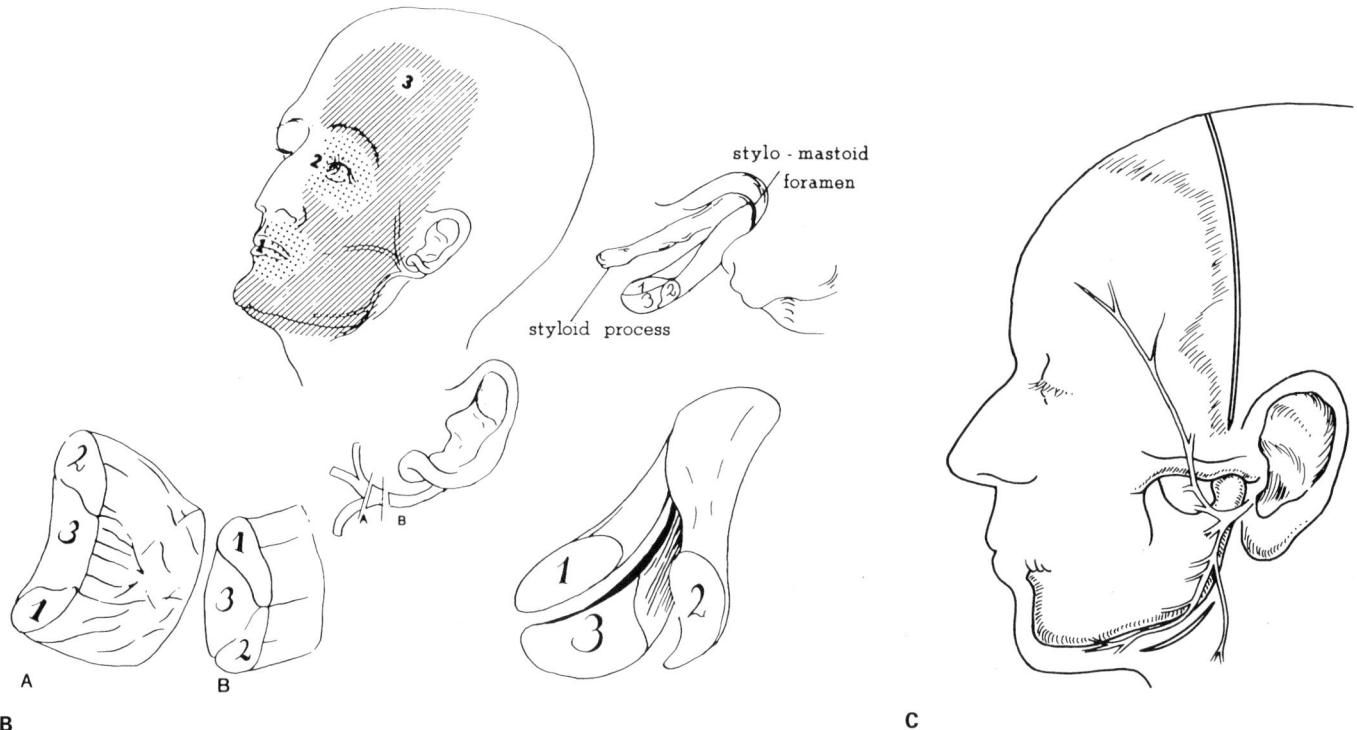

Fig. 2.30 The facial nerve. B After leaving the stylomastoid foramen, the facial nerve enters the parotid gland and breaks up into branches supplying the muscles of the face. **C** The standard coronal scalp incision should be sited so as to spare the frontal branch of the facial nerve; submandibular incisions should spare the mandibular branch.

neuroanatomy is well described by Brodal (1981) and by Carpenter & Sutin (1983). The eighth cranial nerve may be injured in fractures of the skull base involving the petrous bone (p. 439).

Ninth (glossopharyngeal), tenth (vagal) and eleventh (accessory) nerves

These supply the striated muscles of the pharynx and larynx; the spinal root of the accessory nerve supplies the trapezius and sternomastoid muscles. The nerve trunks are rarely injured, except in cases of penetrating wounds of the neck. The glossopharyngeal nerve conveys sensation, including taste, from the posterior third of the tongue (Fig. 2.31), and supplies parasympathetic secretomotor fibres (Fig. 2.32) to the parotid salivary gland through the small tympanic nerve and the lesser superficial petrosal nerve (Brodal 1981). These secretomotor fibres have their cells of origin in the inferior salivatory nucleus of the medulla. The visceral distributions of these nerves are chiefly outside the CMF region.

Twelfth (hypoglossal) nerve

This motor nerve is often injured by missile wounds in the region of the mandible. The nerve leaves the skull base through its own deeply placed canal, and runs deep to the internal carotid artery and the jugular vein to the level of the angle of the mandible. Here it passes forward superficial to the internal carotid artery, usually crossing the lingual artery, and then runs deep to the mylohyoid muscle to supply the muscles of the tongue.

Sympathetic innervation

The whole CMF region receives postganglionic, and some preganglionic, fibres from the cervical sympathetic chain, which are distributed through branches of the cranial and upper cervical nerves, and along perivascular plexuses. These fibres innervate blood vessels, sweat glands, salivary glands, and the smooth muscle of the orbital muscles, iris and ciliary body. Ablation of the superior cervical sympathetic ganglion causes immediate pupillary constriction, mild ptosis, and abolition of sweating; there is also vasodilatation, often causing a stuffy nose on the side of the ablation, from vascular dilatation in the nasal mucosa. But injury to this ganglion is unusual in CMF injuries, and damage to the peripheral branches of the sympathetic system is not usually of clinical significance, unless as a sign of a cavernous sinus lesion.

THE SALIVARY GLANDS

Saliva

Saliva is a viscous, colourless liquid produced in volumes of around 1.5 l per day by the major salivary glands and the many smaller glands lying under the oral mucosa.

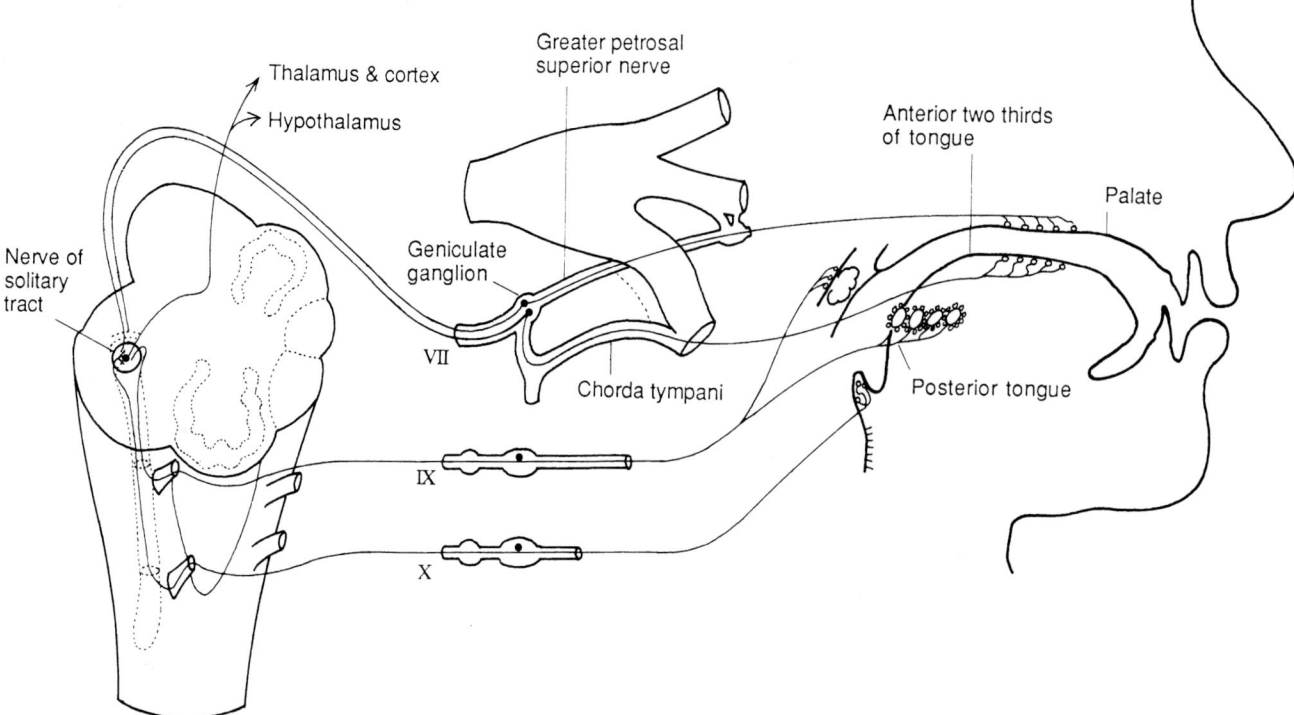

Fig. 2.31 Taste pathways. Chemoceptive cells in the anterior two-thirds of the tongue are supplied by sensory fibres which travel in the chorda tympani nerve; their cells of origin are in the geniculate ganglion, and they establish central connections in the nucleus of the solitary tract. Similar nerve fibres innervate the posterior third of the tongue; they travel centrally in the glossopharyngeal nerve and have their cell bodies in the superior glossopharyngeal ganglion. They also terminate in the nucleus of the solitary tract together with fibres transmitted by the vagus nerve from the epiglottis.

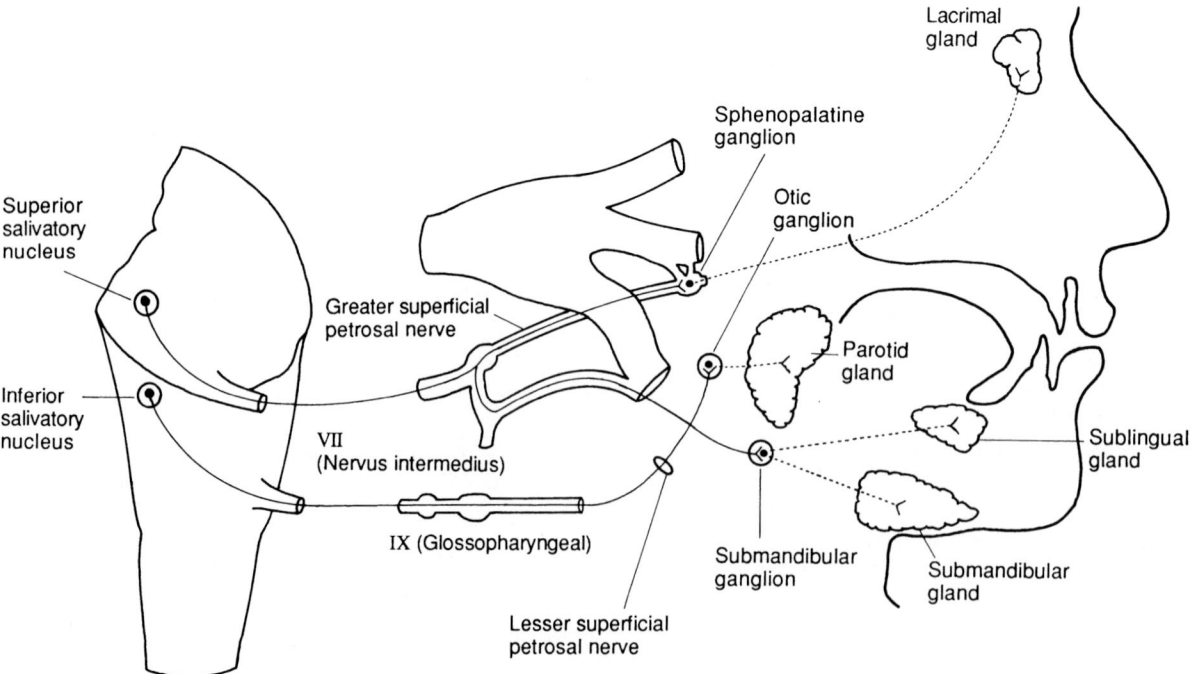

Fig. 2.32 Parasympathetic innervation of the chief salivary glands and the lacrimal gland. Preganglionic fibres arise in the brainstem, travel in the 7th, 9th and 10th cranial nerves and terminate in small peripheral ganglia, from which postganglionic fibres are distributed to innervate secretory cells in the named and unnamed salivary glands and the lacrimal gland.

It has many functions. Saliva assists mastication and swallowing by moistening food and by enzymatic predigestion of starch, and it aids taste perception by acting as a solvent for chemical substances. Saliva moistens the oral lining surfaces, facilitating movements of the mouth in speech and mastication, and helping to maintain oral hygiene in the self-cleansing of the teeth. Moreover, salivary lactoperoxidase has an important antimicrobial role.

Parotid gland

This is a pure serous-secreting gland, which is enclosed in a dense fibrous capsule bound to adjacent structures by the deep investing fascia of the neck. It is lobulated, irregular in shape and wedged into the space bounded anteriorly by the posterior margin of the mandible and posteriorly by the styloid and mastoid processes and their attached muscles. It extends up to the zygomatic arch and the temporomandibular joint, and an extension of the gland lies on the masseter muscle. Within the gland are the external carotid artery, dividing into its terminal branches, and the superficial temporal and maxillary veins, anastomosing to form the posterior facial or retromandibular vein, which usually divides to form the common facial and external jugular veins. The facial nerve enters the gland from its posterior aspect, and divides into upper and lower divisions, which ramify to supply the facial muscles; the nerve lies superficial to these veins, in what is termed the faciovenous cleavage plane. The gland is divided into deep and superficial components by this plane, a cleavage of considerable surgical importance when the facial nerve has to be exposed. The parotid duct forms within the gland, emerges from its anterior aspect, and runs subcutaneously over the masseter to pierce the cheek muscles and enter the oral cavity at the level of the crown of the second molar tooth. The gland and the duct are easily wounded; branches of the facial nerve are often cut at the same time (p. 439).

The parasympathetic secretomotor supply (Fig. 2.32) is derived from the glossopharyngeal nerve: the preganglionic fibres synapse in the otic ganglion and the postganglionic fibres are distributed by the auriculotemporal branch of the mandibular nerve. Injury to these parasympathetic fibres, followed by aberrant regeneration along sympathetic nerves, is thought to explain the finding of facial sweating and flushing on gustatory stimulation, sometimes seen after surgical or traumatic damage to the parotid gland.

Submandibular gland

This has both mucous and serous secretory cells. It lies below and deep to the body of the mandible and comprises superficial and deep components, divided by the posterior border of the mylohyoid muscle. The submandibular duct runs from the deep surface of the gland, under the mylohyoid, to enter the mouth through the sublingual papilla on the side of the frenulum. The gland receives preganglionic parasympathetic innervation from the chorda tympani nerve (see below); the postganglionic relay fibres arise in the submandibular ganglion.

The sublingual gland

This has predominantly mucous secretory cells. It lies beneath the mucosa of the floor of the mouth, medial to the sublingual fossa in the inner surface of the anterior part of the mandible, dorsal to the mylohyoid line. The ducts of the gland drain directly or via the submandibular duct into the mouth. The nerve supply is, like that of the submandibular gland, from the chorda tympani.

MUSCLES

Muscles of facial expression

R. J. Last in his excellent textbook of anatomy emphasizes that the muscles of facial expression are developed from the mesoderm of the second pharyngeal arch (McMinn 1990). During their migration, they drag with them the nerve of that arch, the seventh (facial) cranial nerve. These muscles are part of the panniculus carnosus, the sheet of subcutaneous striated muscles which arises from and inserts into the dermis. In lower mammals this sheet is very extensive; in man, it is largely confined to the muscles influencing facial expression. From a functional viewpoint, the facial muscles are grouped around the orifices of the orbit, the nostrils and the mouth; they provide sphincters to close these orifices and dilators to open them.

Muscles of the eyelids

The orbicularis oculi surrounds the orbital entrance and spreads over the eyelids. It is opposed by two dilator muscles, the levator palpebrae superioris and the occipitofrontalis. The orbicularis oculi comprises two main parts: palpebral and orbital. Some anatomists identify a third lacrimal component (Davies & Coupland 1967).

The palpebral fibres arise from the medial canthal ligament, and arch across both lids in front of the tarsal plates, to form the lateral canthal ligament. These important ligaments are variously designated as palpebral and canthal; the medial ligament is so well defined that it is often termed a tendon, while the lateral ligament is considered by some anatomists to be no more than a raphe of muscle fibres. In this book, the terms medial and lateral canthal ligaments are preferred.

The orbital portion of the sphincter has a wider extent,

and its fibres form loops around the orbit, without interruption on the lateral side; they arise and insert in the nasal part of the frontal bone and the frontal process of the maxilla. The sphincter is opposed by the levator palpebrae superioris, arising from the under surface of the lesser wing of the sphenoid bone just above the optic canal and by the occipitofrontalis, the frontal belly of which runs from the galea aponeurotica of the scalp to insert in the muscles of the orbit and nose. Contraction of the occipitofrontalis elevates the eyebrows and creases the frontal skin; its nerve supply may be damaged by frontal trauma, or iatrogenically in raising a bicoronal scalp flap. The dilator–elevator capacity of this muscle is utilized in brow suspension operations for ptosis (p. 423). The levator palpebrae superioris is supplied by the third cranial nerve, and may be paralysed by injury to that nerve, resulting in a ptosis much more severe than that caused by paralysis of the occipitofrontalis.

The lacrimal or pretarsal fibres of orbicularis oculi are attached to the fascia over the lacrimal sac and insert in the tarsi or interlace in the lateral canthal ligament or raphe; their important role in the blink reflex is described below (p. 76).

Medial canthus

An understanding of the anatomical relationships at the medial canthus is necessary for successful post-traumatic reconstruction: the surgeon must take into account the medial canthal ligament, its relationship to the lacrimal apparatus, its attachments to bone, and its relationships to the orbicularis oculi muscle, skin and conjunctiva. Displacement or detachment of the medial canthal ligament may produce a change in the shape of the palpebral fissure.

The medial canthal ligament (also termed a tendon) is a strong, complex structure (Fig. 2.33). It attaches to the bone of the medial orbit by an element that passes deep to the lacrimal sac, and another more massive component that passes superficial to the sac and inserts into the frontal process of the maxilla. Zide and McCarthy (1983) have described a vertical component to the superficial part of the ligament which inserts into the medial orbital rim adjacent to the nasofrontal suture. The deep portion of the ligament arches, above and below the ampullae of the canaliculi, and inserts into the lacrimal sac behind the posterior lacrimal crest. The strong, thick, superficial part of the medial canthal ligament is attached firmly to the anterior lacrimal crest and extends onto the nasal bone beyond (Rodriguez & Zide 1988). The anterior lacrimal crest protects the lacrimal sac as it nestles in its fossa and the palpable part of the ligament is medial and lies over the bone.

The telecanthus and canthal dystopia which result from damage in this area can be related to severance of all or part of the ligamentous attachment, or to displacement of the bones to which it is attached. The relationship of ligament to lacrimal drainage apparatus is vital when considering diagnosis and treatment of trauma in this area (p. 309 and 582).

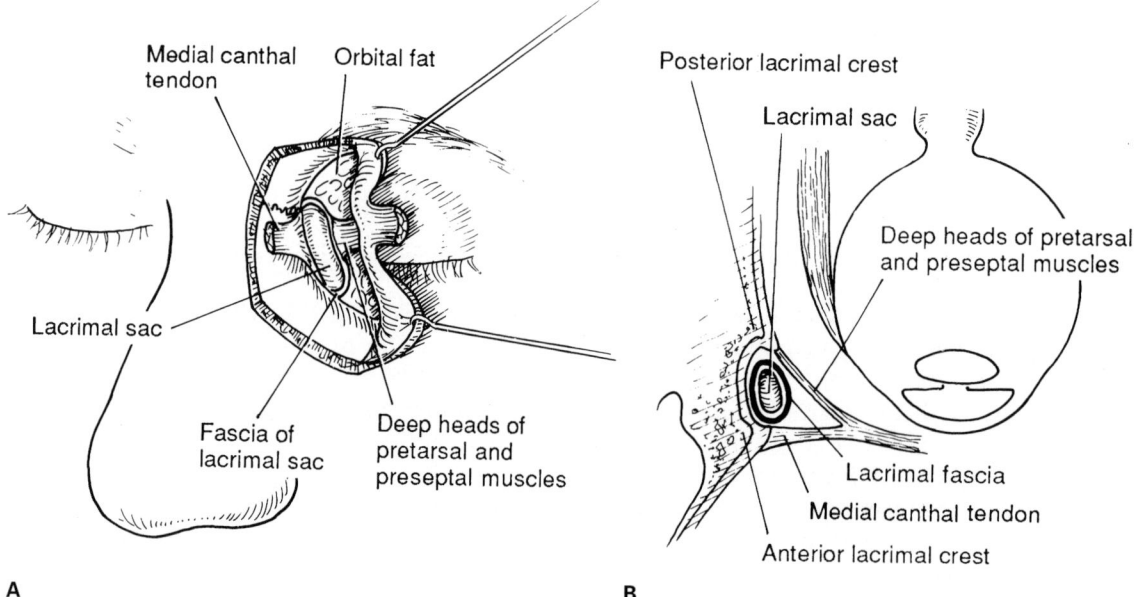

A Medial canthal tendon — Orbital fat — Lacrimal sac — Fascia of lacrimal sac — Deep heads of pretarsal and preseptal muscles

B Posterior lacrimal crest — Lacrimal sac — Deep heads of pretarsal and preseptal muscles — Lacrimal fascia — Medial canthal tendon — Anterior lacrimal crest

Fig. 2.33 The medial canthal ligament. A The medial canthal ligament (tendon) shown with its superficial part peeled back revealing the lacrimal sac. **B** This strong fibrous band is shown attaching to the anterior lacrimal crest and roofing the lacrimal sac; the ligament (tendon) has been divided and its Y-shaped attachment to the tarsal plates is not shown. The preseptal and pretarsal fibres of orbicularis oculi are shown in simplified form lying posterior to the lacrimal sac and attaching to the posterior lacrimal crest. Redrawn from Rodriguez & Zide (1988).

Lateral canthus

The anatomy of the lateral canthal region is not well defined. There is some controversy as to whether or not there is a true ligamentous attachment of the tarsi to the orbital bone or whether there is just a thickening of the periosteum. Couly et al (1976) came down on the side of a definite structure, describing a 'true' ligament, divided into two divergent bundles. The base of this ligament which has the form of a Y, is attached to the external angle of the two tarsi. The bundles diverge, a deep part attaching to the frontal process of the malar bone 2 mm behind the orbital rim, the superficial part continuing over the frontal process and attached to its periosteum. Whitaker (1984) gave some credibility to the existence of the lateral canthal ligament, and others workers in different disciplines, seeing the technical applications of adjustments to this region, make reference to it. In contrast to its medial counterpart its structure is not impressive but in surgical manoeuvres for establishing the correct positioning of the tarsi in relationship to the bone, the lateral canthal ligaments are important none the less.

Muscles of the nostrils

The sphincter of the nostril is the compressor naris, which surrounds the alar cartilages and arises from the maxilla; it is opposed by the dilatator naris, which also arises from the maxilla and is inserted into the ala. The tip of the nose is elevated by the procerus muscle, an extension of the frontal belly of the occipitofrontalis muscle; it is assisted by the levator labii superioris alaeque nasi, and opposed by the depressor septi.

Muscles of the lips and cheeks

The orbicularis oris muscle forms the sphincter of the mouth; the dilators are facial muscles radiating from the lips. The orbicularis oris muscle has fibres which attach near the midline to the upper and lower jaws; these intermingle with fibres of the dilator muscles at the angles of the mouth on each side at a point of convergence called the modiolus, where some fibres actually cross in the form of a chiasma. This modiolus is often difficult to reconstruct after injury.

The buccinator muscle arises from both jaws opposite the molar teeth and from the pterygomandibular raphe (Fig. 2.14). It arises from the whole length of this raphe, interdigitating with fibres from the superior constrictor of the pharynx. The muscle converges on the modiolus, where fibres arising from the raphe decussate. It is pierced by the parotid duct and by the buccal branch of the mandibular nerve, whose fibres supply the muscle. The buccinator is the muscle of the cheek pouch and is lined by adherent mucous membrane; it forms the basis of

a very useful musculocutaneous flap for intraoral reconstruction. It is basically a muscle of mastication, but has other functions.

The dilator muscles of the lips radiate from the orbicularis oris like the spokes of a wheel and are inserted into the lips and the modiolus. When these muscles all contract together, they open the lips to the widest possible extent. Of these radial dilators, the levator labii superioris alaeque nasi arises from the frontal process of the maxilla to insert into the alar cartilage (see above) and the lateral part of the upper lip, which it elevates. The levator labii superioris arises from the inferior orbital margin and is inserted into the remainder of the upper lip, also as an elevator. The levator anguli oris arises from the canine fossa below the inferior orbital margin; it inserts into the angle of the mouth, where it merges with the depressor anguli oris. The zygomaticus minor arises from the zygomaticomaxillary suture and the zygomaticus major further out on the zygomatic bone; both muscles converge on the modiolus. Risorius, a variable muscle derived from the platysma, inserts into the angle of the mouth. The depressor anguli oris arises from the oblique line of the mandible; it is a superficial muscle and passes through the modiolus to insert into the angle of the mouth. It is in part continuous with the levator anguli oris above, and in part with the platysma below. The depressor labii inferioris arises deep to the depressor anguli oris and inserts into the lower lip. The mentalis is a muscle arising from the mandible on each side of the symphysis mentis; its fibres pass downwards through the depressor labii inferioris to insert into the skin of the chin. It is an elevator of the centre of the lower lip and has significance in facial aesthetics and in denture control (McMinn 1990).

All these muscles are supplied by the seventh cranial nerve (see above p. 62). There are many variations, some of them important to the surgeon (Fig. 9.4).

Muscles of mastication

The temporalis muscle originates from the temporal bone and inserts on the apex and medial side of the coronoid process of the mandible (Fig. 2.34). Its functional importance in closing the jaws is considerable. The temporalis muscle is stripped away in the routine bicoronal approach to the craniofacial skeleton (p. 238), and we urge meticulous reattachment to the temporal lines and margins of the temporal fossa. Segments of the muscle can be stripped from the bone and used for reanimation of the face; the blood and nerve supply are preserved. A segment of muscle can be mobilized with a piece of underlying attached calvarium for bony reconstruction of the face (p. 622).

The powerful masseter muscle arises chiefly from the zygomatic arch and inserts on the ramus of the mandible, and assists in closing the jaws. The extensive upper

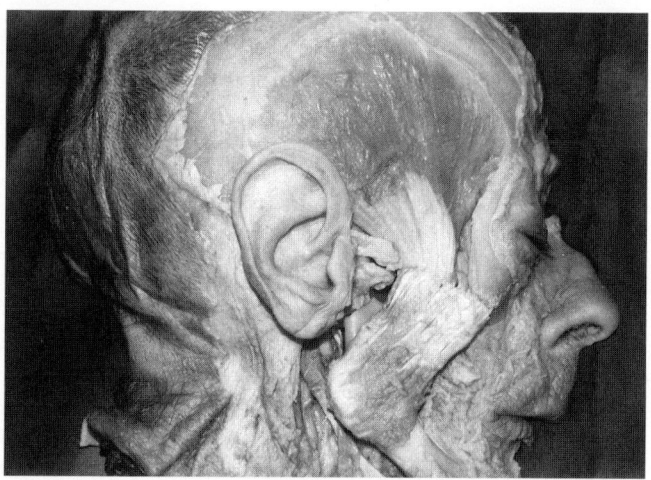

Fig. 2.34 Muscles of mastication. Deep dissection of the face showing the temporalis and masseter muscles. The temporalis fibres converge inferiorly to form a tough ligamentous insertion into the coronoid process of the mandible. Photograph by courtesy of Professor G.C. Townsend, The University of Adelaide.

attachment to the zygoma is of the utmost importance in fractures of this bone and their tendency to displace after correction (p. 315). The pull of the masseter and the pterygoid muscles also influences fractures of the angle of the mandible.

The lateral pterygoid muscle takes origin by two heads, from the infratemporal surface of the greater wing of the sphenoid bone and from the lateral surface of the lateral pterygoid plate. It has a firm round attachment high up to the condylar neck (Fig. 2.5) and to the meniscus of the temporomandibular joint, important in the pattern of displacement of fractures and fracture dislocations of this region. It is the chief agent in opening the mouth.

The medial pterygoid muscle arises from the medial surface of the lateral pterygoid plate and the adjoining palatine bone; it inserts on the ramus and body of the mandible. The medial pterygoid muscle closes the mouth and also moves the mandible in the horizontal plane in side-to-side chewing. The masseter laterally and the medial pterygoid muscle medially enclose the ramus and angle of the mandible.

The digastric muscle with its interesting central tendon bound down to the hyoid bone and its dual innervation from the fifth and seventh nerve assists in the opening of the lower jaw, and also depresses and retracts the chin. It may be used for reconstructive purposes.

Muscles of speech and swallowing

The tongue with its intrinsic and extrinsic musculature, lying in the floor of the mouth and attached to the mandible anteriorly and laterally, helps to form the shape and size of this bone as it develops. McMinn (1990) notes that the intrinsic muscles act in changing the shape of the tongue, whereas the three paired extrinsic muscles stabilize the organ and change its position. Of the extrinsic muscles, the genioglossus arises from the superior mental spine of the mandible, the hyoglossus from the body and greater horn of the hyoid bone; these muscles are likely to be detached or destroyed in avulsive injuries of the anterior mandible. The smaller styloglossus muscles are situated more posteriorly and have less individual importance.

The motor supply is by the twelfth or hypoglossal cranial nerve. Loss of sensation and motor supply to the tongue are both clinically significant, as is loss of the mandibular muscular attachment support which may produce a retrodisplacement of the tongue and airway obstruction.

The soft palate consists of the tensor veli palatini

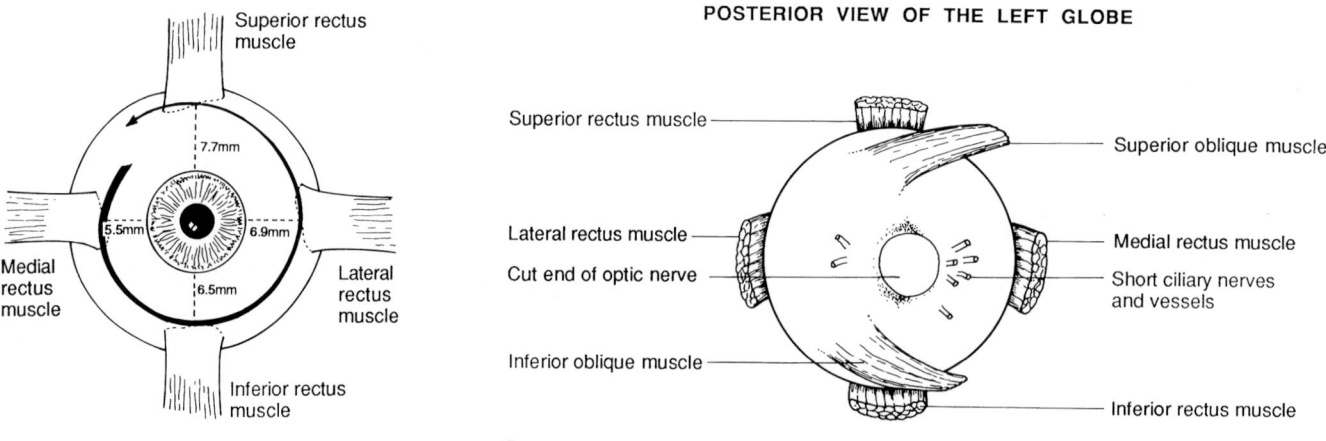

Fig. 2.35 The extra-ocular muscles. The diagram shows the insertions of these muscles. **A** The left eye from in front, showing the four rectus muscles inserting into the globe at varying distances from the limbus, as shown by the spiralling arrow. **B** The left eye from behind, showing the insertions of the two oblique muscles: these are attached lateral to the axis of the globe and posterior to its equator. Also shown are the entry of the short ciliary nerves and veins into the posterior segment of the eye.

muscle, which arises from the scaphoid fossa at the base of the medial pterygoid plate, the spina angularis of the sphenoid and the anterolateral aspect of the cartilage of the eustachian tube. It runs antero-inferiorly and narrows towards the hamulus, where some of its bundles are attached, and widens like a fan towards the centre of the palate. It terminates along the oral side of the aponeurosis which occupies the whole of the anterior third of the velum or directly into it. The levator veli palatini is a cylindrical muscle which arises from the undersurface of the apex of the petrous temporal bone and from the edge of the canal for the passage of the internal carotid artery. Its anterior bundles arise from the posteromedial side and base of the cartilaginous auditory tube. This portion of the Eustachian tube elevates and shifts the soft palate backwards, the muscles of both sides form a sling suspended from the base of the skull. The palatopharyngeus muscle passes from the thyroid cartilage and the adjacent part of the pharyngeal wall through the palatopharyngeal arch to a fan shaped origin from the posterior border of the hard palate. It comprises two parts. The pterygopharyngeal part of the muscle runs from the posterolateral part of the pharynx and attaches to the hamulus and the palatine aponeurosis. The salpingopharyngeal part is the weakest portion: its bundles are attached to the inferior edge of the cartilage of the eustachian tube orifice and blend with the stylopharyngeus muscle (McMinn 1990). The palatoglossus is a slender muscle arising from the transverse bundles of the tongue; it passes up into the palatoglossal arch and inserts fan-wise into the muscles of the soft palate. Together with its opposite muscle it forms the anterior pretonsillar sphincter. The superior pharyngeal constrictor is a quadrangular muscle surrounding from behind and laterally the upper third of the pharyngeal wall. It is the deepest of the pharyngeal constrictors.

Extraocular muscles

Eye movement is controlled by the six striated extraocular muscles which include the four rectus muscles and the two oblique muscles (Fig. 2.35). At the apex of the orbit is the annulus of Zinn which is continuous with the dural sheath of the optic nerve and with periorbital and apical connective tissue. From this annulus arise the rectus muscles. The annulus has an upper tendon (of Lockwood) and a lower tendon (of Zinn). Pathological processes such as trauma may affect all these structures simultaneously, because of their intimate relationship.

Anteriorly, the rectus muscles insert on the globe some 5.5–7.9 mm posterior to the limbus. The medial rectus inserts closest to the limbus; the inferior, lateral and superior muscles insert at increasing distances from the limbus. The superior oblique muscle originates just superior to the annulus and runs forward and becomes tendinous to run through the trochlea which is some 4 mm posterior to the orbital margin and just medial to the supraorbital notch. After passing through the trochlea, the tendon extends in a slightly posterior and lateral direction to fan out inserting on the superior aspect of the globe. The inferior oblique muscle arises from the bone just posterolateral to the nasolacrimal fossa, extending in a similar posterior lateral direction, coursing beneath the inferior rectus and inserting on the inferolateral aspect of the eye. The superior oblique muscle is innervated by the trochlear nerve, and when it contracts the muscle depresses the globe and causes incyclo-version (intorsion or 'wheel-in') of the vertical axis of the eye. The superior oblique has maximum depressing ability when the eye is adducted and maximum rotational ability when the eye is abducted. The muscle also acts as an abductor. The lateral rectus is innervated by the abducent nerve and this muscle abducts the globe. The remaining four extraocular muscles are innervated by branches of the oculomotor nerve. The inferior rectus depresses the globe whilst the medial rectus adducts it and the superior rectus elevates the eye particularly when the eye is abducted. The superior and inferior rectus muscles also act together as adductors. The inferior oblique muscle acts both as an elevator (this is maximal when the eye is adducted) and outward rotator of the vertical axis of the eye, with maximal excyclo-rotation (extorsion or 'wheel-out') occurring in abduction; with the superior oblique it acts as an abductor. Table 2.7 gives the clinical signs of acute paralyses of individual muscles.

The approximate anteroposterior lengths of the rectus muscles and the belly of the superior oblique muscle are 4 cm. Their nerve supply enters at the junction of the posterior and middle thirds of the muscle bellies. The inferior oblique is some 3.5 cm in length; its nerve supply arises from the inferior division of the oculomotor nerve and enters the muscle belly posteriorly after running lateral to the inferior rectus and behind the equator of the globe.

THE EYE AND ITS ADNEXAE

The structure of the eye is very complex (Fig. 2.36): those requiring a full review are referred to such texts as Last (1977). Some aspects of ocular anatomy and physiology require discussion because of their relevance to the pathology and management of eye injuries.

The globe of the eye can be seen as three concentric layers of tissue, each serving a different function. Externally, the fibrous sclerocorneal layer provides structural integrity. Within this layer, the vascular uveal layer (iris, ciliary body and choroid) provides nutrition to the rest of the globe, and especially to the innermost neurosensory layer, the retina.

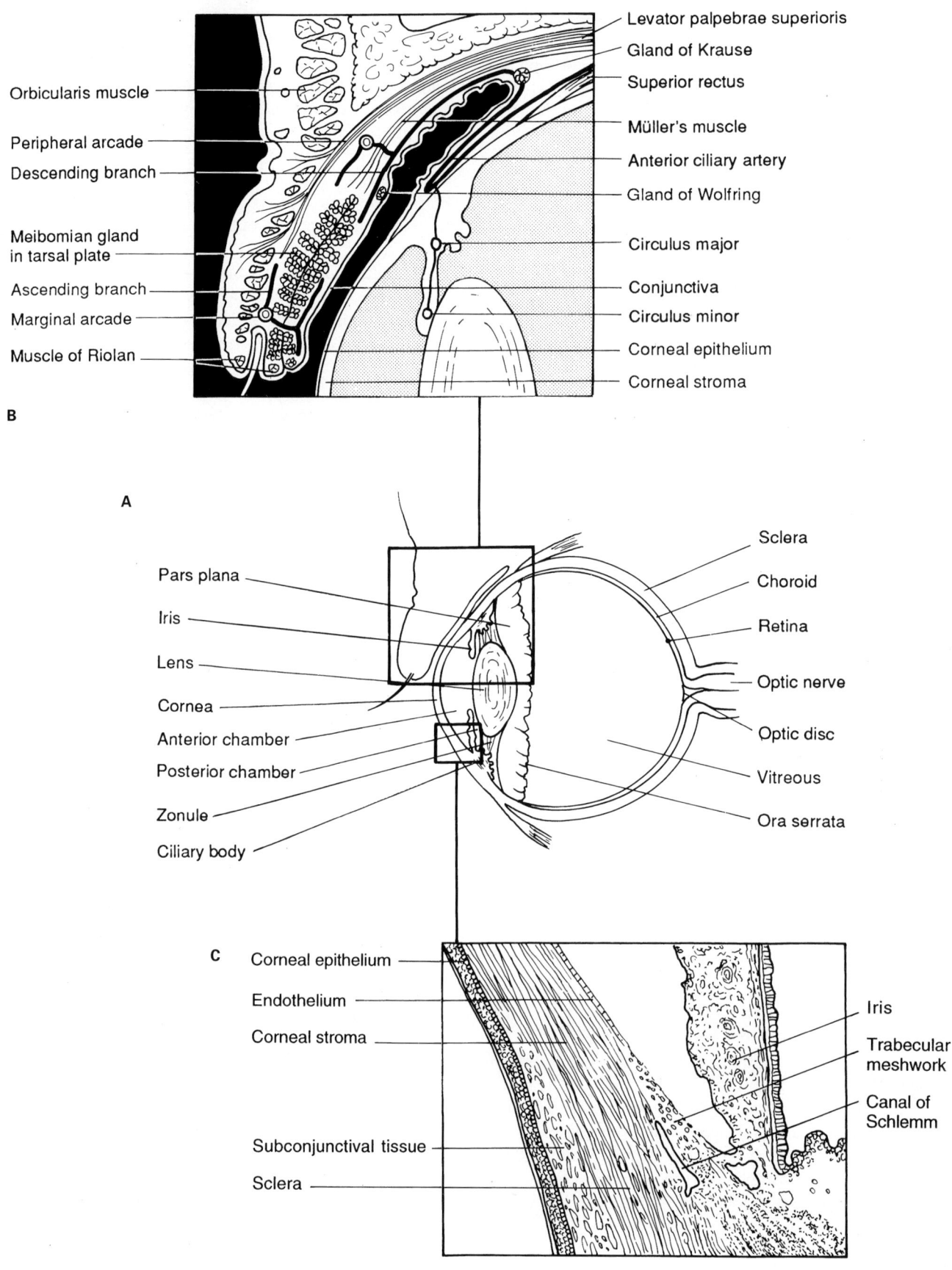

Orbicularis muscle

Peripheral arcade

Descending branch

Meibomian gland in tarsal plate

Ascending branch

Marginal arcade

Muscle of Riolan

Levator palpebrae superioris

Gland of Krause

Superior rectus

Müller's muscle

Anterior ciliary artery

Gland of Wolfring

Circulus major

Conjunctiva

Circulus minor

Corneal epithelium

Corneal stroma

B

A

Pars plana

Iris

Lens

Cornea

Anterior chamber

Posterior chamber

Zonule

Ciliary body

Sclera

Choroid

Retina

Optic nerve

Optic disc

Vitreous

Ora serrata

C

Corneal epithelium

Endothelium

Corneal stroma

Subconjunctival tissue

Sclera

Iris

Trabecular meshwork

Canal of Schlemm

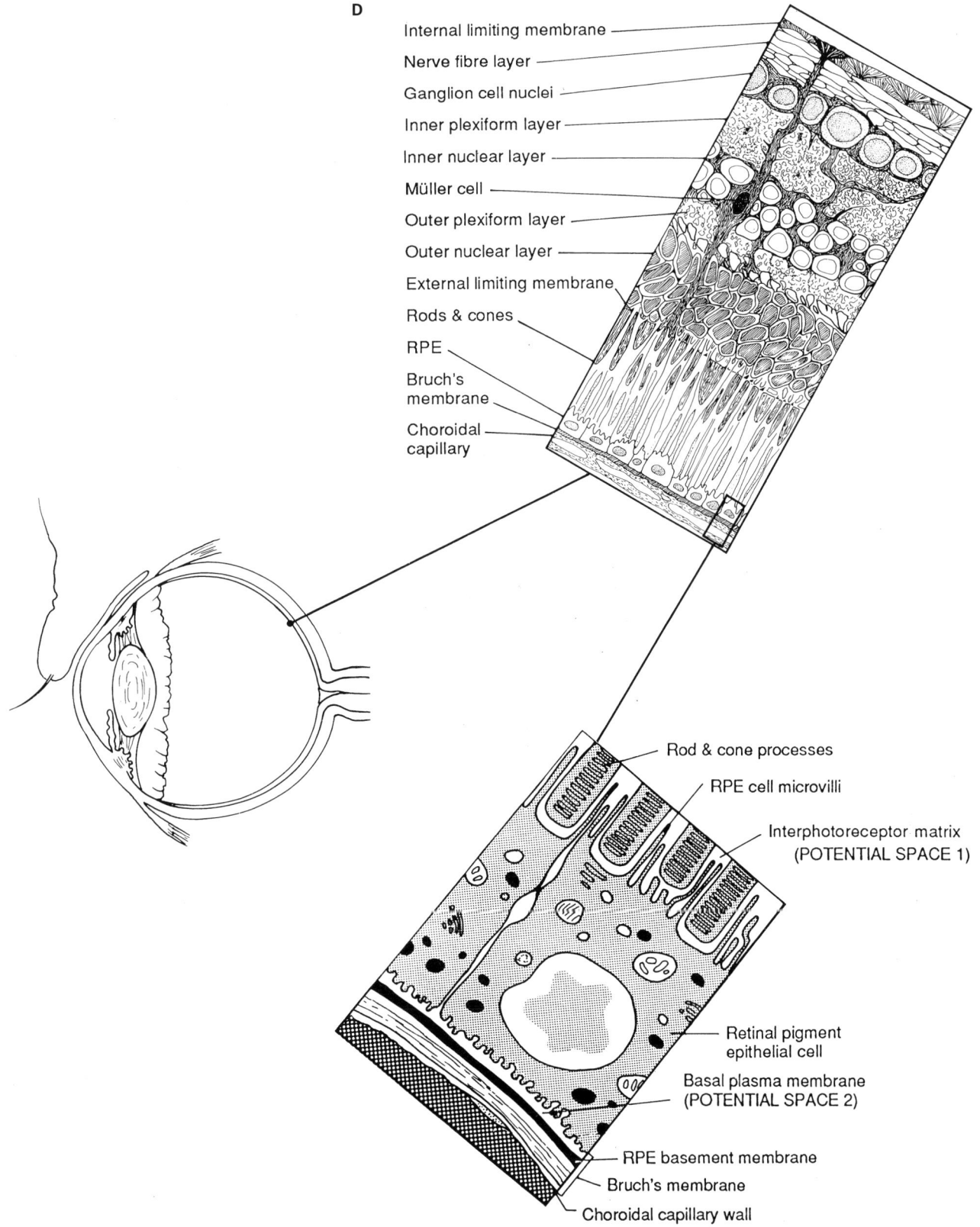

D

Internal limiting membrane
Nerve fibre layer
Ganglion cell nuclei
Inner plexiform layer
Inner nuclear layer
Müller cell
Outer plexiform layer
Outer nuclear layer
External limiting membrane
Rods & cones
RPE
Bruch's membrane
Choroidal capillary

Rod & cone processes
RPE cell microvilli
Interphotoreceptor matrix (POTENTIAL SPACE 1)
Retinal pigment epithelial cell
Basal plasma membrane (POTENTIAL SPACE 2)
RPE basement membrane
Bruch's membrane
Choroidal capillary wall

E

Fig. 2.36 The structure of the eye. A Diagram showing the eyelid and the anterior segment of the eye; the various muscles and glands are shown together with the blood supply of the lid. **B** Schematic diagram of the major anatomical structures of the eye. **C** Diagram showing the transition from sclera to cornea, with the structures in the drainage angle of the eye. **D** Diagram showing the nine layers of the retina, and its membranes. **E** Diagram showing the ultrastructure of a retinal pigment cell in relation to the rod and cone layer (right side) and the choroid (left side).

Table 2.7 Clinical characteristics of paralyses of third, fourth and sixth cranial nerves and of the muscles innervated by them. The signs vary according to the degree of paralysis

Nerve	Muscle	Diplopia	Other signs
Third (oculomotor)	Medial rectus	Horizontal: on gaze to opposite side	Ptosis, fixed dilated pupil, divergent squint; eye may be turned slightly down; paralysed accommodation
	Superior rectus	Vertical: on gaze up	
	Inferior rectus	Vertical: gaze down	
	Inferior oblique	Vertical: on gaze up, with torsional element	
Fourth (trochlear)	Superior oblique	Vertical: on gaze down, with torsional element	Often subtle signs: compensatory head tilt to opposite side, difficulty in looking down
Sixth (abducent)	Lateral rectus	Horizontal: on gaze to same side	Compensatory face turn to same side, weak abduction, convergent squint, worse for distant fixation

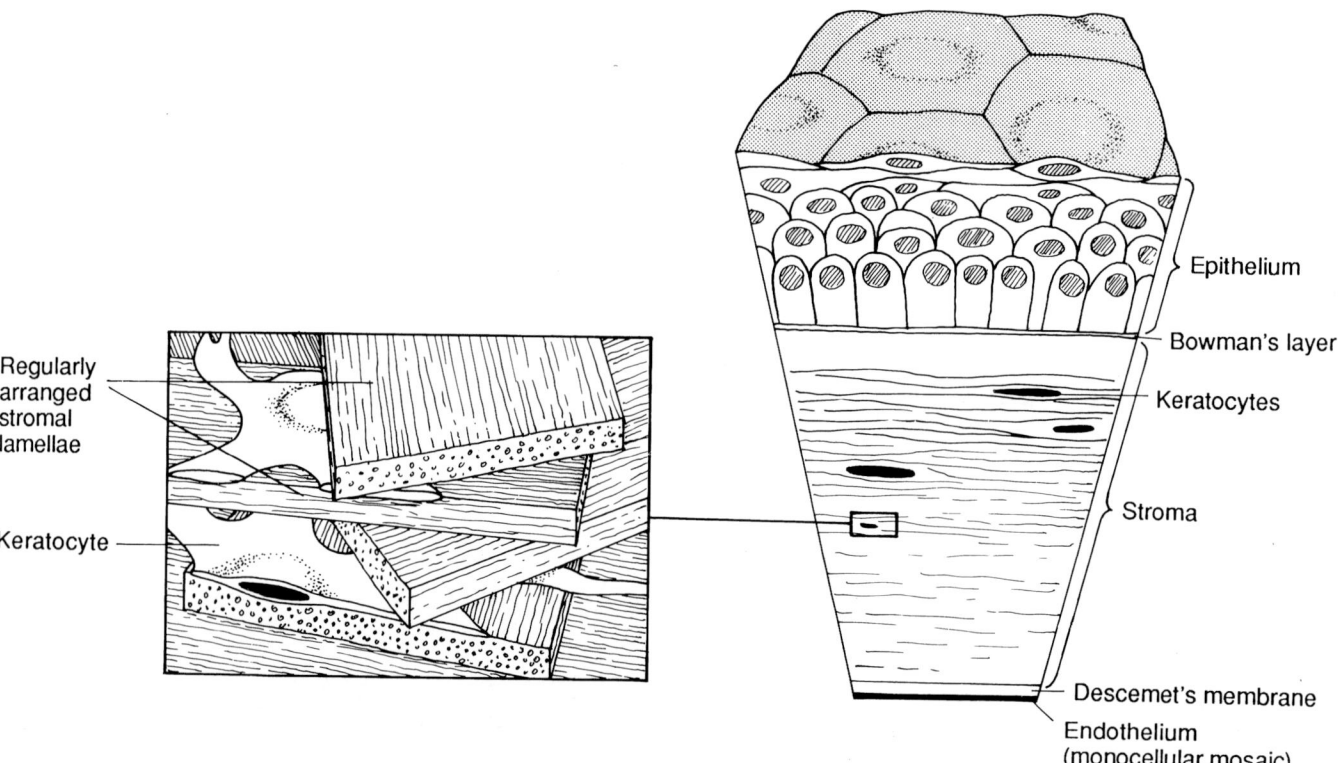

Fig. 2.37 The layers of the cornea. Diagram showing a section of the corneal stroma: the stromal lamellae are arranged regularly in layers. On the inner surface (anterior chamber) there is a monocellular lining layer of endothelial cells, and on the outer surface there is a layer of stratified non-keratinized epithelial cells.

Sclera and cornea

The sclera is composed of collagen and elastic fibres arranged in criss-crossing bundles, with sparse fibroblasts between the fibres. It is about 1 mm thick at the posterior pole of the eye, where the optic nerve enters, and only 0.3–0.4 mm where the rectus muscles insert. The sclera is continuous anteriorly with the cornea, the limbus being the junctional line.

The translucent cornea (Fig. 2.37) is composed chiefly of a stroma of collagen fibrils arranged in regular fashion; between the fibres are stromal cells with fibroblastic capacity. Anteriorly, the cornea is bounded by a layer of non-keratinizing stratified squamous epithelium, resting on Bowman's membrane, which is a homogeneous condensation of the corneal stroma. On electron microscopy, the epithelial cells are seen to have microvilli projecting into the tear film (see below). Posteriorly, the cornea is bounded by a single endothelial layer of hexagonal cells, resting on Descemet's membrane, a basement membrane containing elastic fibrils. The cornea is thinnest (about 0.5 mm) centrally and thickest where it joins the sclera.

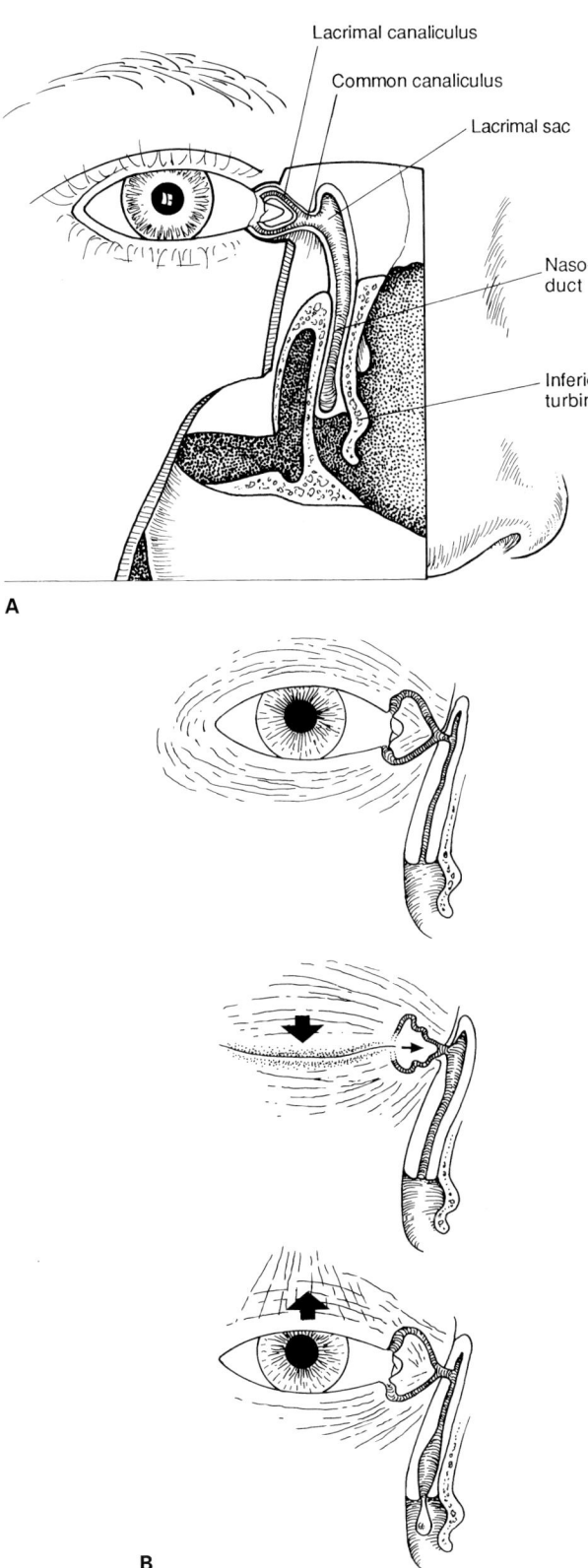

A

B

TEAR FILM

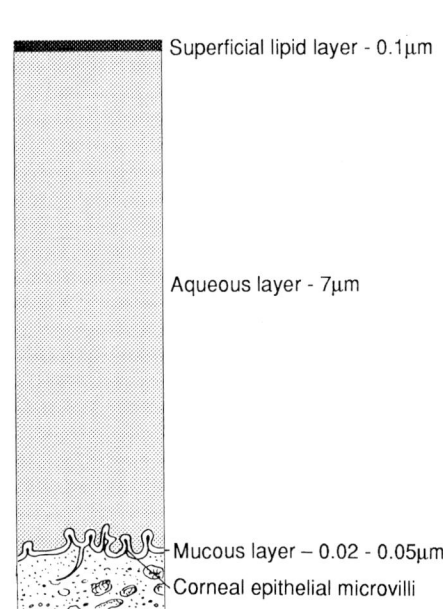

Superficial lipid layer - 0.1µm

Aqueous layer - 7µm

Mucous layer – 0.02 - 0.05µm
Corneal epithelial microvilli

C

Fig. 2.38 The lacrimal apparatus. A Cut-away diagram showing the tear drainage system from the conjunctival sac to the nasolacrimal duct entering the inferior meatus of the nose. **B** Diagram showing the active lacrimal pump mechanism, motored by the orbicularis oculi muscle and involving the lacrimal diaphragm. Upper diagram: with the lids open, the puncta are in contact with the lacrimal pool — the tears tend to collect medially. The canaliculi remain patent as the lacrimal sac collapses. Middle diagram: with eyelid closure, tears are milked to the medial side. The deep heads of the pretarsal muscle contract, shortening the canaliculi and closing their ampullae. At the same time the deep heads of the preseptal muscles pull the lacrimal diaphragm laterally, thereby creating negative pressure within the sac. Lower diagram: as the lids re-open, the lacrimal diaphragm returns to its relaxed position, thereby collapsing the lacrimal sac and propelling the tears into the nasolacrimal duct. The canaliculi reopen to admit more tears and the cycle is repeated. **C** The tear film on the cornea: microvilli of corneal epithelial cells protrude into the tear film, which is a complex sandwich of mucous, aqueous and lipid layers, less than 8 m thick.

It is the major refracting structure in the eye, providing three-quarters of the optical power of the eye as a lens system.

The cornea is wholly avascular, deriving nutrition chiefly from the aqueous humor; the corneal stroma is hydrophilic, and attracts water, glucose and other requirements to maintain the active metabolic requirements of the cellular elements, especially the epithelial cells. Oxygen is also obtained by diffusion, externally through the tear film, internally from the aqueous. The thickness of the cornea, and also its transparency, relate to the water content; dehydration of the cornea causes thinning and loss of normal lucency. The intraocular pressure, in adults normally 16–20 mmHg, is also important in maintaining corneal clarity, and excessive pressure causes corneal oedema.

The cornea is sensitive to pain, touch and cold (Walsh & Hoyt 1985); it is innervated by the ophthalmic division of the trigeminal nerve, through the long ciliary nerves. It has been argued that in some individuals, the lower part of the cornea is innervated by the infraorbital nerve; Rowbotham (1939) found no evidence for this, but our clinical observations suggest that this may still be still an open question.

Uveal layer

The iris is pigmented, reducing light scatter, and contains a diaphragm of constrictor and dilator smooth muscle fibres which represents the effector component of the pupillary light reflex. The vascular ciliary body produces the aqueous humor, which fills the anterior segment of the eye and is absorbed through the trabecular meshwork into the canal (or canals) of Schlemm, which drains through collecting channels into the conjunctival veins (Fig. 2.36C). The ciliary body also contains smooth muscle, acting on the lens through the suspensory zonule in reflex accommodation.

The choroid, also pigmented, is highly vascular and provides nutrition to the outer two thirds of the retina; it also rids the retina of metabolic waste products, and acts as a heat sink.

The lens lies behind the iris and is suspended from the ciliary body by the fibres of the zonule. It is the variable part of the dioptric power of the eye, and has the capacity to absorb ultraviolet light. The lens is composed of tightly packed epithelial cells which elongate to produce long prismatic lens fibres, contained within a capsule 2–20 μm thick and made of an elastic, collagen-like substance. Like the cornea, the lens is nourished by diffusion from the aqueous humor, and also from the vitreous body; also like the cornea, the lucency of the lens depends on its hydration. Throughout life the epithelial cells of the lens are forming new lens fibres by mitotic division, and like all mitotically active cells they are sensitive to radiation: this is the basis of radiation cataract (p. 186).

The vitreous body occupies the posterior segment of the globe, a volume of about 4 ml. It is a hydro-gel containing 99% water: nevertheless it is in a dynamic metabolic state, providing nutrition to the lens and to the retina, and also mechanical support. The junctional surface between the vitreous and the retina is the internal limiting lamina of the retina, a basement membrane delimiting the internal layer of the retinal glial cells and a layer of dense collagen fibrils.

Retina

This comprises two layers, the outer pigmented epithelial layer, and the inner neuroepithelial layer (Fig. 2.36D,E). Between these layers is a potential space, and it is here that separation occurs when the retina is detached (p. 403). The retina is a most complex structure, containing not only light-sensitive rods and cones, but also neurons engaged in visual processing. The most sensitive part of the retina is the macula, whose centre — the foveola — is situated some 3 mm temporal to the optic disc; the retina varies in thickness, being thinnest at the foveola, and thickest where the retinal nerve fibres enter the optic nerve.

Blood supply

The eye is supplied by branches of the ophthalmic artery, the central artery of the retina, the long and short posterior ciliary arteries and the anterior ciliary arteries. These anastomose, but effectively the retina is dependent solely on its central artery. The retinal neuroepithelial cells are vulnerable to anoxia, but less so than might be supposed. Böck et al (1963) found that ischaemia for 6 min obliterated the electroretinogram, but even after 60 min, recovery of vision was possible; total irreversible loss of retinal function was established after 120 min. This finding of recovery after prolonged retinal ischaemia is supported by recent experimental studies in a monkey model (Young et al 1992).

The eyelids and lacrimal apparatus

The firm yet flexible nature of the eyelids (Fig. 2.36B) is given by the tarsal plate, the skeleton of the lid. The tarsal plates are composed of fibrous tissue; the upper plate is more prominent, and receives fibres of the aponeurosis of the levator palpebrae superioris, and also smooth muscle fibres which arise from that muscle and are under sympathetic innervation. The tarsal plates are connected to the circumference of the orbit by the orbital septum, and at their ends, they are attached to the lateral and medial palpebral ligaments. Each tarsal plate contains some 30 Meibomian glands, which open on the lid margin and secrete the oily element in tears. The lids are covered anteriorly by thin skin with lax, easily distensible subcutaneous tissue; posteriorly, they are covered by the conjunctiva, a stratified columnar epithelium containing goblet cells which contribute to the tear film. The lid margin, the free edge of the lid, has anteriorly the row of eyelashes, and posteriorly the row of orifices of the Meibomian glands: the 'grey line' between these rows is an important landmark in the surgery of the eyelid. There are some 150 lashes on the upper eyelid and about half that number on the lower lid; each lash is a typical short stout hair growing from a follicle that contains a sebaceous gland adding sebum to the tears. At the medial end of each eyelid is the lacrimal punctum, draining tears through the lacrimal canaliculi into the lacrimal sac, and so through the nasolacrimal duct into the inferior meatus of the nasal cavity (Fig. 2.38). The bulk of the tears goes by this route; the rest (some 25%) is lost by evaporation. Tear flow is promoted by gravity, capillary attraction and the massaging action of the orbicularis oculi (Zide & Jelks 1985).

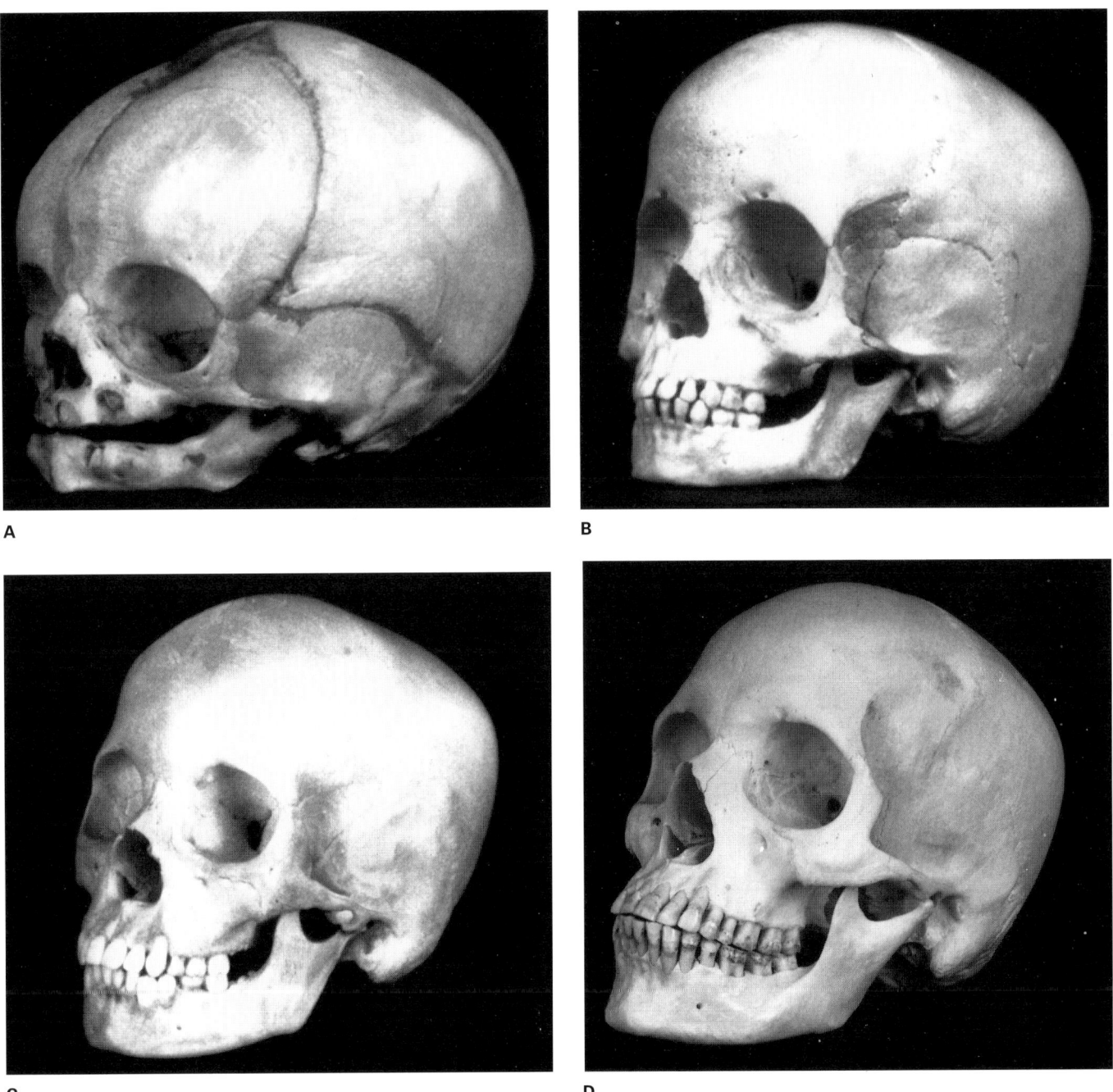

Fig. 2.39 Growth changes in the skull. Skulls in lateral oblique view, demonstrating the changing proportions between cranial vault and facial skeleton with growth. The older skulls have been reduced to the approximate size of the foetal skull. **A** Late foetal or early postnatal skull. **B** Child's skull. **C** Adolescent skull. **D** Adult skull.

The blink and the tears

The tear film is said to be made up of three layers, a superficial oily layer, an aqueous layer, and a layer of mucus opposed to the microvilli of the corneal epithelial cells (Fig. 2.39C). Each has a specific function. The oily layer helps to prevent tear spillage. The mucus promotes adherence to the corneal epithelium. The aqueous layer, in bulk the largest, has nutritive and excretory functions, as described above, and is essential in maintaining corneal hydration; it is secreted by the lacrimal gland and other accessory glands which open into the conjunctival fornices. It is thought that the accessory lacrimal glands maintain tear secretion at a basal level, while the lacrimal gland proper responds to corneal irritation or emotional stimuli. The tear film is spread by the blink, and this is essential to maintain comfort and optical clarity. The normal blink is produced by contraction of the pretarsal fibres of orbicularis oculi, combined with relaxation of the levator muscle and contraction of the superior rectus muscle (Bell's phenomenon); forced lid closure is effected by the orbital component of orbicularis oculi. During normal blinking, the lower lid remains almost stationary, while the upper lid closes like a blind, with a final zipper-like narrowing of the palpebral fissure from lateral to medial canthus: the action helps to move tears toward the lacrimal puncta. In man, the normal blink rate is about 25/min, each blink taking about 0.3 s.

GROWTH OF THE FACE

Early development

The face of a young child is not simply the miniature of the adult face; the face does not have the same proportions between the various regions or parts at all stages of growth (Fig. 2.39). In one of the earliest X-ray cephalometric studies, Broadbent (1937) showed that whereas the cranial vault and the orbits are approximately of adult size as early as the age of 10 years, the facial skeleton continues to enlarge until growth ceases after about 21 years only minor growth continuing thereafter. During the first year of life, both the calvarial and facial components of the skull increase in size by about 30%; in the adult, however, the calvarial skeleton is about 60% greater than its neonatal size, whereas the facial skeleton has enlarged by some 93%. The transformation from neonatal to adult proportions involves a general displacement of the facial skeleton away from the cranial vault in a downward and forward direction; furthermore, mandibular growth tends to outpace maxillary growth, so that the facial profile becomes straighter with age. Thus, the forehead of the child is relatively more prominent — and thus more vulnerable — than the lower facial structures, whereas the mandible is less prominent. This can be related to the greater incidence of childhood injuries in the frontal region, and the relative rarity of mandibular fractures (p. 502).

At birth, the fetal chondrocranium has been largely ossified, and membrane bones have formed in the fibrous capsules of the brain and the facial viscera. New bone is formed by osteoblasts adjacent to proliferating cartilage in the synchondroses which separate the components of the cranial base: the spheno-occipital synchondrosis is the chief of these. This process of endochondral ossification likewise takes place in the septo-ethmoid region and in the mandibular condyle. Bone is also produced by osteoblasts in the periosteum and endosteum covering the developing bones and in the sutures that separate them: the calvarial and facial sutures constitute an important mechanism for continuing ossification of membrane bones in response to the tissue-separating effects of growing

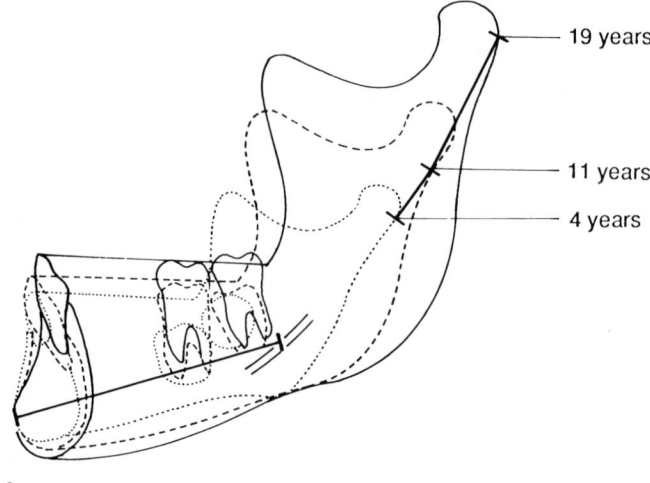

A

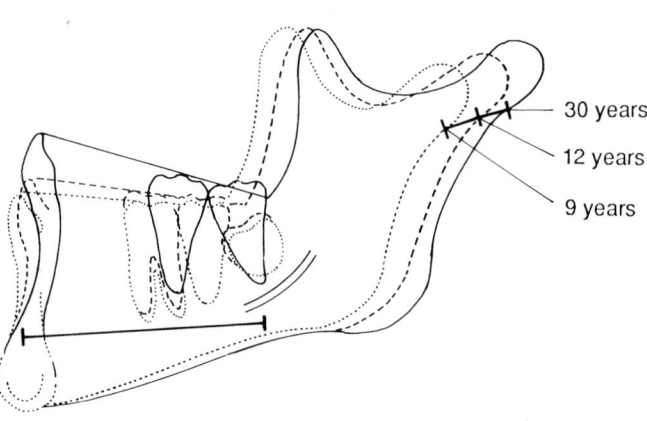

B

Fig. 2.40 Mandibular growth patterns. Mandibular tracings from cephalometric radiographs superimposed on a line joining two stable metallic implants to show remodelling during growth. Anterior rotation in relation to the implant line is shown in **A** and posterior rotation in **B**. In each case there has been resorption along the anterior surface of the ramus and deposition along the posterior. The mandibular border also shows remodelling in conjunction with the anterior rotation. Upward growth of the condyle is accompanied by downward and forward displacement of the mandible relative to the cranial base. Redrawn after Björk & Skieller (1983).

viscera such as the brain, the tongue and the nasal cavity. As growth progresses, and in response to growth requirements, the bones are remodelled. Surface remodelling is effected by a combination of bone deposition by osteoblasts and bone resorption by osteoclasts. This results in changes in the size and sometimes also the shape of the cranial bones.

Bone remodelling and translation

Although these histological mechanisms are well understood, there is controversy over the nature of the dynamic forces that govern the complex process of bone remodelling and translocation of elements of the skull. Enlow

(1982) clarified understanding of these changes by emphasizing the concepts of *drift* and *displacement*. Drift represents remodelling of the borders of growing bones; displacement is seen when a bone moves in response to growth elsewhere, as in the descent of the body of the mandible in response to the upward growth of the condyles. Enlow was also interested in the relationship between bone remodelling and the direction of bone growth. His working hypothesis was that the surface of new bone formation always faces the direction of growth.

Björk, in Copenhagen, used metallic implants placed under the periosteum at various key sites in the maxilla and mandible to study craniofacial growth in children. These implants constituted a stable system of markers of growth. Superimposed serial cephalometric radiographs allowed visualization and quantification of the processes of drift and displacement over time (Björk 1969, Björk & Skieller 1972, 1974, 1976, 1983). Björk was able to show that the maxilla and mandible rotate away from the cranial base during growth, causing changes in the angulation between the anterior cranial base and a line joining two markers. With the face viewed in left profile, anterior rotations occurred when the implant line rotated in a clockwise direction, and posterior rotations when the line turned counterclockwise (Fig. 2.40). Each type of rotation produced characteristic morphological results. Thus, pronounced anterior rotation of the mandible tended to give a closed bite, an anterior facial height short in relation to posterior facial height, and a squarish face; the reverse morphology resulted from pronounced posterior rotation. Despite substantial rotations and remodelling, the basic shape of the mandible remained fairly constant. Björk & Skieller (1977) also showed that the maxilla likewise rotates during growth, and this rotation correlates with that of the mandible; the paths of dental eruption are to some extent determined by these rotations. The implant studies also allowed quantification of the anterior migration of the whole dentition and the associated alveolar remodelling that provides space for the later erupting molar teeth.

Postnatal growth: sites, centres and forces

Earlier workers stressed intrinsic bone growth as a driving force in craniofacial growth, especially endochondral ossification in the spheno-occipital synchondrosis, the septal cartilage, and the mandibular condyles (Scott 1967). Weinmann & Sicher (1947) noted that many sutures are parallel to each other and at right angles to the direction of facial growth downwards and forwards. This was correlated with the older view that sutures also produce a growth force — a view not widely held today: sutural growth is now seen as largely a passive response to expansion of the craniofacial viscera.

Moss (1971, 1972) built on his own and earlier work to formulate his still controversial *functional matrix* theory of craniofacial growth. He saw the head as a structure designed to carry out many functions, notably neural integration, respiration, speech, ingestion and mastication, and the special sensory functions. Each function is exercised by a functional matrix of soft tissues and spaces, and each functional matrix is supported and protected by a micro- or macroskeletal unit. Moss postulated that the growth of skeletal units is subordinate to the growth of the related functional matrices. In this view, the skull bones have no inherent genetic information to direct their growth, which is entirely provided by the functional matrices — the brain, the eyes, and the muscles, teeth, fat and glands.

Growth in the CMF region is still a controversial subject: those interested are referred to the authors cited here and to the series of monographs published by the Center for Human Growth in the University of Michigan, Ann Arbor. Clinicians who manage paediatric injuries must be aware of these controversies. Unquestionably, visceral growth plays a crucial role in determining the morphological appearance of the face, but it is still uncertain whether independent skeletal growth is also a factor.

In the growth of the cranial base, the spheno-occipital synchondrosis is regarded as a major postnatal growth centre: endochondral ossification takes place on both sides of the cartilaginous plate, causing an increase in the length of the skull base posterior to the sella turcica. The synchondrosis closes in females between 11 and 14 years of age, and in males between 13 and 16 years.

The cranial base forms a junctional zone between the calvaria and the facial skeleton, and the growth of these structures is interdependent. The shape of the calvarial vault expresses both the growth of the brain and the growth of the cranial base. The membrane bones of the calvaria are separated by sutures which are sites of bone deposition during the period of rapid brain growth (Fig. 2.41). Sutural growth ceases when the brain ceases to grow, though surface deposition of bone enlarges the calvarial skull for some time into adult life. The sutures fuse at various ages, the metopic suture usually in infancy, the others much later (30–40 years) or never.

There is also little doubt that the form of the skull base influences facial morphology (Björk 1960). Marked flexion of the skull base, measured by the angle between the plane of the clivus and the floor of the anterior cranial fossa (planum sphenoidale), is associated with a low middle fossa, prognathism and a short anterior facial height; conversely, a flat cranial base is associated with the reverse appearance of the face.

The morphology of the upper third of the face and the orbits also relates to the growth of the skull base as well as to the growth of the brain and the eyes (Fig. 2.42). However, the middle third displays a more general growth

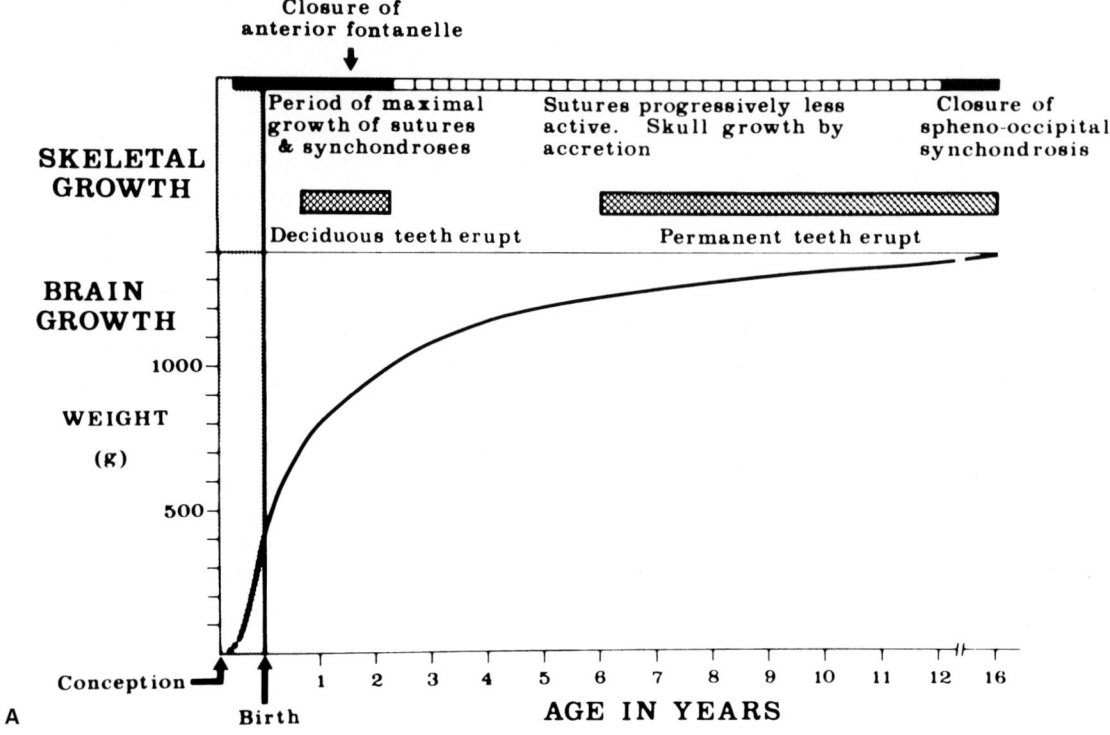

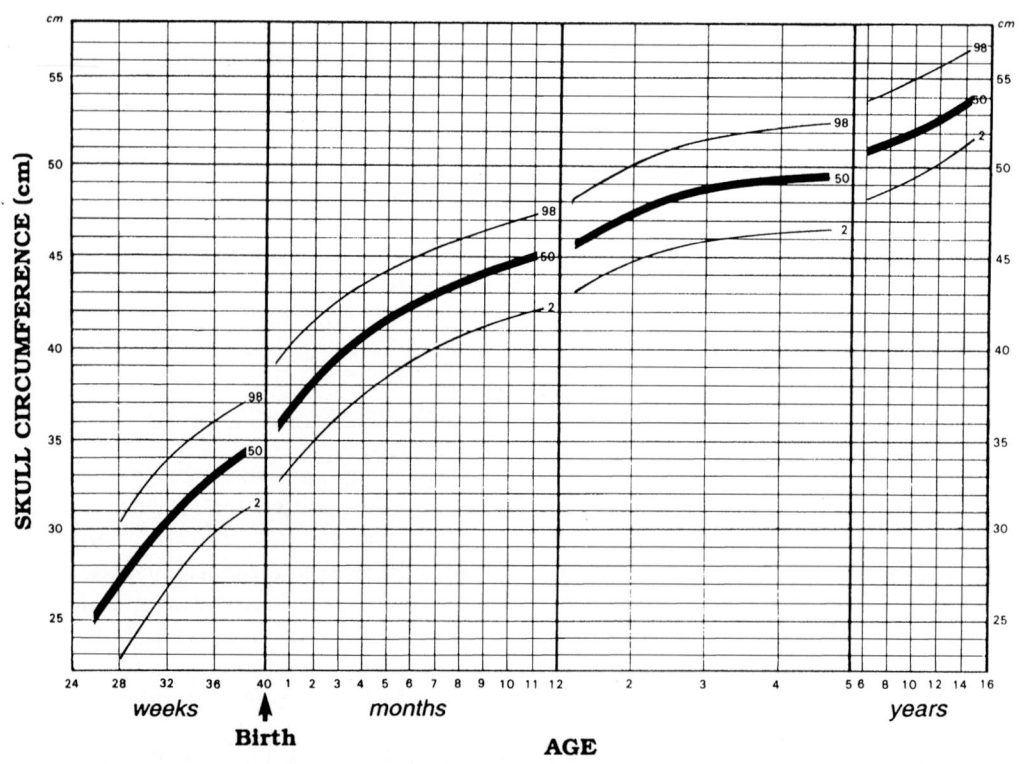

Fig. 2.41 Brain growth in relation to the growth of the skull and the teeth. A Brain mass increases rapidly in utero and during the first 2 years of life; in the same period, calvarial growth is correspondingly fast and takes place especially across the calvarial sutures. By courtesy of Blackwell Scientific Publications. **B** Head circumference of females, in utero, to 12 months, to 5 years, and to 16 years.

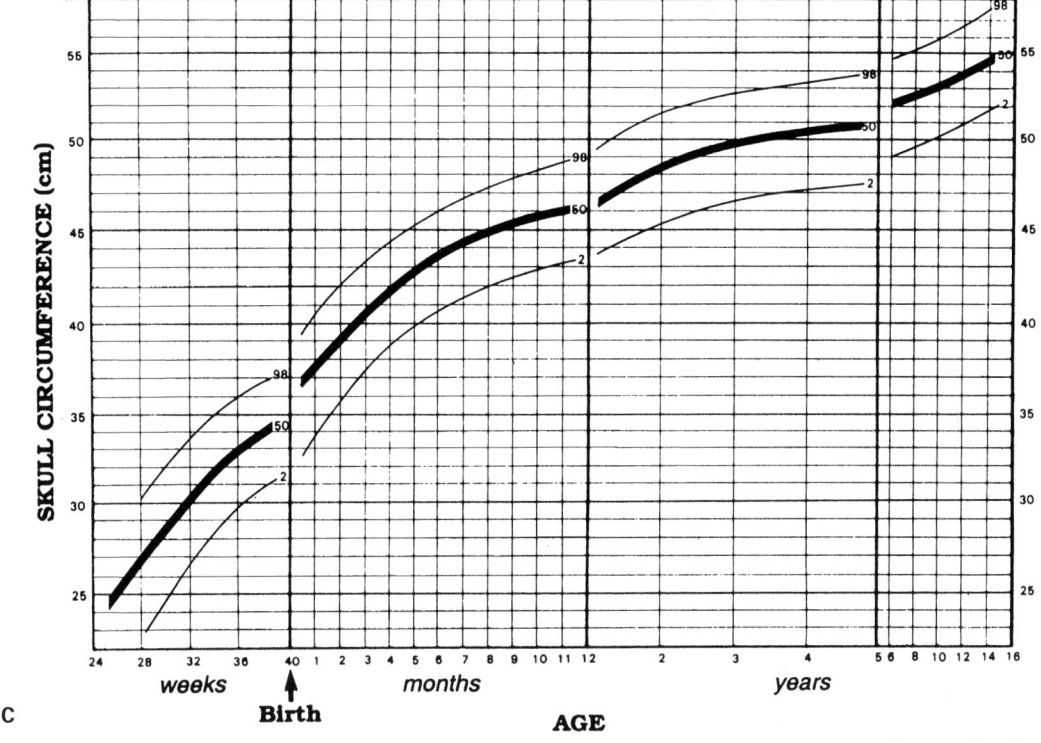

C

Fig. 2.41 Brain growth in relation to the growth of the skull and the teeth. C Head circumference of males, in utero, to 12 months, to 5 years, and to 16 years. For clinical convenience, percentile charts of age-appropriate sections of the skull circumference curve are used. By courtesy of National Health and Medical Research Council of Australia.

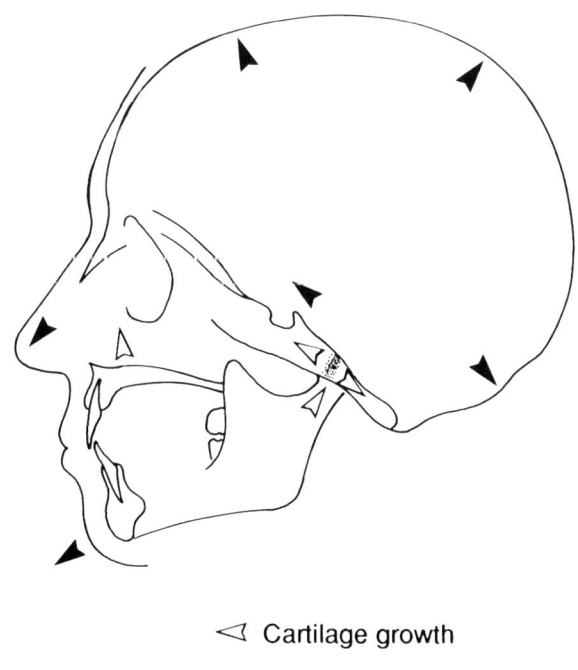

◁ Cartilage growth

◀ Displacement

Fig. 2.42 Craniofacial growth. Displacement of the craniofacial structures with growth and sites of cartilaginous ossification. Redrawn from David et al (1982) by courtesy of Springer-Verlag.

pattern, with greater postnatal growth relative to the growth of the calvaria (see above), and in particular an adolescent spurt. During postnatal growth, the entire facial skeleton is displaced downwards and forwards away from the skull base; the implant studies of Björk & Skieller (1976, 1977) have shown that there is much individual variation in this movement.

The nature of this displacement is in dispute. Most authorities no longer regard growth in the complex system of sutures separating the facial bones as a dynamic force carrying the face down and forwards, though like the calvarial sutures these sutures show continuing deposition of bone during the period of facial growth, and there is concurrent bone remodelling by apposition and resorption on the external and internal surfaces of the maxilla and other facial bones. Bone remodelling is responsible for much of the growth in facial breadth and depth, and in the formation and modification of the alveolar processes to accommodate the primary and later the secondary dentition. Bone remodelling is also involved in the downward relocation of the hard palate — an example of bone drift.

The nasal septum is also involved in this downward and forward displacement. The septum comprises the vertical plate of the ethmoid, the vomer and the septal

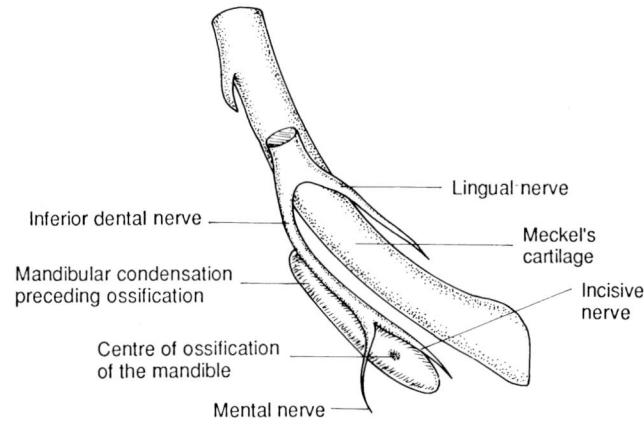

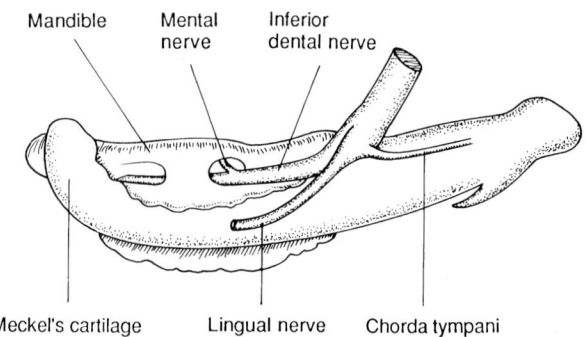

Fig. 2.43 Early development of the mandible. Ossification of the mandible commencing lateral to Meckel's cartilage at the junction of the mental and incisive branches of the inferior alveolar nerve as viewed from above and medially. Redrawn after Scott & Dixon (1978).

cartilage, which is a persisting non-ossified component of the embryonic nasal capsule. There is a site of endochondral ossification at the septo-ethmoid junction, and a site of cartilage proliferation at the septo-vomeral junction. The cartilage retains its osteogenic potential for some time after birth, and bone is deposited along its posterior edge. The time at which septal growth ceases is debatable; Scott (1967) stated that the process ends by the tenth year. The role of the nasal septum is contentious. Is it a primary growth centre, driving the downward movement of the face, or does it respond passively to other growth forces, such as the expansion of oronasal soft tissues and organ spaces? This unsolved question is central in the debate over Moss's functional matrix theory.

Because the teeth must meet in occlusion, growth of the middle third of the face is coordinated with growth of the mandible. Growth changes in the hard palate and maxillary dental arch are also important. During the transitional phase of dental development there are changes in the positions of individual teeth as occlusal relationships are established (Björk & Skieller 1972). As the primary teeth are gradually replaced, there is a decrease in the depth of the dental arch measured from the contact between central incisors to a line tangential to the mesial surfaces of the first permanent molars. This reduction is associated partly with the size differences between the larger primary molars and the succeeding but smaller permanent premolars (Brown et al 1990). Arch breadth increases slightly, particularly in the posterior region, as a result of growth at the midpalatal suture combined with alveolar remodelling, and the incisors become more upright. The mandible is largely formed by membrane bone laid down lateral to Meckel's cartilage, the embryonic skeleton of the first visceral arch; remnants of Meckel's cartilage persist near the symphysis (Fig. 2.43). Secondary growth cartilages appear in the condylar process about 12 weeks after conception; after birth these condylar cartilages persist as a zone of proliferating cartilage cells under the fibrous covering of the articular surface of the temporomandibular joint. Under this zone of proliferation, new bone is formed by endochondral ossification. Thus by generation of new cartilage above, and new bone below, the condylar cartilages gradually add to the height of the mandibular rami, and displace the mandible downwards.

Growth at the condyles and bone remodelling are the main growth processes responsible for the postnatal changes in the size and shape of the mandible. Nevertheless, despite many experimental studies, there is still uncertainty about the role of the condylar cartilage as a primary growth centre. When the condyle is resected experimentally in the monkey, the resulting deformity is limited to the operated side, the other components of the mandible being relatively unaffected; this is also the case when condylar growth is disturbed by injury or disease in early human life, unless bony ankylosis occurs, when gross deformity results (p. 598). Moreover, transplanted components of the rat mandible do not show the independent growth capacity exhibited by transplanted epiphyseal cartilages, unless the transplanted component includes some of the ossified ramus (Koski 1971). These observations suggest that the mandibular condyle is not a primary growth centre but a compensatory structure maintaining correct relationships between the functional components of the temporomandibular joint as the face enlarges.

Bone remodelling is also crucial in postnatal growth of the mandible. Deposition and resorption of bone preserve the shape of the mandible and are also responsible for the development of the alveolar processes under the stimulus of the emerging teeth. Although the symphyseal region remains relatively unchanged with age, there is extensive remodelling elsewhere. Resorption along the anterior border of the coronoid process provides room for the eruption of the third molar teeth; on the other hand, deposition along the superior border increases its height. Remodelling also occurs along the lower border of

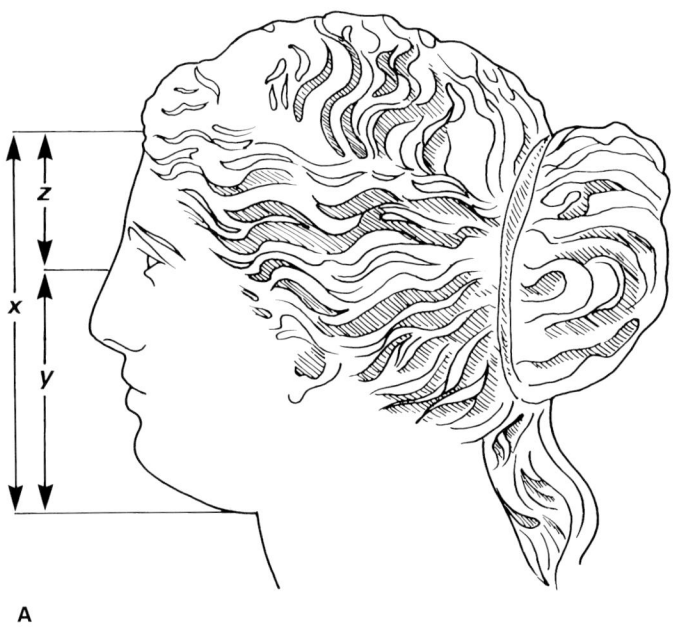

A

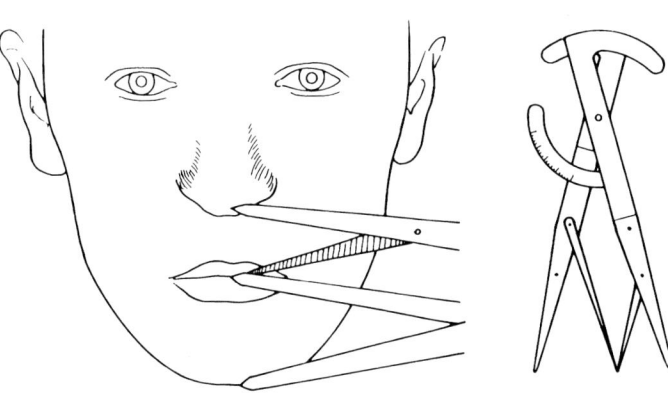

B

Fig. 2.44 Classical aesthetics and the 'golden section'. The Greek
ideal of facial beauty was expressed in geometrical terms; the ratio
1.0:1.618 was seen by some as the ideal (golden) proportion. **A** In this
profile drawn from a Hellenistic statue, this proportion is almost
achieved in the relations of the hair line – the pupil – the junction of
chin and neck. In establishing the soft-tissue landmarks, there is much
imagination and even fantasy. In the classical Greek profile, there is an
almost unbroken line from the forehead to the nose, with very little
indentation at the nasion. Greek sculptors stressed gender differences
in the rounder female chin and jaw line. **B** The golden section and the
golden dividers: Ricketts has designed dividers to establish the ideal
proportion of 1.0:1.618 in assessing the dimensions of the face from
hairline – tip of nose – mouth line – chin point. Redrawn from Powell
& Humphreys (1984) by courtesy of Thieme Medical Publishers, Inc.

the body and the posterior border of the ramus, preserving
the basic shape of the mandible and its relations with
the growing sub- and retromandibular tissues. Though
increase in the breadth of the skull base may be a contributory factor, growth of the width of the mandible is
predominantly due to remodelling — bone drift again!

AESTHETICS OF THE FACE

Ideal proportions

Aesthetics is the science and art of sensual perception.
Greek philosphers defined it as harmony, balance and
proportion, expressed most subtly in the 'golden section':
the concept of subdividing an object so that the smaller
part is to the greater as the greater is to the whole.
This formula for beauty implies that all beautiful things,
including the face, are divisible into parts expressing
the golden relation 1: 1.618 (Fig. 2.44). As a measure of
beauty, this proportion still has its champion: Ricketts
(1981, 1982) has designed a golden divider to ensure that
facial landmarks are related in this way. Some medieval
artists used the magical number 7; others used the
number 5. In the Renaissance, Leonardo da Vinci expressed facial proportions in geometric terms; Converse
(1977) has shown that these remain relevant in art and
in aesthetic surgery, and modern artists still take from
Leonardo the rule that the distance between each eye is
the width of one eye. This rule has been formulated in
the vertical division of the frontal face into fifths, each the
width of the eye from canthus to canthus (Powell &
Humphreys 1984); in the deformity of hypertelorism, the
intercanthal distance is greater (telecanthus) than one-fifth
of the face, and conversely smaller in hypotelorism. The
search for the mathematical basis of beauty has persisted
so that we still analyse faces using cephalometric X-ray
pictures and tracings from these, and relate normal populations to the abnormal, both beautiful and ugly. Nevertheless, aesthetic surgeons who make adjustments of the
facial skeleton to beautify normal faces do so on intuitive
appreciations and on the wishes of their patients as well
as on cephalometric norms (Rosen 1992; Munro 1992).

Measurement

Anthropometry is concerned with the measurements of
points on the face itself. Measurement has grown to be
very sophisticated, and may be made on 3-D images
obtained from CT scans or 3-D wire diagrams from
biplanar cephlometrics; the production of CAD/CAM
(see p. 549) models of faces is a natural progression
of the search for the mathematical secrets of beauty. Hard
tissue proportions are embodied in the many cephalometric analyses available. Steiner's S-curve and -line correlate
soft-tissue points of the nose, lips and chin; Holdaway's
H-angle endeavours to relate hard tissue to soft tissue.
Fig. 2.45 shows these, and two other profile relationships, which we have found helpful in surgical planning.
Powell & Humphreys (1984) have analysed the beautiful
profile in terms of the following soft-tissue geometric
relationships: the nasofrontal, nasofacial, nasomental, and
mentofacial angles, and the nasomental line. For each,

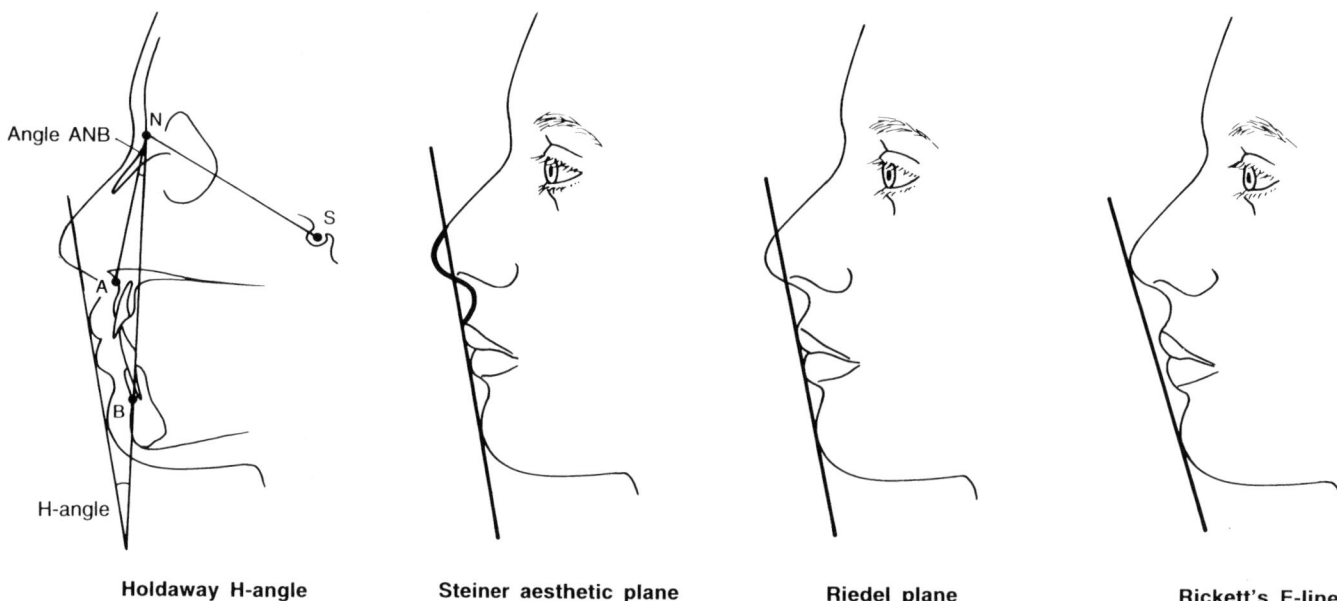

Fig. 2.45 Aesthetic geometry in the profile. In planning surgical reconstructions that will affect the profile, geometric concepts of the ideal adult profile are used. **A** Holdaway's H-angle: bone – soft tissue. Lines are drawn from the nasion N to the supramentale point B (deepest point in outer mandibular concavity) and the subspinale point A (deepest point in outer premaxillary concavity). The H line is drawn tangential to the soft tissue of the chin and upper lip; it makes an angle H with the line B. When the angle between NA and NB is 1–3°, the angle H ought to be 7–9°.
B Steiner's aesthetic soft-tissue plane. The lower border of the columella and the upper lip form a lazy S curve (heavy line in profile): a line is drawn from the middle of the S to the chin. The lips should lie on this line. **C** Riedel's soft-tissue plane. The upper lip, lower lip and chin should lie on a straight line. Redrawn from Powell & Humphreys (1984) by courtesy of Thieme Medical Publishers, Inc. **D** Rickett's soft-tissue E-line. A line from the nasal tip to the chin should be about 4 mm anterior to the upper lip and about 2 mm anterior to the lower lip.

norms have been derived from supposedly beautiful models, celebrities and patients.

Value judgements

There are many different ideas about the essentials of beauty, ranging from Hogarth's 'smooth serpentine line' to Francis Bacon's need for some element of strangeness, perfect symmetry being boring; the Miss Universe contests give much support to Bacon's view. Kant believed in simplicity, and this view periodically surfaces in aesthetic fashions. Some modern psychologists believe that aesthetic judgments are the result of a whole pattern of experiences at a particular time — the total experience. The total experience necessarily involves the brain behind the eye of the beholder if beauty is to be 'in the eye of the beholder'. The beholders, with few exceptions, include the persons themselves.

Freudian psychologists have related beauty to potential sexual function. Vigorous young men and healthy young women present the strength of one and the child-bearing potential of the other. These views have been roundly attacked by Schopenhauer and more recently by Simone de Beauvoir and her followers; but they seem to have relentless persistance. What also persists is the connection between goodness and beauty — an everyday assumption in modern film and television.

When the Scottish philosopher David Hume (1711–1776) threw his weight behind the concept that beauty is in the eye of the beholder, there was an imperative need to examine the eye of the beholder both in individuals and in the societies that mould them, in which there is infinite variety. If to some extent the face that we see (other than our own in the mirror) is a vehicle for personal projections, then there is an argument for examining the mind behind the eye of the beholder. Impressionist painters gave us every opportunity to use our eyes and our imaginations, and the surrealists such as Magritte show us some of the disturbances that may emerge.

Race provides a great variety of aesthetic ideals. There are significant variations of facial form and colour between the major human races, and within each of these are superimposed local cultural and personal preferences (Vistnes & Eskenazi 1991). Concepts of beauty vary radically on a national and cultural basis, and underlying these ethnic stereotypes are the desires and prejudices of the individual.

Trauma and aesthetics

In the setting of recent trauma, the aesthetics of the face may be disrupted in many ways; integument, bone, contour and muscle function may all be deformed or destroyed. With the exception of injury occuring in infancy and early childhood, it is the change that has been wrought that is important in planning treatment. The results of the treatment to correct the deformity produce a wide range of feelings in the affected individual, the family and the community. It is always helpful to have some idea of the appearance of the individual before the trauma, especially in a severely injured patient.

Aesthetic reconstruction is very complex, dealing as it does with bone, muscle, fat, skin and all the specialized structures of the face including the eyes, the nose, and the very special functions involved in movement, such as facial muscular action and eyelid closure, down to the beautiful lines of the lips with its vermillion and white roll borders. In trauma the problem for the treating team is not how to agree on the aesthetic ideal as visualized by the patient and then to conceptualize and deliver it. It is the problem of restoration where possible, as close as possible, to the pre-existing appearance as known to the patient. The aim is restoration not only of self-image but of body-image, so the problems of aesthetics that come into so many other aspects of cosmetic contouring of the craniofacial skeleton are set against a need to return the patient to the former self. This puts the use of measurements against objective standards raised from particular populations into perspective. The demanding requirement to restore the patient to the former self does indeed require some knowledge of the mensuration of ideal facial form but it is not necessary to have more than a reference to this as the emphasis is on restoring the former self.

An excellent up-to-date perspective of aesthetics in facial skeleton surgery is given by Rosen (1992) with expert commentary by Munro. Ricketts (1991) and Barkovic (1991) provide similar up-to-date references from the orthodontic point of view.

REFERENCES

Abbott J R, Moore M H, David D J 1992 The influence of the maxillary canine on mandibular fracture. J Craniofac Surg 3: 141–144

Amaral D G 1987 Memory: anatomical organization of candidate brain regions. In: Mountcastle V B, Plum F, Geiger S R (eds) Handbook of physiology: section 1. The nervous system. American Physiological Society, Bethesda, Vol 5, Ch 7

Barkovic K 1991 Cephalometry and assessment of craniofacial form of proportions. In: Ousterhoud D K (ed) Aesthetic contouring of the craniofacial skeleton. Little, Brown & Co., Boston

Beck E McLardy T, Meyer A 1950 Anatomical comments on psychosurgical procedures. J Ment Sci 96: 157–167

Björk A 1960 The relationship of jaws to the cranium. In: Lundström A (ed) Introduction to orthodontics. McGraw-Hill, London, pp 104–140

Björk A 1969 Prediction of mandibular growth rotation. Am J Orthodont 55: 585–599

Björk A, Skieller V 1972 Facial development and tooth eruption. An implant study at the age of puberty. Am J Orthodont 62: 339–383

Björk A, Skieller V 1974 Growth in width of the maxilla studied by the implant method. Scand J Plast Reconst Surg 8: 26–33

Björk A, Skieller V 1976 Postnatal growth and development of the maxillary complex. In: McNamara J A (ed) Factors affecting the growth of the midface. Center for Human Growth and Development University of Michigan, Ann Arbor, pp 61–99

Björk A, Skieller V 1977 Growth of the maxilla in three dimensions as revealed radiographically by the implant method. Br J Orthodont 4: 53–64

Björk A, Skieller V 1983 Normal and abnormal growth of the mandible. A synthesis of longitudinal cephalometric implant studies over a period of 25 years. Eur J Orthodont 5: 1–46

Blanton P L, Biggs N L 1969 Eighteen hundred years of controversy: the paranasal sinuses. Am J Anat 124: 135–147

Blinkov S M, Gabibov G A, Tcherekayev V A 1986 Transcranial approaches to the orbital part of the optic nerve: an anatomical study. J Neurosurg 65: 44–47

Böck J, Bornstein H, Hommer K 1963 Die Wiederbelebungszeit der menschlichen Netzhaut. Eine elektrographische Studie. Graefe Arch Ophthalmol 165: 435–451

Bradley J C 1975 A radiological investigation into the age changes of the inferior dental artery. Br J Oral Surg 13: 82–90

Broadbent B H 1937 The face of the normal child. Angle Orthod 7: 188–207

Brodal A 1981 Neurological anatomy in relation to clinical medicine, 3rd edn. Oxford University Press, New York

Brown T, Townsend G C, Richards L C, Burgess V B 1990 Concepts of occlusion: Australian evidence. Am J Phys Anthropol 82: 247–256

Caldicott W J H, North J B, Simpson D A 1973 Traumatic cerebrospinal fluid fistulas in children. J Neurosurg 38: 1–9

Carpenter M B, Sutin J 1983 Human neuroanatomy, 8th edn. Williams & Wilkins, Baltimore

Converse J M 1977 Introduction to plastic surgery. In: Converse J M (ed) Reconstructive plastic surgery. Saunders, Philadelphia, Vol 1, Ch 1

Cooter R D, David D J 1989 Computer-based coding of fractures in the craniofacial region. Br J Plast Surg 42: 17–26

Couly G, Hureau J, Tessier P 1976 The anatomy of the external palpebral ligament in man. J Maxillofac Surg 4: 195–197

Crompton M R 1971 Hypothalamic lesions following closed head injury. Brain 94: 165–172

Daniel P M, Prichard M M L, Treip C S 1959 Traumatic infarction of the anterior lobe of the pituitary gland. Lancet 2: 927–930

David D J, Poswillo D, Simpson D 1982 The craniosynostoses. Causes, natural history, and management. Springer, Berlin, p 25

Davies D V, Coupland R E 1967 Gray's anatomy. Descriptive and applied, 34th edn. Longmans, London

Deuschle F M 1969 Some annotations on the anatomy of the maxillofacial region. Otolaryngol Clin N Am, June Issue: 243–249

Diamanti J A 1991 A study of tooth emergence in South Australian children with particular reference to a sample exhibiting agenesis of the permanent first molar. Research report for B.Sc. (Dent) degree, University of Adelaide

Dusoir H, Kapur N, Byrnes D P, McKinstry S, Hoare R D 1990 The role of diencephalic pathology in human memory disorder. Evidence from a penetrating paranasal brain injury. Brain 113: 1695–1706

Duvernoy H 1991 The human brain. Surface, three-dimensional sectional anatomy and MRI. Springer, Wien

Enlow D H 1982 Handbook of facial growth, 2nd edn. Saunders, Philadelphia

Eveleth P B, Tanner J M 1976 Worldwide variation in human growth. Cambridge University Press, Cambridge, pp 207–277

Fain 1980 La role percussive des traumatismes du massif facial sur l'etage anterieur de la base du crâne. Rev Stomatol Chir Maxillofac 81: 31–43

Farmand M, Gottsauner A 1991 Endoskopische Befunde der Kieferhöhle bei frischen Mittelgesichtsfrakturen. Fortschr Kiefer Gesichtschir 36: 27–30

Fox J L, Falik J L, Shalhoub R J 1971 Neurosurgical hyponatremia: the role of inappropriate antidiuresis. J Neurosurg 34: 506–514

Garn S M, Werthheimer F, Sandusky S T, McCann M B 1972 Advanced tooth emergence in Negro individuals. J Dent Res 51: 1506

Gentry L R, Manor W F, Turski P A, Strother C M 1983 High resolution CT analysis of facial struts in trauma: 1 Normal anatomy. Am J Roentgenol 140: 523–532

Graff-Radford N R, Tranel D, Van Hoesen G W, Brandt J P 1990 Diencephalic amnesia. Brain 113: 1–25

Gruss J S, Mackinnon S E 1986 Complex maxillary fractures: role of buttress reconstruction and immediate bone grafts. Plast Reconstr Surg 78: 9–22

Haines D E, Harkey H L, Al-Mefty O 1993 The 'subdural space': a new look at an outdated concept. Neurosurgery 32: 111–120

Har-Shai Y, Fukuta K, Collares MV et al 1992 The vascular anatomy of the galeal flap in the interparietal and midline regions. Plast Reconstr Surg 89: 64–69

Heinze J 1969 Cranial nerve avulsion and other neural injuries in road accidents. Med J Aust 2: 1246–1249

Jeeves M A, Simpson D A, Geffen G 1979 Functional consequences of the transcallosal removal of intraventricular tumours. J Neurol Neurosurg Psychiat 42: 134–142

Jend H H, Jend-Rossman I 1984 Sphenotemporal buttress fracture. Neuroradiology 26: 411–413

Kempe L G 1980 Topical organization of the distal portion of the facial nerve. J Neurosurg 52: 671–673

Koski K 1971 Some characteristics of cranio-facial growth cartilages. In: Moyers R E, Krogman W M (eds) Cranio-facial growth in man. Pergamon Press, Oxford, pp 25–138

Lang J 1983 Clinical anatomy of the head. Neurocranium, orbit, craniocervical regions. Springer, Berlin

Last R J 1977 Wolff's anatomy of the eye and orbit, 7th edn (revised). Lewis, London

Lee M M C, Low W D, Chang K S F 1965 Eruption of the permanent dentition of Southern Chinese in Hong Kong. Arch Oral Biol 10: 849–861

Leighton B C 1968 Eruption of deciduous teeth. Practioner 200: 836–842

Luce E A 1984 Maxillofacial trauma. Curr Probl Surg 21: 1–68

Lysell L, Magnusson B, Thilander B 1962 Time and order of eruption of primary teeth; a longitudinal study. Odont Revy 13: 217–234

Malcolm L A, Bue B 1970 Eruption times of permanent teeth and the determination of age in New Guinea children. Trop Geogr Med 22: 307–312

Maniscalco J E, Habal M B 1978 Microanatomy of the optic canal. J Neurosurg 48: 402–406

Manson P N, Hoopes J E, Su C T 1980 Structural pillars of the facial skeleton: an approach to the management of Le Fort fractures. Plast Reconstr Surg 66: 54–62

Marano S R, Fischer D W, Gaines C, Sonntag V K H 1985 Anatomical study of the superficial temporal artery. Neurosurgery 16: 786–790

McMinn R M H 1990 Last's anatomy. Regional and applied, 8th edn. Churchill Livingstone, Edinburgh

Millen J W, Woollam D H M 1962 The anatomy of the cerebrospinal fluid. Oxford University Press, London

Moran D T, Jafek B W, Rowley J C 1991 The ultrastructure of the human nasal mucosa. In: Laing D G, Doty R L, Breipohl W (eds) The human sense of smell. Springer, Berlin

Moss M L 1971 Ontogenetic aspects of cranio-facial growth. In: Moyers R E, Krogman W M (eds.) Cranio-facial growth in man. Pergamon, Oxford, pp 109–124

Moss M 1972 Twenty years of functional cranial analysis. Am J Orthod 61: 479–485

Munro I 1992 Perspectives in aesthetic surgery, Vol 2, pp 1–25

Nabeshima S, Reese T S, Landis D M D, Brightman M W 1975 Junctions in the meninges and marginal glia. J Comp Neurol 164: 127–170

Noback C R, Strominger N L, Demarest R J 1991 The human nervous system. Introduction and review, 4th edn. Lea & Febiger, Philadelphia

Parkinson D 1984 Arteries of the cavernous sinus (letter) J Neurosurg 61: 203

Penhall B 1992 The mylohoid ridge and endoalveolar crest: an anatomical and clinical study with reference to preprosthetic surgery. MDS thesis, University of Adelaide, Adelaide

Pogrel M A, Dodson T, Tom W 1987 Arteriographic patency of the inferior alveolar artery and its relevance to alveolar atrophy. J Oral Maxillofac Surg 45: 767–770

Pollock R A 1992 Nasal trauma: pathomechanics and surgical management of acute injuries. Clin Plast Surg 19: 133–147

Powell N, Humphreys B 1984 Proportions of the aesthetic face. Thieme, New York

Renn W H, Rhoton A L 1975 Microsurgical anatomy of the sellar region. J Neurosurg 43: 288–298

Ricketts R M 1981 The golden divider. J Clin Orthodont 15: 752–759

Ricketts R M 1982 The biologic significance of the divine proportion and Fibonacci series. Am J Orthod 81: 351–370

Ricketts R M. 1991 The science and art of aesthetic recontouring of the face. In: Ousterhout D K (ed) Aesthetic contouring of the craniofacial skeleton. Little, Brown & Co., Boston

Riu R, Le Den R, Gourlaoven A 1960 Contribution a l'étude du role des sinus paranasaux. Laryngol Otol Rhinol (Bordeaux) 81: 796–839

Rodriguez R L, Zide B M 1988 Reconstruction of the medial canthus. Clin Plast Surg 15: 255–262

Rosen H M 1992 Perspectives in aesthetic surgery, Vol 2, pp 1–25

Rowbotham G F 1939 Observations on the effect of trigeminal denervation. Brain 62: 364–380

Rowe N L, Killey H C 1955 Fractures of the facial skeleton, Livingstone, Edinburgh

Scott J H 1967 Dento-facial development and growth. Pergamon Press, Oxford

Scott J H, Dixon A D 1978 Anatomy for students of dentistry, 4th edn. Churchill Livingstone, Edinburgh, p 357

Shipley M, Reyes P 1991 In: Laing D G, Doty R L, Breipohl W (eds) The human sense of smell. Springer, Berlin, Ch 2

Sicher H M, Du Brul E L 1975 Oral anatomy, 6th edn. Mosby, St Louis

Simpson D A 1952 The efferent fibres of the hippocampus in the monkey. J Neurol Neurosurg Psychiat 15: 79–92

Stammberger H 1991 Functional endoscopic sinus surgery. The Messerklinger technique. Decker, Philadelphia

Stephens R B, Stilwell D L 1969 Arteries and veins of the human brain. Thomas, Springfield

Sturla F, Absi D, Buquet J 1980 Anatomical and mechanical considerations of craniofacial fractures: an experimental study. Plast Reconstr Surg 66: 815–820

Sumner D 1976 Disturbances of the senses of smell and taste after head injuries. In: Vinken P J, Bruyn G W (eds) Handbook of clinical neurology. North-Holland, Amsterdam, Vol 24, Part 2, Ch 1

Tow P M, Lewin W 1953 Orbital leucotomy (isolation of the orbital cortex by open operation). Lancet 2: 644–649

Vistnes L M, Eskenazi L B 1991 Cultural aspects of beauty. In: Ousterhout D K (ed) Aesthetic contouring of the craniofacial skeleton. Little, Brown & Co., Boston

Volchansky A, Makings E 1984 A new mandibular landmark? J Dent 12: 221–224

Walsh K W 1978 Neuropsychology. A clinical approach. Churchill Livingstone, Edinburgh

Walsh K W 1985 Understanding brain damage. A primer of neuropsychological evaluation. Churchill Livingstone, Edinburgh

Walsh & Hoyt's Clinical Neuro-ophthalmology, 4th edn, 1985, Miller N R (ed). Williams & Wilkins, Baltimore, Vol 2

Weinmann J P, Sicher H 1947 Bone and bones. Fundamentals of bone biology. Kimpton, London

Whitaker L A 1984 Selective alteration of palpebral fissure form by lateral canthopexy. Plast Reconstr Surg 74: 611–619

Whitty C W M, Lewin W 1960 A Korsakoff syndrome in the post-cingulectomy confusional state. Brain 83: 648–653

Winternitz W W, Dzur J A 1976 Pituitary failure secondary to head trauma. Case report. J Neurosurg 44: 504–505

Xuereb G P, Prichard M L M, Daniel P M 1954a The arterial supply and venous drainage of the human hypophysis cerebri. Q J Exp Physiol 39: 199–217

Xuereb G P, Prichard M L M, Daniel P M 1954b The hypophysial portal system of vessels in man. Q J Exp Physiol 39: 219–230

Young V L, Gumucio C A, Lund H, MacMahon R, Ueda K, Pidgeon L 1992 Long-term effect of retrobulbar haematoma on the vision of Cynomolgus monkeys. Plast Reconstr Surg 89: 70–76

Zide B M, Jelks G W 1985 Surgical anatomy of the orbit. Raven Press, New York

Zide B M, McCarthy J G 1983 The medial canthus revisited: an anatomical basis for canthopexy. Ann Plast Surg 11: 1–9

Epidemiology

D. A. Simpson   A. J. McLean

INTRODUCTION

The craniomaxillofacial (CMF) region is defined for our purposes as the whole face from the chin to the coronal suture, together with the underlying viscera and skeletal structures (Fig. 2.1). The epidemiology of injuries in this anatomical region is of practical importance from several viewpoints, not least in planning trauma services. The injuries are often complex, involving more than one functional system; they are likely to need coordinated management by specialists in two or more disciplines. The number of cases in a region is therefore important in the organization of the regional trauma service, and especially in justifying the formation of a multidisciplinary craniofacial unit, since this relatively complex team needs a substantial workload to function efficiently (p. 678). Aetiological trauma data are also necessary from the viewpoint of preventive public health. Changes in the causes of CMF injuries can reflect societal problems of many kinds, and trauma surgeons who see increases in the incidence or severity of CMF injuries are well placed to give warning of these and to call for preventive measures.

EPIDEMIOLOGY OF CMF INJURY

Case identification

For epidemiological and aetiological studies, there are difficulties in identifying cases of CMF trauma in records and statistical publications. This is because impacts in the area may damage not only the facial skeleton and integuments, but also the eyes and the brain, structures whose great functional importance justifies separate identification in hospital records and similar sources of injury data.

The International Classification of Disease (ICD) is used throughout the world for statistical purposes and has great value in epidemiological research, though clinicians have been rather slow to use it. The ninth revision (ICD9: World Health Organization 1977) lists facial injuries under the following headings:

N802: Fracture of face bones, with fourth digit identification of fractures of the nasal bones, mandible, malar and maxillary bones, orbital floor, and other facial bones.
N830: Dislocation of jaw.
N873: Other open wounds of head, a category including dental fractures and soft-tissue wounds of the face and mouth; fourth and fifth digits giving more exact anatomical locations are included in a clinical modification of the code.
Burns (N941) of the scalp, face and neck are identified and subclassified according to depth; burns of the mouth are separately identified (N947.0).

Thus, trauma in the mid- and lower facial region is well identified in this code. However, ICD9 does not identify fractures of the anterior fossa except in the general categories of fractures of the skull vault (N800) and base (N801). The optic nerves are listed as N950; other cranial nerves appear as N951, with fourth digit identification of individual cranial nerves, though not of the olfactory nerve, one of the nerves most often injured in CMF trauma. The cerebral injuries which often dominate the clinical presentation of impacts in the CMF region are coded separately (N850–854). Head injuries involving transient loss of consciousness are listed as concussion (N850), but in the clinical modification (ICD9-CM) of the code, the concept of concussion is extended to include cases with prolonged unconsciousness. Intracranial bleeding appears confusingly in two categories, distinguished by the presence or absence of skull fracture: Jennett & Frankowski (1990) have noted the practical difficulties in this. Penetrating injuries of the eyeball (N871) and its adnexae (N870) are adequately identified but the late complications of ocular injuries are listed elsewhere. The tenth revision (ICD 10: World Health Organization 1992) uses an alphanumeric coding. Fractures of the skull vault (S02.0) and skull base (S02.1) are identified without anatomical subclassification; the individual facial bones (S02.2–9) are identified less minutely than in ICD9. Cranial nerve injuries (S04), injuries of the eye and orbit (S05; S01.1), and injuries of the intracranial contents (S06) are coded in a compact and convenient form, and it is now possible to identify cerebral oedema, diffuse or focal cerebral injury and the different types of intracranial haematoma, in accordance with modern concepts of the neuropathology of head impacts (see Chs 5 and 13). Head injuries with loss of consciousness are also better identified. Burns and corrosions of the head, face and neck (T20), and of the mouth (T28.0) are identified much as in ICD9, and there is also provision for separate coding of burns of the eye (T26).

A coder skilled in the use of ICD9 can prepare data suitable for a reasonably exact and detailed anatomical categorization of most types of CMF injury. Unfortunately, in hospital practice, injury coding is often incomplete, or even incorrect. This is especially true of multiple injuries, where secondary injuries not seen as life-threatening may not be coded at all. Thus, hospital statistics may not give a full picture of the prevalence of the diagnostic categories that represent the CMF trauma workload of a craniofacial unit or of the equivalent services in centres that do not have such a unit. Hospital coded data may also be inadequate for clinical studies and audits; many maxillofacial surgeons, neurosurgeons and ophthalmologists prefer to use data bases taken from unit log books or departmental records. The inadequacies of ICD-based data for coding cerebral injuries appear to have been remedied in ICD10, but we have as yet no experience of this system in clinical coding. In the USA, a multiaxial coding system called SNOMED has been proposed as an alternative to ICD, but this system is said to be too complicated for clinical use (Pollock & Evans 1993). In the UK, the Read Clinical Classification has received governmental approval; it has the merit of automatic cross-reference to the ICD system.

It should be possible to use the data collected by health authorities to study the aetiology of CMF trauma. Both ICD9 and ICD10 list causes of injury under separate codes in great detail; provided that coding is efficient,

hospital records collated by national or regional health authorities give useful population-based data on injury causation. Unfortunately efficient indexing of external causes is not always achieved by coders whose business is the cost of injuries; Klopfer et al (1992), in a recent US study of eye injuries, found ICD coding of external cause in only a quarter of their sample of hospital discharges. Clinical reports on CMF injuries may also be incomplete from this viewpoint, since they are usually published for purposes other than epidemiology; moreover, they are often selected because of some special interest in a particular field of trauma management. The formation of injury surveillance registers will doubtless clarify many uncertainties; at present, the world picture of CMF trauma has to be collated from many sources, some of which are not reliable.

Population-based incidence rates

There have been several attempts to quantify head injuries in defined populations, but most of these have been primarily concerned with craniocerebral trauma and have excluded or only partially considered facial injuries. An exception is the study by Selecki et al (1981), which surveyed all cases of 'neurotrauma' hospitalized in the Australian state of New South Wales (population 4 960 000) in the year 1977. Neurotrauma was taken to include all injuries to the head, spine and peripheral nervous system, as identified by the version (ICD 8) of the International Classification of Disease then in use. In the year under study, there were 3982 admissions with the primary diagnosis of facial fracture, representing 17.7% of all admissions for neurotrauma or 25.1% if head injury admissions only are considered. Thus, this study indicated a minimum incidence of 80 CMF injuries per 100 000 population at risk. Large as this number is, it is certainly too small because the diagnostic category 'facial fracture' excludes an unknown but surely not insignificant number of other head injuries with involvement of the anterior cranial fossa and/or frontal bone, and doubtless also a number of cases in which facial fractures were present but not coded as the primary diagnosis. The data also exclude those facial fractures, chiefly nasal fractures, not admitted to hospital. We have no data for eye injuries in our community; in the USA, it appears that the annual hospital admission rate is 29.1 per 100 000 population, the eye injury being the principal diagnosis in nearly half (Klopfer et al 1992).

Age and sex

In all the series reviewed by us, and in our own experience, the victims of CMF injury have been predominantly young men. The peak age incidence is usually in the decade 20–29, though no age is exempt (Fig. 3.1). Children

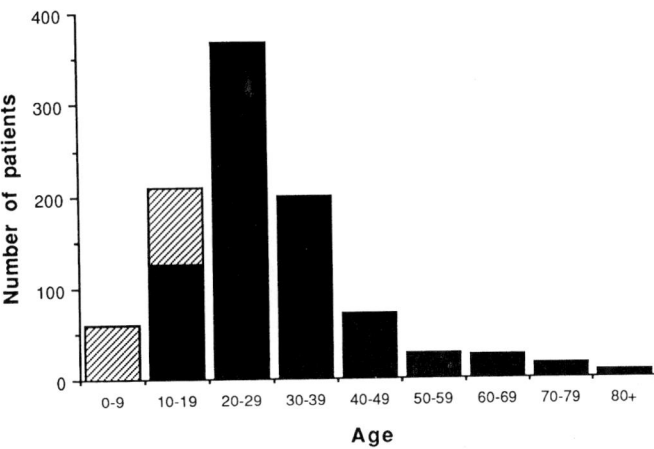

Fig. 3.1 Age distribution of fractures of the facial skeleton. Age distribution in 839 cases of facial fractures admitted to the Royal Adelaide Hospital, 1989–1992 (black bars) and 145 cases of facial fractures admitted to the Adelaide Childrens' Hospital in the same 3 year period (hatched bars). The series are not strictly comparable as the adult series excludes an uncertain number of fractures of the nose

(1–14 years) constituted 12.2% of our combined series of facial fractures and 15.6% of our series of anterior fossa fractures selected for neurosurgical management; there were fewer old people (⩾ 60 years) in these series — 5.0% and 3.4% respectively. The incidence of paediatric cases in the first series would be even lower if nasal fractures were excluded. The male:female ratio is commonly about 4:1, being higher with more severe injuries: in our series of adult facial fractures the ratio was 4.25:1, but 6:1 in our series of anterior cranial fossa fractures needing neurosurgical management.

AETIOLOGY OF CMF INJURIES

Causes of injury

In considering these, it is important to take into account the society in which the injury occurs, because trauma is a mirror of socio-economic conditions. The spectrum of trauma causation often changes over time, favourably in response to preventive public health measures, adversely as communities suffer from increases in endemic or pandemic violence. Also, for the reasons given above, it is difficult to get an overall picture of the causes of CMF trauma in different parts of the world from official statistics. One must therefore look at hospital-based clinical studies giving the causes of injury in various components of the region. But in many of these studies, the causes are poorly described, especially with respect to different categories of road users. Nevertheless, recent reports from developed countries show very similar trends.

In most North American and European communities not involved in war or large-scale insurgency, the two leading causes of CMF injury are road crashes and assault. Falls, sporting accidents, and industrial accidents

are important but less common causes. The relative importance of road trauma and injuries from assault varies, but it appears that in most Western societies, road crashes are becoming fewer and assaults more numerous. Reports from trauma services in the USA (Scherer et al 1989), Europe (Andersson et al 1989, Brook & Wood 1983, Dimitroulis & Eyre 1991, Neumann 1991), Australia (Allan & Daley 1990) and New Zealand (Hammond et al 1991) show that assault is now the leading single cause of fractures of the middle and lower face, accounting for 38–70% of cases admitted to hospital. However, the dominance of assault must be qualified. In most of these reported series, fractures of the upper third of the face are excluded: in reports on this small but important group of injuries from the USA (Lee et al 1987) and Europe (Ioannides et al 1984), some 70% of cases were due to road crashes. Serious maxillary fractures of Le Fort type and panfacial fractures are likewise usually due to road crashes. It is also pertinent that many of the centres reporting very high proportions of CMF injury from assault are reflecting behaviour in depressed urban societies; reports from rural areas and smaller towns in the USA (Cook & Rowe 1990, Schroeder 1989) show a much lower proportion of assaulted patients, as did Bochlogyrus (1985) from Münster, a city once notorious for religious violence but now a peaceful university town in proximity to fast road traffic. In Greece also, road crashes caused 57% of all cases of middle and lower third fractures admitted to a large oral/maxillofacial unit, assault being responsible for only 9%; this series excluded nasal fractures which were treated by plastic surgeons (Zachariades & Papavassiliou 1990). The trauma spectra in Asian and African countries are less well reported, but rapid motorization is a major public health problem in developing countries, and it is not surprising that in western Nigeria (Abiose 1986) and Saudi Arabia (Brown & Cowpe 1985) road crashes are the leading cause, at least in admissions to large hospitals.

Eye injuries have special epidemiological features. Even in highly motorized societies, injuries caused in sport and play may be more numerous than those due to road accidents (Canavan et al 1980), though road accidents account for a disproportionately large number of injuries resulting in blindness. Work-related eye injuries figure prominently in some reports, often resulting from flying metal missiles striking eyes not protected by safety spectacles. Assault is a prominent cause of eye injuries in communities with a high level of endemic aggression. Zagelbaum et al (1993) found that assault accounted for 28% of 584 eye injuries treated in a New York City trauma centre, as against only 13% occurring at work and 4% related to sports.

Our own experience is reflected in Tables 3.1 and 3.2. Table 3.1 summarizes a recent prospective study of 839 facial fractures referred to us over a 3 year period

Table 3.1 Facial fractures in an adult general hospital, 1989–1992

	No. of cases as (%)
Road traffic accidents	158 (18.8)
Assault	430 (51.3)
Sports-related	137 (16.3)
Falls	81 (9.7)
Gunshot	6 (0.7)
Industrial	13 (1.5)
Others	14 (1.7)
Total	839 (100)

Table 3.2 Anterior cranial fossa fractures (all ages) referred for neurosurgical management

	No. of cases as (%)
Road traffic accidents	168 (70.9)
Assault	7 (3.0)
Sports-related	10 (4.2)
Falls	18 (7.6)
Gunshot	6 (2.5)
Industrial	10 (4.2)
Others	9 (3.8)
Unknown	9 (3.8)
Total	237 (100)

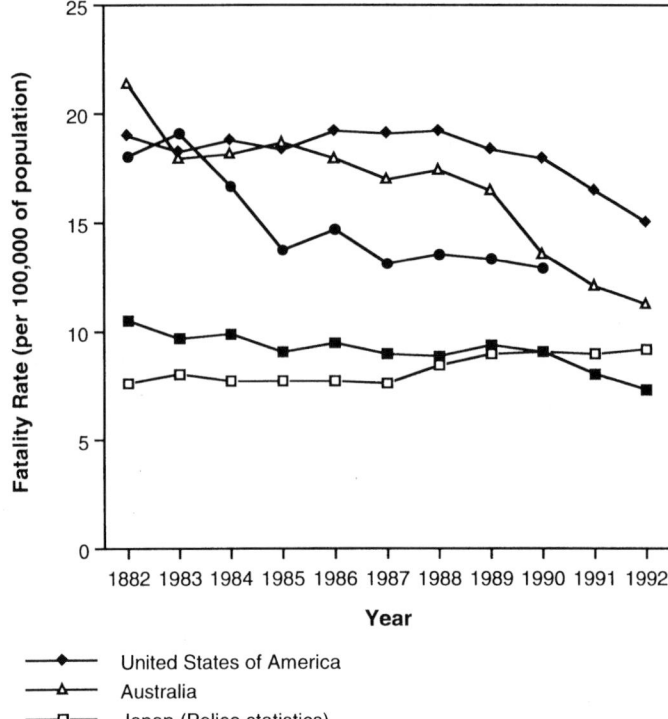

- United States of America
- Australia
- Japan (Police statistics)
- West Germany
- United Kingdom

Fig. 3.2 Trends in the incidence of road fatalities. Since 1982, there has been a downward trend in the rate of deaths from road crashes in the USA, Australia, West Germany, the UK and other developed countries. This has not been seen in Japan, where there has been a slight rise in recent years. [Sources of data: USA: National Highway Traffic Safety Administration, Fatal Accident Reporting System; includes deaths within 30 days of accident. West Germany: Economic Commission for Europe; includes deaths within 30 days of accident. Because of epidemiological changes resulting from the reunification of Germany, data after 1990 are not given. Japan: National Police Agency data; Ministry of Welfare figures are > 10% higher as police figures exclude deaths after 24 h. UK: Department of Transport; includes deaths within 30 days of accident. Australia: Department of Transport & Communications; includes deaths within 30 days of accident.]

in our chief adult general hospital. In this series, assault, chiefly with fists or blunt weapons, was the leading cause (51.3%) and road crashes accounted for only 18.8%. During the same period, 145 cases of facial fracture were managed in an associated paediatric hospital; the causes of injury in this series are less well established, but the proportion of cases due to road crashes was a little larger. Table 3.2 gives data from a retrospective review of 237 cases of anterior fossa fracture (all ages) referred for neurosurgical management over a period of some 35 years; in 89 (37.6%) there were additional fractures in the lower face (Table 13.2). In this series, road crashes were the cause in a large (70.9%) majority.

Our experience of CMF trauma is derived from a reasonably affluent, highly motorized society with a low use of firearms for homicidal purposes, and a fondness for outdoor sports. The national per capita consumption of alcohol is high, ranking in 1989 as highest among English-speaking countries and fifteenth in the world; however, as in other developed countries, there has been a fall in the per capita alcohol consumption in the last decade. Alcohol is a factor in the causation of many CMF injuries: in our series of facial fractures, we found alcohol to be involved in about one-third of all road crashes and more than half of all assaults. Nevertheless, consumption of alcohol has been declining since 1980, and this may be a factor in the very gratifying fall in road deaths over the same period (Commonwealth Department of Health, Housing and Community Services 1992). Australia is

unusual in having a history of early and enthusiastic community support for many safety measures, especially road safety (Simpson & McLean 1988); however the downward trend in road fatalities has been seen also in the USA and some other developed countries (Fig. 3.2). This national background must be taken into account in considering the data cited in later chapters.

Road crashes

Car occupants, motor cyclists and pedal cyclists often suffer injuries in the CMF region, especially in frontal crashes. Pedestrians may also be injured in this part of the body, though our studies of pedestrian fatalities suggest that the first head impact, which is likely to be most

Table 3.3 Impact sites in three series of fatal head injuries in road crashes*

Impact site	Vehicle occupants	Pedestrians	Motor cyclists
Frontal/facial	14 (34%)	27 (23%)	34 (46%)
Lateral	20 (49%)	33 (28%)	13 (17%)
Occipital	3 (7%)	16 (14%)	8 (11%)
Multiple	4 (10%)	40 (35%)	19 (26%)
Total in series	41 (100)	116 (100)	74 (100)

* Cases where the impact site(s) could not be identified are excluded. (Unpublished data from NH & MRC Road Accident Research Unit, Adelaide.)

injurious, is usually in another cranial site (Ryan et al 1989). Table 3.3 sets out the impact sites in the three chief categories of road crashes, established in autopsied cases.

Two questions arise from this high incidence of CMF injuries in road crashes. Are certain categories of road user especially at risk? And are certain types of CMF injury especially characteristic of road crashes? Unfortunately, many surgical series fail to specify the type of road user, while accident analysts often fail to give data relating to the type of injury. Nevertheless, the answer to both questions is a qualified yes.

In our clinical experience of CMF injuries, the different categories of road user are represented roughly in the proportions expected from the statistics of fatal road injuries of all types in our community, with the exception of pedestrians, who represent a smaller proportion. It is generally agreed that extensive panfacial fractures are typically the result of impacts seen when car drivers strike the steering wheel or column in severe frontal crashes. In the past, penetrating injuries of the frontal lobes and eyes were very frequently due to impacts on the windscreen in frontal crashes (Fig. 3.3A,B), but the use of laminated glass has almost eliminated these injuries, and for a pedestrian, the windscreen is now one of the least threatening parts of an oncoming car (Fig. 3.3C). Upper third facial injuries are usually due to vehicular accidents: this is evident in our data and in the small Dutch series reported by Ioannides et al (1984). Middle third fractures, especially those of Le Fort type, are most often caused by road crashes: impact with the steering assembly is often responsible (Table 3.4). Lower third (mandibular) fractures are often seen in road crash victims, either as isolated injuries or as part of panfacial trauma.

Preventive measures have affected the incidence of CMF injuries among car occupants in several developed countries. Seat belt usage has dramatically reduced the risk of fatal injury, but not the risk of CMF injuries among drivers. Afzelius & Rosen (quoted by Rutherford et al 1985) in Sweden could not show a fall in the overall number of facial fractures, though they did find that seat belts reduced the number of serious fractures of the

Le Fort type. In the UK, Rutherford et al (1985) carried out a major study of hospital attendances before and after the introduction of mandatory use of seat belts. Table 3.5 gives data for the chief CMF injuries in the year preceding compulsory belt use, and the percentage change in the following year. It is notable that brain injuries (not all from impacts in the CMF area) were nearly five times more numerous than facial fractures, and six times more numerous than eye injuries. Seat belt legislation was associated with a large fall in the total number of brain injuries, but disconcertingly a rise in the number of serious (AIS $\geqslant$ 3) brain injuries. This appeared to be because belts gave good protection to car passengers, but increased the risk of impact of the driver's head on the steering wheel. This finding appears to give powerful support to the use of airbags, at least on the driver's side. A report from the USA has compared the benefits of airbags and automatic seat belts: it appeared from this that drivers of cars equipped with an airbag had a 24% lower risk of an injury severe enough to need hospital admission, and a lower rate of moderate–severe head injury (Insurance Special Report A-38 1991). Rutherford's study showed a striking reduction in the number of eye injuries, confirming earlier Australian studies on the benefits of seat belts from this viewpoint.

Motor cyclists are at relatively high risk of impact in the CMF region (Table 3.3) and have undoubtedly benefited from helmets (Fig. 3.4A,B). Convincing evidence for this has come from epidemiological studies comparing the risks of death in helmeted and unhelmeted motor cyclists. The pioneer Australian study by Foldvary & Lane (1964) was dramatically confirmed when a number of US states repealed legislation mandating the use of helmets, in deference to partisans of so-called civil liberty. In almost all of these States there was a sharp rise in deaths among unhelmeted motor cyclists, and it was possible to show that riding unhelmeted carries an increased risk of death of 28 ± 8% (Evans & Frick 1988); Wagle et al (1993) and other writers have found no compensating reduction in the risk of spinal injury. Mandatory use of helmets was introduced in South Australia in 1967 and full-face helmets became popular in the 1970s; Vaughan (1977) showed that these reduce the risk of facial injury. Pedal cyclists may also suffer impacts in the CMF area, though less often than motorcyclists; indeed, Fife et al (1983) found only one major (AIS $\geqslant$ 3) facial injury in 173 fatal bicycle accidents. Pedal cycle helmets are now widely used, and have been made mandatory in most Australian states (McDermott 1992). The helmets now in general favour do not fully protect the frontal region (Williams 1991) but give valuable protection to much of the calvarial vault (Fig. 3.5). The benefits and limitations of helmets are further discussed in Chapter 4.

Alcohol is a leading cause of road crashes in countries

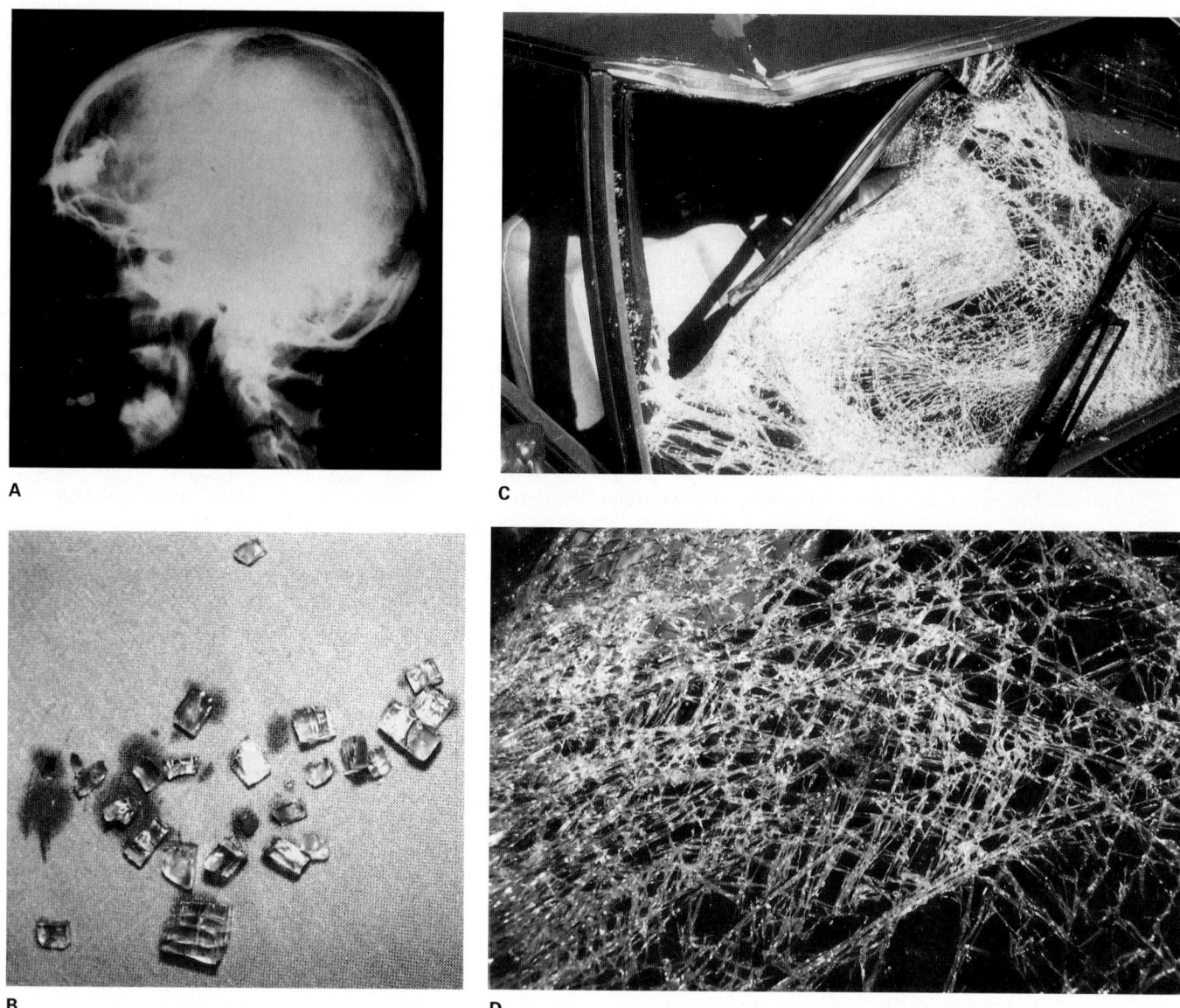

Fig. 3.3 Windscreen injury: injury control by laminated glass. Windscreens made of toughened glass were formerly a frequent cause of craniofacial wounds. The advent of laminated glass has greatly reduced the risk of blindness and brain injury from windscreen impacts.
A Toughened glass embedded in the frontal lobe of a car driver. **B** Typical fragments of toughened glass, removed at operation. **C** Typical star fracture of laminated glass: a pedestrian's head struck in the centre of the windscreen. It was softer than the roof rail (arrow). **D** Close view: the glass is shattered but the lamina of plastic prevents the fragments from breaking loose.

Table 3.4 Fracture sites and aetiology in 839 cases of facial fractures admitted to an adult general hospital

	Assault	Road traffic accidents	Sports	Falls	Other
Frontal	1	2	0	1	2
Orbit	60	4	14	6	4
Zygoma	121*	27	66*	30*	8
Nasal	43	15	10	5	3
Maxilla	8	4	1	3	1
Mandible	170*	44*	40*	32*	13
Le Fort, panfacial and other complex facial fractures	27	62*	6	4	2
Total no. of patients	430	158	137	81	33

* Indicates the two major sites in each aetiological category.

Table 3.5 Numbers of injuries among 8237 hospital attenders, with percentage effect of mandatory seatbelt legislation*

Injury	No. of injured persons				% effect
	Driver	FSP	RSP	Total	
Brain					
Minor	606	296	151	1053	−36.6%
Severe	32	22	13	67	+7.5%
Total	638	318	164	1120	−33.9%
Facial fracture					
Minor	130	52	36	218	
Severe	4	7	0	11	
Total	134	59	36	229	−7.4%
Eye (all types)	98	53	14	164 (?5)	−33.5%

* Simplified from Tables 28, 29 and 39 of Rutherford et al (1985).
FSP = front seat passenger; RSP = rear seat passenger.

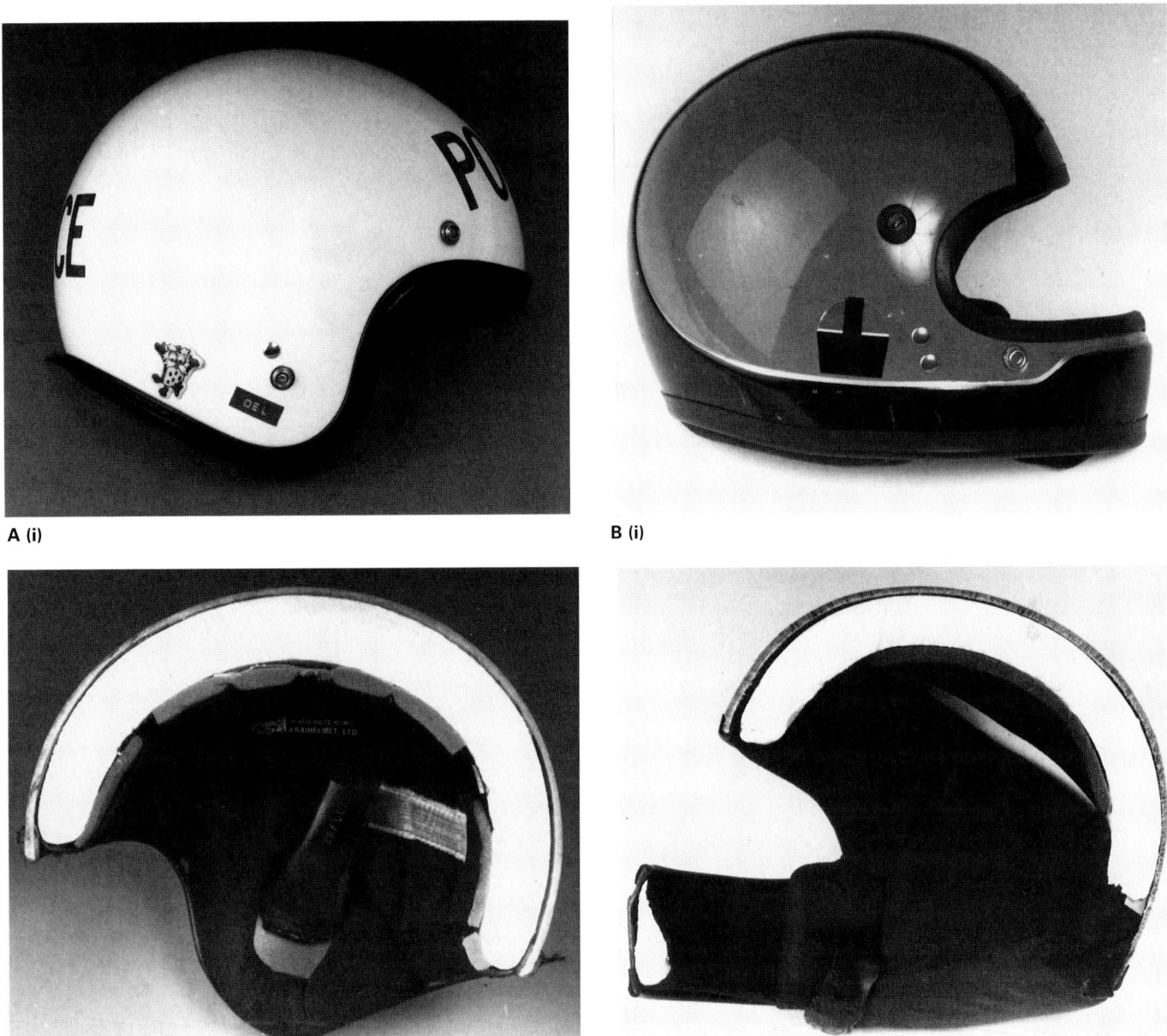

A (i)

B (i)

A (ii)

B (i)

Fig. 3.4 Motorcyclists: injury control by helmets. Most protective helmets embody an outer shell, usually of fibre glass or polycarbonate, an inner lining of expanded polystyrene foam and retentive straps. The shell is designed to resist penetration, and its capacity to do so is tested by a standardized sharp impact; the shell spreads the impact load over a wider area and prevents the foam from shattering. The inner lining is designed to absorb impact energy by deforming and is tested by a standardized blunt impact. The retentive system must also pass tests intended to ensure that the straps will not break or cause obstruction to the airway. Helmets passing these tests are usually massive (1.0–1.8 kg), and are resented by some motorcyclists. **A** (**i**) Open-face helmet. This gives a good field of vision and is well ventilated. In many tropical countries, this pattern is very popular. (**ii**) In section. **B** (**i**) Full-face helmet. This provides protection for the face by an extension of the shell, backed by polystyrene foam. (**ii**) In section.

in which alcohol is an accepted social drug, such as the USA and Australia. The role of alcohol consumption as a cause of road crashes is too well known to require elaboration; the risk of a road crash bears a very striking relation to the blood alcohol level (Fig. 3.6). In a recent Australian survey of 1071 car drivers and motorcycle riders who were admitted to hospital after road crashes and underwent mandatory blood alcohol analysis, O. T. Holubowycz (personal communication) found that 26.2%

had levels in excess of 80 mg/dl and the incidence of this excess among 199 injured pedestrians was even higher. In fatal road crashes, the proportion is higher, both in Australia and in many other countries with similar cultures. Evans (1991) reviewed data from 15 US states, and concluded that in the period 1983–1985, 55.2% of single car fatalities were attributable to alcohol; in multiple car crashes, he found that alcohol could be blamed in about 45%. Evans identified alcohol as the single largest

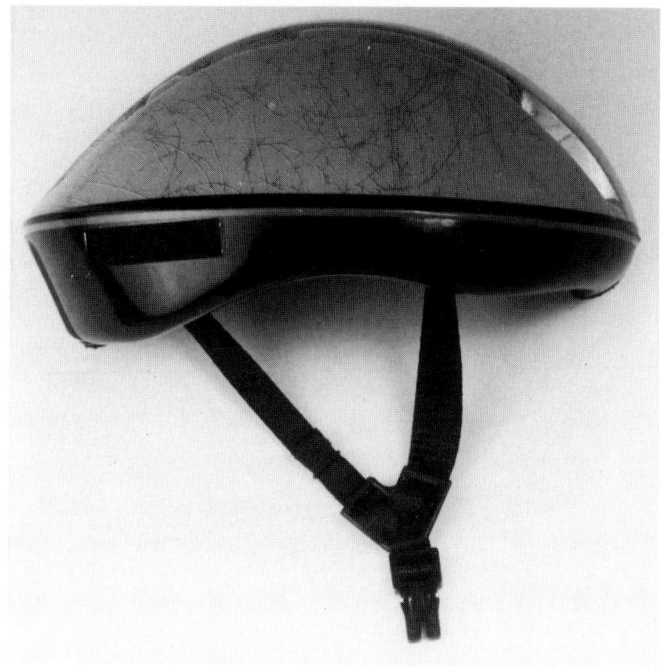

i

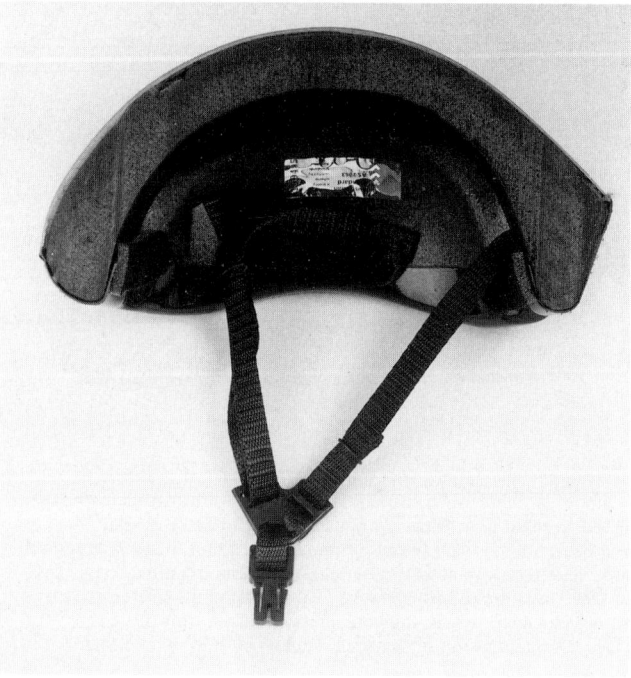

ii

Fig. 3.5 Pedal cyclists: injury control by helmets. (**i**) Pedal cycle helmets are expected to absorb the energy of a blunt impact and is tested accordingly. Some designs of pedal cycle helmet have a shell tested to resist penetration, but penetrating injuries are rare in pedal cyclists, and some authorities accept helmets with no protective shell, or with a microshell and wide openings for ventilation. These helmets perform well in tests of energy absorbtion, and are popular because of light weight (~300 g) and comfort in hot weather. (**ii**) In section.

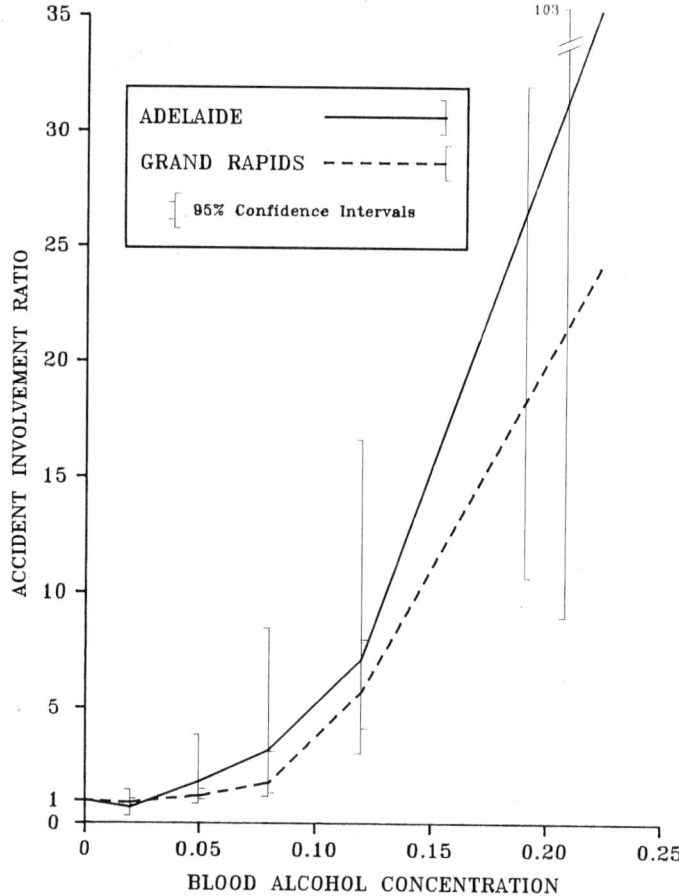

Fig. 3.6 Accident involvement ratio and the driver's blood alcohol level. Case control studies have shown that beyond a blood alcohol concentration of ~0.05% (50 mg/dl) the risk of crash involvement rises with increasing blood alcohol concentration. In two of these, performed in Grand Rapids (Michigan, USA) by Borkenstein et al (1964) and in Adelaide (South Australia) by McLean et al (1980), blood alcohol levels in crash-involved drivers were compared with matched control drivers not involved in accidents. The graphs show that crash-involved drivers were 30 times more likely to have alcohol levels in excess of 0.15% (150 mg/dl) than matched control drivers.

contributing factor in car crashes, and the factor offering most potential for reduction. Even in countries in which alcohol consumption is discouraged for religious or other reasons, reports suggest that alcohol is a factor in many road crashes (Mekky 1984). The significance of other recreational drugs is less obvious, but cannot be dismissed.

Other transportation accidents

In the past, seafaring men often suffered head injuries and facial fractures, but today better safety at sea and smaller crews have made marine accidents an infrequent source of CMF injuries. Aviation accidents have attracted much attention in recent years, but cases surviving with CMF injuries are not numerous. Air crashes, parachuting accidents and ground impacts with propeller or rotor blades are likely to inflict very high energy impacts, and in cases seen by us, the injuries are often bizarre.

Assaults

In brawls and domestic beatings, fists and feet are the usual weapons. The biomechanics of such injuries are considered in Chapter 4; here it is only necessary to note that in our data, the bones commonly fractured by fist blows are the mandible, the zygoma and orbit, and the nasal bones, in that order. This relatively lower incidence of nasal fractures probably reflects hospital admission and referral practice: in our hospitals, these fractures are often treated by ENT surgeons. Maxillary fractures of the Le Fort type require greater brutality, and may result from kicks with boots (p. 113). Eye injuries may result from assault with blunt objects as well as from from a variety of sharp objects; in a recent US study of penetrating eye injuries due to assault, fists were responsible for nearly 20% of these vision-threatening injuries (Dannenberg et al 1992b).

Assaults with the fists or feet are especially seen among men in the lower sociometric groups but women are also often victims, and so are infants. In our experience, infants subjected to battery rarely show facial fractures, though fractures of the skull vault are common; however, facial bruises and tears of the buccal surface of the lips at the alveolar margin often result from blows to the mouth of a crying infant, and serious eye injuries have also been reported (Elner et al 1990; Greenwald et al 1986 — see p. 403).

Extemporized blunt weapons such as bottles and saucepans are often the cause of CMF injuries. In some tribal Australian communities, purpose-designed clubs called nulla-nullas are often used in domestic altercations; baseball clubs are used in urban aggression in parts of the USA (Berlet et al 1992) and in countries to which that tine game has spread. Clubs most often strike the vault of the head, but facial and ocular injuries are also seen.

Sharp weapons such as broken bottles or glasses come conveniently to hand in drunken brawls, and can cause extensive facial lacerations. Knife wounds are rare in our practice, but common in some cultures. De Villiers (1975) has given an elegant account of a large series of cranial stab wounds from South Africa: of 93 craniocerebral injuries, 32 were frontal or orbital.

Alcohol and unemployment have been incriminated as factors in the increasing number of CMF injuries due to assault over the last decade; Shepherd et al (1990a,b) carried out a controlled study of the aetiology of violence in Bristol, and found evidence to support the role of alcohol but not of unemployment. Shepherd & Farrington (1993) have stressed the need to see violence as a public health problem requiring multidisciplinary research.

Falls

These are common causes of injury, though reflex responses by the arms often save the CMF region, and the site of head impact is often lateral or occipital rather than frontal or facial. Children in multi-story tenement buildings may fall from unsecured windows or down staircases; the child's head is relatively larger than the adult's, and calvarial head injuries are very common. In our paediatric series, falls were the cause in some 11% of cases of facial fractures. Adults may fall when drunk, or from ladders or scaffolds. It is usually stated that a fall from more than the person's height can cause serious injury, provided that the struck surface is hard, and this has been our experience (Manavis et al 1991); however, infants and young children often survive falls from up to 3 m and falls from less than 1 m rarely cause serious neurological effects unless complicated by extradural haematomas. The elderly are very prone to fall, from unstable gait, impaired proprioception and poor vision, and may suffer serious head injuries, often complicated by acute or chronic subdural haematomas; facial fractures, especially of the mandible, are also common.

Industrial accidents

These are not numerous in communities in which modern safety standards are enforced. In many reports of 'work-related' injuries (e.g. Iizuka et al 1990) the numbers of industrial injuries are indeed inflated by inclusion of assaults on employees, and road crash victims hurt when on the way to work; our data class as industrial accidents only those which happen at the workplace and are directly related to the work being done, such as explosions and injuries from machinery. Deaths from work-related accidents in Australia were reviewed by Harrison et al (1989). The average annual incidence of workplace deaths in a 3 year period was 4.75 per 100 000 employed persons. The injuries in more than one-third of deaths were due to impacts by moving objects, such as tractors and earth-moving machinery, falling rocks and timber. Impacts of this type often strike in the CMF area. Of the deaths, 22.3% were due to brain injuries and 18.2% to multiple injuries often including brain injuries. In many developing countries, industrial accidents are more numerous and may take forms unfamiliar in Western practice: for example, Sekhon (1975) described compression injuries of the brain and scalp avulsions from bullock-powered cane crushers in rural India. Underground mining has always been a dangerous occupation, and CMF injuries still occur when safety precautions are ignored (Fig. 22.4).

In many countries, eye injuries figure prominently in statistics of industrial accidents, especially in industries where foreign body damage to the cornea is likely. Safety goggles should make this a rare event, but Liu et al (1990) reported a reprehensible neglect of this simple precaution in a series of cases admitted to Moorfields Eye Hospital in London. In the USA, the National Eye Trauma System, a data bank of penetrating eye injuries (Dannenberg et al 1992a), recorded 635 work-related injuries of this type; the activity most often reported as responsible was hammering on or with a metal object, and there was a very low use of safety glasses (6%).

Sport

The prevalence of facial fractures due to sport and other recreations varies with the nature of community pastimes. National or regional predilections for particular sports affect the epidemiology of CMF trauma: some years ago, a report from Ireland gave sport as the leading (36.8%) cause and this was attributed to the violence seemingly inherent in hurling (O'Donoghue et al 1979). Children often suffer injuries in sports and in playgrounds; sports of all types, playground accidents and horse riding accounted for > 20% of facial fractures in our paediatric series. Football is an international cause of CMF injury. Allan & Daly (1990) reported a 19% incidence of sport-related injuries in a series of mandibular fractures: this was in New South Wales, where rugby football is played, a game involving even more body contact than soccer or Australian Rules football, and played without the helmets that protect American footballers. Rugby was the leading cause of dental and facial fractures in a series of 132 sport-related injuries from the UK, with soccer not far behind; rugby is especially apt to cause zygomatic and mandibular fractures (Hill et al 1985). The use of mouthguards in these body contact sports, and in boxing, has reduced the risk of orofacial injury and probably also of concussive cerebral injury; the evidence for this is reviewed by Chapman (1990). In all forms of football, concussive cerebral injuries are common though usually of minor severity; in soccer, the practice of heading the ball may have serious cumulative effects on the brain (Ryan 1991). Some football injuries are inflicted deliberately, and thus represent more or less covert assaults; in a survey of 72 cases of football-related facial fractures, Lim et al (1993) noted that in 11%, the victims identified a deliberate intent to injure.

Baseball, cricket, hockey and other small-ball games may cause CMF injuries; cricket was second to rugby football in the UK series cited above. Blow-out fractures of the orbit have for long been associated with ball impacts over the eye, justifying the increasing use of helmets with visors, or polycarbonate goggles, in these sports (Jones 1987); while squash and other racket-propelled balls are especially prone to damage the eye, even the larger balls used in cricket and baseball may impact directly on the orbital contents and cause ocular damage

(Jones & Tullo 1986). It has been said that golf and cricket are particularly dangerous to young children who are hurt as spectators, standing too close or not watching the game.

The horse continues to figure as a cause of CMF injuries of various types, often very serious (Ilgren et al 1984). Since riding is now usually recreational, these injuries are often termed sporting; many are due to kicks rather than falls (Lim et al 1993). The general use of helmets has made falls less injurious, but young children playing near horses continue to appear as victims in most series. Boxing, wrestling and martial arts, somewhat surprisingly, contribute few cases of serious facial skeletal injuries, even in communities that favour these sports. Boxers do suffer nasal fractures frequently, but these are often not admitted to hospitals and so escape record. Boxing is, however, responsible for a small number of very severe injuries from impact in the CMF region. These include:

1. Acute subdural haemorrhage — sometimes fatal
2. Chronic encephalopathy with dementia and parkinsonian motor impairments
3. Retinal detachment.

The use of boxing helmets does not appear to have mitigated the risks of this sport to any significant degree (Ryan 1991).

Snow and ice sports, swimming and diving sports may also cause CMF injuries. It is stated that in these sports, children are especially apt to suffer injury, presumably from inexperience; however, in Austrian winter sports the peak age incidence of midfacial fractures was 21–30 years (Puelacher et al 1991).

Gunshot wounds

It is usual and convenient to list peacetime gunshot wounds (GSW) in a separate category, whether the injury is sustained in a homicidal assault, attempted suicide or accident.

More than in any other category of CMF injury, the incidence and types of wounds caused by firearms are determined by social and historical conditions. In peaceful communities with few firearms, incidences are low. World Health Organization (1989) statistics show that in Japan the suicidal rate is high (18.7 per 100 000 population) but the homicide rate is very low (0.75 per 100 000 population). Japan has an admirable tradition of gun control (p. 5) and in keeping with this, Lester (1990) found that in 1980 only 3.6% of Japanese homicides were by shooting and the use of firearms in suicide was also rare. In the USA on the other hand, both the homicide and suicide rates are high, being 8.5 and 12.7 per 100 000 respectively in 1987. In Lester's study, firearms were used in 64% of US homicides, and in the majority of suicides; reflecting this, US neurosurgical literature contains many studies of civilian gunshot wounds of the head and face. In Australia, the suicide rate is a little higher than in the USA, but the homicide rate is much lower (1.9 per 100 000 population). It is estimated that there are firearms in about a quarter of all Australian households, the proportion being higher in country areas; Snowdon & Harris (1992) recently found that firearms are used in about 40% of all homicides and in a somewhat smaller proportion of suicides. In a review of data from 20 countries, Lester (1990) found a clear relation between the firearm suicide rate and legal restrictions on the availability of firearms, but such restrictions did not greatly affect the overall community suicide rate, as other means of suicide were used. Nevertheless, the consequences of unsuccessful suicidal attempts with firearms are so appalling that restrictive gun laws can be justified if they do no more than reduce the number of persons surviving blinded and with frontal lobe damage.

Our own experience with GSW wounds in the CMF region is chiefly derived from unsuccessful suicidal wounds and from accidents, either in hunting or in the home, where carelessness may allow children access to sporting rifles. Review of the recent literature suggests that the incidence of facial GSW is not very large even in communities with a reputation for violent behaviour. Nevertheless these are usually very serious injuries, and no surgeon should forget that at any time he may be obliged to treat the effects of an outburst of war, terrorism or individual paranoia.

From the epidemiological view, wartime GSW reflect many factors: the weapons of the combatants, the intensity of fighting, the terrain and the degree of involvement of civilians. Medical services are also relevant, since the experience of clinicians will relate to whether cases reach them soon or late: in some recent wars, army personnel were likely to reach neurosurgical care much sooner than civilians. The CMF region is often injured in war, though much less often than the trunk and extremities. US statistics from the Second World War show that wounds of the head and face accounted for 7.4% and 7.6% of all non-fatal wounds respectively, though for a larger (36.2%) proportion of deaths (Reister 1975). In Chapters 4 and 5, the theoretical and clinical importance of the type of missile is stressed; however, it is not easy to obtain data on the frequency of the various types of missile causing CMF injuries. In the US casualties in the World War II, explosive shells accounted for 57.5% of non-fatal wounds in all sites and for about the same proportion of all battle deaths. In the Korean war, shell fragments accounted for less than half of all penetrating brain wounds coming to operation (Meirowsky 1965). In the war in Vietnam, the proportion of head wounds by fragments was higher for US troops: in two large series, fragments caused some 80% of 1455 penetrating wounds of the brain (Hammon 1971) and 74% of 2795 maxillo-

facial injuries (Tinder et al 1969). By contrast, Andrews (1968) in the same conflict found that 58% of his maxillofacial missile wounds were due to bullets: his cases were Vietnamese service personnel, perhaps involved in engagements of a different type. Wartime eye injuries are also usually due to metallic fragments or grit from explosions. Polycarbonate visors and goggles were used in the Kuwait war (1991) and are said to have been very successful in preventing these injuries. The recent widespread use of landmines, which send small missiles with an upward trajectory (Fig. 13.1), is today causing many wounds in the CMF area, frequently accompanied by leg and torso injuries; children are often the victims.

A low incidence of bullet injuries is today characteristic of overt war: not so in the wounds inflicted in revolts, repressions and gang warfare. Such conflicts are more likely to be fought with small arms and fragmentation missiles are less often seen; in the Irish troubles, bullet wounds have predominated (Byrnes et al 1974). The choice of weapons relates both to the ferocity of the combatants and to the generosity of their suppliers, but little ingenuity is needed to make an explosive device and it should be noted that home-made bombs sometimes generate radiolucent non-metallic missiles, which are prohibited in formal war. The squalid murders of gang warfare are also chiefly perpetrated with pistols and rifles, though there are enormous cultural and economic variations in the patterns of communal violence (Levy et al 1993).

The use of large plastic or rubber bullets in riot control has created a new category of missile trauma; in a study of 123 persons injured by such missiles, Ritchie (1992) found that nine were struck in the facial region.

Facial burns

It is usual and convenient to consider burns as a separate epidemiological entity. Data are usually readily obtainable from hospital data, as the diagnosis is obvious and the affected region likely to be well documented. It has been noted that ICD10 coding distinguishes three regions within the CMF area; there is practical importance in giving burns of the eye separate consideration.

The head and neck are exposed parts of the body and are often injured by explosions, flames, and scalds from hot liquids. The face and scalp may also be burned by electric current, either from the electric flash, or by conduction of current to the skin and the underlying bone or cartilage. Chemical burns of the face may be caused by strong acids or alkalis, or by other chemical agents such as phenols; children may swallow such fluids and sustain chemical burns of the mouth, pharynx and oesophagus.

Facial burns are most often the result of domestic accidents; the young and the elderly are especially at risk. Thermal trauma may be seen in road crashes and in war, especially in ships, aircraft and military vehicles. Burns are common in primitive communities, especially where cooking is done in wooden or grass huts, as in parts of Australia and New Guinea. But burns are also very frequent in developed countries.

MacAfee et al (1991) reviewed recent experience in the USA and found that thermal burns of the head and neck occurred in 50–60% of all victims of burning admitted to hospital. Facial burns were found either alone or in combination with burns elsewhere in the body in 45% of 939 patients admitted to a regional burns unit in California (Wachtel et al 1981); in these patients, the scalp was burned in 13%, the eyelids in 14%, the eyes in only 1%, the ears in 16%, the nose in 15% and the neck in 33%.

Our experience of burns of the head and neck is discussed in Chapter 17. It is based chiefly on work in a specialized adult burns unit serving a population of about 1.5 million people. During the 10 year period 1981–1990, this unit admitted on average 156 patients per year. The male:female ratio was about 4:1. The unit accepts patients from the age of 15 and above; the average age was 25 years, and the two largest age groups were in the ranges 16–24 and 65–74 years. Of these victims of severe burns, the face was involved in 43.5% — an annual average of 68 cases. Scalds were the cause of thermal injury in 45%; other causes included explosions, flame burns and fires in closed spaces such as houses and motor vehicles. In most cases, other parts of the body were also involved: in only 2% was an isolated injury in the head/neck area recorded. Deep burns resulted from direct contact burns with such objects as a hot exhaust muffler box, or a hot domestic iron used in an assault, or from contact with electric power lines in road accidents or agricultural activities.

The spectrum of causes is somewhat different in childhood; in our associated paediatric burns unit, which admits some 120 cases annually, scalds accounted for some 54% of all thermal injuries.

Bites

Human and animal bites cause many soft-tissue injuries in the facial region, and larger animals may damage or avulse skeletal structures. Human bites are inflicted in brawls, or in sexual violence, or in child abuse; in some societies, this is a frequent cause of disfiguring facial injury (p. 495). Dog bites are common in those societies in which dogs are kept as domestic pets or for protection, and small children are especially likely to be bitten in the facial region, whereas an adult attacked by a dog is usually bitten in the arm or leg. Karlson (1984) reported on a series of hospital-treated facial bites in Wisconsin, USA; the great majority of victims were under 15 years old, and the incidence was highest in the age group 0–4 years,

where the incidence of serious injury was also highest. Karlson estimated an annual incidence of 152 facial bites per 100 000 children at risk. Our experience is similar: a hospital-based accident surveillance study suggested a rate of 280 dog attacks per 100 000 children aged 0–12 years, the peak incidence being again in the age group 0–4 years (South Australian Health Commission 1991). In this age group, most (90%) of the serious bites were in the facial region. Certain breeds of dog are especially likely to bite children: in the study cited, bull terriers, German shepherd dogs and Dobermans were together responsible for more than half of all attacks on children, this being 4–5 times more than would be predicted from the number of these dogs on the register. In the UK, mauling of children by pit bull terriers has aroused concern, and in 1991, legislation was passed to enact stringent control of these dogs.

In some parts of the world, bites by the larger carnivores and by large herbivores (horses and camels) are important as causes of ablative facial injury. Sharks and crocodiles occasionally attack the face and head, but it is unusual for the victims to survive. In some developing countries, facial rat bites are a common nuisance; sleepers are attacked, and eyelids may be injured (Wykes 1989). Birds often peck the heads of children, and penetrating eye injuries have been reported; it has been said that some birds defend themselves by pecking at the adversary's eyes (Horsburgh et al 1992).

EPIDEMIOLOGY AND THE TRAUMA AUDIT

Injury severity

This is an important datum in trauma epidemiology, and it is still more relevant in auditing the efficiency of trauma management. ICD9 and ICD10 do not code injury severity. The Abbreviated Injury Scale (AIS: 1990) was designed to quantify severity in case of road trauma, and has since been extended to penetrating wounds. The AIS gives a severity rating from 1 (minor) to 6 (maximum) for injuries in the various parts of the body. Table 3.6 lists the severity ratings of the chief categories of CMF injury. To take into account the cumulative effect of multiple trauma, the AIS has been extended to give the Injury Severity Score (ISS). For the purposes of this rating, the body is divided into six regions. The ISS is the sum of the squares of the AIS rates of the three most severely injured body regions: thus, an adult with brief amnesia due to 'concussion' (AIS 2), a fractured maxilla of Le Fort III type (AIS 3) and a fracture of the shaft of the femur (AIS 3) would score $4 + 9 + 9 = 22$. The maximum ISS value is 75; a score of 6 in any region is automatically assigned an ISS rating of 75. The AIS and ISS have been extensively used in trauma epidemiology

Table 3.6 Injuries in the CMF region, with their AIS gradings (Abbreviated Injury Scale 1990)

Injury	AIS grade
Scalp or facial laceration	
Minor	1
Major (> 10 cm long and into subcutaneous tissue)	2
Blood loss > 20% vol.	3
Intracranial injury	
Cerebral contusion (graded according to size, depth, volume, and number)	3–5
Diffuse axonal injury	5
Intracranial haematoma — extradural, subdural, and/or intracerebral (graded according to size with modification for age ⩽ 10 years)	4–5
Cerebral oedema or swelling (graded according to severity in CT or other pictures)	3–5
Skull fractures	
Skull base (± CSF leak)	3
Skull base — comminuted or with loss of brain tissue	4
Skull vault — closed, simple, linear	2
Skull vault — compound, depressed ⩽ 2 cm	3
Skull vault — compound, with loss of brain tissue, massive depressed > 2 cm	4
Fractured mandible	
Closed, body or ramus	1
Subcondylar	2
Open/displaced/comminuted (all sites)	2
Fractured maxilla	
Closed	1
Le Fort I or II	2
Le Fort III	3
With blood loss > 20% vol.	4
Fractured orbit	
Closed	2
Open/displaced/comminuted	3
Fractured nose	
Closed	1
Open/displaced/comminuted	2
Fractured zygoma	2
Fractured tooth	1
Eye injuries	
Abrasions, lacerations	1
Rupture of globe	2

and accident research, but have definite limitations (Copes et al 1988; Ross et al 1990). For prehospital management decisions (triage) and for trauma management evaluation, more practical measures have been devised. The Trauma Score allocated up to 16 points for conscious level (1–5), respiratory rate (0–4), respiratory expansion (0–1), systolic blood pressure (0–4) and capillary refill (0–2). This measure has been criticized, especially as a field guide, and various modifications have been suggested: at present there is no unanimity on the best measure. The issues have been reviewed by Champion, who has done much to clarify thinking on the quantification of trauma and to develop effective trauma systems in the USA (Champion et al 1990a). He and his colleagues in the Washington Hospital Center combined the Trauma Score, the ISS, the patient's age and the type of injury (whether blunt or penetrating) to give the measure called TRISS, which combines the trauma score with the ISS; it has been correlated with the probability of survival.

Champion et al (1990b) have since reported on a new and more complex characterization of trauma, ASCOT, which is thought to correlate better with data on survival derived from a study of the outcomes in some 150 000 patients. These measures can be used to audit the quality of trauma management.

Audits

Surgical audits are generally agreed to be essential in assuring an acceptable quality of surgical care. They are also necessary in comparing the results of different methods and systems of treatment. In practice, surgical audits range from simple case reviews, often guided paternally by the unit chief, to computerized statistical analyses of key data from large case series, in which the TRISS or other characterizations can be used to identify and to count those cases in which unpredicted death, or unexpected recovery, suggests that management may have been worse or better than the norm. Between these extremes, many surgeons audit their cases prospectively, using purpose-designed software programs, of which at least 20 are now available commercially; some of these are discussed by Pollock & Evans (1993). It seems likely that in the future, clinical audits will be based on ICD-coded hospital data, which are already widely used for administrative purposes. Surgeons, especially trauma surgeons, must ensure that records are coded accurately and quickly and that complications are recorded. Data relating to trauma deaths are of great importance both in auditing the quality of treatment, and in planning or evaluating preventive measures; an adequate autopsy is essential. In most states of the USA, autopsies on cases of trauma deaths are not mandatory (Champion et al 1990b). In the UK, in Australia, and in many European countries, autopsies are usually performed on the victims of lethal trauma, despite occasional protests; in many developing countries, this is regrettably not the case.

Trauma logistics

CMF trauma incidences and prevalences are very relevant in planning trauma services. The trauma load, the population density and other demographic factors must be taken into account, together with the economic resources of the community, when a case is being made for establishing a Level 1 trauma service with an affiliated craniofacial unit or similar specialized service able to care for CMF trauma. Constant attention must be given to changes in incidences of particular types of trauma; in developed countries, there has been a worldwide fall in the incidence and severity of road trauma over the last two decades, and the implications of this are now under study. These issues are discussed in Chapter 23.

REFERENCES

Abbreviated Injury Scale (1990) Association for the Advancement of Automotive Medicine, Des Plaines, IL

Abiose B O 1986 Maxillofacial skeleton injuries in the western states of Nigeria. Br J Oral Maxillofac Surg 24: 31–39

Allan B P, Daly C G 1990 Fractures of the mandible. A 35-year retrospective study. Int J Oral Maxillofac Surg 19: 268–271

Andrews J L 1968 Maxillofacial trauma in Vietnam. J Oral Surg 26: 457–462

Andersson L, Hultin M, Kjellman O, Nordenram Å, Ramström G 1989 Jaw fractures in the county of Stockholm (1978–1980) Swed Dent J 13: 209–216

Berlet A C, Talenti D P, Carroll S F (1992) The baseball bat: a popular mechanism of urban injury. J Trauma 33: 167–170

Bochlogyrus P N 1985 A retrospective study of 1521 mandibular fractures. J Oral Maxillofac Surg 43: 597–599

Borkenstein R F, Crowther R F, Shumate R P, Ziel W B, Zylman R 1964 The role of the drinking driver in traffic accidents. Department of Police Administration, Indiana University

Brook I M, Wood N 1983 Aetiology and incidence of facial fractures in adults. Int J Oral Surg 12: 293–298

Brown R D, Cowpe J G 1985 Patterns of maxillofacial trauma in two different cultures. A comparison between Riyadh and Tayside. J R Coll Surg Edinb 30: 299–302

Byrnes D P, Crockard H A, Gordon D S, Gleadhill C A 1974 Penetrating craniocerebral missile injuries in the civil disturbances in Northern Ireland. Br J Surg 61: 169–176

Canavan Y M, O'Flaherty M J, Archer D B, Elwood J H 1980 A 10-year survey of eye injuries in Northern Ireland, 1967–1976. Br J Ophthalmol 64: 618–625

Champion H R, Copes W S, Flanagan M E, Sacco W J 1990a Injury severity scoring. In: Border J R, Allgöwer M, Hansen S T, Rüedi T P (eds) Blunt multiple trauma. Dekker, New York, Ch 13

Champion H R, Copes W S, Sacco W J et al 1990b The major trauma outcome study: establishing national norms for trauma care. J Trauma 30: 1356–1365

Chapman P J 1990 Orofacial injuries and international rugby players' attitudes to mouthguards. Br J Sp Med 24: 156–158

Commonwealth Department of Health, Housing and Community Services 1992 Studies on drug abuse in Australia 1992. Australian Government Publishing Service, Canberra

Cook H E, Rowe M 1990 A retrospective study of 356 midfacial fractures occurring in 225 patients. J Oral Maxillofac Surg 48: 574–578

Copes W S, Champion H R, Sacco W J, Lawnick M M, Keast S L, Bain L W 1988 The Injury Severity Score revisited. J Trauma 28: 69–77

Dannenberg A L, Parver L M, Brechner R K, Khoo L 1992a Penetrating eye injuries in the workplace. The National Eye Trauma System Registry. Arch Ophthalmol 110: 843–848

Dannenberg A L, Parver L M, Fowler C J 1992b Penetrating eye injuries related to assault. The National Eye Trauma System Registry. Arch Ophthalmol 110: 849–852

De Villiers J C 1975 Stab wounds of the brain and skull. In: Vinken P J, Bruyn G W (eds) Handbook of clinical neurology. Injuries of the brain and skull. North-Holland, Amsterdam, Vol 1, Part I, Ch 24

Dimitroulis G, Eyre J 1991 A 7 year review of maxillofacial trauma in a central London hospital. Br Dent J 170: 300–302

Elner S G, Elner V M, Arnall M, Albert C M 1990 Ocular and associated systemic findings in suspected child abuse. Arch Ophthalmol 108: 1094–1101

Evans L 1991 Traffic safety and the driver. Van Nostrand–Reinhold, New York

Evans L, Frick M C 1988 Helmet effectiveness in preventing motorcycle driver and passenger fatalities. Accid Anal Prev 20: 447–458

Fife D, Davis J, Tate L, Wells J K, Mohan D, Williams A 1983 Fatal injuries to bicyclists: the experience of Dade County, Florida. J Trauma 23: 745–755

Foldvary L A, Lane J C 1964 The effect of compulsory safety helmets on motor-cycle accident fatalities. Aust Road Res 2: 7–24

Greenwald M J, Weiss A, Oesterle C S, Friendly D S 1986 Traumatic retinoschisis in battered babies. Ophthalmology 93: 618–625

Hammond K L, Ferguson J W, Edwards J L 1991 Fractures of the facial bones in the Otago Region 1979–1985. NZ Dental J 87: 5–9

Hammon W M 1971 Analysis of 2187 consecutive penetrating wounds of the brain from Vietnam. J Neurosurg 34: 127–131

Harrison J E, Frommer M S, Ruck E A, Blyth F M 1989 Deaths as a result of work-related injury in Australia, 1982–1984. Med J Aust 150: 118–125

Hill C M, Crosher R F, Mason D A 1985 Dental and facial injuries following sports accidents: a study of 130 patients. Br J Oral Maxillofac Surg 23: 268–274

Horsburgh B J, Stark D J, Harrison J D 1992 Ocular injuries caused by magpies. Med J Aust 157: 756–759

Iizuka T, Randell T, Güven O, Linqvist C 1990 Maxillofacial fractures related to work accidents. J Craniomaxillofac Surg 18: 255–259

Ilgren E B, Teddy P J, Vafadis J, Briggs M, Gardiner N G 1984 Clinical and pathological studies of brain injuries in horse-riding accidents: a description of cases and review with a warning to the unhelmeted. Clin Neuropathol 3: 253–259

Insurance Special Report A-38 1991 Driver injury experience in 1990 models equipped with air bags or automatic belts. Highway Loss Data Institute, Arlington, Virginia

Ioannides C, Freihofer H P M, Bruaset I 1984 Trauma of the upper third of the face. J Maxillofac Surg 12: 255–261

Jennett B, Frankowski R F 1990 The epidemiology of head injury. In: Vinken P J, Bruyn G W, Klawans H L (eds) Handbook of clinical neurology. Elsevier, Amsterdam, Vol 57 Ch 1

Jones N P 1987 Eye injuries in sports: an increasing problem Br J Sports Med 21: 168–170

Jones N P, Tullo A B 1986 Severe eye injuries in cricket. Br J Sports Med 20: 178–179

Karlson T A 1984 The incidence of facial injuries from dog bites. J Am Med Assoc 251: 3265–3267

Klopfer J, Tielsch J M, Vitale S, See L-C, Canner J K 1992 Ocular trauma in the United States. Eye injuries resulting in hospitalization, 1984 through 1987. Arch Ophthalmol 110: 838–842

Lee L F, Wagner L K, Lee Y E, Suh J H, Lee S R 1987 The impact-absorbing effects of facial fractures in closed-head injuries. An analysis of 210 patients. J Neurosurg 66: 542–547

Lester D 1990 The availability of firearms and the use of firearms for suicide. Acta Psychiatr Scand 81: 146–147

Levy M L, Masri L S, Levy K M et al 1993 Penetrating craniocerebral injury resultant from gunshot wounds: gang-related injury in children and adolescents. Neurosurgery 33: 1018–1025

Lim L H, Moore M H, Trott J A, David DJ 1993 Sports-related facial fractures: a review of 137 patients. Aust NZ J Surg 63: 784–789

Liu C, Davison C, Kuling R 1990 Eye protection in the metal work industry (letter). Br Med J 301: 931

MacAfee K A, Zeitler D L, Mayo K 1991 Burns of the head and neck. In: Fonseca R J, Walker R V (eds) Oral and maxillofacial trauma. Saunders, Philadelphia, Vol 2, Ch 26

Manavis J, Blumbergs P C, Scott G et al 1991 Brain injury patterns in falls causing death In: Proceedings of International IRCOBI Conference on the Biomechanics of Impacts. International Research Council on Biokinetics of Impacts. Bron, France, pp 77–88

McDermott F T 1992 Helmet efficacy in the prevention of bicyclist head injuries. World J Surg 16: 379–383

McLean A J, Holubowycz O T, Sandow B L 1980 Alcohol and crashes. Identification of relevant factors in this association. Commonwealth of Australia: Department of Transport, Office of Road Safety: External report CR 11

Meirowsky A M 1965 Penetrating wounds of the brain. In: Meirowsky A M (ed) Neurological surgery of trauma. Office of the Surgeon General, Dept of the Army, Washington, DC

Mekky A 1984 Road traffic accidents in rich developing countries: the case of Libya. Accid Anal Prev 16: 263–277

Neumann H-J 1991 Gibt es einen Wandel in der Atiologie von Gesichtsschadelfrakturen? Fortschr Kiefer Gesichtschir 36: 9–11

O'Donoghue G M, Vaughan E D V, Condon K C 1979 An analysis of the pattern of facial injuries in a general accident department. Injury 11: 52–61

Pollock A, Evans M 1993 Surgical audit, 2nd edn. Butterworth–Heinemann, Oxford

Puelacher W, Röthler G, Strobl H, Toifl F, Waldhardt E 1991 Mittelgesichtsfrakturen im traumatologischen Krankengut der Innsbrucker Abteilung für MKG-Chirurgie von 1982–1988 unter besonderer Berücksichtigung der Wintersportverletzungen. Fortschr Kiefer Gesichtschir 36: 15–17

Reister F A 1975 Medical Statistics in World War II: Medical Department. United States Army: prepared and published under the direction of Richard R Taylor, the Surgeon General, United States Army. Office of the Surgeon General, Dept of the Army, Washington, DC

Ritchie A J 1992 Plastic bullets: significant risk of serious injury above the diaphragm. Injury 23: 265–266

Ross S E, O'Malley K F, Stein S, Spettell C M, Young G 1990 Abbreviated Injury Scaling (AIS-85) of head injury as a prognostic tool for functional outcome. In: Proceedings 34th Annual Conference Association for the Advancement of Automotive Medicine, Des Plaines, IL, pp 433–441

Rutherford W H, Greenfield T, Hayes H R M, Nelson J K 1985 The medical effects of seatbelt legislation in the United Kingdom. Department of Health and Security, Research Report no. 13. HMSO, London

Ryan A J 1991 Protecting the sportsman's brain (concussion in sport). Annual guest lecture 1990, London Sports Medicine Institute. Br J Sports Med 25: 81–86

Ryan G A, McLean A J, Vilenius A T S, Kloeden C N, Simpson D A, Blumbergs P C 1989 Head impacts and brain injury in fatally injured pedestrians. In: Proceedings of International IRCOBI Conference on the Biomechanics of Impacts. International Research Council on Biokinetics of Impacts, Bron, France, pp 27–37

Scherer M, Sullivan W G, Smith D J, Phillips L G, Robson M C (1989) An analysis of 1423 facial fracture in 788 patients at an urban trauma center. J Trauma 29: 388–390

Schroeder W A 1989 Maxillofacial trauma in two rural level II trauma centers. Missouri Med 86: 35–39

Sekhon G S 1975 Head injuries caused by cane crushing machines ('Kohlu injury'). In: Vinken P J, Bruyn G W (eds) Handbook of clinical neurology. North-Holland, Amsterdam, Vol 23, Part 1, Ch 27

Selecki B R, Ring I T, Simpson D A, Vanderfield G K, Sewell M F 1981 Injuries to the head, spine and peripheral nerves. Report on a study. NSW Government Printer, Sydney

Shepherd J P, Farrington D P 1993 Assault as a public health problem: discussion paper. J R Soc Med 86: 89–92

Shepherd J P, Robinson L, Levers B G H 1990a Roots of urban violence. Injury 21: 139–141

Shepherd J P, Shapland M, Pearce N X, Scully C 1990b Pattern, severity and aetiology of injuries in victims of assault. J R Soc Med 83: 75–78

Simpson D, McLean A J 1988 Neurotrauma: the Australian experience (editorial). Surg Neurol 29: 166–167

Snowdon J, Harris L 1992 Firearm suicides in Australia. Med J Aust 156: 79–83

South Australian Health Commission 1991 Injury surveillance monthly bulletin 29. The Health Commission, Adelaide

Tinder L E, Osborn D B, Lilly G E, Salem J E, Cutcher J L 1969 Maxillofacial injuries sustained in the Vietnam conflict. Milit Med 134: 668–672

Vaughan R G 1977 Motor cycle helmets and facial injuries. Med J Aust 1: 125–127

Wachtel T W, Frank D H, Frank H A 1981 Management of burns of the head and neck. Head Neck Surg 3: 458–474

Wagle V G, Perkins C, Vallera A 1993 Is helmet use beneficial to motorcyclists? J Trauma 34: 120–122

Williams M 1991 The protective performance of bicyclists' helmets in accidents. Accid Anal Prev 23: 119–131

World Health Organization 1977 Manual of the international statistical classification of diseases, injuries and causes of death. WHO, Geneva

World Health Organization 1992 International statistical classification of diseases and related health problems. Tenth revision ICD-10. WHO, Geneva

Wykes W N 1989 Rat bite injury to the eyelids in a 3 month-old child. Br J Ophthalmol 73: 202–204

Zachariades N, Papavassiliou D 1990 The pattern and aetiology of maxillofacial injuries in Greece. A retrospective study of 25 years and a comparison with other countries. J Craniomaxillofac Surg 18: 251–254

Zagelbaum B M, Tostanowski J R, Kerner D J, Hersh P S 1993 Urban eye trauma. A one-year prospective study. Ophthalmology 100: 851–856

Mechanisms of injury

D. A. Simpson   A. J. McLean
Contributing author: I. O. W. Leitch

INTRODUCTION

Mechanical injury results when a part of the body suffers deformation beyond its limits of tolerance. The severity of the injury will depend on the magnitude of the causative force, but also on other factors, notably the time-base of its action. When the force is due to an impact, it is usually necessary to know the impact duration, the acceleration imparted by it to the part of the body struck, and the rate of acceleration change. The surface area on which the impact strikes is also very relevant.

There is much practical importance in studying and if possible quantifying the forces that cause craniomaxillo-facial (CMF) injury. Engineers must do so, to calculate the limits of tolerance of the head in various types of accident; on such calculations are based design standards relating to car and aircraft safety, helmets and other aspects of injury prevention. Surgeons who see injuries in clinical settings will better understand the pathology of these injuries if they can visualize the impact forces that caused the injury: failure to do so when confronted by some unfamiliar cause of a wound, such as a high velocity missile, has often led to errors in management (Owen-Smith 1981). However, the anatomy of the head is very complex: skin, bone and brain have very different physical properties, and the calculation of the effects of real-life impacts is a difficult and controversial undertaking (Ryan et al 1989, Simpson et al 1991). Information derived from animal experiments and from simulated accidents using anthropometric dummies can be extrapolated to give rough estimates of the tolerance of the human head, but such estimates can be misleading. Cadaver experiments are more reliable, especially with respect to skeletal structures, but cannot reproduce the effects of injury on the function of the brain. Efforts are being made to correlate the data from all the available experimental sources and to match these with data from clinicopathological studies. Surgeons and pathologists working in accident services can advance this process of synthesis very greatly by collecting accurate data on impact sites, clinical effects and autopsy findings. Radiological evidence is also invaluable. This chapter reviews some of the data on the mechanisms of CMF injury due to impacts from various causes; in Chapter 5, these mechanisms are related to the injuries produced. The Standard International (SI) units commonly used to quantify impacts are given in Appendix I; in the context of CMF trauma, impact force and acceleration are of chief importance, and to facilitate comparisons these have been expressed wherever possible as kilonewtons (kN) and meters/second per second (m/s^2) respectively.

SKIN INJURIES

The skin of the face and scalp may be lacerated, penetrated, crushed, or avulsed. The facial skin is firmly attached to the underlying tissues, and avulsive injuries are unusual, except as the result of missile impacts or bites. The scalp on the other hand has only a loose attachment to the pericranium and can be avulsed: it has considerable tensile strength, but can be ripped from the head by traction on thick hair when this is caught in machinery.

Skin is easily incised by a knife or penetrated by a bullet. However, the resistance to penetration is not inconsiderable, especially when the skin can yield and stretch (Mendelson 1991). It is not unusual to find that a bullet which has penetrated the skull is brought to rest under the scalp on the opposite side (Fig. 5.18A).

In blunt impacts to the head, the skin of the scalp or face absorbs some of the impact energy. Gadd et al (1970) studied the tolerance of cadaver skin to impacts of different kinds: a window glass edge, aluminium angle edges and flat surfaces were dropped perpendicularly and also at 45° to the skin surface. It was noted that the incised wound produced by a 45° oblique impact was semilunar, because the skin slid away and stretched when first struck. Tolerance to a blunt impact over a relatively large area (25 mm²) was measured in different locations. The scalp proved most resistant to crush injury: marginal damage appeared with a peak impact force of 610 lbs (2.7 kN). This loading is within the estimated tolerance of the underlying frontal bone (see below), and clinical experience confirms that an impact great enough to cause a frontal fracture will usually cause some skin injury in an adult, though often barely detectable. The skin over the zygoma and over the maxilla, containing more fat, was less resistant and showed obvious crush damage at peak impact forces of 168 lb (0.7 kN) and 338 lbs (1.5 kN) respectively. Skin has an important protective effect as padding over the skull bones. In cadaver studies, the presence of facial skin added 50% to the kinetic energy needed to fracture the zygomatic bone (Schneider 1985); however, the difference in peak forces (1.07 and 1.16 kN) was much less. Melvin & Evans (1971) found that the protective effect of scalp was greater when the impacting agent had a large surface area; it also increased greatly with oblique impacts. In their experiments, the scalp absorbed 6–13% of the impact energy. There is an unpredictable variation in the strength of the skin; in cadaver experiments it has therefore been necessary to remove the skin and substitute a standard skin surrogate material.

FACIAL SKELETON

Any fracture, however small, is evidence that the bone has been deformed beyond its limit of tolerance. A localized impact of moderate severity may result in a fracture restricted to a single bone. But more frequently, the fracture also involves adjacent bones, since the bones of the calvaria and the face — with the exception of the mandible — are linked by intricate sutures, and in the adult these are strong and rigid. The resulting fracture pattern expresses the anatomy of the skull, especially the anatomy of the facial struts and buttresses described in Chapter 2 and the unique honeycombed structure of the facial skeleton and the paranasal air sinuses. It is usual to divide the face into three parts, the components of which react to impacts in different ways, and the nature of the resulting injuries depends as much on the mechanical

properties of the skeleton in that area as on the characteristics of the impacting force.

Upper third of the facial skeleton

The chief component is the frontal bone. It is a strong and relatively thick plate of bone, often the site of impacts. In adult life, the frontal convexity is usually at least 5 mm thick and greater thicknesses are not uncommon. However, the orbital plates are much thinner: 1–2 mm at most, and in some areas less. The strength of a plate is proportional to the cube of its thickness: if the frontal convexity and the orbital roof were flat and homogeneous plates of bone respectively 5 and 1 mm thick, the convexity would be not 5 but 125 times stronger. In reality, the frontal bone, like other calvarial and facial bones, is not homogeneous: it is a sandwich of two plates, the inner and outer tables, separated by a variable amount of cellular diploe (Fig. 2.2), and in the midline it is pneumatized to a variable extent by the frontal sinus. These considerations complicate simplistic comparisons of impact strength. Moreover, the frontal convexity and the orbital roofs are usually stressed in different ways. Frontal impacts are likely to be perpendicular to the convexity surface, but in planes more or less tangential to the deeply placed orbital roof: hence fractures of the convexity are usually fissures or areas of depression, while the orbital roof often buckles upwards into the frontal lobe, as does the ethmoid bone where it is part of the floor of the anterior cranial fossa (Fig. 4.1). The orbital roof may also buckle downwards into the orbit, as one form

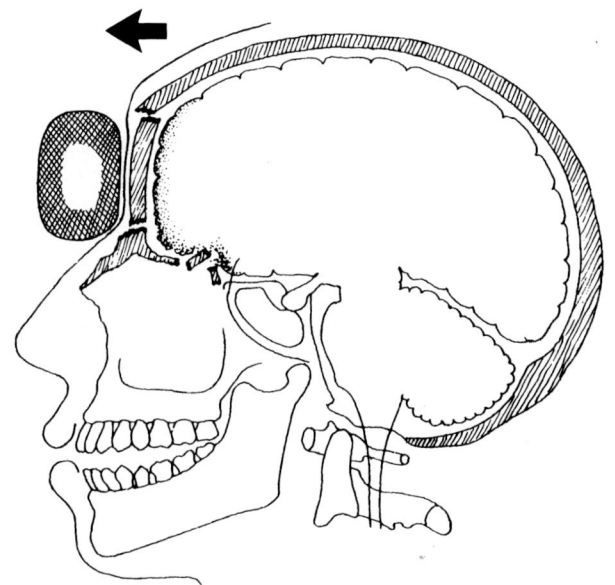

Fig. 4.1 Frontal impact causing depressed fracture. The diagram shows a central frontal impact causing a depressed frontal fracture with buckling in the posterior ethmoid region. More typical is a lateral frontal impact, causing buckling of the orbital roof.

of so-called blow-in fracture (pp. 104 and 327). Tvete (1980) studied basal fractures in tomograms of 21 frontal and nine frontolateral impacts: he found both transverse and parasagittal fracture lines with each type of impact, often running across the orbital roof to remote parts of the skull base. However, the orbital roof is sometimes stressed by a direct impact, as when a missile or sharp object pierces it through the orbit from below (see Fig. 13.12). Hodgson and co-workers at Wayne State University studied the effects of impacts on cadavers in a series of papers reviewed by Schneider (1985). Force was applied to the outer part of the supraorbital ridges: frontal fractures resulted when the force was in the range 4.19–9.12 kN, and these fractures often radiated into the orbital roof on one or both sides. Unlike bones in the middle third of the face (see below), the frontal bone responded as part of the whole calvaria; this implies a greater effect of the impact on the brain. Nahum (1975) also studied frontal impacts on cadavers, the impactor having a 25 mm² circular area and the impact site being a midline area in front of the coronal suture; the duration of the impact pulse was varied by placing crushable nickel foam over the impactor tip. Tolerance, as defined by the appearance of linear fractures, was in the range 800–1600 lbs (3.56–7.12 kN); female skulls were more fragile. In these and other studies, the duration of the impact did not appear to affect the limit of tolerance and peak impact force was considered to be a satisfactory measure of tolerance.

Middle third of facial skeleton

This is a complex of bones and cartilages organized in the system of buttresses described in Chapter 2; in adults it is extensively pneumatized. Some of the components have been studied individually. The zygoma is a flat bone, some 5 mm in maximum thickness. It is supported medially by the lateral wall of the orbit and the lateral wall of the maxillary sinus; although these are very thin plates of bone, their long axes make T-junctions with the zygoma, thus reinforcing the zygoma against lateral impacts. Posteriorly, the zygoma joins the thin zygomatic arch of the temporal bone, which has no internal skeletal support. Hodgson, in the series of cadaver studies already mentioned, and also Nahum (1975), found that impacts on the zygoma and the zygomatic arch in situ caused fractures at relatively low peak forces: in Nahum's tests, the arch failed under forces in the range 208–475 lbs (0.93–2.12 kN) and the body at a somewhat higher range of forces, males being in general at the higher end of the range. Yoganandan et al (1991) have confirmed and amplified these findings in a cadaver study of impacts on the zygoma with steering wheels. The threshold force for fracture by an ordinary steering wheel was 1.4 kN, and somewhat higher with an energy-absorbing wheel;

higher impact forces caused more extensive fractures of the midface. Interestingly, this study did not show an association between bone mineral content and severity of facial fracture.

The maxilla, a box-like bone, has been harder to assess as an entity; Nahum (1975) tested its thin anterior wall and found that this shattered at quite low force loadings, in the range 150–300 lbs (0.67–1.34 kN).

The thin nasal bones are supported laterally by the frontal processes of the maxilla and posteriorly by the septal cartilage. They are very easily fractured; in the cadaver studies by Nyquist et al (1986) cited below, nasal fractures occurred with impact energies well below those needed to fracture other facial bones; in cadavers with only nasal fractures, the mean force was 2.77 kN, but the authors emphasized that this was not a threshold figure, as the nose was fractured in all their experiments and they did not evaluate the lower limit of nasal tolerance. Nahum (1975) gave a tolerance range of 25–75 lbs (0.11–0.33 kN), but admitted that the test series was not extensive. The direction of the impact force is of relevance in determining the nasal distortion (p. 333). In a recent experimental study of nasal impacts, Murray et al (1986) emphasized that the resilient nasal septum is important in determining the nature of the deformity. These authors remarked that the nose is a stronger structure than experimental figures of force tolerance would suggest, because the cited studies have recorded forces applied to a very small area; this is true, but it also remains true that the nose is the most exposed and most fragile part of the facial skeleton.

Tests of the tolerance of the midface as a whole have been done to quantitate the forces of real-life impacts against the steering-wheel and other car interior structures. It has been shown (Schneider 1985) that if force is distributed evenly over the whole face by a form-fitting moulded block, then the facial skeleton will stand very high loadings (>13 kN) without fracturing: under such circumstances, much of the impact force would presumably be transmitted to the head as a whole — and to the brain. Fortunately for car drivers, the actual impacting agents usually load a restricted area of the face, which absorbs much of the impact energy (see below). Two recent cadaver studies have assessed the effects of impact by a metal bar simulating a steering wheel. In a series of unembalmed adult cadavers, Nyquist et al (1986) found that the threshold for serious facial fractures (excluding broken nasal bones) was 3.07 kN. Cesari et al (1989) reassessed the facial tolerance level. Their study is of special clinical interest because it considered impacts at two midface levels — the nasion and the maxilla below the nose. Blows on the nasion sometimes gave classical Le Fort III fractures, or fractures of the nasal and frontal bones, at peak forces of 1.80–3.76 kN, whereas blows below the nose at lower peak forces only broke the nasal spine. Stanley & Nowak (1985), in a cephalometric study of cadaver facial impacts, stressed the importance of the angle of impact in relation to the horizontal buttresses of the facial skeleton. Impacts on the nasion at 30–60° above the horizontal (Fig. 4.2) are likely to cause a Le Fort III fracture (craniofacial disjunction). Horizontal impacts along the Frankfurt base line (Fig. 4.3) can cause Le Fort II (pyramidal) fractures, while direct horizontal or angular blows at the level of the upper teeth, but

below the anterior nasal spine, are likely to cause Le Fort I (horizontal maxillary) fractures (Fig. 4.4). The level at which an impacting force strikes the face may also influence significantly the risk of brain injury. Lee et al (1987) demonstrated that patients with upper facial fractures are at the greatest risk, whereas trauma restricted to the midface or lower face was less likely to cause brain injury presumably because the facial skeleton absorbs energy.

The orbit is often fractured indirectly as part of a midface fracture, or by impacts on the zygoma. The lateral or medial wall of the orbit may buckle inward, causing an area of bony depression: this form of blow-in fracture (p. 327) may impinge on the orbital contents, causing some form of ophthalmoplegia. The orbit may also be fractured by an impact directly on its anterior aspect, by an impacting agent large enough to exert force on the orbital contents without penetration, such as a ball > 50 mm in diameter, or a fist. Converse et al (1977) have very convincingly explained the resultant 'blow-out' fracture(s) of the floor or medial wall as the effect of hydraulic pressure transmitted through the semifluid orbital contents (Fig. 4.5). However, Fujino (1974) has shown that similar fractures can be produced by impacts on the orbital rim in the absence of any orbital contents; presumably this is by downward buckling of the orbital floor. Both explanations of this common fracture could be correct.

MANDIBLE

The lower third of the face is a simpler unit and its mechanical properties are more easily tested; however,

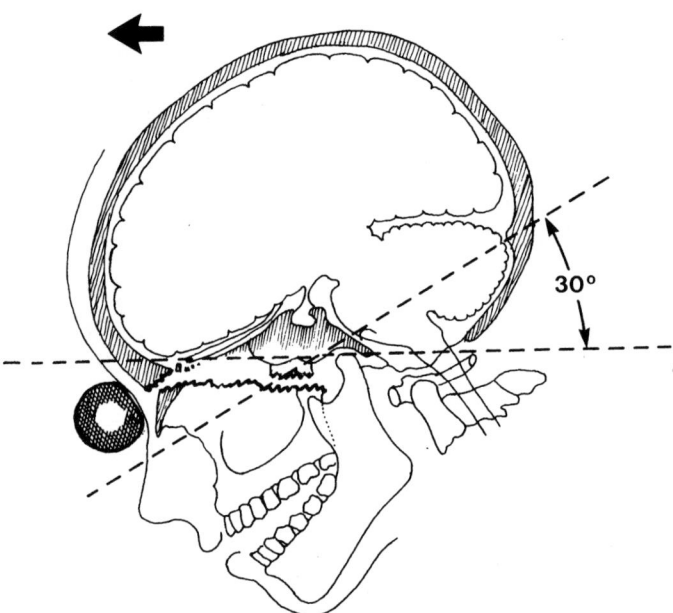

Fig. 4.2 Facial impact causing Le Fort III fracture. Impacts with a vector at an angle 30° above the orbitomeatal plane tend to shear the facial skeleton away from the skull base.

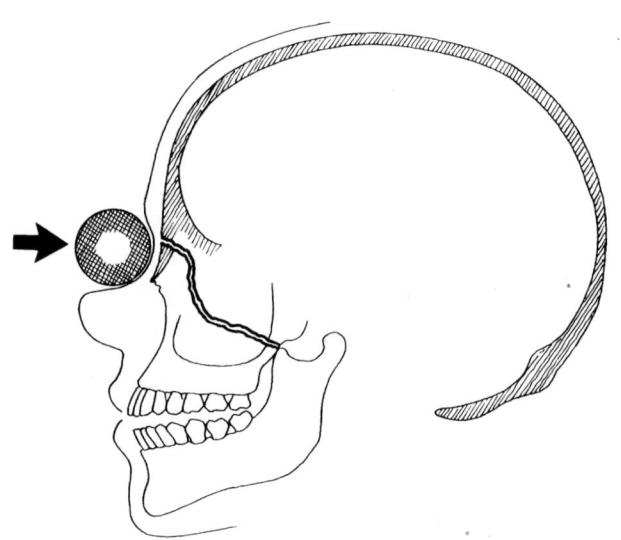

Le Fort II (Pyramidal)

Fig. 4.3 Facial impact causing Le Fort II fracture. Impacts whose vector is in the horizontal (orbitomeatal) plane tend to detach the central component of the midface.

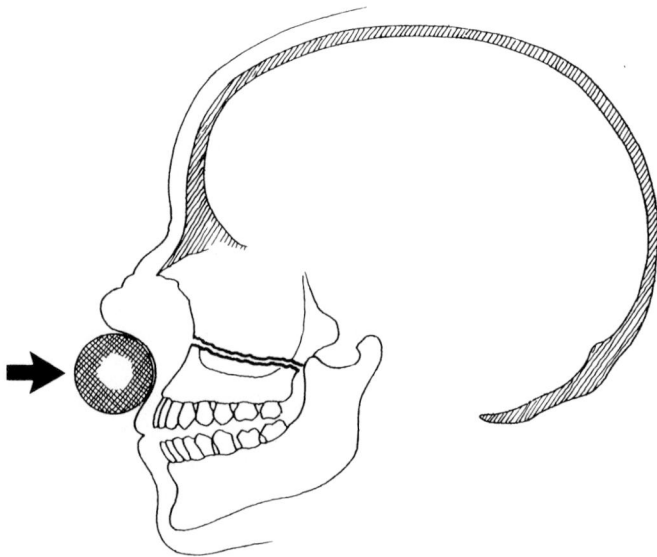

Le Fort I (Horizontal)

Fig. 4.4 Facial impacts causing Le Fort I fracture. Impacts striking below the anterior nasal spine tend to detach the hard palate and maxillary alveoli from the rest of the midface.

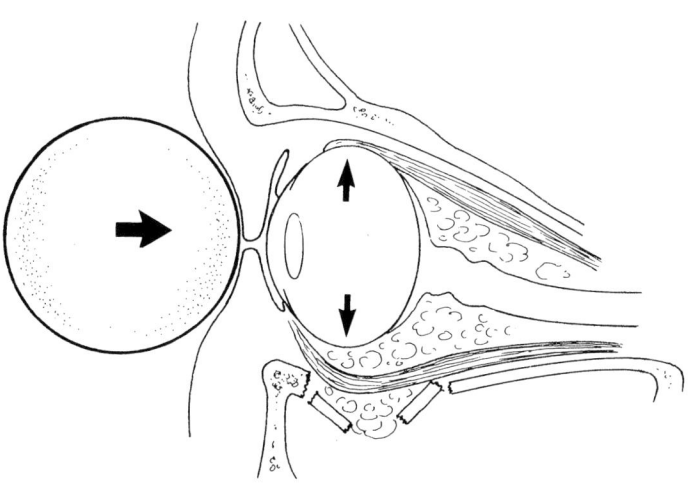

Fig. 4.5 Blunt impact on the orbital contents causing blow-out fracture. A blow by a ball or fist may disrupt the orbital floor. Redrawn after Converse et al (1977).

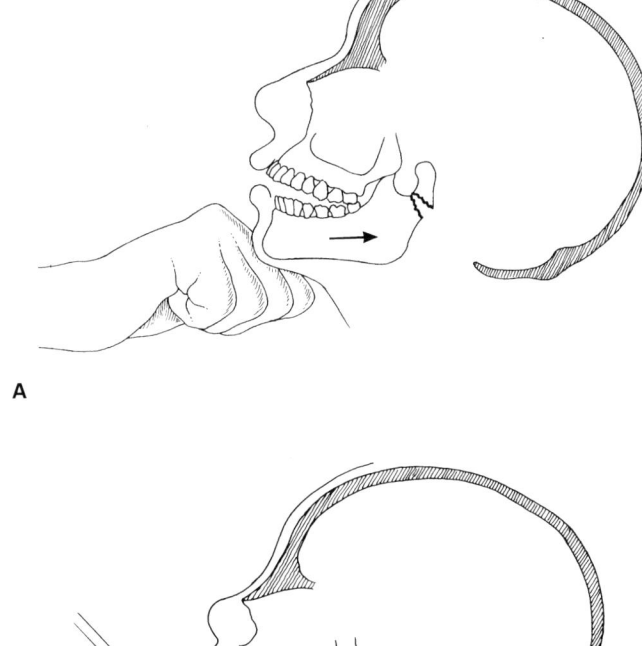

Fig. 4.6 Blunt chin impact to the chin causing mandibular fracture. A In an adult, a punch in the submento-vertical direction may cause unilateral or bilateral subcondylar fractures of the mandible. **B** In a child under 3 years, a fall on the point of the chin may cause a crush fracture of the condyle (s).

its mobility in relation to the rest of the facial skeleton introduces complications in impact analysis and the actions of the masticatory muscles affect the deformities resulting from fractures, so that it is harder to deduce the site of impact from the fracture.

Huelke (1961) carried out a series of cadaver studies of mandibular impacts, including stress coat studies to identify areas of maximum stress: these were found to be the subcondylar region and the mental foramen (Schneider 1985). These are regarded as anatomical points of weakness, though Huelke was not able to confirm that this is true of the mental foramen. Hodgson (1967) also studied mandibular impacts and found that fractures occurred with forces in the range 1.60–2.67 kN. Nahum (1975) looked at the effects of anteroposterior impacts in the region of the symphysis planes. With different force directions in relation to the horizontal plane, impacts could cause fractures either in the symphysis, body or subcondylar region (Fig. 4.6A). Subcondylar fractures appeared with forces in the range 135–550 lbs (0.60–2.45 kN), fractures of the symphysis after higher impact forces (850–925 lbs, 3.78–4.12 kN). It has been argued teleologically that the relative weakness of the subcondylar region is beneficial since a fracture here is preferable to a dislocation of the condyle into the middle fossa (Georgiades 1977). Lateral impacts on a large area of the mandibular body caused transverse fractures, the impact forces varying over a wide range (184–765 lbs, 0.82–3.40 kN). Again, lower levels of forces caused fractures in females.

Cadaver studies of CMF skeletal injury have been valuable in preparing designs for safer car interiors. They are clinically of some importance in understanding the radiological evidences of CMF fractures and in correlating these with external signs of impacts. However, the impact forces listed above should be viewed with caution. The cadavers studied were often elderly; in the old, the limits of skeletal tolerance and even the fracture patterns may not be the same as in healthy young adults. Certainly these experiments cannot be extrapolated to the paediatric age group. The mechanisms of paediatric CMF injury have received little experimental study, but anatomical and clinical experience suggest that impact tolerance and fracture patterns show age-related differences in infants and children. In early life, the calvarial bones are much thinner than in adults and their internal architecture is different: they contain haemopoietic marrow and the diploic bone is not fully modelled in the cellular compartments seen in mature calvarial bone (Fig. 2.2). When struck, the infant's frontal bone dents and the child's frontal bone suffers a depressed fracture (p. 511), under force loads which to our knowledge have not yet been quantified but which seem to be much less than those needed to cause fractures in adults. Similarly the child's facial skeleton is elastic, and contains haemopoietic marrow in the cancellous bone; it is incompletely pneumatized (Fig. 2.10) and it is covered by soft tissues which are usually thicker than in adults, giving better padding (Manson 1988).

Anatomical differences are especially evident in the growing mandible. In the infant and young child, the angle between the ramus and the body of the mandible is more obtuse than in the adult: impacts on the chin are likely to load the condyle in the axis of the ramus, and the condyle, which is in part formed of growing cartilage, may be crushed (Fig. 4.6B). The long-term implications of mandibular immaturity are explored in Chapters 11 and 19 (pp. 282 and 504).

This consideration of the mechanisms of facial fracture has emphasized that the components of the facial skeleton have impact tolerance limits: when these are exceeded, a more or less serious facial fracture results. There is an important corollary to this: in inflicting this skeletal injury, energy is absorbed which might otherwise be transmitted to the brain. Both theoretical considerations and clinical experience suggest that for impacts of a given severity, there is an inverse relation between facial skeletal injury and brain damage (Lee et al 1987). The facial skeleton, and especially its middle and lower thirds, can therefore be regarded as a protective crumple zone. This protective capacity is seen in a different form in the upper third of the face: the frontal convexity is much more resistant to penetration, but does transmit impact force to the whole calvaria, and so to the brain. (An exception may be made for the anterior wall of the frontal sinus, which may fail under a localized impact without transmission of clinically significant force to the whole head.) Nevertheless, there is reason to believe that the upper third of the face has better impact tolerance than other parts of the calvarial skull (p. 15). It is certainly the most impact-resistant part of the facial skeleton, followed by the mandible and the zygoma; the nasal bones have least impact resistance and are most often fractured.

BRAIN

The brain is often injured by impacts in the CMF region. Impacts in the upper third of the face may penetrate or indent the frontal bone and directly injure the underlying brain. This is likely to happen when the impact has high kinetic energy applied to a small surface area, or when the impacting agent strikes thin bone such as the roof of the orbit or nose. (Fig. 4.7). Localized brain injury can result from acute deformation of the overlying skull without dural penetration: contusions of the cerebral cortex are often seen under linear skull fractures, and in infants the skull can undergo injurious deformation without fracture. There are no conceptual difficulties in understanding the mechanisms of these contact brain injuries: both the indentation and the subsequent recoil are obvious causes

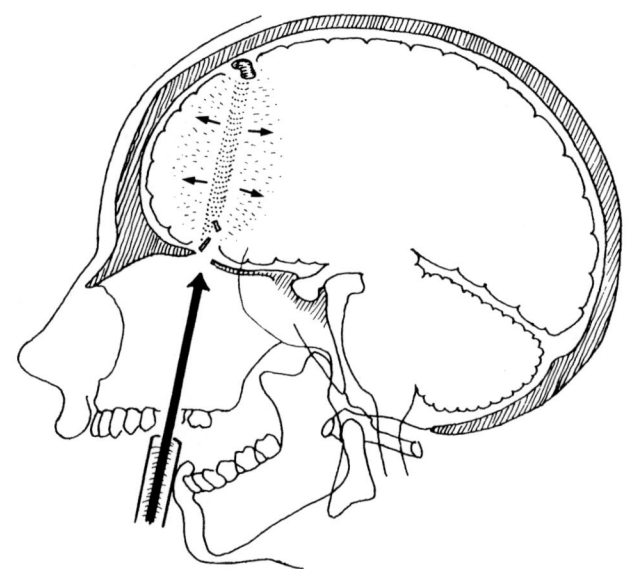

Fig. 4.7 Missile wound of frontal region. A bullet fired through the thin bone of the anterior fossa may penetrate the brain, making a primary wound track or cavity. Energy imparted laterally causes a temporary expansion of the primary cavity (secondary cavity: dotted lines) in the brain, increasing tissue disruption.

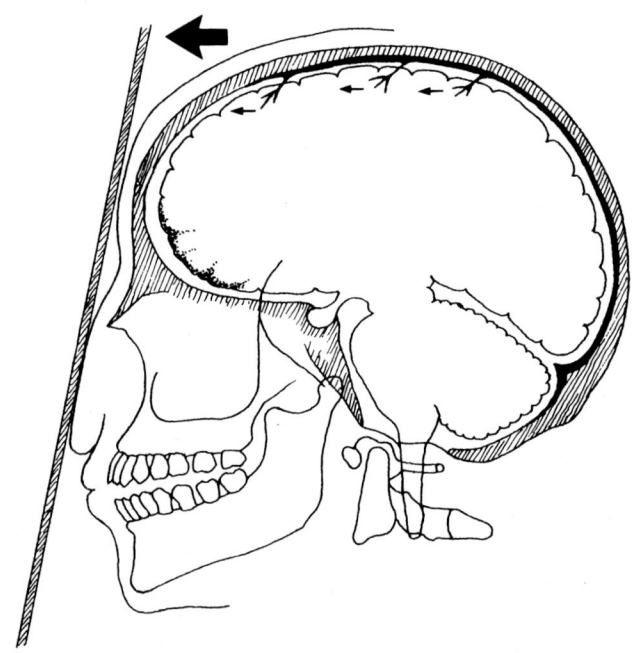

Fig. 4.8 Frontal impact causing inertial brain damage. Blunt impact by the moving head against a flat surface can cause inertial brain damage. This may take the form of frontal and temporal contusions, rupture of bridging veins and subdural bleeding (small arrows), or diffuse axonal damage. Impacts in the sagittal plane are less detrimental than lateral impacts.

of injury to the underlying cortex. But in the majority of cases, the brain sustains injury in the absence of skull penetration or significant local deformation, often in parts of the brain remote from the impact site (Fig. 4.8). An extreme example is seen in boxing, where an impact on the chin may cause loss of consciousness or even rupture of a major cerebral vessel and death (Unterharnscheidt 1975).

The mechanisms of brain injury in such closed head injuries have been much discussed and many fruitful experimental studies have been carried out. Cadaver studies have been useful, but cannot reproduce the physiological effects of brain injury, or indeed the microscopic pathology. Human volunteers have given useful data, but only within the limits of survival — though these have been taken dangerously far by the celebrated Col. John P. Stapp (p. 25). Animal experimentation, especially on anaesthetized primates, has therefore been indispensable.

The phenomenon of ultimate concern is the response of the brain of the living human to impact to the face or calvarial vault. Brain injuries can be readily studied by neuropathological methods in fatal cases. In vivo, neuroradiology — CT or MRI scan — provides a relatively crude though clinically valuable indication of the location and extent of brain injuries. In contrast, the physical characteristics of the impact to the head are far more difficult to estimate after the event. When the impacting object has been identified, and can be examined, some information of value in the estimation of the severity of the impact may be obtained, particularly if the object itself has been deformed (see below). In some situations, such as a fall from a known height, a reasonably accurate estimate can be made of the velocity with which the head strikes the ground. Similar estimates of impact velocity can sometimes be made by careful reconstruction of evidence available after a road crash. When combined with information on the characteristics of the object struck, the impact velocity can yield an estimate of the force of the impact.

It is now generally agreed that a major cause of brain injury is tissue deformation induced by acceleration imparted to the whole head. When the head is struck, the skull is accelerated; the brain shows inertia and suffers shear strains of different types. An identical sequence of *inertial injury* is seen when the moving head hits a rigid object and is abruptly decelerated. The physicist Holbourn (1943, 1945: see p. 25) concluded that the most injurious type of acceleration must be rotational. The brain is an incompressible jelly-like substance; it has only limited capacity to move within the rigid calvarial box, and Holbourn discounted the significance of linear acceleration under these circumstances. He emphasized the importance of the compartmenting structures within the skull, notably the falx and the sphenoidal ridges, and produced a model of brain injury (Fig. 4.9) that showed the stresses resulting from angular acceleration producing shear strains maximal in the vicinity of these ridges, in sites corresponding to the distribution of contusional damage after blunt impacts (p. 138). The presence of irregularities in the orbital bone surfaces can be seen as an augmenting factor in the causation of inferior frontal and temporal contusions.

Not all workers accepted Holbourn's concept of the primacy of rotational or angular acceleration. Movement of the brain inside the skull does occur: the brain lies within the smooth-surfaced dural envelope, to which it is anchored by bridging veins dorsally, and ventrally by a number of structures such as the pituitary stalk and the cranial nerves. Avulsion of these tethering structures

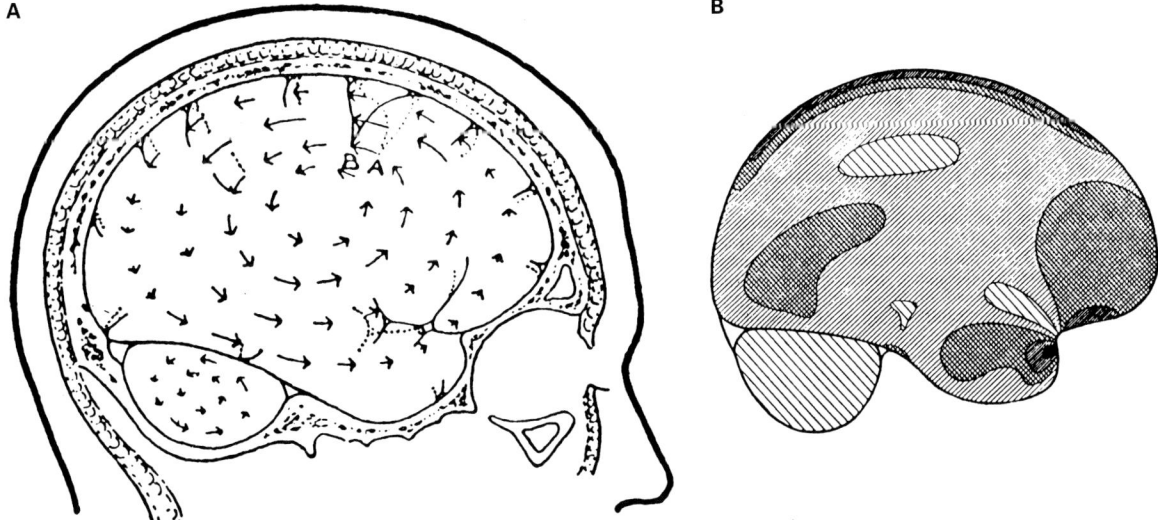

Fig. 4.9 Accelerational injury of the brain. Holbourn conceived angular or rotational acceleration as the chief cause of brain injury. **A** In rotational movement of the head after impact, the skull and brain do not move together: lagging of the brain takes the form of whirling movement (arrows). **B** Gelatine model of the brain showing distortion (darker shading) when the model is rotated in the sagittal plane as by an occipital impact. Distortion is maximal in the temporal and subfrontal regions. From Holbourn (1945) by courtesy of the *British Medical Bulletin*.

(see below) is clinically quite common, suggesting that linear or translational brain movement may be a factor in injury causation. Moreover, the open foramen magnum allows adjustment of intracranial pressure: it has been argued that when the head suffers an impact, a craniospinal pressure gradient is set up and pressure waves are transmitted to the lower brainstem. Gurdjian et al (1968) saw this as a mechanism for causing shear stresses in the brain stem. Other workers, notably in Sweden, saw shock waves as a mechanism for causing cavitation lesions in the brain substance, evident to neuropathologists as contusions (p. 138). Later research has discounted both craniospinal pressure gradients and cavitation induced by shock waves as significant causes of acute primary brain injury (Stålhammer 1990).

Ommaya (1985) and others have endorsed the importance of rotational or angular acceleration, but have also found evidence to support the role of linear or translational acceleration as a cause of some focal lesions. Experimental studies by Gennarelli (1983) have strongly reinforced the importance of angular acceleration. By devising primate experimental models in which either linear or angular acceleration can be produced in various planes and at various speeds, Gennarelli and his colleagues have been able to produce the chief pathological lesions seen in acute closed head injury. Linear (translational) acceleration produced contusional brain damage without the physiological effects of 'cerebral concussion'. At high angular acceleration generated in a short time interval (rise time < 10 ms) and applied in the sagittal plane, acute subdural haematomas were produced: these were usually lethal and survival with prolonged coma was not seen (Gennarelli & Thibault 1982). But when angular acceleration in the coronal plane was generated over a longer rise time, diffuse axonal injury (p. 139) with coma was regularly and predictably the outcome, and the duration of coma was roughly proportional to the magnitude of the acceleration. These findings suggest that inertial stress induced by acceleration will reproduce virtually all of the primary effects of closed head injury.

The limits of brain tolerance have been explored in cadavers, in animal experiments, in human volunteers and in real-life accidents (Gurdjian 1972); anthropomorphic dummy heads have also been used to model and extend the data. These limits are conveniently expressed in units of acceleration (g or m/s^2: see Appendix I), since the acceleration can be measured by attaching accelerometers to the head or the head surrogate. Two markers of brain injury threshold have been used: skull fracture in cadavers and loss of consciousness in accidents and experiments. The use of a skull fracture as a marker needs no justification. The use of loss of consciousness as evidence of significant brain injury is also reasonable. When the loss is transient (< 5 min) and followed by complete clinical recovery, it has been assumed that there is no structural

brain damage, and in the past the term concussion was given to this seemingly benign effect of head impact. But modern thinking places concussion in a spectrum that extends to include diffuse structural brain damage and even death; it is therefore proper to regard loss of consciousness, however brief, as evidence of an injury that may be beyond the limits of tolerance. In these terms, the limits of human brain tolerance are thought to be reached by peak accelerations of 150 g (1470 m/s^2). This corresponds to a force of about 6 kN transmitted to the cranium (Haley et al 1983).

However, the duration of the impact pulse is of great importance in determining tolerance. This is expressed in the well-known Wayne State University (WSU) Tolerance Curve (Fig. 4.10) which shows that shorter pulse durations are better tolerated, whereas longer (> 10 ms) accelerations may be injurious well below 100 g. The data embodied in the WSU tolerance curve have been used in the development of the Head Injury Criterion (HIC) which, though often criticized, still remains the measure of risk of head injury in car crash testing.

This book is primarily concerned with impacts in the CMF region, in many of which brain damage may result from force applied to the frontal region, or transmitted through the facial skeleton. It is therefore pertinent to ask how relevant are these limits of tolerance in the context of CMF trauma. In fact, the original WSU data were derived from frontal impacts in cadavers, and they are therefore directly relevant to injuries of the upper third of the face; the effects of injuries to the lower face are attenuated by the mechanisms discussed above. There is a good deal of evidence to suggest that Percivall Pott (p. 15) was right in thinking that impacts in the frontal

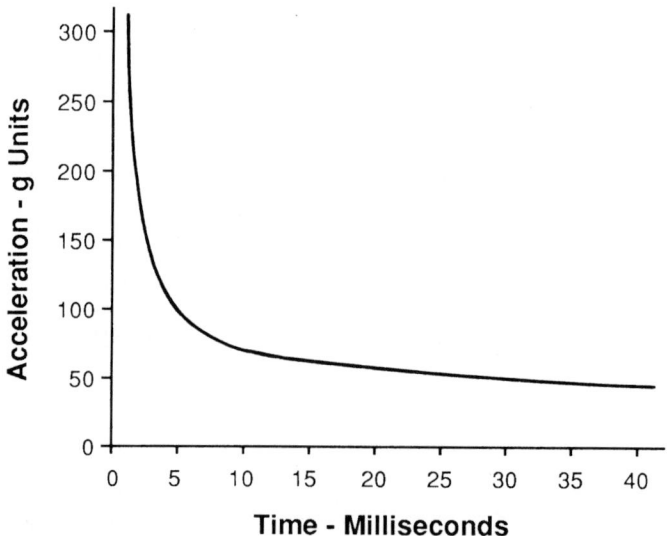

Fig. 4.10 The Wayne State University Tolerance Curve. Above the curve, head impacts are likely to cause significant brain injury (Gurdjian 1972).

region are less injurious than lateral and occipital impacts. Our own clinicopathological studies (Simpson et al 1991) suggest this, and there are several possible explanations. The mechanical properties of the frontal skull may be responsible. Nahum and coworkers (quoted by Melvin & Evans 1971) found that in the frontal region, impact force needed to produce a fracture was twice that needed in the temporoparietal region. It is also possible that the brain is less vulnerable to acceleration in the sagittal plane: this was one of the most interesting findings in the experiments by Gennarelli and coworkers cited above. There is need for further research, but at present the HIC seems the best available measure of the limits of tolerance to frontal impacts.

CRANIAL NERVES AND PITUITARY STALK

The cranial nerves are often injured in association with other CMF injuries (p. 136). The mechanisms have received surprisingly little attention. When nerve injury is seen in association with a penetrating injury, no difficulties arise in interpretation, but nerve damage after blunt impact can pose problems. Two mechanisms are postulated: stretch or traction, and compression.

The peripheral nerves have some elasticity and considerable tensile strength, which is due to the connective tissue perineurium. But they suffer disruption if stretched by more than 30% of their length, or even less. It seems likely that the cranial nerves, like the spinal nerve roots, are relatively less able to tolerate traction in their subarachnoid course, where their perineurial sheaths are less well developed. Certainly, operative experience suggests that the fine filaments of the olfactory nerve are easily avulsed, and the fourth (trochlear) nerve is also easily damaged in surgical dissections around the midbrain. It is postulated that the frequent occurrence of anosmia after occipital impacts represents traction–avulsion by movement of the brain in the sagittal plane. Anosmia is also common after frontal impacts. In such cases, it is uncertain whether traction should be postulated: in some, the cribriform plate is fractured and the olfactory filaments could be torn at the fracture site. Traction is also postulated in some cases of injury to the third, fourth and sixth cranial nerves. Heinze (1969) found autopsy evidence of avulsion of rootlets of these nerves, in the absence of skull fracture; the chief site was the junction with the brainstem.

Many authors have favoured tensile or shear stress as a mechanism of optic nerve injury. The optic nerves are anchored in the optic canal, and the pathological findings (p. 418) accord well with the concept that the nerve is stretched or sheared in this region, perhaps especially at its intracranial end. Tomei et al (1990) have shown experimentally in a guinea-pig model that a 30 g tensile loading at a strain rate of 200 ms will cause axonal injury in the optic nerve: this experiment was not designed as a model of human optic nerve injury, but it does show that axons in the optic nerve are vulnerable to tension. Damage to the pituitary stalk could also result from traction. Although there is an abundant literature on post-traumatic diabetes insipidus and anterior pituitary failure from infarction of the adenohypophysis (p. 57), the mechanism or mechanisms have not been clearly defined (Treip 1984); traction seems very likely in some cases.

Peripheral nerves are sensitive to compression, especially if prolonged; Nitz & Matulionis (1982) found that rat peripheral nerves subjected to tourniquet compression at only 300 mmHg showed ultrastructural damage after 30 min, and marked loss of myelin after 3 h. Compression seems the likely mechanism in those cases in which a fracture is close to the injured nerve. Branches of the trigeminal nerve are often injured in association with facial fractures; the infraorbital nerve and the inferior dental nerve may be compressed within their respective canals. The optic nerve is also sometimes found to be compressed by a displaced fragment of bone: Gonzalez et al (1990) reported a case of permanent blindness from intrusion of a piece of the greater wing of the sphenoid after an impact on the zygomatic bone. It is harder to provide a satisfactory explanation when there is an optic nerve lesion without radiologically visible fracture in the canal. Jend & Jend-Rossmann (1984) reported cases showing an association between fractures of the sphenotemporal buttress and optic nerve injury without fracture of the optic canal; their case reports suggest that these fractures were due to impacts in the frontolateral region, and we have seen cases with a similar association of optic nerve damage and frontolateral impact site. In such cases, it is possible that force transmitted through the skull has caused transient compression of the nerve in the optic foramen, with elastic recovery of the bone. Anderson et al (1982) performed holographic interferometric studies on dried skulls, and concluded that force applied to the supraorbital ridge was transmitted to the region of the optic foramen; this may explain why blindness due to optic nerve damage sometimes results from relatively minor impacts in this site, especially in children (p. 418).

EYE

The eye and its adnexae may be lacerated or incised by sharp objects or missiles. The eye can be damaged, even ruptured, by a blunt object small enough to enter the orbit. The lids, cornea and conjunctiva may be injured by direct impact. The globe itself is a robust structure, cushioned by muscles and by intraconal and extraconal fat, but its limits of tolerance can be exceeded: when it is impacted with sufficient force, it deforms and expands at its equator, and the outcome may be a scleral rupture (Fig. 4.11). Less severe deformation may result in internal

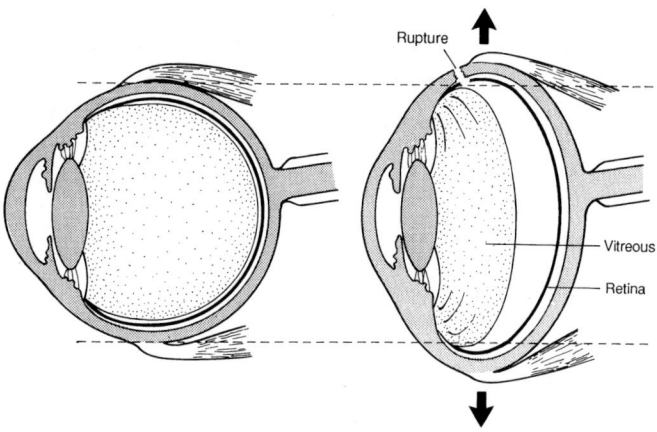

Fig. 4.11 Blunt impact on eyeball causing scleral rupture. An impact on the cornea may rupture the sclera at the equator (arrows); detachment of the vitreous body and the retina may result. Drawn after Maguire & Benson (1986).

damage, notably retinal detachment by traction on the collagenous fibres anchoring the vitreous to the anterior border of the retina (Maguire & Benson 1986). Antero-posterior compression may also damage the attachment of the ciliary body and the drainage angle (Fig. 2.36C), possibly causing secondary glaucoma (p. 413). Green et al (1990) carried out experiments on the macaque monkey in which force was applied to the globe alone: a force developing energies in the range 2.08–3.56 J consistently caused a blow-out fracture of the orbital floor, but also ruptured the globe in about a quarter of the experiments.

EXTRACRANIAL INJURIES

Impacts on the frontal bone and the facial skeleton may cause serious damage in structures outside the CMF region by inducing hyperextension of the head on the neck. In a series of 36 fatal brainstem lacerations, 26 (72%) had evidence of impact on the face or on the frontal aspect of protective helmets; it appeared that these impacts had fractured the skull base or dislocated the atlanto-occipital joint by inducing violent hyperextension (Simpson et al 1989). Frontal impacts may also cause hyperextension dislocations and/or fractures of the cervical spine (Kazanjian 1983). Of more relevance in this book, acute hyperextension may load the carotid arteries in the neck. These arteries are anchored in the skull base and in the chest; sudden axial loading may result in arterial injury and even rupture (p. 145). This is believed to be one cause of extracranial thrombosis of the internal carotid artery by blunt trauma, the other being direct impact on the neck. However, these conjectured mechanisms of arterial injury have not yet been validated experimentally.

CAUSES OF IMPACTS IN CMF REGION

Falls

From the biomechanical viewpoint, the calculation of head impact force and acceleration is simple in the case of a free fall. Given that the height of the fall and the nature of the struck surface are known, the velocity at impact (v) is given by the formula:

$$v = \sqrt{2\,gh}$$

where g is the acceleration of gravity and h the height of the centre of gravity of the body from the struck surface The linear head impact acceleration (a) is given by the formula:

$$a = v\sqrt{K/m}$$

where K is the combined stiffness of the head and the impacting surface — a measure derived experimentally — and m the effective mass of the head. From these relatively simple calculations, Manavis et al (1991) concluded that the impact-induced linear accelerations in 18 fatal falls were in the range 2000–7000 m/s², or about 200–700 g.

In real falls, the clinical outcome depends on the height and on the part of the head that strikes the ground. In the series of fatal falls studied by Manavis et al (1991), there was only one case of impact on the frontal aspect of the head: the others were all lateral or occipital. In non-fatal falls, the protective effect of the facial skeleton and the primitive reflex extension of the arms presumably reduce the impact acceleration of the head to a level that is tolerable by the brain.

Road crashes

The outcome of a road crash depends on the velocity of the head at impact, on whether the head strikes a hard surface, and on whether that surface is flat, angular or sharp. The anatomical site of the impact is also of critical importance, not only because some parts of the face are more vulnerable than others, but also because the degree of angular acceleration imparted to the head depends on the torque, and hence on the relation of the impact vector to the centre of gravity of the head.

Car occupants may suffer head impacts from some part of the car interior, or less commonly by an intruding object; if not properly restrained, the car occupant may be ejected and strike the road surface or some other external object. Penetrating injuries by impact over a small area have been seen when the head or face struck a dashboard knob; better design of car interiors has made this unusual, and today most injuries in car occupants are due to blunt impacts by surfaces which may be relatively unyielding (in engineering terms 'stiff') such as the steel pillars of

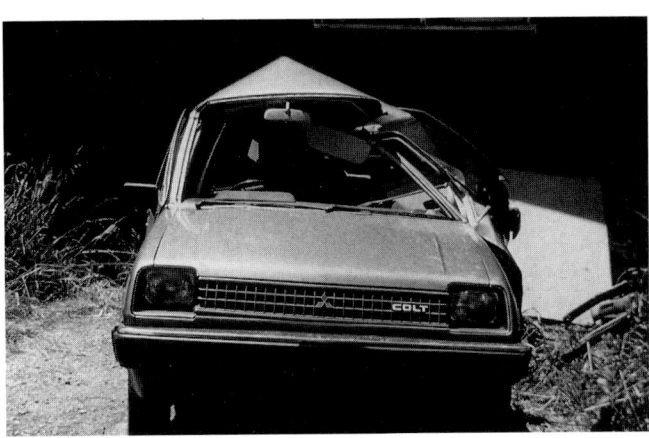

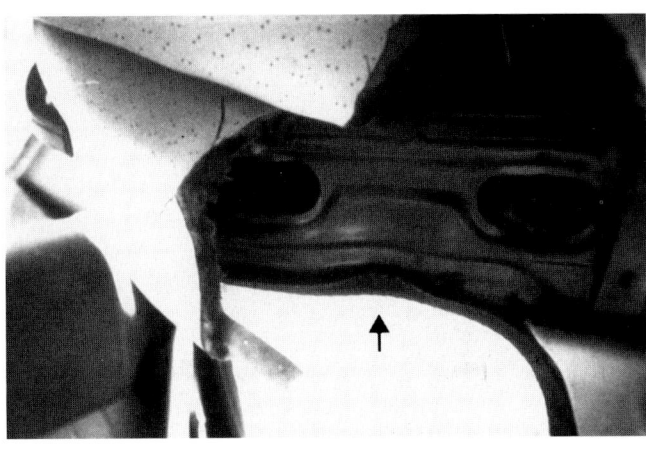

A

B

Fig. 4.12 Estimation of linear and angular impact accelerations in a case of frontal impact. It is sometimes possible to estimate linear and angular acceleration caused by head impacts in road crashes, provided that the relevant data have been obtained by accident investigation and examination of the head impact site. **A** A 17-year-old man lost control of his car which struck a tree on the left side; from accident site investigation and the deformation of the car, the impact velocity was estimated at 43–50 km/h. **B** His head hit an intruding roof rail at an estimated velocity of 45 km/h. The roof rail was deformed by the impact. The stiffness of the roof rail was classed as 'hard' (estimated stiffness 600 000 N/m) from car structure data; the stiffness and mass of the head were estimated from the driver's age and assumed mass. It was then possible to deduce the maximum linear acceleration of the head: $a = 4300$ m/s^2, or about 440 g. The impact site was in the left frontal region and it was possible to estimate the offset of the force vector from the centre of gravity of the head. From this was deduced the maximum angular acceleration of the head: $a = 30\,000$ rads/s^2 Simpson et al (1991).

the car frame, or capable of reducing the impact force by deformation. Such head- or face-friendly surfaces are the padded dashboard and (somewhat surprisingly) the windscreen, if this is composed of laminated glass (Fig. 3.3). Ryan (Simpson et al 1991) tried to estimate the accelerations in car crashes that resulted in death or serious brain injury from impacts in the frontal area by calculations which take into account the stiffness of the impacted structure as well as the velocity of the head when struck and the site of the impact. It was estimated that linear accelerations were in the range 1000–6600 m/s^2 (102–670 g), while angular accelerations were in the range 6600–50 000 rad/s^2. While these estimates are open to criticism, those for linear acceleration accord quite well with experimental studies on cadavers.

For a pedestrian or unhelmeted motor- or pedal cyclist, the outcome of a road crash may depend on whether the head strikes the yielding sheet metal of the bonnet, or some relatively sharp structure, or the unyielding road surface. A properly designed helmet reduces the risks of both sharp and blunt impacts. Most helmets have a hard outer shell of fibreglass or polycarbonate, designed to resist penetration, and penetrating brain injuries are now rare in motorcycle crashes, except when the helmet is shattered. Protective helmets also have an inner layer of expanded polystyrene foam, designed to crush under force and so to reduce the acceleration imparted to the

brain to a tolerable level (Fig. 4.13A). Kingsbury & Rohr (1981) showed that standard motorcycle helmets retain this capacity to cushion impact forces as high as 20 kN.

Published data on helmet performance do not always give information on whether helmets were properly secured; experience has shown that failure to secure helmets is not unusual in injured motorcyclists so that the helmet may fly off at the first impact. Clearly there are limits to the protective value of a helmet (Fig. 4.13B), even when it is properly secured. In real-life motorcycle crashes, fatal brain injuries are often seen when the inner liner is crushed, presumably because its capacity to absorb impact energy has been exhausted. However, it is of concern that serious or even fatal head injuries are sometimes seen in the absence of any evidence of liner crush in CT scans of the helmet (Cooter 1990). Protective helmets are designed to pass tests which measure the capacity of the helmet to reduce linear acceleration, and it is possible that these give insufficient attention to the importance of rotational acceleration in brain injury causation.

Full-face helmets are designed to protect the facial skeleton as well as the brain (p. 89). Cooter et al (1988) have suggested that the provision of facial protection may predispose to skull base fractures (Fig. 4.13D), but this possibility does not detract from the proven overall benefits of helmet use (Simpson et al 1989).

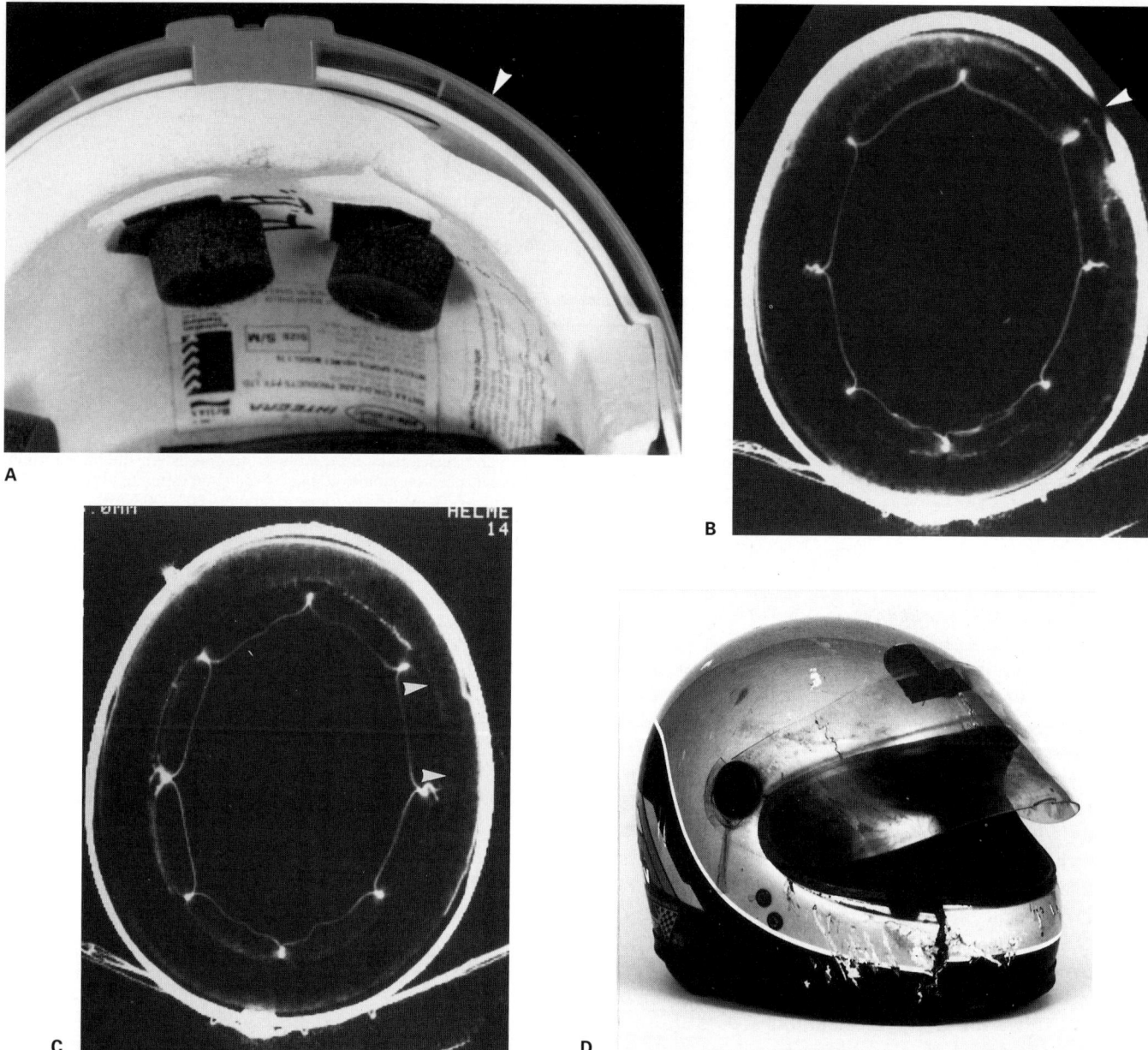

Fig. 4.13 Injury control by helmets: limitations of protection. Helmets are designed to withstand penetration and to reduce the energy of blunt impacts to a level within the tolerance of the brain. Nevertheless there are limitations to the protection given by the helmets now in use, and these are sometimes evident in road crashes at relatively low speeds. **A** Pedal cycle helmet: a young cyclist suffered an impact (arrow) in the occipital region. The foam deformed, presumably absorbing energy, but there was a significant closed head injury. **B** CT scan of helmet: a young pillion rider fell from a motorcycle and was struck in the left frontal region (white arrowhead). There was evidence of damage to the helmet shell, which did not shatter. **C** The scan shows that the helmet liner deformed at the impact site (between arrowheads), no doubt absorbing energy; however, death resulted from a closed head injury with multifocal vascular injuries and severe cerebral swelling. CT has been found to be a useful method of evaluating helmet damage (Cooter 1990). **D** A rider wearing a fibreglass full-face helmet fell from his motorcycle and struck the front of the helmet against a concrete curb. He suffered a skull base fracture and a brainstem tear, and was dead on admission to hospital. There was no evidence of injury to the facial bones. The helmet showed a fracture of the face bar and compression of the energy-absorbing layer in the back of the helmet. It was postulated that impact on the face bar had been transmitted to the skull base, bypassing the energy-absorbing facial bones (Cooter et al 1988).

Boxing and kicking

CMF injuries due to punching are usually left-sided, since a right-handed assailant will tend to strike his adversary on the left side of the face. The punch of a skilled boxer can generate a force of 3–3.5 kN (Joch et al 1981) and this will transfer considerable kinetic energy to the target. Peak linear accelerations of 50–159 g and peak angular accelerations of up to 16 000 rads/s^2 were recorded by Pincemaille et al (1986) in gloved boxers trading punches that did not result in loss of consciousness or even disturbances of cerebral evoked potentials. The bare fist can deliver enough force to fracture the strong mandible, and the gloved fist can impart sufficient acceleration to cause rupture of bridging veins and a lethal subdural haematoma. Kicks, especially with booted feet, are capable of inflicting great force: A. T. S. Vilenius (personal communication) has calculated that a footballer's kick could generate a peak impact force as high as 9 kN, enough to fracture the human skull or to give the head a peak acceleration in excess of 200 g. This estimate may be too high; Schwartz et al (1986) studied the accelerations induced in a dummy head (Hybrid II dummy with simulated skin mask) when kicked or punched by experts in karate and found that maximum peak accelerations were in the range 90–120 g. Direct measurements of force were not made in this study.

Impacts in sport

In body contact sports such as the various types of football, the impact forces are comparable to those sustained in assaults, though usually of lesser magnitude, since most players do not inflict grievous bodily harm deliberately (but see p. 94 for a contrary view on this). In ball–bat/club games, the injuries relate to the mass and impact velocity of the striking object and to its surface area, as well as to the impact site. In cricket (Hill et al 1985), it has been stated that some 70% of injuries are due to the ball, which weighs about 160 g and can travel at velocities as high as 30–40 m/s. The cricket ball is hard and its diameter is about 7.4 cm; typically the impact is localized and the victim sustains a facial fracture, or a skull fracture with contusion of the underlying brain, but little or no accelerational injury in the brain as a whole. A lad struck by a cricket ball (Fig. 4.14) suffered a skull fracture, a small intracerebral haematoma, and an extradural clot, but had only little or no loss of consciousness. In baseball, the ball is only slightly smaller than the cricket ball — its weight is about 142 g — but the velocities are of the same order; impact energies are therefore considerable and able to fracture the skull. Tennis balls are a little smaller and much lighter (about 57 g), but also travel fast (up to 40 m/s²); if a tennis ball impacts on the orbit, it will deform and may transmit hydraulic pressure to the orbital floor in the manner described above (Fig. 4.5). A squash ball, smaller and harder, is also a well documented cause of orbital blow-out fracture.

A golf ball weighs about 45 g, and can be driven very fast: velocities as high as 70 m/s are quoted. However, golf ball impacts are not common. In golf, the chief cause of injury is the club, and as golf clubs have relatively sharp edges, the impact force is localized over a small area and a depressed fracture is the likely result. In the series of head injuries due to golfing accidents reported by

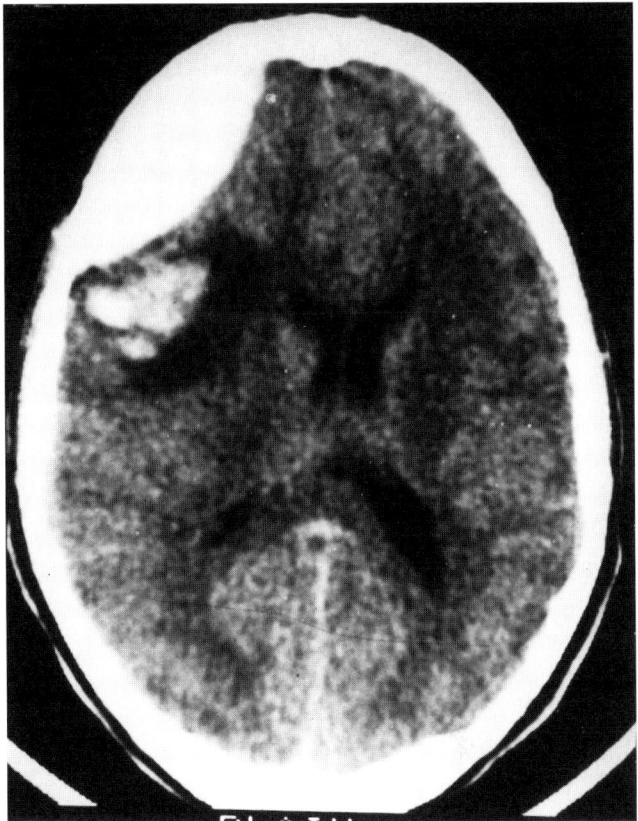

Fig. 4.14 Blunt impact causing frontal extradural haematoma. A boy was hit in the right frontal region by a cricket ball. He was not admitted to hospital. He later developed an extradural haematoma at the point of impact; CT also showed a small intracerebral haematoma.

Smith et al (1991), nine of 11 children had compound depressed fractures.

Bites

The wounds inflicted by human and animal bites are discussed in Chapter 18. The forces developed by larger animals are impressive: Chambers & Payne (1969) stated that guard dogs have a natural bite pressure of 150–200 psi, which can be raised by military training in canine aggression to 450 psi. Wolpoff (1971) has reviewed data on human bite force; it appears that the molars develop maximal forces of the order of 78 kg, or less than 1 kN, and the incisors rather less.

Missile impacts

When a bullet or small shell fragment strikes the head, force is applied to an area that may be only a few millimetres in diameter. Very little acceleration is imparted to the head as a whole, but devastating injury can be inflicted by penetration and tissue disruption, especially if the missile is travelling at high velocity.

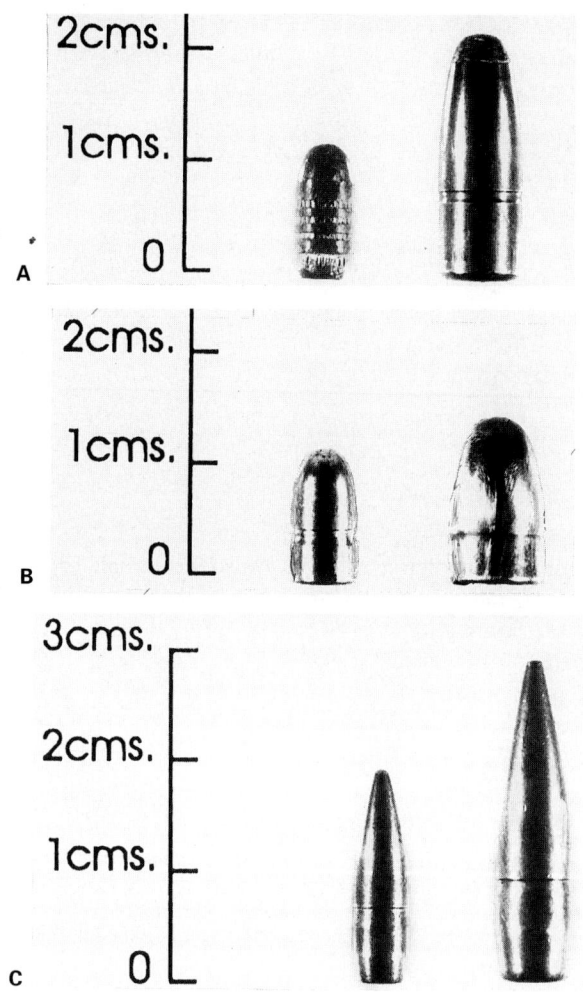

Fig. 4.15 **Bullets in common use. A** Sporting rifle bullets: on left, a .22 in. (5.56 mm) long rifle bullet, made of lead, no jacket; on right, a .303 in. (7.70 mm) hunting bullet, with cupronickel jacket but soft nose of lead. **B** Pistol bullets, with nickel or cupronickel jackets: on left a .25 in bullet, on right a 9 mm ball bullet, used in World War II. **C** Military rifle bullets, with nickel or cupronickel jackets: on left, a version of the small .22 in (5.6 mm) bullet fired by the Armalite or M16 rifle; on right the 7.62 mm NATO rifle bullet.

Figure 4.15 shows some sporting and military bullets in common use today; Table 4.1 sets out their characteristics. The damage resulting from a bullet wound in the CMF region is related to a number of factors:

1. The kinetic energy of the bullet at impact
2. The dimensions of the bullet at impact
3. The wobbling or tumbling of the bullet in flight and after impact
4. The tendency of the bullet to fragment or deform
5. The secondary missiles — teeth, bone chips etc. — which may be set into motion.

The relative importance of these factors is in debate. Excellent accounts of the ballistics of missile wounds are given by Owen-Smith (1981), Fackler (1988) and Mendelson (1991). The muzzle velocity of the bullet has been given great prominence, since it largely determines the impact energy. The impact energy of a missile is calculated by the well-known formula:

$$E = \tfrac{1}{2} MV^2$$

where M is the mass of the missile and V its velocity. Clearly, the velocity is more relevant than the mass: as Table 4.1 shows, the bullet fired by the 5.56 mm Armalite rifle is not much heavier than the .25 in pistol bullet, but because its velocity is so much greater, its impact energy is perhaps as much as 17 times larger. Nevertheless, Fackler (1988) has stressed the importance of other factors, notably the tendency of the bullet to fragment.

A low velocity bullet, fired by a pistol or small sporting rifle, can be lethal at short range. But commonly the wound track of such bullets is narrow and not much larger than the diameter of the bullet, though increased if the elongated bullet is tumbling, or if it has already fragmented. Small sporting rifles and older revolvers fire lead bullets which easily fragment or distort, and some bullets fired from sporting rifles are indeed designed to

Table 4.1 Characteristics of typical missiles used in civil and military shootings

Weapon	Diameter (mm)	Bullet weight (g)	Muzzle velocity (m/s)	Impact energy (J)
Sporting .22 in. rifle	5.56	2.6 (no jacket)	340–380	160
Lee–Enfield WWII .303 in. rifle	7.7	11.7	780	3600
Sporting .303 rifle	7.7	9.5 (jacket, soft nose)	?	?
NATO SLR rifle	7.62	9.7 (jacket)	860	3500
US M16 Colt 'Armalite'	5.56	3.6 (jacket)	980	1700
Automatic pistol (~.38 in.)	9	7.5 (jacket)	270	?270
Pistol (~.25 in.)	6.35	3.3 (jacket)	250	100
12 gauge shotgun	20.5	32	330	?

The data for impact energy at contact range at approximate, and are given to emphasize relative differences in the effects of different missiles. (From various sources.)

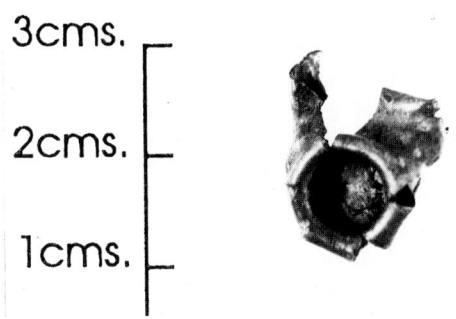

Fig. 4.16 Shooting accident. A soft-nosed hunting rifle bullet (.303 in.) disintegrated after passage through bone and the jagged cupronickel jacket was retrieved from the brain of the victim.

mushroom after impact (Fig. 4.16). Military rifles and automatic pistols fire bullets with a steel or cupronickel jacket and a lead core: these remain intact with lower energy impacts, but may also fragment when they strike at high velocities. In war, the use of bullets deliberately designed or modified to fragment — dum dums — is prohibited by international convention; Sykes et al (1988) give the history of this well-meant prohibition and note that it is not considered to apply with respect to criminals and terrorists, against whom small explosive bullets ('Devastators') have been designed. The modern military SS109 5.56 mm bullet, called the M855 in the USA, has a steel core and an internal structure which ensures a great penetrating power and a capacity to fragment in the tissues, carving out large cavities.

After impact by a high velocity military rifle bullet, damage is usually very extensive, being increased by

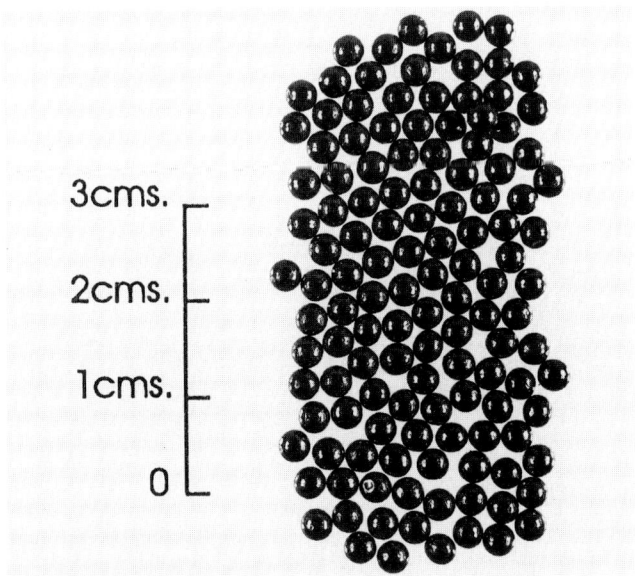

Fig. 4.17 Shotgun pellets. A charge of 128 shotgun pellets, each 3.4 mm in diameter, suitable for shooting birds. Larger shot is used for larger animals. In the past, lead pellets were used; from fear of lead poisoning from shot birds, pellets of mild steel or bismuth are now favoured.

energy imparted to the tissues laterally (Fig. 4.7) and by negative pressure behind the bullet, which sucks material — often contaminated — in its wake. When examined at autopsy, the missile track or primary cavity may be relatively narrow, but at the time of wounding, a much larger secondary cavity can be inferred from studies on gelatine and animal models. Haemorrhages are often seen wide of the missile tract, presumably from sudden stretching when the secondary cavity is formed.

Military rifle bullets are usually lethal when the brain is penetrated, except when the bullet has spent its energy in flight (Fig. 5.19) or by a ricochet (Fig. 5.6C). A high velocity rifle bullet can cause serious brain injury without penetrating: a bullet that grazes the surface of the skull tangentially may cause contusion of the underlying cerebral cortex by energy transmitted through the skull even in the absence of a skull fracture (Dodge 1965). The smaller sporting rifles can also be lethal, especially when fired at short range, but survival is less unusual. When a high velocity bullet strikes the jaws, much loss of tissue may be seen, because the bullet may fragment or project secondary missiles such as bone chips and teeth. Shotgun injuries may also be devastating at close range, because the numerous small balls (Fig. 4.17) fan out and create a massive wound. Both high velocity bullets and shotguns may avulse substantial masses of bone and soft tissue.

Except in suicides or executions the data — especially the firing distance — are usually inadequate for calculations of the impact energy in real-life rifle and pistol shootings. This is even more the case with bombs, mines and shells. It has been said that an 81 mm mortar shell can generate some 600 metal fragments of various sizes and shapes, with initial velocities of up to 800 m/s; the velocities fall off rapidly, and it is impossible to calculate the impact energy in individual cases. Sometimes it is clearly relatively slight and injury occurs only because a vulnerable CMF area is hit. Not all bombs and mines kill by fragmentation: some are packed with spherical steel pellets, and these have been reported to cause brain wounds with a high incidence of intracranial haemorrhage, perhaps from a tendency to rebound from the opposite side of the skull (Nguyen Thuong Xuan, personal communication).

A further and often forgotten cause of injury is the blast of propellent gas. This is seen when a bullet is fired at very close range; it is also seen in the vicinity of a bomb explosion.

Thermal electrical and chemical burns

Thermal injury results when energy is transferred from a hot object, either by contact conduction or by radiation. The tissues vary considerably in their sensitivity to heat, and in their capacity to dissipate it; however, over 44°C cellular death can result from prolonged exposure, and

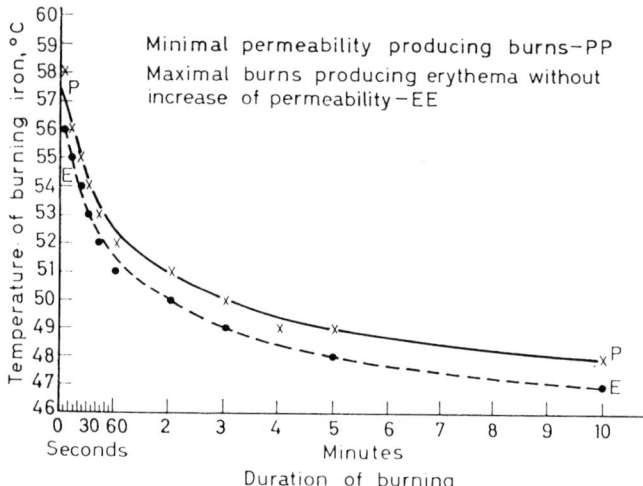

Fig. 4.18 Thermal trauma: the effect of exposure time. The graph shows the relation between the temperature of a heated iron and the duration of application needed to produce threshold burn damage, measured by skin erythema (lower curve) and by increased skin capillary permeability (upper curve). Higher temperatures are tolerated if the exposure time is short. Reproduced from Sevitt (1957) by courtesy of Butterworth.

between 44 and 51°C cellular death doubles with each degree rise in temperature. Experimental studies by Sevitt (1957) showed that the capacity of cells to withstand elevated temperatures is a factor of the duration of exposure as well as the severity of the elevation in temperature (Fig. 4.18); over 70°C, cellular coagulation necrosis results from very short periods of exposure.

Electrical injury is determined by the duration of exposure as well as by the voltage and amperage, the electrical resistance of the tissues, the type of circuit (direct or alternating) and the pathway of current flow. Lightning may have a potential as great as a billion volts; high tension power lines may conduct currents with 1000–100 000 V potentials. Domestic power is supplied at much lower voltages; in the UK and Australia for example, household electrical power is alternating current at 50 Hz with a voltage of approximately 240 V, while in the USA and many other countries a voltage of 110 V (60 Hz) is found satisfactory and less dangerous (Plueckhahn & Cordner 1991). Voltages in excess of 1000 V usually cause soft-tissue destruction, which may extend to deeper structures such as muscles, or to the skull. Intense heat (up to 3000°C) is generated at the point of entry: this causes local charring and mummification. The damage may not appear extensive on the surface, but may include deep areas of necrosis. The electric current may have effects on the whole body not seen with other causes of burning; the electric activity of the myocardium may be disturbed, and there may be neurological effects (p. 488). The electrical resistance of the skin varies, thin moist skin offering less resistance than thick skin; the greater the local resistance, the less the likelihood of severe cardio-respiratory effects but the greater the likelihood of a local burn. Bone has relatively low heat conductivity and is also a poor electrical conductor; cerebral electrical burns (Fig. 17.20) are therefore usually localized and associated with severe burns of the overlying scalp.

Chemical burns represent coagulation necrosis of complex nature (Jelenko 1974). Oxidizing agents such as potassium permanganate and sodium hypochlorite cause protein denaturation. Corrosives, such as strong alkalis (lyes) and phenol, also cause protein denaturation; desiccation and local anoxia are other causes of coagulation necrosis. These detrimental effects can continue, since the chemical agent may remain active for some time; this is often the case when a necrotizing fluid lodges in the conjunctiva (Fig. 17.1).

REFERENCES

Anderson R L, Panje W R, Gross C E 1982 Optic nerve blindness following blunt forehead trauma. Ophthalmology 89: 445–455

Cesari D, Ramet M, Welbourne E 1989 Experimental evaluation of human facial tolerance to injuries. In: Proceedings 1989 International IRCOBI Conference on Biokinetics of Impacts. International Research Council on Biokinetics of Impacts, Bron, France, pp 55–63

Chambers G H, Payne J F 1969 Treatment of dog bite wounds Minn Med 52: 427–430

Converse J M, Smith B, Wood-Smith D 1977 Orbital and naso-orbital fractures. In: Converse J M (ed) Reconstructive plastic surgery: principles and procedures in correction, reconstruction, and transplantation, 2nd edn. Saunders, Philadelphia, Vol 2, Ch 25

Cooter R D 1990 Computed tomography in the assessment of protective deformation. J Trauma 30: 55–68

Cooter R D, David D J, McLean A J, Simpson D A 1988 Helmet-induced skull fracture in a motorcyclist? Lancet 1: 84–85

Dodge P R 1965 Tangential wounds of the scalp and skull. In: Meirowsky A M (ed) Neurological surgery of trauma. Office of the Surgeon General, Dept of the Army, Washington, DC, Ch 13

Fackler M L 1988 Wound ballistics. A review of current misconceptions. J Am Med Assoc 259: 2730–2736

Fujino T 1974 Experimental 'blow-out' fracture of the orbit. Plast Reconstr Surg 54: 81–82

Gadd C W, Nahum A M, Schneider D C, Madeira R G 1970 Tolerance and properties of superficial soft tissues in situ. Proceedings 14th Stapp Car Crash Conference, Paper 700910. Society of Automotive Engineers, New York, pp 356–368

Gennarelli T A 1983 Head injury in man and experimental animals: clinical aspects. Acta Neurochirurg Suppl (Wien) 32: 1–13

Gennarelli T A, Thibault L E 1982 Biomechanics of acute subdural haematoma. J Trauma 22: 680–686

Georgiades N G 1977 Fractures of the condyle. In: Converse J M, McCarthy J G (eds) Reconstructive plastic surgery: principles and procedures in correction, reconstruction, and transplantation, 2nd edn. Saunders, Philadelphia, Vol 2, Ch 24

Gonzalez M G, Santos-Oller J M, De Vicente Rodriguez J C, Lopez-Arranz J S 1990 Optic nerve blindness following a malar fracture. J Craniomaxillofac Surg 18: 319–321

Green R P, Peters D R, Shore J W, Fanton J W, Davis H 1990 Force necessary to fracture the orbital floor. Ophthal Plast Reconstr Surg 6: 211–217

Gurdjian E S 1972 Prevention and mitigation of injury. Clin Neurosurg 19: 43–57

Gurdjian E S, Hodgson V R, Thomas L M, Patrick L M 1968 Significance of relative movements of scalp, skull, and intracranial contents during impact injury of the head. J Neurosurg 29: 70–72

Haley J L, Shanahan D F, Reading T E, Knapp S C 1983 Head impact hazards in helicopter operations and their mitigation through improved helmet design. In: Ewing C L, Thomas D J, Sances A, Larson S J (eds) Impact injury of the head and spine. C C Thomas, Springfield, Illinois

Heinze J 1969 Cranial nerve avulsion and other neural injuries in road accidents. Med J Aust 2: 1246–1249

Hill C M, Crosher R F, Mason D A (1985) Dental and facial injuries following sports accidents: a study of 130 patients. Br J Oral Maxillofac Surg 23: 268–274

Hodgson V R 1967 Tolerance of the facial bones to impact. Am J Anat 120: 113–122

Holbourn A H S 1943 Mechanics of head injuries. Lancet 2: 438–441

Holbourn A H S 1945 The mechanics of brain injury. Br Med Bull 3: 147–149

Huelke D F 1961 The production of mandibular fractures: a study in high speed cinematography. J Dent Res 40: 743–744 (abstract)

Jelenko C 1974 Chemicals that 'burn'. J Trauma 14: 65–72

Jend H H, Jend-Rossman I 1984 Sphenotemporal buttress fracture. Neuroradiology 26: 411–413

Joch W, Fritsche P, Krause I 1981 Biomechanical analysis of punching in boxing. In: Morecki A, Fidelus K, Kedzier K, Wit A (eds) Biomechanics VII-B: Proceedings of the Seventh International Congress of Biomechanics. University Park Press, Baltimore, pp 343–349

Kazanjian L 1983 Classification of simple spinal column injuries. In: Ewing C L, Thomas D J, Sances A, Larson S J (eds) Impact injury of the head and spine. C C Thomas, Springfield, Illinois

Kingsbury H B, Rohr P R 1981 Structural characteristics of motorcycle helmets. SAE Technical Paper Series 810372. Society of Automotive Engineers, Warrendale, Pennsylvania

Lee K F, Wagner L K, Lee Y E, Suh J H, Lee S R 1987 The impact-absorbing effects of facial fractures in closed head injuries. An analysis of 210 patients. J Neurosurg 66: 542–547

Maguire J I, Benson W E 1986 Retinal injury and detachment in boxers. J Am Med Assoc 255: 2451–2453

Manavis J, Blumbergs P C, Scott G et al 1991 Brain injury patterns in falls causing death. In: Proceedings of International IRCOBI Conference on the Biomechanics of Impacts. International Research Council on Biokinetics of Impacts, Bron, France, pp 77–88

Manson P N 1988 Skull and midface injuries. In: Mustarde J C, Jackson I T (eds) Plastic surgery in infancy and childhood, 3rd edn. Churchill Livingstone, Edinburgh, Ch 17

Melvin J W, Evans F G 1971 A strain energy approach to the mechanics of skull fracture. Proceedings 15th Stapp Car Crash Conference, Paper 710871. Society of Automotive Engineers, New York, pp 666–685

Mendelson J A (1991) The relationship between mechanisms of wounding and principles of treatment of missile wounds. J Trauma 31: 1181–1202

Murray J A M, Maran A G D, Busuttil A, Vaughan G 1986 A pathological classification of nasal fractures. Injury 17: 338–344

Nahum A M 1975 The biomechanics of facial bone fracture Laryngoscope 85: 140–156

Nitz A J, Matulionis D H 1982 Ultrastructural changes in rat peripheral nerve following pneumatic tourniquet compression. J Neurosurg 57: 660–666

Nyquist G W, Cavanaugh J M, Goldberg S J, King A I 1986 Facial impact tolerance and response. In: Proceedings 30th Stapp Car

Crash Conference, Paper 861896. Society of Automotive Engineers, Warrendale, Pennsylvania, pp 379–400

Ommaya A 1985 Biomechanics of head injury: experimental aspects In: Nahum A M, Melvin J (eds) The biomechanics of trauma. Appleton-Century-Crofts, Norwalk, Connecticut, Ch 13

Owen-Smith M S 1981 High velocity missile wounds. Edward Arnold, London

Pincemaille Y, Trosseille X, Mack P, Tarriere C, Breton F, Renault B 1989 Some new data related to human tolerance obtained from volunteer boxers. In: Proceedings 33rd Stapp Car Crash Conference. Society of Automotive Engineers, Warrendale, Pennsylvania, pp 177–190

Plueckhahn V D, Cordner S M 1991 Ethics, legal medicine and forensic pathology, 2nd edn. Melbourne University Press, Melbourne, Ch 19

Ryan G A, McLean A J, Vilenius A T S, Kloeden C N, Simpson D A 1989 Head impacts and brain injury in fatally injured pedestrians. In: Proceedings 1989 IRCOBI Conference on the Biomechanics of Impacts. International Research Council on Biokinetics of Impacts, Bron, France, pp 27–37

Schneider D C 1985 In: Nahum A M, Melvin J (eds) The biomechanics of trauma. Appleton-Century-Crofts, Norwalk, Connecticut, Ch 15

Schwartz M L, Hudson A R, Fernie G R, Hayashi K, Coleclough A A 1986 Biomechanical study of full-contact karate contrasted with boxing. J Neurosurg 64: 248–252

Sevitt S 1957 Burns. Pathology and therapeutic applications. Butterworth, London

Simpson D A, Blumbergs P C, Cooter R D, Kilminster M, McLean A J, Scott G 1989 Pontomedullary tears and other gross brainstem injuries after vehicular accidents. J Trauma 29: 1519–1525

Simpson D A, Ryan G A, Paix B R et al 1991 Brain injuries in car occupants: a correlation of impact data with neuropathological findings. Proceedings 1991 IRCOBI Conference on the Biomechanics of Impacts. International Research Council on Biokinetics of Impacts, Bron, France, pp 89–100

Smith R A, Ling S, Alexander F W 1991 Golf related injuries in children. Br Med J 302: 1505–1506

Stålhammer D A 1990 The mechanism of brain injuries. In: Vinken P J, Bruyn G W, Klawans H L, Braakman R (eds) Handbook of clinical neurology. Elsevier, Amsterdam, Vol 57, Ch 2

Stanley R B, Nowak G M 1985 Midfacial fractures: importance of angle of impact to horizontal craniofacial buttresses. Otolaryngol Head Neck Surg 93: 186–192

Sykes L N, Champion H R, Fouty W J 1988 Dum-dums, hollow-points, and devastators: techniques designed to increase wounding potential of bullets. J Trauma 28: 618–623

Tomei G, Spagnoli D, Ducati A et al 1990 Morphology and neurophysiology of focal axonal injury experimentally induced in the guinea pig optic nerve. Acta Neuropathol Berl 80: 506–513

Treip C S 1984 The hypothalamus and pituitary gland. In: Adams J H, Corsellis J A N, Duchen L W (eds) Greenfield's neuropathology, 4th edn. Edward Arnold, London, Ch 16

Tvete S 1980 Frontobasal skull fracture patterns. Fortschr Geb Roentgenstr Nuklearmed 133: 56–58

Unterharnscheidt F J 1975 Injuries due to boxing and other sports. In: Vinken P J, Bruyn G W (eds) Handbook of clinical neurology. North-Holland, Amsterdam, Vol 23, Part 1, Ch 26

Wolpoff M H 1971 Interstitial wear. Amer J Phys Anthropol 34: 205–228

Yoganandan N, Sances A, Pintar F A et al 1991 Traumatic facial injuries with steering wheel loading. J Trauma 31: 699–710

Pathology of injury and repair

D. A. Simpson   J. Abbott
Contributing authors: D. J. David   M. Hammerton
I. O. W. Leitch

INTRODUCTION

The pathology of craniomaxillofacial (CMF) injuries expresses the general pathology of trauma, modified by the structural and functional peculiarities of the CMF region and its component tissues and organs. Of these, the brain, the eyes and the teeth are so specialized that their responses to trauma are in many respects unique: each has its own special pathology. Even for less specialized tissues such as skin and bone, the primary effects of injuries in the CMF region show features that demand individual consideration.

The secondary effects of trauma are very diverse. Some result from acute disorders of normal physiology: the secondary pathophysiology of brain injuries is a subject in itself. Other secondary complications represent microbial colonization, either by organisms normally colonizing epithelial surfaces or by exogenous bacteria; the face, the mouth and the nasopharynx have rich and variable microbial populations.

The reparative processes of the CMF tissues also require individual consideration. As elsewhere in the body, epithelial surfaces and bone heal well; the peripheral nerves of the face regenerate exceptionally well. Cartilage cells and striated muscle fibres have only limited regenerative capacity, but wounds of the facial cartilages or muscles do not as a rule have serious consequences, whereas the complete inability of the neurons of the central nervous system to regenerate is the chief cause of permanent disability from injuries in the CMF region. The processes of repair are mediated by a large number of biologically active chemical substances, of which the proteins identified as specific growth factors are especially important from the surgical viewpoint. Some growth factors are now being used experimentally as therapeutic agents.

In the management of any injury, the surgeon's fundamental aim is to utilize and foster natural healing. When there is massive tissue loss, it may be necessary to supplement local reparative processes by a transplant from elsewhere in the body, or from another individual, or even from another species: reactions to autografts, allografts and xenografts are part of the surgical pathology of trauma. Finally, some injuries are best managed with the help of a surgical implant: the choice and use of implants require understanding of the tissue reactions to foreign materials.

MICROBIAL FLORA

Linton & Hinton (1990) have described the normal flora, or more correctly the microbiota, of surfaces and cavities in the CMF region, notably the skin, the upper respiratory tract and the mouth. They emphasize that the 'normal' resident microbes are constantly supplemented by transient intruders from the environment or from other parts of the body. Ecosystems vary between individuals and in the same individual, according to age and health; severe injury may reduce local or systemic resistance and more virulent organisms may establish themselves. In abnormal environments, such as intensive care units, cross infection may alter the individual's microbiotic ecosystem; invasive procedures may allow intrusion by organisms into cavities which are not ordinarily colonized. Diseases, such as aquired immune deficiency syndrome (AIDS; p. 535), and therapeutic interventions, such as antibiotic therapy, create situations where organisms not usually pathogenic can cause opportunistic infections. Yet, within limits, the composition of the chief regional ecosystems in the CMF region is remarkably constant.

The incidence of infections after wounds of the face and scalp is low compared with wounds in other sites, such as the feet, presumably because the number of endogenous potential pathogens is lower, and also because of the rich blood supply. The facial skin harbours large numbers of coagulase-negative staphylococci, especially *Staphylococcus epidermidis*, which has a predilection for sebaceous glands. Coryneform bacteria are also numerous, especially where the skin sebum content is high. These organisms are weak pathogens, but the skin may also be colonized by coagulase-positive *Staph. aureus*. These often aggressive organisms are especially prevalent in hairy areas, such as the beard and the scalp. The scalp microbiota also includes organisms of little clinical importance, such as the *Pityrosporum* yeasts; these seem incapable of causing infection, even in the favourable environment of a penetrating wound. *Staph. aureus*, on the other hand, is the organism usually responsible for the cerebral infections complicating scalp wounds (Carey et al 1971, de Louvois et al 1977), except when the use of prophylactic antibiotics has fostered gram-negative organisms.

Respiratory tract

The upper respiratory tract harbours a number of separate ecosystems. The anterior nares are often colonized by potentially pathogenic coagulase-positive staphylococci; Wheat et al (1981) quote carrier incidences of 10–50% in healthy populations. The nasopharynx commonly has a normal microbiota of streptococci, especially of the viridans type, and gram-negative cocci. These include many organisms that are not pathogenic, or pathogenic only under favourable conditions. But it is of great clinical importance that *Streptococcus pneumoniae*, *Haemophilus influenzae* and the meningococcus may normally or transiently colonize the nasopharynx. The pneumococcus is the chief cause of meningitis after CMF trauma; repeated attacks of pneumococcal meningitis occurring long after injury (p. 388) may relate to intermittent transient colonization by virulent pneumococci in association with a poorly healed fracture of the anterior cranial fossa. The accessory nasal air sinuses are normally sterile.

Conjunctiva

The conjunctiva is sometimes colonized by *Staph. epidermidis* or by diphtheroids; however, serious pathogens are rarely found except when there is clinical evidence of infection. This paucity of significant conjunctival organisms is attributed to the efficiency of lacrimation and lacrimal drainage: the tears contain lysozyme and other antibacterial agents, and the eyelids, acting like a windscreen wiper, maintain movement of tears to the nasolacrimal duct (p. 74).

Oral cavity

The mouth has an extremely complex microbiota, including yeasts, viruses and protozoa as well as bacteria. The dental age of the individual, the state of dental hygiene and the presence of foreign materials such as dentures are important in determining the composition of the oral microbiota. Notably absent from the normal oral microbiota are coagulase-positive staphylococci and the intestinal gram-negative bacteria. Organisms of potential clinical importance include numerous types of streptococci, including *Strep. milleri*, and anaerobes such as bacteroides; also of clinical interest is the gram-negative facultative anaerobe *Eikenella corrodens*, a coccobacillus found on mucous membranes but capable of causing infection. Yeasts of the candida genus and actinomycetes may assume pathogenic roles in abnormal circumstances. It might be supposed that oral wounds would show a high incidence of infection, but this is not so (Lieblich & Topazian 1991): the oral mucosa has antibacterial defences, including secretory immunoglobulin A, and infection is rare unless there is associated bone injury. Fractures of the mandible are notoriously prone to cause osteomyelitis if not treated effectively; the organisms responsible often include anaerobes which are not easily cultured. Actinomyces species are often found in the normal mouth and chronic actinomycotic infections may complicate orofacial trauma. The human oral microbial population assumes a different significance when man bites man (or woman): some organisms not often seen as wound pathogens may then cause infections in the victim (p. 496). *E. corrodens* is not uncommonly found in infected human bites.

Intestinal tract

Under abnormal conditions, the microbiota of the gut often complicate the management of CMF injuries. After extensive burns and other forms of very severe trauma, the gut mucosa may atrophy, causing breakdown of the mucosal barrier. It is believed that this contributes to the passage (translocation) of gram-negative bacteria and enterococci into the lymphatic system and bloodstream, resulting in septicaemia, endotoxaemia and multiple organ failure (Rush et al 1988). The experimental evidence for this concept is strong, and there is circumstantial support from clinical studies. It is suggested that an insulin-like growth factor (IGF-1) may have a protective effect in maintaining mucosal integrity (Huang et al 1993); epidermal growth factor (EGF) has also been shown to reduce bacterial translocation after severe burn injury in an experimental model (Ahdoot et al 1992, Zapata-Sirvent et al 1993).

SOFT TISSUES

Skin wounds

The general processes of skin wound healing have been much studied and several excellent reviews of the recent literature have been published (Feinberg & Larsen 1991, Cohen et al 1992). Healing follows a sequence of overlapping phases: haemostasis is followed by an inflammatory phase, commonly lasting up to 5 days; this merges into a phase of proliferation and after perhaps 3 weeks to a phase of maturation (Fig. 5.1).

Haemostasis and inflammation

Incised wounds of the face usually heal by primary union (healing by first intention). If the skin edges are not widely separated, they are first coapted by a fibrinous coagulum, formed during the immediate haemostatic response to the injury: blood platelets, tissue thromboplastin and the plasma coagulation factors together mediate the formation of this weak union. Within a few hours, a leukocyte response initiates an antibacterial defence process. Neutrophil polymorphs appear in large numbers in the wound margins, and kill bacteria. It has been supposed that their chief role is to phagocytose organisms, but it appears that their more important function is to liberate proteolytic enzymes and oxygen-derived free radicles, which have microbicidal effects (Wahl & Wahl 1992). Blood monocytes appear, at first in small numbers; they transform to become macrophages, which remove dead tissue and in other ways promote wound healing. After the first few days, the macrophages are more numerous than the polymorphs, which have a much shorter cell half-life; the macrophage is seen as the most important cell in the first stage of wound healing. These leukocyte responses are stimulated by numerous mediator agents released from damaged tissues and from the blood platelets, as well as by activated complement from the plasma (Fig. 5.1). In addition to chemotactic agents derived from tissue breakdown and bacterial action, current opinion emphasizes the roles of cytokines, hormone-like regulators of cellular activity (McKay & Leigh 1991). Of these cytokines, the peptide growth factors appear especially important; some of their sites of action and the abbreviations used to identify them are set out in Fig. 5.1. The platelet-derived growth factor (PDGF) is vital in promoting the cellular response to injury (Ross et al 1986); however, it is only

one of an array of growth factors contained in the platelets and believed to be important in wound healing. The mast cells, very numerous in the subcutaneous connective tissues, liberate histamine and chemotactic substances (leukotrienes). Blood vessels dilate under the influence of histamine and other agents; endothelial cells alter in morphology and begin to proliferate under the stimulation of mitogenic agents, including the fibroblast growth factors (FGF: Schweigerer et al 1987), of which seven have been identified (Werner et al 1992). Lymphocytes and macrophages become active in defence mechanisms; they produce lymphokines and monokines, active agents among which the interleukins have been shown to stimulate the local cellular inflammatory responses as well as the systemic metabolic response to injury. Interleukin-1 (IL-1), which is produced by activated macrophages, is especially important in the inflammatory response, and also has a role in epidermal regeneration.

Concurrently, and also in response to mediator agents, epithelial cells (keratinocytes) become active. Keratinocytes in the basal layer of the epidermis at the wound edges show amoeboid movement: they proliferate by mitosis and grow into the wound gap. The agents responsible for this include epidermal growth factor (EGF), keratinocyte growth factor (KGF: Werner et al 1992) and other cytokines; Lynch et al (1989a) have shown that two of these, one of the transforming growth factors (TGFβ) and an insulin-like growth factor (IGF-1), act only in synergy. However, epithelial growth does not provide wound cover until there is a substrate of granulation tissue.

The formation of granulation tissue begins only a little after the leukocyte reaction. Capillary buds grow into the wound, together with a migration of fibroblasts and lymphocytes. This inflammatory response is chemically mediated, being promoted by a cascade of mediator agents including PDGF which stimulates fibroblast growth as well as leukocyte migration, and the transforming growth factors (TGFα and β) which have many actions, including the stimulation of collagen formation (Jeffrey 1992). Lymphocytes have many roles in wound healing, not all of which are yet understood; the T-lymphocytes produce agents promoting fibroblast proliferation.

Proliferation

The inflammatory phase is followed by the second or proliferative phase of wound healing. Epithelialization, fibroblastic activity and deposition of collagen dominate this stage. Epidermal cells migrating into the wound meet other epidermal cells and establish continuous epithelial cover; they then cease to migrate and by continued mitosis they establish a mature stratified epidermal layer. When migration ceases, the keratinocytes lay down a new basement membrane composed of type IV collagen.

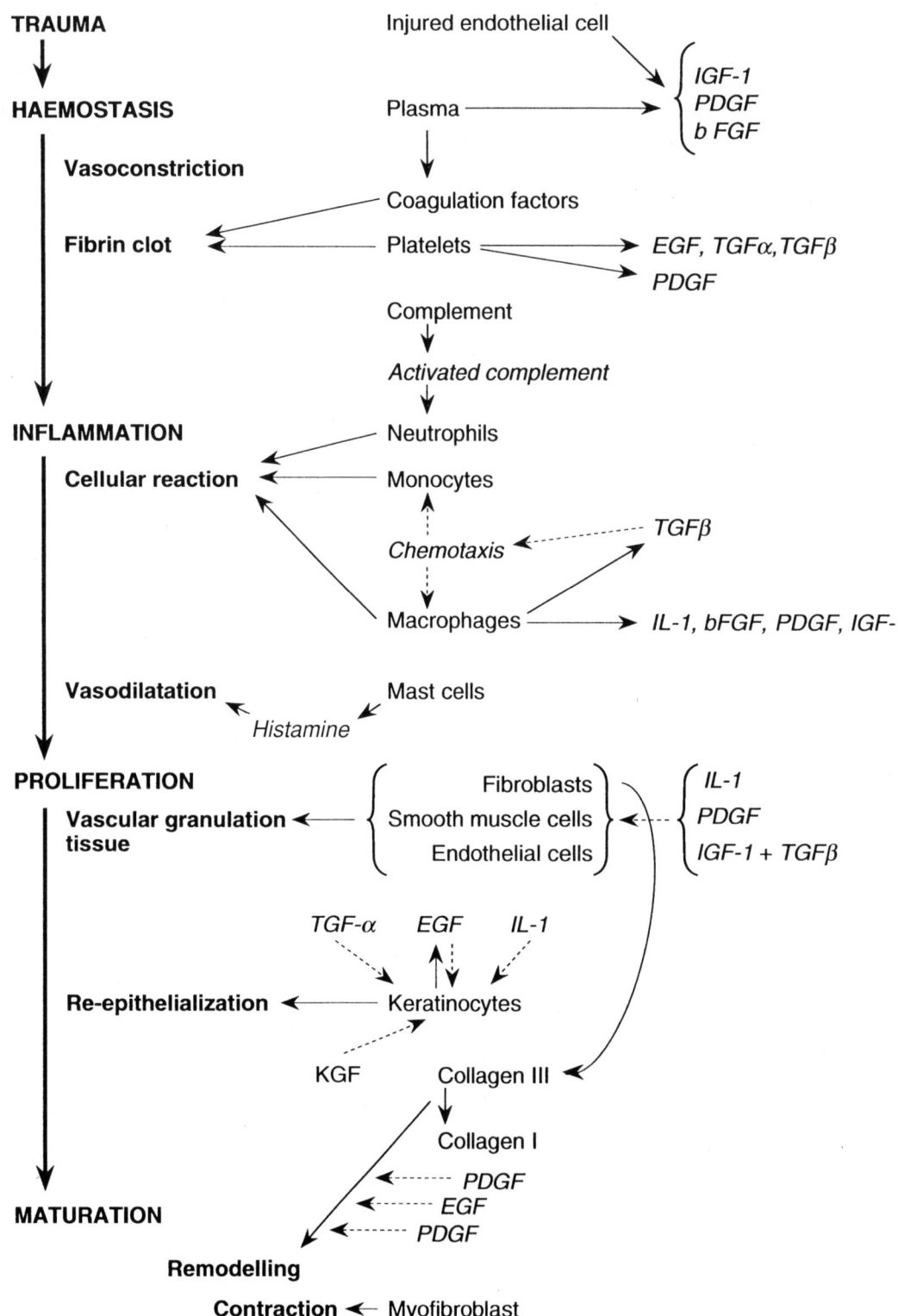

Fig. 5.1 Skin wound healing: the roles of chemical mediators. Schematic summary of skin wound healing; the phases of healing overlap, and the linear sequence given in the diagram is an oversimplification. Some of the many chemical mediators are shown in italics: *EGF*, epidermal growth factor; *b-FGF*, basal fibroblast growth factor; *IGF-1*, insulin-like growth factor; *IL-1*, interleukin, *KGF*, keratinocyte growth factor; *PDGR*, platelet derived growth factor; *TGFα, TGFβ*: transforming growth factors.

The fibroblasts secrete extracellular matrix; they lay down collagen in the form of an unorganized gel as early as the second day after injury. Initially, collagen of the embryonic type III is deposited in the extracellular matrix. Collagen formation is promoted by the growth factor TGFβ but retarded by glucocorticoids.

Maturation

This is the third stage of healing and continues for some months. In the deeper layers of the wound, cross-linked type I collagen replaces type III collagen, and gives a stronger union. Estimates of wound tensile strength depend to some extent on the technique of measurement chosen; after the third or fourth day, strength increases, but it is stated that as late as 3 weeks, skin wounds commonly have only a third of their normal tensile strength. Collagen fibres are remodelled and tensile strength increases, though experimental wounds in aponeurotic tissue are said to be less strong than normal controls even a year later (Douglas 1963). The wound becomes less vascular, by regression of newly formed capillaries; however, larger vessels are formed, giving better flow of blood across the line of the healed wound. The wound becomes a scar and maturation of the scar may continue for some years. Maturation and scar shrinkage are unpredictable processes, variable both in time and in extent; this unpredictability explains the occasionally disappointing aesthetic result of some reconstructive surgical procedures, especially in the orbital region (p. 573).

Complications

The idealized process of primary wound healing is seen after surgical incisions in the face and scalp, and many clean accidental wounds follow a similar course. However, facial injuries due to blunt impact may be bruised or abraded; there may be implanted foreign matter (Fig. 5.2A). Abrasion of the epidermis and even of the dermis is often seen, and this may lead to delayed wound healing (healing by second intention). The abraded surface is covered by a fibrinous coagulum, which hardens as a scab. Epithelialization may then result from cellular migration from the margins of the abraded area, or from residual skin appendages such as sweat glands and hair follicles under the scab. This process is facilitated by contraction of the injured area: fibroblasts (Darby et al 1990) in the granulating wound develop the contractile properties of smooth muscle cells and the action of these so-called myofibroblasts (Guber & Rudolph 1978) reduces the area to be covered by epithelial cells. However, the process of contraction may have adverse aesthetic and functional effects (p. 475). Wound contraction is more effective in young tissues (Catty 1965).

The general processes of wound healing can take different forms in various parts of the CMF region. Scalp wounds usually heal well, unless there is impairment of blood supply, when areas of marginal necrosis may be seen: this is especially likely if the wound is closed under tension, for the scalp has less elasticity than the facial skin (Fig. 5.2B). Incised wounds of the face also heal well; however, facial abrasion and tissue loss can lead to an unsightly scar, as can indriven foreign matter. Explo-

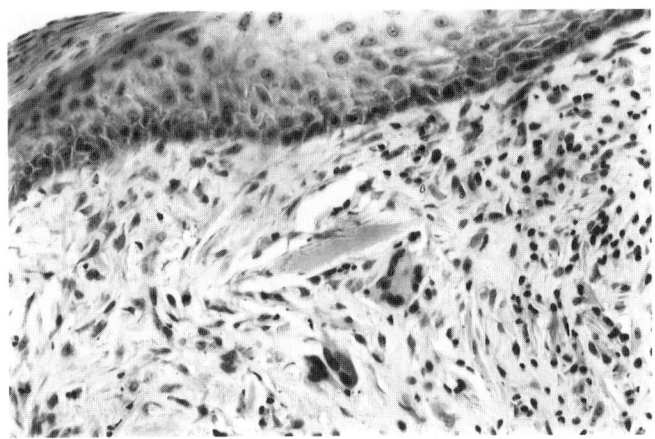

A

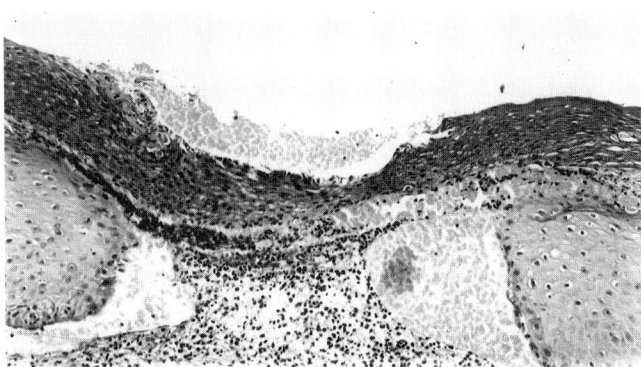

B

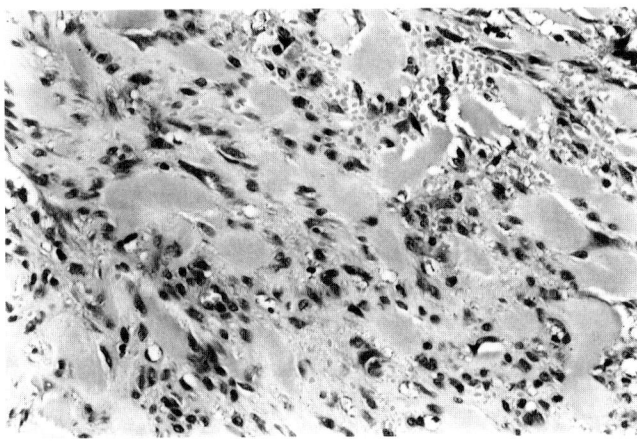

C

Fig. 5.2 Abnormal healing in skin wounds. These biopsies show various complications in wound healing, all of which can result in delayed healing and/or ugly scars. **A** Inflammatory reaction, with giant cells in relation to a foreign body; the overlying epithelium is thickened. Haematoxylin and eosin (H&E), × 169. **B** Dehiscence: a layer of dead epidermis covers the separated edges of healthy epidermis and a cellular exudate has formed in the centre of the wound. H&E, × 73. **C** Subcutaneous keloid: bundles and sheaves of coarse collagen, with many fibroblasts. H&E, × 169.

sions can drive grains of earth or debris into the skin causing permanent tattooing. Keloid formation (Fig. 5.2C) represents an abnormal and excessive overgrowth of fibrous tissue in a wound; keloid tissue is characterized by nodules of vascular and fibroblastic hyperplasia, with poorly organized bundles of collagen (Murray & Pinnell 1992), often including large hyalinized fibres. Keloid formation is not especially common in the CMF region, but is by no means rare.

Facial burns

Thermal or chemical injury causes denaturation of cellular proteins and consequent cellular necrosis (p. 115). Depending on the intensity and duration of the injurious event, the cells may suffer immediate coagulative destruction, or may appear intact but undergo delayed death, or may show reversible swelling (Sevitt 1957). Necrosis is first evident in the tissue layer closest to the injurious agent, normally the epidermis (Fig. 5.3); if exposure is prolonged, as when an unconscious accident victim lies

against a hot structure, the considerable protective capacity of the epidermis is destroyed and deeper tissues undergo necrosis — first the dermis and then muscle, bone and even brain. In a superficial skin burn, keratinocytes in the outer layers of the epidermis die, but the basal cell layer remains intact (Fig. 5.4A). The subcutaneous capillary plexus shows vasodilatation, evident as erythema, but there is no blister formation. The epidermis regenerates in a few days and the erythema subsides. In deeper burns, both epidermis (Fig. 5.4B) and dermis (Fig. 5.4C, D) are involved. Tissue damage evokes an outpouring of inflammatory mediators which increase capillary permeability, allowing escape of serum to form oedema fluid. This may separate viable from non-viable tissue; in partial thickness (second degree) burns, oedema fluid raises a blister by separating necrotic or partly necrotic epidermis from living dermis. When the blister ruptures, the protein-

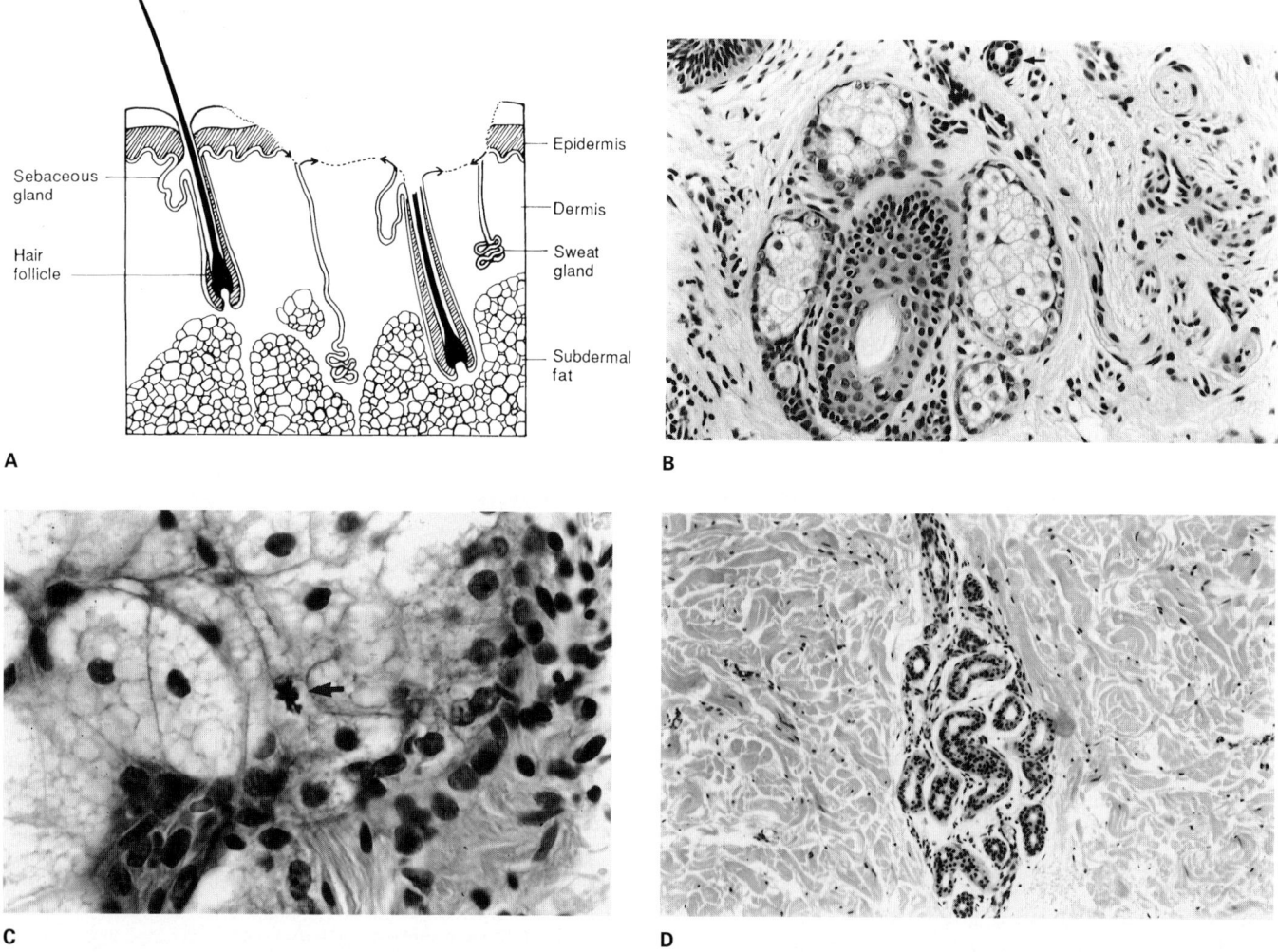

Fig. 5.3 The skin: thermal defence in depth. The epidermis constitutes a significant barrier against thermal and chemical injury; the epidermal glands and hair follicles provide mitotically active cells for regeneration of the epidermis if this has been destroyed. **A** Diagram of a skin burn, showing the layers and the chief sources of epithelial regeneration. **B** Hair follicle, surrounded by sebaceous glands; a single coil of a sweat gland is shown at the top of the field (arrow). H&E, × 169. **C** One of the cells in a sebaceous gland is in mitosis (arrow). H&E, × 507. **D** Sweat gland deeply placed in the dermis. H&E, × 85.

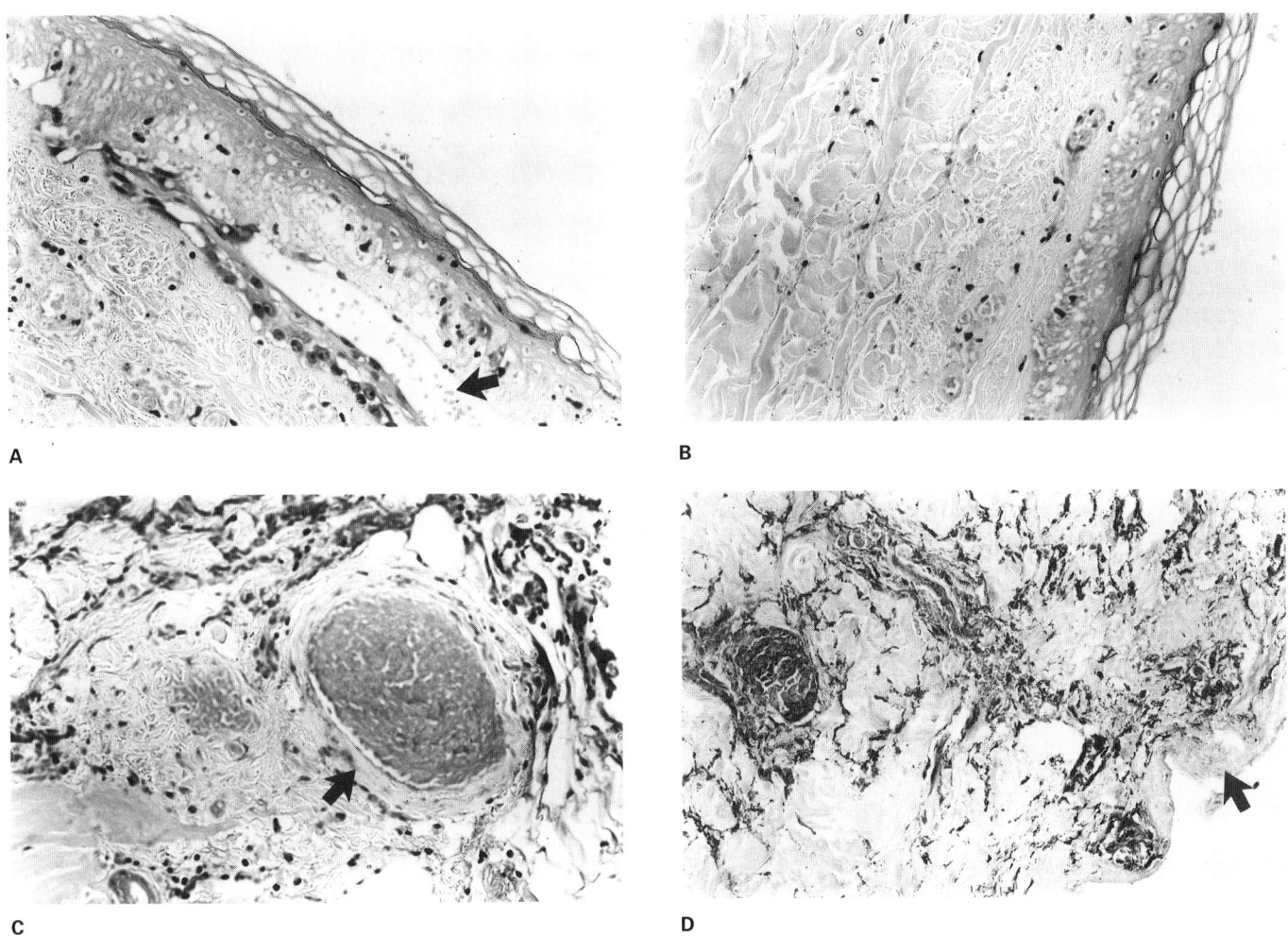

Fig. 5.4 Skin burns. These biopsies show types of burn, several days after injury. **A** Superficial burn, with blister formation (arrow); the basal epithelial layer has survived and is beginning to regenerate. H&E, × 146. **B** Deeper burn, with necrosis of whole epidermis and some of the dermis. H&E, × 146. **C** Necrosis of hair follicle (arrow) and adjacent glandular tissue. H&E, × 146. **D** Deep burn, with necrosis of epidermis (arrow) and underlying dermis; the hair folllicles and glands are almost unrecognizable. H&E, × 146.

aceous fluid leaks out and the dermis is exposed, typically as a moist surface with intact pinprick sensation and intact capillary circulation. Such burns will usually heal spontaneously. Modern biologically compatible dressings allow more rapid re-epithelialization and give better cosmesis and function. More severe burning destroys an increasing depth of dermis. In a full-thickness burn all epithelial structures are lost and the dermal collagen shows coagulation necrosis, losing its normal eosinophilia and fusing into coarse strap-like bands (Fig. 5.4D). There may be complete capillary stasis, and secondary thrombosis may be seen. Between these extremes, there may be burns of intermediate depth, in which a few epidermal structures are preserved, resulting in slower or incomplete re-epithelialization. In deep burns, the collagen necrosis results in formation of a slough or eschar.

A burn is a three-dimensional wound, often involving a considerable area and extending to varying depths. Jackson (1953) distinguished a central zone of coagulation surrounded by a zone of capillary stasis; in his experiments the vascular stasis led to an increase in the necrotic zone, and this is in accord with the clinical observation of progressive increase in the area of non-viable tissue 3–5 days after the burn. Surrounding the zone of stasis was a zone of inflammatory hyperaemia. Later research has amplified these findings. The hyperaemic zone is the result of the liberation of vascular mediators such as histamine, serotonin and vasoactive kinines. When the inflammatory reaction subsides, normal healing begins in the hyperaemic zone. Robson et al (1979) studied the progressive loss of dermal perfusion in the zone of vascular stasis, and demonstrated that thrombosis was the cause of the increase in the area of coagulation. This process is thought to begin with platelet thrombo-embolism which causes venous obstruction in the presence of continued pulsatile arteriolar flow. Robson et al (1979) have implicated prostaglandins, especially thromboxane A_2 as one cause of the intradermal vascular shutdown. The progress of necrosis in the zone of stasis can be partly arrested by wound cooling (Boykin & Molnar 1992), and by a biologically compatible dressing such as porcine skin (Zawacki 1974).

Electrical burns have unique characteristics. Necrosis is intense at the point of entry, but may extend deeply along tissue planes in an unpredictable way. Fig. 17.20 shows the effects of a severe electrical burn in the frontal region:necrosis of the scalp and skull, thrombosis of the underlying sagittal sinus and of smaller vessels in its vicinity, and necrosis of areas of the dura mater. In this case, it was noteworthy that the inflammatory reaction, though quite strong on the surface of viable dura mater, showed no sign of invasion of the necrotic dura nearly 4 weeks after the burn.

Superficial burns heal rapidly: the epidermis regenerates from mitosis in the basal layer, or if this is destroyed, from squamous cells in the surviving hair follicles, sebaceous glands and sweat glands (Fig. 5.3B–D); Boykin & Molnar (1992) quote work indicating that the hair follicles are the chief source of epidermal regeneration. It appears that the process is promoted by EGF and transforming growth factors. Deeper burns with destruction of the epidermal glands and hair follicles must heal by second intention (see above). Granulation tissue forms, and collagen is laid down: this contracts under the influence of myofibroblasts, and the scar is then epithelialized by migration of epidermal cells from the periphery. This process is retarded by overlying eschar. Slow healing predisposes to hypertrophic scar formation and an ugly secondary deformity often with considerable functional loss (p. 486). Modern burn management includes early tangential excision of eschar to accelerate the healing process and to minimise wound contraction.

Skin grafts

In the routine procedure of split-skin grafting, an area of normal skin is cut to give a sheet of epidermis, with a variable amount of the underlying dermis (Converse et al 1977); a medium thickness split-skin graft is 0.016 in. (0.4 mm) in depth. The graft is secured on the denuded area to be covered whether this be a granulating burn, an area of exposed pericranium or an area of cancellous bone. Survival depends initially on nutritional support by serum exuded from the capillaries in the denuded tissue. Permanent survival depends on vascular connections between the dermal elements in the graft and the host tissue, and these appear within 48 h of graft application. Capillary buds and later fibroblasts invade the deeper layers of the graft, and within 7–10 days both vascular supply and drainage are established. The nature of this critically important process of revascularization is reviewed by Converse et al (1977). The stratum corneum

of the graft is usually desquamated in the second week. Klein & Rudolph (1972) showed that the collagen components of a skin graft are rapidly replaced by new collagen locally synthesized during the last 4 weeks. New collagen is laid down, and this contracts under the influence of myofibroblasts. The process of wound contraction may result in shrinkage of the grafted area and an ugly appearance; Rudolph et al (1992) have reviewed evidence showing that myofibroblastic activity is inhibited by a surviving skin graft. The success of the process of grafting depends on maintaining contact between graft and host tissue: this is lost if the graft moves, or if bleeding takes place under the graft. Infection, especially by *Strep. pyogenes* or *Pseudomonas pyocyaneus*, may also cause graft failure. Full-thickness skin grafts, denuded of fat, are less rapidly revascularized, but have the merit that they are less apt to contract or to become pigmented.

Skin allografts, whether taken from a living donor or from a cadaver, are invariably rejected, unless taken from an identical twin. The grafted skin is at first accepted and invaded by capillaries, but after 2–4 weeks the host lymphocytes recognize tissue incompatibility and the graft becomes necrotic. Cadaver skin has nevertheless been much used as a temporary dressing to cover a large area of burned skin. Alternatively, autogenous keratinocytes can be grown in tissue culture, the growth being accelerated with EGF, and may then be used to cover a large area, perhaps in conjunction with other types of skin graft. Hansbrough (1990) and Boykin & Molnar (1992) have reviewed current work on cadaver skin and other substitutes for autogenous skin grafts.

Striated muscle

If a muscle is lacerated or severely contused, the sarcolemmal sheaths of the muscle fibres are disrupted, and the fibres undergo necrosis and are removed by macrophages. Two types of reparative process may then follow. Under favourable conditions, true regeneration of new muscle fibres takes place. Long ago, Le Gros Clark (Clark 1960) noted that if the endomysial connective tissue tubes were preserved, buds of sarcolemmal proliferation might regenerate new muscle fibres. It is now known that this regeneration represents the activation of satellite cells lying within the muscle fibre; they are transformed into myoblasts and finally into mature contractile muscle fibres (Lehto & Järvinen 1991). However, repair by fibrous tissue is more usual. In facial muscular lacerations, the divided ends of the cut muscles are almost always separated and unite by scar tissue. Fibroblastic activity fills the gap between the muscle ends and they are joined by a collagenous scar: a reduced contractile capacity results, especially if there is also damage to the innervation of the muscle. This may affect the aesthetics of facial expression.

Adipose tissue

This has very limited regenerative power. Damaged fat cells liberate their contents and these are removed by phagocytosis; in orbital injuries, loss of tissue fat may result in permanent recession of the globe. The inability of fibrofatty tissue to regenerate effectively is also seen in the cheeks: damage to a cheek pad can result in loss of the normal contour of the face.

SKELETAL TISSUES

Bone

Fracture types

Fractures of the facial skeleton and calvaria take many forms and these can be extremely complex. However, two main fracture types are traditionally identified: linear — with or without displacement — and depressed. In a depressed fracture, an area of bone is detached and driven in below the normal anatomical surface. One can identify a third type of penetration fracture, in which a missile or sharp object pierces bone, leaving a bone defect.

Linear fracture

Linear fractures, usually without displacement, are often seen in the calvarial bones (Fig. 5.5A). Blunt impacts in the frontal region may crack the strong frontal bone and propagate linear fractures running into the temporal bone or the roof of the orbit; more posterior frontal impacts may diastase the coronal suture, again with linear extensions. Mandibular fractures are usually linear (Fig. 5.6A) and occur in sites of structural weakness; the action of the powerful masticatory muscles often causes displacement. Linear fractures are also often seen in the maxillary complex, running along the lines of weakness identified by Le Fort (p. 18); these are usually associated with some degree of displacement.

Depressed fracture

These fractures result from localized overload (p. 102). An area of bone is driven in, and displaced into the underlying soft tissues. Such fractures often result from impacts on the frontal bone (Fig. 5.5B), the depressed fragment(s) being driven into the brain or the frontal air sinus. Fractures of the zygomatic bone are also usually depressed: the slender arch breaks and the body of the bone is driven into the temporalis muscle, with variable infracturing of the lateral wall. Blow-out fractures of the floor of the orbit are depressed by force transmitted through the orbital contents (p. 104); depressed fractures of the orbital wall (Fig. 5.6B) or roof may be caused

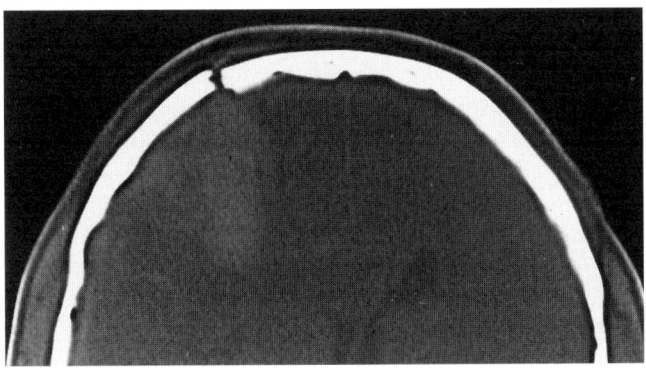

A

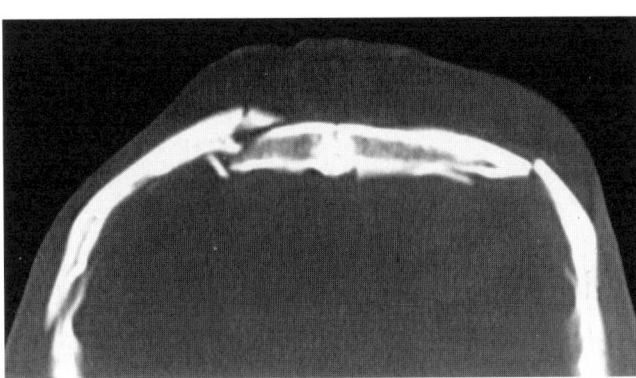

B

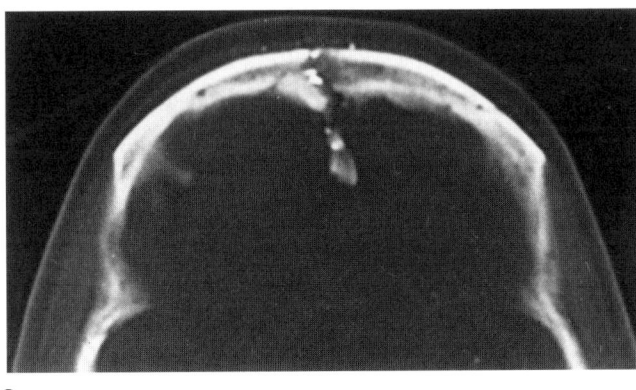

C

Fig. 5.5 Fracture patterns in the calvaria. A CT scan: linear fracture in frontal bone. There was an underlying cortical haematoma. **B** CT scan: depressed fracture, with shattering of bone at medial margin of depression. There was extensive frontal contusion. **C** CT scan: frontal penetrating bullet wound with indriven bone chip.

by buckling. Missile wounds sometimes cause depressed fractures, when the missile has a low impact velocity, or when it strikes the skull tangentially.

Penetration fracture

The penetrating or perforating wounds inflicted by bullets are characterized by a round bone defect, often not much larger than the bullet; numerous small chips of shattered

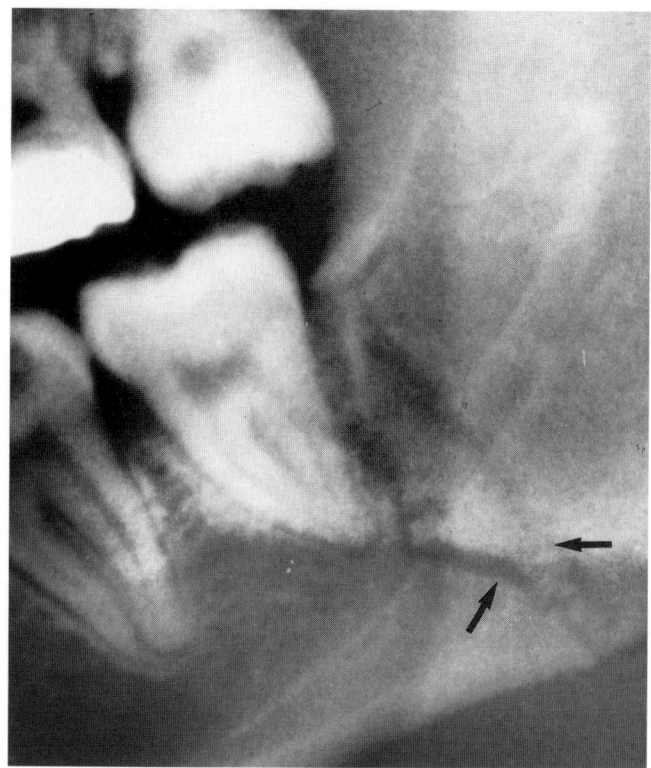

A

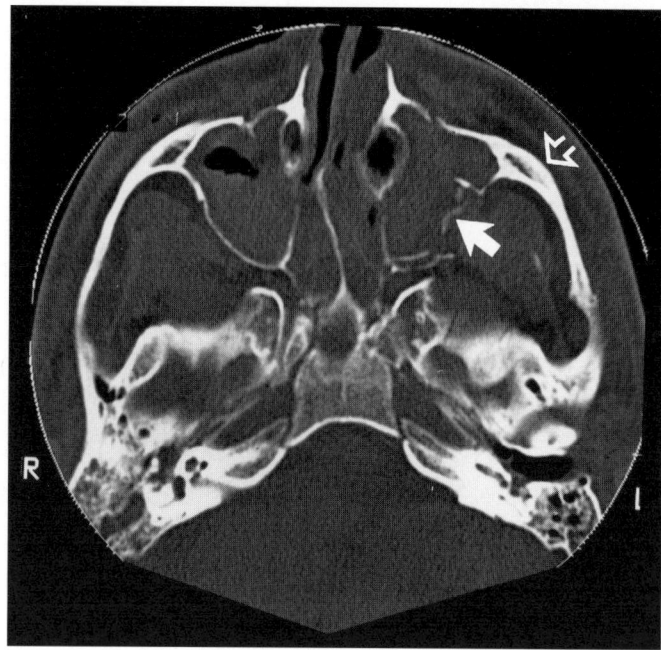

B

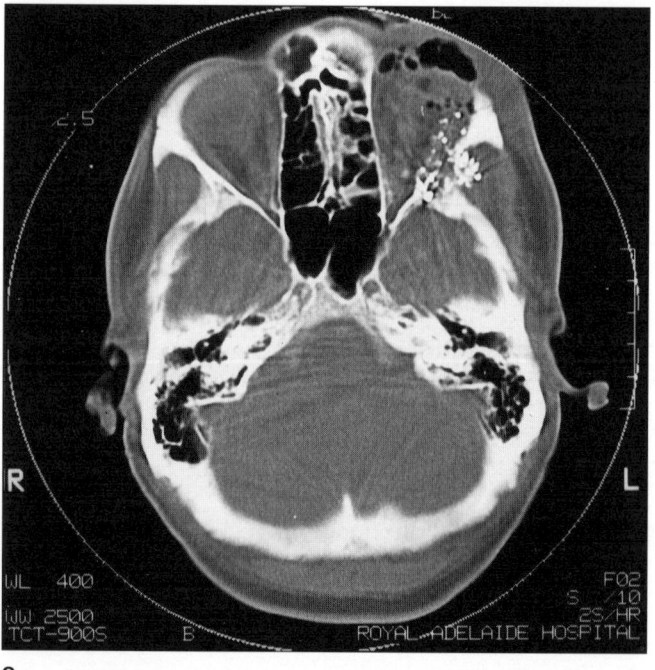

C

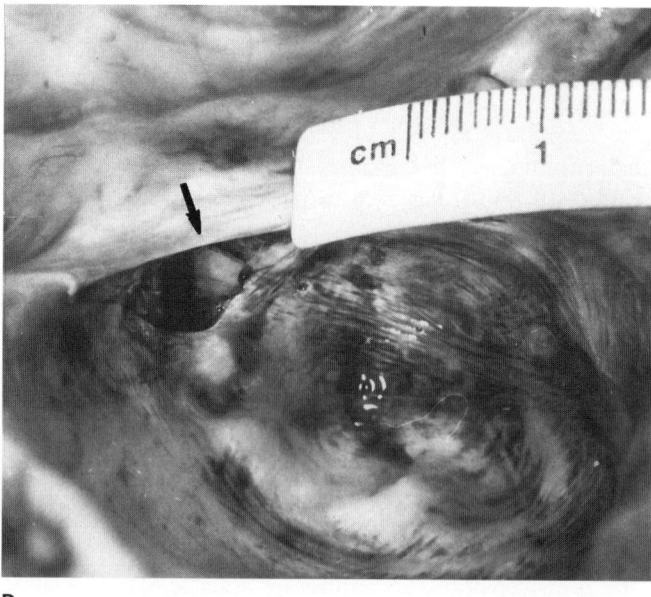

D

Fig. 5.6 Fracture patterns in the facial skeleton. A OPG: linear fracture (arrows) in the mandible. **B** CT scan: depressed fracture (arrow) in the maxilla, buckled by a blow (open arrow) on the malar eminence. **C** CT scan: penetrating wound of orbit by fragmented hunting rifle bullet. **D** Autopsy (same case): the arrow points to a small fracture in the posterolateral wall of the orbit, below the sphenoidal ridge. By courtesy of Dr C. Manock.

bone are driven deeply into the brain or facial soft tissues (Figs 5.5C and 5.6C,D). Very high energy missiles leave a larger bone defect, but these are usually lethal.

Bone healing

Whatever the fracture pattern, the healing process expresses the general tendency of bone to reconstitute unless there are adverse local or systemic conditions. Although most parts of the facial and calvarial skeleton differ from the long bones in embryological origin, there is no reason to think that the healing processes are qualitatively different: facial fractures tend to unite more rapidly than most long bone fractures, but this can be attributed to their small size and good local vascularity (Phillips & Rahn 1992).

Bone healing may take two forms: primary, or direct, and secondary, or healing by callus. Direct bone healing is further classified as contact and gap healing, according to the distance between the bone edges.

Primary bone healing

This is seen when the bone edges are in good apposition and immobile (Spiessl 1989). If there is less than 0.1 mm between the edges, it is usual to speak of contact healing (Fig. 5.7A); if the distance is 0.1–1 mm, the process is termed gap healing (Fig. 5.7B). Two phases are recognized: an initial inflammatory phase and a later phase of remodelling. In the first, which is analoguous to the inflammatory phase of healing of a skin wound, there is a proliferation of capillaries, osteoblasts and osteoclasts from the edges of the fractured bones: the endosteum, the haversian canals and the periosteum all contribute. Osteoblasts lay down new bone; osteoclasts remodel surviving compact and trabecular bone.

In contact healing, the process is direct: bridges of new bone extend from one bone surface into holes reamed out of the opposite face, so that continuous haversian systems are established. Rahn (Spiessl 1989) has visualized this process very elegantly in scanning electron micrographs taken after separation of the bone edges: wedges of new bone are seen projecting to engage in reciprocal pits in the opposite bone face. Contact healing is nevertheless associated with initial osteoporosis and loss of structural strength.

When the gap between the edges is too wide to allow direct union of haversian systems (osteons), the interspace is filled with osteogenic granulation tissue, in which trabeculae of bone are laid down, often in a plane parallel to the fracture line. In the second stage of bone healing, the process of remodelling, these trabeculae are converted into lamellar bone. Gap healing is slower than contact healing, but ultimately as strong.

Secondary bone healing

This is seen when the bone edges are not fully immobilized (Fig. 5.7C). Bleeding into the fracture site forms a haematoma which is invaded by blood vessels, macrophages and fibroblasts. It appears that the haematoma fluid develops osteo-inductive capacities (Mizuno et al 1990). Collagen is laid down and there is an influx of cells capable of osteoblastic and chondroblastic activity. Variable amounts of fibrocartilage and osteoid appear and glue the bone edges together. As the blood supply improves, the cartilage becomes calcified and finally ossified as a mass of callus joining the bone ends with increasing rigidity. In the stage of remodelling, the callus is converted into cortical and trabecular bone and the structure of the bone at the fracture site is restored.

Regulation of bone healing

Bone healing is apparently promoted and regulated by a cascade of growth factors; PDGR and IGF-1 are considered to be important (Lynch et al 1989b). Proteins present in bone matrix evidently stimulate local cellular activity; one of these, known as bone morphogenetic protein, is potent in inducing new bone formation (see p. 134). Bioelectric forces also play a local role in the process, while systemic parathormone appears to modulate the formation and release of growth factors (Mohan & Baylink 1990).

Bone healing in the CMF region

In this region, both types of bone healing may be seen. Calvarial fractures unite by the primary or direct process: the intact bone edges slowly generate new bone. This is accompanied by a transient increase in vascularity evident in X-ray pictures as osteoporosis. A similar process is seen in depressed calvarial fractures: pieces of detached bone undergo avascular necrosis, appearing abnormally dense, with surrounding osteoporosis in the intact bone (Fig. 5.8). Even untreated depressed fractures of the skull vault heal in this way: the depressed fragment is eventually fully incorporated, still in the depressed position, with the tables and diploe reconstituted. Similar primary union is seen in facial fractures and osteotomies: Thaller & Kawamoto (1990) have shown full reconstitution of lamellar architecture in biopsies of middle third facial fractures. Indeed, the thin well-vascularized plates of facial bone commonly unite rapidly by contact or gap union.

Only in fractures of the mandible has union after callus formation been a common finding, and this of course expresses the difficulty of achieving complete immobility of the fractured mandible. Rowe & Killey (1955) illustrated the process of secondary healing in a series of biopsies of mandibular fractures. First, the fracture haematoma was invaded by monocytes, followed by fibroblasts depositing collagen, which effected fibrous union after 3 weeks. Primary callus was evident at 6 weeks: the authors saw this as woven bone, though their beautiful micrographs suggest that some cartilage may have been present. Later remodelling created lamellar bone. Rever et al (1991) have found that experimental fractures in the rabbit zygoma show an intermediate phase of cartilaginous union before eventual complete bony union. Modern methods of miniplate fixation (p. 237) should achieve primary union in all facial fractures.

Fracture complications

These include non-union, mal-union and infection. In the CMF region, fractures of the mandible are especially likely to show these complications, but fractures in other parts of the facial and calvarial skeleton may also exhibit abnormal healing patterns.

Non-union

This may result from displacement of bone fragments and interposition of soft tissue (Fig. 5.9). This is seen especially in the roof and floor of the orbit: herniations of brain and orbital contents respectively prevent reconstruction of the skeletal anatomy. Herniations of brain and/or leptomeninges will prevent bone healing in the skull base; Linell & Robinson (1941) showed in autopsy material that this failure of healing in the vicinity of one of the paranasal air sinuses is a cause of delayed meningitis (p. 147). In infants and young children, pulsating leptomeningeal herniations may actually expand a fracture line, constituting a growing fracture (p. 511). Growing fractures are usually seen in the parietal region, but have been reported in the frontal bone. Non-union of mandibular fractures, when not due to infection, may be due to poor blood supply, as in the edentulous mandible, or to failure in immobilization (Spiessl 1989).

Mal-union

This is basically the result of failures in reduction and fixation of fractures; these are discussed in Chapter 11.

Infection

This is no longer a common event in developed countries, but may always occur if wounds in the CMF area are neglected. Infected cranial fractures can be complicated by spreading osteomyelitis, and by infection in the extra-dural space; extradural abscess is potentially a serious condition, since it can lead to subdural and/or cerebral

suppuration (p. 147). However, the intact cranial bone usually resists infection though ischaemic fragments of bone are likely to be sequestrated.

Osteomyelitis of the mandible is always a threat, since fractures of this bone are often compound into the mouth (Fig. 5.10). The older literature contains many references to such infections; Rowe & Killey (1955) identified dead teeth or tooth roots, foreign material and delayed treatment as aetiological factors. Haematoma formation has also been cited as a cause (Bochlogyros 1985). Devitalized bone is also likely to be infected; the rich blood supply of the mandible makes bone necrosis unlikely in civilian practice, though missile wounds with extensive tissue loss and devitalization may be complicated by sequestration of infected bone fragments.

Bone grafts

Free grafts of autogenous bone are routinely used in the repair of facial fractures (p. 331) and calvarial bone defects (p. 548); vascularized bone transfers are increasingly used in the repair of gunshot wounds of the mandible when a large segment of tissue is lost (p. 626). The process of bone transplantation is therefore of fundamental importance in CMF trauma surgery.

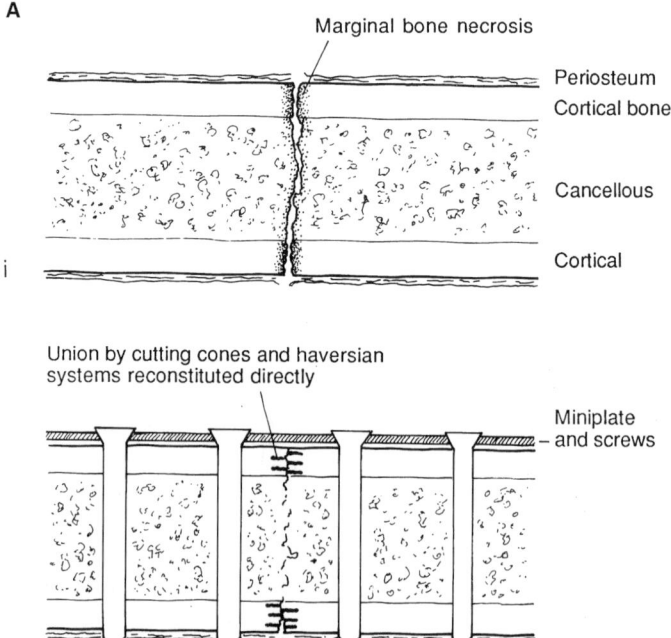

Fig. 5.7 Types of bone healing after fracture. A Contact healing: (i) The bone ends are in contact. There is some bone necrosis at the margins, but little haematoma formation. (ii) The fracture is immobilized by a plate. Osteoclasts ream out new haversian systems in the apposed bone surfaces, and bridges of new bone unite the fragments. The periosteum is reconstituted.

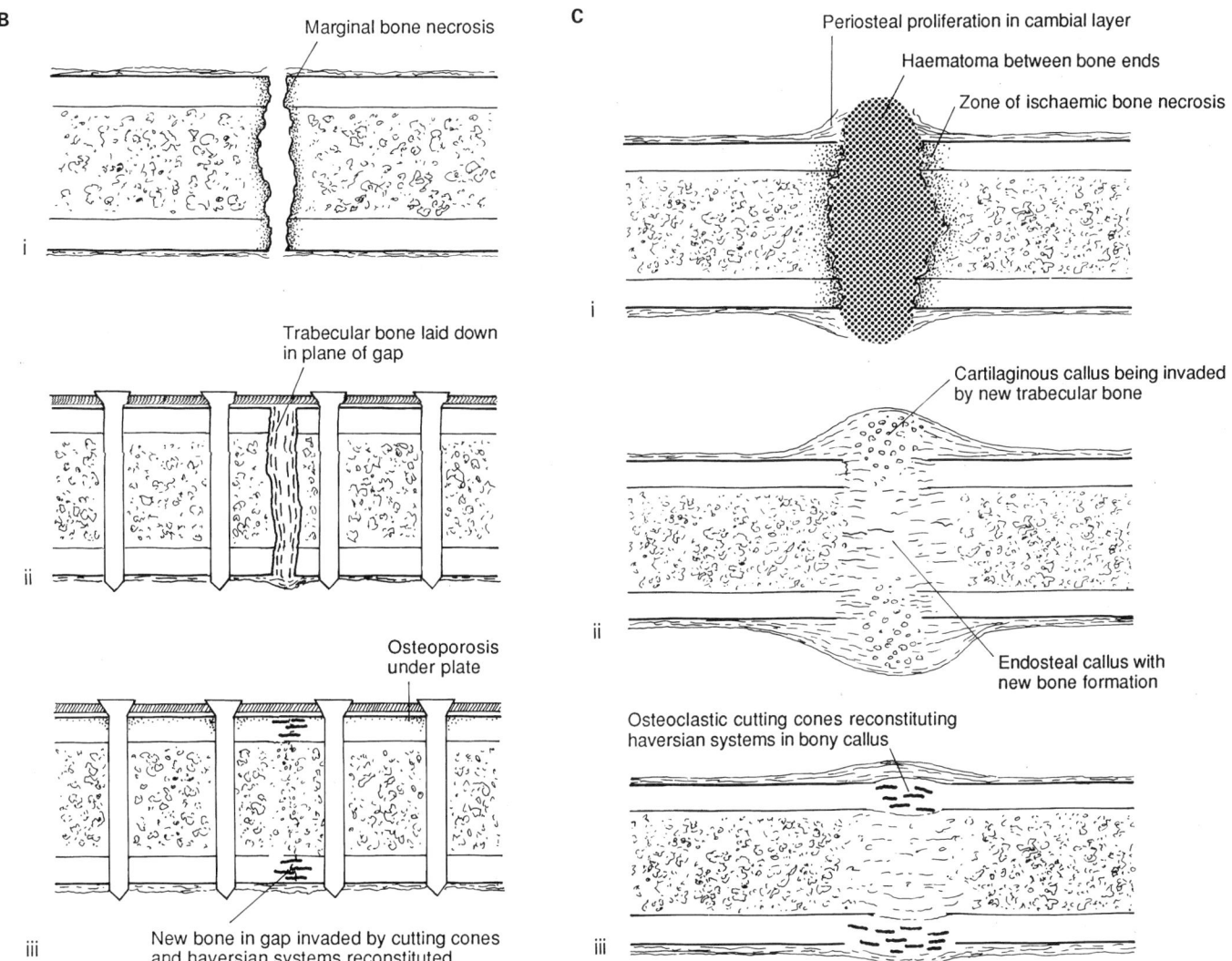

Fig. 5.7 Types of bone healing after fracture. B Gap healing: (i) The bone edges are separated by a narrow gap. (ii) The fracture is immobilized by a plate. The gap is filled by trabeculae of new bone, formed in osteogenic granulation tissue. (iii) The new bone is remodelled into haversian systems in the cortex, and trabecular bone in the medulla or diploe. **C** Healing by callus formation: (i) The bone edges are separated by a haematoma. The fracture is not immobilized. (ii) The haematoma is converted to granulation tissue; osteoid and cartilaginous callus forms, especially around the fracture site. (iii) The callus ossifies and is remodelled into cortical and medullary bone.

We use grafts of iliac crest, rib and calvarial bone. These are as a rule composed of both cancellous and cortical bone. Cancellous bone is rapidly and reliably accepted and incorporated into the host bone by the process known as creeping substitution (Burchardt 1983). The transplanted bone has no blood supply, and most of its cellular elements die before the graft undergoes neovascularization, though some osteoblasts on the periphery of the graft may survive to join with cells from the host tissue — usually a fracture site or cranial defect — to form new bone. Granulation tissue from the host tissue forms around the graft, and mesenchymal cells in the granulation are induced to become the precursors of osteoblasts and osteoclasts. The process of bone induction is governed by growth factors derived from the grafted bone as well as from the host tissue; Urist et al (1983) have stressed the role of bone morphogenetic protein, which is present in demineralized bone matrix and able to induce bone and cartilage in ectopic sites. When cells with osteogenic capacity have been induced, the process known as osteoconduction begins. The marrow spaces of the transplanted cancellous bone are invaded by new blood vessels, and osteoblasts deposit appositional new bone on the trabeculae of dead graft bone. For a period, living and dead bone coexist, and the graft actually appears in radiographs to be denser than normal bone. (Fig. 5.8B shows this in a piece of replanted calvarial bone.) Later, osteoclasts remove the dead bone, and eventually the cancellous graft is entirely replaced by new bone. The process of bone conduction appears to be faster in young persons.

Cortical bone is often used to give structural strength

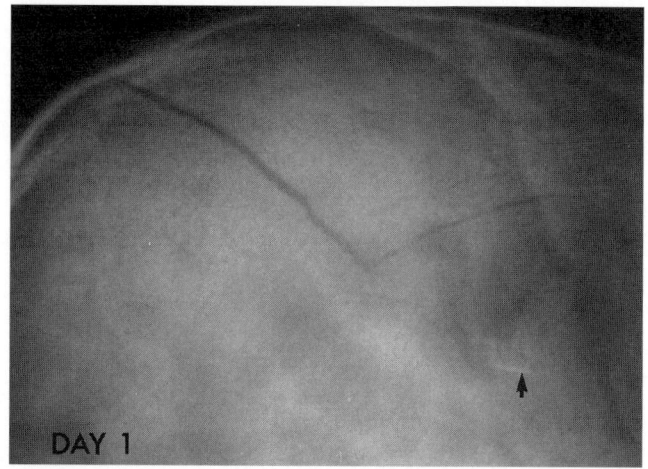

A

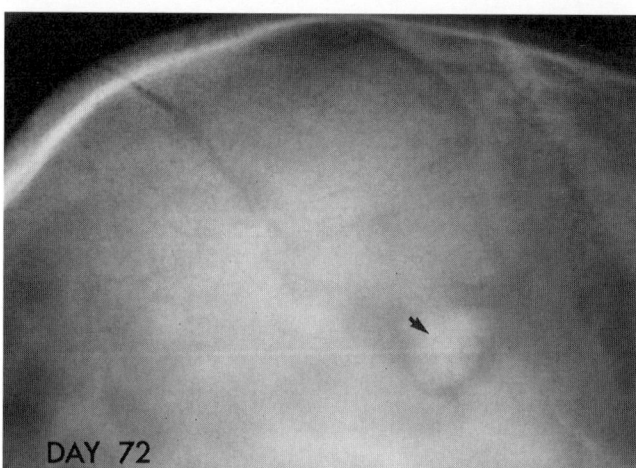

B

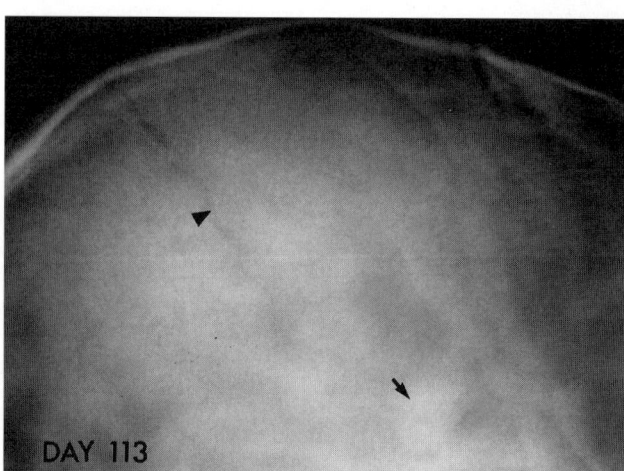

C

Fig. 5.8 Healing in a depressed calvarial fracture. A child aged 8 was hit with a cricket bat; he sustained a depressed fracture in the parietal region, and a small extradural haematoma. After some delay, the fracture was elevated and the clot was evacuated. The bone fragments were replaced. **A** Day 1 (before operation): the edge of a depressed fragment (arrow) is seen as a white line. **B** Day 72: the depressed fragment (arrow) appears hyperdense, and is surrounded by hypodense bone. **C** Day 113: The depressed fragment (arrow) is less dense and appears to be incorporated with the rest of the calvaria. The linear fracture (arrow head) is largely but not wholly united.

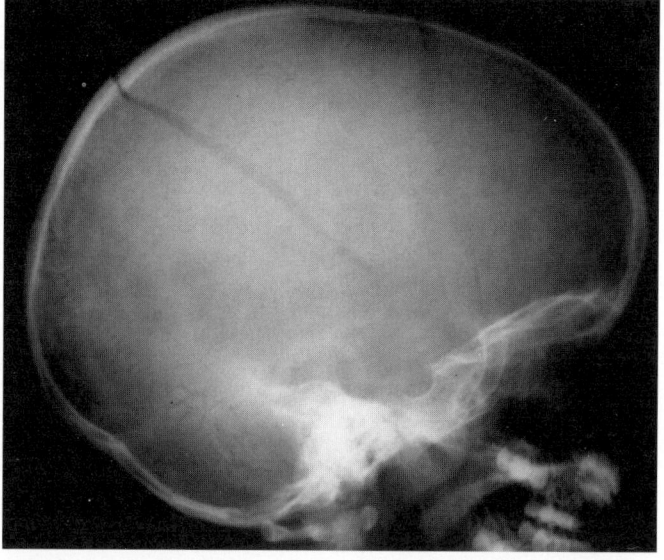

A

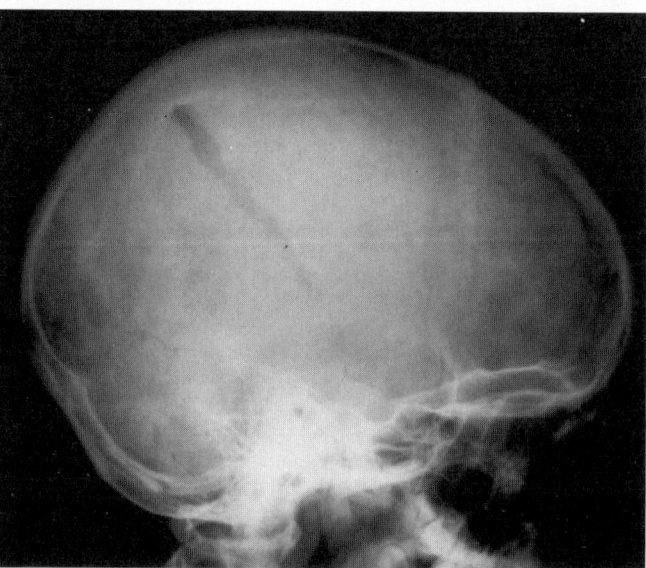

B

Fig. 5.9 Partial healing of a linear calvarial fracture. Fracture of parietal bone in a boy injured at the age of 3 years. **A** The fracture shows some separation of the edges soon after injury. **B** At the age of 10 years, the fracture edges (arrow) show failure of healing and slightly increased separation. There was no palpable defect or pulsation. There was complete healing in the midline.

or a smooth contour. The incorporation of cortical bone is slower. First, osteoclasts ream out the haversian canals of the graft, which are then revascularized; during this process, the graft loses density and strength. New bone is then laid down and the graft is partially replaced by creeping substitution; however, some of the dead cortical bone is incorporated and remains permanently in the reconstituted structure. Manchester (1972) showed that a large graft of cancellous and cortical iliac bone, used to replace an excised hemimandible, may survive and behave like living bone, healing when osteotomized and showing

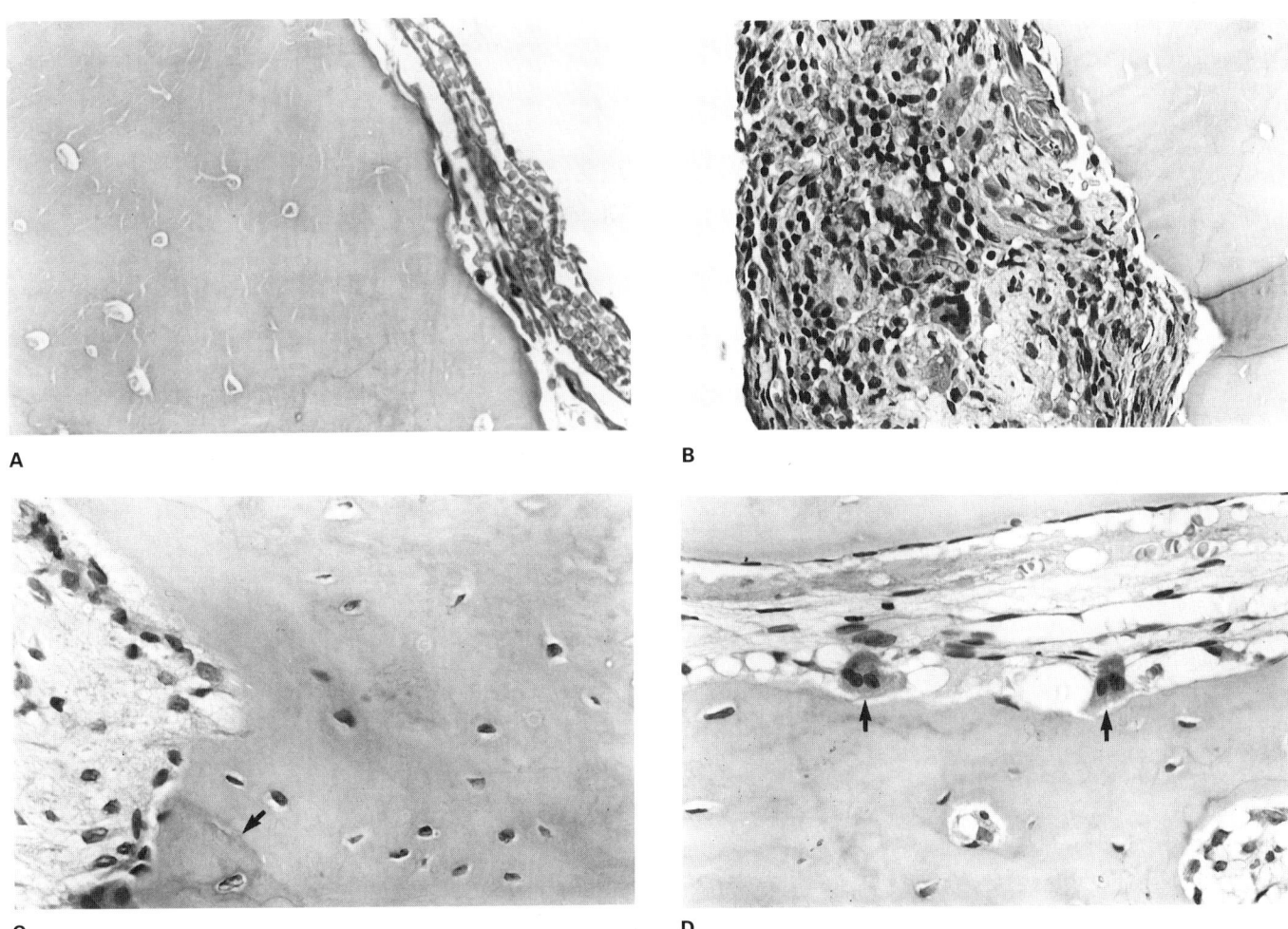

Fig. 5.10 Cellular activity in an infected mandibular osteotomy. Biopsies show stages of bone necrosis and repair. **A** Sequestrum of necrotic bone: empty lacunae containing no osteocytes; very little cellular activity on the surface of the bone. H&E, × 210. **B** Chronic inflammatory granulomatous reaction H&E, × 210. **C** Osteoblasts laying down new bone; arrow indicates older bone being remodelled. H&E, × 210. **D** Two osteoclasts remodelling living bone. H&E, × 210.

trabecular remodelling. He attributed the success of such large grafts to rapid revascularization in the absence of haematoma formation. This emphasizes the importance of the state of the host bed in which the graft is placed. In the facial region, the soft tissues are normally very vascular, and in general bone grafts survive well if firmly fixed. This is not always so with bone grafts placed in calvarial defects, perhaps because the adjacent diploe is often poorly vascularized.

It is sometimes convenient to use autogenous bone preserved by freezing, as when a craniotomy flap has been removed because of brain swelling. In such grafts, the osteocytes are presumably dead, but osteo-inductive factors such as bone morphogenetic protein may survive. Frozen autografted bone is usually accepted, though we have seen resorption of such grafts under circumstances in which a fresh graft would probably have survived. At one time, we sterilized such preserved autografts by gamma irradiation: most of the grafts underwent resorption and this is in accord with the observation that bone

morphogenetic protein and other bone growth factors are destroyed by irradiation (Marx & Stevens 1991).

When a bone graft is vascularized by microsurgical anastomosis, the transplanted bone survives unless the period of ischaemia is too long. Östrup & Frederickson (1974), in their pioneering experimental study of mandibular reconstruction with a vascularized rib, found that many grafted osteocytes did die, presumably from ischaemia, but no massive bone necrosis took place and the graft formed abundant new bone. The general success of vascularized bone grafts confirms that the process of incorporation is more direct and more rapid than with free autogenous grafts.

Since the supply of autogenous bone is limited, efforts have been made to promote bone union by cadaver bone grafts. These allografts are immunologically active and may be rejected, but the allogeneic bone can act as a resorbable supporting matrix, especially if used in conjunction with an agent able to induce new bone formation, such as autogenous bone or bone marrow. Marx

& Stevens (1991) give an excellent account of the use of cadaver bone in conjunction with autogenous cancellous bone to repair mandibular defects, but we have not used this method. Nor have we used deproteinized animal bone for CMF injuries: the use of this material, in conjunction with autogenous marrow grafts, has been reviewed by Salama (1983). Oberg & Rosenquist (1994) have described the osteogenic effects of implants of allogeneic bone from which antigens had been extracted, combined with hydroxyapatite: exuberant bone overgrowth appeared, presumably from the action of bone morphogenetic protein. Preparations of purified bone morphogenetic protein are being used clinically to promote retention of surgical implants in the facial skeleton (Sailer & Kolb 1994).

Cartilage

Mature cartilage has very little reparative capacity and most wounds involving cartilage unite, if at all, by fibroblastic activity. On the other hand, cartilage is very tolerant of ischaemia. In the CMF region, several types of cartilage are found, and it is likely that their reparative capacities are somewhat different. Hyaline cartilage is found in the nose and nasal septum, and the external ear contains yellow elastic cartilage; incised wounds of these structures unite only by fibrous scar tissue. The articular surfaces of the temporomandibular joint (TMJ) and its disc are fibrocartilaginous; wounds of the joint may be filled with fibrous tissue from the joint capsule, and this may be transformed into cartilage to re-establish the original joint surface. Robinson (1993) has shown this in the marmoset: small lesions in the mandibular condylar cartilage were first filled with collagen fibres and then with normal-seeming cartilage. It appeared that the new chondrocytes were derived from precursor cells in the periosteum, rather than from the adjacent uninjured condylar cartilage. This reparative capacity is not seen in other cartilaginous joints; it is unclear whether it is relevant in the recovery of the TMJ after trauma.

The cartilages of the nose and ear may be damaged in facial burns. There is only a thin layer of subdermal tissue between skin and cartilage, and the subcutaneous vasculature is intimately related to the perichondrial blood supply; thermal skin injury may be associated with necrosis of the cartilage and secondary deformity (p. 479).

Cartilage grafts

Free grafts of autogenous rib cartilage, or combined rib bone and cartilage, are used in repair of some CMF injuries, especially those involving the temporomandibular joint (p. 287). Cartilage, an avascular tissue, usually survives well, unless unable to obtain nutrition by diffusion from the surrounding tissues or exposed by skin breakdown or absence of the mucoperichondrium. However,

sculpting cartilage to meet an aesthetic need may unbalance tensions within the graft, which may then warp; the literature on this is briefly reviewed by Wornom & Buchman (1992). Cartilage cadaver grafts have been used, but cartilage has some immunogenic capacity and it appears that cartilage allografts are less satisfactory than autogenous grafts (Burwell 1985).

Teeth

The teeth have limited reparative capacities, even in young persons, and certain types of localized injury may lead to destruction of the entire tooth and even to spread of infection to the underlying bone.

Dental fractures

These are common injuries, young permanent upper incisors being especially at risk; the fracture can involve the palatal, incisal or proximal surfaces of the tooth. Andreasen (1981) classified dental fractures on an anatomical basis:

1. Crown infraction: crack involving only enamel, with no loss of tooth substance.
2. Crown fracture:
   a. uncomplicated
      — involving enamel only (Fig. 5.11A)
      — involving enamel and dentine, but not the pulp (Fig. 5.11B)
   b. complicated — involving enamel, dentine and pulp (Fig. 5.11C)
3. Crown–root fracture:
   a. uncomplicated — involving enamel, dentine and cementum but not involving pulp
   b. complicated — involving enamel, dentine, cementum and pulp (Fig. 5.11D)
4. Root fractures — involving dentine, cementum and pulp (Fig. 5.11E)
5. Subluxation: tooth loose but not displaced
6. Luxation: tooth displaced into the alveolar bone (intrusive), or partially avulsed (extrusive), or displaced laterally
7. Exarticulation — tooth completely avulsed.

Fractures involving only the enamel present minimal risk to the pulp or periodontal tissues. When the fracture involves the dentinal layer, bacteria invade the dentinal tubules. The prognosis for the tooth then depends largely on the extent of the fracture: a fracture involving only a small exposure of dentin, such as a mesio- or disto-incisal edge fracture, is less likely to go on to necrosis than a fracture going deeply into the dentine.

After a fracture complicated by pulp exposure, blood clot, fibrin and inflammatory cells may be present on the pulpal surface (Fig. 5.12A). If treatment is delayed for

CROWN FRACTURES

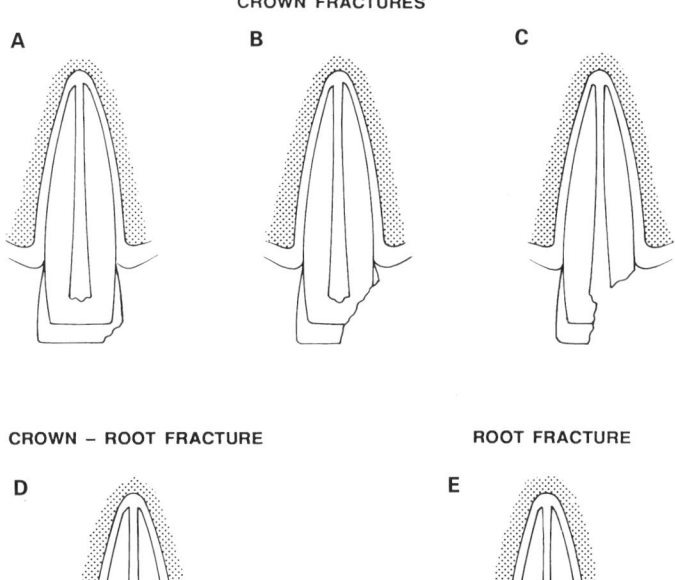

Fig. 5.11 Types of dental fractures. A Uncomplicated crown fracture, confined to the enamel. **B** Uncomplicated crown fracture, involving enamel and dentin but not the pulp. **C** Complicated crown fracture, involving the pulp. **D** Complicated crown-root fracture, involving the pulp. **E** Root fracture. Redrawn after Andreasen (1972).

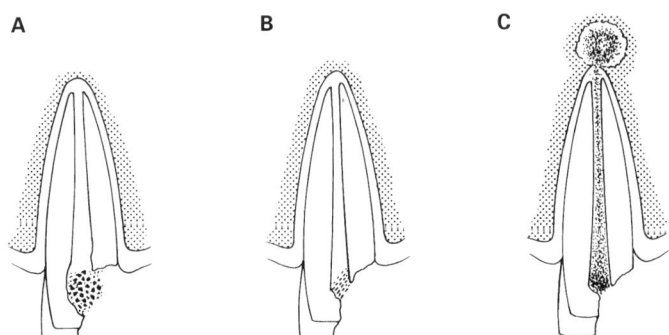

Fig. 5.12 Complications of dental fractures. A Granuloma formed in pulp cavity. **B** Calcific bridge closing the fracture and sealing the pulp cavity. **C** Bacterial infection in the pulp cavity, giving rise to an apical abscess. Modified after Andreasen (1972).

a few days, the exposed pulp usually develops a hyperplastic mass of exudate rich in fibrin, cells and antibodies. This defence reaction may be followed by sealing of the exposed dentinal tubules by a calcific layer (Fig. 5.12B); secondary dentine may be formed in the pulp cavity, and the tooth may be saved. However, the formation of plaque on exposed dentinal tubules may lead to diffusion of microorganisms through these tubules into the pulpal tissue: a deeper inflammatory response is now established

under the surface of the fracture, which can spread to the periapical tissues and beyond as osteomyelitis of the jaw. The dental defence mechanism can be frustrated if there is excessive bleeding, separation of the pulp tissue from the pulp wall at the moment of fracture, and/or fluid build-up under pressure in the pulp chamber.

Pulp injuries

The pulp occupies the central cavity of the tooth, and is enclosed by dentine. Although the cells lining this cavity can be regarded as mesenchymal connective tissue, they carry out a number of vital functions. During the developmental period, the pulp mesenchyme has cells (odontoblasts) which are capable of producing dentine. In the adult tooth, these cells continue to produce physiological dentine, and if the tooth is traumatized, a reparative process begins, whereby secondary dentin is laid down under the site of the assault. This may go on to obliterate the pulp chamber.

The dental pulp responds to injury by manifesting all the classical signs of inflammation: dilation of blood vessels, transudation of serum and extravascular migration of leukocytes within the pulp chamber. The presence of extravascular exudates in the confined space of the rigid pulp chamber results in increased pressure and pain from stimulation of pulp nerves and nerve endings. If the process is mild in nature and of short duration, the pulp tissue will usually recover; in severe cases, the pulp may undergo necrosis and the tooth may be lost.

Bacterial invasion follows traumatic exposure of the pulp. The pulp tissue reacts in a protective manner, but the resulting inflammatory processes may continue and lead to pulp necrosis and apical abscess formation (Fig. 5.12C). Young teeth have a large pulp chamber which has considerable capacity to survive injury. However, it is important in dealing with injuries of young teeth having incomplete root development to ensure that pulp vitality is protected. The treatment of pulp exposure is discussed on p. 349.

Dental and alveolar resorption

Severely traumatized teeth may occasionally undergo resorption (Fig. 5.13). This peculiar dystrophy of the pulp tissue results in massive destruction of the dental hard tissues. The process begins in the pulp and spreads laterally through the dentine; in all probability, the internal resorption of the dentine, as in other hard tissue resorptions, is the work of macrophages and multinucleate giant cells, indistinguishable from osteoclasts (Fig. 5.10D). The lost dentine is replaced by chronic inflammatory tissue. The process may or may not result in loosening and loss of the affected tooth; appropriate endodontal therapy may prevent this, though in the case of Fig. 5.13 this treatment was unsuccessful.

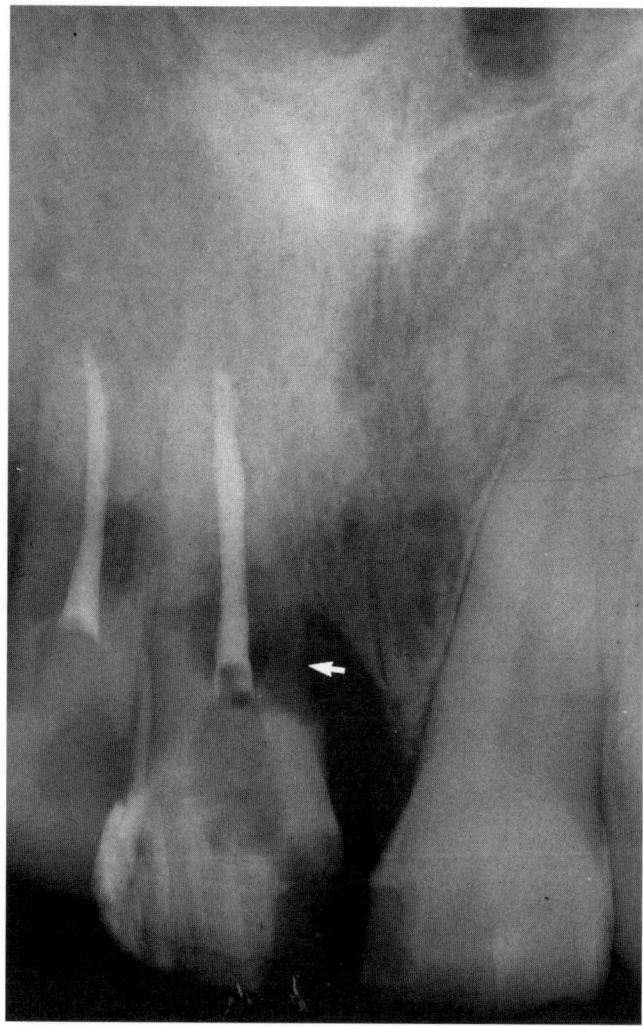

Fig. 5.13 Severe resorption following endodontic treatment of fractured teeth. Radiograph showing maxillary incisors and canine teeth in an adult, some time after crown fractures. In the two incisor teeth, the fractures had opened the pulp; gutta percha was inserted in the hope of saving the tooth, but dramatic resorptive changes appeared in the mid root regions (white arrow) and in the alveolar bone. In the canine fracture, the pulp was not opened.

In adults, loss of teeth by trauma or extraction results in resorption of the dental alveolus. This is especially important in the anterior maxilla following the loss of one or more teeth. This bone resorption can jeopardize aesthetic tooth replacement by fixed bridgework, and may also prevent the insertion of dental titanium implants to hold replacement tooth crowns. Bone grafting may be necessary to augment the alveolus before placing an implant (p. 637).

GLANDULAR TISSUES

Salivary glands

These glands are often contused or lacerated; the parotid gland is especially vulnerable. The chief complications of parotid injury are pseudocyst formation and salivary fistula. It appears that permanent obstruction of the parotid duct leads to atrophy of the secretory cells (Landau & Stewart 1985). Harrison & Garrett (1976) showed this in the cat: parotid duct ligation caused severe progressive glandular atrophy, but ligation of the submandibular and sublingual ducts caused less striking changes. Parasympathetic denervation also induces some degree of glandular atrophy.

NEURAL TISSUES

Cranial nerves

First cranial nerve

The olfactory system is complex (p. 57). The olfactory tract and bulb are part of the central nervous system; they are often contused or lacerated in association with frontal lobe damage and have no capacity to regenerate. The olfactory filaments are peripheral nerves and are said to have some capacity to regenerate, at least in the monkey (Monti-Graziadei et al 1980); this may explain the rare but well-documented recovery of olfaction after closed head injury.

Second cranial nerve

The optic nerve is a component of the central nervous system and has no capacity to regenerate. The optic nerve and chiasm are often damaged in cases of CMF trauma; they may be lacerated, contused or rendered ischaemic. The end result of such injuries is optic atrophy and demyelination. The pathology of optic nerve trauma has been well reviewed by Walsh & Hoyt (1982–1991) and by Kline et al (1984) but is still controversial. Several surgeons have ventured to biopsy damaged nerves soon after loss of sight, and the appearances have been variously interpreted as indicative of ischaemic necrosis due to damage to the pial vascular supply of the nerve, or to axonal shear damage. Crompton (1970) found evidence of one or both processes in 37 of 84 autopsied cases, but concluded that it was impossible to distinguish between them in histological material. The clinical implications of this uncertainty are discussed in Chapter 14 (p. 420).

Nerve regeneration

The remaining cranial nerves are often injured in association with CMF trauma; they are peripheral nerves with Schwann cell sheaths, and they are capable of regeneration. Seddon (1972) and Sunderland (1978) devised classifications of peripheral nerve injury, using terms which express the loss of continuity of the components of the nerve. Table 5.1 gives the classification and nomenclature popularized by Seddon, though he did not coin the

Table 5.1 Classification of nerve injuries (after Seddon 1972)

Characteristics	Neurotmesis	Axonotmesis	Neurapraxia
Pathology	Continuity lost in all elements	Epi- and perineurium and Schwann sheaths preserved; axons interrupted	Nerve in continuity; selective focal demyelination of larger axons
Clicincal	Complete paralysis	Complete paralysis	Motor paralysis; often sensory sparing
Treatment	Nerve suture	Expectant	Expectant
Recovery	1–2 mm/day; likely to be imperfect	1–2 mm/day; usually perfect	Perfect

elegant names neurotmesis, axonotmesis and neurapraxia. If the axon is transected, as in both neurotmesis and axonotmesis, then it degenerates distally in its whole course: the classical Wallerian degeneration. The proximal axon degenerates to the first node of Ranvier, and sometimes further if there has been severe trauma, as in a gunshot wound. The cell body of the parent neuron shows loss of Nissl substance, but usually survives and synthesizes the proteins necessary for axonal regeneration. The distal axon shows swelling and clumping of mitochondria; the axoplasmic reticulum breaks up and the neurofilaments fragment. The myelin sheath also breaks down and the degenerating fragments are removed by macrophages. The Schwann cells along the course of the degenerating axon swell and undergo mitotic division under the stimulus of a mitogen or mitogens produced by the degenerating axon or its sheath.

The Schwann cells form tubes and cords extending distally from the point of nerve section. It appears that these cells form or attract neuronotrophic substances, of which nerve growth factor (NGF) is the best studied (Taniuchi et al 1988). Under the stimulus of such chemoattractive agents, axons sprout from the proximal stump of the nerve and form multiple small unmyelinated fibres, one of which — all being well — finds a Schwann cell tube, enters it and grows toward the target structure at a rate usually estimated as 1 mm/day. Eventually, the target structure (muscle fibre, gland or sensory terminal) is reinnervated and function is restored.

The success of this remarkable process depends on the nature of the injury: in axonotmesis, as in a crushed nerve, full regeneration is often seen, whereas in neurotmesis recovery will be prevented if the severed ends are not apposed or if there is local sepsis. Age, the nature of the nerve and other factors also influence the degree of recovery. Not rarely, regenerating axons take aberrant paths, and reach inappropriate muscle fibres or secretory cells.

In facial injuries, the nerves likely to be injured are the facial nerve, a predominantly motor nerve, and the trigeminal nerve which is for practical purposes a sensory nerve, since its motor component is deeply placed and only injured by penetrating trauma. The third, fourth and sixth cranial nerves are often injured in closed head injuries.

The facial nerve may be divided or less often crushed at any point in its course. It has a remarkable capacity to recover, if the ends are in continuity. But the complex anatomy of the facial nerve (p. 62) makes aberrant regeneration a common sequel of CMF injuries involving that nerve; mass facial muscular action, gustatory sweating (Frey syndrome) and lacrimation (crocodile tears) may be disfiguring consequences (p. 441). Misdirected axonal regeneration may also follow injury of the oculomotor nerve (p. 405).

The branches of the trigeminal nerve are likely to be injured when traversing bony canals or grooves: damage to the supraorbital, infraorbital and inferior dental nerves are commonly associated with facial fractures of various types. The trigeminal ganglion and its main branches are sometimes injured in skull base fractures. McGovern et al (1986) have reported a case of trigemino-abducens synkinesis after a severe CMF injury, which appeared to represent aberrant regeneration of trigeminal motor axons into the proprioceptive innervation of the abducent nerve (p. 415).

Sensory nerve recovery is often less than perfect, but may be masked by lateral ingrowth by the terminals of intact nerves supplying the neighbourhood of the denervated area. If nerve regeneration is not achieved, there will be a neuroma at the point of section, composed of axon end bulbs and proliferating Schwann cells and fibroblasts; these neuromas may be painful, but their importance as a cause of chronic post-traumatic facial pain is in doubt (p. 660).

Nerve grafts

Autogenous nerve grafts are used to repair gaps in the inferior dental nerve, usually iatrogenic, and in facial nerve repair. The grafted nerve provides tubes of living Schwann cells to guide the regenerating axons to the distal nerve trunk. To survive, the graft must be revascularized from the proximal and distal nerve stumps and from the host bed within a few days: if this does not happen, the graft undergoes ischaemic necrosis. The facial tissues are very vascular, and with good microsurgical technique excellent results are usually obtained with free grafts. However, for the long transfacial anastomoses used to reinnervate the facial nerve from the opposite side, a microvascularized graft from the saphenous nerve has been used (Kärcher et al 1989) and increasing use is being made of this method of promoting regeneration.

There is an extensive literature on nerve allografts, but at present these are not recommended.

Meninges

The dura mater is of great importance in cranial trauma. The outer layer is osteogenic and participates in the repair of fractures of the calvaria and skull base; in infants and young children, large calvarial bone defects may close spontaneously if the dura is intact. There is some debate on the capacity of older subjects to achieve this spontaneous regeneration. Kent & Misiek (1991) give 6 years as the upper age limit; we have seen substantial reossification in adolescents, especially when the pericranium is intact, but agree that this is not always evident.

Haemorrhages from arteries and veins in the outer layer of the dura can give rise to extradural haematomas (see below); if these do not cause serious cerebral compression, they are invaded by fibrovascular tissue and absorbed, or less often encapsulated by fibrous tissue and even bone from the dura mater. The inner layer of the dura (p. 36) is also capable of considerable fibrovascular activity in response to subdural bleeding, forming the inner and outer membranes seen in chronic subdural haematomas (p. 524).

The dura is a valuable barrier against infection; tears or penetrating dural wounds usually require surgical closure to reconstitute the barrier. Incised wounds of the dura mater heal well if the edges are coapted. However, dural healing may be deficient if leptomeninges and brain tissue are interposed between the edges of the dural tear (see below), or if the tear is in proximity to a cerebrospinal fluid cistern. Dural defects are closed by a neomembrane formed from the adjacent soft tissues rather than from the edges of the torn dura, and this may constitute a false meningocele. The arachnoid and pia mater are almost always torn in penetrating wounds of the dura, and participate with it in forming a fibroglial meningocerebral scar.

Dural grafts

Autogenous fascia or pericranium is often used to close dural defects; in a few months the graft usually appears to have fused with the rest of the dura. Allografts of freeze-dried (lyophilized) cadaver dura mater have been used for some 40 years (Campbell et al 1958), and with

considerable success; the process of lyophilization eliminates the immunogenicity of the transplant. The transplanted collagen hyalinizes and is slowly removed and replaced by new collagen; after a few months the graft appears incorporated. However, Brown et al (1992) have reported seven cases of progressive dementia and death from Creutzfeld–Jakob disease after implants of this allograft, and we have ceased to use it. Xenografts of freeze-dried porcine dermis have been used to repair dural defects (O'Neill and Booth, 1984), and it appears that the grafted collagen was not rejected.

Brain

It is usual to distinguish between closed and open head injuries, and this distinction is especially relevant in the neuropathology of impacts in the CMF region. In closed head injuries, primary brain damage is inflicted by acute tissue deformation due either to acceleration imparted to the whole head (Fig. 4.8), or to force acting locally at the impact site (Fig. 4.1): the resulting brain lesions may be diffuse or focal. In open head injuries, localized primary brain damage may be inflicted by something that penetrates the protective capsule of the brain, the skull and meninges (Fig. 4.7). Both types of injury may be complicated by secondary pathological processes, such as cerebral compression or anoxia; in open head injuries, there is the additional risk of microbial infection. In the CMF region, open brain injuries are common and often serious; they may involve the paranasal air sinuses, and may give rise to cranionasal fistulas (p. 376).

Closed brain injuries

The primary effects of blunt head impact have been well reviewed by Adams (1992). Focal effects include contusions and lacerations. Frontal impacts commonly cause haemorrhagic contusions in the frontal lobes, especially in the polar and orbital cortex; the temporal poles may also be injured. Thus, CMF injuries are likely to be complicated by frontotemporal brain damage; contrecoup occipital damage is very unusual except after impacts incompatible with survival. The probable mechanisms have been discussed (p. 106).

Contusions

Small contusions are typically collections of red blood cells, often grouped around a small vessel running at right angles to the surface of the cortex. Larger haemorrhagic contusions may extend into the white matter, and subarachnoid bleeding is also often seen. The red cells remain intact for a day or more and then show lysis; there is a macrophage reaction and deposition of bilirubin. There is neuronal death in the contused area and eventu-

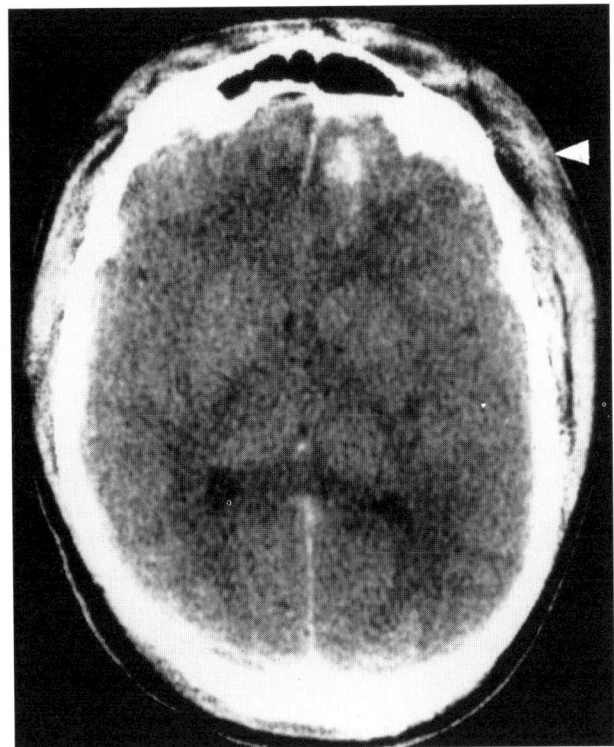
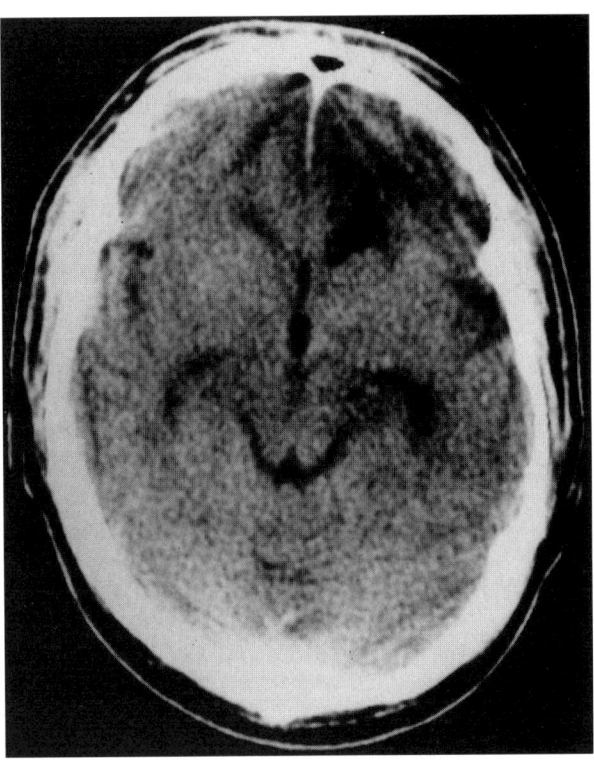

Fig. 5.14 Contusional brain injury from frontal impact. A-26-year-old man fell from a slowly moving car and struck his head in the left frontal region. He sustained a left-sided linear skull fracture and was drowsy. **A** CT 24 h after injury showed multiple hyperdense lesions in the left frontal lobe, presumably haemorrhagic contusions. Scalp swelling was evident at the site of impact (white arrowhead). **B** CT 6 weeks later showed extensive bilateral low density lesions in the frontal white matter; these presumably represent axonal destruction and gliosis. There were permanent changes in personality.

ally replacement by astrocytic gliosis, often stained yellow by the bilirubin. The site of an old contusion is evident as an area of atrophy, typically at the convexity of a convolution and stained yellow or brown.

The sequential changes in a cerebral contusion are mirrored in radiological images. In computerized tomograms (CT), the haemorrhagic components of the contusion are obvious as hyperdense masses ((Fig. 5.14A), while the associated oedema and later gliosis appear as hypodense areas (Fig. 5.14B). Magnetic resonance images (MRI) also visualize contusions well, and the progressive degradation of haemoglobin gives changing appearances that relate to the age of the lesion (Table 7.5).

Lacerations

These are areas of disruption of brain and meninges; they are seen especially in association with depressed skull fractures, but may also be caused by violent movement of the brain. The junction of the pons and the medulla is often the site of a laceration, or even a complete pontomedullary transection; this injury sometimes follows high velocity impacts in the CMF region (Simpson et al 1989) and usually results in instant death, though smaller lesions are compatible with prolonged survival (p. 212).

Diffuse brain injury

The diffuse effects of blunt head impact include damage to axons, dendrites vessels and glia. Widespread axonal damage presumably from shearing stresses, is termed diffuse axonal injury (DAI). The axonal lesions are often multifocal rather than diffuse, and there are sites of predilection, notably the corpus callosum and the superior cerebellar peduncle (Fig 5.15). Similar impacts may cause multifocal or diffuse vascular injury (DVI), and again there are sites of predilection: these include the corpus callosum and the superior cerebellar peduncle, but also the parasagittal cortex and the basal ganglia. It is not yet known whether the distribution of DAI lesions is related to the site of the causative impact; however, it is clear that DAI is often seen after impacts in the CMF region. In life, DAI can be inferred on clinical grounds, but cannot be verified radiologically, whereas the larger (5–10 mm) lesions of DVI can usually be seen in CT or MRI scans. It is often assumed that DVI ('tissue tear haemorrhage') is a marker of DAI, and that non-haemorrhagic lesions seen in MRI scans are areas of DAI (p. 210). These assumptions are often correct, but the correlations between radiological pathology and histopathology need fuller documentation. Damage to glial

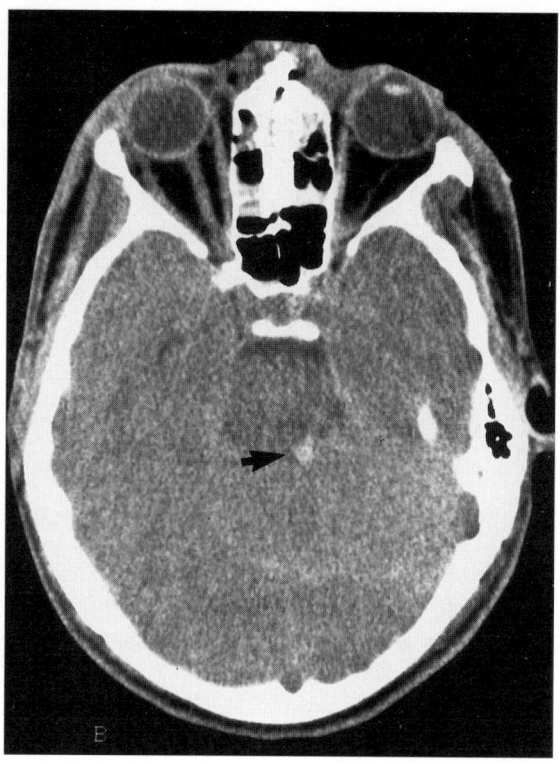

A

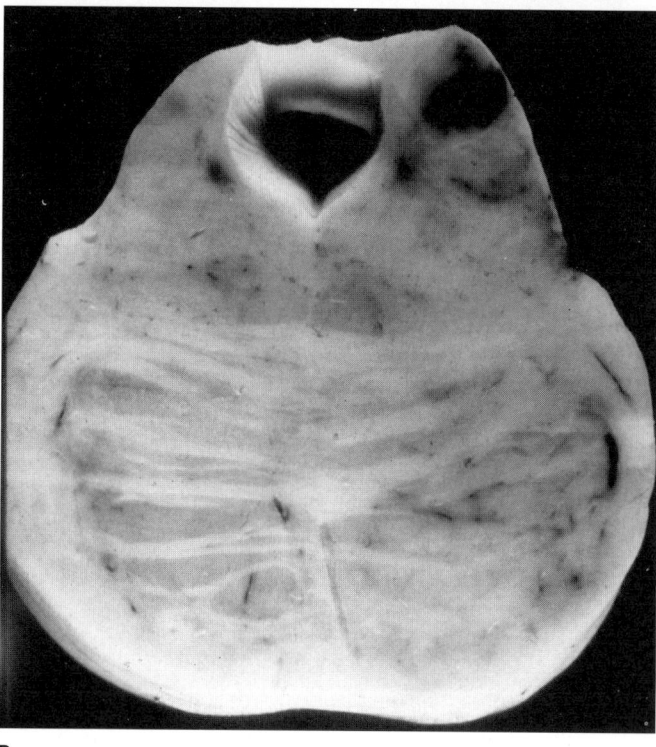

B

Fig. 5.15 Vulnerable sites: the midbrain. The attachment of the superior cerebellar peduncle to the lower midbrain appears to be a vulnerable site in diffuse brain injury: both vascular and axonal damage are often seen in this area. **A** CT in young adult hurt in motor cycle accident: the hyperdense lesion (arrow) is presumably a haemorrhage. Note the absence of the perimesencephalic cisterns: a sign of raised intracranial pressure, though it may also result from subarachnoid bleeding. **B** Similar lesion in autopsied case.

cells may accompany DAI (Blumbergs & Wainright 1988); the clinical significance of diffuse glial injury remains to be explored.

Minor head injuries

Clinicopathological correlation is more difficult in cases of closed head injury caused by less severe impacts since autopsy evidence is rarely available and radiological evidence of damage may be absent. The pathology of minor head injuries is still largely unknown, but minimal lesions of DAI type are demonstrable (Oppenheimer 1968), and the upper brainstem is the probable site in cases of transient loss of consciousness ('concussion'). P. Blumbergs (personal communication) has also noted a high incidence of lesions in the fornices after minor head injury.

Open brain injuries

These are characterized by focal penetration of the meninges and brain, with variable remote damage. At the point of focal penetration, there is a cerebral laceration, usually with some haemorrhage.

A distinction is made between brain wounds made by depressed skull fractures, penetrating brain wounds and perforating ('through-and-through') brain wounds. This distinction expresses the size of the impacting object and its kinetic energy. A large, relatively blunt object will depress a large area of bone (Fig. 5.5B), and the underlying brain will be contused and often lacerated, but unless the impact force is very great, damage will be confined to the impact site. Smaller objects with high kinetic energy will penetrate the bone (Fig. 5.5C), and if the kinetic energy is not attenuated at the initial impact, there is likely to be deep penetration and widespread brain damage.

Missile brain wounds

If the penetrating agent is a bullet or shell fragment, there will be a track of brain destruction; if the missile has very high energy, there will be extensive local cavitation causing deformation and bleeding wide of the missile track (Fig. 5.17A). High energy missiles may also cause contusional damage in remote parts of the brain and even fractures of the skull base by transmitted force; this is seen especially in the thin bones of the orbital roofs (Strich 1976, Allen et al 1982). The autopsy on President Lincoln (p. 17) showed shattered orbits, supposedly from this mechanism. The initial effects of mechanical disruption are increased by haemorrhage, oedema and loss of vascular autoregulation, combining to produce raised intracranial pressure (ICP) with all its consequences.

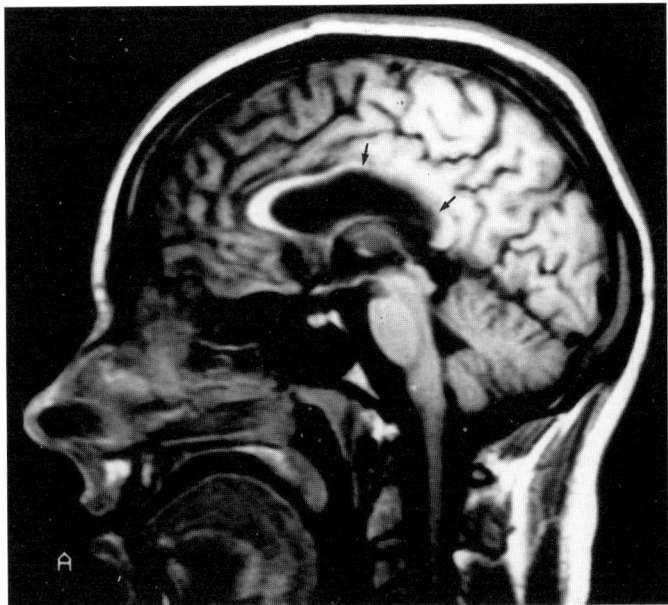

A

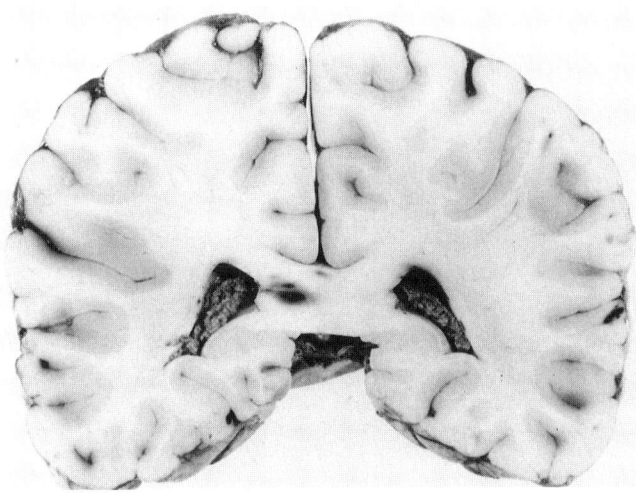

B

Fig. 5.16 Vulnerable sites: the corpus callosum. The corpus callosum may be injured in closed head injuries; haemorrhagic lesions and diffuse axonal damage are often seen. **A** MRI 8 years after a severe closed head injury with residual intellectual and behavioural disabilities. Between the arrows, the body of the corpus callosum is barely visible: in coronal views, it was seen as a thin band. **B** Haemorrhagic lesion in splenium of corpus callosum in a 12-year-old boy hit by a car; it is likely that this was a survivable head injury, death being due to an intra-abdominal haemorrhage.

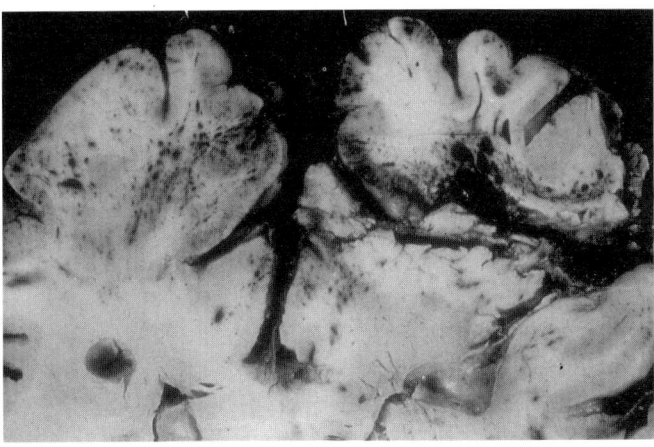

A

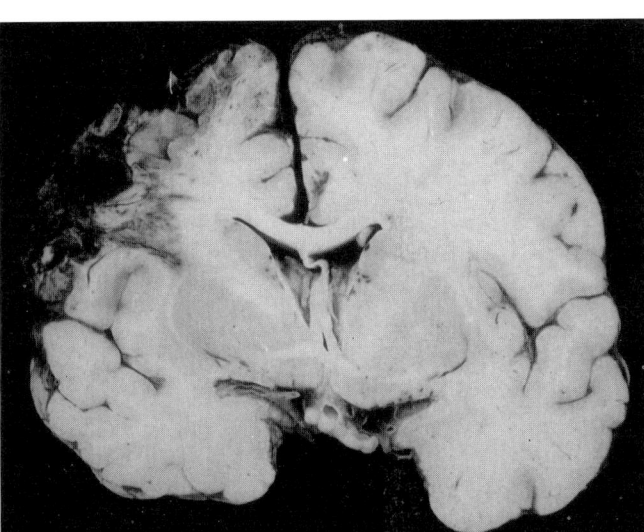

B

Fig. 5.17 Missile wounds of the brain. A Perforating frontal suicidal wound with widespread haemorrhages: the bullet traversed both frontal lobes. Many satellite haemorrhages are seen; these are not directly in the track of the bullet, and result from acute deformation. **B** Tangential wound, with contusion of the cortex; bone chips were driven in from the calvaria.

For surgical purposes, craniocerebral missile wounds are categorized as penetrating, perforating and tangential. In a penetrating wound, the missile penetrates the scalp, the skull and the dura, but does not leave the head (Fig. 5.18A): there is no exit wound. In a perforating wound, the missile traverses the brain ('through and through') and has both entry and exit wounds (Fig. 6.2). A missile wound is described as tangential when it grazes the skull but does not penetrate it: the skull may or

may not be fractured, and the brain may be damaged by transmitted energy (Fig. 5.17B). Missile wounds may be complicated by intracerebral or subdural haemorrhage, sometimes of delayed onset; Hadas et al (1990) have reported cortical laceration and acute subdural bleeding after a tangential pistol wound without breach of the calvarial bone.

Metallic fragments and even entire bullets may remain in the brain. Lead and iron fragments are usually fixed in a chronic fibroglial scar (Fig. 5.18B,C); missiles containing copper are more toxic and evoke a local inflammatory reaction (see below). Large bullets may remain mobile in a cyst or in the ventricular system, changing position according to the posture of the head (Fig. 5.19).

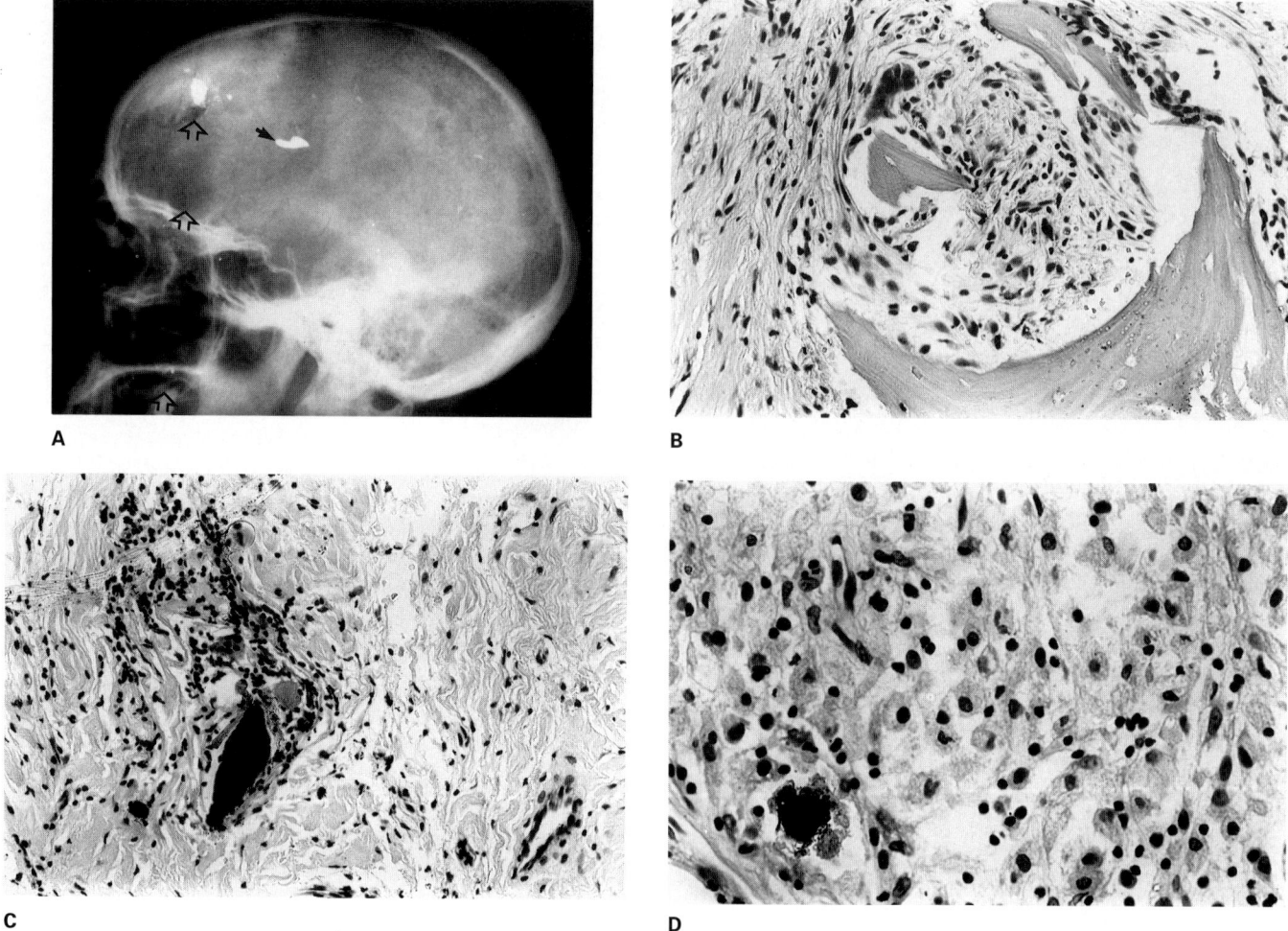

Fig. 5.18 Penetrating brain wound: histology of a meningocerebral scar. A 39-year-old man fired a .22 in lead bullet through his chin into his brain. He survived. The missile track was explored (probably unnecessarily) 5 weeks after wounding. **A** Plain skull radiograph showing missile track (open arrows) in skull, with large fragment of lead bullet lying subcutaneously. The deeper fragment (solid arrow) was embedded in the vicinity of the falx. **B** Biopsy of scar tissue around the deep fragment: a bone chip with cellular reaction, including a giant cell. H&E, × 171. **C** Biopsy in same area: black material, probably carbon from propellant. H&E, × 171. **D** Biopsy of cerebral tissue near the deep fragment: foamy macrophages and a fragment of black material. H&E, × 342.

Histopathology of brain injury

Whatever the cause of injury, the microscopic appearances are dominated by neuronal death and its consequences. Neurons in the central nervous system have very little reparative capacity. If an axon is severed or a neuronal cell body ruptured, then the entire neuron dies; there may even be trans-synaptic degeneration of other neurons deprived of functional stimulation. The axon undergoes degeneration in its whole length, as do the dendrites. The synaptic terminals swell and become argyrophilic. The axis cylinder becomes fragmented, and light microscopy shows globular and fusiform masses which stain pink with eosin and black with reduced silver stains (Fig. 5.20A); electron microscopy shows that these masses are electron-dense and composed of degenerating neurofibrils, mitochondria and other organelles. These

axonal changes are seen by light microscopy 3 or 4 days after injury or even earlier; recent neuropathological studies in our laboratory (P.Blumbergs, personal communication) have shown that immunochemical stains for Alzheimer precursor protein (APP) show swollen axons at an earlier stage after injury than the silver stains. These may represent interference in fast axoplasmic transport. Electron microscopy (Povlishock et al 1989) has shown in experimental studies that the axon may be intact in the first few hours after injury, but later swells and fragments. (This finding raises hopes that early use of neuroprotective drugs may preserve axons). Concurrently, the neuronal body loses its Nissl substance and the cytoplasm becomes homogeneously eosinophilic (Duchen, 1992). The myelin sheath at first looks unaffected, but after several weeks, it begins to fragment, at first near the point of injury and along the whole length of the fibre. The

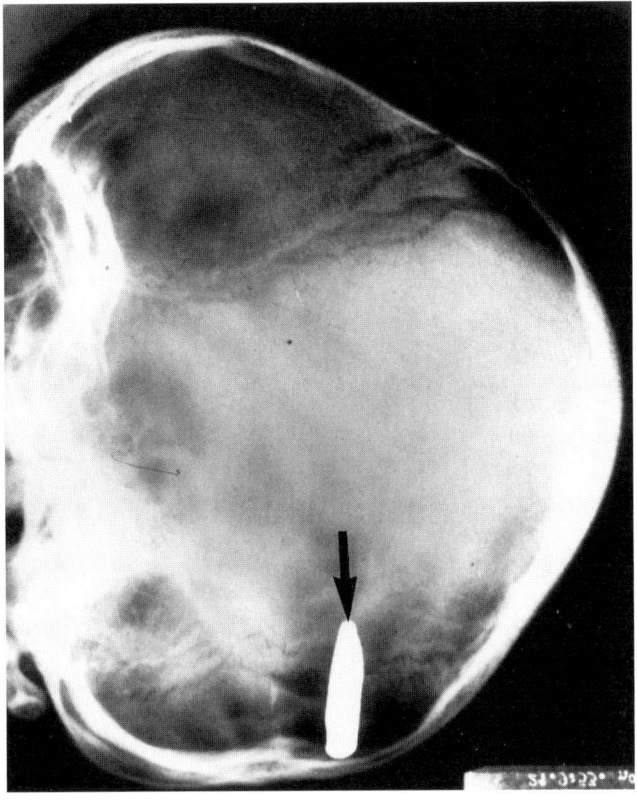

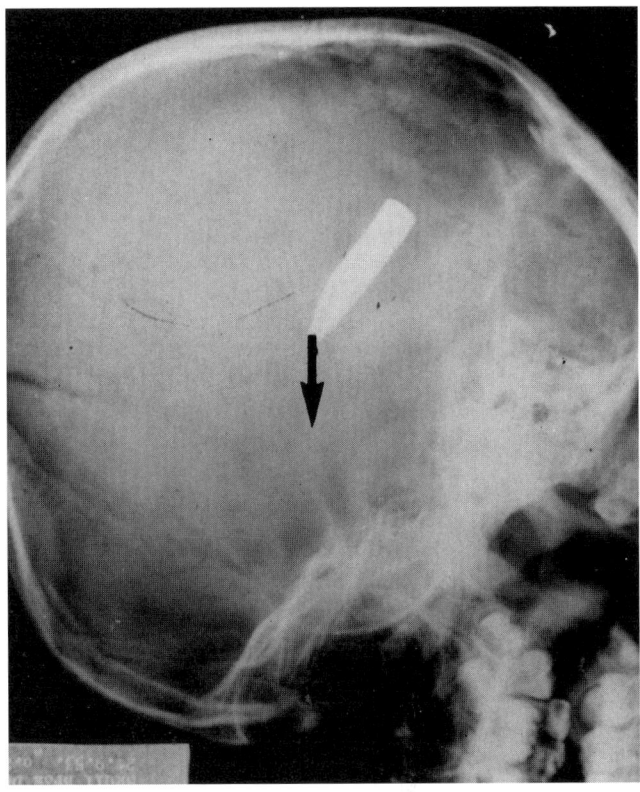

A

B

Fig. 5.19 Migrating bullet. Military rifle bullet in the brain of a young child, hit at long range by a random shot in the occipital region. **A** In the brow up position, the bullet lies near the point of entry. **B** In the brow down position, the bullet has moved forward into the lateral ventricle. Arrows point down.

myelin changes its chemical structure and becomes stainable by the Marchi stain; later there is a further breakdown to simple lipids which can be stained by ordinary fat stains. Eventually the entire neuron usually disappears. This process of relentless degeneration is seen in the brain and also in the optic nerve and olfactory tract; it underlies the permanent neurological and opthalmological disabilities so often seen after CMF trauma. But some qualifications can be made. A neuron may survive a distal axonal injury if its functional activity is maintained through a collateral branch proximal to the point of injury. A neuron deprived of its input will survive if its functional activity is maintained by other inputs; it may even obtain more inputs by the sprouting of new synapses from intact neurons, though the significance of this process in clinical recovery is still uncertain.

The inflammatory response to brain injury is very different from what is seen in other tissues. Polymorphs are seen in penetrating wounds but are inconspicuous in closed brain injuries. Macrophages appear in large numbers when there is necrotic neural tissue (Fig. 5.18D). Some of these macrophages are circulating monocytes from the circulating blood (Imamoto & Leblond 1977), and some are thought to be mobilized microglial cells, though the evidence for this metamorphosis is question-

able. These cells phagocytose the products of degenerating myelin and other debris and soon become stuffed with lipid material. Somewhat later, astrocytes respond to the injury: they multiply by mitosis as early as 10 days after injury and lay down glial fibrils in the damaged areas. It is probable that the activity of astrocytes is stimulated and regulated by growth factors; Lipton (1989) has reviewed possible roles of these in promoting favourable interactions between glial cells and injured neurons. Eventually, after months or years, the site of injury and the course of the degenerated fibre systems are identifiable by an increased glial population as well as by absence of neurons and their processes. Fibroblasts play little part in the reparative processes of clean brain wounds, but appear in great numbers when an abscess forms: the walls of chronic abscesses are densely collagenous. Fibroblasts are also active in meningeal and meningocerebral scars.

Secondary complications of head injury

These include:

1. Intracranial haemorrhage — extradural, subdural and intracerebral
2. Brain swelling
3. Hypoxic brain damage

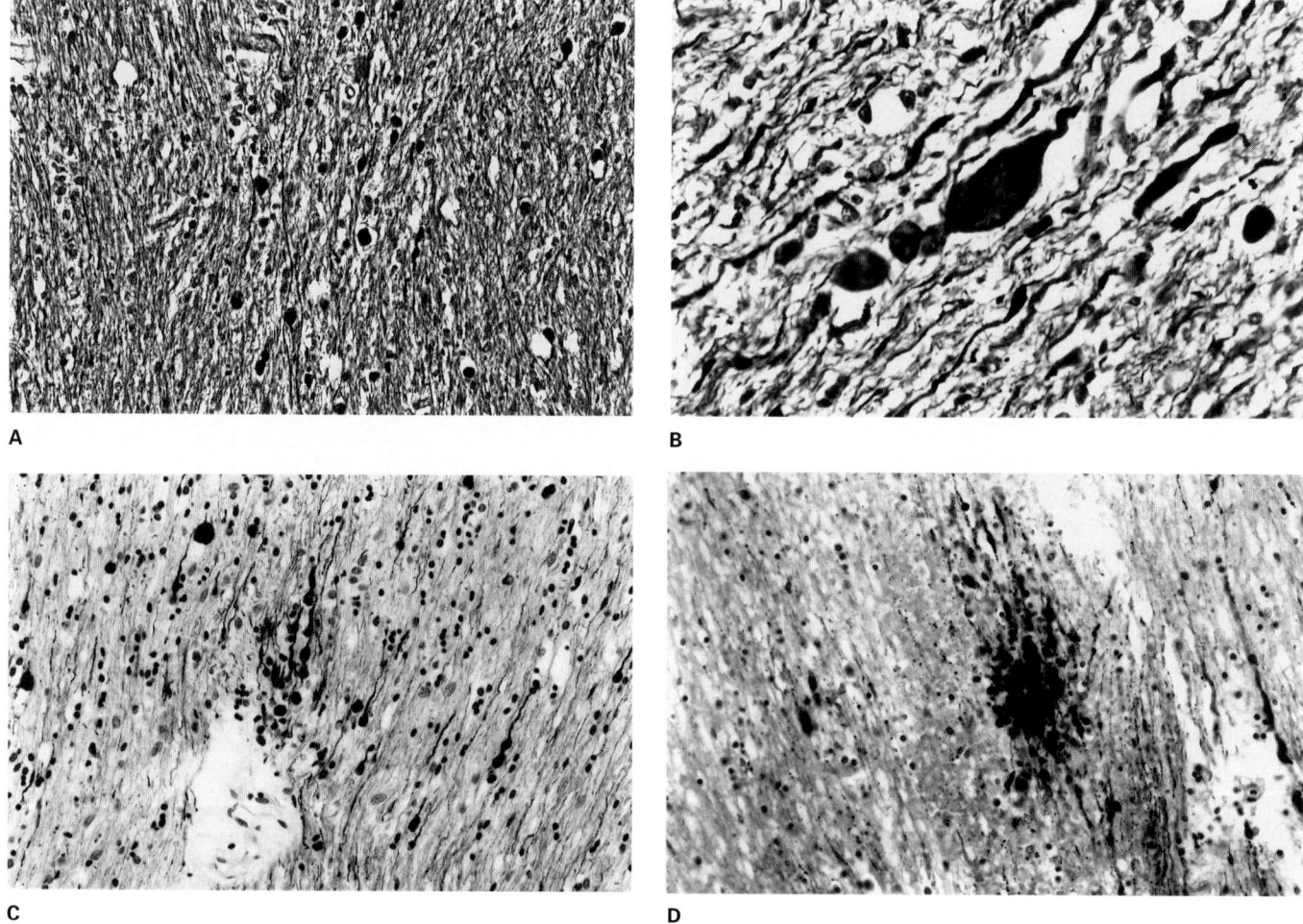

Fig. 5.20 Diffuse axonal injury in the corpus callosum. A 15-year-old boy died 5 days after a road accident. Sections taken from the corpus callosum show typical axonal degeneration. **A** Palmgren's silver impregnation; the dark globular masses represent degenerating axons. × 167. **B** The same: higher power view showing a large fusiform mass of degenerating axon. × 342. **C** Immunochemical stain for neurofibril protein (phosphorylated: NFP-P): the dark balls represent degenerating axons. × 167. **D** Immunochemical stain for Alzheimer precursor protein (APP): the mass of degenerating axons is well defined from the surrounding corpus callosum. × 167. All three stains show abnormal material derived from degenerating axons. In the two immunochemical stains, the degenerating axons are clearly distinguished from the remainder of the corpus callosum; identification of the lesion is easier than in the classical silver stains. The changes demonstrated by the APP stain are evident at a relatively earlier time after injury; indeed, they may be seen in cases surviving less than 1 h.

4. Arterial injury — traumatic thrombosis, false aneurysm formation and carotid–cavernous fistula
5. Infection — cerebral abscess, subdural abscess, pyogenic thrombophlebitis and leptomeningitis; extradural abscess and cranial osteomyelitis are less serious forms of infection
6. Obstructive hydrocephalus.

The clinical implications of these life-threatening complications are discussed in Chapter 13. Here it is appropriate to review briefly their pathology and to discuss to what extent general neuropathological descriptions apply to the complications seen after the frontal impacts which cause CMF injuries.

Extradural haemorrhage

Extradural haematomas of clinical importance usually result from injury to a meningeal artery. In our experience, a substantial minority of extradural haematomas are located in the frontal or subfrontal area. Most of these result from off-centre frontal impacts. In our series of 366 cases of extradural haematomas of all types (Jones et al 1993), 11.4% were classed as frontal and the percentage was higher in children (Molloy et al 1990). Commonly, these frontal haematomas result from tears of relatively small branches of the middle meningeal artery, and are less rapid in onset, hence less serious, than temporal or subtemporal extradural haematomas (Fig. 4.14).

Subdural haemorrhage

Subdural haematomas of clinical importance may result from injury to a bridging cortical vein, or from bleeding related to a severe cerebral contusion. Subdural haemorrhage is not especially common after frontal impacts, but can occur. The presentation may be acute or chronic; the chronic haematomas of elderly persons are rare as sequels of CMF injury (p. 524).

Intracerebral haemorrhage

Intracerebral haematomas may complicate both closed and penetrating injuries. Severe closed frontal impacts may cause deep frontal or basal ganglionic arterial bleeding; the striate arteries appear to be the usual source. Missile wounds usually cause some intracerebral bleeding, and sometimes this is severe enough to constitute a space-occupying lesion.

Brain swelling

This is a common and often lethal complication of severe brain injury. Localized swelling is a usual pathological concomitant of contusions. Diffuse hemispheric brain swelling is a common complication of acute subdural haematomas; it may also be seen in association with hyperacute extradural haemorrhage and around missile tracks (Carey et al 1990). Under the light microscope, the white matter is most obviously affected: myelin stains show pallor in the vicinity of a contusion, and the myelin sheaths are seen to be swollen vacuolated and beaded (Miller & Adams 1992). However, the histopathological examination of brain swelling is often uninformative, and the best understanding of this very important complication has come from clinical and experimental studies.

Brain swelling may represent true oedema in the sense of extravascular fluid collection, or vasodilation attributable to failure of autoregulation. North & Reilly (1990) recognize several forms of cerebral oedema:

1. Vasogenic oedema, where a protein-rich transudate passes into the extracellular space through a dysfunction of the blood–brain barrier in the cerebral capillaries. This process is increased by increased intravascular pressure and/or increased cerebral blood flow due to hypercarbia or hyperpyrexia. It is the most important form of post-traumatic oedema.
2. Cytotoxic oedema, where fluid accumulates within the cell bodies of neurons, glial cells and endothelial cells, because of failure of cell membrane mechanisms, as in anoxic or ischaemic states.
3. Hydrostatic oedema, where fluid transudes from the ventricles into the periventricular white matter as a result of increased intraventricular pressure — this is also called interstitial oedema. Hydrostatic oedema is also seen after the evacuation of a large intracranial clot, when increased intravascular pressure is suddenly transmitted into an unprotected, possibly damaged, capillary bed. Hyperemic vascular engorgement due to an increase in cerebral blood volume may result from

loss of the autoregulatory functions of the cerebral vasculature, especially the arterioles. This is said to be especially common after head impacts in children; the evidence for this is considered in Chapter 19.

Cerebral hypoxia

This is is a common complication of severe head injury and has many causes. After CMF injuries, airway obstruction is often seen and may convert a recoverable brain injury into irreversible brain damage. Arterial hypotension may occur after a severe brain injury or as the result of blood loss from a maxillofacial wound; this may impair cerebral tissue perfusion. Raised ICP may have the same effect. The most obvious early microscopic sign of neuronal anoxia is loss of Nissl substance and eosinophilic cytoplasmic change; later, neuronal outfall is seen, typically in such vulnerable areas as the hippocampal cortex and the cerebellar Purkinje cell layer.

Arterial injury

Injury of small cerebral arteries is a common effect of closed head injury, but damage to larger arteries is relatively unusual. However, the internal carotid artery is vulnerable in its cervical course and within the skull. In both sites, the arterial injury may complicate the management of other CMF injuries. An impact in the neck may crush the internal carotid artery in its extracranial course, perhaps against the vertebral column. Giannotti & Gruen (1992) report an association between displaced mandibular fracture and damage to the underlying internal carotid artery; we have not seen this association, nor does it appear in the large series of carotid injuries reviewed by Krajewski & Hertzer (1980), though these authors mention a case associated with temporomandibular dislocation. The internal carotid artery may also be stretched or even ruptured by violent hyperextension of the head, often a consequence of impact in the CMF area. In both types of arterial injury, the pathological findings include a fracture of the intima, possibly rupture of the media, and thrombosis. Occlusion of the artery, or secondary embolism from the thrombosis, may cause cerebral infarction (Fig. 5.21).

Carotid–cavernous fistula

The internal carotid artery may also be injured within the cavernous sinus, as a result of a fracture of the skull base. The artery is fixed at its point of entry into the cavernous sinus, and also where it leaves the sinus anteriorly; it is susceptible to shearing stresses between these points of fixation. Transverse fractures of the sphenoid bone are especially likely to cause intracavernous arterial injury, and the injured artery may rupture into the cavernous

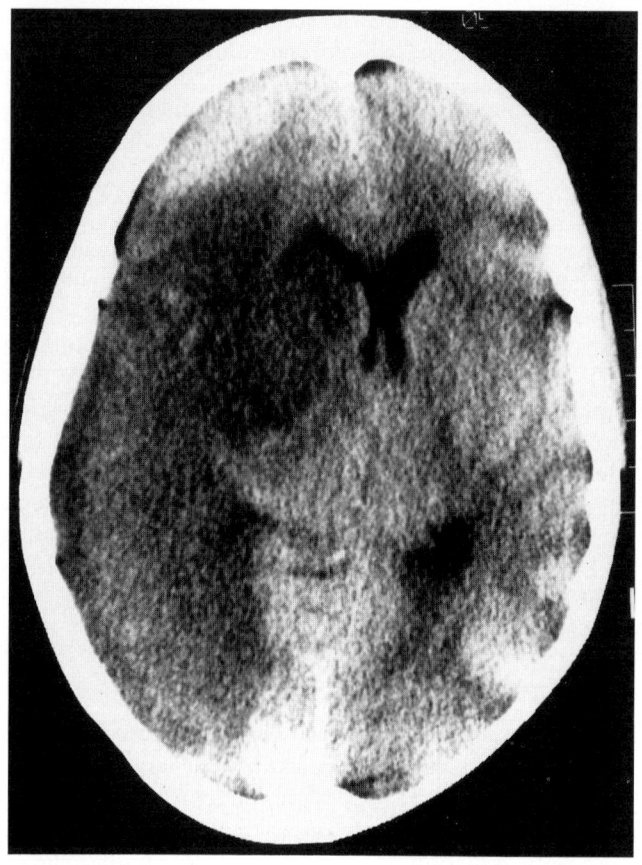

A

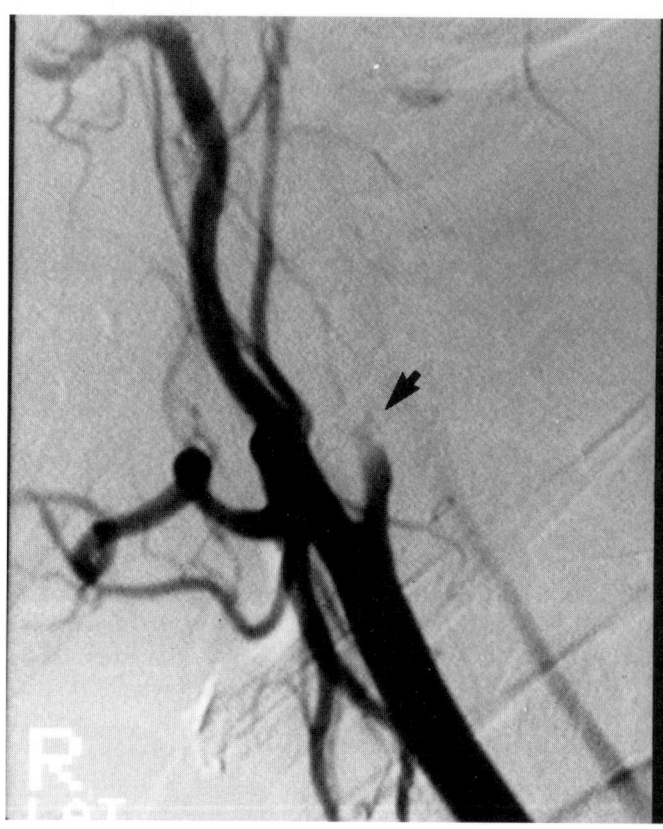

B

Fig. 5.21 Carotid thrombosis: ? a seatbelt injury. A-28-year-old car driver was injured in a head-on crash. She was wearing a lap-sash belt. There was bruising in the neck but initially she appeared neurologically intact. A few hours later, she developed a left sided hemiplegia. **A** CT showed extensive low density change in the right cerebral hemisphere, suggesting massive infarction. **B** Angiography showed obstruction of the right internal carotid artery. She remains very severely disabled.

sinus. In some reported cases, there has been a rent in the anterior part of the artery within the sinus; in others, the artery has been totally transected. Under these circumstances, there is a high-flow leak of arterial blood into the cavernous sinus. When one of the small intra-cavernous arterial branches of the artery is torn (p. 47), there may be a low-flow leakage from both ends of the torn artery (Parkinson 1965).

The pathological effects of a carotid–cavernous fistula can be dramatic. The regional draining veins dilate under arterial pressure, and may rupture into the nasal cavity or the subarachnoid space. This however is unusual; more often, the arteriovenous fistula produces proptosis and other visual symptoms. The visual effects of carotid–cavernous fistulae include impaired extraocular muscle action, hypoxic retinopathy and secondary glaucoma (Jorgenson & Gutthoff 1985). The flow dynamics and surgical management of these lesions are discussed on p. 392.

Traumatic aneurysm

Penetrating wounds may easily injure large arteries, and traumatic aneurysms may form at the site of the arterial wound. These are false aneurysms, and have been described after both missile and knife wounds (de Villiers 1975).

Cerebral abscess

A suppurative infection may result from implantation of microbes in the brain substance in a penetrating wound or by secondary spread from infection outside the brain. Thrombophlebitis is a possible mechanism of spread from a local source of infection, and haematogenous seeding can occur as a result of post-traumatic septicaemia. Implanted foreign bodies are a well-attested cause of brain abscess (Fig. 13.12).

The first response to cerebral infection is a migration

of circulating polymorphs into the brain; macrophages and lymphocytes are also mobilized and an area of cerebritis develops, with necrosis of brain tissue. Macrophages ingest the products of degeneration, especially lipoid material. Continued bacterial growth in the necrotic area and continued response by leukocytes generate pus. If the infection is contained, and does not spread or burst into the lateral ventricle, granulation tissue forms around the purulent cerebritis; fibroblasts appear, presumably migrating from the adventitia of small blood vessels, and form a collagenous abscess capsule. Astrocytes also lay down a fibrillary gliosis.

Brain abscesses resulting from externally compound skull fractures are most often due to staphylococcal infection, but many other organisms have been reported, including clostridia; brain abscesses complicating fractures of the skull base may give more diverse microbial cultures (Table 5.2). The reported increase in infections by gram-negative infections may result from prophylactic antibiotic medication (Rish et al 1981).

Subdural abscess

This form of intracranial suppuration, also known as subdural empyema, is rare as a sequel of penetrating brain injury. It is an extremely dangerous infection, spreading and pocketing over the surface of the cortex and often loculating between the cerebral hemispheres in relation to the falx. Vasculitis may cause infarction of the underlying cortex and sometimes this leads to survival with devastating brain damage. The literature on post-traumatic subdural abscess is too scanty to comment on the bacteriology; in two cases of ours, a blunt frontal impact of no great severity was followed by aggressive extra-

and subdural infection due to a multiplicity of organisms, suggesting pre-existing paranasal sinusitis (p. 390).

Extradural abscess

Extradural pyogenic infection is usually found in association with cranial osteomyelitis (see above), and has also been seen as a sequel of operative repair of compound frontal fractures (p. 372). The dura mater is a good barrier against the spread of infection to the leptomeninges, and extradural infection is usually far less serious than subdural infection.

Acute leptomeningitis

Bacterial meningitis is a frequent complication of fractures involving the paranasal air sinuses. Table 5.2 gives the bacteriological findings in 31 cases of meningitis in a series of 238 cases of anterior fossa fractures treated by us. In this series, the chief organism was *Strep. pneumoniae*, and the infection was often fulminating, though the overall mortality was low.

It cannot be too strongly emphasized that these infections can occur many years after injury (Simpson et al 1990). Fractures involving the skull base may never heal if a protrusion of brain has been driven into the fracture line. The poor healing of fractures in the vicinity of the paranasal air sinuses is familiar to neurosurgeons exploring the anterior fossa in cases of post-traumatic meningitis and was well shown histologically in autopsy material by Linell & Robinson (1941), but is often forgotten by persons who are reassured by the cessation of a leak of cerebrospinal fluid (CSF). In our series, the longest latent period between injury and meningitis was 10 years, but we know of longer intervals.

Cerebral thrombophlebitis and venous sinusitis

These conditions are not often seen as complications of CMF injury; Krayenbuhl (1967) reported on a series of 73 cases of cerebral and venous sinus thromboses of all kinds, and in only three was trauma seen as an aetiological factor. Nevertheless, pyogenic cortical thrombophlebitis is sometimes seen as a sequel of post-traumatic extradural or subdural infection; it may lead to cerebral abscess formation. Septic cavernous sinus thrombosis has been reported as a sequel of infected facial wounds or post-traumatic infections of the ethmoid or sphenoid sinuses, and also as a complication of facial surgery (p. 391); however, even in the pre-antibiotic era, trauma does not appear to have been a frequent cause of this deadly infection. It may be associated with meningitis and cerebral venous infarction. Septic thrombosis of the superior

Table 5.2 Meningitis and brain abscess complicating anterior fossa fractures (from Simpson et al 1990)

Organism	Meningitis	Meningitis abscess	Cerebral abscess
Streptococcus pneumoniae	22 (1 died)	1	–
Other streptococci	2	–	–
Neisseria meningitidis	1	–	–
Haemophilus influenzae	3	–	–
Staphylococcus aureus	–	–	2
Streptococcus + Bacteroides	–	–	1
Pseudomonas spp.	1	–	1
Enterobacter	1	–	–
Mixed	–	–	1 (died)
Unknown	1 (died)	–	–
Total	31	1	5

sagittal sinus appears to be even rarer as a complication of CMF injury, though it may follow frontal sinusitis; we have seen thrombosis of this sinus in a case of deep frontal electric burn, but the histology of the sinus suggested that the thrombosis was due to the burn rather than to secondary infection (Fig. 479).

Post-traumatic hydrocephalus

Obstructive hydrocephalus is sometimes seen after severe closed head injury. It seems likely that the cause is blockage of CSF circulation by the breakdown products of traumatic bleeding into the ventricular system or the subarachnoid space; the site of blockage is presumed to be the arachnoid villi, though occasionally post-traumatic aqueduct obstruction is seen. Obstructive ventricular dilatation must be distinguished from ventricular dilatation due to cerebral atrophy.

Raised ICP and internal cerebral displacements

These are life-threatening complications of many types of CMF injury. A mass lesion complicating a frontal impact, whether acute (e.g. an extradural clot) or chronic (e.g. a frontal lobe abscess), may expand within the cranial cavity. A small expanding mass is at first accommodated by two mechanisms: CSF is displaced into the spinal canal, and venous blood is displaced from the cerebral veins into the general extracranial circulation. When the mass exceeds a critical volume, these compensatory displacements are insufficient and ICP rises. The pathophysiology of raised ICP has been reviewed by North & Reilly (1990).

Severe and sustained elevation in ICP can impair cerebral blood flow (CBF). In any vascular bed, blood flow is dependent on the gradient between arterial and venous pressures, and on the vascular resistance to flow. Since the cerebral veins are thin-walled and collapsible, venous pressure and ICP are closely related: in practice, sagittal sinus venous pressure is 1–2 mmHg lower than ICP. So the relation can be expressed by the equation:

$$CBF = \frac{\text{arterial pressure} - ICP}{\text{cerebrovascular resistance}}$$

Normally, total CBF is maintained at a fairly constant rate (about 50 ml/100 g brain tissue/min) by variations in vascular resistance: these variations express the ability of the cerebral arterioles to dilate or contract in response to the local metabolic demands of the brain. This mechanism is termed autoregulation. When ICP rises, autoregulation causes arteriolar dilatation, and this, together with neurogenic reflex arterial hypertension, will maintain cerebral perfusion. But if ICP reaches an extreme height, or if autoregulation fails, then the cerebral resistance vessels dilate passively and CBF falls. Experimental studies

suggest that neuronal activity ceases when CBF is less than 12 ml/100 g brain tissue/min (Astrup 1985). With very high ICP, flow through the internal carotid artery ceases altogether and this is a recognized sign of brain death (p. 231).

Often, the effects of post-traumatic mass lesions are due to internal cerebral displacements rather than to a general elevation in ICP. The cranial cavity is compartmented by the falx and the tentorium. An expanding haematoma or localized area of brain swelling may displace the cingular gyrus under the falx (subfalcine herniation). More seriously, the medial temporal lobes may be displaced through the tentorial hiatus (transtentorial herniation: Fig. 2.28). The midbrain may be compressed and the quadrigeminal cistern may be obliterated — a danger sign in the CT scan (p. 209). Laterally placed mass lesions characteristically cause medial and downward displacement of the ipsilateral temporal lobe, with compression of the ipsilateral third nerve and pupillary paralysis, but the frontal haemorrhages and brain swelling more characteristic of impacts in the CMF area are likely to cause symmetrical transtentorial herniation. A rare but very serious effect of transtentorial herniation is kinking and occlusion of one or both posterior cerebral arteries: this can result in bilateral occipital infarction and cortical blindness. With more advanced downward displacement, the vessels supplying the brainstem may be stretched: areas of ischaemia and small haemorrhages may appear in the midbrain and pons. This usually means that the process is clinically irreversible. For the pathologist, these secondary effects of a mass lesion must be carefully distinguished from primary brainstem haemorrhages which represent an element in diffuse vascular injury: these haemorrhages are more likely to be in the dorsal tegmentum and in the superior cerebellar peduncles. Finally, the expansion of the intracranial contents may squeeze the cerebellar tonsils into the spinal canal: this is tonsillar herniation.

THE EYE

Ocular injuries

The globe of the eye may suffer primary damage from a penetrating agent (Fig. 5.22) or from blunt violence (Fig. 5.23); the eye may also suffer secondary effects of injury to some part of the visual apparatus, such as the aqueous drainage, the blood supply of the retina or the blink mechanism and the lacrimal system. The eye may also be injured by thermal energy, radiation, or chemical agents, especially alkalis. The pathology of ocular trauma is well discussed by Iyer & Rowland (1993).

The eye is unique in possessing a transparent optical pathway which focuses light on the light-sensitive photoreceptors in the retina. To maintain the transparency of

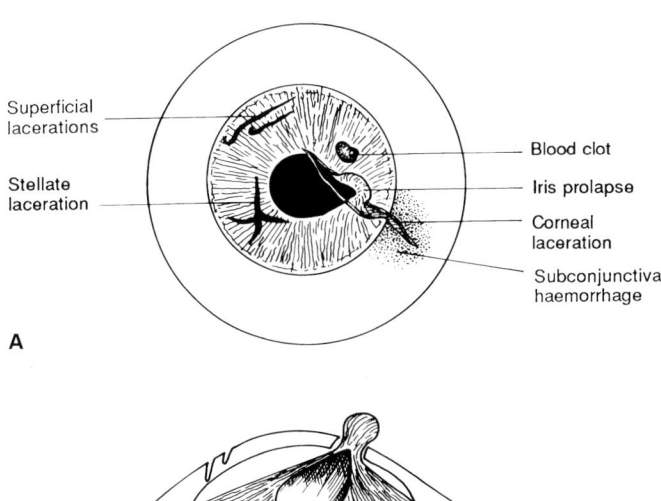

Fig. 5.22 Corneal laceration. A Composite diagram showing the effects of penetrating (sharp) trauma to the anterior segment: superficial non-perforating, shelving corneal lacerations; stellate laceration; perforating corneal laceration with iris and prolapse leading to distorted pupil, associated hyphaema (i.e. blood clot in anterior chamber) and subconjunctival haemorrhage. **B** The same in section.

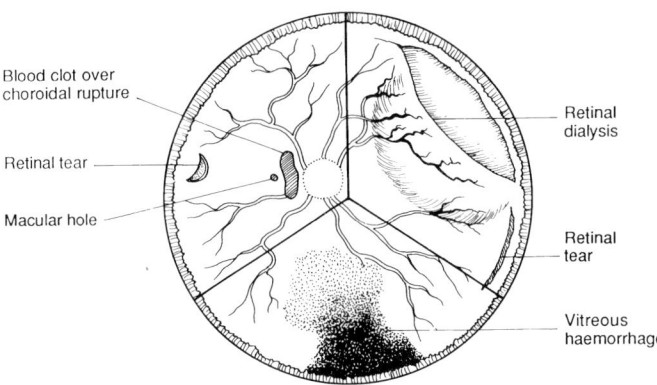

Fig. 5.23 Blunt trauma to posterior pole of the eye. Composite diagram showing: detachment of the iris from its insertion (dialysis), with a distorted pupil; blood in the anterior chamber (hyphaema); cataract formation in the lens.

this optical pathway the structures through which light travels are predominantly avascular. The effects of injury and also the effects of healing processes will in most instances produce changes in the clarity of the optical pathway or induce alterations in the lens system (cornea and crystalline lens). The unique hypovascularity of the globe renders it excessively sensitive to infection and slows normal healing processes. Moreover, the globe is enclosed in a corneo-scleral skeletal envelope and is isolated by a physiological blood–ocular barrier: it is thus relatively sequestered from the immune reactions of the body as a whole. The neural tissues of the retina and optic nerve have very little reparative capacity: indeed the effects of injury and of healing on the ganglion cell axons which form the optic nerve are as adverse as those of the brain.

The basic healing processes of coagulation, inflammation, proliferation of fibrovascular tissue and surface cells and tissue remodelling occur in all sites of the eye after injury. These processes are modified in the avascular zones. Thus there is little in the way of haemostasis around corneal wounds; however, the composition of the aqueous in the anterior chamber undergoes secondary changes after penetrating injury, developing a high protein content and fibrin clot, and this, combined with the swelling of corneal stromal fibres, prevents excessive leakage of aqueous.

Cornea

The cornea can be damaged primarily from an impact or a burn, or secondarily from injuries of the lids, conjunctiva and limbal region. Distortion of the normal lamellar arrangement of the collagen fibres in the cornea produces scarring and refractive changes such as astigmatism which may be progressive. Scarring in the optical axis of the eye will produce reduced vision or glare and light intolerance.

When the cornea is lacerated epithelial cells are damaged for a variable distance from the anterior aspect of the wound edge. Stromal keratocytes are transected and endothelial cells are destroyed or dislodged from the posterior aspect of the wound (Matsuda & Smelser 1973). The corneal epithelial layer can regenerate itself by mitotic division and cell migration over the denuded part of the cornea; regeneration is faster if the basement membrane is intact (Khodadaust et al 1968). Undamaged epithelial cells aggregate and after a brief refractory period migrate towards the wound edge (Buck 1979). The origin of these cells is the limbal stem cell population; their migration is guided by the topographical features of the epithelium and eyelids and by chemical messengers (Cameron et al 1988). Limbal stem cells are of great importance in corneal epithelial healing; ischaemia of the limbal region, often produced by alkali injury, is one of the most important factors in predicting the outcome of such injuries. Corneal healing will not be satisfactory if the limbal region is severely damaged.

The migration continues over exposed Bowman's membrane until the cells meet the physical barrier of corneal stroma, fibrin clot or healthy endothelium. When migration is complete, further mitotic cell division occurs and the corneal epithelium is reconstituted. If Bowman's membrane is intact, this process leaves no scar. If this membrane, which does not regenerate, is damaged, the epithelium is restored, but there may be a corneal nebula in the injured area. Wounds of the corneal stroma are repaired by fibroblastic proliferation. The corneal keratocytes have a long refractory period: after several days the keratocytes repopulate the wound area and begin producing new collagen which lacks the original sheathing. The new collagen is not arranged in the highly organized fashion of undamaged cornea and therefore does not provide complete clarity. The corneal endothelium has little capacity to restore itself. Defects in the endothelial layer may be covered by migration and stretching of the remaining cells. The migration extends over Descemet's membrane as a monolayer of cells and mitosis is very limited. Generally the endothelium regenerates and heals poorly and this may lead to persistent corneal oedema. In future, agents such as EGF, TGFα and -β and fibronectin may be used in promoting corneal healing (Schultz et al 1992); zinc and other trace metals as well as vitamins may also have a role in this.

Perforating wounds of the cornea may be complicated by prolapse of the contents of the globe, forced out by the intraocular pressure: uveal tissue or the lens capsule may be trapped in the corneal wound, and this will prevent healing (Fig. 5.24). The prolapsed tissue may be welded to the cornea by granulation tissue invading the cornea, or corneal epithelium may migrate through the wound into the anterior chamber of the eye; if this invading epithelium obliterates the filtration angle of the anterior chamber, then aqueous drainage is blocked and glaucoma is the outcome. Penetrating wounds of the cornea may also lead to bacterial infection — a corneal abscess or hypopyon. Blunt injury of the cornea may cause internal damage to the endothelial layer, allowing aqueous to be forced into the corneal stroma, which becomes hazy. When the cornea has been significantly damaged and there is distortion of the usual lamellar collagen fibrils as well as disturbances of the limbal anatomy, blood vessels grow into all layers of the cornea. These abnormal blood vessels contribute to the healing process but naturally have an undesirable effect on vision in that they increase the opacity of the cornea.

Sclera

Perforation of the sclera heals well unless complicated by extrusion of uveal tissue; healing involves the formation of vascular granulation from the choroid and/or the episcleral layer, followed by scar formation. Blunt violence to the globe may rupture the sclera, sometimes at the site of impact, sometimes elsewhere, perhaps at the thin equator of the globe (p. 72), perhaps at the limbus. As a rule, the eye is destroyed by an impact severe enough to cause scleral rupture. The sclera heals mostly from the fibrovascular components of the episclera and uveal tract.

Iris and ciliary body

The iris may be damaged both by penetrating and non-penetrating trauma (Figs 5.22 and 5.23). Bleeding results, and the red cells may sink to the lower part of the anterior chamber as a compact mass or hyphema. This eventually absorbs, but if the hyphaema is large the cornea may be

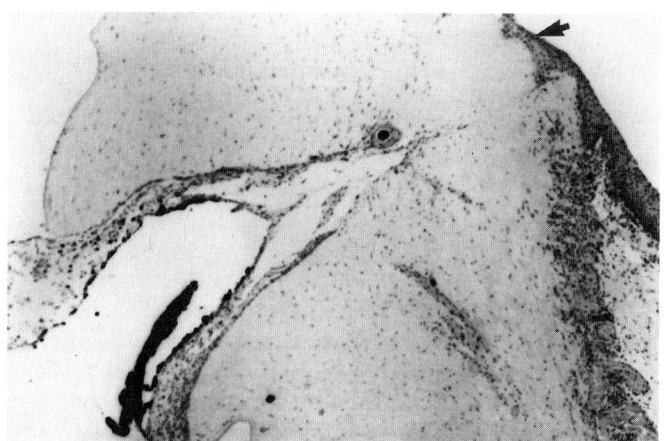

A

B

C

Fig. 5.24 Penetrating eye injury: iris synechia. The iris has herniated into a traumatic cleft in the cornea in the limbic region. Healing of the cornea is prevented. **A** The herniation of iris tissue extends deeply into the corneal stroma; the corneal epithelium (arrow) is intact. H&E, × c. 35. **B** Iris tissue, which contains much pigment, is applied to the lacerated cornea. Descemet's membrane (arrow) shows no sign of regeneration. H&E, × c. 83. **C** Island of corneal epithelium in the corneal laceration, presumably a traumatic inclusion cyst. H&E, × c. 165. By courtesy of Dr Prema Iyer.

stained. Bleeding into the aqueous can lead to glaucoma, especially if the bleeding recurs.

Trauma to the iris may cause alterations in pigmentation and loss of the posterior pigmented epithelial layer leading to a translucent iris. There may also be alterations in the muscular structures of the iris producing irregularities in the size and shape of the pupil. There may be functional changes in that the pupil does not constrict normally to light (traumatic mydriasis). These changes, although relatively minor, may affect vision by inducing optical aberrations and by reducing the eye's tolerance of glare. Dialysis of the iris occurs if the iris is torn from its root; generally this is not of major clinical importance, though it increases sensitivity to glare and occasionally causes diplopia. Traumatic inflammatory responses may produce adhesions of the iris to the cornea or lens (anterior or posterior synechiae), and also secondary glaucoma and cataract. In severe contusive injuries the iris root and the anterior chamber angle may be cleft, producing angle recession. The fibrous reparative tissue may then impede aqueous outflow and produce secondary glaucoma.

Lens

In most instances, the lens responds to trauma by becoming opaque. This may be as a result of direct injury to the lens or may be a secondary effect of forces such as those of electrocution or shock waves, producing damage to the mitotically active lens epithelium and perhaps inducing structural changes in the lens proteins. The lens has little reparative capacity. A small perforation of the lens capsule will heal, but a larger tear admits aqueous into the lens substance: the lens fibres swell and usually fragment, and the lens becomes opaque. Blunt violence may tear the attachments of the lens to the zonule; the lens may be partially or totally dislocated.

Posterior segment trauma

The prognosis for posterior segment trauma is generally bad. Blindness frequently results from fibrovascular and glial proliferation within the vitreous cavity, causing retinal detachment and ciliary body damage leading to a blind hypotonic eye.

Blunt injury to the globe causes deformation (Delori et al 1969). This can lead to posterior pole and vitreous changes remote from the impact site (Fig. 5.25). This may be seen as retinal oedema or retinal tears. Vitreo-retinal traction may cause retinal breaks, most commonly dialyses. Horseshoe tears may occasionally be found, most frequently in the upper nasal quadrant. There may also be mechanical fragmentation of the retina.

In contusion injuries of the posterior segment there is hyperaemia and dilatation of the choroidal vessels at

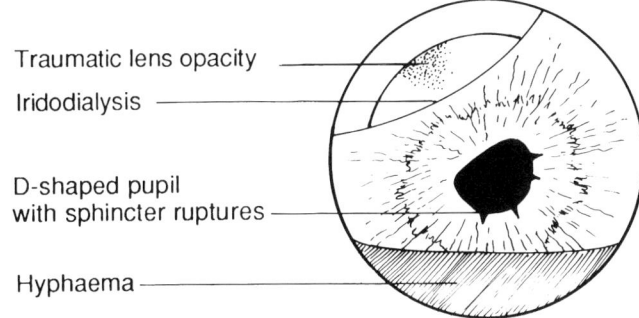

Fig. 5.25 Blunt trauma to posterior segment. Composite diagram showing some of the effects of blunt trauma as seen by ophthalmoscopy: retinal tears; a traumatic hole in the macula (likely to cause loss of acuity and a central scotoma); a small blood clot obscuring a choroidal rupture through the maculopapillary bundle (likely to cause central visual loss); retinal detachment (dialysis; likely to cause flashes, floaters and a field defect); inferiorly a vitreous haemorrhage.

the impact site, with infiltration of polymorphonuclear leukocytes (Gregor & Ryan 1982); as in other inflammatory reactions, macrophages later become the predominant cell type. Subretinal haemorrhage may result from rupture of choroidal vessels; these may bleed into the vitreous. Subretinal blood is replaced by fibrocellular membranes resulting from proliferation of the retinal pigment epithelium. Intravitreal proliferation may be stimulated by serum-derived proteins such as fibronectin, PDGF, complement and interleukin-1. These substances are chemotactic for retinal pigment epithelial cells, fibroblasts and glial cells (Campochiaro et al 1984, Glaser et al 1987).

When severe penetrating trauma produces gross tissue disruption or expulsive choroidal haemorrhage, there is little potential for visual recovery. Penetrating trauma involving the vitreous and the lens produces cataract and vitreous haemorrhage, with fibrovascular ingrowth into the vitreous which produces membranes of a contractile nature. Ultrastructural studies have revealed cells with the characteristics of myofibroblasts (p. 123) embedded in the matrix of collagen-like fibrils within the vitreous at 2–6 weeks following injury (Cleary et al 1980). These cells are contractile fibroblasts, which proliferate from the pigmented and non-pigmented cells of the ciliary epithelium. They extend into the vitreous cavity along the surface of the detached posterior vitreous.

By 4–6 weeks after the injury, multilayered epiretinal membranes occur on the posterior retina; subretinal membranes may also occur. With these membranes may be associated areas of subretinal haemorrhage and proliferation of retinal pigment epithelium. The retina heals very poorly but occasionally there may be some visual recovery: this depends on the degree and severity of retinal damage and the persistance of haemorrhage and oedema, which delay the establishment of retinal layer continuity.

The contractile properties of intravitreal membranes are responsible for the development of tractional retinal detachment. Using microstrain gauges, forces of 30–100 mg were generated by these membranes (Kirmani & Ryan 1985).

Secondary complications of eye injuries

These include:

1. Raised intraocular pressure (glaucoma)
2. Infection
3. Sympathetic ophthalmitis.

Raised intraocular pressure

Secondary glaucoma may be due to direct damage to the anterior chamber angle and trabecular meshwork with fibrovascular tissue distorting the normal aqueous outflow channels and producing a rise in pressure. This may result from anterior chamber inflammatory reactions, debris from red blood cell breakdown, and accumulations of inflammatory and phagocytic cells in the anterior chamber angle, blocking the trabecular meshwork.

Raised intraocular pressure may also arise after lens rupture. Phakolytic and phakoanaphylactic glaucoma and uveitis occur when the lens capsule has been ruptured and cataract has formed, releasing lens proteins into the general circulation. This complication was first described by Verhoeff (Shingleton et al 1991); it is characterized by polymorphonuclear leukocytes, eosinophils and giant cells in the presence of lens matter. Lens proteins normally enjoy an immunologically sequestered position within the lens capsule: the inflammatory reaction to released lens protein may block aqueous drainage through the trabecular meshwork. Secondary glaucoma results in cupping of the optic disc and thinning of the nerve fibres, which may go on to optic atrophy (Fig. 5.26).

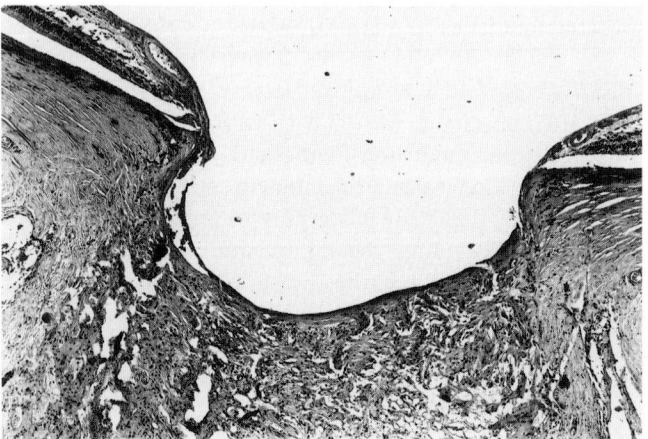

Fig. 5.26 Post-traumatic glaucoma. The optic disc is deeply cupped; the optic nerve shows evidence of atrophy. H&E, × 50. By courtesy Dr Prema Iyer.

Infection

Microbial infection may be implanted in the eye by a penetrating wound, especially when a foreign body has been introduced. A wide range of organisms may be responsible; since the eye is immunologically isolated, its antimicrobial defences are not strong and even bacteria and fungi of low virulence can establish a severe endophthalmitis (p. 410). The infection may at first be localized, but is likely to spread throughout the eye (panophthalmitis). There is hyperaemia of the uveal tissues, with an effusion of leukocytes and serum; this tends to pool in the lower part of the anterior chamber (hypopyon). The posterior chamber may also be affected, and destruction of the retina may result.

Sympathetic ophthalmitis

This devastating complication of ocular injury can lead to complete blindness of the uninjured as well as the injured eye. It is a delayed inflammatory reaction in the uveal tract, usually seen some weeks after perforating injury of the iris, ciliary body or lens capsule. The histological features were described long ago by Fuchs (1905). The whole uveal tract, the choroid especially, is infiltrated by lymphocytes, epithelioid cells and some giant cells; the epithelioid and giant cells may phagocytose pigment (Fig. 5.27). Eosinophils are also seen. Nodular aggregations form on the inner surface of the choroid (Dalén–Fuchs nodules). Lymphocytes form a mantle on the perforating posterior ciliary vessels and vortex veins. Electron microscopy and immunohistological staining show that Dalén–Fuchs nodules are transformed retinal pigment epithelial cells (Jakobiec et al 1983); mature nodules contain depigmented retinal epithelial cells, histiocytes and a few lymphocytes. As the disease advances, the immunological and ultrastructural properties of the uveal infiltrate change, the helper/inducer subset of T lymphocytes being replaced by suppressor/cytotoxic cells (Kaplan et al 1986).

The cellular infiltration spreads out into the extraocular tissues along vascular and neural pathways. The inflammation goes on to diffuse atrophy and fibrosis of the choroid, gliotic destruction of the retina and finally complete disorganization of the globe. The onset is insidious and the course is often remittent.

Both the histopathological appearances and the results of animal experimentation strongly suggest that sympathetic ophthalmitis is a cell-mediated hypersensitivity response to antigens liberated by damaged uveal tissue. The relatively normal lymphoid cell distribution in the peripheral blood suggests that the condition is a localized and not a systemic disease (Müller-Hermelink et al 1984). The eye, as Medawar (1948) showed, is a privileged site, exempt from many immune reactions; however, it is believed that ocular perforation allows intraocular antigens

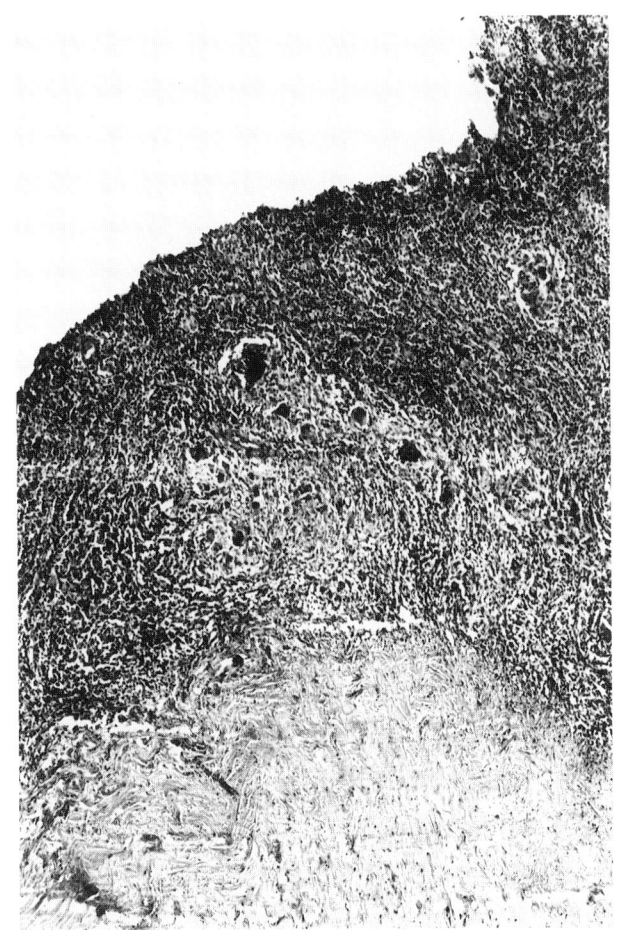

Fig. 5.27 Sympathetic ophthalmitis. The choroid is expanded by a diffuse granulomatous inflammatory infiltrate containing lymphocytes, plasma cells, epithelioid cells and multinucleate giant cells. H&E, × 50. By courtesy of Dr Prema Iyer.

to reach regional lymph nodes, inducing immunopathological responses within the eye. This concept explains the absence of sympathetic ophthalmitis after non-penetrating trauma, however severe, and after retinal detachment or photocoagulation (Rao et al 1979).

Wacker et al (1975) have identified three distinct antigens: S and P antigens from the retina and U from the membrane of Bruch in the choroid. It is now believed that the P antigen is identical with the visual pigment rhodopsin. Experimental studies in guinea-pigs have shown that as little as 5–10 µg of the S antigen will produce a granulomatous panuveitis with histological features similar to those of sympathetic ophthalmia. HLA A-11 antigens appear to be a genetic marker for increased susceptibilty to sympathetic ophthalmitis complicating ocular perforation (Reynard et al 1983).

Corneal grafts

Cadaver corneal allografts are widely used; because the cornea is to a considerable extent immulogically privileged, the risks of rejection are much less than with other tissue allografts. Nevertheless, there are immunogenic cells in corneal grafts, and if these come into contact with host cells then rejection is likely. Previous corneal vascularization or infection may result in graft failure (Coster & Williams 1989); when done for post-traumatic corneal opacities the risk of rejection is not inconsiderable (p. 407).

TISSUE REACTIONS TO FOREIGN MATERIAL

Causes of implantation

Foreign material may be implanted by accident or surgical intention. Accidental implantation is seen when earth, road material, wood, windscreen glass, bullets or shell fragments are driven into the tissues. Such implants are often contaminated with bacteria. Surgical implants, on which there is a vast literature (see Kent & Misiek 1991), are used in many of the procedures discussed in this book.

Histopathology

Unless wholly biocompatible, implanted foreign matter excites a cellular reaction and a chronic inflammatory state may develop. It appears that the macrophage is the chief cell mobilized in response to foreign material, followed by a fibroblastic response. Macrophages can engulf small particles, but if the material is resistant to enzymic dissolution, the macrophages beome less active as phagocytes, and assume an epithelioid appearance. Multinucleated giant cells are characteristic of a foreign body reaction (Fig. 5.2A): they are formed by coalescence of macrophages. Sometimes, a giant cell may contain a fragment of silica or some other exogenous material. The histological picture may be complicated by reactions to implanted microorganisms or by an immune response. The presence of continuing low-grade microbial infection may attract polymorphs; lymphocytes and plasma cells suggest an immune response. But the typical response to an irritative foreign body is the macrophage–giant cell reaction; non-irritative foreign bodies evoke a protective fibroblastic response and become encapsulated.

Accidental metallic implants

The materials often accidentally implanted include some which are extremely irritative or even toxic.

Copper

Of the metals likely to be implanted, copper — used as a jacket in some bullets (p. 114) — is probably the worst (Wigle 1992). Copper ions pass into the tissues and form toxic salts; in the eye or the brain, this can cause severe neuronal destruction (Sights & Bye 1970).

Lead

Lead salts may be toxic, but lead in the tissues forms an oxide which is well tolerated, and lead missiles are encapsulated by fibrous tissue without much local tissue damage (Fig. 5.18). In the past, shotgun pellets were made of lead, and rare cases of systemic lead toxicity have been recorded when large numbers of pellets are implanted (Stromberg 1990).

Iron

Iron salts are much less toxic, but iron and mild steel, used in shell casings, corrode in the tissues and can cause a local inflammatory reaction. Iron fragments in the eye may cause progressive retinal destruction (siderosis bulbi). Corrosion is increased by electrolytic action, and this is especially seen when two dissimilar metals are in proximity.

Surgical implants

These must be fully biocompatible. Tests for biocompatibility begin with in vitro chemical screening tests for cytotoxic agents, followed by tests in cell cultures (Kent & Misiek (1991). Animal experimentation is then necessary before clinical trials. Even when an implant material is approved, surgeons who re-explore the tissues in the vicinity of an implant should obtain a biopsy if there is any suspicion of an unusual reaction, as manufacturing errors or adventitious contamination can occur. A surgical implant should not excite a prolonged macrophage/giant cell response, and is usually encapsulated in collagenous fibrous tissue with a smooth lining of flattened cells apposed to the implant surface. Fig. 5.28 shows such appearances in biopsies from the vicinity of tantalum and titanium implants: tantalum is now little used, but titanium is now employed in many CMF procedures.

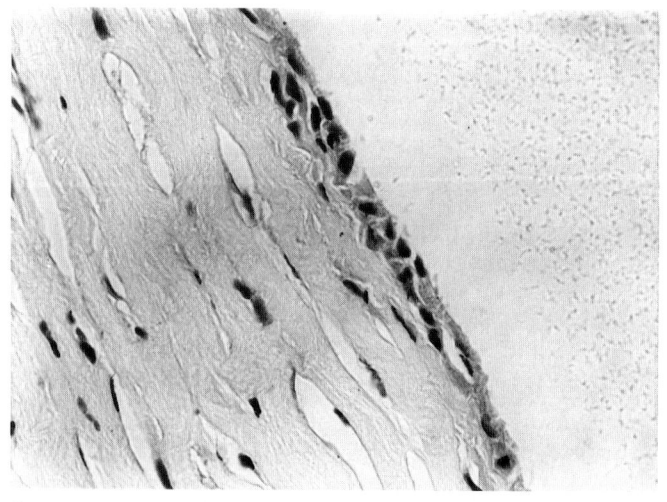

A

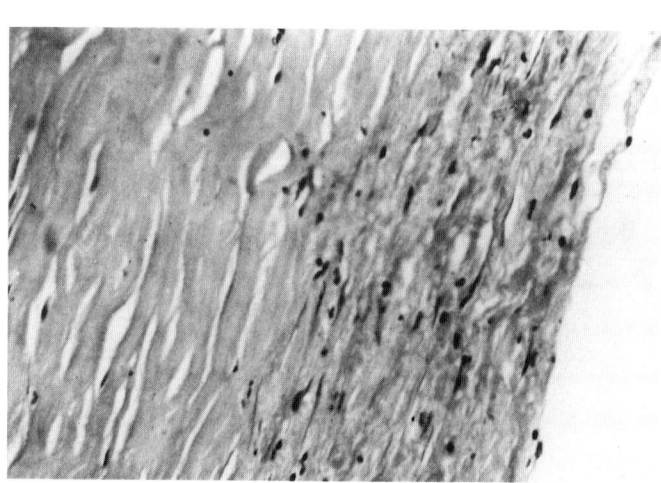

C

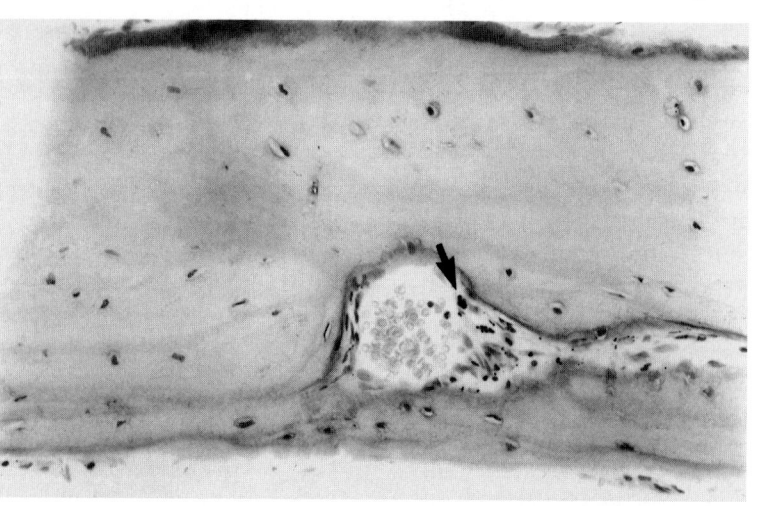

B

Fig 5.28 Tissue reactions to biocompatible implants.
A A tantalum plate became infected and was removed. The biopsy, taken from an uninfected area, shows a collagenous membrane encapsulating the plate; there is a layer of fusiform or multangular cells in contact with the plate. H&E, × c. 163. **B** A titanium plate was removed after 6 years because a dermal sinus formed in one of the plate holes. The plate was found to be well integrated into the skull and bone had grown over its edges: biopsy of thin bone on the outer surface of the plate showed normal appearances. Some black pigment, presumably titanium dioxide, was present in a cavity (arrow) within the new bone. H&E, × 190. **C** In the same case, biopsy from the inner surface of the scalp in contact with the plate showed layers of flattened fibroblasts, with no evidence of giant cell reaction to the titanium. H&E, × c. 82.

The requirements for a surgical implant relate to its purpose, and go far beyond biocompatibility: strength and other mechanical properties, ease of sterilization and handling in the theatre, colour, radiolucency, and cheapness may all be relevant.

Plastics and ceramics

Of the plastic materials used for implants in the CMF region, methyl methacrylate polymer is reasonably well accepted by the tissues, but monomer left after the process of polymerization can excite a strong reaction, often with a serous effusion. Silicone rubber is still less likely to evoke an adverse tissue response, though over time calcification may form over the implant, and occasionally materials used in the preparation of the implant may be irritative. Polyethylenes have been used in facial reconstruction for many years. Polyethylene implants evoke a fibroblastic reaction and if the implant is porous, it will be invaded and fixed by fibro-vascular proliferation. Porous high-density polyethylene (Medpor®) is now widely used to replace aesthetic deficiencies in the facial skeleton, and appears to be well tolerated (p. 563). However, polyethylenes are not recommended as load-bearing or protective implants.

Polytetrafluoroethylene (Teflon®) has been much used as an implant. It is inert chemically and is well tolerated, though the initial tissue response is inflammatory, with a giant cell reaction. Proplast® is a porous bone-like composite, in which polytetrafluoroethylene is the chief ingredient. In the original Proplast, carbon fibres were used to give the mechanical properties of bone; in later variants, aluminium hydroxide or hydroxyapatite has replaced the carbon fibre. When implanted, Proplast evokes a cellular response and its pores are invaded by granulation tissue; this is later replaced by fibrous tissue, or in favourable situations by osteoid or in the case of Proplast–hydroxyapatite by mature bone. Unfortunately, it has been found that Proplast® Teflon® may evoke a local osteolytic reaction, and the use of this substance is now in question, especially in a load-bearing structure (Feinerman & Piecuch 1993). Hydroxyapatite is the chief mineral element in bone and has therefore obvious attractions; it is now available for use in implants. Porous or dense ceramics of hydroxyapatite have been used as bone substitutes in cranioplasty and for other purposes; their clinical utility is at present uncertain. Coralline hydroxyapatite has proved satisfactory in our hands as an orbital implant after enucleation of a blind eye, unless complicated by infection (p. 408).

Metals

Many metals have been used as implants in the surgery of the face and calvaria. At present, the chief in use are 316L stainless steel, titanium and the cobalt–chromium–molybdenum alloy Vitallium®. All are well tolerated in clinical practice. The Swiss AO/ASIF (p. 26) form of 316L steel typically contains 62.5% iron, 17.6% chromium, 14.5% nickel, 2.8% molybdenum and minor amounts of other elements (Disegi 1992). This steel is paramagnetic and does not move or become heated in the course of MRI; however, it is dense in X-ray images, as is Vitallium. Both the 316L stainless steel and Vitallium resist corrosion by forming a protective surface film of chromium oxide. Titanium has been used by us for some 30 years chiefly because it is relatively radiolucent (Simpson 1965); it is very well accepted by the tissues. In modern CMF surgery, titanium is used as mesh, plates, miniplates, screws and neurosurgical haemostatic clips. When implanted, a film of titanium dioxide forms over the surface of the metal and this makes the implant very resistant to corrosion. Usually titanium implants are encapsulated in fibrous tissue, with very little inflammatory reaction. Pigmented masses of titanium dioxide are sometimes seen in the tissues near an implant, but at present there is nothing to suggest that these are irritative or otherwise detrimental (Rosenberg et al 1993). In favourable conditions, bone grows over the implant and may incorporate it. This integration of bone and titanium has been seen with titanium cranioplasty plates (Fig. 5.28), and is the basis for the use of titanium in osseo-integrated implants to support external prostheses (p. 637). For some purposes titanium is too soft, but titanium–aluminum–vanadium alloys are harder and are said to be as well tolerated.

Even metals or metallic alloys showing good biocompatibility will corrode if subjected to continued abrasion, as in joint prostheses. Corrosion is also likely if the implant is in proximity to a dissimilar metal: this can happen when a surgeon ignorantly places a dissimilar screw in an implanted plate, but it may also occur if a piece of a dissimilar tool is broken off or cold-welded on the surface of the implant. We have advised the use of titanium-tipped screwdrivers to minimize this risk (Simpson 1965).

Concern must arise at the possibility of a carcinogenic reaction to a surgical implant, especially in children. Altobelli (1992) cites 11 reported cases of malignant tumours arising in relation to metallic implants, most of which contained chromium. Chromates and chromium alloys, and also nickel, have shown carcinogenicity in animal experiments. Friedman & Vernon (1983) have reported a case of oral squamous-cell carcinoma developing in relation to a mandibular staple supposedly made of titanium–aluminium–vanadium alloy, but this was a permucosal implant associated with much local irritation; so far it seems that no case associated with commercially pure titanium has been reported.

REFERENCES

Adams J H 1992 Head Injury. In: Adams J H, Duchen L W (eds) Greenfield's neuropathology, 5th edn. Edward Arnold, London, Ch 3

Ahdoot D Y, Hansborough J F, Zapata-Sirvent R L 1992 Effects of epidermal growth factor administered after burn injury on bacterial translocation. Clin Res 40: 53A (abstract)

Allen I V, Scott R, Tanner J A 1982 Experimental high velocity head injury. Injury 14: 183–193

Altobelli D E 1992 Implant materials in rigid fixation: physical, mechanical, corrosion, and biocompatibility considerations. In: Yaremchuk M J, Gruss J S, Manson P N (eds) Rigid fixation of the craniofacial skeleton. Butterworth–Heinemann, Boston, Ch 5

Andreasen J O 1972 Traumatic injuries of the teeth, 1st edn. Munksgaard, Copenhagen

Andreasen J O 1981 Traumatic injuries of the teeth, 2nd edn. Munksgaard, Copenhagen

Astrup J 1982 Energy-requiring cell functions in the ischemic brain: their critical supply and possible inhibition in protective therapy. J Neurosurg 56: 482–497

Blumbergs P C, Wainwright H 1988 Glial fibrillary acidic protein in traumatic brain injury. Clin Exp Neurol 25: 164 (abstract)

Bochlogyros P N 1985 A retrospective study of 1521 mandibular fractures. J Oral Maxillofac Surg 43: 597–599

Boykin J V, Molnar J A 1992 Burns scar and skin equivalents. In: Cohen I K, Diegelmann R F, Lindblad W J (eds) Wound healing. Biochemical and clinical aspects. Saunders, Philadelphia, Ch 32

Brown P, Preece M A, Will R G 1992 'Friendly fire' in medicine: hormones, homografts and Creutzfeldt–Jakob disease. Lancet 340: 24–27

Buck P C 1979 Cell migration and repair of mouse corneal epithelium. Invest Opthalmol Vis Sci 18: 767–784

Burchardt H 1983 The biology of bone graft repair. Clin Orthop 174: 28–42

Burwell R G 1985 Bone and cartilage. General principles of grafting. In: Rowe N L, Killey J L (eds) Maxillofacial injuries. 2nd edn. Churchill Livingstone, Edinburgh

Cameron J D, Hagen S T, Waterfield R R, Furcht L T 1988 Effects of matrix protein on rabbit corneal epithelial cell adhesion and migration. Curr Eye Res 7: 293–301

Campbell J B, Bassett C A L, Robertson J W 1958 Clinical use of freeze-dried human dura mater. J Neurosurg 15: 207–214

Campochiaro P A, Jerdan J A, Glaser B N 1984 Serum contains chemo-attractants for human retinal pigment epithelial cells. Arch Ophthalmol 102: 1830–1833

Carey M E, Young H, Mathis J L, Forsythe J 1971 A bacteriological study of craniocerebral missile wounds from Vietnam. J Neurosurg 34: 145–154

Carey M E, Sarna G S, Farrell J B 1990 Brain edema following an experimental missile wound to the brain. J Neurotrauma 7: 13–20

Catty R H 1965 Healing and contraction of experimental full thickness wounds in the human. Br J Surg 52: 542–548

Clark W E, Le Gros 1960 The tissues of the body, 4th edn. Oxford University Press, London

Cleary P E, Minckler D S, Ryan S J 1980 Ultrastructure of traction retinal detachment in Rhesus monkey eyes after a posterior penetrating ocular injury. Am J Ophthalmol 90: 829–845

Cohen I K, Diegelmann R F, Lindblad W J 1992 Wound healing. Biochemical and clinical aspects. Saunders, Philadelphia

Converse J M, McCarthy J G, Brauer R O, Ballantyne D L 1977 Transplantation of skin: grafts and flaps. In: Converse J M (ed) Plastic reconstructive surgery, 2nd edn. Saunders, Philadelphia, Ch 6

Coster D J, Williams K A 1989 Surgical manoeuvres to reduce the impact of corneal allograft rejection. Dev Ophthalmol 18: 156–164

Crompton M R 1970 Visual lesions in closed head injury. Brain 93: 785–792

Darby I, Skalli O, Gabbiani G 1990 Alpha-smooth muscle actin is transiently expressed by myofibroblasts during experimental wound healing. Lab Invest 63: 21–29

Delori F, Pomerantzeff O, Cox M S 1969 Deformation of the globe under high speed impact: its relation to contusion injury. Invest Ophthalmol 8: 290–301

De Louvois J, Gortvai P, Hurley R 1977 Antibiotic treatment of abscesses of the central nervous system. Br Med J 2: 985–987

De Villiers J C 1975 Stab wounds of the brain and skull. In: Vinken P J, Bruyn G W (eds) Handbook of clinical neurology. North-Holland, Amsterdam, Vol 23

Disegi J A 1992 Magnetic resonance imaging of AO/ASIF stainless steel and titanium implants. Injury 23 Suppl 2: S1–S4

Douglas D M 1963 Wound healing and management. Livingstone, Edinburgh

Duchen L W 1992 General pathology of neurons and neuroglia. In: Adams J H, Duchen L W (eds) Greenfield's neuropathology, 5th edn. Edward Arnold, London, Ch 1

Feinberg S E, Larsen P E 1991 Healing of traumatic injuries. In: Fonseca R J, Walker R V (eds) Oral and maxillofacial trauma. Saunders, Philadelphia, Vol 1

Feinerman D M, Piecuch J F 1993 Long-term retrospective analysis of twenty-three Proplast®-Teflon® temporomandibular joint interpositional implants. Int J Oral Maxillofacial Surg 22: 11–16

Friedman K E, Vernon S E 1983 Squamous cell carcinoma developing in conjunction with a mandibular staple bone plate. J Oral Maxillofac Surg 41: 265–266

Fuchs E 1905 Ueber sympathisierende Entzündung nebst Bemerkungen über seröse traumatische Iritis. Archiv Ophth 61: 365–456

Giannotti S L, Gruen P 1992 Vascular complications of head trauma. In: Barrow D L (ed) Complications and sequelae of head injury. American Association of Neurological Surgeons, Park Ridge, Illinois, Ch 3

Glaser B N, Cardin A, Biscoe B 1987 Proliferative vitreoretinopathy. The mechanism of development of vitreoretinal traction. Ophthalmology 94: 327–332

Gregor Z, Ryan S J 1982 Combined posterior contusion and penetrating injury in the pig eye. II. Histological features Br J Ophthalmol 66: 799–804

Guber S, Rudolph R 1978 The myofibroblast. Surg Gynecol Obstet 146: 641–649

Hadas N, Schiffer J, Rogev M, Shperber Y 1990 Tangential low-velocity missile wound of the head with acute subdural haematoma: case report. J Trauma 30: 358–359

Hansbrough J F 1990 Current status of skin replacements for coverage of extensive burn wounds. J Trauma 30 Suppl: S155–160

Harrison J D, Garrett J R 1976 Histologic effects of ductal ligation of salivary glands of the cat. J Path 118: 245–254

Huang K F, Chung D H, Herndon D N 1993 Insulinlike growth factor 1 (IGF-1) reduces gut atrophy and bacterial translocation after severe burn injury. Arch Surg 128: 47–53

Imamoto K, Leblond C P 1977 Presence of labelled monocytes, macrophages and microglia in association with a stab wound of the brain after an injection of bone marrow cells labelled with ³H-uridine into rats. J Comp Neurol 174: 255–280

Iyer P, Rowland R 1993 Ophthalmic pathology. Churchill Livingstone, Edinburgh

Jackson D M 1953 The diagnosis of the depth of burning. Br J Surg 40: 588–596

Jakobiec F A, Marboe C C, Knowles D M et al 1983 Human sympathetic ophthalmia. An analysis of the inflammatory infiltrate by hybridoma-monoclonal antibodies, immunochemistry and correlative electron microscopy. Ophthalmology 90: 76–95

Jeffrey J J 1992 Collagen degradation. In: Cohen I K, Diegelmann R F, Lindblad W J (eds), Wound healing. Biochemical and clinical aspects. Saunders, Philadelphia, Ch 10

Jones N R, Molloy C J, Kloeden C N, North J B, Simpson D A 1993 Extradural haematoma: trends in outcome over 35 years. Br J Neurosurg 7: 465–471

Jorgensen J S, Gutthoff R F 1985 24 cases of carotid–cavernosus fistulas: frequency, symptoms, diagnosis and treatment. Acta Ophthalmol Suppl (Copenh) 173: 67–71

Kaplan H J, Waldrep J C, Chan W C 1986 Human sympathetic ophthalmia. Immunologic analysis of the vitreous and uvea. Arch Ophthalmol 104: 240–244

Kärcher H, Eskici A, Zwittnig P 1989 The vascularized cross-face nerve graft. In: Riediger D, Ehrenfeld M (eds) Microsurgical tissue transplantation. Quintessence, Chicago

Kent J N, Misiek D J 1991 Biomaterials for cranial, facial, mandibular, and TMJ reconstruction. In: Fonseca R J, Walker R V (eds) Oral and maxillofacial trauma. Saunders, Philadelphia, Vol 2

Khodadoust A A, Silverstein A M, Kenyon K R, Dowling J E 1968 Adhesion of regenerating corneal epithelium: the role of basement membrane. Am J Ophthalmol 65: 339–348

Kirmani M, Ryan S J 1985 In vitro measurement of contractile force and transvitreal membranes formed after penetrating ocular injury. Arch Ophthalmol 103: 107–110

Klein L, Rudolph R 1972 ^{3}H-collagen turnover in skin grafts. Surg Gynecol Obstet 135: 49–57

Kline L B, Morawetz R B, Swaid S N 1984 Indirect injury of the optic nerve. Neurosurgery 14: 756–764

Krajewski L P, Hertzer N R 1980 Blunt carotid artery trauma. Report of two cases and review of the literature. Ann Surg 191: 341–346

Krayenbuhl H A 1967 Cerebral venous and sinus thrombosis. Clin Neurosurg 14: 1–14

Landau R, Stewart M 1985 Conservative management of posttraumatic parotid fistulae and sialoceles:a prospective study. Br J Surg 72: 42–44

Lehto M U, Järvinen M J 1991 Muscle injuries, their healing process and treatment. Ann Chir Gynaecol 80: 102–108

Lieblich S E, Topazian R G 1991 Infection in the patient with maxillofacial trauma. In: Fonseca R J, Walker R V (eds) Oral and Maxillofacial Trauma. Saunders, Philadelphia, Vol 2

Linell E A, Robinson W L (1941) Head injuries and meningitis. J Neurol Neurosurg Psychiat 4: 23–31

Linton A H, Hinton M H 1990 The normal microbiota of the body. In: Parker M T, Collier L H (eds) Topley and Wilson's principles of bacteriology, virology and immunity, 8th edn. Edward Arnold, London

Lipton S A 1989 Growth factors for neuronal survival and process regeneration. Implications in the mammalian central nervous system. Arch Neurol 46: 1241–1248

Lynch S E, Colvin R B, Antoniades H N 1989a Growth factors in healing. Single and synergistic effects on partial thickness porcine skin wounds. J Clin Invest 84: 640–646

Lynch S E, Williams R C, Polson A M et al 1989b A combination of platelet-derived and insulin-like growth factors enhances periodontal regeneration. J Clin Periodontol 16: 545–548

Manchester W M 1972 Some technical improvements in the reconstruction of the mandible and temporomandibular joint. Plast Reconstr Surg 50: 249–256

Marx R E, Stevens M R 1991 Reconstruction of avulsive maxillofacial injuries. In: Fonseca R J, Walker R V (eds) Oral and maxillofacial trauma. Saunders, Philadelphia, Vol 2

Matsuda H, Smelser G K 1973 Electron microscopy of corneal wound healing. Exp Eye Res 16: 427–442

McGovern S T, Crompton J L, Ingham P N 1986 Trigemino-abducens synkinesis: an unusual case of aberrant regeneration. Aust NZ J Ophthalmol 14: 275–279

McKay I A, Leigh I M 1991 Epidermal cytokines and their roles in cutaneous wound healing. Br J Dermatol 124: 513–518

Medawar P B 1948 Immunity to homologous grafted skin, fate of skin homografts transplanted to the brain, to subcutaneous tissue and to anterior chamber of eye. Br J Exp Pathol 29: 58–69

Miller J D, Adams J H 1992 The pathophysiology of raised intracranial pressure. In: Adams J H, Duchen L W (eds) Greenfield's neuropathology, 5th edn. Edward Arnold, London, Ch 2

Mizuno K, Mineo K, Tachibano T, Sumi M, Matsubara T, Hirohata K 1990 The osteogenetic potential of fracture haematoma: Subperiosteal and intramuscular transplantation of the haematoma. J Bone Joint Surg Br 72B: 822–829

Mohan S, Baylink D J 1990 Bone growth factors. Clin Orthop 263: 30–48

Molloy C J, McCaul K A, McLean A J, North J B, Simpson D A 1990 Extradural haemorrhage in infancy and childhood. Child's Nerv Syst 6: 383–387

Monti-Graziadei G A, Karlan M S, Bernstein J J, Graziadei P P C 1980 Reinnervation of the olfactory bulb after section of the olfactory nerve in monkeys (Saimiri sciureus). Brain Res 189: 343–354

Müller-Hermelink H K, Kraus-Mackiw E, Daus W 1984 Early stage of human sympathetic ophthalmia. Histologic and immunopathologic findings. Arch Ophthalmol 102: 1353–1357

Murray J C, Pinnell S R 1992 Keloids and excessive dermal scarring. In: Cohen I K, Diegelmann R F, Lindblad W J (eds) Wound healing. Biochemical and clinical aspects. Saunders, Philadelphia, Ch 30

North J B, Reilly P L 1990 Raised intracranial pressure. A clinical guide. Heinemann, Oxford

Öberg S, Rosenquist J B 1994 Bone healing after implantation of hydroxyappatite granules and blocks (Interpore 200®) combined with autolyzed antigen-extracted allogeneic bone and fibrin glue. Experimental studies on adult rabbits. Int J Oral Maxillofac Surg 23: 110–114

O'Neill P, Booth A E 1984 Use of porcine dermis as a dural substitute in 72 patients. J Neurosurg 61: 351–354

Oppenheimer D R 1968 Microscopic lesions in the brain following head injury. J Neurol Neurosurg Psychiat 31: 299–306

Östrup L T, Frederickson J M 1974 Distant transfer of a free living bone graft by microvascular anastomosis:an experimental study. Plast Reconstr Surg 54: 274–285

Parkinson D 1965 A surgical approach to the cavernous portion of the carotid artery. Anatomical studies and case report. J Neurosurg 23: 474–483

Phillips J H, Rahn B A 1992 Bone healing. In: Yaremchuk M J, Gruss J S, Manson P N (eds) Rigid fixation of the craniomaxillofacial skeleton. Butterworth–Heinemann, Boston

Povlishock J T, Kontos H A, Ellis E F 1989 Current thoughts on experimental head injury. In: Becker D P, Gudeman S K (eds) Textbook of head injury. Saunders, Philadelphia

Rao N A, Wacker W B, Marak G E 1979 Experimental allergic uveitis. Clinicopathologic features associated with varying doses of S Antigen. Arch Ophthalmol 97: 1954–1958

Rever J, Manson P N, Randolph M A, Yaremchuk M J, Weiland A, Siegel J H 1991 The healing of facial bone fractures by the process of secondary union. Plast Reconstr Surg 87: 451–458

Reynard M, Shulman I A, Azen S P, Minckler D S 1983 Histocompatibility antigens in sympathetic ophthalmia. Am J Ophthalmol 95: 216–221

Rish B L, Caveness W F, Dillon J D, Kistler J P, Mohr J P, Weiss G H 1981 Analysis of brain abscess after penetrating craniocerebral injuries in Vietnam. Neurosurgery 9: 535–541

Robinson P D 1993 Articular cartilage of the temporomandibular joint:can it regenerate? Ann R Coll Surg Engl 75: 231–236

Robson M C, Del Becarro E J, Heggers J P 1979 The effects of prostaglandins on the dermal microcirculation after burning, and the inhibition of the effect by specific pharmacological agents. Plast Reconstr Surg 63: 781–787

Rosenberg A, Gratz K W, Sailer H F 1993 Should titanium miniplates be removed after bone healing is complete? Int J Oral Maxillofac Surg 22: 185–188

Ross R, Raines E W, Bowen-Pope D F 1986 The biology of platelet-derived growth factor. Cell 46: 155–169

Rowe N L, Killey H C 1955 Fractures of the facial skeleton. Livingstone, Edinburgh

Rudolph R, Vande Berg J, Ehrlich H P 1992 Wound contraction and scar contracture. In: Cohen I K, Diegelmann R F, Lindblad W J (eds) Wound healing. Biochemical and clinical aspects. Saunders, Philadelphia, Ch 6

Rush B F, Sori A J, Murphy T F, Smith S, Flanagan J J, Machiedo G W 1988 Endotoxemia and bacteremia during hemorrhagic shock. the link between trauma and sepsis? Ann Surg 207: 549–554

Sailer H F, Kolb E 1994 Application of purified bone morphogenetic protein (BMP) in cranio-maxillo-facial surgery. BMP in compromised surgical reconstructions using titanium implants. J Craniomaxillofac Surg 22: 2–11

Salama R 1983 Xenogeneic bone grafting in humans. Clin Orthop 174: 113–121

Schultz G, Chegini N, Grant M, Khaw P, Mackay S 1992 Effect of growth factors on corneal wound healing. Acta Ophthalmol 70 Suppl 202: 60–66

Schweigerer L, Neufeld G, Friedman J, Abraham J A, Fiddes J C, Gospodorowicz D 1987 Capillary endothelial cells express basic fibroblast growth factor, a mitogen that promotes their own growth. Nature 325: 257–259

Seddon H 1972 Surgical disorders of the peripheral nerves. Churchill Livingstone, Edinburgh

Sevitt S 1957 Burns—pathology and therapeutic applications. Butterworth, London

Shingleton B, Hersh P, Kenyon K (eds) 1991 Eye trauma. Mosley Year Book, Sydney

Sights W P, Bye R J 1970 The fate of retained intracerebral shotgun pellets J Neurosurg 33: 646–653

Simpson D 1965 Titanium in cranioplasty. J Neurosurg 22: 292–293

Simpson D A, Blumbergs P C, Cooter R D, Kilminster M, McLean A J, Scott G 1989 Pontomedullary tears and other gross brainstem injuries after vehicular accidents. J Trauma 29: 1519–1525

Simpson D A, David D J, Reilly P L 1990 Fractures of the anterior cranial fossa: the craniofacial approach. Asian J Surg 13: 23–31

Spiessl B 1989 Internal fixation of the mandible. A manual of AO/ASIF principles. Springer-Verlag, Berlin

Strich S 1976 Cerebral trauma. In: Blackwood W, Corsellis J A N (eds) Greenfield's neuropathology, 3rd edn. Edward Arnold, London, Ch 9

Stromberg B V 1990 Symptomatic lead toxicity secondary to retained shotgun pellets:case report. J Trauma 30: 356–357

Sunderland S 1978 Nerves and nerve injuries, 2nd edn. Livingstone, Edinburgh

Taniuchi M, Clark H B, Schweitzer J B, Johnson E M 1988 Expression of nerve growth factor receptors by Schwann cells of axotomised peripheral nerves: ultrastructural location, suppression by axonal contact, and binding properties. J Neurosci 8: 664–681

Thaller S R, Kawamoto H K 1990 A histologic evaluation of fracture repair in the midface. Plast Reconstr Surg 85: 196–201

Urist M R, Delange R J, Finerman G A M 1983 Bone cell differentiation and growth factors. Science 220: 680–686

Wacker W B, Donoso L A, Kalsow C M 1977 Experimental allergic uveitis; isolation, characterisation and localisation of a somble uveitopathological agent from bovine retina. J Immunol 199: 1949–1958

Wahl L M, Wahl S M 1992 Inflammation. In: Cohen I K, Diegelmann R F, Lindblad W J (eds) Wound healing. Biochemical and clinical aspects. Saunders, Philadelphia, Ch 3

Walsh F B, Hoyt W F 1982–91 Clinical Neuro-ophthalmology, 4th edn. Williams & Wilkins, Baltimore, Vol 3, pp 2369–2386

Werner S, Peters K G, Longaker M T, Fuller-Pace F, Banda M J, Williams L T 1992 Large induction of keratinocyte growth factor expression in the dermis during wound healing. Proc Natl Acad Sci USA 89: 6896–6900

Wheat L J, Kohler R B, White A 1981 Treatment of nasal carriers of coagulase-positive staphylococci. In: Maibach H I, Aly R (eds) Skin microbiology. Relevance to clinical infection. Springer, New York, Ch 7

Wigle R L 1992 The reaction of copper and other projectile metals in body tissues. J Trauma 33: 14–18

Wornom I L, Buchman S R 1992 Bone and cartilaginous tissue. In: Cohen I K, Diegelmann R F, Lindblad W J (eds) Wound healing. Biochemical and clinical aspects. Saunders, Philadelphia, Ch 23

Zapata-Sirvent R L, Hansborough J F, Wolf P, Grayson L S, Nicolson M 1993 Epidermal growth factor limits structural alterations in gastrointestinal tissues and decreases bacterial translocation in burned mice. Surgery 113: 564–573

Zawacki B E 1974 The natural history of reversible burn injury. Surg Gynecol Obstet 139: 867–872

Systematic clinical assessment

J. Trott   R. Cooter
Contributing authors: J. Crompton   J. Tomich

INTRODUCTION

In the evaluation of the patient with craniomaxillofacial (CMF) trauma, it is wise to develop a method of quick initial clinical assessment that includes all the relevant body systems. This should:

— give an overall picture of the patient's injuries and their pathophysiological effects
— initiate early cardiopulmonary resuscitation
— allow early referral to appropriate specialists for management of life-threatening or serious injuries in any part of the body
— permit informed decisions on the priorities of investigation and treatment of the CMF injury.

The various specialists will make their assessments in whatever depth and detail seems necessary. In this chapter, our routine specialist clinical examinations are described; in practice, these examinations are often curtailed, less often expanded, according to the clinical findings. Some components of these examinations should never be omitted and the surgeon who handles CMF trauma single-handed must be competent in a wide range of clinical skills.

Organization

In the emergency room the doctor who makes the crucial first assessment must be experienced in the management of trauma. The modern trauma centre provides an organizational system that ensures that a suitably experienced person is available immediately. Preferably, the assessment is initiated by a surgeon or an intensivist with a special interest in trauma, able to mobilize a trauma team when this is required, and to act as team coordinator for triage in cases of multisystem injury. Facial injuries should be assessed early by an experienced surgeon with a developed interest in maxillofacial trauma management. When a cerebral injury is evident, a neurosurgical evaluation is imperative, and should be performed by a surgeon with considerable experience in neurotrauma management. Ideally, any trauma system should provide a neurosurgeon to see an unconscious patient at very short notice; indeed, this is a requirement for designation by the American College of Surgeons (1986) as a Level I Trauma Centre. In remote places, this may be impossible, but modern telecommunications (p. 222) should be used to provide a neurosurgical opinion when the cerebral injury is life-threatening. Similarly, an ophthalmological consultation should be available at short notice.

Initial assessment

The history

The emergency assessment includes a careful history, not always compiled immediately, since there may be more urgent needs to be met. The patient, if awake and orientated, is the most reliable historian. If not, then any witness to the events before or after the injury may give valuable evidence on the mechanisms of injury, the likely area injured, and the course of events since the injury was inflicted, including confirmation of pre and/or post-traumatic amnesia of the patient. For medicolegal reasons, it is wise to document the informant's name clearly and accurately, and to note the time and date of the interview. Ambulance officers are especially valuable as trained witnesses; relatives and friends may be able to give details of the patient's general health and past medical history. Specific enquiries should be made about previous conditions such as hepatitis and HIV seropositivity; the nutritional status should be determined, and also the alcohol intake, both around the time of the injury, and in ordinary day-to-day life. A history of blood coagulopathy, high blood pressure, cardiac disease, epilepsy or cerebral disorder may be very relevant. Drug consumption and drug allergies should be recorded. The use of spectacles, dentures or protective head-wear, e.g. motorcycle helmet, should be recorded in all cases of craniofacial injury (Cooter 1990).

Airway, breathing and circulation

Assessment of these vital functions is the first priority, and is discussed in detail in Chapter 8. Further assessment is not attempted until the cardiopulmonary systems are stabilized to the satisfaction of the assessing surgeon or intensivist.

As soon as possible, a chart is prepared to record at appropriate intervals:

— respiratory rate, rhythm and depth
— heart rate — preferably by electrocardiograph
— blood pressure and pulse pressure — if necessary from a cannula in the radial artery
— temperature.

Conscious level

This is the next most important part of the initial evaluation. The examiner notes and charts the patient's eye opening, best verbal response, and best motor response, according to the Glasgow Coma Scale (GCS). Figure 6.1 gives the expected levels in a fully conscious adult and the various levels of impairment for each type of response, according to the 14-point version of the GCS (Jennett & Teasdale 1981), which does not distinguish between normal and abnormal flexion as separate levels in the best motor response category. Although the 15-point scale is accepted as the basis of international comparative studies, the simpler 14-point scale is more easily understood by staff who have no special neurological training.

Infants and very young children cannot achieve the adult norms for verbal and motor responses even when fully conscious and cooperative; after a frightening injury, no cooperation may be given and the level of response will be still lower. Under the age of 5 years, the conscious level is therefore a less helpful guide to cerebral function. However, the Paediatric Glasgow Coma Scale (Fig. 19.10) can be used to monitor conscious levels in a realistic way: this scale sets norms for the best verbal and motor responses that are appropriate for different ages (Simpson

et al 1991). The value and limitations of this scale are discussed in p. 513.

Pupillary light reflexes, diameter and size are recorded on the same serial chart.

Head-to-toe examination

A systematic method should be developed to give a quick but accurate assessment of the injured patient from head to toe. The method is a matter of personal preference, but should include all the relevant body systems. Gloves, a mask and eye protection should be worn if there is a chance that the examiner will come in contact with body fluids from the injured person, as is usually the case in accident victims.

If the patient is conscious, areas of pain, swelling and loss of function will be reported; in the confused or unconscious patient, these must be looked for methodically. Clothes must be removed, and skin lesions noted: lacerations, abrasions, haematomas, burns and areas of skin loss are described and recorded on a body chart. Photographs, perhaps with a polaroid camera, are useful for more exact recording; this is especially important when the injury has forensic implications (Fig. 6.2). The face, ears, tongue and mouth are inspected; particular attention is given to small punctate wounds that may be associated with deep penetration (Fig. 6.3). The facial skeleton and the overlying soft tissues are then systematically palpated (see below). The pupillary reactions to light are tested with a strong narrow-beam torch. The cervical spinous processes are palpated for deformity, tenderness or swelling. The conscious patient is asked to lift the head and demonstrate a normal range of neck movement; the unconscious patient is assumed to have a potentially serious neck injury until this has been excluded by X-ray (Davidson & Birdsel 1989). The anterior and posterior aspects of the chest are inspected: bruising and abnormal chest movements are noted. With the patient supine, the sternum is pressed, to elicit pain or even crepitus from a fracture of the sternum or ribcage. It is important to auscultate the lungs and heart. Reduced breath sounds, with a hollow percussion note, may indicate a pneumothorax, while reduced breath sounds and a dull percussion note suggest a haemothorax. Diminished cardiac sounds may indicate haemopericardium, and an abnormal bruit may point to intrinsic cardiac damage. With the patient lying on one side, the thoracic and lumbar spines are palpated, and tenderness or deformity is noted. Observation of the abdomen may reveal local or general distention, bruising, or lack of movement on respiration. Tenderness or rigidity is sought from methodical palpation from quadrant to quadrant; the abdomen may be percussed to elicit dullness, perhaps indicative of a haemoperitoneum. Auscultation of the bowel sounds is carried out: absent sounds may mean a ruptured viscus. The pelvic girdle is inspected for

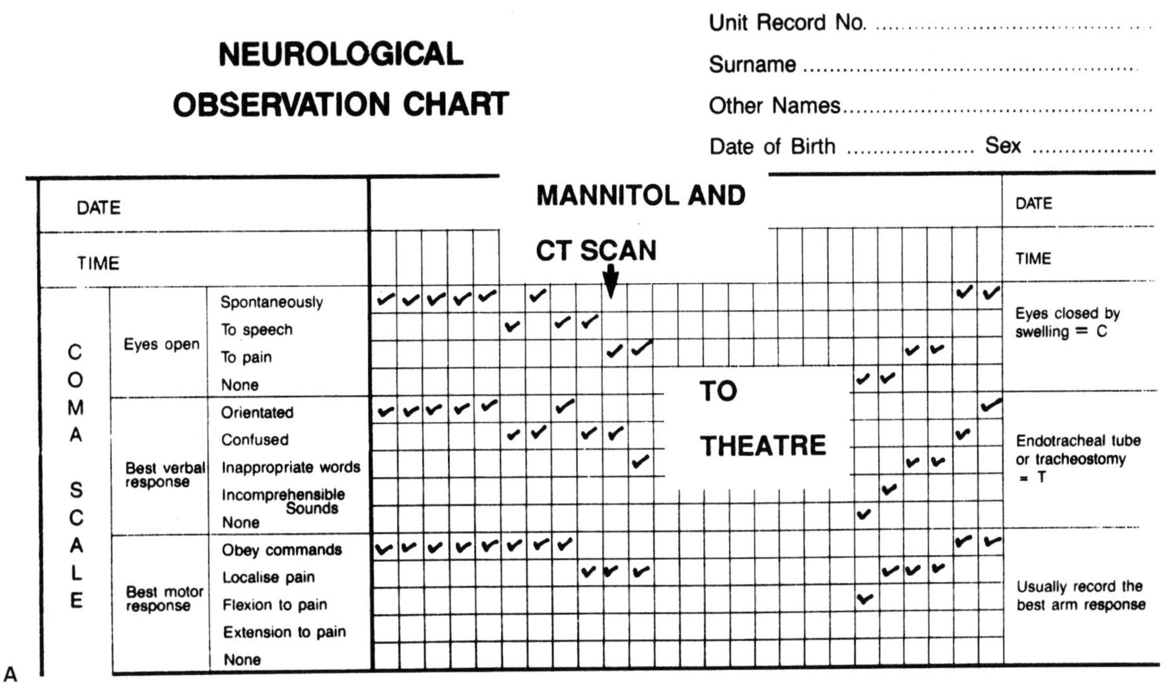

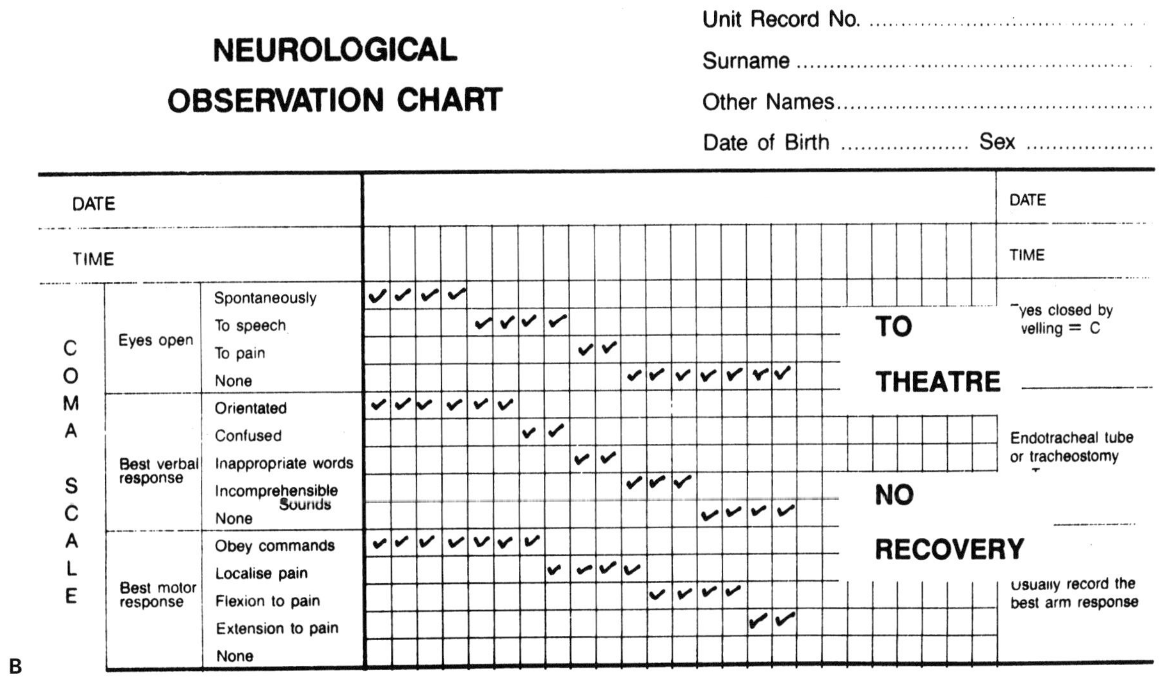

Fig. 6.1 Glasgow Coma Scale. The figure shows deteriorating conscious level in two hypothetical cases. The 14-point scale is used; in the 15-point version of the scale, the motor responses distinguish between normal and abnormal flexion. **A** Deterioration was evident when the conscious level fell from a Coma Score of 14 to 10. CT scan showed the lesion, and an operation was done with a good outcome. **B** Deterioration was evident, but no action was taken until the Coma Score was 4: the patient was in decerebrate rigidity and operation was unsuccessful.

bruising or swelling. Transverse compression or distraction of the iliac crests may cause pain, or reveal abnormal movement, indicative of a pelvic fracture. Inspection of the perineum may show bruising. If appropriate a rectal examination is performed. If the patient can pass urine, it is tested for blood. The limbs are inspected for bruising, laceration or deformity; the patient able to cooperate is asked to put each limb in turn through a normal range. If the patient is not cooperative, then each limb is methodically put through a full range of movement, any sign of a fracture or joint injury being noted. The tendon and plantar reflexes are tested.

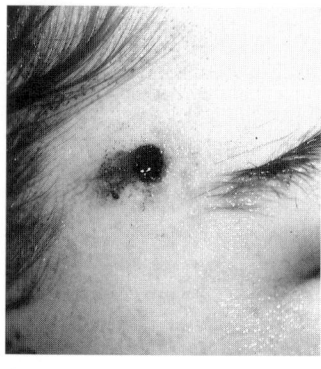 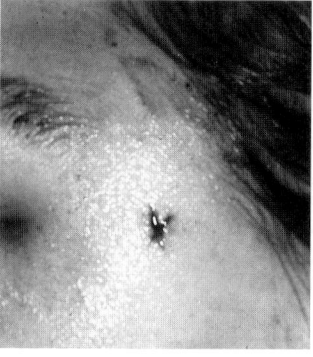

A   **B**

Fig. 6.2 Photographs of the face for forensic use. A young woman was thought to have shot herself with a .22 in rifle. Photographs were taken before the wounds were excised. **A** wound of entry in right temple, showing powder burns suggesting very close range. **B** wound in left temple, suggesting exit by a small lead fragment. At operation, the wounds were excised and sent for histological investigation; the finding of powder material in the tissues was confirmatory evidence of a point-blank shot. All such photographs should be clearly labelled and the negatives kept in safety.

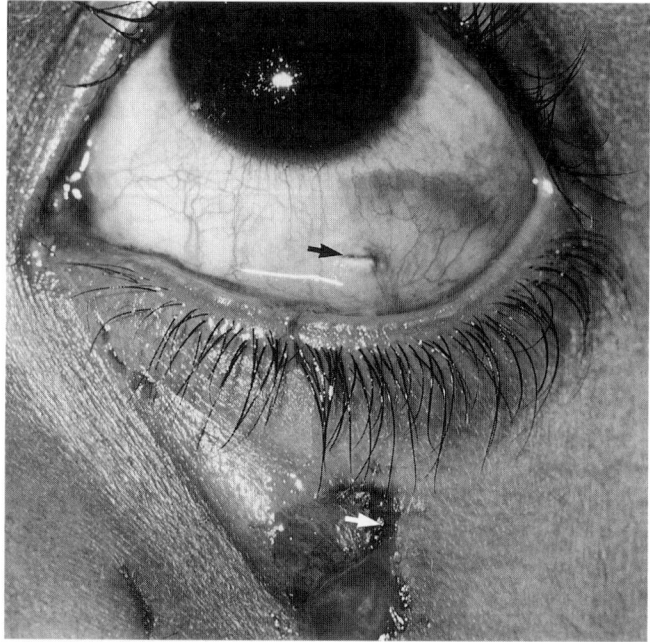

Fig. 6.3 Penetrating wound of the eyelid. A child ran a twig into the lower eyelid (lower arrow). When the eyelid was lifted, a penetrating wound of the sclera was seen, with vitreous prolapse (upper arrow).

This head-to-toe examination will detect most though not all injuries, and will point towards further investigations. If evidence of injury is found, then the affected area is examined in more detail by the appropriate specialist. Each discipline has its own routine for systematic assessment; the timing and scope of these depends on the degree of urgency of the case, and often resuscitation must be given priority. The definitive examination may have to be deferred until the injured person is in the ward, or even in the outpatient department when the problem

is of minor degree, though this practice can lead to the embarrassment of the late discovery of some injury of considerable importance.

Face and facial skeleton

The patterns of bruising, lacerations, and contour changes are usually obvious and can be depicted diagrammatically or photographed (Fig. 6.4). Inspection may show abnormal discharges (e.g. blood, cerebrospinal fluid, saliva), or abnormal movements of the eyes, jaws, or muscles of facial expression. In all facial injuries it is of particular importance that the eyes be inspected and vision tested by confirming that the patient can count fingers with one eye covered. If there is gross eyelid swelling, Desmarres' retractors (see below) may be used to allow an assessment of the integrity of the globe; this needs skill and care. The pupillary light reflexes are again tested, both to direct and consensual stimuli. The muscles of mastication are tested by asking the patient to open and close the jaws; the masseters can be felt to contract when the teeth are clenched. If this causes pain, it may be a clue to a jaw fracture. Damage to facial sensory nerves is identified by assessing light touch perception in the relevant zones. Specific regions of interest include the forehead (supratrochlear and supraorbital nerves), the cheek and upper lip (infraorbital nerve) and the lower lip (mental nerve). To assess the sensation in teeth (superior and inferior alveolar nerves) the patient is instructed to palpate them with a sweeping action of the tongue. Facial nerve function may be tested by brow elevation, eye closure, smiling and pursing the lips or whistling; in uncooperative patients, a grimace may be elicited by supraorbital pressure (see below).

A systematic method of clinical evaluation with a

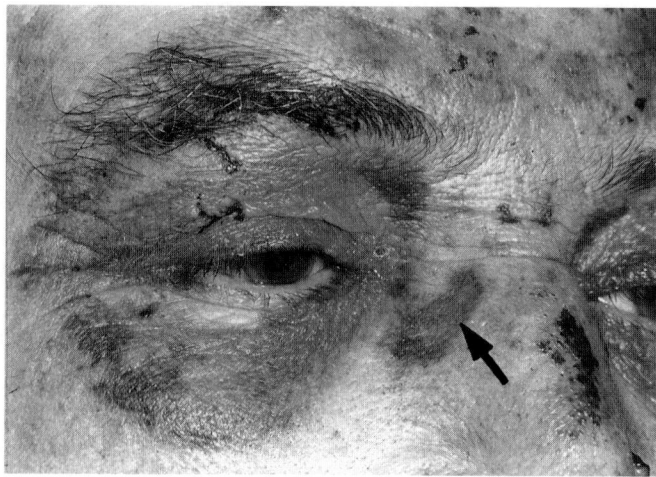

Fig. 6.4 Signs of spectacle impact. The pattern of abrasions and bruising is typical of impact on a spectacle frame, often associated with fractures of the orbital rim. From Cooter (1990).

specific palpation sequence is recommended (Fig. 6.5: Cooter 1990). In this method of palpation, the cervical spine is first examined for obvious neck injury and this manoeuvre precedes palpation of the scalp for lacerations or haematomas. The mastoid region is closely inspected for bruising (Battle's sign) as this may indicate a skull base fracture. The examiner then stands behind the patient with the patient's head held back, and any asymmetry of facial prominences or midline deviation is identified. Much information about facial bone integrity can be gained from direct palpation through the overlying soft tissue.

An attempt is made to examine sequentially the topography of each zone from the frontal bone down to the mandible (Fig. 6.5). Particular emphasis is placed on the orbital rims because many facial fractures have an associated orbital component; even with gross eyelid swelling this thin mobile skin can be gently compressed and the underlying bones palpated. The pattern of inferior orbital margin displacement may help to differentiate simple zygomatic fractures (in which the lateral aspect of the inferior rim is usually depressed) from mid-face pyramidal fractures or nasomaxillary fractures (in which the medial aspect of the rim is sunken). Medial canthal ligament integrity may be assessed by applying lateral traction on the lateral canthus and then checking for normal eyelid bow-stringing, which occurs when the medial canthi are intact. The mandible is initially examined with the patient's mouth slightly opened: the posterior rami, angles, lower border and symphyseal regions are first palpated externally. By applying compression medially at each mandibular angle simultaneously, pain is elicited at a fracture site anteriorly. With active mandibular excursions the condylar movements are easily palpated by placing an examining finger (with the pulp anteriorly directed) into each external auditory meatus. For the intraoral examination a gloved finger is used to palpate each alveolar ridge and the hard palate. Dentoalveolar injuries are recorded on a dental chart. The anterior wall of the maxilla and the zygomaticomaxillary junction are also palpable through the buccal sulcus. Abnormal movements of the mid-face can be elicited by grasping the maxillary alveolar ridge (not the incisors) and applying rocking movements whilst palpating the face with a free hand (Fig. 6.5H). Specific areas to palpate include:

— the anterior maxillary wall adjacent to the piriform aperture: movement occurs if there is a horizontal maxillary fracture of the Le Fort I type.
— the nasofrontal junction and the inferior orbital margins: movement at both of these regions occurs in pyramidal midfacial fractures of the Le Fort II type.
— the zygomaticofrontal sutures and the nasofrontal junction: mobility at both locations is present in craniofacial disjunctions of the Le Fort III type.

Neurological examination

The emergency examination (see above) establishes the level of consciousness, the pupillary status, and the limb movements; in conscious patients, vision should be checked by covering each eye successively and asking if the examiner's face looks normal. If possible, fundoscopy is done, chiefly to look for the presence or absence of early retinal haemorrhages.

A definitive neurological examination needs time — usually about an hour — and also tools. These include:

— ophthalmoscope and otoscope
— test types to estimate close and distant visual acuities, suitable both for literate and illiterate persons
— pins with white or coloured heads
— smell and taste bottles
— age-appropriate dysphasia test objects
— high (1024 Hz), medium (512 Hz) and low (128 Hz) frequency tuning forks
— a percussion hammer
— sensory testing materials, including disposable needles, cotton wool, and a two-point discriminator (Fig. 6.6A)
— possibly some simple tests for grading reading capacity and non-verbal intelligence.

In the ideal trauma service, these tools are always available in the chief trauma ward; in the real world, the prudent neurosurgeon carries a personal set in a handbag.

The examination begins with inspection. Signs of impact trauma anywhere in the head area are noted and recorded (see above). Fluid leakage (blood and/or cerebrospinal fluid) from the nostrils or external auditory canal is noted and if possible a sample is sent for immuno-chemical examination (p. 368). If there is orbital swelling, it is auscultated to detect a bruit. Auscultation of the carotid arteries may also be done.

If the patient is unconscious or confused, the GCS level is again noted, and a limited neurological examination is undertaken. If the patient is conscious and cooperative, a definitive assessment can be carried out.

The history is reviewed, with attention to any items not earlier recorded. If there was a period of altered consciousness, the period of amnesia is documented: the patient is asked to remember the last clear event before the accident and the first clear event after it. In young children, these recollections are rarely reliable. Later, a relative is interviewed to corroborate and expand the patient's story, and to give an assessment of the patient's mood and insight.

Speech is assessed during the narration of the history. The patient is always asked which hand is preferred, though it must be remembered that many left-handed persons have full or partial left hemisphere dominance. If there is any reason to suspect injury to the dominant hemisphere, the patient is asked to name a series of

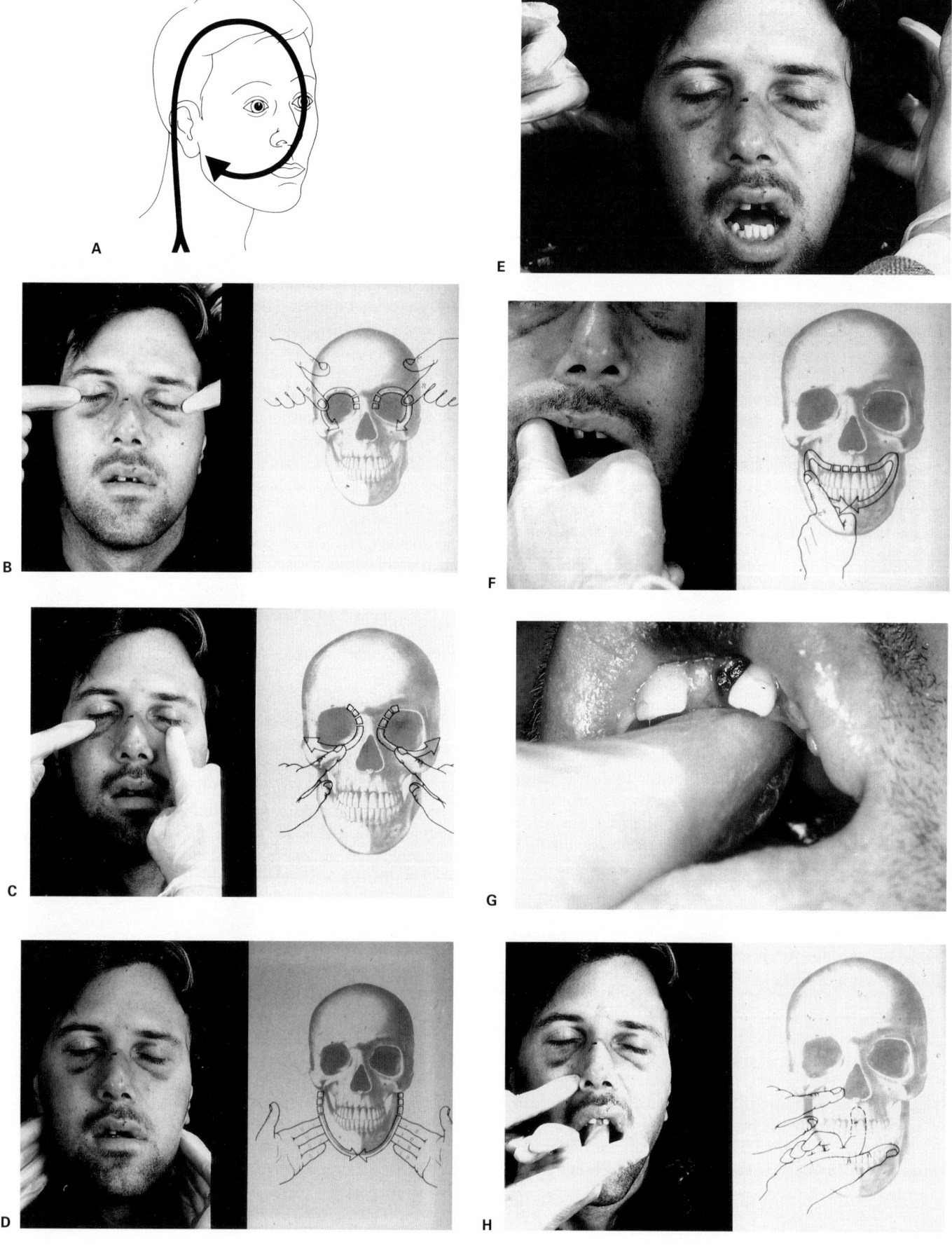

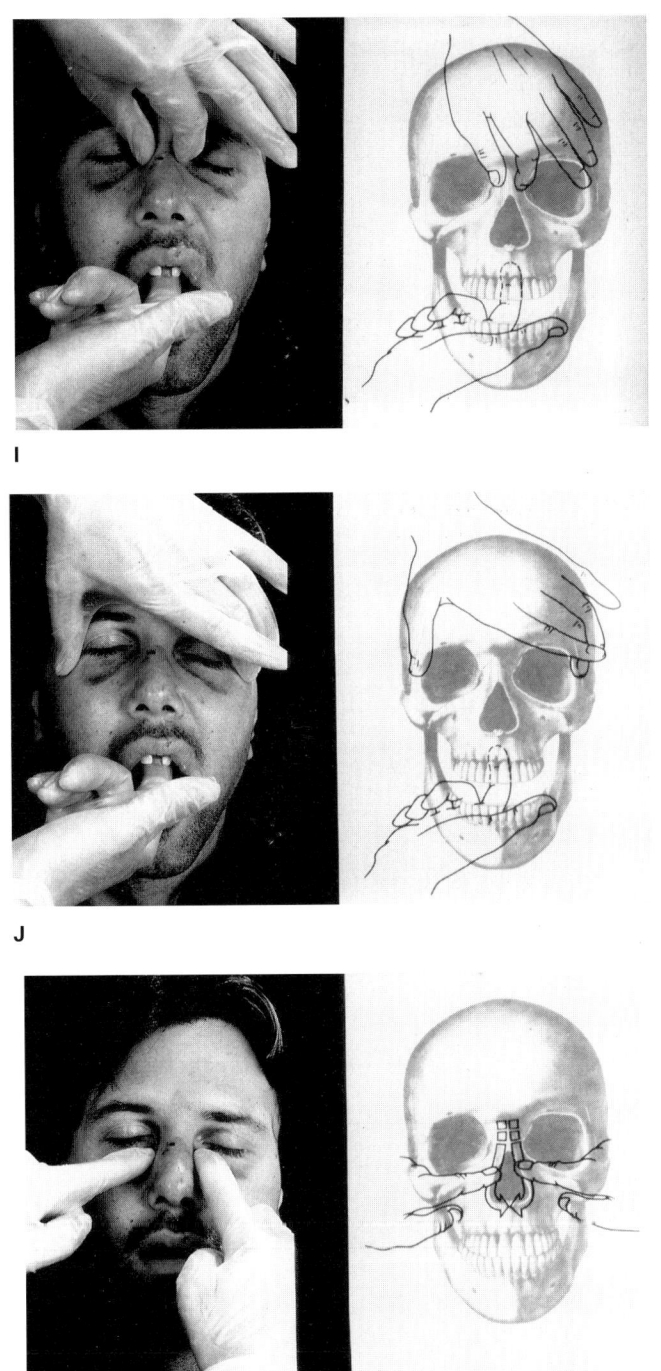

I

J

K

Fig. 6.5 The 'P' sequence of craniofacial palpation. Cooter (1990) has described a systematic sequence of examination by palpation. **A** Palpation begins with the neck, works around the head and then moves down to the mouth. **B** From behind the lateral superior and orbital margins are palpated. **C** From in front of the patient the medial and inferior orbital margins are felt. **D** The mandible is systematically palpated from in front. **E** The mandibular condyle is felt to assess translocation with mouth opening. **F** Intraoral palpation is performed with gloved fingers. **G** Midface mobility is sought with an examining finger on the maxillary alveolar margin, not on the crowns of the incisors. **H** Palpation for a suspected Le Fort I fracture. **I** Movement at the nasofrontal suture with palatal pressure is indicative of a Le Fort II fracture. **J** Le Fort III fracture is associated with separation of the midface from the skull base. **K** Nasal and nasomaxillary palpation seeks tenderness or deformity from fractures of the nose or maxilla.

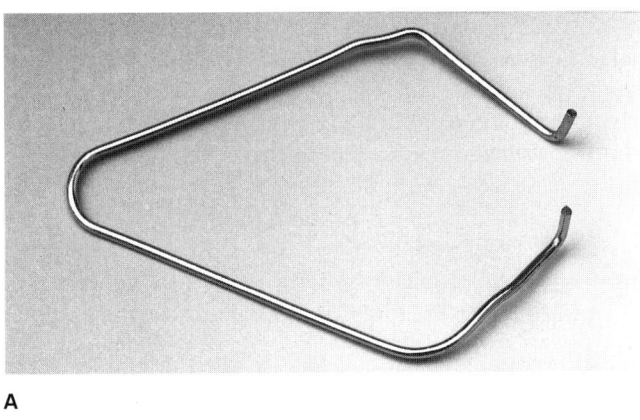

A

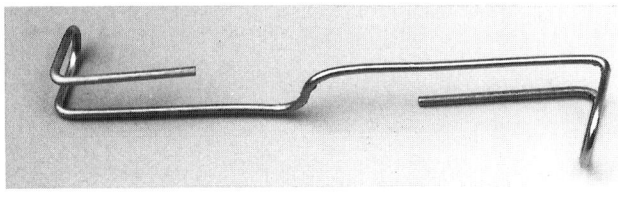

B

Fig. 6.6 Uses of a paper clip. A large glider clip is bent with pliers into: **A** a two-point sensory discriminator, to assess fine sensation on the lips or fingers; **B** a Desmarres' eyelid retractor.

5–10 test objects of increasing complexity: for adults, the final challenge can be the parts of a watch and for children a toy hippopotamus. This test for nominal dysphasia can also be used to test recent visual memory, by asking the patient to recall as many as possible of the objects immediately after the naming test; 8/10 is a good score. Other standard tests of memory include recall of a test name, address and flower after 5 min and timed serial subtraction of 7 from 100. Intelligence testing is left to the neuropsychologist (p. 654), but it may be helpful to check literacy with an age-graded word list (p. 513) and to estimate non-verbal intelligence by some simple method suitable for quick clinical testing. We have used the Raven coloured matrix test (Raven 1986), but many other tests are available. In CMF injuries affecting the upper third of the face, a good assessment of speech, intelligence and also mood is of paramount importance since the frontal lobes are often injured.

Vision is always assessed in CMF injuries, though the depth and scope of assessment vary with the nature of the injury. Covering one eye may lead to a subjective discovery of visual loss or blurring; the Snellen and reading test types quantitate this. For illiterates, the STYCAR toys provide a simple and quick way of estimating visual acuity (Sheridan 1976). Peripheral visual fields are tested by confrontation with the examiner's fingers as stimulus; central fields can be tested with a small (2–5 mm) white or red object, such as the head of a mapping pin, or a bead on a black stick; it is also possible to assess the central fields very effectively by asking the patient to fix on the examiner's nose and to say if any feature is missing or blurred. The optic fundi are examined; normal appearances are an important baseline in assessing abnormalities detected later. Retinal haemorrhages may be an important sign of raised intracranial pressure, especially if not seen in the initial examination. Papilloedema is an unusual finding soon after acute CMF trauma, but may appear after a few hours or more usually days (Selhorst et al 1985).

In the early period after a CMF injury, it is unwise to paralyse the pupils even with a short-acting mydriatic, because the pupillary light reflex is an important monitor of transtentorial herniation and other complications of cerebral injury; full fundoscopy may therefore be left to the ophthalmologist to be done at a later time.

The sense of smell is also of great importance in CMF injuries involving the anterior cranial fossa (Fig. 6.7). Tar or phenol is a good strong test odour, but must be complemented by a milder odour such as coffee or cloves; each nostril is tested separately, and to exclude guessing, the patient is warned that the test bottle may be empty. A more objective system of smell testing is provided by the University of Pennsylvania Identification Test* (Doty et al 1984). This 'scratch and sniff' test is self-administered; the patient scratches a series of odorants embedded in microencapsulated crystals located on paper strips in booklets (Fig. 6.7B) and identifies the smell from a multiple choice questionnaire. This quantitative smell test will permit the examiner to determine whether there is normal olfaction, microsmia, anosmia or malingering.

Taste is rarely of importance, but may be worth testing when there is a facial paralysis; each side of the tongue is tested with strong syrup or salt solution. In our experience, electric stimulation of taste has not been very helpful. However, Schirmer's test of lachrymation is a very useful test in facial paralysis: thin strips of filter paper are placed in the conjunctival sac for 30 seconds, and the extent of saturation is measured (Fig. 6.8A,B).

Hearing is checked by whispering words or numbers into each ear; if deafness is found, the 1024 or 512 Hz tuning fork is used to distinguish inner and middle ear deafness by the Weber and Rinne test. A Barany noise box can be used to mask hearing, though in routine quick testing it is acceptable to mask by a finger gently rubbed in a circular manner over the meatus to generate a repetitive noise. An ENT consultation is obtained if hearing is impaired (see below).

The remaining cranial nerves are then tested, as described in the examination of the face, though often in more detail. The eye movements are tested in lateral, vertical and oblique planes, and note is made of diplopia (Table 2.7), squint or nystagmus. Minor degrees of nystagmus can be detected by watching the fundus with an

*A version of this is commercially available from Sensonics Inc, 125 White Horse Pike, Haddon Heights, New Jersey 08015, USA (Fax: 609 547 5665)

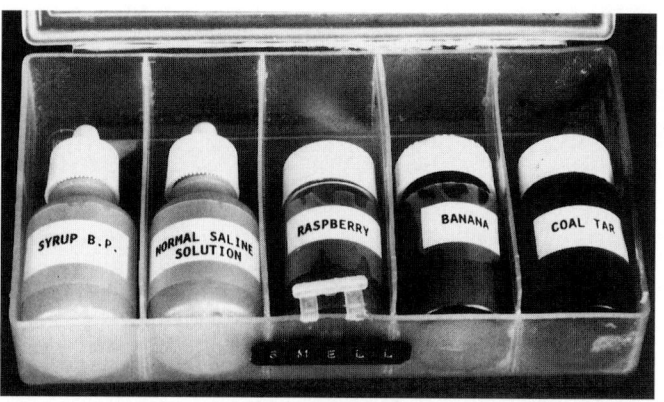

A

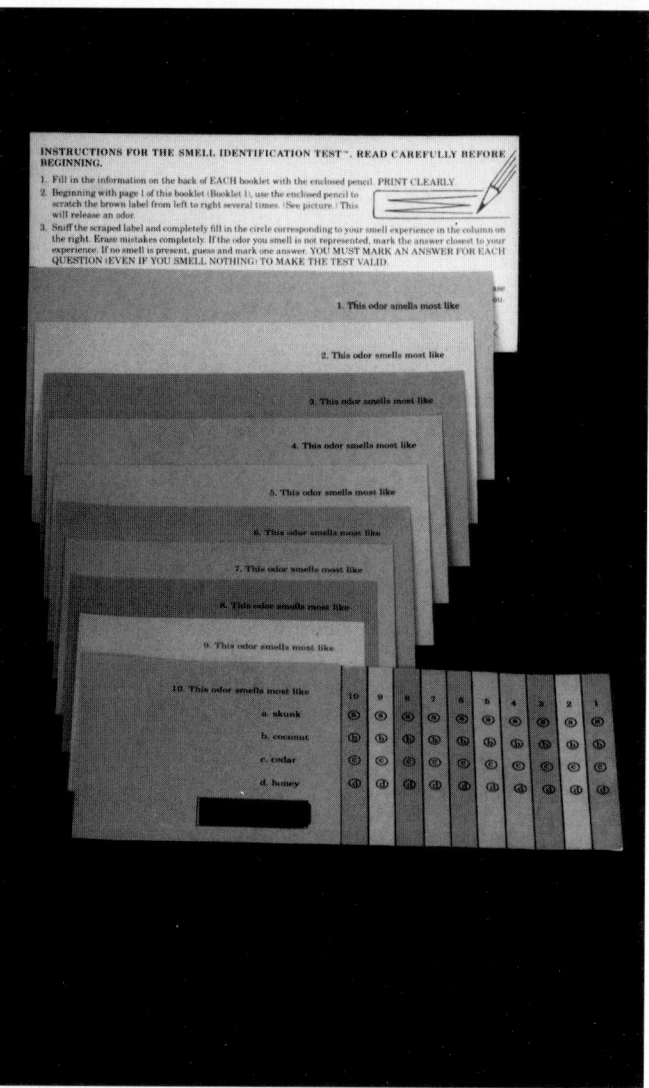

B

Fig. 6.7 Testing smell and taste. A Set of smell and taste bottles. Tar is an excellent test odour, remaining strong for a long time. Raspberry and banana are often identified by children; in adults, cloves and coffee may be better. Sweet and salt solutions are usually enough for taste testing; quinine can be used if a bitter taste is needed. **B** For precise tests of smell, the University of Pennsylvania Smell Identification Test (UPSIT) is strongly recommended.

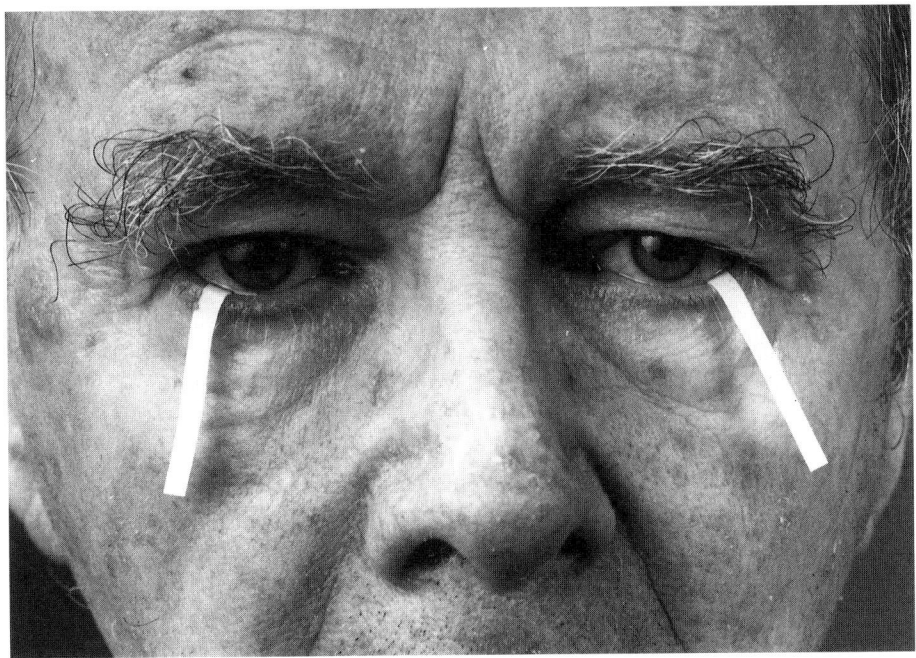
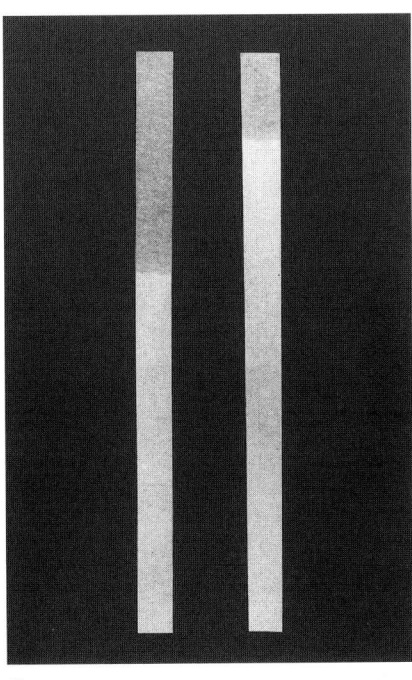

A

B

Fig. 6.8 Schirmer's test for tear secretion. A Strips of filter paper are placed in each conjunctival sac for exactly 30 s. **B** The extents of saturation are compared.

ophthalmoscope in a darkened room when fixation by the other eye has been masked. The corneal reflex is tested with a wisp of cotton wool or face tissue; mild trigeminal hypaesthesia may be brought out by two-point testing on the lips. The motor component of the facial nerve is tested as described above; an emotional facial weakness of upper motor neuron type may be brought out by watching the spontaneous smile. If there is any facial weakness, it is most important to know when it developed and whether it has increased: late onset facial weakness usually recovers spontaneously (p. 439). In unconscious patients, unless in deep coma, the facial movements can be elicited by painful pressure on the supraorbital nerve or temporo-mandibular joint. The lower cranial nerves are tested, though rarely affected in CMF injuries.

Limb motor function is tested with respect to muscle tone, power against graded resistance, and coordination; in the convalescent phase after a head injury, quantitative measures of limb function, such as the Purdue pegboard test (p. 663) are useful, and for these consultation with a specialist in occupational therapy is advisable. The tendon and plantar reflexes are again tested.

Sensation, except in the trigeminal area, is rarely affected in CMF injuries, and a full sensory examination is needed only if there is some associated spinal or brainstem injury.

Ophthalmological examination

This assesses both the state of the eyeball and its neural connections. The optic and ocular motor nerve fibres together amount to some 42% of all the fibres in the cranial nerves (Bruesch & Arey 1942), and their central connections are established in many parts of the brain: the neurophthalmological examination is therefore a good screening test of cerebral function. In some cases the ophthalmological examination precedes the neurosurgical examination and may even supersede it, but more often both specialties are concerned and the examinations are complementary.

The history of the causative accident often indicates the likely nature of the injury. Thus, impact with a ball or fist is likely to cause a blow-out fracture of the orbital floor or medial wall (p. 104), perhaps with impaired ocular motility, intraocular bleeding and traumatic mydriasis; a windscreen or side-window impact suggests a perforation of the globe by glass. Previous visual disabilities may be relevant. Congenital or longstanding blindness or aniso-coria may be overlooked; persons with such abnormalities should be encouraged to have the condition engraved on a wrist bracelet (p. 529).

In a conscious patient, the presence of vision is confirmed by covering each eye (see above). If the patient can count the examiner's fingers, he/she is asked to read a reduced Snellen chart at 3 m and the acuity for each eye is recorded; if the patient cannot see the chart, the ability to count fingers at whatever range is recorded; if this also is impossible, then the examiner records perception of hand movements or accurate projection of light or awareness of any light at all, as successive stages towards total blindness. In a semiconscious patient, the presence of at least some vision can be predicted if the patient flinches when suddenly exposed to the bright light of an ophthalmoscope. An intact pupillary light reflex confirms the integrity of the afferent visual pathway to the midbrain and the efferent pathway via the third nerve to the pupillary sphincter. If the patient is conscious but without spectacles to correct distance vision, a reasonably accurate estimate of refracted vision can be obtained with a pinhole aperture.

The size, shape and equality of the pupils are recorded. If the patient is conscious, then accommodation should be controlled by asking the patient to fix on a distant object while the pupillary light reflexes are checked with a bright light. This prevents 'contamination' of the light reflex by a reflex constriction of the pupil caused by accommodation. Each eye is tested with the other eye masked: this detects the presence or absence of the direct and consensual light reflex in each. The bright light is also swung repeatedly from one eye to the other: a relative afferent pupillary defect, due either to retinal or optic nerve pathology, will be detected if the pupils show relative dilatation when the light is shone on one eye, but normal constriction when the other eye is tested. This sensitive test should never be omitted, and if a relative afferent pupillary defect is found, the examiner should ask for the patient's subjective estimate of the brightness of the light on each side. Accommodation may also be tested by asking the patient to fix on a distant object and then on a near object; the pupils constrict in close fixation and in convergence.

Colour vision can be tested with the Ishihara plates, or with a selection of coloured pencils, held before each eye in turn to give a comparative evaluation of optic nerve function on each side.

Visual field assessment by confrontation has been discussed; the examination can be refined by asking the patient to count the examiner's fingers in each quadrant. These very rapid screening tests will detect and localize the majority of visual field defects, especially those in the eye, optic nerve, and optic chiasm (Fig. 2.27). Homonymous defects from lesions in the optic tract or visual cortex should also be detected, but these are less often seen after CMF injury. Interestingly, patients are often unaware of peripheral homonymous field defects. Quantitative perimetry is useful for permanent record. A variety of excellent computerized perimeters is available, offering a selection of programs that can be used according to the ability of the injured person to concentrate for whatever time-span is needed for the test. Obtunded patients may be able to sustain concentration for the few minutes needed in a rapid screening test, but not for more detailed tests. It must be emphasized that field tests are subjective and influenced by many factors; one should not rely solely on any one visual field test, and defects found by computerized perimetry should always be checked by simple confrontation.

Visual pursuit movements (slow following movements) are tested by asking the patient to follow a pencil torch light moved in the cardinal gaze positions (Fig. 6.9) The position of the light reflected from the torch on the cornea should normally be symmetrically placed over each pupil. Asymmetry of the position of this corneal light reflex will indicate an impairment of ocular motility. Saccadic movements are tested by asking the patient to look left, right, up and down; convergence is tested by asking the patient to follow the torch or a finger towards the tip of the nose.

In the unconscious or semiconscious patient, the vestibular ocular reflexes are tested. To elicit the doll's eye response, the examiner first makes sure that there is no likelihood of injury or other pathology in the cervical spine. The head is then turned from side to side, and then up and down, to see whether the eyes move in the reverse direction: this gives a measure of brainstem reflex function and may also unmask paralysis of one or more of the external ocular muscles. The vestibular ocular reflex responses to cold water irrigation of the external auditory meati may also be tested if the ear drums are known to be intact. Unilateral cold water induces horizontal nystagmus with the fast movement away from the side tested; unilateral warm irrigation gives the reverse fast movement and bilateral warm irrigation gives vertical nystagmus with the fast phase downwards. Caloric testing is unpleasant and may cause vomiting, but it is nevertheless a valuable procedure, especially as one of the battery of tests used to establish brainstem failure or death (p. 230).

Eye movements are tested by asking the patient to fix on a distant object, and then on an object in each of the cardinal gaze positions; this may elicit diplopia and/or ocular misalignment. The cover test is used when there is ocular misalignment: in each movement, each eye is covered in turn. If there is no change in the ocular misalignment in the various positions after covering, then concomitant squint can be diagnosed; this is usually due to a childhood squint and no diplopia is experienced. Midbrain trauma sometimes causes an incomitant squint, such as convergence or divergence paralysis or convergence spasm. If the ocular misalignment changes in different gaze positions, then the cause is either incomitant or paralytic strabismus. With an incomitant strabismus, a forced duction test is performed to distinguish between a mechanical or muscular problem or a neurological defect. Topical anaesthetic drops (amethocaine 1%) are instilled, and the eyes are then mechanically moved to determine the range of movement, and to detect any muscular tethering. Some use a cotton bud to move the eye, but we like a suction cap which fixes to the cornea. A negative forced duction test in the presence of an incomitant squint suggests a skew deviation from brainstem injury, but a

THE OCULAR MUSCLES AND GAZE POSITIONS

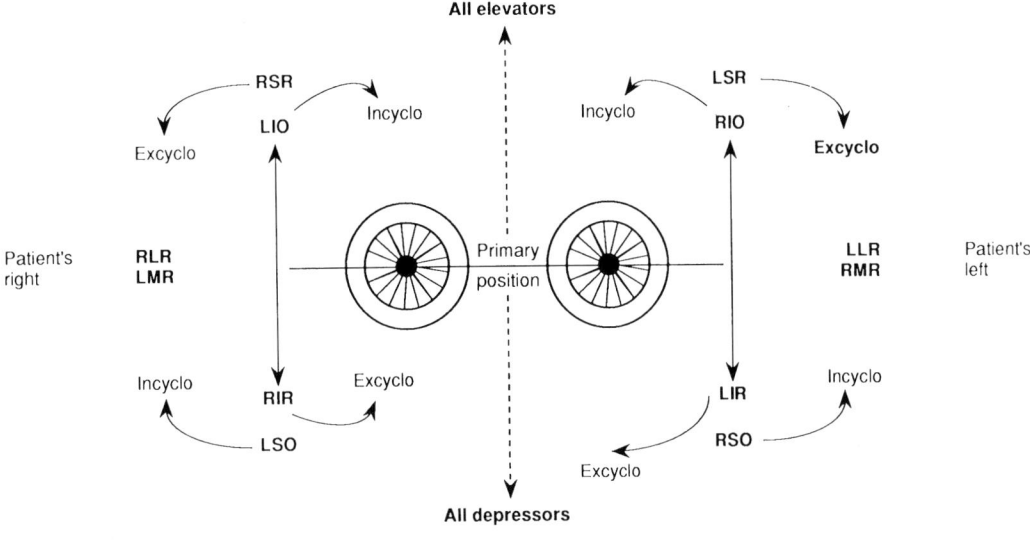

LEGEND: **RSR** = Right superior rectus muscle   **RLR** = Right lateral rectus muscle   **LMR** = Left medial rectus muscle

        RIR = Right inferior rectus muscle   **LIO** = Left inferior oblique muscle   **LSO** = Left superior oblique muscle

Fig. 6.9 Actions of the extraocular muscles. The diagram shows the different extraocular muscles used in the various positions of gaze. The muscles producing torsion of the globe (incyclo- and excyclo-torsion) are shown.

positive response suggests entrapment or some other restriction of one of the external ocular muscles.

Paralytic strabismus is a common and important finding after CMF trauma: it is due to injury of the third, fourth or sixth cranial nerve, alone or in combination (p. 414), and requires full evaluation. The clinical findings and the nature of the diplopia are usually diagnostic (Table 2.7); accurate measurement of the angle of the strabismus requires specialized examination with orthoptic equipment such as a synoptophore or Hess chart. The position of each globe should be assessed relative to the other eye, by holding a ruler under the eyes and seeing whether the inferior limbus of each eye is at the same level; the ruler also allows one to measure the distance from the centre of each pupil to the midline of the nose. Proptosis or enophthalmos should also be noted and if possible measured with a plastic ruler or other instrument pressed against the lateral orbital margin; trauma to the orbit may make this impossible.

The state of the eyelids and the corneal reflex should be assessed (see above); inadequate tear secretion or impaired blinking is a threat to the integrity of the cornea. A perforating wound of an eyelid means a perforating ocular wound until proved otherwise (Fig. 6.3). A subconjunctival haemorrhage may hide a perforating wound; any conjunctival wound should be explored in the theatre, if necessary under anaesthesia. Glass may produce multiple shelving corneal lacerations; even with a slit lamp it may be hard to determine whether one of these penetrates the cornea. Inspection under cobalt blue light after

instillation of topical fluorescein sodium 2%, with light pressure on the globe if necessary, will reveal a leak of aqueous fluid from a penetrating corneal wound (Seidel's test). Slit lamp examination will reveal a minute hyphaema, and may show splits in the sphincter of the pupil, a cause of traumatic mydriasis to be distinguished from the pupillary dilatation due to third nerve paralysis. Distortion of the pupil may point to adhesions (synechia) resulting from a perforation or from scar tissue.

Often, chemosis of the conjunctiva and lids may make ocular examination very difficult or even impossible. Instillation of a drop of topical anaesthetic may allow the insertion of Desmarres' lid retractors, or a paperclip bent into a similar shape (Fig. 6.6B); this may enable one to use a hand-held slit lamp.

Fundus examination is essential, but may be difficult if the pupils have been constricted by systemic opioid medication. For reasons set out earlier, pupillary dilatation by a mydriatic (e.g. tropicamide 1%) should not be done until the risk of cerebral complications is past. Intraocular pressure should also be measured, especially when there has been intraocular bleeding.

ENT examination

The emergency examination includes inspection of the pinna, the post-auricular area and the external auditory meatus. The tympanic membrane is examined with an otoscope; if the meatus is filled with clot or debris, it is cleared, preferably by aspiration under micro-otoscopic vision. If there is any fluid that could be CSF, a sample is taken for immunochemical analysis.

Hearing may have already been tested with tuning forks as part of the neurological examination, but retesting will usually be done. This will show whether there is any significant hearing loss, and whether such loss is neuro-sensory, or due to a middle ear lesion, or of mixed type. When life-threatening problems have been dealt with, more discriminating otological investigations may be indicated. To evaluate deafness and/or tinnitus, one may want:

— audiometry for bone conduction, air conduction and speech
— impedance audiometry
— evoked response audiometry (Gibson 1982), giving a measure of function in the cochlea, the brainstem and the auditory cerebral cortex
— in cases of giddiness with or without nystagmus, electronystagmography (Barber & Stockwell 1980) and the vestibular caloric responses may be needed.

Rhinoscopy, or telescopic nasendoscopy, should show any laceration or disruption of the vestibular skin or nasal mucosa, or any sign of a septal haematoma; CSF rhinorrhoea may be detected when not externally obvious.

Oral and dental examination

The range of dental injury associated with CMF trauma is wide and extends from minor enamel fractures to crown—root fractures, luxation injuries, and complete avulsions of teeth from their sockets. Loss of pulp vitality is a complication of many of these injuries. More severe impacts can cause dento-alveolar fractures and soft-tissue damage. Fractures of both the maxilla and the mandible are likely to cause difficulty in occluding the teeth.

The dental assessment is thus often of great importance, and in some cases it is urgent, since avulsed teeth should be replanted within 30 min of injury (p. 353). However, dental examination may be impeded by haematomas in the floor of the mouth, or by restrictions of mouth opening, or by concentration of attention on more urgent injuries.

The methodology of examination is set out in Chapter 12. Here, it is important to emphasize that the trauma evaluation should include a dental assessment if there is any likelihood of intraoral injury, and this should be done urgently if replantation is possible. Recording the post-traumatic dental status is important from the medicolegal viewpoint, and unrecorded injuries may be blamed on some member of the trauma team, such as the anaesthetist. The dental examination includes evaluation of both the hard and soft tissues of the oral cavity, and assessment of facial swelling and lacerations. Tooth fractures and mobile teeth are noted and described; loose tooth fragments and dentures are removed, and the opportunity is taken to clean the mouth with a chlorhexidine mouthwash. Where there are lip lacerations and missing incisal edges of anterior teeth, soft-tissue radiographs are necessary to detect tooth fragments embedded in the lips, and a chest radiograph is also ordered to exclude inhaled objects such as teeth, dislodged restorations or fragments of a denture.

Laboratory investigations

In cases of severe CMF trauma, or if there is any reason to suspect blood loss or antecedent anaemia, the haemoglobin and haematocrit levels are ordered, and blood is sent for grouping and possible matching. In any head injury in which there is the likelihood of alcohol consumption, the blood alcohol level should be urgently measured. Some clinicians are reluctant to do this without the patient's consent; in South Australia, the investigation is legally obligatory for all victims of road crashes who are admitted to hospital. Even in countries not enacting this, the investigation can be justified because of its proven importance in evaluating disturbed consciousness (Jagger et al 1984). Other haematological and biochemical tests will be demanded by a history of previous disease, e.g. diabetes mellitus (p. 537), and if the patient is unconscious it is advisable to obtain baseline investigations of the electrolyte status and osmolality, and the blood gas levels.

Radiological investigations

These are discussed in Chapter 7. It should not be necessary to say that X-ray investigations are ordered on the basis of the clinical assessment, and not as reflex responses to a reported diagnosis; too often, unthinking use of diagnostic procedures results in waste of time and money. Ideally, a full clinical assessment is done before a systematic plan of radiological investigation is prepared. But in certain clinical situations, the emergency examination may indicate the need for some procedure as soon as possible. Thus, the comatose patient will usually require a computerized tomogram (CT) of the head as soon as possible, unless there is such rapid deterioration that immediate operation is needed (p. 385); arrangements for the scan may be made while the clinical examination is being completed. Similarly, the eye examination may raise the possibility of a perforating wound or an intraocular foreign body and call for urgent decision on the choice of the best procedure; CT scanning may best show intraocular air or metal, magnetic resonance imaging may best image wood, and ultrasonography may be appropriate to show the integrity of the posterior segment (p. 406). The clinical examination leads to the radiological procedure, which may reciprocally call for revision or extension of the clinical examination.

REFERENCES

American College of Surgeons 1986 Hospital and prehospital resources for optimal care of the injured patient. Bull Am Coll Surgeons 71: 4–12

Barber H O, Stockwell C W 1980 Manual of electronystagmography, 2nd edn. Mosby, St Louis

Bruesch S R, Arey L B 1942 The number of myelinated and unmyelinated fibres in the optic nerves of vertebrates. J Comp Neurol 77: 631–665

Cooter R D 1990 Craniofacial fracture patterns. MD thesis. Department of Surgery, The University of Adelaide

Davidson J S, Birdsel D C 1989 Cervical spine injury in patients with facial skeletal trauma. J, Trauma 29: 1276–1278

Doty R L, Shaman P, Kimmelman C P, Dann M S 1984 University of Pennsylvania smell identification test: a rapid quantitative olfactory function test for the clinic. Laryngoscope 94: 176–178

Gibson W P R 1982 The use of auditory evoked potentials for the estimation of hearing. In: Halliday A M (ed) Evoked potentials in clinical testing. Churchill Livingstone, Edinburgh, Ch 9

Jagger J, Fife D, Vernberg K, Jane J A 1984 Effect of alcohol on the diagnosis and apparent severity of brain injury. Neurosurgery 15: 303–306

Jennett B, Teasdale G 1981 Management of head injuries. Davis, Philadelphia

Raven J C 1986 Coloured progressive matrices. H K Lewis, London

Selhorst J B, Gudeman S K, Butterworth J F, Harbison J W, Miller J D, Becker D P 1985 Papilledema after acute head injury. Neurosurgery 16: 356–363

Sheridan M 1976 Stycar vision tests. NFER, Windsor

Simpson D A, Cockington R A, Hanieh A, Raftos J, Reilly P L 1991 Head injuries in infants and young children: the value of the Paediatric Coma Scale. Child's Nerv Syst 7: 183–190

CHAPTER 7 | Diagnostic imaging

B. Clark   A. Abbott   A. Whyte

INTRODUCTION

Diagnostic imaging, particularly radiological investigation, should not be performed until a detailed clinical examination has been done, and a plan of investigation has been formulated. Standard radiographic projections are usually the essential first step; if indicated, images using other modalities such as computed tomography (CT) and magnetic resonance imaging (MRI) can then be obtained. However, in some emergency situations, this sequence is not followed, and time is saved by proceeding at once to an investigation which is most likely to give definitive diagnosis. Pathria & Blaser (1989) have given an excellent overview of imaging in craniofacial fractures.

Before the advent of CT, radiological imaging of craniomaxillofacial (CMF) trauma was regarded as difficult because of the problems often encountered in obtaining good quality standard radiographic films of the injured patient, and complex because of the intricate anatomy of the region. CT allows imaging of most injuries with minimal superimposition of structures. The CT data can be displayed to show both bone and soft tissue in selected planes and in three-dimensional (3D CT) reconstructions. We first began to use 3D CT reconstructions in 1980 (Hemmy et al 1983), as did other major centres (Marsh & Vannier 1983, Gillespie et al 1987), and the usefulness of 3D CT reconstructions in patient management has grown with their improved quality.

The indiscriminate use of modern imaging techniques can incur needless cost and radiation dosage and therefore there must be a systematic plan of investigation designed to be both informative and parsimonious.

This chapter discusses the logistics and facilities, imaging modalities and techniques, and clinical applications.

LOGISTICS AND FACILITIES

The patient

The patient may have sustained a CMF injury with any degree of severity ranging from a fractured nose or mandible, to a panfacial fracture with coma and multiple extracranial injuries. The injury may be life-threatening, for example a cervical spinal injury, or a compromised airway. A blocked nose may make certain radiological postures difficult. Impaired consciousness may preclude placing the patient in the supine position until the airway has been secured. These immediate and often urgent problems are discussed in Chapter 8; here, it is only necessary to stress that the timing of diagnostic imaging must be related to the patient's condition as a whole. This demands good communication between the clinician, the radiologist and the radiographer.

Staff

A team of radiographers, radiologists and specialist surgeons gathered in a well-established multidisciplinary unit can offer the clinical experience of many years. Ideally, such a team is armed with the best diagnostic facilities that can be procured, and honed by regular clinico-radiological meetings. Such experience and such facilities are rarely if ever available in the radiological departments of smaller or less specialized centres, yet it is often to such departments that the victim of a CMF injury is first referred. This emphasizes the need for an integrated community trauma system that uses the craniofacial trauma unit to the best advantage (p. 677).

Location of service

Patient handling on arrival in hospital should be optimized by an appropriate hospital layout of casualty, ward, operating theatre and radiology department. In some centres, radiological facilities are sited in the emergency suite, adjacent to a dedicated operating theatre; where this is not the case, there must be provision for rapid transfer to and from the radiology department, if necessary under anaesthesia.

Anaesthesia for imaging

In a restless or uncooperative patient, it may be impossible to obtain satisfactory images. This difficulty often arises in cases of head injury or alcoholic intoxication, and in frightened children; general anaesthesia may then be necessary. The decision to use general anaesthesia in an unprepared, recently injured person should not be taken lightly; it is sometimes better to defer the investigation until the patient is more cooperative. Alternatively, the radiological investigation can be done under anaesthesia as part of a planned sequence of procedures leading up to a definitive operation. In either strategy, the benefits and dangers of delay or intervention must be discussed by the clinicians and radiologists concerned. The principles and techniques of anaesthesia after CMF injury are discussed in Chapter 10.

The imaging request form

A standardized request form on which the referring doctor indicates apppropriate clinical details is mandatory. It cannot be overemphasized how important a detailed written request is to the radiologist; this is so even when there can be a verbal dialogue between surgeon and radiologist. For example, our CT request form incorporates a frontal outline diagram of the craniofacial skeleton with twenty horizontal lines traversing it from chin to vertex. On this, the surgeon can indicate graphically the extent of scanning needed.

The imaging report

Patterns of CMF injuries can be extremely complex and this presents problems for the radiologist who needs to summarize the findings succintly in the form of a radiological report. A standardized reporting sheet in which individual facial and calvarial bones are detailed is advisable to expedite the rapid and systematic review of the injury and also to facilitate research. Dialogue between clinician and radiologist is also important. Together, the written report and the verbal discussion give optimal efficiency in diagnosis leading to appropriate patient management and lower patient morbidity.

Teleradiology

Teleradiology denotes the transmission of any kind of diagnostic image from one location to another. This can be between hospitals in the same city or from a remote part of the country to a city, or internationally. By this means, clinico-radiological consultation can be made over variable distances and appropriate patient management expedited. Especially in large countries such as Australia, teleradiology has the potential to transform the early management of critically ill and injured patients who are remote from specialist centres. Remote assessment and diagnosis by specialists may avoid expensive and unnecessary transfer of patients. Bidgood & Staab (1992) give a good overview of this subject.

IONIZING RADIATION MODALITIES

Standard radiographic projections

Plain film technique and radiological anatomy have been well described by Merrell et al (1968a,b), Dolan & Jacoby (1978) and Meschan (1978). Standard views of the facial skeleton and the calvarial skull are still used, additional options being added if necessary. These standard views are designed to maximize the yield of information from the minimum number of films, and so to minimize X-ray dosage. The standard films are analysed in the light of the expected fracture patterns; in modern practice the surgeon and the radiologist then go on to consider CT scanning, additional plain views now having little place.

The clinician needs to keep in mind the two basic facial topographic lines to which X-ray beam angulation is related in standard radiographic technique: the radiographic base line or canthomeatal line, drawn from the centre of the external auditory meatus to the outer canthus of the eye, and the interpupillary line.

These two lines constitute the transverse facial plane. The routine standard radiographic films are taken in relation to this plane, though the experienced radiographer may not rigidly adhere to the precise beam angles given in this chapter when there is variation in the shape of the head — this is part of the radiographer's art! Preference is given wherever possible to postero-anterior views to minimize radiation dosage to the eyes as well as to give better definition of the facial skeleton.

Five standard views may be required:

- Lateral view
  — Brow-up
  — Standard

- Caldwell view
- Walters view
- Submento-vertical view
- Towne's view.

As a general view, it is better to overexpose plain films taken for CMF injuries, as cranial fractures are likely to be missed if the film is too 'white'. A 'black' film can be scrutinized for fractures with a bright light, whereas an underexposed ('white') film cannot be so assessed.

Lateral view: brow up

The X-ray beam is horizontal; correct laterality is indicated by superimposition of both mandibular rami, orbital roofs and sphenoidal surfaces (Figs 7.1 and 7.2).

This view is used to show air-fluid levels in the paranasal air sinuses or within the cranial vault (Fig. 7.2B). A vertical grid is used to avoid a spurious appearance of fluid. A fluid level in an air sinus may indicate a cerebrospinal fluid (CSF) leak, though pre-existing sinus disease may give a similar appearance; blood and tears may also form fluid levels in the sinuses. A fluid level or gas bubble in the cranial cavity may signify a cranionasal or craniomastoid fistula (Fig. 13.8). Vault fractures are often seen, though care is needed to distinguish these from vascular markings or cranial sutures. The same film gives a lateral view of the cervical spine, but a formal cervical spine view should be done if — as in all unconscious head injuries — there is need to exclude cervical trauma (p. 225). A good assessment of the lateral view has been given by Daffner et al (1983) who stressed that it is often not exploited

to its full potential: in an era of 'hi-tech' imaging, sight should not be lost of the usefulness of plain films, and they should be systematically examined for fractures and displacements.

Standard lateral view

This should be centred on the malar region (Fig. 7.1). The standard view may be employed when there is complete clinical confidence that the anterior fossa is intact.

Aim of lateral view: apart from visualizing fluid levels in the skull or sinuses, this view shows in profile the frontal calvarial surface, the cribriform plates, the anterior and posterior walls of the frontal sinuses, the hard palate, the maxillary and mandibular dental arches, the posterior and anterior walls of the antra, and the heights of the orbits (and therefore their floors and roofs) and antra, and the malar struts. The lateral view also shows Dolan's square (Fig. 7.3), a useful aid in demonstrating fractures causing displacement in the midfacial region.

Caldwell view

A postero-anterior view with 15° X-ray beam angulation caudad to the CM line (Fig. 7.4).

Aim of Caldwell view (Fig. 7.5): to project the floor of the orbit just above (or at the level of) the petrous bones, so that the orbital floors are seen clearly. The Caldwell view is ideal for showing the orbital margins, especially the medial orbital walls and floors, superior orbital fissure and zygomaticofrontal suture and the frontal regions generally, together with the maxillary alveolus and upper dental arch, the piriform nasal aperture, the bony nasal septum, the lesser sphenoid wing and the innominate (oblique orbital) line. The orbit height should equal the antral height.

Waters view

A postero-anterior view with 37° X-ray beam angulation caudad (Fig. 7.6).

Aim of Waters view (Fig. 7.7): to project the petrous bones below the floors of the antra, and so to allow clear visualization of the sinuses and other neighbouring structures. It is par excellence the view to show the midface, including the maxilla and its sinus, the zygoma and the orbital rim and floor. This is probably the most informative single film for facial fractures. One should beware of 'pseudo-fracture' lines due to the anterior and posterior superior alveolar neurovascular channels (Dolan & Hayden 1973).

Submento-vertical (base or axial) view

An anteroposterior view taken with the CM line vertical and parallel with the film, the X-ray beam being angled

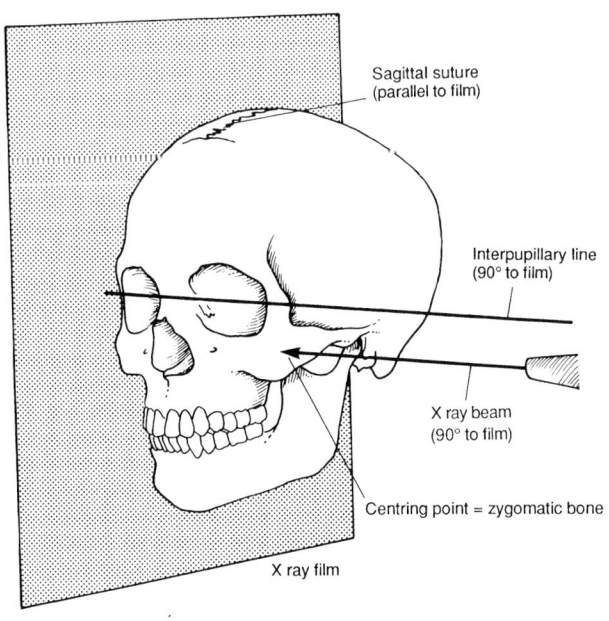

Sagittal suture
(parallel to film)

Interpupillary line
(90° to film)

X ray beam
(90° to film)

Centring point = zygomatic bone

X ray film

LATERAL FACIAL BONES

Fig. 7.1 Lateral skull radiograph: the projection. The diagram shows the standard lateral facial view.

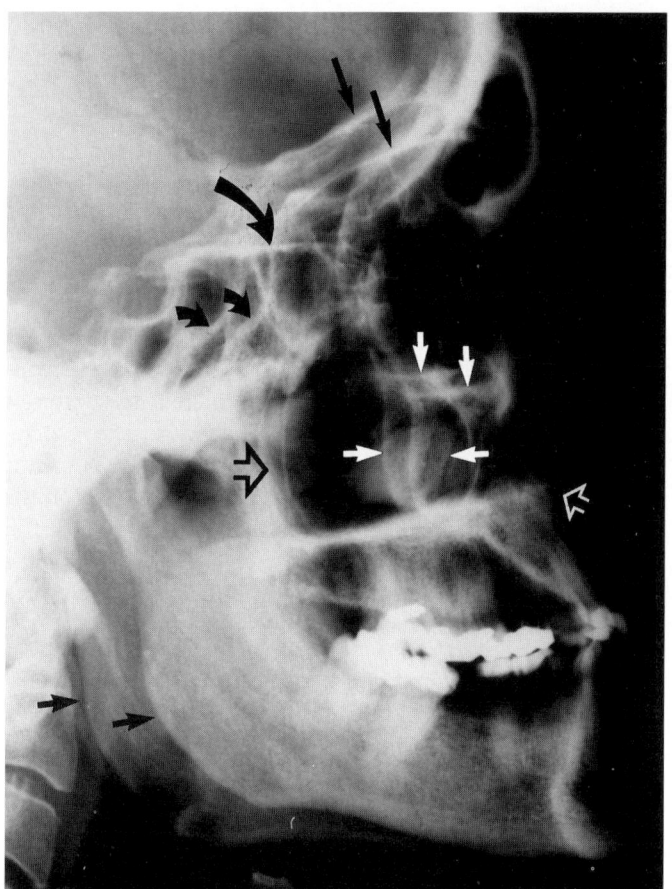

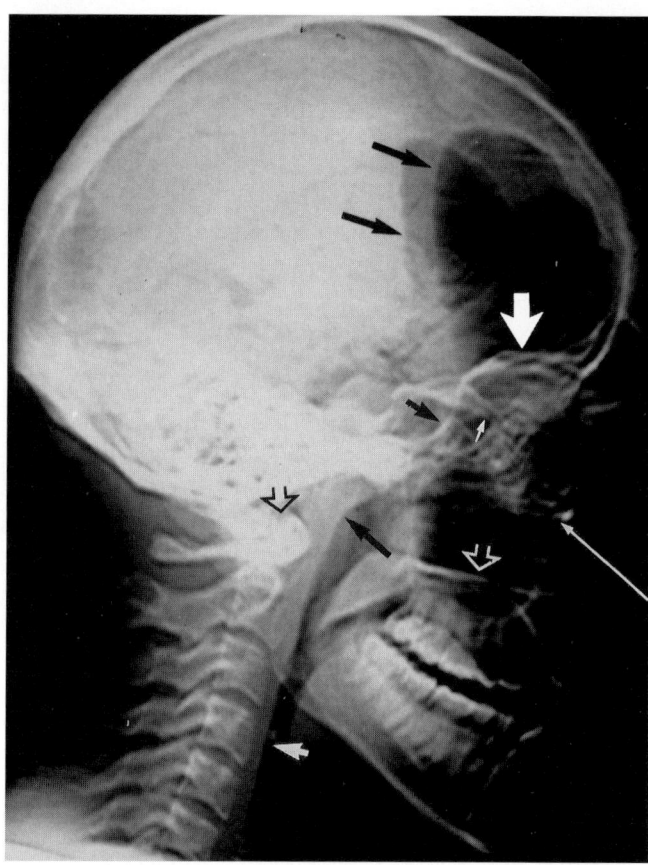

A

B

Fig. 7.2 Lateral skull radiograph: the landmarks. A This is not a true lateral view as indicated by lack of superimposition of orbital roofs (long straight black arrows), mandibular rami (short straight black arrows), floors of orbits (vertical white arrows) and sphenoid wings (short curved black arrows). Due to this, one of the malar struts (horizontal white arrows) is separated from the contralateral one (which is anterior to it on the film) and, therefore, any displacement due to trauma cannot be assessed. The more posterior malar strut corresponds to the higher orbit floor. Open black arrow shows the separation of the posterior walls of both maxillary sinuses, and overlies the pterygomaxillary fissures and pterygoid plates. Open white arrow indicates site of anterior nasal spine, seen well by bright illumination, as are the nasal bones. Note the large anteroposterior diameter of frontal sinuses with prominent glabella. Large black curved arrow indicates junction of planum sphenoidale and cribriform plate. Sinuses appear clear with no fluid levels. **B** This horizontal film shows two fluid levels due to pneumocephalus. No bony injury is seen. This is a true lateral view as the orbital roofs (large solid white arrow) and halves of mandible superimpose, together with the greater sphenoid wings (small black arrow) which form the anterior bony limits of the middle cranial fossae. A small white arrow indicates the line formed by the cribriform plate. Behind the greater wings of sphenoid is the sphenoid sinus, behind which is the pituitary fossa, and above which is the planum sphenoidale. Hard palate (open white arrow) is well seen with soft palate posterior to it. The posterior nasopharynx wall (inferior long black arrow) may be swollen in spheno-occipital skull base fractures (beware adenoids in children). Long white arrow indicates orbital floors. The prevertebral thin soft-tissue stripe (intermediate white arrow) may be swollen by haematoma/oedema in a cervical spinal injury. The gentle curve of the normal cervical spine should be assessed by following the continuous line formed by the posterior aspects of the vertebral bodies and by the anterior aspects of the spinous processes. Vertebral bodies and neural arches should be assessed for fractures. The atlanto-odontoid joint gap (open black arrow) should not be > 3.5 mm in an adult (5.0 mm in the child).

5° (Fig. 7.8). Cervical spine injury must be excluded before this view is obtained.

Aim of base view (Fig. 7.9): to show walls and posterior surfaces of maxillary sinuses, lateral orbital walls, zygomatic arches, arch of mandible, temporomandibular joints, ethmoidal sinuses and mastoid air cells.

Towne's view

An anteroposterior view taken with the CM line at right

angles to the film, the interpupillary plane being parallel to the film; the X-ray beam is angled 30° in caudad direction (Fig. 7.10).

Aim of Towne's view (Fig. 7.11): this is not a classic facial bone view but is included for completeness, as it is one of the major views performed for head injuries. However, the zygomatic arches can be quite well seen, as are the mandibular rami and condylar necks. In fact the condyles and necks can be well seen on modified, coned views in this projection. The primary aim is to 'reveal' the

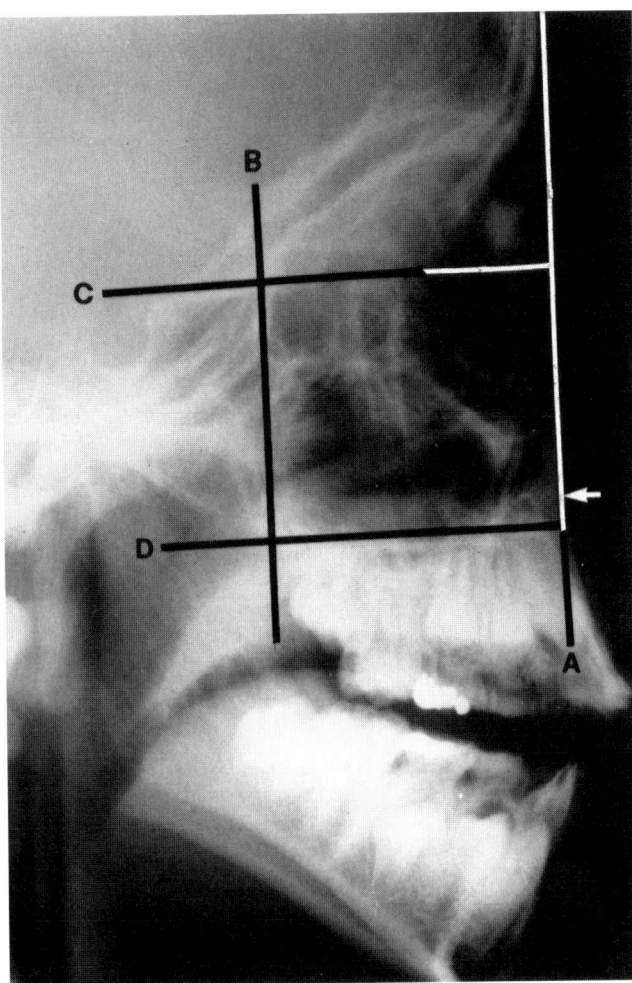

Fig. 7.3 Dolan's square in the lateral view. The square is formed from four lines. Line A connects the frontal sinus surface and anterior hard palate and should parallel the posterior vertical line B connecting the sphenoid wing and posterior edge of hard palate. Line C along the planum sphenoidale/cribriform plate should parallel line D along the nasal surface of the hard palate. Facial fractures (and developmental defects) may deform the square. White arrow indicates anterior wall of maxilla which should be scrutinized for fracture. Note malar struts posterior to this.

lower parts of the occipital bones (which are obscured on the Caldwell view) so that fractures are not missed (bearing in mind the general advice that overexposed 'black' films are better for fracture assessment). The dorsum sellae is projected over the foramen magnum. The lambdoid sutures may be diastased with trauma. The petrous bones are well seen. The transverse occipital lucencies corresponding to the grooves for the transverse venous sinuses are usually obvious. A 'slit' Towne's view was used prior to CT scanning to assess the size of the internal auditory canals.

Additional views

Additional views for mandibular fractures (see below)

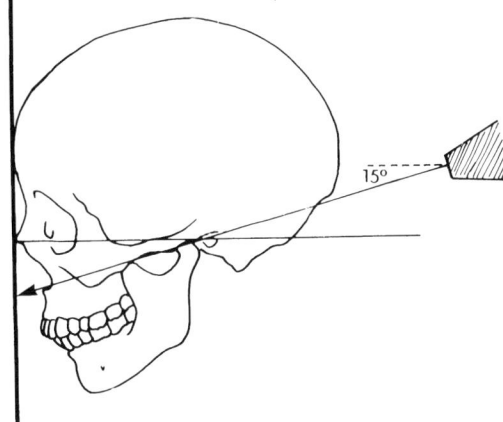

Fig. 7.4 Caldwell view: the projection. The diagram shows the 15° postero-anterior view.

include lateral oblique films (to highlight the anterior body, ramus angle and condyle), a true postero-anterior view, a slit Towne's view, and occlusal films (p. 348). However, clinical diagnosis supplemented by an ortho-pantomogram will often be sufficient.

Nasal bone fractures are best seen on an under-penetrated coned lateral view, allied with coned axial views. A fractured anterior nasal spine is also seen on the lateral view; this finding is important, as it may indicate that there is significant nasal septum damage.

If a fracture of the skull base is thought to involve the petrous temporal bones, special mastoid and petrous views may be needed; these are described in standard radiographic textbooks. However, thin section CT using a bone algorithm is now the examination of choice.

Cephalometry

We routinely use the cephalostat, combined with the OPG, in assessing residual deformity when corrective surgery is contemplated (see Ch. 21). Anteroposterior, lateral and basal views are obtained, the whole head being shown on each film to give the maximum number of craniofacial reference points for measurement of morphological changes before and after operative correction. We insist on scrupulous cephalostat technique so that there are no variations between examinations in the same patient. When the lateral view is taken, it is essential that the patient has the posterior teeth in contact and the mandible in maximum retrusion. A facial filter is used to show the lateral soft-tissue profile as well as the bone profile; the lips must be relaxed and not pursed or in a grimace.

Sialography

Sialography is occasionally necesary in facial trauma. The

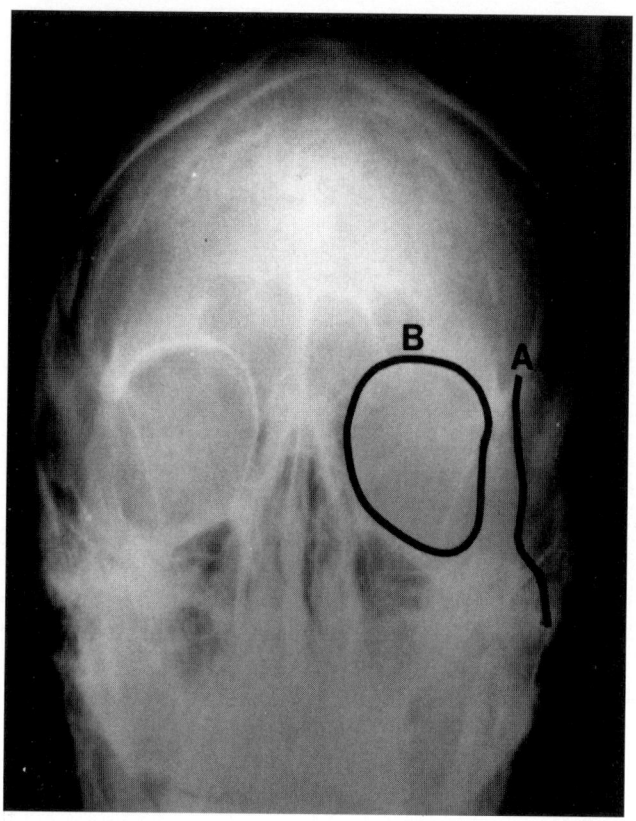

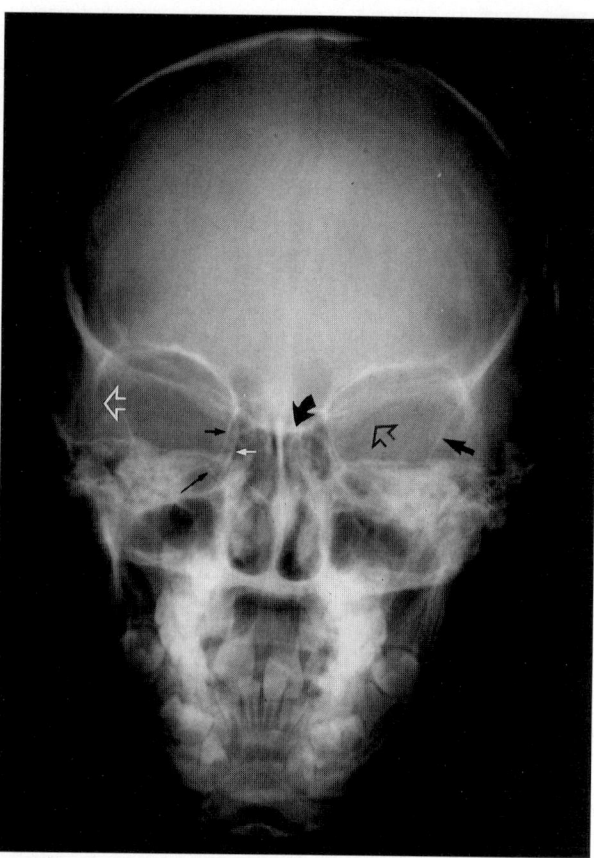

A

B

Fig. 7.5 Caldwell view: the landmarks. A This is a steeply angled Caldwell, projecting the petrous ridges well below the orbit floors. The lateral line follows the orbital process of the frontal bone, the surface of the orbital process of the zygoma, and the superior zygomatic arch. The line of the orbital margin is obvious: on a straighter Caldwell, two lines form the lower medial orbital margin: the line of continuity follows the more medial line (the posterior lacrimal crest). **B** In this case, the petrous ridges are projected over the lower orbits. This makes assessment of the floors of the orbits difficult. Otherwise the orbit margins are well seen. The zygomaticofrontal sutures are poorly defined; the right one is indicated by an open white arrow. The piriform nasal aperture is well seen, as well as the bony nasal septum. Note the 'double' medial orbital margin on the right due to the (medial) posterior lacrimal crest (small white arrow) and the (lateral) lamina papyracea (small black arrow). The left superior orbital fissure (open black arrow) divides the (superomedial) lesser sphenoid wing from the (inferolateral) greater wing. The curved black arrow indicates the combination of the left planum sphenoidale and fovea ethmoidalis; the arrow overlies the left frontal sinus whose density should be roughly that of the orbit. This is also a good view for the ethmoidal sinuses. The innominate (oblique orbital) line is shown (larger straight black arrow) and is the orbital process of the sphenoid bone. The heights of orbits roughly equate to the maxillary sinuses. A long thin black arrow shows the right foramen rotundum. Note displaced upper right central incisor due to trauma.

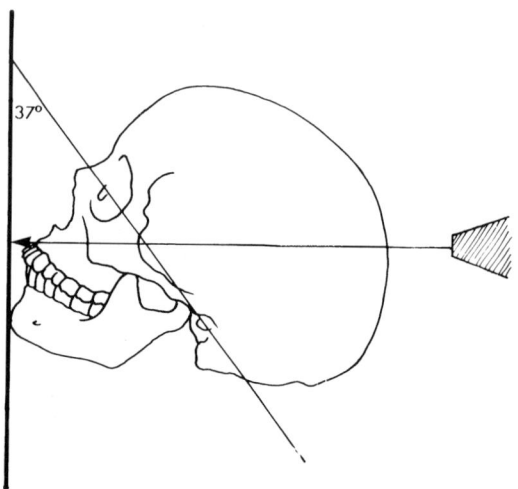

Fig. 7.6 Waters view: the projection. The diagram shows the 37° occipitomental view.

technique involves injection of a contrast agent into a salivary duct. Oily agents have been used in the past but they can produce chemical irritation of the tissues with extravasation, and water-soluble agents are now preferred. A metal cannula is used attached to a long catheter which can be left in the duct after injection. The injection can be combined with screening. Sialography is usually done to visualize the parotid duct, which may be lacerated or transected. Lateral/oblique, lateral and frontal views are standard; a CT examination can be employed.

Dacryocystography

Conventional dacryocystography is done by injection of water-soluble contrast via a fine cannula and catheter into one of the two puncta, usually the lower. Occipitomental and lateral radiographs are taken during the injection.

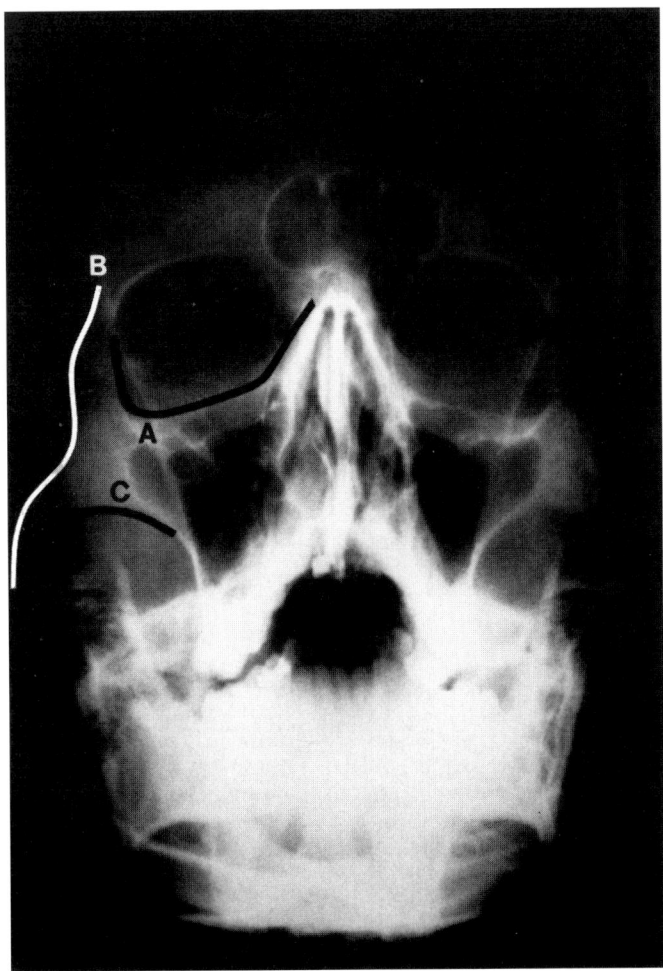

A

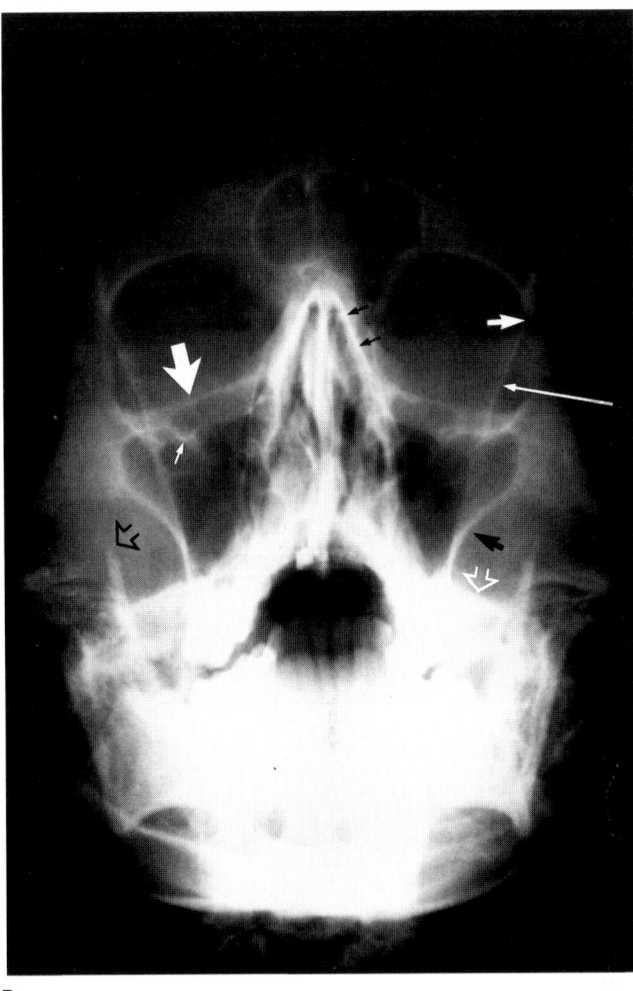

B

Fig. 7.7 Waters view: the landmarks. A Imaginary lines of continuity have been drawn; these should be smoothly continuous lines. Line A: resembles a pair of half-frame reading glasses and extends from the inner aspect of the zygoma and maxilla, frontal process of maxilla and the nasal bone arch. Line B: extends from outer aspects of zygomaticofrontal suture, along the upper border of the zygomatic arch, curving medially to the glenoid fossa of the temporomandibular joint. Line C: extends from the root of the zygoma along the inferior border of the zygomatic arch, lateral wall of maxilla, to the dento-alveolar margin. Lines B and C enclose an area resembling a side view of an 'elephant's head and trunk'.
B This view can be coned down to give the classic paranasal sinus view. Note how the left petrous ridge (open white arrow) is projected just below the maxillary sinus, allowing good assessment of the lateral wall of the maxilla (small solid black arrow) for a possible fracture. The zygomatic bones with their processes are well seen, also the zygomaticofrontal sutures. The inferior orbital margins are sometimes difficult to assess, appearing as a double line here (due to the oblique ray); the superior of the two lines is the actual margin (large white arrow). The infraorbital canals are seen (short white arrow). The nasal bones are well seen 'end-on' with no displacements (two tiny black arrows). The piriform aperture is seen rather obliquely and the bony nasal septum is better assessed on the Caldwell view. The frontal and maxillary sinuses are well seen but the ethmoids are not (best seen on the Caldwell). The orbital margins overall are well viewed. Oblique orbital (innominate) lines are noted (long white arrow). A reasonable view of the maxillary dental arch is obtained and the symmetry of the mandible is noted; the coronoid process is indicated (open black arrow).

Modifications of this basic technique include magnification (macrodacryocystography: Hurwitz et al 1975, 1976), tomography, and subtraction; these supplementary techniques improve the detail of the imaging of the lacrimal system.

Angiography

Intracranial, facial and cervical angiography, perhaps combined with embolization (p. 228), may occasionally be needed to locate and treat traumatic or pre-existing vascular lesions, such as arterial laceration, intimal tears, thrombosis, aneurysm and arteriovenous fistulae, e.g. carotid–cavernous. The carotid arteries are usually catheterized via the femoral artery. Magnetic resonance angiography now has an important part to play in the diagnosis of vascular injury.

Conventional tomography

If CT is available, conventional tomography is out-dated; CT offers soft tissue contrast, improved bone detail,

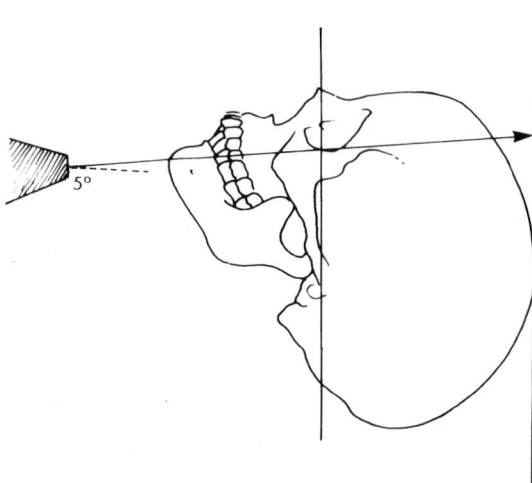

Fig. 7.8 Basal view: the projection. The diagram shows the submento-vertical view.

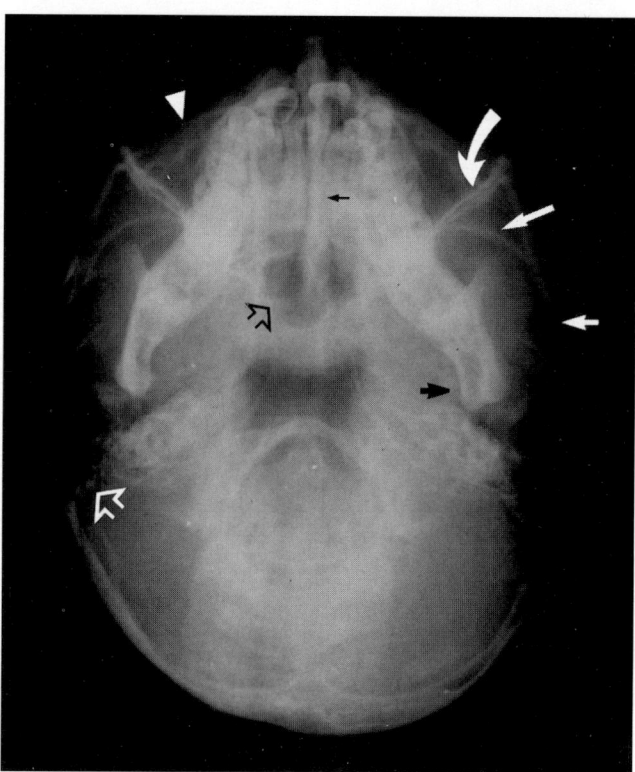

Fig. 7.9 Basal view: the landmarks. This is rarely requested now in the context of acute facial injury. It is a difficult and potentially dangerous view to take and CT has rendered it almost redundant. However, a base view is still done as part of a cephalostat series for a follow-up study. It shows asymmetry well. If rather underexposed, the zygomatic arches (short white arrow) are well seen together with lateral wall of maxillary sinuses and orbits (curved white arrow). A posterior displacement of the anterior maxilla (white arrowhead) and inferior orbital margin may be shown. The relationship of condyles (large black arrow) to articular fossae is quite well seen, as is displacement of the coronoid process. Medial tilting of a fractured condyle may be well seen. The greater wings of sphenoid forming the anterior limits of the middle cranial fossae and the posterior walls of orbits are well seen (long white arrow). The bony nasal septum (small black arrow) posterior ethmoid and sphenoidal sinuses (open black arrow) are always seen. The mastoid air cells should be compared for possible opacification due to bleeding in cases of temporal bone fracture (open white arrow).

and lower radiation dosage. The raw data obtained by CT in the axial (transverse) plane can be reformatted to give various tissue planes, notably the coronal or parasagittal planes; the reformatted images give poorer spatial resolution than conventional tomography but are sufficient for most clinical needs. The advantages of CT have led to the supersession of pluridimensional tomography (Zilkha 1982; Brant-Zawadzki et al 1982; Cooper et al 1983).

However, one form of non-computed tomography has enormous practical value, namely orthopantomography (OPG), also known as panoramic radiography (Fig. 7.12). This investigation has revolutionized the radiography of the jaws and teeth. If the patient's condition permits, an OPG should always be obtained when damage to the mandible, temporomandibular joint or teeth is suspected. The OPG gives a good overall view of the mandible, and by altering centering levels when the film is taken, one can highlight the maxilla or the temporomandibular joint. Misdiagnosis is nevertheless possible: there is variable tomographic blurring of the image in the incisor area, which can mask a subtle fracture, and overlying linear lucencies from the airways can mimic a fracture. Significant traumatic distortion of the mandible will distort the image because the bone is no longer in the plane of focus. Although often diagnostic in its own right, the panoramic radiograph can be viewed as a screening study, supplemented by views such as intraoral, lateral oblique or postero-anterior radiographs, when greater detail is needed. The OPG shows the vertical extent and density of alveolar bone and also the proximity of the inferior dental neurovascular bundle and the antra; these findings are helpful in planning where to site a fixation plate, or in a patient for whom osseo-integrated alveolar implants may be suitable (p. 637).

Computed tomography

CT is a major diagnostic tool in CMF surgery and of great importance in presurgical assessment, planning and evaluation. CT provides an unimpeded visualization of the cranial skeleton and the surrounding soft tissues: this greatly facilitates the understanding of the spatial relationship between disrupted and normal structures, including the brain and the larger intracranial blood vessels as well as the calvarial and facial bones.

In standard diagnostic CT, where the prime concern is the display of a specific area of interest, the scanned region will be restricted to that area. However, for diagnostic imaging of patients with panfacial craniofacial trauma, an overview is very useful and a scan of the

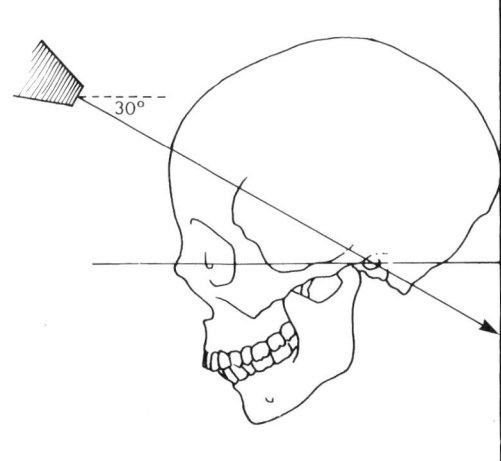

Fig. 7.10 Towne's view: the projection. The diagram shows the 30° oblique half-axial view.

entire head is usually required, from chin to cranial vertex. Modern scanners can achieve this very rapidly.

CT is rapidly evolving. Advances in computers, X-ray tube cooling, generators, and detector technology are reducing scan times and radiation doses, while image quality and fidelity are improving.

Digital storage of the CT data permits retrieval for later use, when advantage can be taken of technological improvements. This is a significant gain, because with better analytical systems, greater use can be made of past data to understand better the various forms of CMF trauma.

To maximize the clinical and research benefits of the CT radiographic examination standardized scanning protocols should be followed (David et al 1990, Herman 1991). These ensure that the most useful data are collected and facilitate comparison between scans so that experience is gained in interpreting the images. The standard protocols also allow comparable information to be collected by different machines to form a database for ongoing research. The adherence to protocols renders the procedure routine and increases efficiency. Special circumstances may arise where the CT scanning procedure needs to be modified but the protocol will act as a guide to the quality required.

The following factors should be considered when establishing scanning protocols:

- Patient positioning and stabilization
- The request form
- Scanning procedure
- Photography of slice data
- Two-dimensional (2D) CT scanning
- Three-dimensional (3D) CT reconstructions
- Storage
- Artefacts.

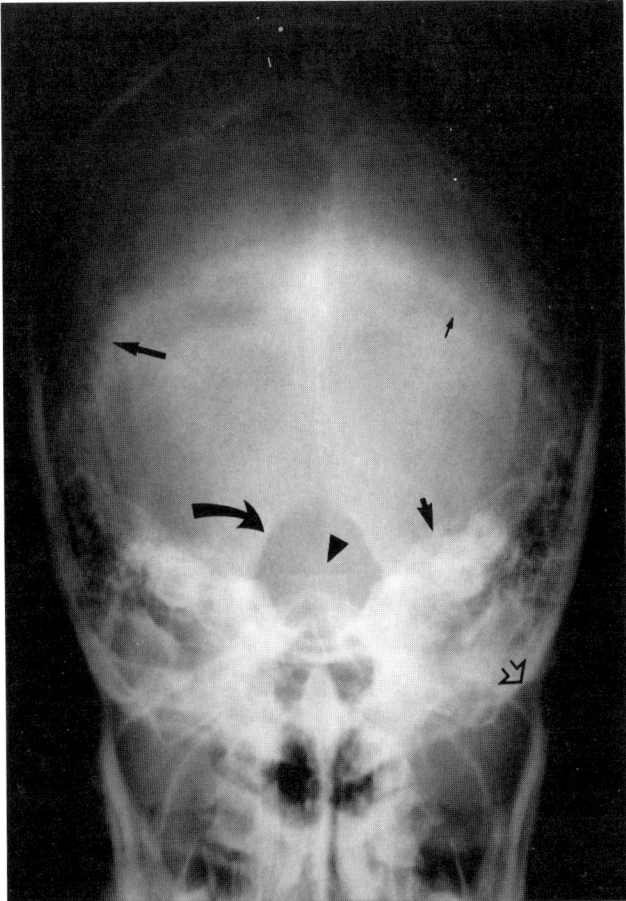

Fig. 7.11 Towne's view: the landmarks. The occipital bone is well seen, forming the margin of the foramen magnum (curved arrow). Fractures around the posterior part of this foramen must not be mistaken for normal sutures in this area, seen in the young, or a persisting metopic suture (which will 'traverse' the margin of the foramen). The dorsum sellae (arrowhead), right lambdoid suture (large straight arrow) and groove for the left transverse sinus (small arrow) and the left petrous ridge (intermediate arrow) are all indicated. The left mandibular condyle (open arrow) and its neck and associated ramus are also seen. Although the density of the occipital bone is good for appraisal, the cranial vault and zygomatic arches are 'blacked-out' and need assessment using a bright light.

Patient positioning and stabilization

For each CT examination, care needs to be taken to ensure that the patient does not move. It is necessary to sedate or give general anaesthesia to young children and other patients whose cooperation cannot be assured.

In general the patient's head should be centred and not rotated within the head holder and aligned so that the orbitomeatal line (Frankfort Horizontal Line) is perpendicular to the floor. An exception is when direct coronal scanning is indicated, either supine or prone, provided the patient can tolerate this procedure. Positions are maintained by the use of straps.

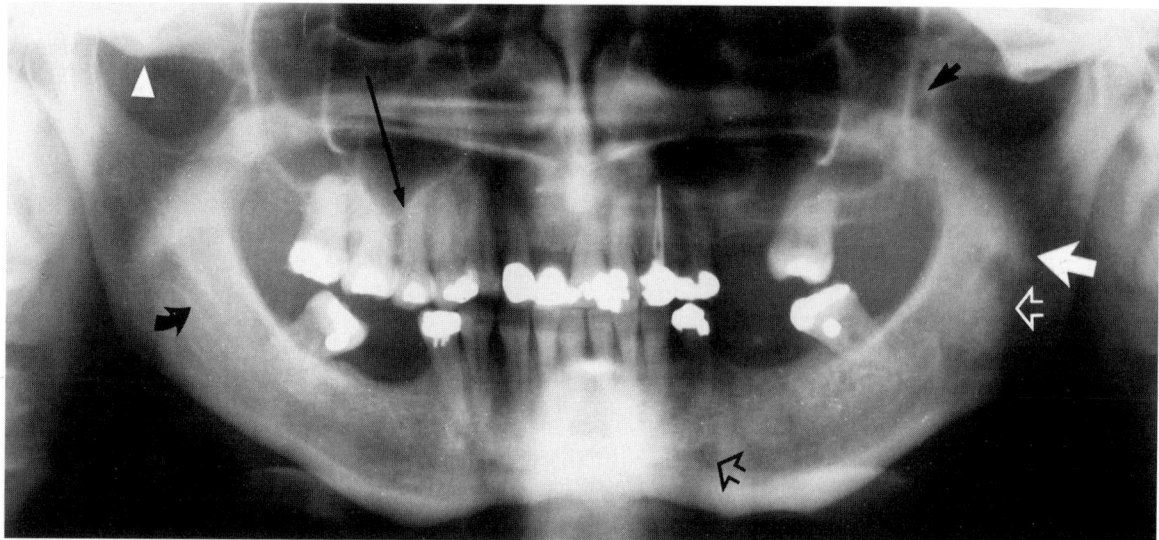

Fig. 7.12 Orthopantomogram. This shows overall tomographic blurring — a subtle undisplaced fracture could be missed (particularly of condyles or symphysis). This technique is prone to midline blurring/opacification but modern machines give much improved images and a splendid overall display of dentition. The state of the alveolar bone should be noted and the relationship of maxillary teeth to adjacent maxillary sinuses (long black arrow). Any suspect unclear area is examined by intraoral films. The position of teeth relative to the inferior dental canal is noted (curved black arrow). Open black arrow indicates the mental foramen. Caries, periapical lucencies, periodontal disease and extractions, restorations and root fillings should be commented upon. Sinus disease, such as a mucus retention cyst may be noted, also the position of the zygomatic arches and the temporomandibular joint articulation. Soft palate (solid white arrow), back of tongue (open white arrow), pterygomaxillary fissure separating posterior wall of maxillary sinus from the pterygoid plates (small black arrow) and zygomatic arch (white arrowhead) are seen.

The request form

The examination may be vitiated by incomplete information. Clinical details are needed to guide the CT technician and radiologist to carry out an appropriate primary investigation. Repeated examinations to clarify the findings of the initial scan are costly, time-consuming and an irradiation hazard; if possible, they should be avoided. The standardized request form described above is intended to do this.

Scanning procedure

The scanning procedure should be standardized and will depend on the nature of the injury and on the available facilities. The nature of the trauma will influence the extent of the scan, and the resolution, slice thickness and slice separation required. Often high resolution is required for the principal region of interest, while a lower resolution will suffice for surrounding regions: the trade-off is resolution against scan time and radiation dose.

The quality of 3D CT reconstructions depends largely on the thickness and separation of the acquired slice data. At the Women's and Children's Hospital, Adelaide, a GE HiSpeed Advantage helical CT scanner is now used. The standard protocol is helical scanning with a pitch of one and a bream of 3 mm. Intermediate slices are created retrospectively to provide effectively 3 mm slices at a

separation of 1.5 mm. When optimum bone demonstration is needed, for example in visualizing the orbits, temporomandibular joints and petrous bones, 1 mm slices are used. Appendix II gives our protocols for orbital trauma (midfacial fracture, blow-out orbital fracture, frontal fracture), occlusal trauma (midfacial and/or mandibular fracture) and panfacial fracture.

In the past, we used International General Electric CTT 8800 scanners, and many of the illustrations in this book were obtained with one of these scanners, or with a now obsolete first generation scanner. Such scanners are still giving good service in many parts of the world; their disadvantages include a long scan time and a long reconstruction time. Helical (spiral) CT scanning, brought into clinical service in 1989, is currently state-of-the-art CT imaging. The helical data set is acquired by moving the scan table at a constant speed while the X-ray tube in the gantry rotates continuously during radiation exposure. Crucial to the technique has been the development of the slip-ring gantry, which permits continuous rotation unhindered by electric cables. This gives fast acquisition of a seamless set of data on a given volume of the body with no spatial or temporal gap, reducing the risk of missing a small lesion by partial volume averaging. We have found helically acquired 3D images superior to non-helical, and see this as now the dominant CT technology; the advantages and limitations are well described by Heiken et al (1993).

2D slices

Viewing 2D CT slice data is a well-established method of assessing facial fractures, particularly those of the middle third of the face. Facial fractures are often complex, defying any short description. The best way to visualize a fracture is to scan at right angles to the bony plane that contains the fracture. An alternative course is to reformat the acquired slice data into the desired plane (Fig. 7.13), but this does to some extent degrade the image, depending on the scanning technique: the thinner the slices, the better are the reformats. Although CT usually shows fracture lines with great elegance, scanning in two planes may be needed to define clearly the line of injury; the axis of the scan can be adjusted to optimize the chance of detecting fractures in certain planes. Thus, direct CT scanning in the coronal plane is needed to show a blow-out fracture of the orbital floor (p. 329) to best effect. Sometimes a fracture line cannot be followed in continuity in the CT scan, and its presence can only be inferred from adjacent but unconnected fracture lines, or from soft-tissue changes such as emphysema. This is probably because the fractured bones, after springing apart on impact, have rebounded to their normal configuration. In such cases, soft tissue injury may be greater than would be expected from the appearances of the bones.

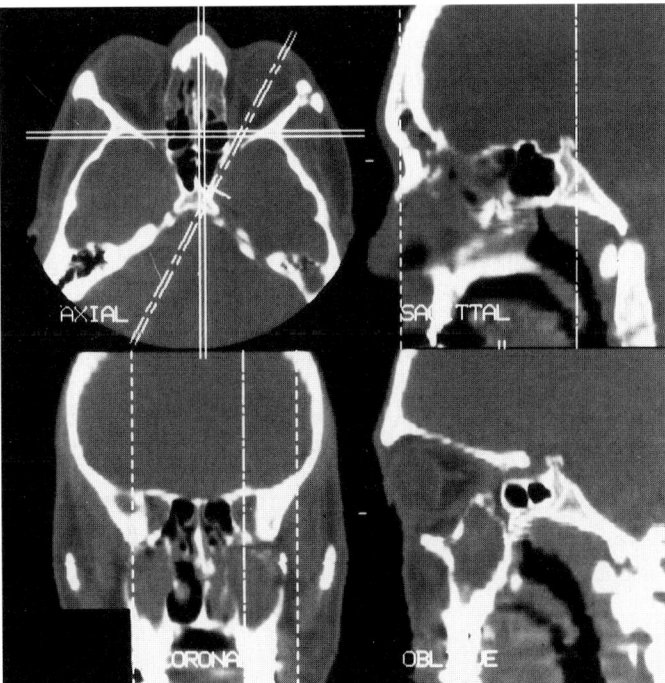

Fig. 7.13 Examples of various CT reformats. Top left: illustrative axial CT section through orbits obtained as part of an axial study of the facial skeleton with three reformation cursors shown (coronal through posterior orbits, oblique sagittal along optic nerve and a midsagittal). The resultant three reformats are shown. Thus, images have been produced without further scannings of the patient but at some sacrifice in detail.

Gentry et al (1983) used high resolution, thin section CT scans of the normal and traumatized anatomy of the face in studies of six cadaver heads to elaborate Le Fort's experimental categorization of fractures of the face (p. 18). They divided the facial skeleton into an inter-communicating system of bony struts or arches in horizontal, sagittal and coronal planes (Fig. 2.15D). When evaluating the CT images of these bony struts there should also be assessment of the adjacent soft-tissue structures (Tables 7.1–7.3). Johnson (1984) described the CT findings in maxillofacial trauma in the light of Gentry's classification, with an additional category of combined plane fractures and with the accompanying soft-tissue injuries (Table 7.4).

Axial CT scanning is now virtually indispensable in managing the severe craniocerebral injuries so often associated with impacts in the CMF region, both for immediate evaluation and in the detection of complications (p. 368). CT scanning after intravenous contrast injection is rarely used in the investigation of facial trauma, and is avoided if possible in acute craniocerebral trauma. However, in diagnosing complications such as brain

Table 7.1 Struts of the horizontal plane (From Gentry et al 1983)

Strut/component	Associated structures
Superior:	
Fovea ethmoidalis/ cribiform plate	Olfactory nerves, dural plate, anterior and posterior ethmoidal nerve and artery, nasal branch of anterior ethmoidal nerve and artery
Orbital roof	Levator palpebrae muscle, superior rectus muscle, superior oblique muscle, optic nerve, structures of anterior cranial fossa
Middle:	
Zygomatic arch	Parotid gland, coronoid process of mandible
Orbital floor	Infraorbital nerve and artery, inferior rectus muscles, inferior oblique muscle, globe
Inferior:	
Hard palate	Incisive foramen, greater and lesser palatine nerve and artery, soft palate

Table 7.2 Struts of the sagittal plane (From Gentry et al 1983)

Strut/component	Associated structures
Median:	
Nasal septum	Nasopalatine artery and nerve
Parasagittal:	
Medial maxillary sinus wall	Nasolacrimal duct, maxillary sinus ostium
Medial orbital wall	Medial rectus muscle, superior oblique muscle, trochlea, anterior and posterior ethmoidal nerve and artery
Lateral:	
Lateral alveolar ridge	Canine, molar, premolar teeth
Lateral maxillary sinus wall	Posterior superior alveolar nerve and artery
Lateral orbital wall	Inferior orbital fissure, superior orbital fissure, lateral rectus muscle, lacrimal gland, structures of middle cranial fossa

Table 7.3 Struts of the coronal plane (From Gentry et al 1983)

Strut/component	Associated structures
Anterior facial:	
Frontal	Supraorbital nerve and artery, lacrimal gland, frontal sinus, anterior cranial fossa
Zygomaticofrontal	Lateral canthal ligament
Nasofrontal	Lacrimal sac, medial canthal ligament/lacrimal crest, nasofrontal duct
Anterior maxillary sinus wall	Anterior superior alveolar nerve and artery, infraorbital nerve and artery
Anterior alveolar ridge	Incisor teeth
Posterior facial:	
Posterior maxillary sinus wall	Internal maxillary artery, pterygopalatine ganglion, pterygomaxillary fissure, pterygopalatine nerve and artery
Pterygoid plates	Skull base, maxillary nerve, torus tubarius, sphenopalatine nerve and artery, posterior nasopharynx

Table 7.4 Combined plane injuries (From Johnson 1984)

A. Fronto-ethmoid complex fractures
   1. Disruption of medial canthal ligament, resulting in telecanthus and epiphora
   2. Injury of the lacrimal sac
   3. Compromise of the nasolacrimal duct

B. Zygomaticofrontal (trimalar) fractures
   1. Soft-tissue injuries described with fracture of lateral struts and orbital floor
   2. Injury to the globe and/or lens

abscess (Fig. 13.12) and subdural empyema (Fig. 13.13) and in the detection of carotid–cavernous fistula, contrast is necessary.

3D CT reconstructions

For the planning and evaluation of CMF injuries, the acquired CT slices, usually axial, can be used as input to programs that produce life-like 3D representations of the skeleton and/or soft tissue, referred to as 3D CT reconstructions. These representations can be viewed from any direction. The 3D CT reconstructions greatly facilitate the surgeons' understanding of the patient's morphology and represent a significant advance in understanding the anatomy of facial fractures (Hemmy et al 1983, Vannier et al 1984, Gillespie et al 1987, Levy et al 1992, Zinreich 1992). The 2D slices indicate the extent and precise nature of the facial injuries, and the 3D CT reconstructions simplify the overall visual perception and facilitate surgical management planning. The two most common approaches to the creation of 3D CT reconstructions are surface and volume rendering.

Surface rendering involves binary segmentation of the data by setting a threshold such that voxels whose X-ray absorption coefficients (density or Hounsfield number) exceed this threshold are included, whereas those voxels whose coefficients are less than the threshold are excluded from the reconstruction. The external surface of the retained voxels is subsequently determined and displayed. However, there is always a trade-off with threshold selection: for example, if the threshold is too low in selecting for bone reconstructions, soft tissue will be included and this may mask skeletal areas of interest. On the other hand, if the threshold is too high, thin bone is not included, giving the appearance of holes, sometimes called pseudoforamina. By referring back to the original slice data it can be determined whether the bony plate is intact. To visualize the relationship between soft tissue and underlying bone, or contrast medium, the appropriate 3D CT surface reconstructions can be merged.

With the other technique, known as volume rendering, a range of voxel densities is displayed so the risk of selecting a threshold that potentially excludes tissues of interest is very much reduced. To view skeletal material, for example, the low density voxels are made more transparent. The low densities associated with soft tissues remain visible and the relationship between bone and soft tissue is apparent.

While 3D CT reconstructions have many applications in facial trauma these should be used as an adjunct to the original 2D axial slices and other reformats for accurate overall assessment. 3D CT reconstructions well demonstrate displaced fractures, depressed fractures, alterations in the shape of the orbit and the sinuses, and subtle surface asymmetry, but undisplaced fractures are seen poorly if at all.

Photography of CT images

The photography of the acquired slice data, reformats and 3D CT reconstructions should be standardized to streamline the investigation and to ensure that the clinician receives all the images that are required. Through the region of principal interest (the high resolution area as described above) every acquired slice should be filmed. Elsewhere, every second or third slice is usually recorded. Depending on clinical requirements two complete sets of films can be produced: one set to look specifically at bone and the other set to look at soft tissue.

The quality of the image as reproduced on film should be assessed using the grey level display placed to one side of each frame to assess possible loss of image definition. If all grey levels cannot be clearly seen then this is indicative of maladjustment of the photographic equipment.

Storage

The research benefits and the potential for further clinical use of the data dictate that the original slice data are retained. Normally this is done on magnetic tape or optical disk.

Artefacts

Artefacts can appear in the original slices, arising from a number of sources, some of which can be readily minimized by good technique. Thus, the radiographer should ensure that there is no patient movement during the scanning procedure, and should remove metallic objects such as jewellery. Non-removable metallic objects such as dental amalgams, physical processes such as beam hardening, and signal processing effects like edge effects also give rise to artefacts that degrade the fidelity and appearance of the images. Wherever possible 'CT-friendly' titanium should be used surgically as it introduces minimal artefacts into CT scan images compared to stainless steel and cobalt–chrome alloys. The reader is referred to general CT textbooks for detailed descriptions relating to appearance and formation of artefacts.

Nuclear scanning

Radioisotopes have a limited role in the evaluation of CMF trauma. When suitably labelled with an appropriate chelate, compounds containing technetium, such as [^{99m}Tc] methylene diphosphonate, provide physiological imaging of the skeleton. Following intravenous injection of the radionuclide, the initial vascular and blood pool images demonstrate the soft-tissue hyperaemia of repair which provides an indication of the potential for fracture union. The delayed images, which are normally obtained 2 h following injection of the isotope, demonstrate the osteoblastic healing response.

In a healthy bone which has been fractured, hyperaemia of repair is detectable at 8–12 h after injury. Evidence of bone turnover at the fracture site is usually present in delayed images 12 h to 3 days after the fracture has occurred. Radioisotope bone scans are therefore extremely sensitive in the detection of fractures.

There is little indication for nuclear medicine evaluation in uncomplicated maxillofacial trauma: the anatomical detail of bone scans is poor compared with other imaging modalities such as standard radiographic projections or CT.

Bone scans may be of some value in detection of occult fractures and also in detection of facial fractures as part of the general skeletal assessment of non-accidental injury in children. In these situations, medicolegal implications are of importance. However, it is in the evaluation of fracture complications that nuclear medicine has a definite role, and especially in the diagnosis of non-union and osteomyelitis. Non-union of mandibular fractures is a not infrequent problem due to the relatively poor vascularity of this bone which is almost entirely dependent on the inferior dental artery (p. 49). The vascular supply of the mandible declines with age and the thin edentulous mandible of an elderly patient is at particular risk of non-union. (In contrast non-union of midface fractures is uncommon because of the rich vascular supply in this region.) Non-union appears in standard radiographic projections as eburnated, rounded bone margins at the fracture site. A bone scan shows absence of the hyperaemia of repair normally seen on the early images at the fracture site. The delayed images demonstrate increased activity within the fracture margins corresponding to increased turnover in the eburnated bone due to rubbing secondary to mobility at the fracture site. This pattern in an isotope bone scan indicates that the fracture will not heal: other measures, such as bone grafting, should be considered.

Osteomyelitis complicating midface fractures is rare, but less uncommon in the mandible. The isotope bone scan typically shows increased activity in both the blood pool and delayed images. This could be confused with the normal response to fracture healing shortly after a fracture has occurred. However, in uncomplicated healing, the initial blood pool phase declines from days to weeks after the injury while persistent uptake is present at the fracture site for 12–18 months. To confirm infection, additional nuclear medicine studies utilizing an isotope which accumulates in white blood cells can be performed; labelling with gallium citrate or indium may be used for this purpose. Nuclear bone scans may also be helpful in assessing abnormalities of the mandibular condyle, such as growth arrest or avascular necrosis.

There are other specialized applications of nuclear imaging. Pertechnetate (^{99m}Tc) eyedrops are used for isotope dacrocystography in cases of post-traumatic epiphora. Isotope dacryocystography is performed by instilling the eyedrops on the cornea in the supine position; a gamma camera is used to follow movement, or absence of movement, down the nasolacrimal duct. The applications are described below (p. 197).

Isotope cisternography was once much used in the diagnosis of CSF rhinorrhoea and other CSF leakages. In this procedure, a radioactive agent is injected by lumbar puncture, and a gamma camera is used to image the flow of CSF in the subarachnoid space and into the nasal cavity if there is a cranionasal fistula. The intrathecal radiopharmaceutical agent favoured by us has been [^{99m}Tc] diethylenetriaminepenta-acetic acid (DTPA). Cisternography by CT scanning after intrathecal injection of a radiological contrast agent has largely superseded isotope cisternography, but the two methods are sometimes combined. The indications and methods are discussed on p. 201.

Positron emission and single photon emission tomography

Positron emission tomography (PET) provides a measure of regional cerebral metabolism; glucose metabolism is usually studied. The high cost of this examination, and the associated logistic problems, have made it unavailable to us.

Single-photon emission tomography (SPECT) provides a cheaper alternative. This technique utilizes a technetium-based radiopharmaceutical ([^{99m}Tc]hexamethylpropyleneamineoxime: HMPAO) together with CT. HMPAO is taken up by the cells of the brain, and hence gives an estimation of cerebral blood flow (CBF) which is based on brain cell activity. Regional distribution does not alter for several hours; imaging can therefore be performed at a convenient time after injection of the radiopharmaceutical.

Since patterns of regional CBF usually reflect cellular metabolic activity or demand, SPECT has promise in defining areas of impaired brain function after head injury. P. L. Reilly (personal communication) has compared SPECT and CT scans in 10 patients comatose after acute head injuries: SPECT showed some 40% of the lesions seen in CT scans, but also showed a number of focal areas of presumed physiological impairment that were not evident in CT scans (Fig. 19.16). The utility of SPECT in cases of chronic brain damage is also being explored.

Radiation dose

All the modalities discussed above involve radiation by X-rays or gamma-ray photons, and therefore all have the potential to damage tissues. In the CMF area, the target organ of chief concern is the lens of the eye, and more peripherally the thyroid gland. Although the use of CT scanning entails a relatively low dose, repeated examination or bad technique could result in a dosage above the threshold for radiation induction of a cataract (Siddle & Sim 1990). Radiation dose is multifactorial, and depends among other things on the scanner model and the technique. Machine radiation dose, which is measured in mGy (1 Gy = 100 rads), relates also to the type of X-ray detector and the X-ray source/detector geometry. This multifactorial causation may lead to problems in selecting an appropriate CT scanner with respect to its potential radiation dosage (Poletti et al 1984), especially in children: the dose may vary even in individual versions of the same model. With modern CT scanners, it is possible to lower the dosage by reducing the milliamperage to between 80 and 120. This is now standard practice and gives adequate bone detail in the CMF region, though the soft-tissue contrast may suffer. The technique of scanning with overlapping slices, described above, does produce an increased dose. Manufacturers may give statistics on the dose delivered by an X-ray machine, but these should be read with caution as the craniofacial techniques to be used may deliver different doses; it is better, when the machine is purchased, to measure dosage in the indicated procedures, and to check it from time to time. Actual figures are very reassuring to colleagues, patients and parents. It has been suggested (Dalrymple et al 1973, Martin & Harbison 1972) that the threshold dose for cataract is about 4 Gy; the incidence of radiation cataracts is proportional to dose, duration of exposure and age, and single doses of 2 Gy or fractionated doses of 4 Gy can cause cataracts. Measurements of the dose to the lens with different CT scanners have given levels well below this figure (Siddle et al 1990). In the worst case to be envisaged, with maximum factors for current and voltage, together with the use of overlapping slices, coronal slices, and intravenous contrast, a dose to the lens of 1 Gy is possible: this could reach the threshold level. However, it should be clearly understood that in routine clinical practice the dose to the lens is likely to be less than 0.05 Gy per axial examination. Russell (1984) has given a good overview of the possible dangers in X-ray diagnosis and Cobb (1993) discusses CT in relation to radiation doses.

The nuclear scans described above do not result in high or prolonged levels of radioactivity in the body. The half-life of technetium is short (6 h), and a high photon flux is achieved by doses well within permissible dosages.

NON-IONIZING MODALITIES

Magnetic resonance imaging

At present, our chief use for MRI in craniofacial trauma is to depict injury to the intracranial contents in the subacute and late phases, but there are other important fields for MRI, such as the eye and the orbital contents (Mafee & Peyman 1987, Mafee et al 1987) and the temporomandibular joint (Kaplan et al 1987). MRI is also finding applications in the diagnosis of retropharyngeal and parapharyngeal haematomas, and in imaging vascular lesions, such as carotid–cavernous fistulas and aneurysms. Gentry (1989) has defined the roles of MRI in trauma of the face and brain.

Makow (1989) gives a good account on the physics of this modality. The advantages over CT include exquisite soft–tissue contrast, non-ionizing radiation, and multiplanar capability. Disadvantages include slow scan times, relatively poor bone detail, incompatibility of some life-support systems in the zone of high field strength magnets (Barnett et al 1988), high cost and the potentially dangerous effect on ferromagnetic materials implanted in the body (Crues & Shellock 1988).

CT remains our primary tool in diagnosing acute brain trauma because of its rapidity, and its ability to show the presence and location of intracerebral and extra-cerebral haemorrhage, bony fractures, compressed ('tight') brain, ventricles and subarachnoid space. These findings may dictate urgent surgical or medical intervention, and the CT scan is now almost indispensable in the management of cerebral injuries. The chief deficiency of CT in diagnosing intracranial trauma is in visualizing non-haemorrhagic cortical lesions, axonal shearing injuries and small infarcts; as a rule, these are not visible on CT but may be visible on MRI (Hesselink et al 1988).

Ultrasound

Diagnostic sonography has become a very important imaging tool and its uses continue to proliferate. Its place in imaging the effects of CMF trauma is limited, in our practice, to the intracranial contents in paediatric cases before closure of the anterior fontanelle, and to the eye, for which it is very useful.

In examining the eye, a high frequency 7.5 or 10 MHz 'small parts' probe is used, through a thick layer of sonographic gel or a pad placed over the closed eye; the patient is supine. Alternatively, a waterbath may be used, when the eye can be open. The entire globe is scanned in the axial and sagittal planes, and relevant images are selected for record by films. Scanning during eye movement may demonstrate mobility of detached membranes, a dislocated lens or a foreign body.

A traumatized eye must be scanned with great care; pressure should be applied as little as possible. Open wounds of the eye and the surrounding tissues are contraindications to sonography.

Mensuration using an independent workstation

For acute trauma little quantification is usually undertaken, though measurements of intracranial displacements are often made on 2D CT scans. The imaging modalities are chiefly used by clinicians to define the qualitative extent of injury in relation to anatomical features. Quantitative mensuration plays a greater role in assessing post-traumatic deformity prior to further surgery and for postoperative evaluation; this is evident in the planning and appraisal of corrections of orbital dystopias (p. 566).

Independent high performance graphics workstations provide an environment removed from the data sources which allows detailed analysis of digital diagnostic image data. The decision to invest in such additional equipment depends on the following considerations:

- The clinical need for additional interactive examination of the data
- Whether the images and the software available on the scanner are sufficient to provide all of the required clinical information
- Whether the data are to be used for research purposes where programs may need to be modified to extract additional required information
- The cost relative to the benefits for clinical management and research.

An independent workstation allows greater advantage to be taken of the continuing developments in technology and imaging software.* Data can be loaded from different scanners, and from different imaging modalities (e.g. CT, MRI, PET), and examined and analysed in a similar fashion; the digital data produced by the different systems can be integrated for the same patient. The ability to integrate the complementary information allows for a more complete analysis and interpretation of the data. This has obvious advantages in the clinical evaluation of patients.

In our unit several networked Silicon Graphics workstations (4D/220, Indigo Elan and Indigo2 XZ) are in routine clinical and research use. The software package Persona, developed by our research unit, allows detailed analysis and interpretation of medical image data.

Persona provides an interactive environment for rapid simultaneous viewing of the original slice data, orthogonal and oblique reformats, and 3D CT reconstructions. Knowledge of precise location within the data volume is achieved by displaying the 'active marker' position in all views. Stereoscopic viewing dramatically enhances understanding of the 3D geometry. Predefined landmark prompts are subdivided according to anatomic region to simplify the determination of the positions of anatomical landmarks. These landmarks can then be used to provide distance and angle information regarding the shape of anatomical regions. In addition, the measurement tool can be used to provide this information for points that are not predefined anatomical landmarks. Colour coded wireframe models can be created using the identified landmarks. These can be overlaid on the 3D reconstructions and/or the 2D reformats and are used to facilitate pre- and postoperative comparisons. In addition boundaries in the volume data can be defined using contours and surface meshes for area and volume determination; for example, for measurement of ventricular size, haematoma size and determination of the extent of post-traumatic enophthalmos (Bite et al 1985, Manson et al 1986). Selected area density statistics are also useful for determining whether a collection of fluid contains blood.

The 3D volume data can be used for the production of solid models for subsequent fabrication of custom designed prostheses. First, the position of the custom-designed prosthesis and the extent of the region requiring modelling are determined in planning sessions with the clinician, technician and scientist. Full presurgical planning is essential. If other prosthetic elements are to be added a later date, consultation with suitable specialists should occur at this stage as to the requirements. There are several options for production of the solid model.

---

* Suitable software products include Analyze distributed by Mayo Medical Ventures, Centre Place (4), Mayo Clinic, Rochester, MN 55905, USA; VoxelView distributed by Vital Images, 505 N Fourth Street, Iowa 52556, USA; Persona distributed by Maptek, 210 Glen Osmond Road, Fullarton, South Australia 5063.

Contours for each slice can be produced through the region with a spacing equal to that of the thickness of the plastic sheet. These can be laser-cut or printed onto transparencies for use as templates for hand cutting. However, if available, stereolithography or selective laser sintering techniques are preferable because the potential introduction of errors is minimal.

Independent workstations can also be used for mock surgery: the manipulation and cutting of bone segments on a computer. This is valuable for estimating positional shifts, bone requirements and assessing the potential outcome of various surgical scenarios.

The independent workstation environment with custom software has enabled us to provide better solutions to difficult clinical problems. At present, measurements from 3D image modalities are performed generally only in the larger craniofacial institutions which incorporate active imaging research groups (Abbott et al 1990, Cutting et al 1986, 1987, Marsh et al 1986, Udapa & Herman 1991).

CLINICAL APPLICATIONS

Mandibular fractures

Mandibular imaging includes a panoramic view (OPG), postero-anterior and slit Towne's view, lateral obliques, intraoral views (periapicals and occlusals) and possibly a CT scan.

Mandibular fractures have sites of predilection: the chief sites are the angle/ramus and the body, in roughly equal frequency, followed in decreasing order by the condyle, the symphysis and the coronoid process — the rarest site in our experience. The mandible reacts to trauma as a bony ring and there are often two or more coexisting fractures, e.g. symphysis + bilateral condylar fractures, or body + contralateral subcondylar. Dental and alveolar injury should be noted; involvement of a tooth root makes the fracture compound. The occlusion is checked; malocclusion may be absent in condylar fractures. An apparently unstable fracture of the body should be indicated. Other unstable fractures must also be identified: these include comminuted fractures, displaced subcondylar fractures and angle fractures in an unfavourable plane.

Fractures of the ramus, angle and body are relatively easy to detect. Undisplaced fractures of the mandible can be missed on the panoramic image due to tomographic blurring. Spurious fracture lines can be created by air above the tongue and other superimposed lucencies. The symphysis can also be a difficult area due to bony overlap or tomographic blurring. Skilled clinical assessment and appropriate imaging request details will help to avoid missing a fracture.

Intracapsular fractures are more common in young children. These fractures can appear as a dense and compressed condyle in standard radiographic projections, when CT alone may make the true diagnosis.

Although it is not our routine to ask for a CT scan in isolated mandibular injury, the mandible must be included in the CT scan when assessing associated mid-facial injuries (Fig. 7.14); useful preoperative information concerning the mandible is often discovered. Such information may be extremely helpful to the surgeon when considering open reduction and internal fixation. Knowing the precise geometry of a fracture determines the optimal surgical approach and results in minimal stripping of bone for internal fixation; this promotes healing under stable conditions, and avoids intermaxillary fixation.

In late cases radiology can be used to show a pseudarthrosis or malunion as a sequel of an untreated or inappropriately treated unstable mandibular fracture. Such complications, and also possible supervening infection, are monitored by panoramic radiographs. Infection will produce lucency around the fracture and fixation devices, perhaps with a periosteal reaction; sclerosis may be a later finding. Sequestra should be noted. Isotope bone scanning has a place in the investigation of malunion, growth arrest, avascular necrosis and osteomyelitis.

Temporomandibular (TMJ) joint injuries

The acute pathology of the injured TMJ includes true (intracapsular) condylar fracture, acute haemarthrosis, and internal joint derangement. A normal TMJ may be painful in consequence of contralateral damage — a diagnostic trap. Delayed joint problems include osteoarthritis, condylar hypoplasia in the young, condylar avascular necrosis and TMJ ankylosis (p. 594). TMJ assessment may be needed after a surgical procedure such as arthroplasty, perhaps with a prosthesis.

The joint has been notoriously difficult to image and significant injuries can be missed; Coombs (1992) has given a good overall account of the problems associated with TMJ injury. Study of the TMJ has in the past called for lateral oblique views with jaw open and shut, other customized plain views, single or double-contrast arthrography, pluridirectional tomography, CT combined with arthrography, and MRI. In general, CT scanning is indicated for bony problems and MRI for soft-tissue problems although there is overlap in the utility of the two modalities.

In CT scanning of suspected bony abnormalities, we utilize thin (1–2 mm thick) slices in axial and/or other planes such as coronal and sagittal (Fig. 7.14B). Reformats can be done in planes parallel, or at right angles to, the oblique transverse plane of the condyles, albeit at the expense of some detail. 3D CT reconstructions can be very useful, particularly in visualizing medially displaced condyles, hypoplastic condyles (which may mimic hemifacial microsomia), ankylosis and osteochondral grafts.

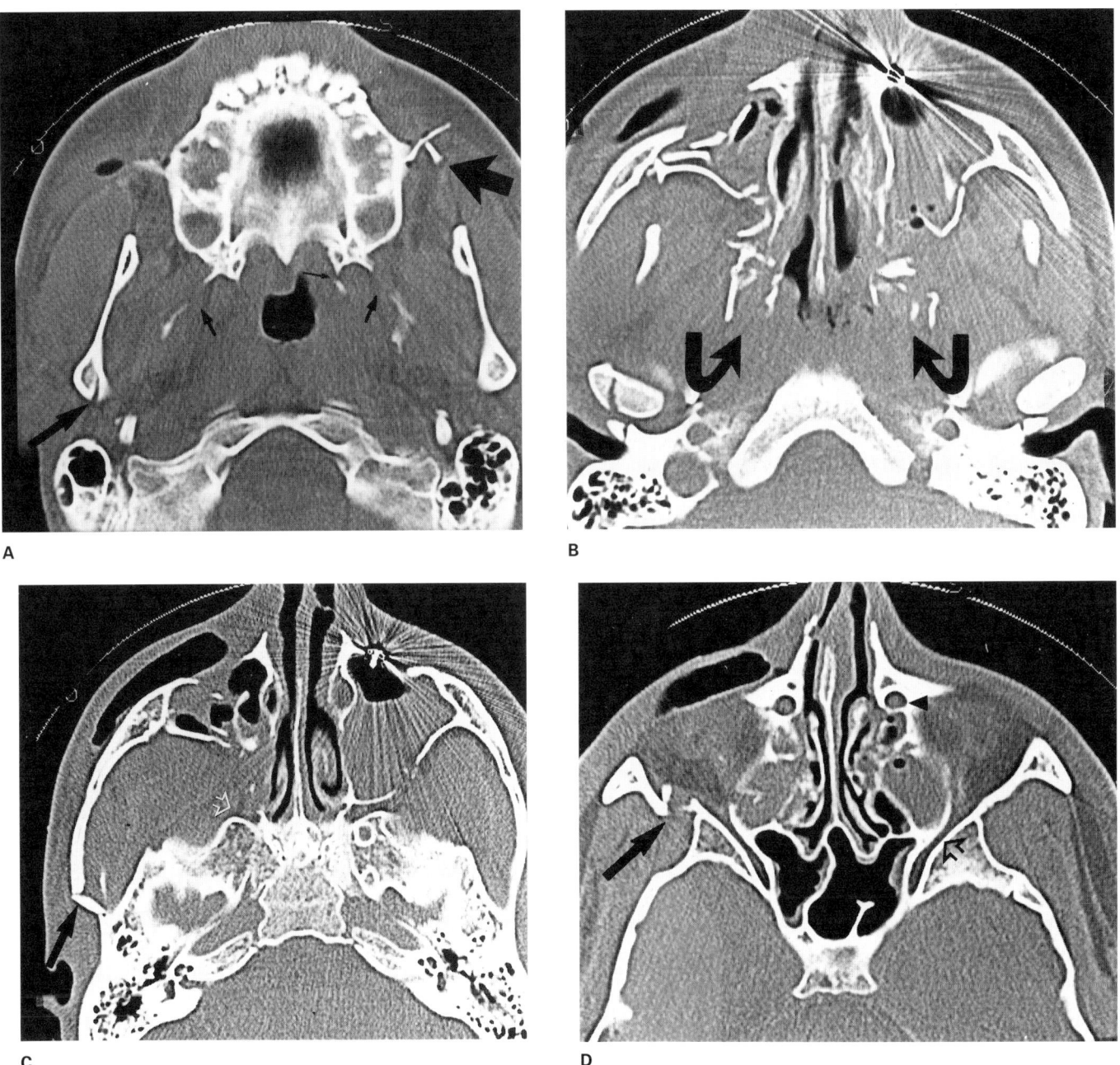

Fig. 7.14 Fracture of mandibular condyle with multiple facial fractures. A Low axial CT section shows fractures of pterygoid plates, an essential finding in Le Fort fractures, also a sagittal fracture of the right condylar neck and a comminuted fracture in the region of the lower margin of the left zygomaticomaxillary suture. **B** A higher section shows the intracapsular component of the right mandibular condyle fracture. There are fractures of the anterior and lateral walls of maxillary sinuses and nasal septum. Fractures of pterygoid plates are confirmed. Metallic artefact on the left is due to a surgical screw — not titanium! There is a further fracture of posterior wall of left maxillary sinus. **C** A section higher than **B** shows gross widening of the right pterygomaxillary fissure (with attendant danger of haemorrhage) due to anterior disruption. Traumatic emphysema of right cheek and a fracture of the posterior right zygomatic arch are seen. Note the asymmetry of zygomatic arches — of great importance to the surgeon. A coronal scan confirmed comminution and depression of the right orbit floor. **D** Highest of all four sections shows fracture of the right lateral orbital wall found in both zygomaticomaxillary complex and Le Fort III fractures. Fractures of nasal bones are present. Note intact nasolacrimal ducts and normal posterior portions of inferior orbital fissures.

Associated temporal bone fractures are studied by thin section CT at the same time.

Post-traumatic internal derangements of the TMJ can be investigated by arthrography, MRI and direct sagittal CT scanning. Choice will depend on the expertise of the radiologist and the availability of equipment. The best procedure at present available is the MRI scan, which gives exquisite soft-tissue detail and does not entail irradiation (Katzberg et al 1986, Westesson et al 1987a,b, Hasso et al 1989). MRI views can be done with the jaw

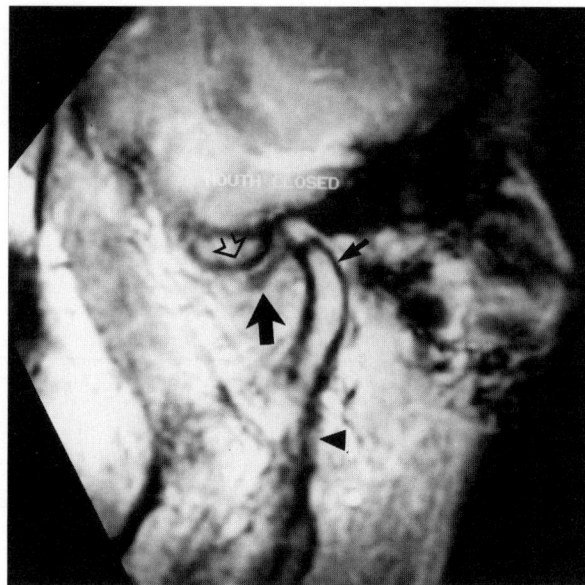

Fig. 7.15 MRI scan showing derangement of the temporo-mandibular joint (TMJ). Sagittal T1-weighted gradient echo MRI scan of left TMJ, part of a kinematic series; mouth closed. Shows anterior subluxation of the articular disc (large black arrow), in relation to articular eminence (open black arrow), condyle (small black arrow), and posterior ramus (black arrow head).

open and shut, and this so-called dynamic scanning is our preferred method, giving some assessment of functional anatomy as well as visualization of structure (Fig. 7.15).

Arthrography also provides a dynamic study of the TMJ meniscus and is as accurate as MRI in diagnosing meniscal derangements. The chief disadvantages of arthrography in comparison with MRI are its discomfort for the patient and its poor capacity to show the internal structure of the meniscus. It is however the only procedure able to visualize the meniscal perforations seen in advanced internal derangements of the TMJ; these are diagnosed when contrast leaks from one compartment to the other through the perforated meniscus.

CT scanning is not as accurate as MRI or arthrography in the diagnosis of internal derangements. In CT scanning, the sagittal plane is optimal; the meniscus can be made to stand out on the CT console or film as a high density structure, and its position can be examined in the open and shut positions of the mouth. MRI has been found very useful in investigating failure of a temporo-mandibular prosthesis (Kneeland et al 1987).

Midface injuries

The midface is an area of the highest complexity and its imaging by high resolution CT has revolutionized the diagnosis and therefore the management of facial injuries. A more critical approach to the analysis of facial fracture management, and the collateral development of advanced internal fixation techniques, has generated the need for very detailed preoperative imaging. Our standard CT scan plane has been axial and if coronal reformats were inadequate in demonstrating injuries in the coronal plane then direct coronal scanning was done provided the patient could tolerate the procedure. Direct coronal scanning is being used with increasing frequency due to shorter scan times possible now. Coronal images appeal visually, as such full frontal views mimic the surgeon's approach to the patient.

3D CT reconstructions are important because they ensure that even subtle deformity of the normal facial morphology is readily recognized, by allowing it to be viewed from multiple aspects. The surgeon, when assessing a Le Fort fracture, looks for a 'key' to restore the vertical height of the midface (Assael 1993). Bringing the maxillary teeth into normal occlusion with the teeth in an intact mandible restores the projection and width of the midface. Establishment of the vertical dimension is then possible by restoration of at least one of the four major midface supporting buttresses: the two piriform rims and the two zygomatic buttresses. Once a single buttress is restored to its pre-injury position, and given two intact condyles and a correct dental occlusion, then the plane is defined that can restore the position of the midface before injury. Once the first buttress position is restored by internal fixation, it will serve as the key to the restoration of the vertical height of the remainder of the face. Direct coronal scans or reformats are very useful in identifying the key buttress.

If all the midface buttresses are too comminuted to act as a key, a lateral cephalometric radiograph can be used with objective measurements to enable the restoration of the vertical height of the face to an arbitrary mean. An improperly positioned maxilla will result in an impaction malunion, readily visible on CT scanning and in cephalometric films. Other CT findings which influence the surgical plan include traumatic abnormalities in the nasal septum, anterior nasal spine fractures, comminution of the palate, and bone or a tooth in a sinus.

Although midfacial fractures often involve more than one bone, it is convenient to consider the details of radiographic investigation of individual bone injuries.

Maxillary injuries

Isolated maxillary fractures are uncommon. The antero-lateral wall of the maxillary sinus may be fractured by direct force. Such a fracture is often hard to see in plain films, and may be confused with a normal marking; if the fracture edges overlap, the film may show a linear density (Merrell et al 1969). An opaque sinus is of course not necessarily evidence of a fracture in its wall. Axial CT best shows these anterior maxillary fractures, though if the edges are impacted, the presence of an injury can only be surmised; in general, coronal CT best shows fractures of the maxilla.

Fractures of the anteromedial antral wall can damage the nasolacrimal duct (Unger 1992), producing epiphora and chronic dacrocystitis. Fractures a little more posterior, as in some Le Fort fractures, can impede drainage of the maxillary antra leading to chronic sinusitis or mucocele formation.

Maxillary alveolar fractures are best seen in occlusal films and in the OPG; they are likely to be associated with displaced teeth and with fractures of the mandible. The radiological visualization of the alveolar elements of the jaws is also relevant in the expanding field of dental implantology (Abrahams 1993). This requires precise mapping of the alveolar bone, perhaps distorted as a late sequel to trauma. Several types of implants are available — rootforms, blades and subperiosteal implants; in making a choice, the height, width and quality of residual alveolus need to be assessed, together with the adjacent maxillary sinuses and inferior dental canals. The OPG and CT scan play a crucial role in this assessment.

The three classic midfacial fracture patterns described by Le Fort in 1901 (pp. 18 and 293) are relatively uncommon, especially in pure form. Asymmetry is virtually the rule, combinations of Le Fort fractures being often found on opposite sides (Fig. 7.16). The fracture lines may be hard to identify, especially when extreme force results in such extensive comminution as to defy precise classification — the so-called panfacial injury (p. 336).

The Le Fort I fracture is a horizontal fracture separating the maxillary alveolus and palate from the superior part of the maxilla, through the walls of the maxillary sinus, creating the 'floating palate'. The lateral radiograph may show a fracture of the anterior maxillary wall and disruption of the pterygoid plates, which are fractured in all Le Fort fractures. An anterior open bite is not uncommon, due to palatal shift: the palate is pushed posterior to line B in Dolan's square (Dolan & Jacoby 1978: see Fig. 7.3).

The Waters view may show fractures of the lateral and medial walls of the maxilla, the vomer and the borders of the piriform aperture. Coronal CT scans show this fracture to best effect, axial scans less well even when reformatted in the coronal plane. The coronal CT scan is therefore the preferred investigation, if the patient's condition makes it possible.

The Le Fort II fracture, if bilateral, is termed the piriform fracture. In the midline it involves the nasion, crosses the ethmoidal complex, the inferior orbital fissure, inferior orbital rim and the posterolateral wall of the maxilla. Bilateral pterygoid fractures are present. The lateral orbital walls and zygomatic arches are intact. This fracture is best seen in a coronal CT scan; this can be combined with an axial study. Where a coronal scan is not feasible, an axial study alone is done, with coronal reformats. Reformats tailored to suit the injury are always done, such as oblique sagittal reformats parallel with the optic nerves through the orbits; these show the orbital floor well. As for all the Le Fort fractures, 3D CT reconstructions are always done. The plain lateral view may show alteration in Dolan's square; the Waters view shows separation of the central piriform fragment, fractures of the lateral maxillary walls and inferior orbital margins, and fractures in the region of the nasion.

The Le Fort III fracture: in this injury, the facial skeleton separates from the skull base–craniofacial disjunction (Fig. 7.16). Starting in the nasofrontal area, the fracture extends across the ethmoid bone to the region of the inferior orbital fissure, then laterally through the lateral wall of the orbit, the zygomatic bone and the pterygoid region. Often the whole face drops, and in plain frontal radiographs the orbits appear to be tall. The plan of CT diagnosis is as described for other Le Fort fractures.

Orbital fractures

Orbital fractures may occur in isolation, or may be associated with other injuries, such as Le Fort II or III fractures, or a zygomaticomaxillary complex fracture. Isolated orbital fractures may involve the orbital rim, the walls or the floor.

The orbital rims are well seen in the combined Waters and Caldwell views. The inferior orbital margin is often hard to identify; on the Waters view, it is seen above the orbital floor, and usually appears thicker. The rim may disappear as the result of rotation and detachment of the inferior orbital rim. This injury can simulate a blow-out fracture; the distinction can be made by CT, especially by coronal scanning or paraxial reformatting. 3D CT reconstructions beautifully demonstrate the orbital margins, allowing easy comparison between the two sides and identifying subtle asymmetries not seen in axial slices.

Fractures of the orbital walls are usually inferior and/or medial blow-out fractures (p. 326), or fractures of the lateral wall associated with a zygomatic fracture. Blow-out fractures are termed pure when the rim is spared, and impure when it is involved.

In inferior blow-out fractures, the orbital floor is fractured posteriorly, medial to the infraorbital groove, with inferior displacement of a fragment or fragments; if the displaced fragment is large, there may be enophthalmos and diplopia. The orbital contents can herniate into the maxillary antrum if the periosteum and bony floor are disrupted: the herniation involves primarily the posterior inferior pad of fat, lying between the periosteum of the orbital floor and the inferior rectus and inferior oblique muscles (Figs 7.17 and 7.18). This pad has a rich venous plexus and many fibrous strands running from the extraocular muscles and the periosteum; oedema, bleeding and dislocation of the pad of fat may lead to restriction of the eye movements from tension in the inferior rectus

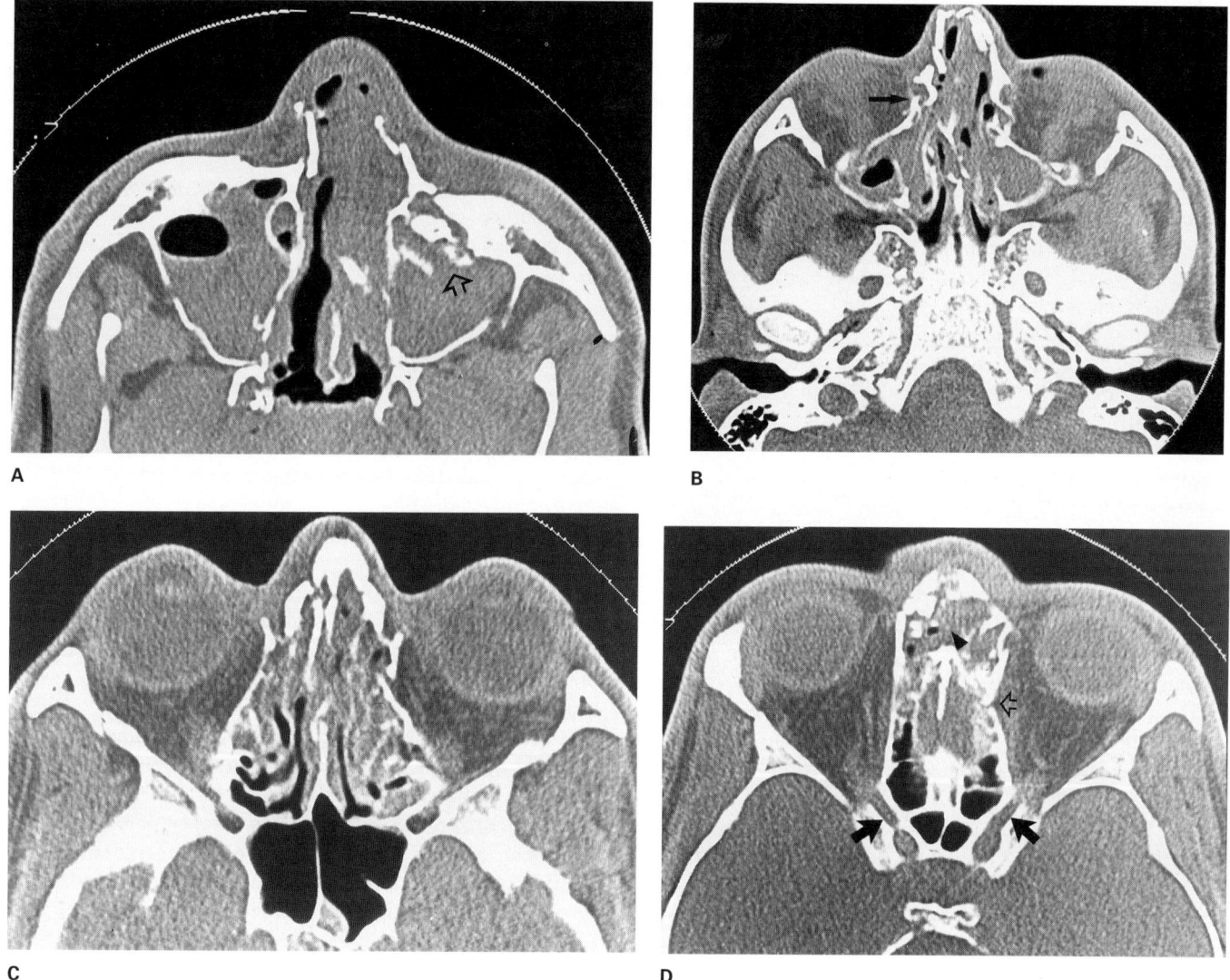

Fig. 7.16 Le Fort III fracture. Le Fort III fracture with 'smash': injury element, fractured left zygomatic and left medial orbit 'blow-out' fracture. **A** Lowest axial CT section shows fracture of right medial pterygoid plate (probably also on left), fractures of anterior, lateral and medial walls of both maxillary sinuses, fractures and displacements of the frontal processes of maxillae, both nasal bones, bony nasal septum. The floor of the left orbit appears fragmented (open arrow) and depressed (and needs coronal reformats or a direct coronal scan to fully detail). Fluid level in right maxillary sinus. **B** Higher axial CT section. A fracture of the posterior wall of the origin of the right nasolacrimal duct is shown (arrow), and of the posterior left zygomatic arch. **C** Higher axial CT section shows some depression of the anterior naso-ethmoidal complex with opaque ethmoidal sinuses. Fractures of the lateral orbit walls. **D** Highest axial CT section shows medial deviation of the medial wall of the left orbit (open black arrow) which can produce enophthalmus. Comminution around the region of the foramen caecum (black arrowhead) may well involve the frontonasal ducts (frontal recesses). The optic canals (solid black arrows) are intact.

muscle, and so cause diplopia. Actual muscle entrapment is believed to be less common.

The medial orbital blow-out fracture through the thin lamina papyracea is less often seen, and may occur in association with a fracture of the floor (Fig. 7.19). However, it is likely that in the past these fractures were often missed, especially before the advent of CT; in our experience this has indeed been the fracture most often missed. It is important to search for the medial wall fracture in acute orbital injury, as persisting enophthalmos complicating such a fracture may be hard to treat at a later stage (p. 559).

Anterior orbital injury may lacerate the lacrimal sac or the proximal part of the nasolacrimal duct. Injury to the lacrimal drainage system may be indirect, resulting from avulsion of the medial canthal ligament, the integrity of which is necessary for satisfactory drainage (p. 66). CT will not show this injury but it may be inferred if the CT shows bony injury of the anterior lacrimal crest. This avulsion produces telecanthus, epiphora and chronic dacrocystitis. Entrapment of the medial rectus muscle is rare — indeed, we have not seen it.

Much information can be gained from standard radiographic projections of the orbital region (Hammerschlag

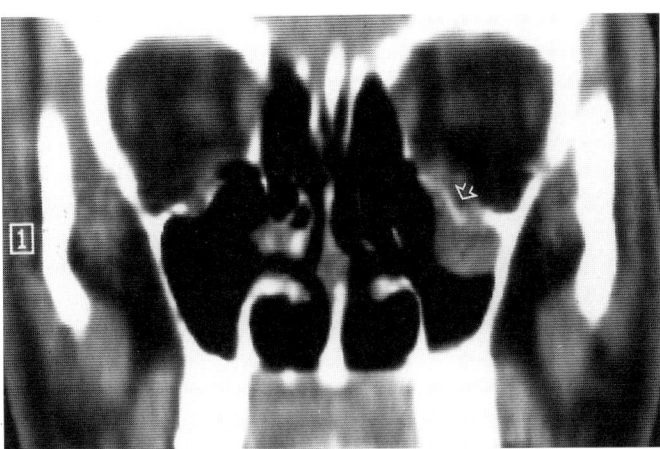

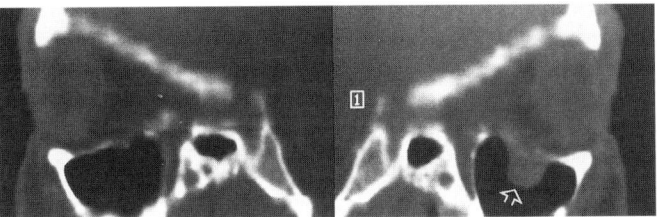

Fig. 7.17 Inferior orbital blow-out fracture: CT diagnosis.
A Direct coronal CT section shows the 'tear-drop' of intraorbital fat herniated into the left maxillary sinus with associated inferior tilting of the bony floor of the orbit (open white arrow). The inferior rectus is probably in a normal position; if significantly displaced, it may pull the medial rectus down as well — an indirect sign. The herniation of soft tissue was observed on the axial view but bony disruption was not clearly suggested. **B** Oblique sagittal CT reformat through orbits parallel to optic nerves. This clearly shows the left 'tear-drop' (open white arrow).

et al 1982). In a blow-out of the floor, the Waters view will usually show a 'tear drop' of herniated soft tissue in the roof of the maxillary sinus; however, this may be obscured if the sinus is opacified by blood. The Waters view may also show a fragment of depressed bone (Merrell et al 1969). In a medial blow-out fracture, the ethmoid air cells are opacified, and sometimes one may see medial displacement of the lamina papyracea on the Caldwell view.

CT will show unequivocally both the soft-tissue damage and the fractures. If an inferior blow-out fracture is suspected either clinically or from plain films, a direct coronal scan is done, or a coronal reformat is obtained from a thin-slice axial study. The scan plane is at right angles to the plane of the orbital floor, and the extent of the scan is taken from the orbital rim to clear the apex of the orbit. This scan will also show a fracture of the medial wall, and a zygomaticomaxillary complex fracture. The slices are filmed with suitable magnification and at both soft tissue and bone windows. Other reformats can also be done; the oblique reformat through the eye, lens and optic canal is particularly useful to show the orbital floor.

Direct oblique sagittal CT scanning is reported to give better visualization of the inferior rectus muscle (Ball 1987). Whereas axial CT scanning is not very useful to visualize a blow-out fracture of the floor, it will show a blow-out of the medial wall well; an axial scan taken in a plane parallel to the cribriform plate may usefully amplify the coronal scan to give the surgeon a bird's eye view of the orbit in planning to insert bone grafts in the medial orbital wall.

Particular attention should be directed to the optic nerve itself and the optic canal. Fractures of the canal often have sinister significance; the optic nerve may be contused, or compressed by bony fragments and/or intra-orbital haematoma, or even transected. Coronal and oblique sagittal CT scans are needed to visualize this region, because the nerve has a serpiginous course. MRI has a definite place in visualizing the optic nerve, but is of little value in delineating the bony canal.

CT scan may show pathological abnormalities within the orbit, and this may be very helpful when orbital swelling prevents external examination. There may be a sub-periosteal orbital haematoma, which can become a chronic haematocele and may then require drainage. Orbital dystopia is well seen on 3D CT reconstructions. Post-traumatic hypertelorism is well shown on coronal and axial 2D CT images, from which measurements can be made.

Encroachment on the superior orbital fissure by bone, haematoma or foreign body can produce a superior orbital fissure syndrome involving the third, fourth, sixth and ophthalmic division of the fifth cranial nerves.

Although air is not uncommonly seen trapped under the eyelids in the injured patient, this finding should be distinguished from orbital emphysema, which implies that air has escaped from the ethmoid or maxillary sinuses — sometimes under tension (Fig. 7.20).

3D CT reconstructions are not very useful in showing orbital fractures, and one should be aware of partial voluming effects in thin but intact orbital plates; 3D reconstructions may, however, be needed to visualize adjacent fractures. 3D volumetric display can provide estimates of orbital volume as well as area measurements, and these can be useful in planning the treatment of enophthalmos. Sagittal MRI scans are very useful to delineate the soft tissues, including the inferior rectus muscle.

Since the decision to explore the isolated fracture of the orbital floor is rarely taken at once, the CT investigation may be deferred for up to 10 days to allow blood to be cleared from the maxillary sinus: this gives optimal visualization of the orbital floor by air contrast.

Fractures of the lateral orbital wall are often combined with zygomatic fractures with diastasis or displacement at the zygomaticofrontal suture and the zygomaticosphenoid suture. The lateral wall is best seen in axial CT scans

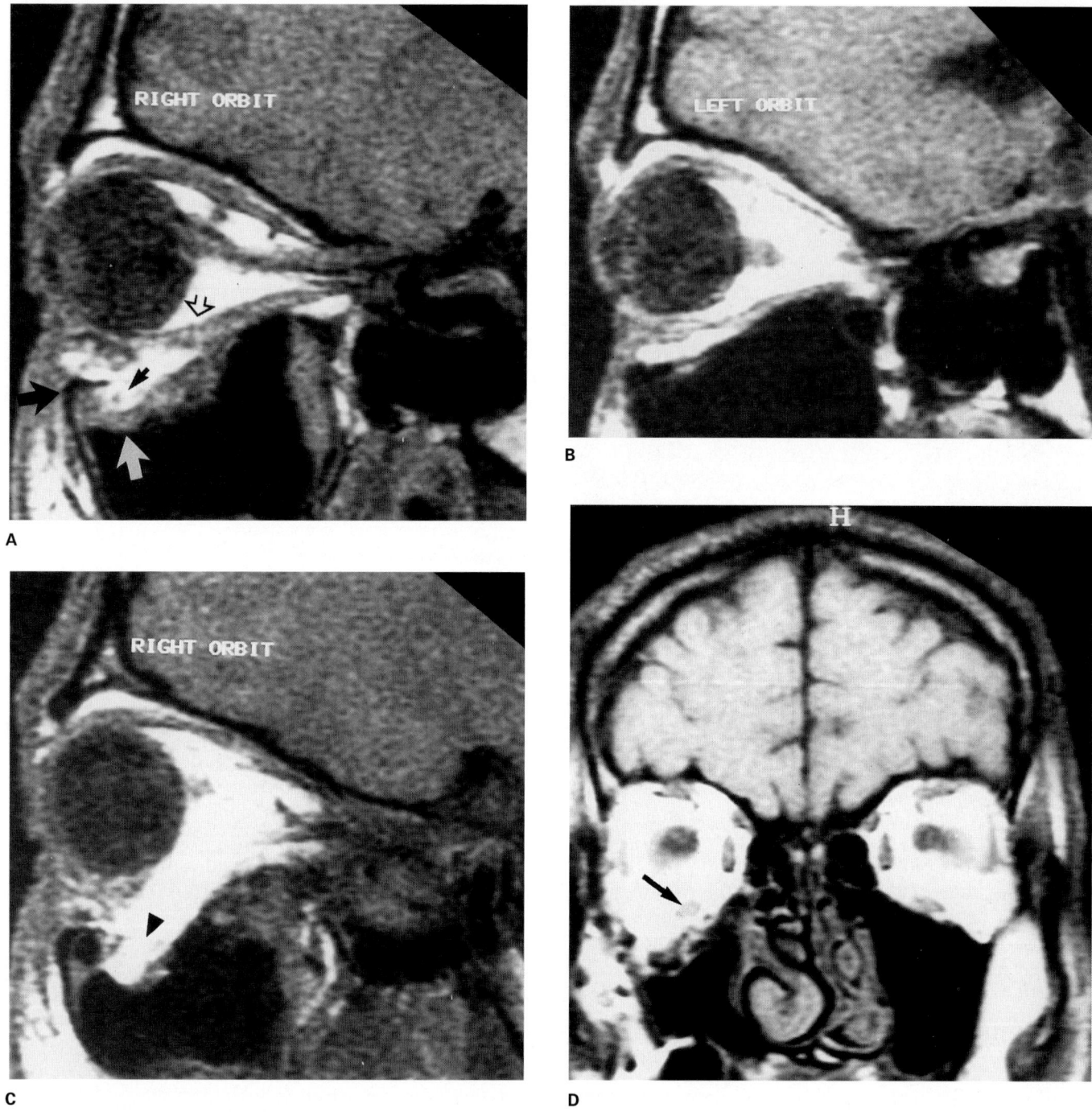

Fig. 7.18 Inferior orbital blow-out fracture: MRI diagnosis. A Oblique sagittal T1 spin echo MRI. High signal of right orbital fat (white). A little herniation of intraorbital fat (small black arrow) into the maxillary sinus behind an intact inferior orbital margin. There is associated thickening of the sinus mucosa (white arrow). The inferior rectus muscle does not appear compromised and is in normal position (open arrow). Large black arrow indicates anterior wall of the maxilla. **B** Similar MRI section through normal left orbit for comparison with **A**. **C** Similar MRI section to **A** but rather more lateral showing greater herniation of intraorbital fat (white high signal) into sinus. **D** Coronal T1 spin echo MRI through orbits shows inferior fat herniation on the right. Note normal position of the right inferior rectus muscle (arrow).

where a fracture can be confused with the normal zygomaticosphenoid suture. The lacrimal gland may be damaged. The orbital apex may also be involved by a fracture, and this may extend to the superior or inferior orbital fissure with possible neurovascular damage. For this

region, thin CT sections (1.0 mm abutting slices with the GE High Speed Advantage scanner) are advised; usually axial scanning is appropriate.

Fractures of the orbital roof are usually caused by a severe frontal or frontolateral impact, and often involve

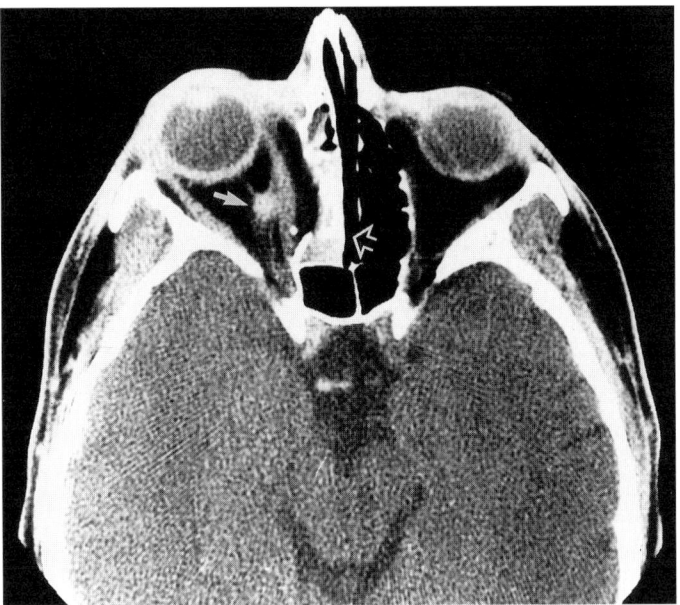

A

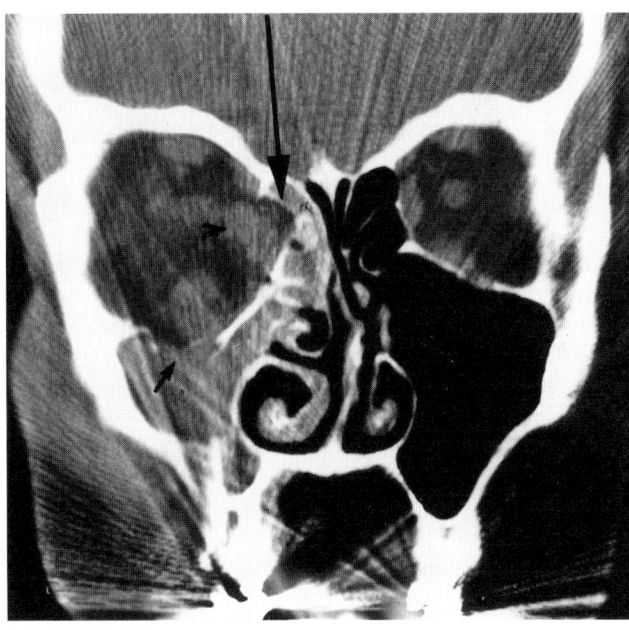

B

Fig. 7.19 Combined inferior and medial orbital blow-out fractures. A Axial CT section shows medial deviation of the right lamina papyracae in association with opaque ethmoidal sinuses (open white arrow) on the same side. The ipsilateral medial rectus looks plump (? contused) and there is a localized soft-tissue density (closed white arrow) on its lateral aspect (? haematoma). **B** Direct coronal CT section. This is degraded by artefact due to dental amalgams. The medial deviation of the right medial orbital wall (long black arrow) is clearly seen but is associated with depression of the orbital floor as well (small black arrow). The medial rectus is identified (arrow head) with some apparent haematoma around it. Intraorbital fat has 'invaded' the region of the ethmoidal sinuses. The medial blow-out injury has been under-reported in the past.

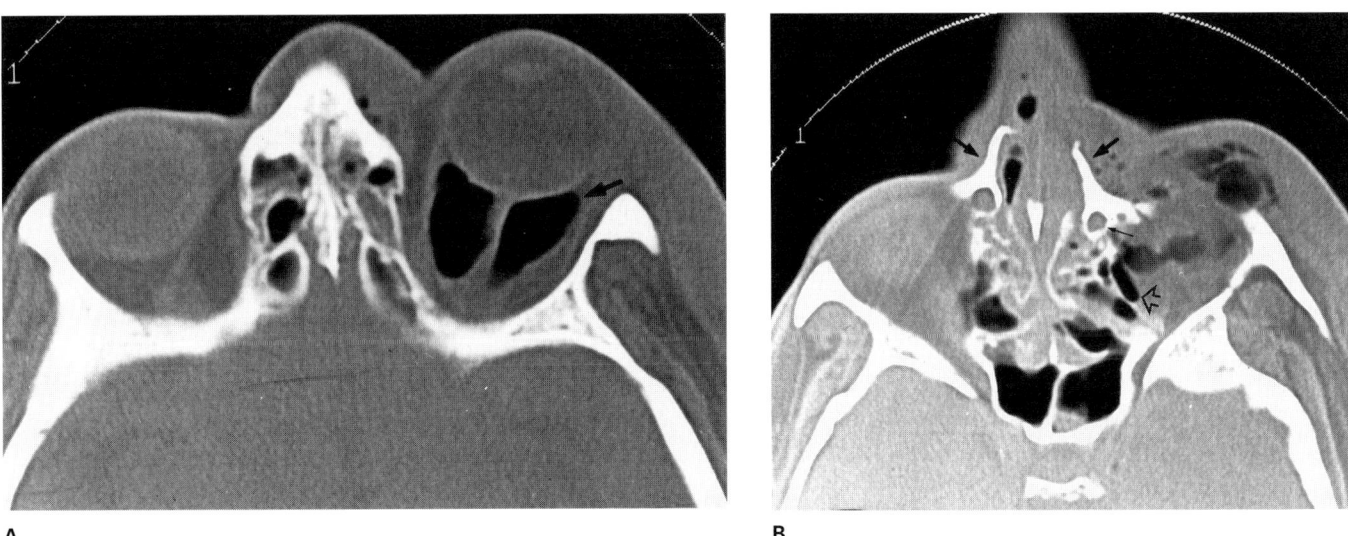

A

B

Fig. 7.20 Orbital emphysema associated with fracture of nasoethmoid complex. A Axial CT section shows left proptosis with much intraconal air (arrow). The proptosis was due to the air under tension, and was thought to need surgical relief. There was no significant intraorbital haematoma or bony encroachment. Opaque ethmoidal sinuses are noted with some concertinaing and some irregularity of the lamina papyracea on each side due to the posterior force delivered. **B** Lower axial CT slice shows fractures involving the naso-ethmoidal complex. Although both frontal processes of the maxillae are depressed (black arrows), this is greater on the left side. The left nasolacrimal duct (thin black arrow) is also seen to be more posterior. A small amount of intraorbital emphysema (open black arrow) is seen adjacent to both the ethmoidal sinuses and the superior limit of the maxillary sinus on the left.

the superior orbital rim; the fracture may extend to the cribriform plate (Fig. 7.21). Isolated roof fractures may result from a penetrating wound or by extension from a distant impact point; superior blow-out and blow-in frac-

tures have been described. Curtin et al (1982) reported two cases of orbital roof blow-out fractures involving the frontal sinuses. Standard plain radiographs will usually be done, but CT is the investigation of choice (optimally

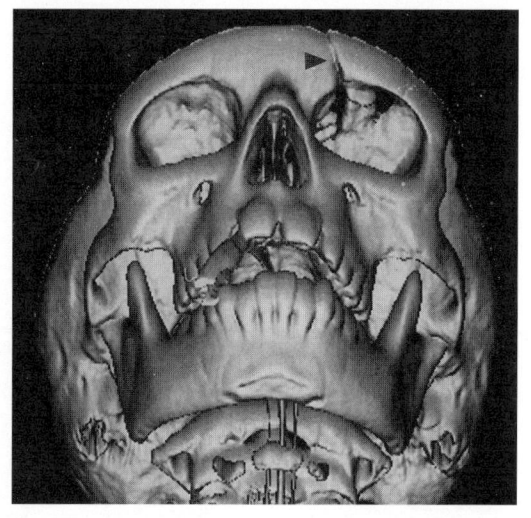

A

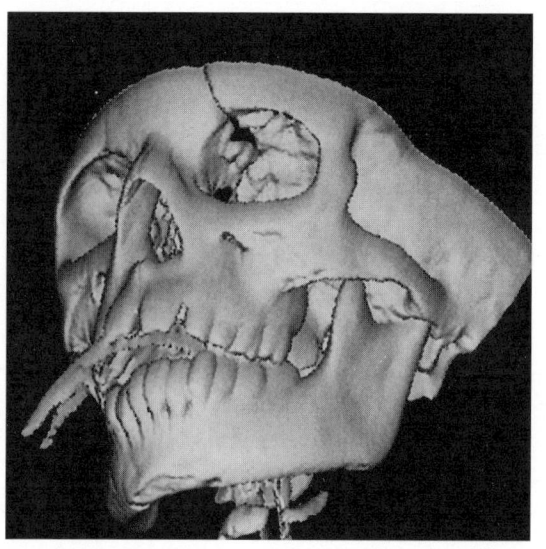

B

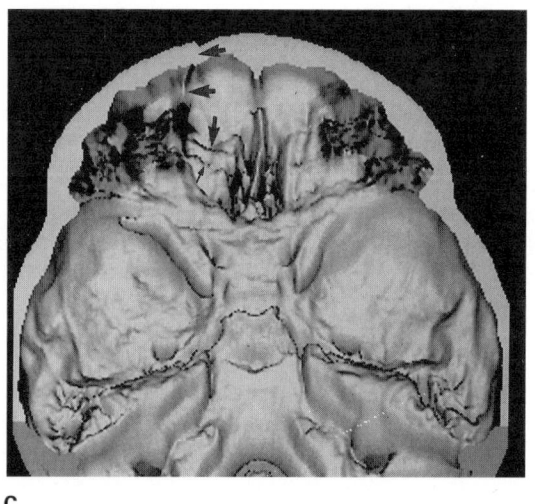

C

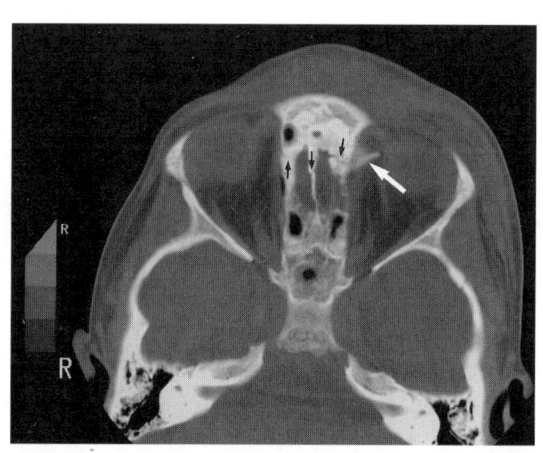

D

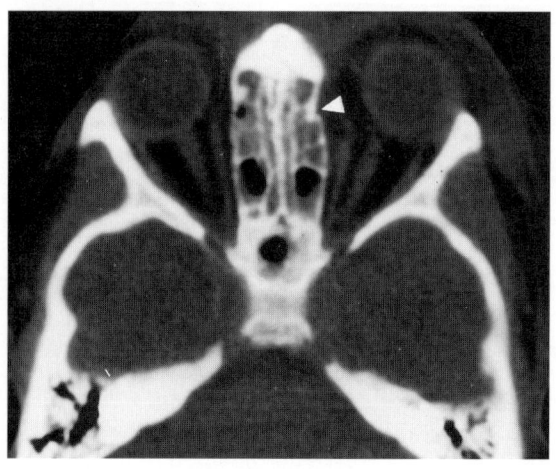

E

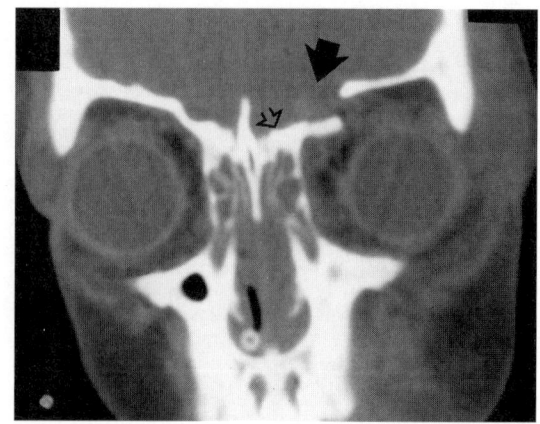

F

Fig. 7.21 Fracture of orbital roof with naso-ethmoid involvement. Plain X-ray indicated a fracture running vertically, involving the medial superior orbital margin on the left. **A** Bone 3D reconstruction (Waters-type projection) confirms this fracture (arrowhead) involving the frontal convexity and orbital roof. Note exquisite overall portrayal of facial morphology. **B** Lateral oblique bone 3D shows better the course of the fracture with some associated bony deformity of the medial orbital roof. **C** Oblique bird's-eye bone 3D shows slight malalignment of frontal convexity fracture which extends as shown by large black arrows. The transverse component involves the orbital plate and fovea ethmoidalis; another transverse fracture is present just posterior to this (small arrow). **D** Axial CT shows fracture (three black arrows) traversing both the right and left fovea ethmoidalis (and therefore the cribriform plates), with a depressed medial orbital plate of frontal bone on the left (white arrow). Very subtle tilting of naso-ethmoidal complex. **E** Axial CT section shows fracture (arrowhead) indenting anterior left lamina papyracea, with twisting of naso-ethmoidal complex anteriorly to the left. Opaque anterior and middle ethmoidal sinuses. **F** Coronal CT shows depression of medial orbital roof (solid black arrow) and apparent flattening of the fovea ethmoidalis (open arrow) with opaque ethmoidal sinuses. The left eye is displaced laterally. Low left frontal lobe haemorrhagic contusion is poorly seen on this CT bone setting.

in the coronal plane) to show the fractures, the orbital contents and the brain.

Ocular lesions

Injuries of the globe may be visualized in CT or MRI scans obtained to assess the orbit and its contents. The eye may be shown to be collapsed or deformed by rupture or by an adjacent displaced fragment of bone. Dense vitreous haemorrhage may be seen on CT, but vitreous haemorrhages, lacerated or dislocated lenses and retinal detachments are better seen by ultrasound.

High resolution real-time sonography, performed after clinical evaluation, is a good method of imaging many acute and chronic injuries of the globe, although MRI is said to be the examination of choice for intraocular haematomas (Mafee and Peyman 1987, Mafee et al 1987). Sonography is contraindicated if an open wound of the eye has been diagnosed or suspected (p. 187).

The anterior chamber of the eye is normally a sono-lucent space and haemorrhage (hyphaema) is seen as diffuse echogenicity. Trauma may collapse the anterior chamber, or alternatively an iridocorneal angle cleavage (p. 417) may lead to an increase in its depth, often associated with post-traumatic glaucoma.

Trauma may cause fragmentation or dislocation of the lens and the degree of these injuries can be defined by ultrasound. Dislocations are usually posterior, and may be subtle or very obvious. Post-traumatic cataracts are seen as increased echogenicity of the lens substance and its boundary echoes.

The posterior chamber of the eye is usually not well imaged by sonography. Vitreous haemorrhage may be difficult to detect during the first days after injury; only a few low amplitude echoes may be apparent. As the haemorrhage matures and organizes, echogenicity increases dramatically; with eye movement, the haemorrhagic debris moves freely and settles with gravity in the dependent part of the globe. Between 2 and 8 weeks after injury, the remnants of the haemorrhage gradually disappear, leaving vitreous membranes which are thick but usually mobile. These membranes may later retract, causing a traction detachment of the retina (p. 152).

Trauma may also cause retinal or less commonly choroidal detachment at an earlier stage. When the retina detaches, it remains attached at the optic nerve head posteriorly and the ora serrata anteriorly; fluid, sometimes containing echogenic blood, accumulates between the retina and the choroid, and may be visualized by sonography (Fig. 7.22). The retina may be detached in its entirety or in a local area; it is at first thin and mobile, but in chronic detachments the layers are thicker and immobile. Chronic retinal detachments may assume a funnel-shaped configuration.

The optic nerve may be visualized by ultrasound at the posterior aspect of the globe, as a hypoechoic band surrounded by the echogenic retro-orbital fat. MRI is the method of choice in imaging the optic nerves, in conjunction with CT scanning to demonstrate the anatomy of the optic canals (p. 423). Location of intraocular or intra-orbital foreign bodies is often necessary. MRI has only a limited role: most foreign bodies are metallic, and if ferromagnetic, the foreign body may move when scanned, causing further damage. If not metallic, foreign bodies give on MRI a weak or absent signal in T1 and T2 weightings, resembling cortical bone or emphysema. CT is therefore the examination of choice. However, MRI is useful if the foreign body is known to be non-metallic and associated with laceration or hypotony of the globe, when ultrasound is unwise; multiplanar MRI may be superior to CT in relating a non-metallic foreign body to the wall of the globe.

Lacrimal drainage

Lacrimal obstruction is most often seen at the junction of the lacrimal sac with the nasolacrimal duct; lacrimal fistulas are usually from the sac to the skin. Dacryocystography may be required (p. 178). For exact diagnosis, conventional radiological dacryocystography is needed, isotope dacryocystography (p. 185) is a useful functional test, but does not give anatomical detail.

Nasal and naso-orbito-ethmoid injuries

Nasal bone injuries may occur in isolation or with other bone injury. De Lacey (1977) considered that X-ray views of suspected isolated nasal fractures are unnecessary, and stated that bony depression of the nose is best assessed clinically. However, radiological confirmation of the clinical diagnosis may be requested.

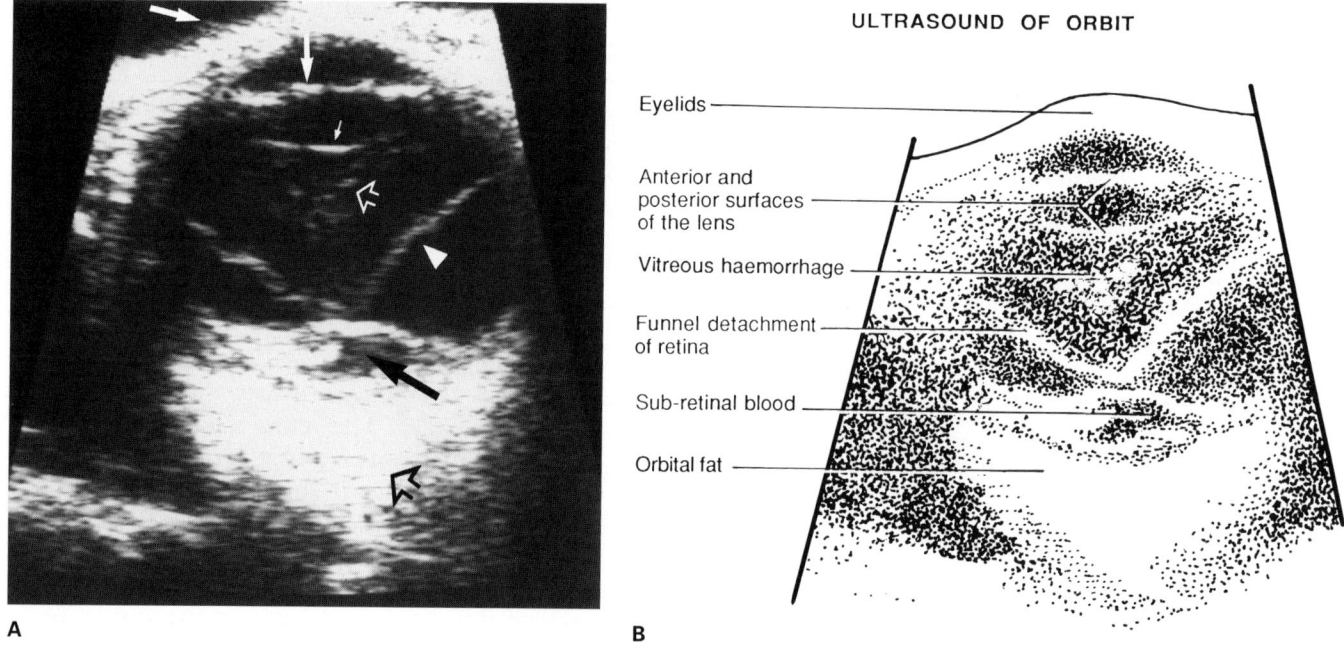

ULTRASOUND OF ORBIT

Eyelids

Anterior and posterior surfaces of the lens

Vitreous haemorrhage

Funnel detachment of retina

Sub-retinal blood

Orbital fat

A   B

Fig. 7.22 Sonogram of retinal detachment. A Standard ultrasonic study of the eye. **B** Diagram showing the findings: a large chronic retinal detachment.

The coned underpenetrated lateral view is best to demonstrate the commoner transverse nasal fracture. Longitudinal fractures may be seen in the same view, but must be distinguished from normal grooves, namely the paired nasomaxillary and nasociliary nerve grooves. These grooves are less sharply defined than fracture lines. The Waters view is best to show disruption of the bony nasal arch, or coned axial views may be preferred.

Nasal cavity injuries are studied routinely by CT as part of the assessment of the paranasal sinuses. Sinonasal radiological anatomy assessment has developed apace over the last decade, harnessed to improvements in CT scanners and to demands for fine detail as a basis for functional endoscopic sinus surgery in the treatment of chronic sinus disease. The ENT surgeon routinely requires a direct coronal study with fine cuts through the ostiomeatal complex, the key area in the pathogenesis of chronic naso-sinusitis (Fig. 2.8). Axial slices are optional but often add useful information. These requirements for preoperative anatomical imaging have been described by Mafee (1993).

The imaging of the traumatized lateral nasal wall has been described in discussing maxillary injuries; the difficult but vitally important task of imaging the cribriform plate is considered below. The floor of the nasal cavity is the palate, termed the inferior horizontal facial strut by Gentry et al (1983). The palate is well assessed by coronal CT. Fractures of the palate often receive scant mention; they are usually longitudinal and may involve the incisive or palatine foramina, with possible haematoma formation. Oronasal fistulas are rare.

The midsagittal strut is the nasal septum. This is frequently damaged and may be lacerated, fractured or dislocated. A resultant septal haematoma can be missed clinically and should be looked for in CT scans. Damage to the anterior nasal spine should also be assessed because it may be associated with septal damage. Failure to diagnose and evacuate a septal haematoma may lead to deviation or perforation of the septum secondary to septal cartilage resorption at the site of the septal haematoma.

The imaging of complex naso-orbito-ethmoid injuries (p. 308) has been made much easier by the advent of high definition CT scanning in the coronal plane, with axial and other reformats. The cribriform plate and the olfactory fossa on each side are best seen on coronal CT images; it is important to identify fractures of these midline structures in view of the possibility of leakage of CSF and the potential risk of delayed meningitis. It is our view that radiological demonstration of a severe fracture in this region may be presumptive evidence of a cranionasal fistula unlikely to heal without surgical repair (p. 378). Damage to the inferior aspect of the frontal lobes must be looked for in soft tissue scans, optimally done in the coronal plane. Opaque foreign bodies here and elsewhere can be well located by CT, although MRI also has a place in the identification of foreign material. especially wood (p. 369). Identification of fractures along the course of the anterior ethmoidal artery should alert to the possibility of significant bleeding.

Zygomatic injuries

These are the most common midfacial fractures after fractures of the nasal bones. Complex zygomatic fractures involving the orbit (p. 317) are more often seen than isolated fractures of the zygomatic arch. Isolated arch fractures are often depressed: commonly three fracture lines are seen, with depression of the two central fragments (Freimanis 1966). The depression may compromise the movement of the coronoid process, and delayed fibrosis may also limit jaw opening.

In diagnosing zygomatic fractures by plain X-ray, the excellent review by Dolan & Jacoby (1978) is very helpful, as are the observations of Daffner (1983) on the lateral view of facial fractures. The Caldwell view is best to show disruption of the frontozygomatic suture and disjunction between the zygoma and the greater wing of the sphenoid bone. The Waters view displays the zygomatic arch, the orbital rim, the orbital floor and the lateral maxillary wall; the arch is also well seen in an underpenetrated base view. Depression and rotation are best assessed from the overall evaluation of all four basic plain films. The zygoma must be assessed at each point of junction with the maxilla, sphenoid, frontal and temporal bones.

Clinical and plain radiological examinations often give an accurate picture of a zygomatic injury, but we also perform a CT scan to give the maximum possible information (Fig. 7.23). Axial scans with 5-mm-thick slices overlapping at 3 mm intervals are routinely obtained from the maxillary teeth to a level above the orbits. Both 2D and 3D CT recontructions are always done, 3D being especially helpful to show depressions and rotations of the zygoma, to compare the two zygomatic arches, and to clarify the diagnosis where the fracture is severely separated. After operative reduction of a zygomatic fracture, it is our routine to document the state of the reduction by plain radiographs and a 3D CT scan where necessary, both to define the surgical procedure and to provide a postoperative baseline; cephalostat radiographs may also be useful.

Pterygopalatine fossa injuries

This is a region of particular interest because of its deep central and posterior position in the face and its structural importance in facial trauma. It is a small triangular space with a multitude of connections situated between the upper posterior wall of the antrum and the upper anterior aspect of the pterygoid plates; it is therefore situated between the anterior and posterior parts of the posterior coronal strut of Gentry et al (1983: see Fig. 2.15D). The space is just below the orbital apex, at the junction of pterygomaxillary and infraorbital fissures. It is a focus of complex neurovascular anatomy. It is associated with five foramina, namely, the foramen rotundum, the pterygoid canal, the pharyngeal canal, the sphenopalatine foramen, and the pterygopalatine canal. Trauma to this area can damage the maxillary artery, the maxillary nerve, the pterygopalatine nerve and a large venous plexus. Retropharyngeal haematomas are common and may lead to respiratory compromise; as clinical detection may be difficult, radiological appreciation of the problem is vital. Other vascular injuries such as thrombosis or pseudoaneurysm of the maxillary artery can occur. Neural compression can produce complex acute neurological problems or chronic facial pain due to compression of fifth nerve branches. Trauma can obstruct the distal eustachian tube leading to otitis media. The area must sometimes be explored: a technique for transantral ligation of the maxillary artery is described on p. 227. There are therefore many reasons for wishing to image this space. It is poorly shown in standard radiographic projections, and is best assessed in axial CT scans (Fig. 7.14), in 2D and 3D subregioned reconstructions, and by MRI.

Calvarial injuries

These may be imaged by standard lateral, posteroanterior and Towne's plain views, or by CT scanning. There is dispute on the need for a routine skull X-ray sequence after any head impact. In several large series of head injury, the incidence of significant bony abnormalities has been shown to be low, and the diagnostic value of the plain skull radiograph has been questioned. Masters et al (1987) attempted to carry out a follow-up study of 7035 cases of head injury; although the study failed to trace nearly half of these patients, the authors were able to show that the omission of routine skull radiographs was unlikely to have affected the outcome in patients identified as at low risk of serious complications by clinical criteria.

However, there are some strong and well-recognized indications for imaging the head. These include:

- Altered level of consciousness — especially when this persists after resuscitation
- Focal neurological signs or symptoms
- Open scalp or frontal cutaneous wound potentially associated with deeper penetration
- Clinical suspicion of a fracture of the vault or the base
- Persisting headache.

If there is any evidence of clinical deterioration, these indications become absolute and imperative, and an urgent neurosurgical consultation should if possible be obtained.

If a CT scanner is available, these indications warrant a scan. It is now usual to proceed immediately to CT scanning in any case with the above indications, and especially in unconscious patients. A rapid CT scan is done to scrutinize the intracranial contents for any intracerebral or extracerebral lesion; at the same time, the facial skeleton can be surveyed very quickly on modern scanners. However, if there is no scanner at hand then plain skull radiography is often a useful second-best, especially if the surgeon intends to proceed at once to an operative intervention.

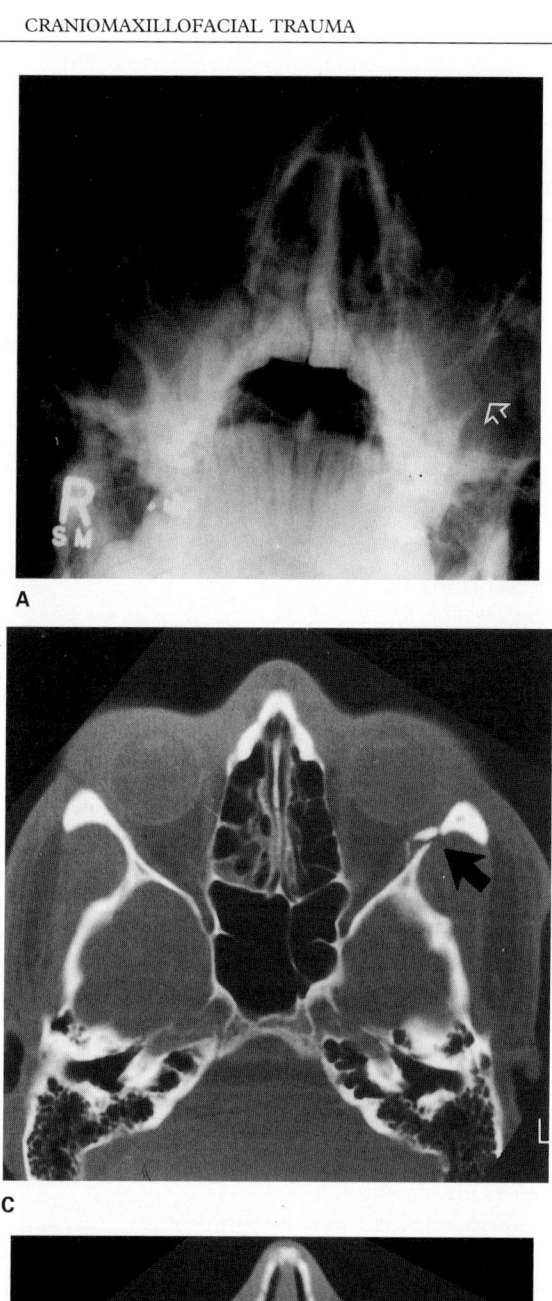

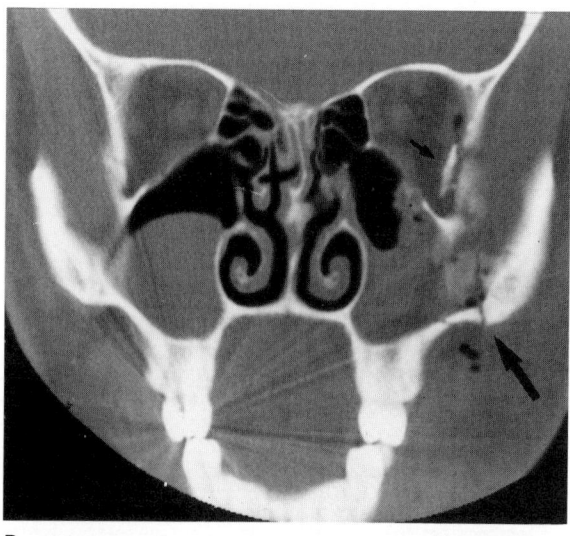

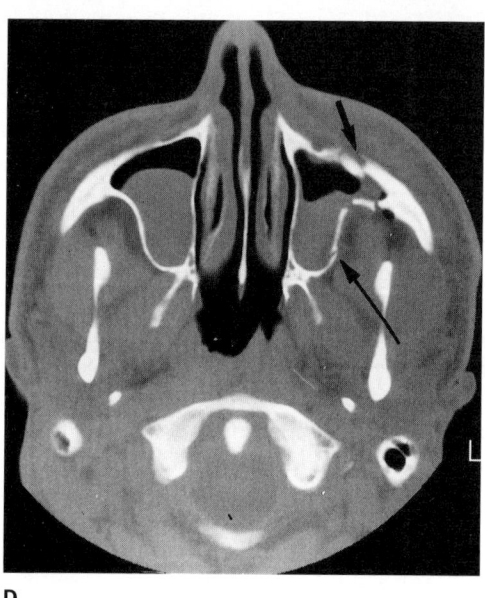

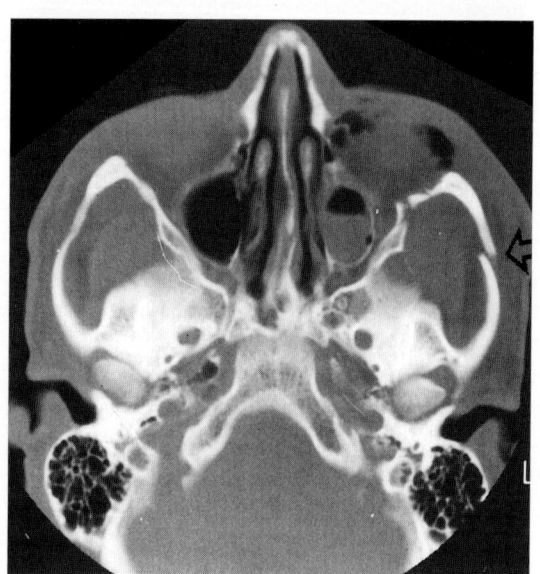

Fig. 7.23 Zygomatic fracture with orbital involvement. A Oblique tilted Water's view. There is discontinuity of the lateral wall of the left maxillary sinus (arrow) on the side of the facial injury. **B** Direct coronal CT section shows a fracture fragment (small arrow) in the left lateral orbital cavity adjacent to the zygomaticosphenoidal junction, some apparent discontinuity of the left orbital floor and a fracture of the lateral sinus wall (large arrow). Some left orbital and cheek emphysema is present together with presumed left maxillary haemosinus, and an incidental right maxillary sinus mucocele). **C** Axial CT section shows comminuted fracture of left lateral orbit wall (arrow). Large fragment corresponds to that seen in **B**. **D** Axial CT showing fracture at zygomaticomaxillary junction (thick black arrow), and lateral wall of maxillary sinus with depression (thin arrow). **E** Axial CT shows fracture of mid-zygomatic arch on left (arrow). Associated orbital emphysema and fluid level (presumed blood) in left maxillary sinus. Only mild asymmetry of the zygomatic arches.

The CT scan may fail to detect linear skull fractures, especially a fracture running parallel to the plane of the scan. When the finding of a skull fracture is of medicolegal consequence, plain skull radiographs may be needed, and in some centres, these are used as a screening measure before deciding to employ the CT scanner, since the finding of a skull fracture increases the risk of an intracranial haematoma by about 400 times (Jennett 1980). If a CT scan is the first procedure, the lateral scout CT image of the skull, and perhaps also a frontal scout film, should be studied for a fracture line. It is important to view the CT console image so that window level and width can be adjusted to give the optimal settings for bone appraisal. If the CT scan was done to visualize the brain, the bones will not be seen to good effect, and although a set of films on bone settings will be obtained for a record, their diagnostic quality will not be so good as that of a study on the CT monitor with varying settings of window width and level.

Frontal sinus fractures

These have been classified as anterior or posterior wall fractures and fractures involving the frontonasal drainage system (p. 37). The fractures may involve one or both sinus walls; they may be linear or comminuted, non-depressed or depressed. Complications include pneumocephalus, CSF rhinorrhoea and blockage of the frontal sinus drainage with sinusitis or retention mucocele.

Plain lateral and Caldwell views usually show these fractures. But CT provides more detailed information, and is very useful to the surgeon, especially in showing fractures involving the posterior wall of the sinus. Associated fractures through the ethmoid air cells and orbital roof are often combined with injury of the frontonasal drainage; this can only be inferred, as fractures in the vicinity of the frontal recess or frontonasal duct are rarely seen even with CT.

The CT findings have been well described by Olson et al (1992), who stressed the strong association of fractures of the frontal sinuses with fractures of adjacent structures, such as the orbit, the naso-ethmoid region, the maxillary sinuses and the neurocranium (Figs 7.24 and 7.25); fractures of the posterior sinus wall may be complicated by frontal extradural haemorrhage or infection. Harris et al (1987) have shown the value of CT in frontal sinus trauma involving the drainage of the sinus.

Cerebrospinal fluid rhinorrhoea

Post-traumatic CSF rhinorrhoea (p. 376) may result from a fracture of the posterior wall of the frontal sinus or more commonly from an ethmoidal fracture involving the cribriform plate and the adjacent ethmoid air cells; a sphenoid fracture may also be responsible, or a petrous

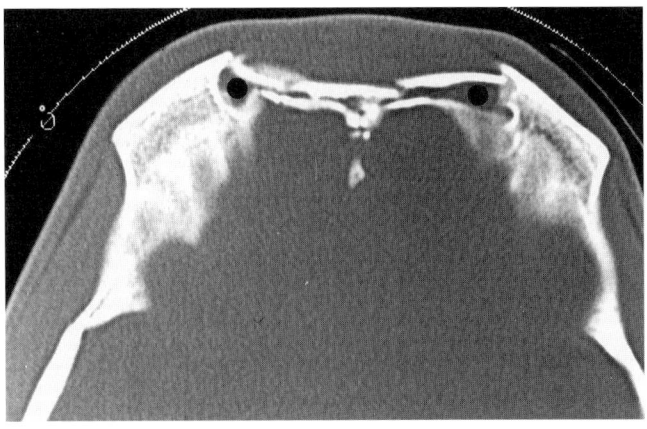

A

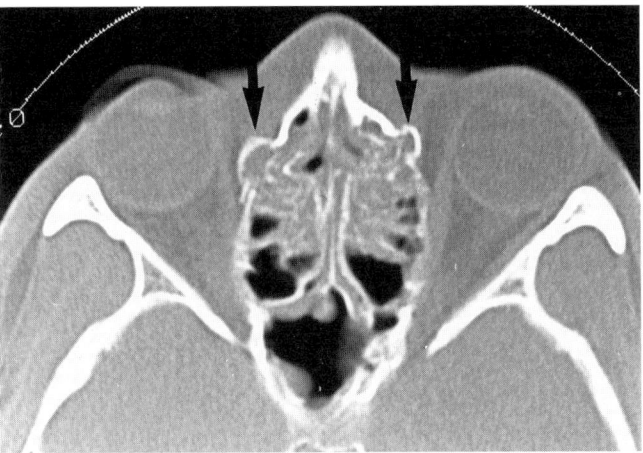

B

Fig. 7.24 Fractures of both walls of frontal sinus. A Axial CT section shows posterior displacement of anterior and posterior walls of frontal sinuses which are opaque (black circles). Note tip of crista galli in the midline. No convincing intracranial abnormality was shown but pneumocephalus, haemorrhage and contusion must be looked for. Infective complications and retention mucoceles secondary to blockage of the frontonasal duct are late complications of such injuries. **B** Lower axial CT section indicates posterior concertining of the naso-ethmoidal complex with subsequent traumatic hypertelorism.

temporal fracture causing CSF leakage into the eustachian tube. It is surgically important to visualize the fracture site, and to determine the degree of separation of the bone edges, since this relates to the likelihood of spontaneous healing. If the rhinorrhoea persists, it may be studied by intrathecal injection of a non-ionic water-soluble radiographic contrast, to locate the site of the causative dural tear. When the ethmoid site is suspect, the CT scan is performed in the coronal plane, with the patient prone using 1.0- or 1.5-mm-thick abutting slices. It is important to obtain a plain scan before injecting the contrast, to allow distinction between a small amount of leaking contrast and an area of dense cortical bone. It is pointless to do this test unless the patient is actively leaking. A similar technique is used to pinpoint CSF leak in fractures of the tegmen tympani.

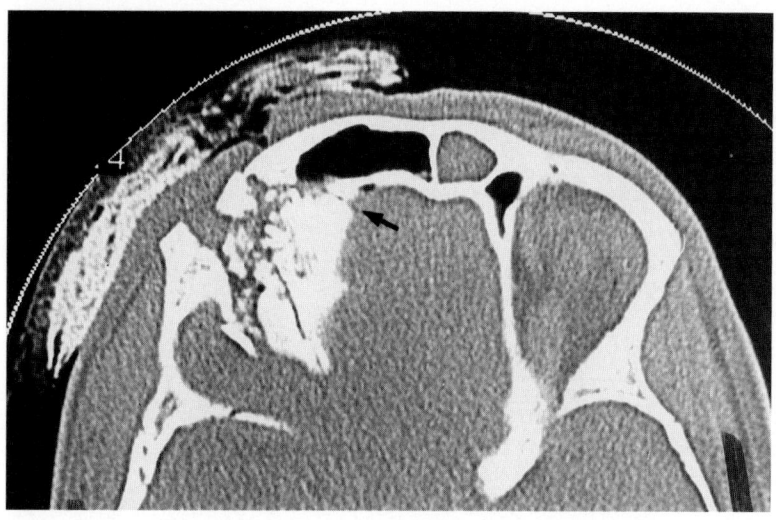 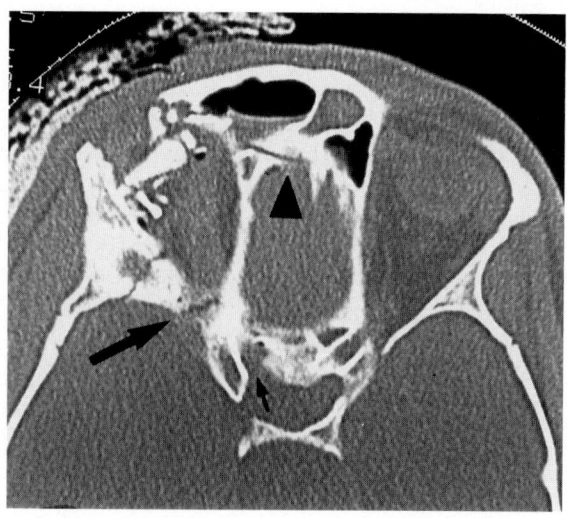

A   **B**

Fig. 7.25 Complex fracture of orbital roof. A Axial CT section through level of right orbit roof shows fracture of the roof with much comminution, and disruption of the superior orbital margin. One fracture line (arrow) involves the posterior wall of the frontal sinus, with potential for meningitis. A small bubble of intracranial air is noted behind the same sinus. **B** Axial CT section through upper orbital cavities shows further extent of fractures. An anterior fracture (black arrowhead) runs transversely across the fovea ethmoidalis and cribriform plate — both possible sources for meningitis. The medial of the two more posterior fractures runs approximately where the lesser wing of sphenoid and orbital process of frontal bone join (large arrow); this runs adjacent to the anterior aperture of the optic canal which is seen more posteriorly (small arrow) and may therefore compromise the nerve. Note fluid level in the right frontal sinus, an opaque left frontal sinus, and that the fracture is compound. Patient also had a right medial blow-out fracture and a vitreous haemorrhage.

We have also used intrathecal injection of [^{99m}Tc] DTPA or other radioactive isotope in the diagnosis of CSF leakage. The delineation of the leak point is sometimes excellent, and the scan may be complemented by examination of the radioactivity of pledgets placed in the nose or in the region of the eustachian tube. However, CT delineation is more convincing, and more likely to give precise identification of the site of the fracture. Neither form of imaging gives positive findings unless there is actual leakage at the time of the examination, and in many cases of intermittent CSF rhinorrhoea this is not the case. In our practice, neither procedure is routinely used, and most operations for CSF rhinorrhoea are done on clinical indications and on the radiological findings without the use of contrast. Farrell & Emby (1993) have reported on a series of 30 cases of post-traumatic meningitis: with coronal CT scans they were able to demonstrate fractures in all cases, and in 28 these fractures corresponded with the sites of dural tears found at operation.

Petrous temporal fractures

Trauma to this bone is mentioned here although outside the general scope of this book, because petrous fractures are clinically important and may be associated with CMF injury (Dolan 1989, Schwartz & Harnsberger 1992). The petrous bone can be damaged by force transmitted from the mandibular condyle, or by fractures extending from the occipital or squamous temporal bone. The petrous bone is a robust structure, and a substantial impact force may be sustained without an obvious fracture line on CT scanning.

The majority of petrous fractures are longitudinal — that is, parallel with the petrous ridge. They should not be confused with normal sutures. A CT scan frequently shows the fracture (Figs 7.26 and 7.27). Blood may be seen in the middle ear cleft and mastoid air cells, and damage to the auditory ossicles may occur.

In a minority of cases of petrous fracture, the fracture is transverse — across the long axis of the petrous ridge. These fractures are more likely to be associated with sensorineural hearing loss or vertigo due to damage to cochlea, vestibule or semicircular canals and internal auditory canals. Hearing may also be impaired by dehiscence of the round or oval windows. The facial nerve may also be damaged (p. 439).

Petrous fractures may be associated with CSF otorrhoea; on occasion there is CSF rhinorrhoea, from leakage along the eustachian tube into the nasal cavity. Damage to the jugular fossa can lead to jugular vein thrombosis (Fig. 7.28).

Thin-section axial and coronal CT images on bone algorithm on modern scanners exquisitely detail most injuries but much expertise in assessment is required. MRI has a place in the diagnosis of labyrinthine concussion and soft-tissue problems around the ear.

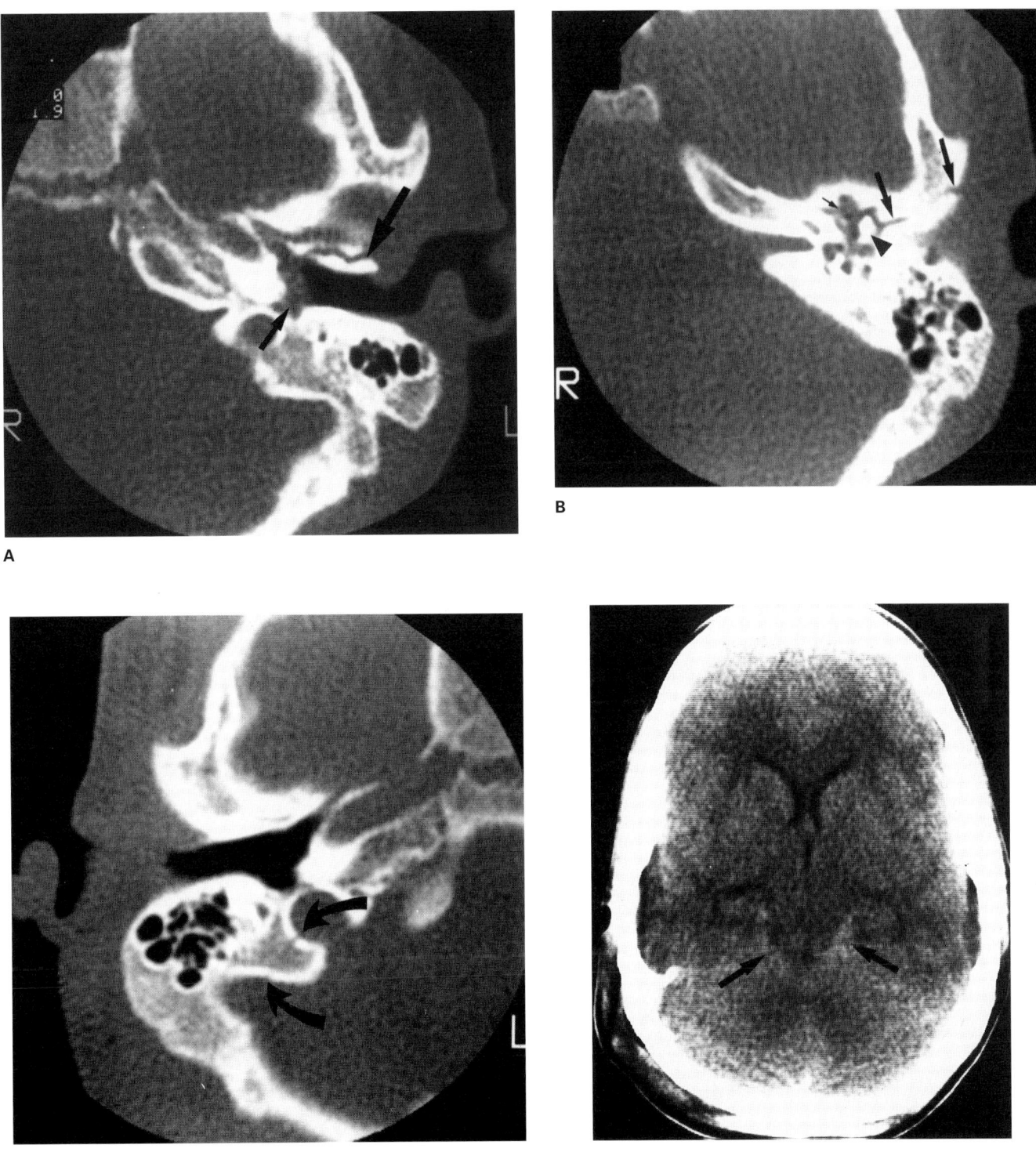

Fig. 7.26 Longitudinal fracture of petrous bone, contralateral fracture involving jugular foramen, and probable brain swelling. A Left axial petrous CT scan shows a haemotypanum (short arrow) and a longitudinal fracture involving the anterior wall of the bony external auditory canal (long arrow). A slightly lower CT section showed air bubbles in the jugular foramen (extravenous), and presumably derived from air within the ear. **B** Higher left axial petrous CT section shows a longitudinal fracture in the roof of the external canal (large arrows). Blood is noted in the epitympanum (small arrow) around the auditory ossicles (arrowhead). Some blood is noted in mastoid air cells. **C** Right axial petrous CT section shows a fracture involving the jugular foramen (anterior arrow) and margin of sigmoid sinus (posterior arrow). Clear middle ear and mastoids. **D** Axial brain CT scan shows obliteration of the ambient cistern (arrows) around the midbrain. The frontal horns appear to be of reasonable size. Subarachnoid blood in the ambient cistern could mimic this appearance, but it is presumptive evidence of raised intracranial pressure. Equivocal low density zones in the temporal lobes may represent contusion.

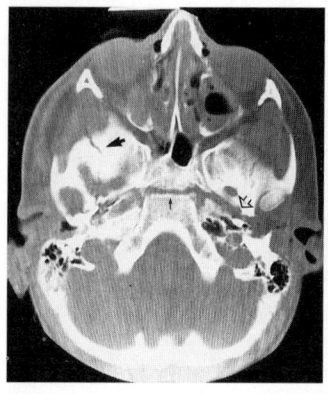 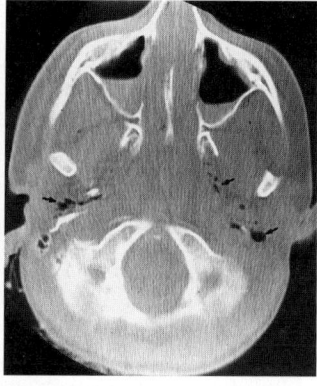

A **B**

Fig. 7.27 Bitemporal fractures with pneumocephalus. A Axial CT section of skull base in a 13-year-old child shows diastasis of right sphenotemporal suture (large black arrow), apparent diastasis of spheno-occipital synchondrosis (small black arrow) and separation along suture dividing left petrous bone from the greater wing of sphenoid (open arrow). Adjacent slices indicated blood in external auditory canals and middle ear clefts. Bilateral longitudinal fractures of temporal bones were diagnosed. **B** Lower axial CT shows air pockets in tissue planes below the skull base (arrows), presumably from the mastoids and/or middle/outer ears. Sections higher up showed air around the circle of Willis and adjacent subarachnoid spaces. Fluid levels in maxillary sinuses noted.

INTRACRANIAL LESIONS

CT is the modality of choice for the initial assessment of acute intracranial trauma. CT is a rapid and non-invasive investigation, readily identifying those lesions which are surgically correctable in the acute phase, and is also able to identify most significant subacute complications, including those occurring in the postoperative phase. A big advantage of CT is the ability to view the brain, the bone of the skull vault and base and the facial skeleton at the same examination. Johnson & Lee (1992) have given a comprehensive account of CT in cerebral trauma.

MRI is more sensitive than CT in imaging the brain; its role in cerebral trauma is described by Sklar et al (1992). Thus, small cortical contusions and small subdural haematomas are well seen by MRI but frequently are not seen on CT. A severe brain injury with multiple punctate cerebral haemorrhages seen on CT (Wilberger et al 1990) is assumed to have more extensive injury present, which would be visible in MRI; our own comparisons with antemortem CT, postmortem MRI and neuropathological examination have shown that both modalities may fail to visualize small haemorrhagic lesions < 5 mm in diameter, but there is no doubt that MRI misses fewer. Gentry et al (1988a,b) have reviewed the distribution of radiopathological features of traumatic lesions and have compared CT and MRI in closed head injury. They emphasized the greater sensitivity of MRI in detecting non-haemorrhagic lesions, including diffuse axonal injury (DAI: see p. 139). Kelly et al (1988) compared MRI with CT in 100 patients and came to similar

conclusions. There is indeed no doubt that MRI is superior to CT in visualizing non-haemorrhagic lesions, especially those presumed to represent DAI, though this assumption should be tested by careful neuroradiological–neuropathological correlation. Nevertheless, in acute head injuries CT is more readily employed, and will detect most of the lesions requiring surgical treatment. MRI is indicated when the neurological deficit exceeds the CT findings and to document late sequels of injury. Magnetic resonance angiography has a role also in visualizing arterial and venous occlusions, post-traumatic arteriovenous fistulas and arterial dissections. Paediatric traumatic neuropathology especially is shown better by MRI than by CT (Sato et al 1989) and this is important in non-accidental injury, not just as a more sensitive detector of lesions but also because MRI may suggest the timing of the trauma (Table 7.5).

The usual CT scanning technique to image cerebral trauma is to take 5-mm-thick abutting axial slices through the posterior fossa and 10-mm-thick slices to the vertex. The scout image is usually a lateral view although a frontal view can be used; this should be scrutinized for signs of injury, such as a skull fracture or a fluid level in a sinus. The individual axial slices must be viewed on the console of the scanner with varying window width and level, as subtle changes, such as thin extra-cerebral collections or low density zones (oedema), can be easily overlooked in the film, and even fractures can be missed. The hard copy, in the form of the film, must include brain settings and bone settings, the latter being used to show bony injury. Fast scanners (1–2 s scan times) reduce the need for anaesthesia.

From the radiological view, the effects of head injury can be classified as extra-axial and intra-axial processes. The extra-axial processes include extradural haematomas (EDH), subdural haematomas (SDH) and subarachnoid haemorrhage. The intra-axial processes include cerebral swelling, infarcts, DAI, multifocal vascular injury (haemorrhagic shear lesions or tissue tear haemorrhages), contusions, intracerebral haematomas and intraventricular haemorrhages. These abnormalities have been discussed in Chapter 5; some of them have very characteristic appearances in CT and MRI scans.

Extradural haematoma

These lesions are usually produced by bleeding from one of the meningeal arteries and are not necessarily associated with a fracture: in our own series of 366 cases, fractures were recorded in 75.1%, the incidence being somewhat lower in children (Jones et al 1993). The site depends on the meningeal branch involved: most are in the temporal region (Fig. 7.29). The extradural haematoma appears in axial scans as a lenticular biconvex mass, shaped by the constraint of dural attachments,

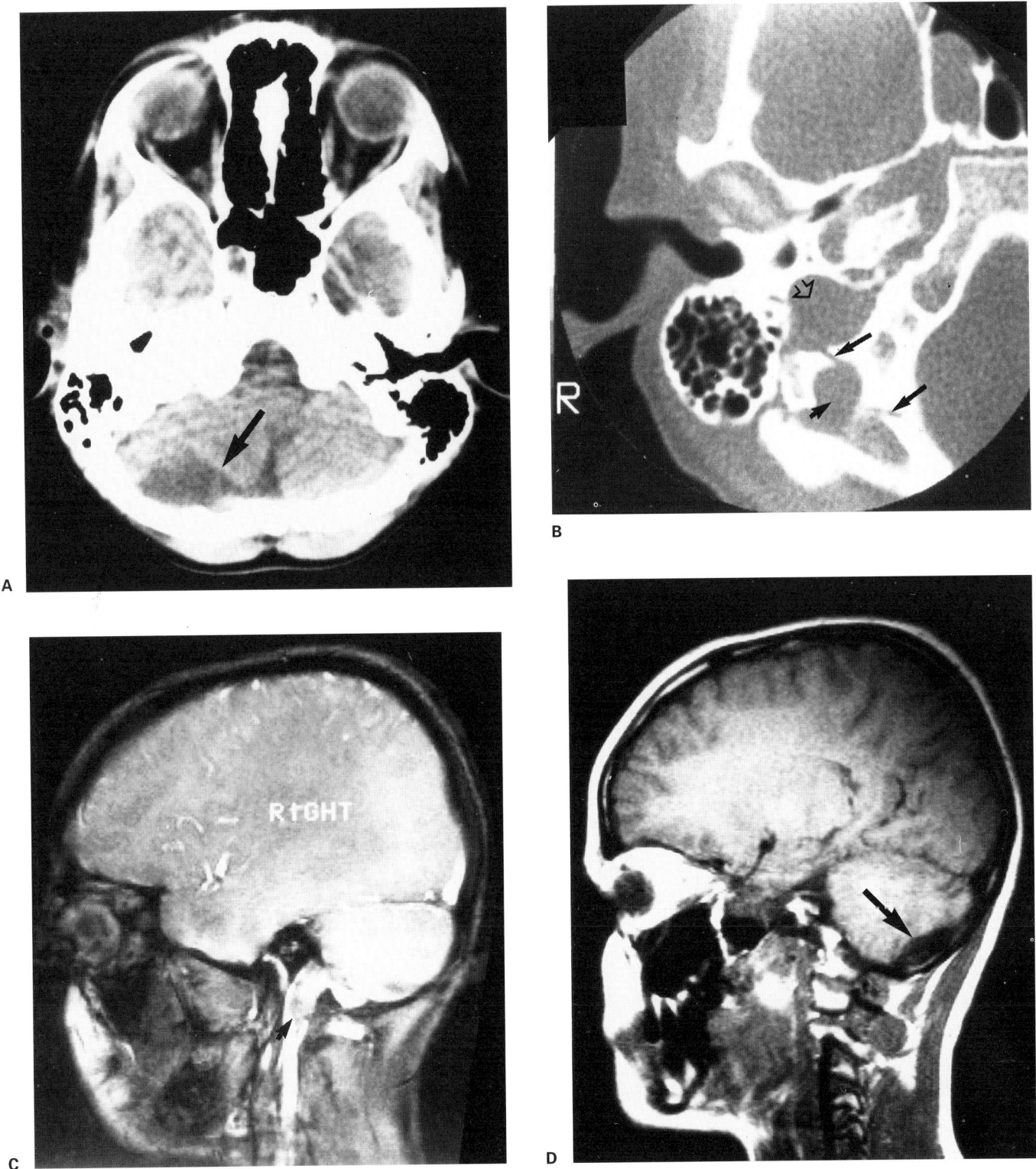

Fig. 7.28 Occipital fracture with subdural hygroma and jugular bulb thrombosis. A 14-year-old boy sustained a severe occipital impact.
A Axial CT section through low posterior fossa on day 2 following head injury shows a low density acute subdural hygroma on the right beneath the cerebellar hemisphere (arrow). No significant mass effect is shown. On bone settings, this section showed a fracture of the occipital bone directly behind the collection. **B** Low axial petrous bone CT section shows a fracture involving the forament magnum and jugular foramen (long black arrows) and the adjacent jugular bulb (open arrow) and sigmoid sinus (short black arrow). The possibility of major venous damage was entertained. **C** Right parasagittal gradient echo fast image steady state precession (FISP) MRI scan. The high signal (white) jugular bulb contains an ill-defined low signal area (grey) consistent with the presence of intravenous clot (arrow). This had not fortunately, propagated proximally. Presumed due to venous damage from adjacent fracture. **D** Parasagittal T1-weighted spin echo MRI section. Note low signal of subdural hygroma (arrow), behaving as cerebrospinal fluid.

Table 7.5 Intracerebral haematomas: changes in MRI signal intensity over time

Age of haematoma	< 24 h (hyper-acute)	24–72 h (acute)	3 days–2 weeks (subacute)	> 2 weeks (chronic)
Pathology	Water and protein present; Fe still in form of oxy-Hb	Hb within red cells is deoxygenated; there is surrounding oedema and serum	Red cell lysis and oxidation of deoxy-Hb to met-Hb, starting at periphery. Speed of process varies	Met-Hb forms haemochromes
T1-weighted signal	Low – intermediate (protein effect)	Slightly hypo- or iso-intense Adjacent tissues: low signal	Hyper-intense	Gradually reduces to iso-intensity with water. Often some hyper-intensity lingers, due to protein
T2-weighted signal (high hyper-intense magnetic field strength >1.0 Tesla)		Hypo-intense Adjacent tissues: hypointense	Hypo- to hyper-intense	Approaches intensity of water (hypo-intense); thin rim of low-intensity haemosiderin

Fe = iron, Hb = haemoglobin.

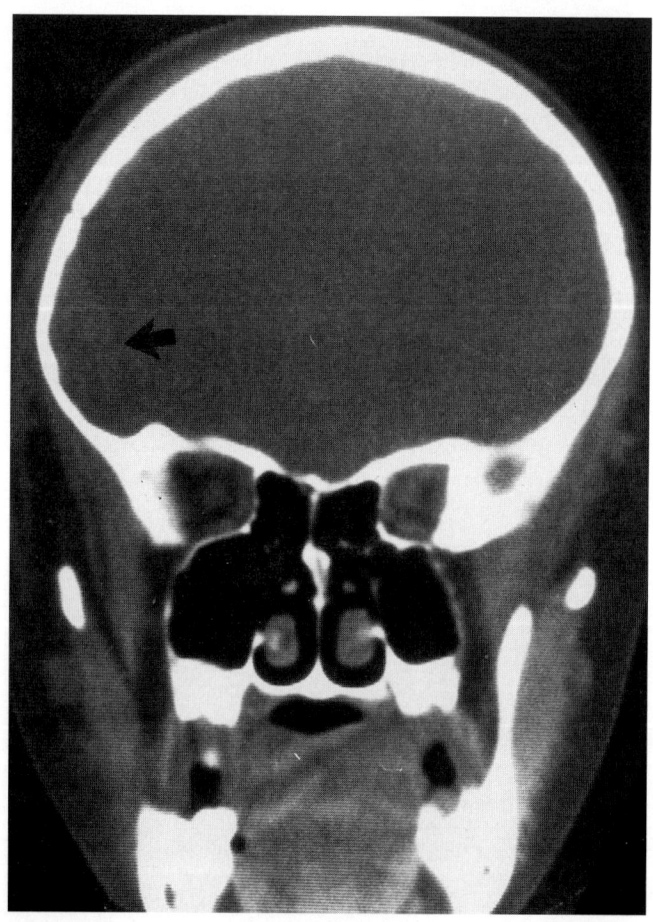

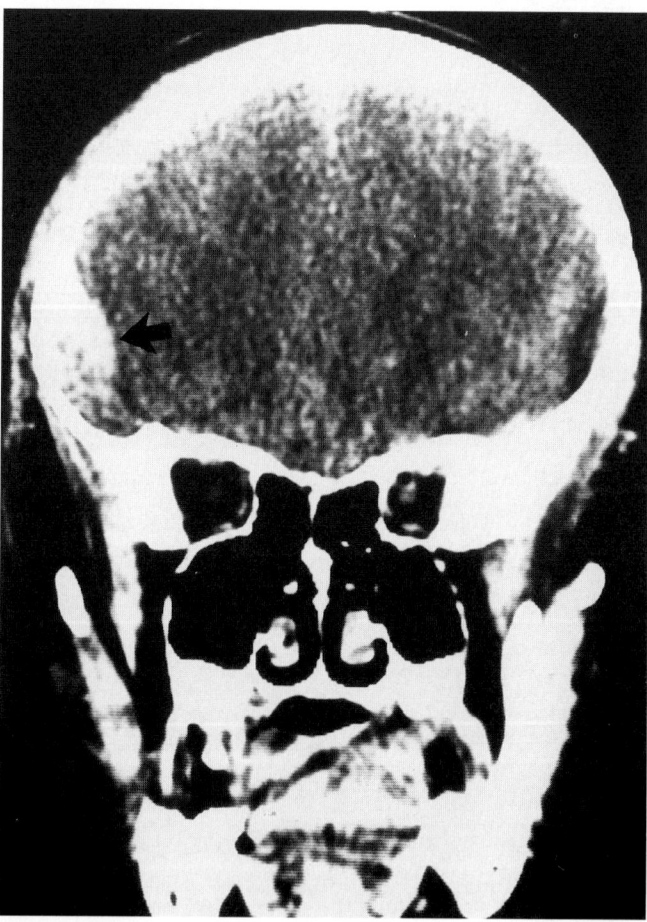

A

B

Fig. 7.29 Acute extradural haematoma. A Coronal CT on settings for facial bone assessment shows a very poorly seen right temporal extradural haematoma (arrow), which could be easily missed. **B** Coronal CT section on brain setting (same level) clearly shows an acute blood collection. This shows the importance of assessing intracranial contents as well as the bony skeleton.

which reduce the expansion of the haematoma. When acute, the haematoma is often uniformly hyperdense (Fig. 7.30), but varying appearances are seen, including a 'swirling' pattern and/or a mass with mixed densities (Norman et al 1977, Zimmerman & Bilaniuk 1982, Petersen & Espersen 1984). These relate to the ratio of clotted to unclotted blood. Uncommonly, gas bubbles are seen in the haematoma — presumed to come either

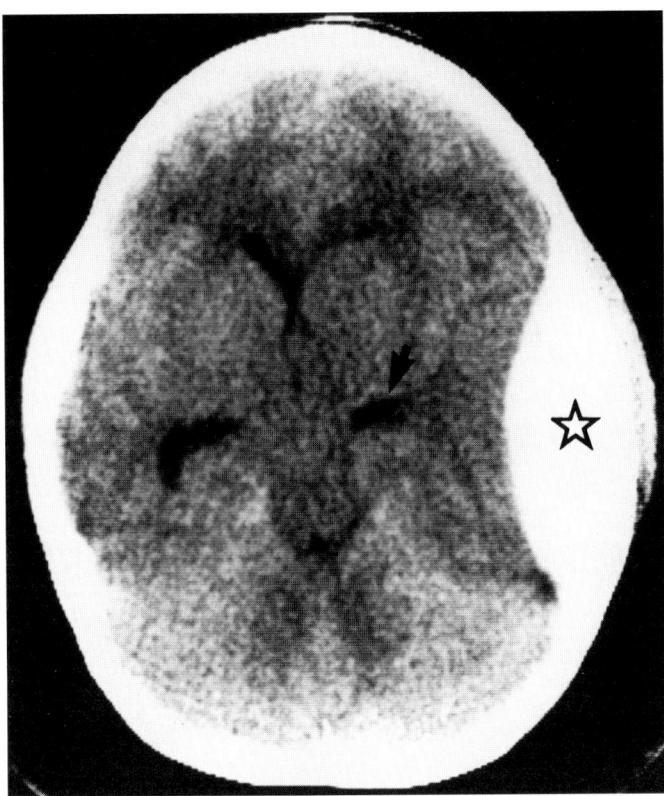

Fig. 7.30 Classic acute extradural haematoma. 'White' acute haematoma (star) deep to left squamous temporal bone, presumably from middle meningeal artery trunk. Left temporal horn (arrow) is distorted and displaced to the right, as are midline structures. The midbrain looks rather distorted.

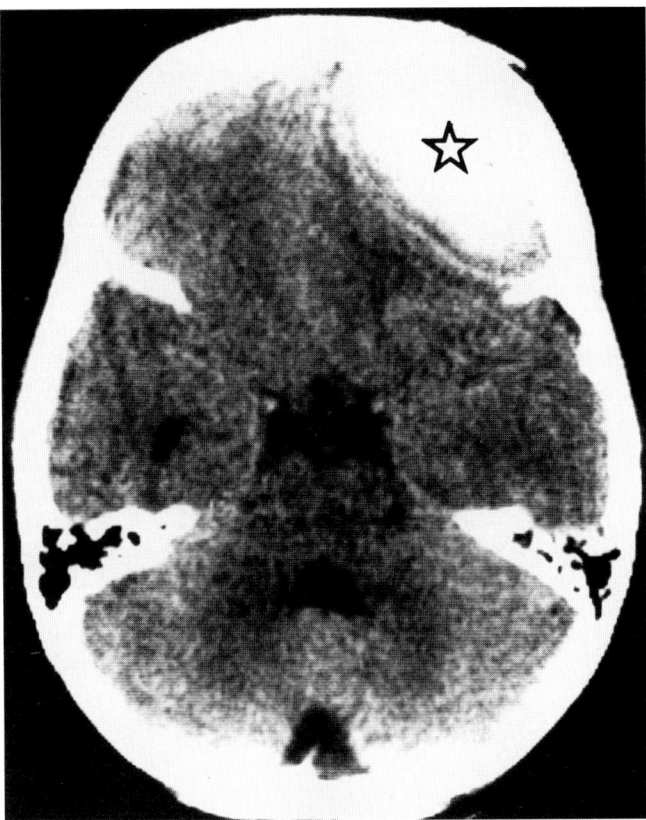

Fig. 7.31 Subacute extradural haematoma. 9-year-old girl was hit on the left side of the forehead and had continuing headache, dizziness and drowsiness. The axial CT section at 13 days shows a haematoma (star) over the roof of the left orbit — a relatively clinically silent area for an extradural bleed.

from a fracture line crossing a paranasal or mastoid air cell, or by gas exchange across membranes. Thin vertex and subtemporal extradural clots can be missed on axial scans; if necessary, these areas should be surveyed with thinner axial slices or by coronal imaging. Posterior fossa extradural collections are uncommon but often very dangerous; they are more likely to occur in children in association with an occipital fracture. Bleeding in the posterior fossa may be from a major venous sinus, emissary vein or diploic space. If the transverse sinus is responsible, the haematoma may traverse it extradurally and thus be both supra- and infratentorial. An extradural haematoma resulting from injury to the superior sagittal sinus crosses the midline in similar fashion. Sometimes a delayed extradural bleed is revealed, not uncommonly following acute decompressive surgery for another lesion. Delayed presentation can be due to low pressure bleeding, and is often seen in a clinically silent area such as the frontal or subfrontal region (Fig. 7.31); in such cases, there may be other types of CMF trauma, and the finding of the haematoma may be made in investigations preparatory to a definitive operative repair of a facial or craniofacial fracture.

Extradural haematoma may be associated with intra-

dural pathology. In the 80 patients reported by Tapiero et al (1984), 68% had other intracranial abnormalities, chiefly contusions or subdural haematomas. This incidence is high; in a series of 109 cases, Simpson et al (1988) found multiple haematomas (subdural, intracerebral, or extradural haematoma in another site) in only 20 (18.3%).

Subdural haematoma

Unlike the extradural space, the subdural space — be it potential or actual (p. 36) — opens readily and there is little if any constraint on the spread of subdural bleeding. Lanksch (1979) claimed that most subdural clots are on the same side as the impact, but that 33% are contrecoup injuries; we have not been able to confirm this. The subdural haematoma is usually seen in CT scans as a crescentic collection over the hemisphere convexity. Subdural collections can also be located on the side of the falx cerebri (interhemispheric collections), with a convex surface on the lateral aspect and a straight medial border; these are common in childhood trauma, including non-accidental trauma (Fig. 7.32). Spread over the tentorium can occur; such a collection can be difficult to distinguish from the tentorial edge itself. Spread under the tentorium

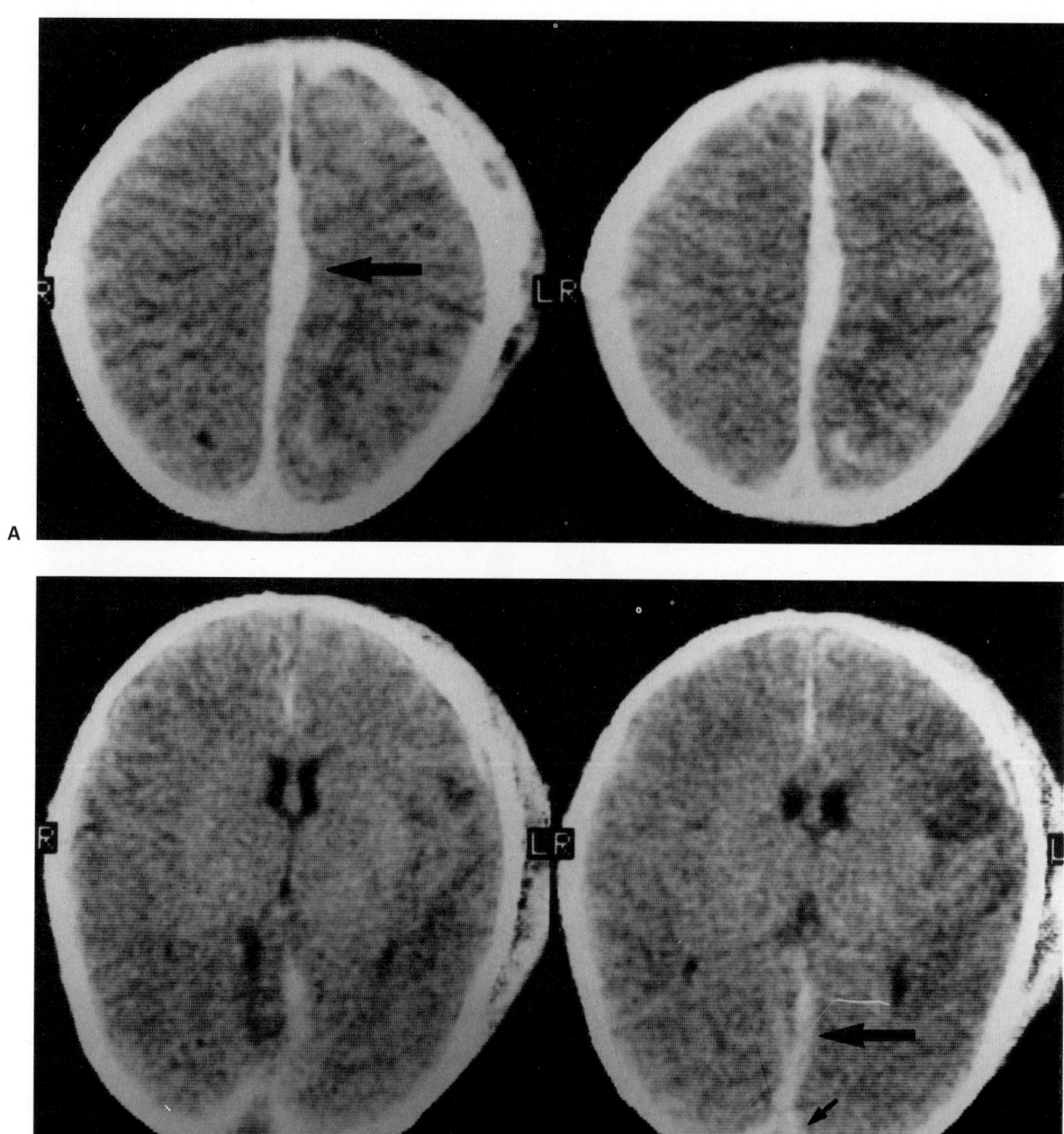

Fig. 7.32 Cerebral swelling and subdural haematoma. An infant sustained non-accidental injury. **A** High axial CT sections show acute left parafalcine sudural haematoma (arrow). A small amount of fresh blood is also noted superficially posteriorly on the left, either cortical contusion or subarachnoid blood in a sulcus. **B** Lower axial CT section (without intravenous contrast) shows the haematoma (large arrow) continued down to the tentorium. Blood on either side of the superior sagittal sinus produces a 'pseudo-delta' sign. Note poor grey/white differentiation associated with constricted ventricles (the 'tight' brain). Thin subdural haemorrhage over left parietal convexity is associated with focal low density of adjacent brain, an overlying fracture and scalp swelling. A late scan indicated severe shrinkage of both cerebral hemispheres, with enlarged ventricles and widened extracerebral spaces.

is less common than a collection above; subdural blood may be seen in both sites together. Subdural blood can outline the superior sinus itself; at the posterior end of the sinus, this gives the 'pseudo-delta' sign (Fig. 7.32B), resembling the filling defect of a thrombosed superior sagittal sinus after intravenous contrast — the true delta

sign. If scanned less than 16 h from trauma, a subdural clot may mimic an extradural haematoma in having a biconvex shape; this was seen in 10/28 patients examined by Reed et al (1986), suggesting that the haematomas may spread over the convexity with the passage of time. Classically hyperdense at presentation, subdural haematomas may vary in density over time. Layering within an acute lesion is seen in acute on chronic haematomas: there is a laminar pattern paralleling the brain surface. Failure of clotting produces dense blood posteriorly (gravitational layering). An inhomogeneous acute appearance probably indicates the presence of unclotted blood, as in some extradural clots. Chronic subdural haematomas appear hypodense on CT, the densities being at or rather above CSF. There is thus a change from an initial high density to a low density, and at some stage the haematoma is isodense with brain. At this stage the collection can be difficult to see; the difficulty is compounded if the haematomas are bilateral and 'balanced', i.e. with little or no midline shift. With modern scanners and an awareness of this potential for diagnostic error, misdiagnosis can be avoided and intravenous contrast is rarely needed now to identify the true surface of the brain. It has been stated that chronic hypodense subdural collections can be difficult to distinguish from the widening of the subarachnoid space often found in communicating hydrocephalus. This has been seen as a diagnostic problem in children with non-accidental injury; however, with a pure subdural collection, the surface of the brain is flattened, whereas an expanded subarachnoid space involves widening of the sulci. The distinction can be very difficult when there is increased fluid content in both spaces. An enhancing dural membrane can be seen in many subdural collections. MRI is a more sensitive indicator of a subdural collection than CT and is useful in picking up small subdural haematomas missed by CT (Fig. 19.16). Residual methaemoglobin and protein in a subdural haematoma result in hyperintensity on T_1-weighted images, whereas CSF in a wide subarachnoid space will be of low intensity. Both subdural fluid and CSF appear hyperintense in T2-weighted images, though the signal from the former may be more variable.

Subarachnoid haemorrhage

This is common after trauma and is visualized in CT scans done in the first few hours. Subarachnoid haemorrhages can vary from focal collections to widespread bleeding around the circle of Willis, around the midbrain, in the major fissures, and convexity sulci. This can lead to vasospasm, just as in cases of ruptured aneurysms. It should be noted that MRI is less successful in showing acute subarachnoid bleeding than CT. Diffuse acute subarachnoid blood may complicate assessment of the degree of brain swelling as the extracerebral subarachnoid cisterns are filled in with blood, mimicking a 'tight brain'; in particular, the quadrigeminal cistern may appear to be obliterated. A follow-up scan will remove this confusion as the subarachnoid blood clears; however, it may be wise to measure the intracranial pressure (ICP) at once in doubtful cases (p. 369).

Brain swelling

This is common after head injury and the increased water content of the brain produces hypodensity of both grey and white matter on CT scanning. The swelling may be global or hemispheric, perhaps in association with an acute extracerebral haematoma, or may be focal in the form of single or multiple areas around intracerebral haematomas or contusions. Swelling is also seen in association with infarction arising from various causes, such as intra- or extracranial vascular injury, coning and displacement of the brain with vascular compression, vasospasm, vascular thrombosis, embolization and systemic hypotension and metabolic disorder. Hesselink et al (1988) have compared CT with MRI of brain contusions, and have emphasized the greater sensitivity of MRI, especially when the contusion is less strongly haemorrhagic.

Cerebral swelling has more than one cause (p. 145) and the distinction between true oedema, oedematous contusion and infarct is almost impossible on CT alone; moreover, differing pathologies can coexist. Various factors must be correlated: the injury time, the neurological status, coexistent bone and soft-tissue injury, and the morphology of the abnormality, which may correlate with a recognizable territory of vascular supply. The presence of a mass effect on the ventricles and/or subarachnoid cisterns is non-specific. Generalized oedema causes a 'tight' brain with narrowed (or absent) ventricles and subarachnoid cisterns and sulci. Gray/white matter differentiation is lost and the brain therefore appears rather hypodense on CT. In children, the swollen brain sometimes appears denser; this is considered to be due to an increase in overall brain perfusion (p. 512). Narrowing or obliteration of the basal cisterns on initial scans is known to correlate positively with raised ICP pressure and is associated with poor outcomes (Toutant et al 1984).

Infarction

This may be produced by arterial or less often venous obstruction, or by both in combination. Direct vascular injury may result from blunt or penetrating injury (p. 145), but the incidence of injury to major cerebral vessels is low (El Gindi et al 1979). Direct vascular occlusion usually causes early infarction, though an embolism from an injured artery may present later. The possibility of damage to the internal carotid artery must be kept in mind: this artery may be damaged in the neck (Fig. 5.21), at the entrance to the carotid canal, within the canal or cavernous sinus, or where the artery penetrates the dura mater adjacent to the cavernous sinus. The skull base should therefore be thoroughly scrutinized for a fracture in any case of infarction in the carotid distribution. The site of the sigmoid sinus and the jugular foramen should also be examined: we have seen a fracture into the jugular foramen which was complicated by jugular bulb thrombosis (Fig. 7.28). Such a venous thrombosis can spread proximally to cause venous infarction of the cerebral hemispheres.

Vascular occlusion may also result from vasospasm or from compression by a brain herniation or mass displacement, and systemic hypoperfusion may cause ischaemia in the territory of a cerebral artery. Intracranial infection may cause arteritis or thrombophlebitis, giving rise to vascular occlusion; subdural empyema is a notorious cause of cortical thrombophlebitis (p. 147). These effects have been described as indirect vascular injury, and may cause arterial or venous infarctions. Mirvis et al (1990) emphasized the importance of brain herniation as a cause of cerebral infarction, especially in the territories of the posterior and anterior cerebral arteries.

Infarcts appear in CT scans as low density areas, and it has been noted that it may be impossible to distinguish these from oedema or contusion on the basis of the CT image alone. Marginal enhancement by intravenous contrast is seen after a variable period, and this may give the diagnosis. Similarly, MRI may show gadolinium enhancement as early as 12 h after onset of infarction. In the past, it has been usual to document the cause of a major post-traumatic infarction by carotid or vertebral angiography, but these procedures have some morbidity, and in our experience have rarely disclosed any treatable cause. MRI angiography is much less invasive; its role has been reviewed by Sklar et al (1992).

Diffuse axonal injury

Diffuse axonal injury, probably due to shear stresses from angular accelation (p. 107), is common after severe closed head injury. MRI will visualize non-haemorrhagic lesions which are thought to represent foci of diffuse axonal damage (Gentry et al 1988a); these lesions are seen in the lobar white matter, the corpus callosum and especially in the splenium (Figs 5.16 and 7.33), the dorsolateral aspect of the rostral brainstem (Fig. 5.15) and the medial lemnisci (Adams et al 1977). The lesions seen in MRI scans are usually less than 1 cm in diameter and are located in the white matter, often at corticomedullary junctions, or in large white matter fibre bundles such as the corpus callosum; they appear as areas of increased signal in T2-weighted MRI images. It has been said that callosal injury indicates a poor prognosis for full functional recovery; it is probably more correct to say that corpus callosum injury is the most easily demonstrable form of DAI, and therefore is seen in most severe cases of that condition. We have also seen callosal lesions in relatively less severe injuries. Haemorrhagic shear lesions (multifocal vascular injury) are shown both by CT and MRI (Figs 7.33 and 7.34), though our autopsy studies suggest that MRI is more sensitive (see above). A normal CT scan after head injury with neurological impairment demands an MRI

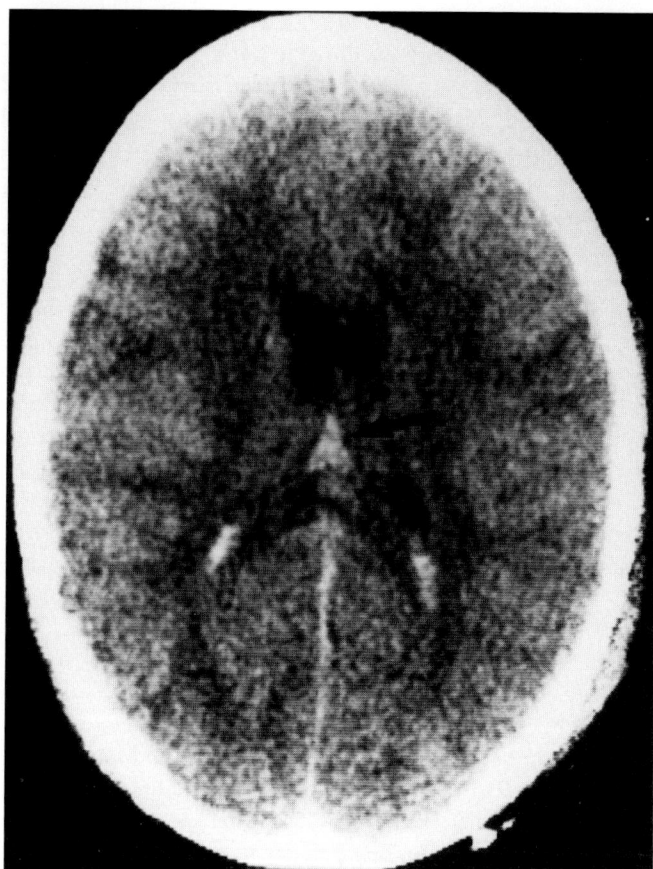

Fig. 7.33 Traumatic haematoma in corpus callosum. Axial CT section shows midline hyperdensity consistant with acute bleeding in the splenium of the corpus callosum or in the subjacent tela choroidea.

scan to show shear injuries. The late effects of head trauma are best evaluated by MRI as part of the definitive assessment of the patient's disabilities (p. 567); this investigation will often show focal or general atrophy which may represent the end result of DAI (Fig. 5.16).

Cortical contusions

These are common and involve the cerebral cortex, often appearing to spare the white matter; the sizes vary, and larger contusions extend into the subjacent white matter. The temporal and frontal lobes are most commonly involved. Contusions are typically haemorrhagic, which increases the chance of detection by CT in the acute phase; however, cortical blood may be difficult to distinguish from overlying skull or from a small extracerebral collection. MRI will easily detect methaemoglobin in the T1 weighted sequences after an appropriate interval (Table 7.5).

Subcortical haemorrhage

Many authors have described traumatic lesions in the

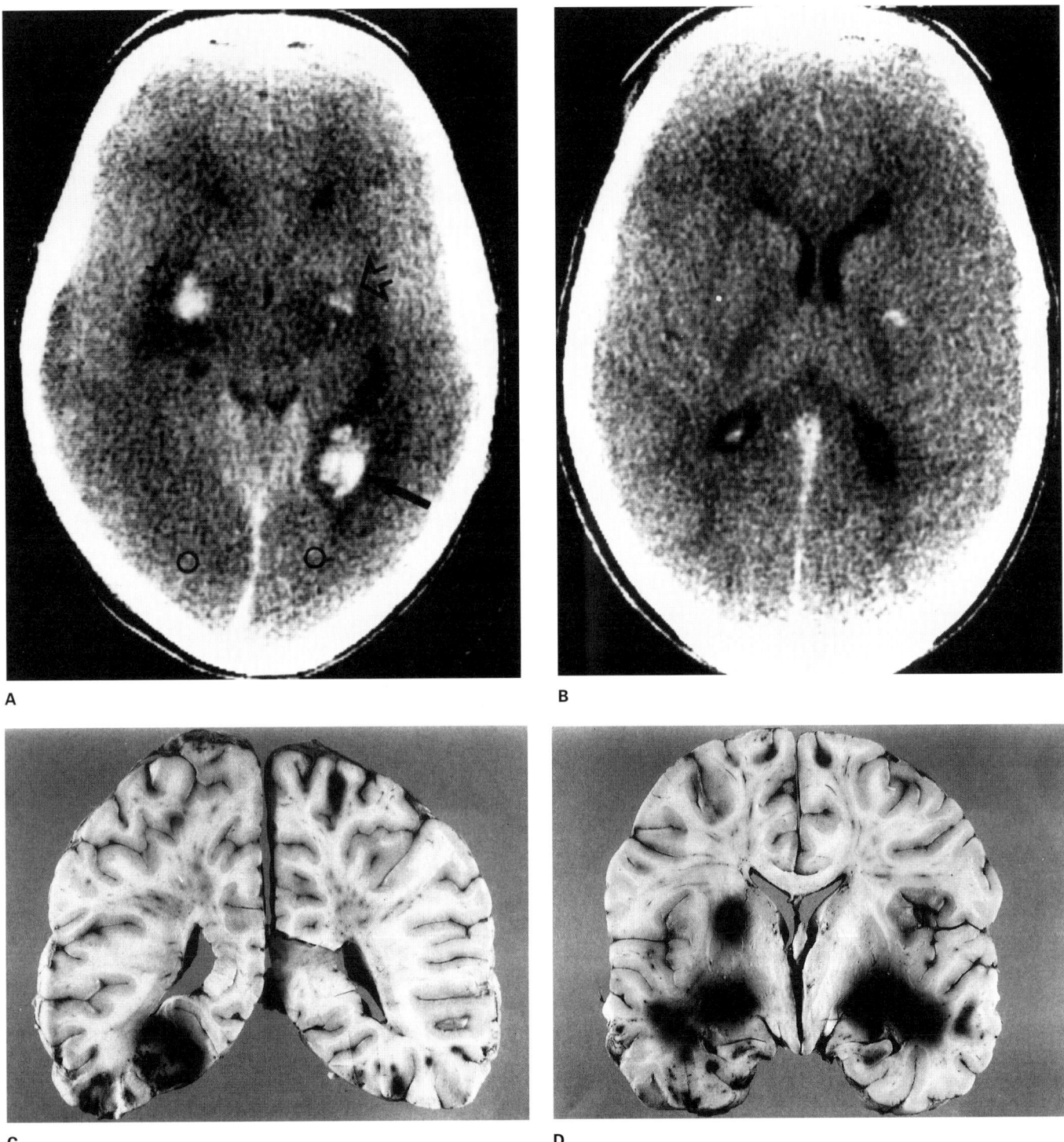

Fig. 7.34 Multiple intracerebral haemorrhages. A boy fell from a motor cycle and was immediately unconscious. **A** Axial CT shows bilateral haematomas, in the basal ganglia (open arrow) and left occipital lobe (solid arrow). Poor grey white differentiation in the occipital lobes (circles) suggests possible occipital infarction from tentorial herniation. However the ambient cistern is preserved. **B** Higher axial CT shows small lesion in the left putamen. **C, D** Autopsy shows bitemporal and basal ganglionic haematomas.

basal ganglia and thalamus. These may be a secondary effect of disruption of small perforating blood vessels; we regard them as a manifestion of vascular shear injury (Fig. 7.34B). Similar lesions in the brainstem have been described by Sklar et al (1992), together with other evidence of diffuse shear injury, in association with stormy clinical courses and evidence of sympathetic hyperactivity. In a few cases, haematomas in the basal ganglia have been large enough to require surgical evacuation; presumably these result from rupture of one of the striate arteries.

Intracerebral haematoma

These may be acute, though occasionally the onset may be delayed by several days or weeks; intracerebral haematomas sometimes present after decompressive surgery, and delayed intracerebral bleeding may follow missile brain injury. CT shows a high-density rounded or irregular collection in the brain parenchyma; it is important, though difficult, to distinguish a haematoma from a haemorrhagic contusion or shear lesion, in which the extravasated blood is interspersed with areas of injured or oedematous brain. Haematomas are often multiple and are predominantly seen in the frontal and anterior temporal lobes; they are often seen in association with haemorrhagic contusions, and may represent continued bleeding in a contusion.

For clinical purposes, resolution of a haematoma is gauged in CT scans by reduction in volume (Dublin et al 1977). Degradation of haemoglobin produces a reduction in density with time, and the changes give clues to the age of the haematoma. The MRI appearances depend on the nature of image contrast (T1 or T2 weighting), the time from onset of the haematoma (allowing change from oxyhaemoglobin to deoxyhaemoglobin to methaemoglobin to haemosiderin), the magnetic field strength and the imaging sequence, such as gradient – echo or spin – echo (Silberstein & Hennessy 1993). On T1 weighting, the haematoma initially may be low signal (black) or iso-intense to brain (grey). Within a few days, it becomes hyper-intense (white). It may remain hyperintense or gradually reduce, to approach CSF in intensity (high signal — white). On T2 weighting with a high field strength, the initial high signal changes within hours and becomes hypo-intense. Around the middle of the first week the haematoma becomes hyper-intense again, later developing a low signal rim of haemosiderin. Table 7.5 sets out these changes in schematic form.

The spatial configuration of an intracerebral haematoma should be kept in mind when assessing CT and especially MRI scans. There are four components: the inner core, the outer core, the rim and the surrounding tissues. The changes indicative of haemoglobin degradation first appear peripherally, and extend to the inner core. The rim seen in MRI scans of chronic haematomas is haemosiderin. The changes seen in the surrounding tissues, both in CT and in MRI, represent vasogenic oedema in brain adjacent to the haematoma.

A primary cerebral haemorrhage causing trauma by inducing a fall or an accident when driving may be confused with a traumatic haemorrhage, and the distinction is often difficult or impossible. Gomori et al (1985) discussed MRI findings in 20 patients in this context.

Intraventricular haemorrhage

CT will easily pick up large amounts of blood in the ventricular system but small amounts in the dependent occipital horns or fourth ventricle may be missed unless closely scrutinized.

Brainstem lesions

Lesions in the pons, midbrain and medulla oblongata are usually associated with a severe initial impairment of consciousness. Injury is either primary or secondary. The commonest primary damage is diffuse axonal injury and is usually part of generalized white matter shear injury; in fatal cases, gross brainstem tears are seen, and occasionally smaller tears may be compatible with survival. We have found diagnostic MRI signs in a small ponto-medullary tear (Blumbergs et al 1991) in a patient who lived for some 4 weeks; longer survival has been reported.

Secondary brainstem damage results from high ICP, herniation and brain distortion, hypotension and ischaemia. Secondary Duret haemorrhages (p. 148) are centrally placed midline tegmental haematomas in the rostral pons and midbrain, probably due to stretching or tearing of penetrating arteries as the upper brainstem is caudally displaced during transtentorial herniation (Fig. 2.28). These can be well seen in CT scans when acute, and their anatomy is exquisitely shown in sagittal MRI images (Fig. 7.35).

Open craniocerebral wounds

In comparison with the complex sequence of pathological changes seen after severe closed head injury, the effects of compound skull fractures and penetrating craniocerebral wounds are relatively simple. CT imaging is usually satisfactory for clinical purposes: bone settings visualize fractures, indriven bone chips and missiles, while brain settings show the contusional haemorrhages and oedema often accompanying these injuries. MRI has been little used, since CT scanning is more convenient; in missile wounds, the possibility of a ferromagnetic missile provides a further argument against the use of MRI.

In open brain wounds, the possibility of arterial damage arises; false aneurysms may form, resulting in delayed haemorrhage. We have seen this after a non-penetrating cerebral wound, but it is much more often recorded after a missile wound. For this reason, cerebral angiography should be performed if the trajectory of a missile suggests that a major artery may have been wounded, or of course if a delayed haemorrhage has actually occurred. The role of cerebral angiography is further discussed in Chapter 13 (p. 386).

Delayed effects of brain injury

Almost always, areas of brain damage will continue to swell after an initial acute injury. This must be expected,

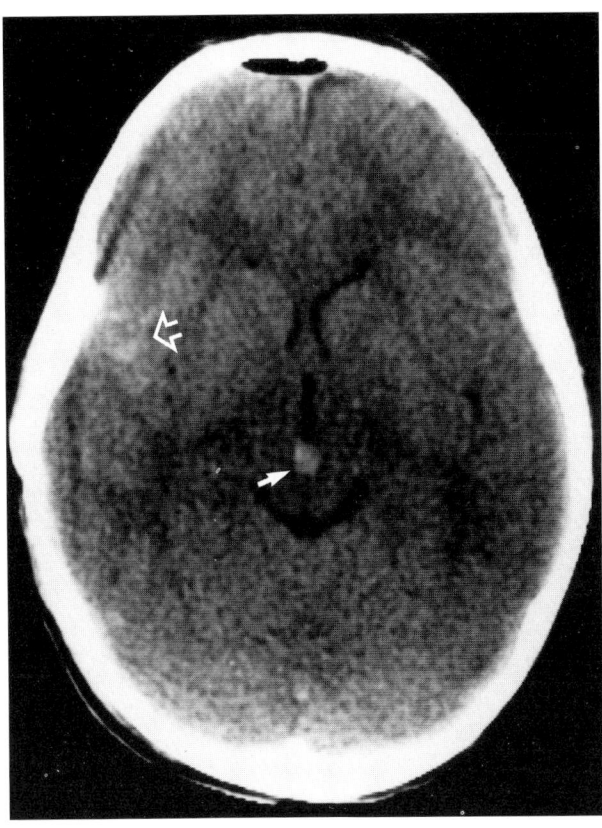

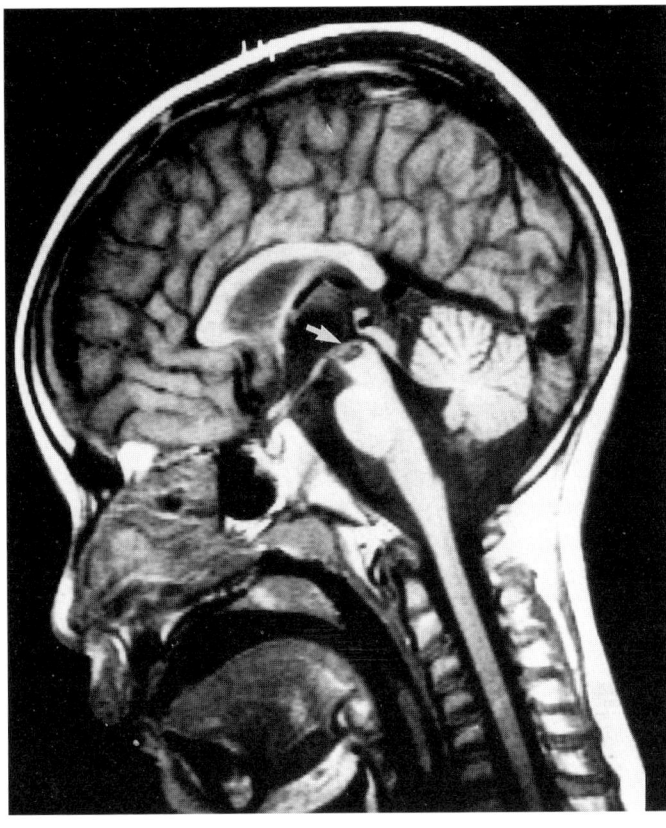

A   B

Fig. 7.35 Acute Duret haemorrhage in midbrain. A Axial CT brain scan shows rounded hyperdensity (solid white arrow) in the region of the posterior third ventricle. The differential diagnosis included acute blood in the third ventricle. Note acute subarachnoid blood in the right Sylvian fissure (open white arrow) which was associated with a comminuted depressed fracture of the overlying vault. There is very subtle asymmetry of the frontal horns. Extracerebral air is noted anteriorly. **B** Midsagittal T1 spin echo MRI section. A discrete low signal rounded lesion (arrow) is present in the upper midline tegmentum of the midbrain, consistent with an acute haematoma (Duret haemorrhage). Note the aqueduct of Sylvius just posterior to the lesion, with the tectum behind that.

though it may to some extent be controlled by appropriate osmolar treatment. A significant number of patients will develop new haemorrhagic lesions, independent of any operative procedure, and there may be deterioration in known lesions. Delayed subdural haemorrhage may appear hours or days after decompressive surgery. Haemorrhage with surrounding oedema frequently develops in areas of contusion, especially in elderly patients with fragile blood vessels. Delayed infarction is another risk. To detect these and other surgically significant complications, it is imperative that CT scans should be repeated in the course of management of a severe head injury. This should be done, not only if there is clinical evidence of deterioration, but also if there is failure to improve.

Infective complications should also be kept in mind, especially after CMF injuries involving the anterior cranial fossa, and after penetrating wounds. From the radiologist's viewpoint, the possibility of an intracerebral abscess, subdural empyema or meningitis will justify the use of contrast enhancement: the typical findings in post-traumatic abscesses are discussed in Chapter 13.

In the investigation of long-term cerebral disabilities, MRI scan is the investigation of choice (Figs 22.2 and 22.3). However, a CT scan is often informative, especially if a scan from the early post traumatic period is available for comparison (Fig. 7.36).

Non-accidental craniocerebral injury in childhood

These injuries are disquietingly frequent in some countries. Although impacts in the CMF area are not especially common, and facial fractures are not often seen, non-accidental injury (NAI) is relevant in this book because it may masquerade as accidental trauma. The hallmark of NAI is injury separated in time and space; CT (Fig. 7.37) and still more MRI scans may be very helpful in indicating the time of injury or injuries. Head injury is certainly very common, with or without skull fractures, and includes the full gamut of cerebral and extracerebral injury described in Chapter 5. Injuries vary from severe brain damage leading to death to an isolated skull fracture; delayed cases often present with enlarging heads due to

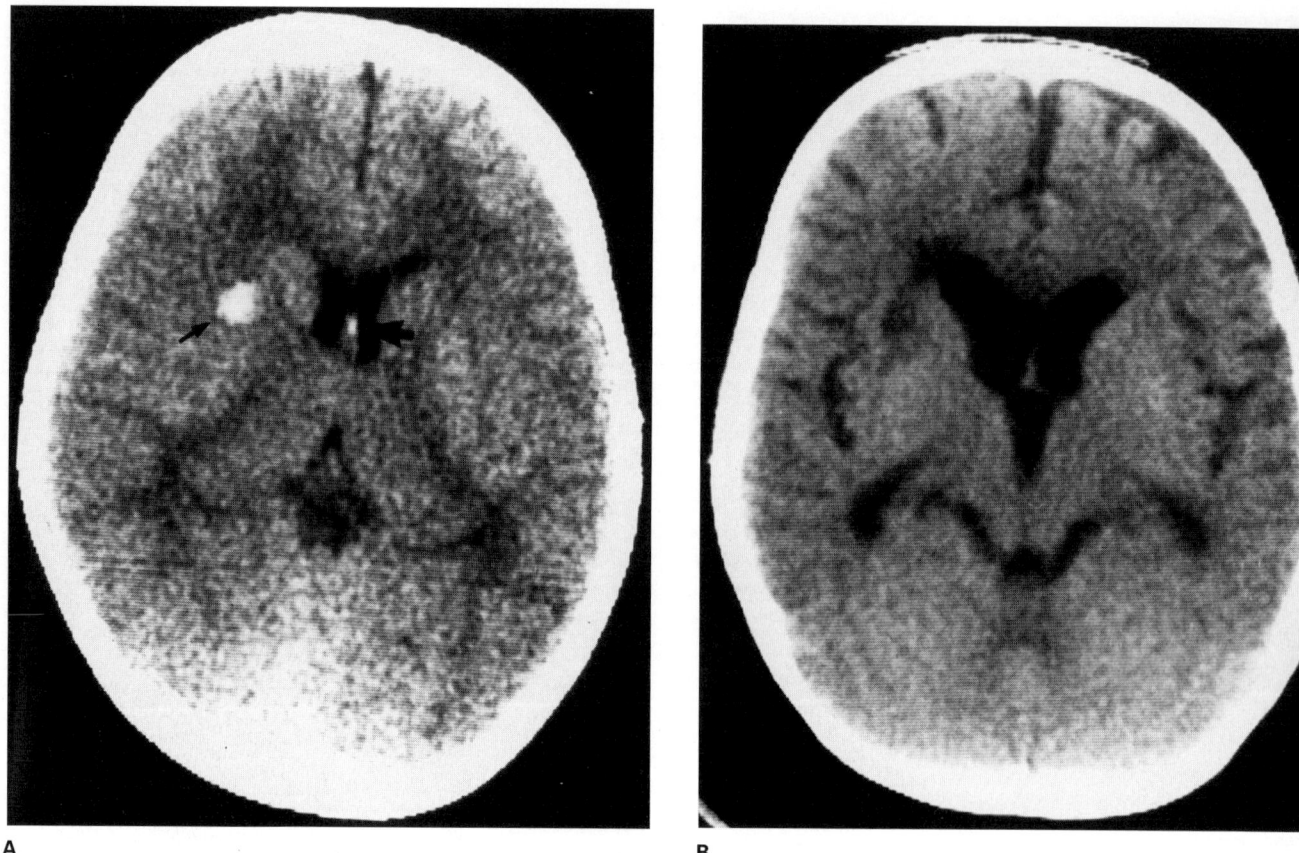

A B

Fig. 7.36 Acute closed head injury with later gliosis. A Axial CT slice shows acute bleed in the anterior limb of the right internal capsule (small arrow) just lateral to the caudate nucleus head and involving lentiform nucleus. Small haematoma in septum pellucidum (large arrow). **B** Axial CT 6 months later shows residual gliosis at the site of original haematoma and also around the tip of the right frontal horn. Cerebral atrophy has resulted in enlarged lateral ventricles and widened subarachnoid spaces.

subdural effusions. MRI has been shown to be superior to CT in diagnosing the lesions characteristic of child abuse (Sato et al 1989). Frequently, small subdural haematomas are missed by CT, especially if parallel to the scanning plane, but not by MRI. These are attributed to rupture of bridging veins, resulting from shaking, though we have reservations about this often-postulated mechanism — more aggressive violence is a probable cause in some cases. Differentiating chronic SDH from the wide arachnoid spaces of communicating hydrocephalus may have critical medicolegal implications. Communicating hydrocephalus is suggested by a symmetric bilateral enlargement of the extra cerebral spaces including the sulci, and MRI shows this well, giving a signal suggesting CSF in these spaces. Subdural haematomas can generally be characterised as such by MRI. In some cases of NAI, there may be so-called malignant cerebral oedema, supposed by some to be peculiar to childhood (Bognanno 1990) and attributed to loss of autoregulation; in this form of brain swelling, MRI findings are surprisingly normal. NAI may also be associated with devastating hypoxic brain damage. Post-anoxic cortical laminar necrosis may be seen on serial CT examinations as serpiginous

enhancement of cortical lesions; the enhancement is presumably due to damage to the blood–brain barrier or to vascular proliferation in the cortex. The diagnosis of NAI is a complex and sensitive clinical issue; for the radiologist, it is important to have a low threshold of suspicion for child abuse.

SUMMARY

CT is the most useful method of detecting and classifying maxillofacial injuries and diagnosing acute intracranial injury. Good standard radiographic projections are still necessary, together with panoramic tomograms and cephalometric radiographs. CT scans in both axial and coronal planes are often the optimal investigation, but reformats from scans performed in the axial plane may be used. 3D CT presentations are useful to define skeletal and soft-tissue displacement and deformity. 3D models can now be created and a proposed operation can be performed as a practice procedure; the use of 3D computer information in the theatre to direct robotized surgical operations on the patient is something for the near future.

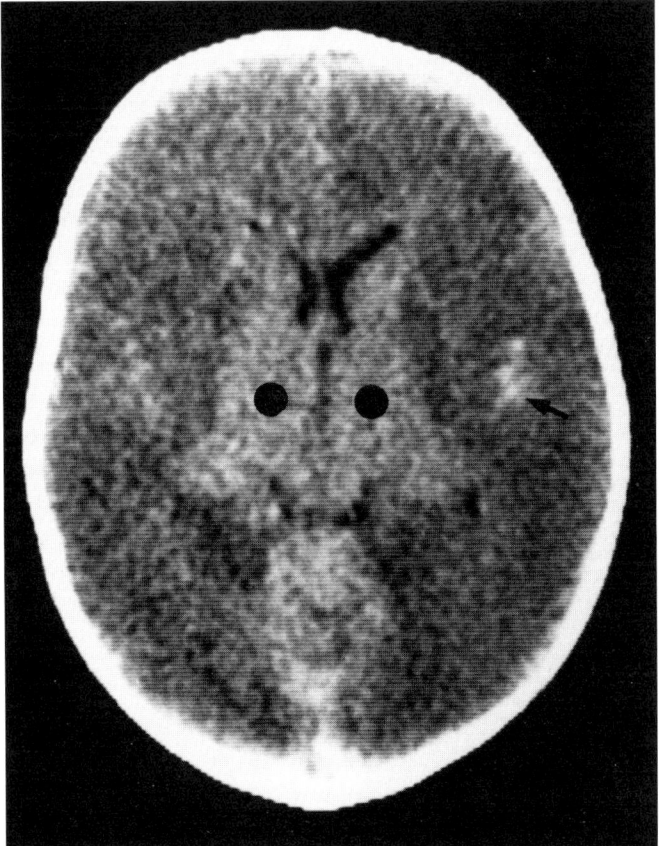

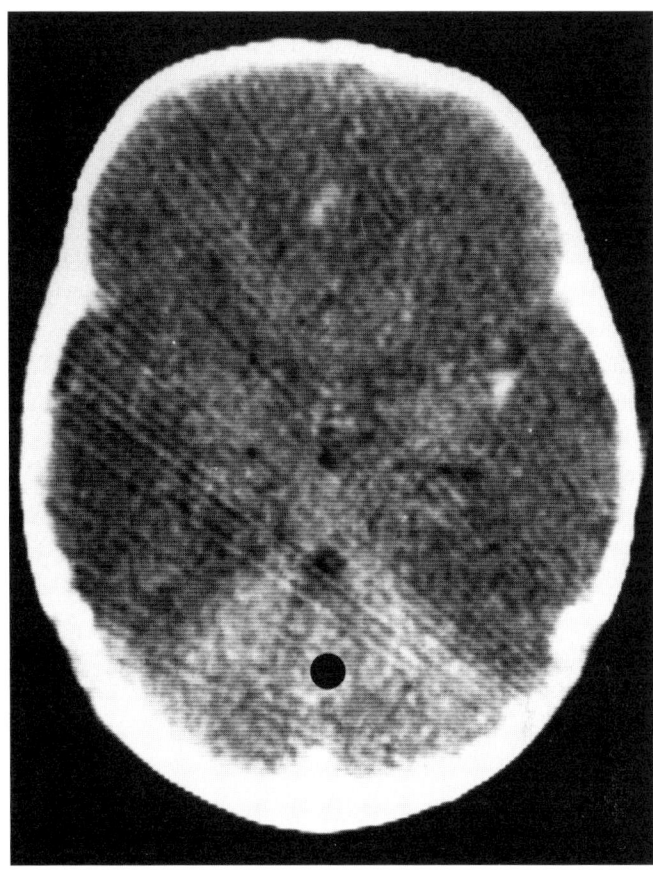

A   **B**

Fig. 7.37 Non-accidental injury with global oedema. A young infant was admitted in coma. **A** Axial CT slice through thalami (black circles) which stand out as relatively dense to the cerebral white matter and cortex. Subarachnoid blood is seen in left Sylvian fissure (arrow). Global cerebral oedema is suggested by the loss of grey/white matter differentiation. The density posteriorly in the midline is probably normal density cerebellum at the tentorial hiatus (although associated subdural haematoma is common in relation to the tentorium). The cerebral sulci are absent, suggesting brain swelling. **B** Lower axial CT section shows the 'white cerebellar' sign (black circle) wherein normal density cerebellum contrasts with oedematous, black, cerebrum.

MRI can be complementary, by exploiting its multi-planar capability and exquisite soft tissue contrast. MRI is very useful in evaluating subacute and chronic intracranial injury, orbital blow-out fractures, orbital and ocular haemorrhage and temporomandibular joint problems. Magnetic resonance vascular imaging is increasingly replacing invasive forms of angiography, but may not be available, especially for missile wounds of the brain or lower face presenting under emergency conditions, when percutaneous catheteric angiography may still be needed.

REFERENCES

Abbott A H, Netherway D J, David D J, Brown T 1990 Application and comparison of techniques for three dimensional analysis of craniofacial anomalies. J Craniofac Surg 1: 119–134

Abrahams J J 1993 The role of diagnostic imaging in dental implantology. Radiol Clin North Am 31: 163–180

Adams J H, Mitchell D E, Graham D I, Doyle D 1977 Diffuse brain damage of immediate impact type. Brain 100: 489–502

Assael L A 1993 Clinical aspects of imaging in maxillofacial trauma. Radiol Clin North Am 31: 209–220

Ball J B 1987 Direct oblique sagittal CT of orbital wall fractures. AJR 148: 601–608

Barnett G H, Ropper A H, Johnson K A 1988 Physiological support and monitoring of critically ill patients during magnetic resonance imaging. J Neurosurg 68: 246–250

Bidgood W D M Staab E V 1992 Understanding and using teleradiology. Semin Ultrasound CT MR 13: 102–112

Bite U, Jackson I T, Forbes G S, Gehring D G 1985 Orbital volume measurements in enophthalmos using three-dimensional CT imaging. Plast Reconstr Surg 75: 502–507

Blumbergs P C, Oatey P E, Sandhu A, Thomas A C, Simpson D A 1991 Pontomedullary tear in a speedboat accident; report of a case with MRI diagnosis. Zentralbl Neurochir 52: 89–93

Bognanno J R 1990 Trauma and mechanical disorders of the brain. In: Cohen M, Edwards M (eds) MRI of children. Decker, Philadelphia, pp 127–153

Brant-Zawadzki M N, Minagi H, Federle M P, Rowe L D 1982 High resolution CT with image reformation in maxillofacial pathology. AJR 138: 477–483

Cobb B J 1993 CT and radiation dose. The Radiographer 40: 27–28

Coombs M I 1992 Temporomandibular joint imaging. Parts I & II. The Radiographer 39: 11–17, 142–148

Cooper P W, Kassel E E, Gruss J S 1983 High resolution CT scanning of facial trauma. Am J Neuroradiol 4: 495–498

Crues J V, Shellock F G 1988 High-field-strength MR imaging and metallic biomedical implants: an ex vivo evaluation of deflection forces. AJR 151: 389–392

Curtin H D, Wolfe P, Schramm V 1982 Orbital roof blow-out fractures. AJR 139: 969–972

Cutting C, Grayson B, Bookstein F L, Fellingham L, McCarthy J C 1986 Computer-aided planning and evaluation of facial and orthognathic surgery. Clin Plast Surg 13: 449–462

Cutting C, Bookstein F L, Grayson B, Fellingham L, McCarthy J G 1987 Three dimensional computer-aided design of craniofacial surgical procedures. In: Marchac D (ed) Craniofacial surgery. Springer-Verlag, Berlin

Daffner R H, Apple J S, Gehweiler J A 1983 Lateral view of facial fractures: new observations. AJR 141: 587–597

Dalrymple G V, Gaulden M E, Kollmorgen G M, Vogel H H 1973 Medical radiation biology. Saunders, Philadelphia, pp 235

David D J, Hemmy D C, Cooter R D 1990 Craniofacial deformities. Atlas of three-dimensional reconstruction from computed tomography. Springer-Verlag, New York

De Lacey G J 1977 Radiology of nasal injuries. Problems of interpretation and clinical relevance. Br J Radiol 50: 412–414

Dolan K D 1989 Temporal bone fractures. Semin Ultrasound CT MR 10: 262–279

Dolan K D, Hayden J 1973 Maxillary "pseudofracture" lines. Radiology 107: 321–326

Dolan K D, Jacoby C G 1978 Facial fractures. Semin Roentgenol 13: 37–51

Dublin A B, French B N, Rennick J M 1977 Computed tomography in head trauma. Radiology 122: 365–369

El Gindi S, Salama M, Tawfik E, Aboul Nasr H, El Nadi F 1979 A review of 2000 patients with intracranial injury with regard to intracranial haematomas and other vascular complications. Acta Neurochir (Wien) 48: 237–244

Farrell V J, Emby D J 1993 Meningitis following fractures of the paranasal sinuses: accurate non-invasive localization of the dural defect by direct coronal computed tomography. Surg Neurol 40: 375–382

Freimanis A K 1966 Fractures of the facial bones. Radiol Clin North Am 4: 341–363

Gentry L R 1989 Facial trauma and associated brain damage. Radiol Clin North Am 27: 435–446

Gentry L R, Manor W F, Turski P A, Strother C M 1983 High resolution CT analysis of facial struts in trauma. 1. Normal anatomy. 2. Osseous and soft tissue complications. AJR 140: 523–532, 533–541

Gentry L R, Godersky J C, Thompson B 1988a MRI imaging of head trauma: review of the distribution and radiopathologic features of traumatic lesions. AJR 150: 663–672

Gentry L R, Godersky J C, Thompson B, Dunn V D 1988b Prospective comparative study of intermediate-field MR and CT in the evaluation of closed head trauma. AJR 150: 673–682

Gillespie J E, Isherwood I, Barber G R, Quayle A A 1987 Three-dimensional reformations of computed tomography in the assessment of facial trauma. Clin Radiol 38: 523–526

Gomori J M, Grossman R I, Goldberg H I, Zimmerman R A, Bilaniuk L T 1985 Intracranial haematomas: imaging by high-field MR. Radiology 157: 87–93

Hammerschlag S B, Hughes S, O'Reilly G V, Naheedy M H, Rumbaugh C L 1982 Blow-out fractures of the orbit: a comparison of CT and conventional radiography with anatomical correlation. Radiology 143: 487–492

Harris L, Marano G D, McCorkle D 1987 Nasofrontal duct: CT in frontal sinus trauma. Radiology 165: 195–198

Hasso A N, Christiansen E L, Alder M E 1989 The temporomandibular joint. Radiol Clin North Am 27: 301–314

Heiken J P, Brink J A, Vannier M W 1993 Spiral (helical) CT. Radiology 189: 647–656

Hemmy D C David D J Herman G T 1983 Three-dimensional reconstruction of craniofacial deformity using computed tomography. Neurosurgery 13: 534–541

Herman G T 1991 Quantitation using 3D images. In: Udupa J K, Herman G T (eds) 3D imaging in medicine. CRC Press, Boca Raton, pp 145–162

Hesselink J R, Dowd C F, Healy M E, Hajek P, Baker L L, Luersson T G 1988 MR imaging of brain contusions: a comparative study with CT. AJR 150: 1133–1142

Hurwitz T J, Welham R A N, Lloyd G A S 1975 The role of intubation macrodacryocystography in management of problems of the lacrimal system. Can J Ophthalmol 10: 361–366

Hurwitz T J, Welham R N, Malsey M D 1976 Intubation macrodacryocystography and quantitative scintillography: the complete lacrimal assessment. Trans Am Acad Ophthalmol Otolaryngol 81: 575–582

Jennett B 1980 Skull x-rays after recent head injury. Clin Radiol 31: 463–469

Johnson D H 1984 CT of maxillofacial trauma. Radiol Clin North Am 22: 131–144

Johnson M H, Lee S H 1992 Computed tomography of acute cerebral trauma. Radiol Clin North Am 30: 325–352

Jones N R, Molloy C J, Kloeden C N, North J B, Simpson D A 1993 Extradural haematoma: trends in outcome over 35 years. Br J Neurosurg 7: 465–471

Kaplan P A, Tu H K, Williams S M, Lydiatt D D 1987 The normal temporomandibular joint: MR and arthrographic correlation. Radiology 165: 177–178

Katzberg R W, Bessette R W, Tallents et al 1986 Normal and abnormal temporomandibular joint: MR imaging with surface coil. Radiology 158: 183–189

Kelly A B, Zimmerman R D, Snow R B, Gandy S E, Heier L A, Deck M D 1988 Head trauma: comparison of MR and CT — experience in 100 patients. Am J Neurorad 9: 699–708

Kneeland J B, Ryan D E, Carrera G F, Jesmanowicz A, Froncisz W, Hyde J S 1987 Failed temporomandibular joint prostheses: MR imaging. Radiology 165: 179–181

Lanksch W 1979 Computer tomography in head injuries. Springer, New York

Levy R A, Edwards W T, Meyer J R, Rosenbaum A E 1992 Facial trauma and 3D reconstructive imaging: insufficiences and corrections. Am J Neuroradiol 13: 885–892

Mafee M F 1993 Preoperative imaging anatomy of nasal-ethmoid complex for functional endoscopic sinus surgery. Radiol Clin North Am 31: 1–20

Mafee M F, Peyman G A 1987 Retinal and choroidal detachments: role of CT and MRI. An analysis of 145 cases. Radiol Clin North Am 25: 487–507

Mafee M F, Putterman A, Valvassori G E, Campos M, Capek V 1987 Orbital space-occupying lesions: role of computed tomography and magnetic resonance imaging. An analysis of 145 cases. Radiol Clin North Am 25: 529–559

Makow L S 1989 MRI: a brief review of image contrast. Radiol Clin North Am 27: 195–218

Manson P N, Grivas A, Rosenbaum A, Vannier H, Zinreich J, Iliff N 1986 Studies on enophthalmos: II. The measurement of orbital injuries and their treatment by quantitative computed tomography. Plast Reconstr Surg 77: 203–214

Marsh J L, Vannier M W 1983 The 'third dimension' in craniofacial surgery. Plast Reconstr Surg 71: 759–767

Marsh J L, Gado M H, Vannier M W, Stevens W G 1986 Osseous anatomy of unilateral coronal synostosis. Cleft Palate J 23: 87–100

Martin A, Harbison S 1972 An introduction to radiation protection. Science Paperbacks, London, p 41

Masters S J, McClean P M, Arcarese J S et al 1987 Skull x-ray examinations after head trauma. Recommendations by a multidisciplinary panel and validation study. N Engl J Med 316: 84–91

Merrell R A, Yanagisawa E, Smith H W, Thaler S 1968a Radiographic anatomy of the paranasal sinuses. I Waters view. Arch Otolaryngol 87: 184–195

Merrell R A, Yanagisawa E, Smith H W, Thaler S 1968b Radiographic anatomy of the paranasal sinuses. II. Lateral view. Arch Otolaryngol 87: 196–209

Merrell R A, Yanagisawa E, Smith H W 1969 Abnormal linear density. A useful x-ray sign in the evaluation of maxillofacial fractures. Arch Otolaryngol 90: 518–525

Meschan I 1978 Radiographic positioning and related anatomy. Saunders, Philadelphia

Mirvis S E, Wolf A L, Numaguchi Y, Corradino G, Joslyn J N 1990 Posttraumatic cerebral infarction diagnosed by CT: prevalence, origin and outcome. Am J Neuroradiol 11: 355–360

Norman D, Price D, Boyd D, Fishman R, Netwon TH 1977 Quantitative aspects of computed tomography of the blood and cerebrospinal fluid. Radiology 123: 335–338

Olson E M, Wright D L, Hoffman H T, Hoyt D B, Tien R D 1992 Frontal sinus fractures: evaluation of CT scans in 132 patients. Am J Neuradiol 13: 897–902

Pathria M N, Blaser S I 1989 Diagnostic imaging of craniofacial fractures. Radiol Clin North Am 27: 839–853

Petersen O F, Espersen J O 1984 How to distinguish between bleeding and coagulated extradural haematomas on the plain CT scanning. Neuroradiology 26: 285–292

Poletti J L, Williamson B D, Le Heron J C 1984 Radiation dosimetry descriptors applied to four CT scanners in New Zealand. Australas Radiol 28: 161–170

Reed D, Robertson W D, Graeb D A, Lapointe J S, Nugent R A, Woodhurst W B 1986 Acute subdural haematomas: atypical CT findings. A J Neuroradiol 7: 417–421

Russell J G B 1984 How dangerous are X-rays? Clin Radiol 35: 347–351

Sato Y, Yuh W T, Smith W L, Alexander R C, Kao S C, Ellerbroek C J 1989 Head injury in child abuse: evaluation with MR imaging. Radiology 173: 653–657

Schwartz J D, Harnsberger H R 1992 Imaging of the temporal bone, 2nd edn. Thieme, New York, pp 247–267

Siddle K J, Sim L H 1990 Radiation doses to the lens of the eye during computerised tomography examination of the orbit, the pituitary fossa, and the brain on a General Electric 9800 Quick CT scanner. Australas Radiol 34: 326–330

Siddle K J, Sim L H, Case C C 1990 Radiation doses to the lens of the eye during computerised tomography of the orbit; a comparison of four modern computerised tomography units. Australas Radiol 34: 323–325

Silberstein M, Hennessy O 1993 Magnetic resonance imaging of central nervous system haemorrhage. Australas Radiol 37: 161–165

Simpson D A, Heyworth J S, McLean A J, Gilligan J E, North J B 1988 Extradural haemorrhage: strategies for management in remote places. Injury 19: 307–312

Sklar E M, Quencer R M, Bowen B C, Altman N, Villanueva P A 1992 Magnetic resonance applications in cerebral injury. Radiol Clin North Am 30: 353–366

Tapiero B, Richer E, Laurent F, Guibert-Tranier F, Caille J M 1984 Post-traumatic extradural haematomas. CT diagnosis and features. J Neuroradiol 11: 213–226

Toutant S M, Klauber M R, Marshall L F et al 1984 Absent or compressed basal cisterns on first CT scan: ominous predictors of outcome in severe head injury. J Neurosurg 61: 691–694

Udupa J K, Herman G T 1991 3D imaging in medicine. CRC Press Boca Raton

Unger J M 1992 Fractures of the nasolacrimal fossa and canal: a CT study of appearance, associated injuries, and significance in 25 patients. AJR 158: 1321–1324

Vannier M W, Marsh J L, Warren J O 1984 Three dimensional reconstruction images for craniofacial surgical planning and evaluation. Radiology 150: 179–184

Westesson P-L, Katzberg R W, Tallents R H, Sanchez-Woodworth R E, Svensson A S 1987a CT and MR of the temporomandibular joint: comparison with autopsy specimens. AJR 148: 1165–1171

Westesson P-L, Katzberg R W, Tallents R H, Sanchez-Woodworth R E, Svensson A S, Espeland M A 1987b Temporomandibular joint: comparison of MR images with cryosectional anatomy. Radiology 164: 59–64

Wilberger J E, Rothfus W E, Tabas J, Goldberg A L, Deeb Z L 1990 Acute tissue tear haemorrhages of the brain: computed tomography and clinicopathological correlations. Neurosurgery 27: 208–213

Zilkha A 1982 Computed tomography in facial trauma. Radiology 144: 545–548

Zimmerman R A, Bilaniuk L T 1982 CT staging of traumatic epidural bleeding. Radiology 144: 809–812

Zinreich S J 1992 3D reconstruction for evaluation of facial trauma. AJNR 13: 893–895

Emergency management

R. M. Edwards   D. J. David
Contributing authors: J. Tomich   M. H. Moore

INTRODUCTION

Craniomaxillary (CMF) injury may be an immediate threat to life. Impacts on the face may completely close the airway at the time of the accident; the obstruction may be due to shattering of the facial skeleton, or to dislodged dentures, or to collapse of the mandibular arch and retroposition of the tongue. Obstruction may appear after an interval of a few hours, as injured tissues swell or burns blister. The resulting hypoxia and hypercarbia may affect the brain, causing confusion and even coma, or worsening in the effects of an associated brain injury.

Severe CMF injuries, especially facial wounds caused by missiles, may bleed, causing hypovolaemic shock and hypotension — another threat to brain function. Associated brain injuries may be life-threatening in themselves, by causing depression in the vital protective reflexes, especially the cough and swallow reflexes. Blood and vomit may be inhaled, and this also promotes hypoxia; massive aspiration of blood is a common finding in cases of maxillofacial injury found dead at the accident site (Arajärvi et al 1986).

CMF injuries are often associated with injuries elsewhere in the body, which may cause hypotension and other disorders of cardiorespiratory function. Major chest injuries were present in 396 (37%) of 1159 fatal head injuries studied by Selecki et al (1981).

All patients with severe CMF trauma need careful cardiovascular, respiratory and cerebral monitoring. Any degree of airway obstruction, hypoxia or hypercarbia is unacceptable, and must be relieved. To achieve this, there must be appropriate emergency care at all stages from the accident site to the intensive care unit. This means skilled staff in an organized trauma service, and every community must accept the need for a trauma service appropriate to its demographic and economic circumstances.

LIFE SUPPORT

First aid at the accident site

Hossack (1972), on the basis of autopsy findings, thought that up to 7% of all road trauma deaths in Australia were due to asphyxia and might have been prevented had someone with basic first aid skills been present at the road side. In England, Hoffman (1982) studied 344 road deaths, half of which were at the accident site, at autopsy there was inhaled blood in many, especially in cases of skull base fracture or maxillofacial trauma, and in 9.3% this appeared to be the chief or sole cause of death. However, Ottoson (1985) studied a similar series of 158 fatalities, and doubted whether the number of preventable deaths was really significant. Whatever the percentage of preventable trauma deaths, there is no doubt that good first aid is desirable, and Canadian experience has shown that intensive community training in first aid has benefits in accident prevention as well as in better injury control (Hunt 1977). In some countries, notably Germany, basic first aid training has been a prerequisite for a driving licence, but it has been questioned whether this is effective (Schneider & Schneider 1987) and an official German survey in 1980 suggested that only 18% of those holding driving licences felt confident to give first aid alone.

The first aider should be able:

1. To open the mouth and remove airway obstruction by dentures or other impacting body
2. To control external haemorrhage by local pressure
3. To place the victim in the lateral position to promote drainage of oral secretions or blood and to allow injured tissues to fall forward by gravity, thus opening the airway
4. To assess other injuries and to provide expired air (mouth-to-mouth) ventilation if necessary and possible: in some CMF injuries, the mouth and nose are completely disrupted
5. To arrange transport to a medical centre able to treat trauma.

These basic skills need to be taught in relation to CMF injuries as well as to other types of injury. To open the mouth and clear the airway without hyperextending the neck, two manoeuvres are useful: jaw thrust and chin lift. In the first, the mandible is thrust forward by pushing the angles on both sides from behind with the forefingers. In the second, the chin is lifted by grasping the symphysis menti with thumb and finger (Fig. 8.1). First aid teachers should prepare the class for the shock of feeling a shattered mandible. Control of haemorrhage is to be done with gentleness in facial wounds, and still more so in scalp wounds with an underlying depressed skull fracture; the use of a spring paper clip to control scalp bleeding can be demonstrated. The value of cardiopulmonary resuscitation should be taught, and the first aider should be warned of the problems arising if there is massive facial trauma. The use of the lateral or semiprone position may be life-saving in some facial fractures, especially if the tongue has lost its mandibular support.

Advanced life support at the accident site and in the ambulance

Good first aid will allow some accident victims to survive the journey to hospital and to arrive in better condition. However, more advanced forms of life support may be needed to deal with the airway obstruction and bleeding often seen in CMF injuries, especially missile injuries of the face and neck. Endotracheal intubation, venous cannulation and cricothyroidotomy or tracheostomy may be life-saving. These procedures may be carried out by a skilled paramedic or by a medical specialist.

In the USA, inspired by wartime experience, paramedic services have been developed to a high standard in many regions. Reines et al (1988) studied the management of multisystem trauma in urban and rural South Carolina: they found that paramedics were present at the accident scene in 93% of urban cases and 80% of rural cases. Life supportive procedures were not always successful: failure was recorded in 33% of attempts at endotracheal intubation and in 12% of attempts at intravenous cannulation. Nevertheless, the authors concluded that advanced life support administered by paramedics had been beneficial in some 85% of cases. In Germany, great emphasis has been placed on hospital-based medical retrieval teams brought to the accident site by helicopter or road ambulance at the request of the police or local ambulance service; Tscherne et al (1990) give a good account of this impressive system, which has been compared favourably with a similar US paramedic retrieval service (Schmidt et al 1992). Medical retrieval teams have obvious merits, and are used selectively in our practice. However, medically staffed teams are relatively expensive, and in rural accidents they are likely to arrive to the acci-

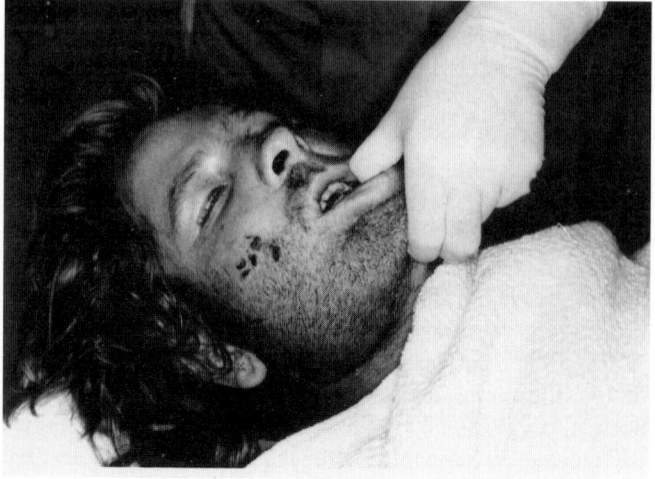 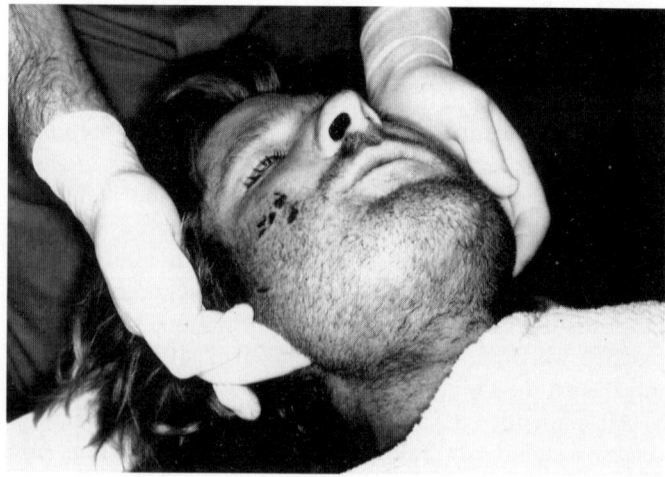

A   B

Fig. 8.1 Airway control in panfacial fracture. A 26-year-old man was found unconscious beside his crashed car. He had panfacial fractures and required jaw support at the accident site to maintain the airway. **A** Jaw thrust. **B** Chin lift.

dent scene later than a locally deployed ambulance. We have often combined both systems: initial management is begun by a rural ambulance team which is joined at the site, or on the road, by the hospital-based retrieval team.

The level of advanced skills that can be developed by an ambulance service depends on the population density and geography of the region, and on its resources of health personnel. A paramedic who rarely cannulates a vein or passes an endotracheal tube should not be expected to give these services to a patient who is shocked and asphyxiated from facial injuries. The paramedic who works in a populous North American urban area is more likely to be able to maintain these skills than is possible in a country such as Australia, where about half the major trauma occurs in isolated, thinly settled country areas: yet it is especially in places remote from a trauma centre that lives may be saved by good primary care. Throughout the world, ambulance services are having to decide whether to train their officers to 'load and go', after only basic first aid, or to provide training in more complex skills in immediate resuscitation, or to rely on medically staffed retrieval teams. The debate is sometimes acrimonious, especially when it raises issues of status and payment. Medical trauma experts should work closely with ambulance services to produce protocols, both logistic and technical, that are appropriate for their localities. Their patients will benefit.

The emergency physician, the flight nurse and the rural medical practitioner need to gain wisdom from experience and skill from practice in procedures. Special courses in Advanced Life Support (ATLS) were introduced by the American College of Surgeons in 1978, and have been very successful in many countries, including Australia; however, they have obvious limitations, and the skills they impart can be lost with the passage of time.

Resuscitation

Accident site airway control must succeed quickly to be justifiable. Endotracheal intubation is not easy at the roadside, or even in an ambulance, and unsuccessful attempts to intubate may leave the victim's airway in worse state, as well causing possibly lethal delay. Similarly, futile attempts at intravenous cannulation can be detrimental. Nevertheless, blood volume restoration before and during transport to hospital may be life-saving. The medical retrieval team can undertake this and in our practice often does; in situations where a retrieval team cannot be provided, a skilled paramedic may have an important role.

Fluid volume replacement

There has been much controversy over the relative merits of crystalloids and colloid solutions in emergency resusci-

tation after trauma (Shoemaker 1976, Lamke & Liljedah 1978, Kox & Gamble 1988). Reviewing the literature, Fischer (1989) has concluded that this controversy is unlikely come to a decisive resolution, and that traumatologists should be skilled in using both types of fluid replacement according to circumstances. We favour the use of colloids — gelatin (Haemaccel), dextran 70 (Macrodex), or 5% normal serum albumen. In experimental animals, haemodilution with colloid solutions is tolerated to a haemoglobin level as low as 4.0 g/dl (Takaori & Safar 1966)

In the emergency situation, the primary need is to restore and to maintain the volume of the intravascular compartment. Colloids remain in the intravascular compartment, whereas sodium is rapidly distributed throughout the extracellular fluid because the sodium pump mechanism effectively pumps sodium ions out of cells. Crystalloid solutions such as normal saline and Hartmann's solution expand the intracellular fluid space; only one-third remains within the intravascular compartment. Hypertonic saline solutions (3% or 7.5%) are more effective in expanding the intravascular space, because they drag water from the extravascular space, giving an expansion greater than the volume of the infusion (Holcroft et al 1987).

Those fluids whose isotonicity depends wholly or partly on dextrose have no place in blood volume expansion; dextrose is rapidly metabolized, leaving only the water infused.

We believe that large volumes of crystalloids are best avoided in patients with a tendency to pulmonary oedema or with a head injury. Admittedly, blood volume expansion by as much as three times the intravascular deficit by infusion of crystalloid solutions is tolerated by young patients. However, the large volume of fluid passing into the extravascular compartment affects both the lung and the brain. In those patients, especially the elderly, in whom the left ventricle is failing as a pump, pulmonary venous pressure will rise and more fluid will be sequestered in the lung. Pulmonary capillaries may have been damaged by aspiration of acid gastric contents or by direct contusion, or later as part of multisystem organ failure. Water, electrolytes, fibrin and even red cells may pass into the pulmonary interstitial space and eventually flood the alveoli. A sticky conglomerate resembling treacle fills the alveoli, and surfactant production may fail resulting in hypoxia and microatelectasis. An increase in the interstitial and intracellular water content is also undesirable in head injuries at risk of cerebral oedema.

These issues should be clearly understood and a simple plan of management should be formulated; in emergency resuscitation, whether at the accident site or in hospital, there is no time for debate. Our preference is to use colloids, in the form of 5% normal serum albumin (sodium 140 mmol/l, chloride 125 mmol/l) or Haemaccel if available; if these are not at hand, crystalloids (normal saline or Hartmann's solution) are used. Haemodilution to 7 g/dl is quite acceptable. Hypertonic saline solution may be a good alternative, especially when there is likely to be a swollen brain. We prefer to replace losses of > 20% of the blood volume with whole blood as soon as possible.

If haemorrhage is massive, transfusion with unmatched blood may be required during transport. Ideally, O Rh– blood should be used; however, if this is not available, O Rh+ blood can be used with little increased risk. Some 50% of unimmunized Rh– individuals will develop anti-Rh antibodies if transfused with Rh+ blood, though this is less likely to happen when the transfusion reaches wash-out magnitude; the risk of later problems in transfusion and in pregnancy must be balanced against the immediate risk of death from exsanguination. But if possible, blood transfusion with whole blood or packed cells is done later after full matching of blood from donors appropriately screened for viral infection.

Monitoring of the circulatory, respiratory and neurological functions (p. 160) is begun at the accident site; the results are recorded and re-evaluated at appropriate intervals. In battle, and after civilian disasters, the accurate recording of such data is especially vital, so that deterioration may be evident to anyone seeing the injured person for the first time at a later stage in management (Fig. 8.2).

The role of the peripheral hospital

Severe CMF trauma needs the facilities of a trauma centre able to give definitive care for all the effects and complications of the injury; intensive care and neurosurgical services, CT scanning and specialized oral – faciomaxillary care are usually essential. When the accident victim cannot be admitted quickly to such a centre, there are important roles for the less well equipped hospital which is nearer to the accident site. Such hospitals should be prepared to provide blood volume replacement, surgical procedures to arrest haemorrhage, correction of airway obstruction, chest drainage and splinting of fractures. These procedures can be carried out during a short stop in the Accident and Emergency Department or even in the ambulance; patients with spinal injuries should be moved as little as possible. However, in country hospitals several hundred kilometres away from the trauma centre, a more prolonged admission may be wise, to allow fuller assessment and stabilization. This is especially prudent when the injured person is unconscious from a head injury: a period of observation may detect a life-threatening condition such as an extradural haemorrhage or a ruptured abdominal viscus. In all circumstances, there should be telephone consultation between the peripheral hospital and the trauma centre, which should have a skilled specialist in intensive care and a neurosurgeon available for

such consultations at short notice (Simpson et al 1988). There should also be a transport system able to get the injured person to the trauma centre as quickly and safely as possible: this may be by road ambulance, helicopter or fixed-wing aircraft.

Inevitably, the quality of trauma management in a peripheral hospital does not always reach the level attainable in a major trauma centre. In a prospective audit of 153 cases of severe neurotrauma referred to Adelaide from country hospitals, Simpson et al (1984) found deficiencies in management in 11 patients; these were chiefly in dealing with cardiopulmonary emergencies. Nevertheless, in Australia and in countries with similar demographic problems (Nordström et al 1989), peripheral hospitals are essential components in regional trauma services. Indeed, in countries where climatic or economic conditions make air transport less readily available, the role of the peripheral hospital may be more ambitious, and may include definitive management of a larger proportion of CMF injuries.

Transport to the trauma centre

In the choice of transport, one must carefully weigh the needs of the injured person against the hazards and costs of transport. While it is useful to have agreed guidelines, it is also important to ensure that there is good communication between the intensivist or surgeon in the trauma centre, the ambulance or air service providing transport, and the medical officer caring for the patient in the peripheral hospital or at the accident site.

Road ambulances are cheap, safe, and capacious. Nevertheless, air transport is often the best way of bringing an injured person to the appropriate trauma centre with speed and — when this is necessary — under intensive care. Helicopters have been used with great success in war, and in populous urban areas where road transport is slow and uncertain; they are invaluable in mountain terrain and at sea (Liskiewicz 1992). We have employed helicopters both for primary transport from the accident site, and more frequently for secondary transfer from a peripheral hospital. However, helicopters are expensive and the accident rate is not inconsiderable, especially when pilots are under pressure to extricate a critically injured person from a difficult place. It is our practice to use road transport in the metropolitan area and for nonurgent transport in the country; helicopters have been used for urgent retrieval in a radius of about 50–200 km. In countries with severe urban congestion, helicopter retrieval is used over much shorter ranges. The single-engined helicopters formerly used were cramped, and unsuitable for in-flight intensive care; larger helicopters with a longer range have been available in recent years. We have found the Bell 412 helicopter very suitable for our purposes.

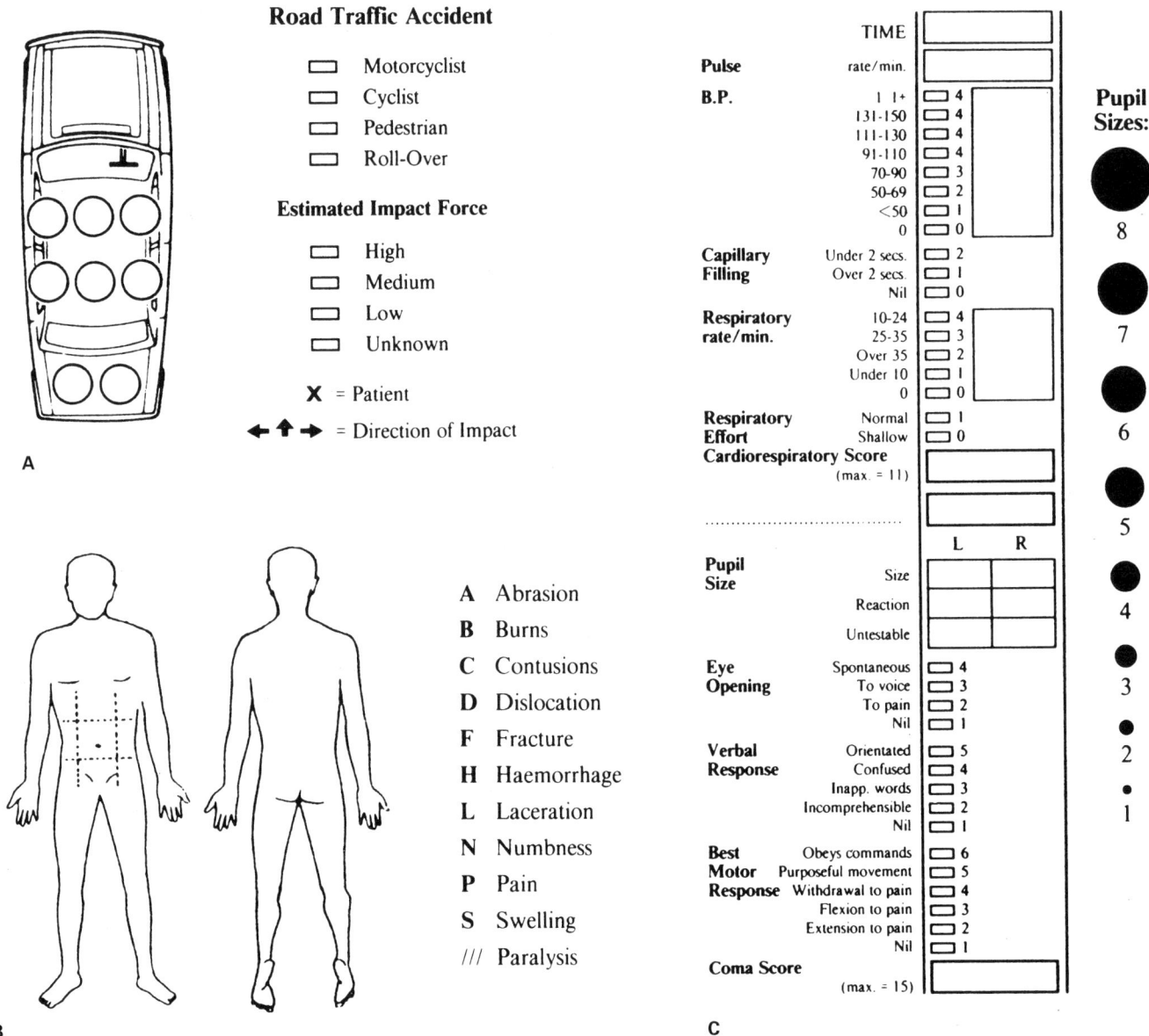

Road Traffic Accident

Motorcyclist
Cyclist
Pedestrian
Roll-Over

Estimated Impact Force

High
Medium
Low
Unknown

X = Patient

← ↑ → = Direction of Impact

A

A Abrasion
B Burns
C Contusions
D Dislocation
F Fracture
H Haemorrhage
L Laceration
N Numbness
P Pain
S Swelling
/// Paralysis

	TIME			
Pulse	rate/min.			
B.P.	1 1+	4		Pupil Sizes:
	131-150	4		
	111-130	4		8
	91-110	4		
	70-90	3		7
	50-69	2		
	<50	1		6
	0	0		
Capillary Filling	Under 2 secs.	2		5
	Over 2 secs.	1		
	Nil	0		4
Respiratory rate/min.	10-24	4		
	25-35	3		3
	Over 35	2		
	Under 10	1		2
	0	0		
Respiratory Effort	Normal	1		1
	Shallow	0		
Cardiorespiratory Score (max. = 11)				

		L	R
Pupil Size	Size		
	Reaction		
	Untestable		
Eye Opening	Spontaneous	4	
	To voice	3	
	To pain	2	
	Nil	1	
Verbal Response	Orientated	5	
	Confused	4	
	Inapp. words	3	
	Incomprehensible	2	
	Nil	1	
Best Motor Response	Obeys commands	6	
	Purposeful movement	5	
	Withdrawal to pain	4	
	Flexion to pain	3	
	Extension to pain	2	
	Nil	1	
Coma Score (max. = 15)			

B

C

Fig. 8.2 Ambulance form recording accident data. Information recorded by an experienced ambulance officer is of great value. Our standard record sheet includes: **A** A diagram of a vehicle with seating positions and provision for identifying other types of road user, also estimates of impact force and site. **B** A simple body diagram to record lesions. **C** Record of vital cardiorespiratory data and Glasgow Coma Scale. Pupillary diameters are in millimetres. Elsewhere on the same record sheet there is space for name and other biographical data, history of incident, ambulance times and details of resuscitation; the record is on two sheets, each with a carbon duplicate.

Fixed-wing air ambulances find an invaluable role in secondary transfer between the peripheral hospital and the trauma centre over long distances; they are also used in international transfers, when a severely injured person is sent to another country for specialist care or to return to his/her place of origin. We have routinely used twin-engined turbopropeller-driven aeroplanes with pressurized cabins for distances in excess of 200 km in cases of head injury requiring intensive care in transit (Simpson et al 1988); the aircraft at present in service are Beechcraft B200 Kingairs, with a usual ground speed of ~400 km/h. Over distances >1500 km, economic considerations may favour the use of a commercial air liner. To transport an unconscious patient needing ventilation, we have deployed a team of one medical specialist and two expert nurses; this necessitated the use of 15 seats, but a chartered jet would have been more expensive. The need for very long range intercontinental transport is unusual, but sometimes does arise when highly specialized treatment is required, or where the injury occurred in some remote place isolated by geography or politico-military events (Spittal et al 1992). Dedicated long-range jet aircraft are ideal for such purposes, and are being used in several parts of the world. We now employ a twinjet Bae 800 for transport over long distances in Australia; this aircraft has a speed of ~800 km/h and for distances > 1500 km it is our preferred means of transport (J. E. Gilligan, personal communication).

If air transport is to be used to retrieve critically injured patients it is important that the retrieval team have appropriate training and equipment. Gilligan (1990), who has been a pioneer in organizing and operating aeromedical services in our region, has emphasized the importance of stabilizing the injured person's physiological state before transport by air. He has listed the ideal requisites for any modality of transport of a severely injured person:

1. Physical safety; flying conditions or enemy action may affect this requirement
2. No abrupt movement in any axis
3. Sufficient space, with an attendant at the head end
4. Adequate supply of gases for life support and energy for the delivery systems: nickel–cadmium batteries are favoured, but must be kept charged
5. Easy embarkation and disembarkation of the injured person
6. Adequate lighting and internal climate control, including cabin pressurization: even in so-called pressurized aircraft, the cabin pressure may be equivalent to 2000–2500 m altitude, and in some circumstances low-level flight may be requested, at the cost of a bumpy flight
7. Tolerable noise and vibration
8. Flying speed appropriate to the degree of medical urgency
9. Minimal secondary transport (e.g. transport by road to or from the airfield)
10. Good communications with the sending and receiving medical centres.

Ideally, the aircraft should be equipped as a mobile intensive care unit; a commercial plane temporarily adapted to transport an injured person is a poor substitute. Even when good in-flight facilities are available, it is best to perform procedures such as endotracheal intubation and intravenous cannulation before leaving the primary hospital. In our air ambulances, the cabins have full facilities for in-flight resuscitation and ventilation, including blood gas analysis, capnography, and oximetry. Arterial and intracranial manometry can be done, using lightweight battery-operated display systems.

Flying to higher altitudes entails lower atmospheric pressure. An eye with a penetrating wound must be presumed to contain air, and in accordance with Boyle's Law this air will expand if atmospheric pressure falls. Since the inelastic eye cannot expand, the intraocular pressure will rise; in the presence of a perforating wound, the increased pressure will force intraocular contents — aqueous, iris, lens, vitreous — out through the wound (Fig. 8.3A,B). When atmospheric pressure rises again,

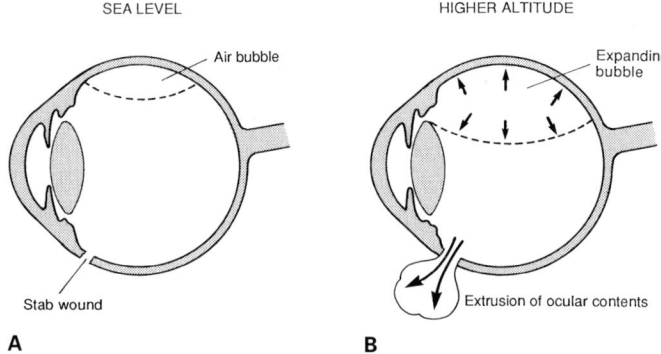

Fig. 8.3 Air in the eyeball: the effect of high altitude flying.
A A penetrating wound of the globe has admitted a bubble of air into the posterior chamber. **B** At low atmospheric pressure, the bubble expands, forcing vitreous and other intraocular contents out of the eye.

as when the plane comes down, the eye will collapse; blindness is the likely outcome. This lesson was first learned in the Korean War (1950–1951); it has been confirmed by primate experiments (Dieckert et al 1986). It is now recommended that penetrating wounds of the eye should not be exposed to atmospheric pressure at altitudes > 650 m, from fear of promoting prolapse of intraocular contents. For penetrating eye wounds, it is wise to avoid low cabin pressures and to maintain cerebral oxygenation in flight with a high flow mask; vomiting should be prevented with an anti-emetic and the eyes should be padded (Colvin 1981). It is also considered that intracranial air could expand in a detrimental way at low environmental pressures; routine skull radiography before flight should exclude this risk, but it is again wise to keep cabin pressures at sea level during flight if an aerocele is a real possibility. The aircraft used by us permit this.

Other possible effects of high altitude flight in an unpressurized aircraft include expansion of the cuff of an endotracheal tube and accelerated flow from an intravenous line, due to expansion of gas in the drip chamber.

Emergency room

This may give the first opportunity to perform the head-to-toe examination described on p. 160, and to take a detailed history. It is often the place where definitive measures to support life are undertaken.

Assessing the airway

Two dangerous associated injuries should be carefully looked for.

Fracture of the larynx

This contraindicates an attempt to pass an endotracheal tube (Schaefer 1991). The signs are:

● hoarseness and stridor

- local bruising and swelling
- loss of the normal laryngeal prominence
- haemoptysis
- surgical oedema
- inability to voice a high 'E'.

Attempts to pass an endotracheal tube may produce complete disruption of the larynx and airway obstruction from dissection into the tissues of the neck by the tube; even in the absence of airway obstruction, the delicate components of the larynx may be damaged. Cricothyroidotomy may have similar dangers, and tracheostomy under local anaesthesia should be considered (Nahum 1969).

Spinal injury

A fracture or dislocation of the cervical spine may be associated with CMF trauma, and attempts to secure the airway may then endanger the spinal cord. Injury to the vertebral column should be assumed until excluded by radiographs, and the neck is immobilized in all unconscious trauma victims. Therefore, if it is at all possible, a lateral X-ray picture of the neck should be taken before endotracheal intubation is attempted. The emergency room should have an overhead X-ray machine for this purpose. However, in cases of CMF injury, airway obstruction is common and cervical spinal injury is not so common, and fear of quadriplegia should not cause delay in clearing the airway if the patient is asphyxiating. Ross et al (1992) found that the chief clinical indicators of an unstable cervical spinal injury are loss of consciousness — even if brief — from head injury, spinal tenderness, and of course neurological signs; fracture or soft-tissue injury of the face did not appear to be a significant warning sign.

In assessing the X-ray picture (Fig. 7.2), care is needed to ensure that all seven cervical vertebrae are seen. In the ATLS (1993) manual, the following guidelines are given to identify significant abnormalities:

A. Alignment
1. Vertebral malalignment > 3.0 mm = dislocation
2. Anteroposterior spinal canal space < 13 mm = cord compression
3. Angulation of an intervertebral space > 11°

B. Bones
1. Vertebral body
   a. Anterior height < 3 mm posterior height = compression fracture
   b. Olique lucency = tear-drop fracture
2. Lack of parallel facets of the lateral mass = possible lateral compression fracture
3. Lucency through the tip of the spinous process = avulsion fracture
4. Atlas and axis (C1 and C2)

   a. Distance between posterior aspect of C1 to anterior surface of odontoid process > 3 mm = dislocation
   b. Lucency through the odontoid process = fracture.

C. Soft-tissue space
1. Widening of the prevertebral space > 5 mm = haemorrhage accompanying spinal injury
2. Loss of prevertebral fat stripe = fracture at same level
3. Widening of space between spinous processes = torn interspinous ligaments and likely spinal fracture anteriorly.

These guidelines are not absolute indicators of trauma and the X-ray findings should be discussed with a radiologist. In a recent prospective study of 453 cases of fractures and subluxations of the cervical spine, Woodring & Lee (1993) found that 61% of unstable fractures and 36% of subluxations were incorrectly diagnosed by plain X-ray examination; indeed, in nearly one third, no abnormality was detected in the standard sequence of plain films.

Securing the airway

Difficulties may arise from:

1. Swollen lips, tongue or floor of the mouth
2. Disruption of teeth and/or jaws
3. Continuing local bleeding, especially interstitial bleeding in the neck — a very dangerous complication of a coagulopathy (Fig. 20.4)
4. Disruption of anterior cranial fossa
5. Trismus.

Trismus due to pain may relax after anaesthesia has been induced, but when the cause is a fracture of the mandibular condyle, the coronoid process, or the zygoma, then it may be impossible to open the jaw. One cannot always predict whether trismus will relax or not. Combinations of these injuries will increase the difficulties: swelling of the tongue and floor of mouth, a comminuted maxilla, gaps in the teeth, and an intact mandible make a particularly bad combination. Several methods of securing the airway are worth consideration in such situations.

Intubation without anaesthesia — 'awake' intubation

The patient may be unconscious from a cerebral injury; if not, light sedation may be given. Laryngoscopy allows damaged tissues to be lifted away from the larynx and posterior wall of the pharynx, after which intubation is often surprisingly easy. Topical anaesthetic may be applied to the larynx; alternatively, laryngoscopy may show that it is in fact safe to induce anaesthesia with thiopentone and a muscle relaxant (suxamethonium) and intubate thereafter.

Intubation under thiopentone and muscle relaxation

This is comfortable for the patient and gives the endoscopist the best possible conditions. But what if a tube cannot be passed? Still worse, what if the paralysed patient cannot be ventilated? *This situation must and can be avoided.*

Pivotal in our thinking has been the case of a 12-year-old lad who was accidentally shot in the mouth with a .22 in. bullet, some 300 km from Adelaide. Teeth were shattered, the hard palate and the mandible were fractured and the tongue was lacerated. However, the boy was initially alert and remained so during transfer to our care by air. When he arrived in the operating theatre 8 h after injury, his airway was compromised by gross swelling. It was decided to perform a tracheostomy under general anaesthesia, with gas induction. However, when placed in the supine position — he had been sitting up — the boy became distressed and uncontrollable. The options were considered and the boy was given pentothal and suxamethonium, but his tongue was so swollen that the larynx could not be seen, and an endotracheal tube was passed blindly. The surgeon then opened the neck, but met with brisk bleeding and signs of asphyxia; the cervical tissues were so swollen that the trachea and the larynx could not be located. The endotracheal tube was felt by palpation, and opened: it proved to be in the oesophagus! By the time the trachea was located and a tracheostomy performed, severe hypoxic brain damage had supervened, and the boy later died. From this case, and others, we have learned the importance of early intubation, before local swelling has developed. But this may not be possible.

Gaseous induction

If the patient can be successfully anaesthetized with O_2 and halothane, the airway can be inspected, and intubation can be accomplished with or without a muscle relaxant. But if the patient is bleeding profusely, or vomiting, gaseous induction may be difficult or impossible. If there is gross disruption of the face, it may not be possible to contain the gas within the face mask. Moreover, in patients with severely compromised airways, complete obstruction may appear when light anaesthesia is induced.

Fibreoptic intubation

It takes only a spot of blood to blind the fibrescope. The instrument is therefore unreliable in acute CMF trauma, though useful later when bleeding is absent.

Tracheostomy under local anaesthesia

This is sometimes regarded as a useful option, and we have done this with success when unwilling to disturb a massive foreign body impaling the face in the region of the temporomandibular joint (Fig. 14.1). But what if an already compromised airway becomes obstructed during the operation? There may be quite severe local bleeding under these circumstances.

Tracheostomy is easy when done electively with a secure airway and quiet ventilation. When there is asphyxia and the patient has not been intubated, the surgeon must grasp the larynx and locate the cricoid cartilage and the suprasternal notch. A midline vertical incision is made between these landmarks. In desperate cases, the midline tissues are then divided and the trachea is opened vertically or preferably with a flap, the first ring being spared. A cuffed tube is inserted, the cuff is inflated, and anaesthesia is induced. Less urgent settings allow the standard procedure of dissection, transection of the thyroid isthmus, and transverse incision of the trachea.

Percutaneous tracheostomy has been recommended as a simpler and quicker means of intubating the trachea; however, even in experienced hands, this method sometimes fails (Ivatury et al 1992) and we have not used it as an emergency procedure, though it has been very satisfactory in elective tracheostomies.

Cricothyroidotomy

This is a most useful option when it is not possible to pass an endotracheal tube, or if the necessary skill to do so is not available. A transverse incision exposes the cricothyroid membrane, which is incised. The opening is dilated and a small (5–7 mm) endotracheal tube is inserted.

The procedure should be used more often. However, there are patients in whom it is difficult to palpate the thyroid and cricoid cartilages, especially when the anatomy is distorted by swelling or haematoma. Open cricothyroidotomy is not recommended in children, in whom it is preferable to insert a large intravenous cannula through the cricothyroid membrane and insufflate oxygen intermittently.

Blind nasotracheal intubation

Blind intubation is potentially dangerous and we do not advise it in patients with CMF trauma until a fracture of the anterior fossa has been excluded: if the floor of the anterior cranial fossa is fractured, a nasal tube may pass through the fracture and enter the brain (p. 251). Moreover, in victims of acute trauma, the stomach may be full of blood and alcohol: the stimulus of pernasal intubation may induce vomiting and the vomit may be aspirated. The stomach can of course be emptied by a nasogastric tube. However, this also is dangerous if there is a fracture of the anterior cranial fossa (p. 383). Also, the stimulus may cause quite violent movement of the head and neck, perhaps endangering the spinal cord if there is an injury of the cervical spine.

Any of these methods of securing the airway may fail; in fact, all may fail. Tragedies are best avoided by anticipating them. If there is any degree of airway obstruction, it must be corrected at once. If there is undue swelling, a tube should be inserted: as time passes, the situation will get worse. A misplaced tube may obstruct one bronchus (Fig. 19.1); this may cause severe pulmonary insufficiency and anoxia, especially detrimental when there is an associated cerebral injury.

Cases of CMF injury with airway obstruction require a senior anaesthetist with experience of acute trauma. Insist on that.

Control of haemorrhage

CMF injuries, especially those in the midface region, may present with exsanguinating bleeding, which must be controlled at once. The bleeding may be from superficial arteries, notably the facial and superficial temporal arteries, or from deep branches of the external carotid artery, especially the maxillary artery (p. 48). Superficial arterial bleeding may be controlled by direct pressure; this is often insufficient, and it is then necessary to explore the wound and to ligate or clip the bleeding vessel (Alexander 1989).

Epistaxis or oropharyngeal bleeding may be controlled by packing.

As a first step, the nasal cavity and nasopharynx are carefully inspected under general anaesthesia. A telescopic nasendoscopy is very useful in doing this. Any obvious bleeding point is cauterized with diathermy, and nasal tamponade is carried out with due care to ensure that the packs can be removed at a later time.

Recurrent bleeding after tamponade may need emergency operation. When the bleeding is thought to come from the lower half of the nasal cavity, the pterygopalatine segment of the maxillary artery can be ligated through an anterior antrostomy (Friedman 1985, Spiessl 1990). A sublabial incision is made, and an opening is made in the anterior antral wall (Fig. 8.4A). The posterior wall of the antrum is removed with a diamond bur in its superomedial wall, exposing the posterior periosteum (Fig. 8.4B). An operating microscope with a 350 mm lens is then used to explore the pterygomaxillary fossa. The periosteum is opened; careful dissection with blunt hooks then exposes the maxillary artery and its descending palatine branch (Fig. 8.4C). These are then ligated with titanium or tantalum clips: three clips are essential to control bleeding in the nose and nasopharynx, on the maxillary artery proximal to the origin of the descending palatine artery, on the descending palatine artery itself (as low as possible), and on the terminal portion of

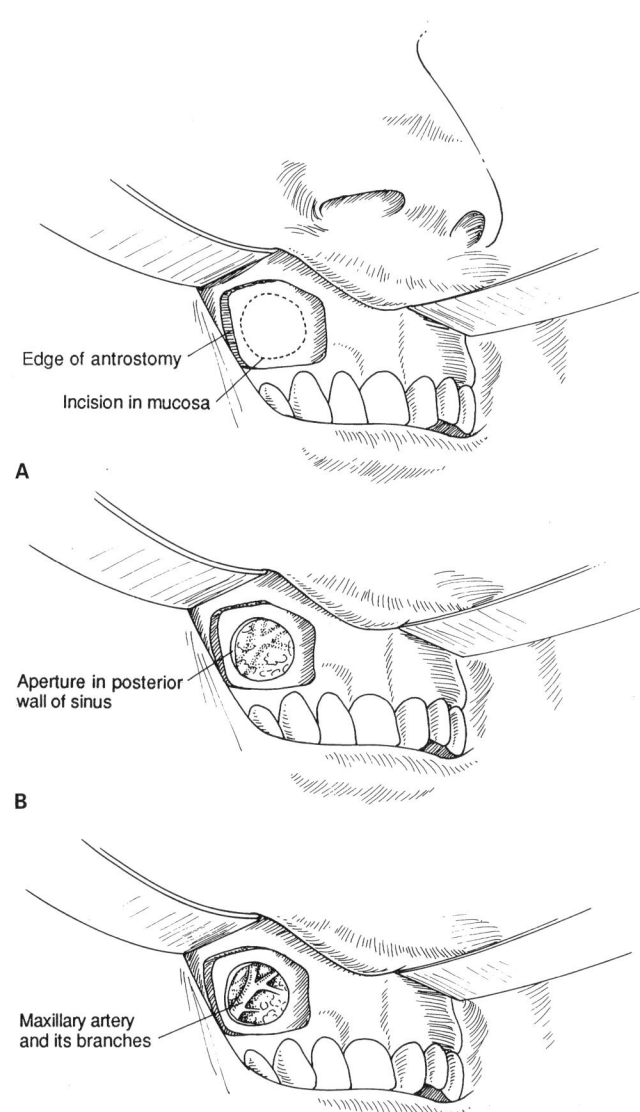

A

Edge of antrostomy

Incision in mucosa

B

Aperture in posterior wall of sinus

C

Maxillary artery and its branches

Fig. 8.4 Transantral exposure and ligation of the maxillary artery. Under endotracheal anaesthesia (not shown), the upper lip is retracted, and a sublabial incision is made, as for a Caldwell–Luc antrostomy. **A** An anterior antrostomy is made above the canine root and enlarged to allow visualization of the posterior wall of the antrum. The posterior mucosa is incised (dotted line). **B** A small bone window is made in the posterior wall of the antrum, exposing the periosteum and beyond this the pterygomaxillary fossa. **C** In the space are the maxillary artery and its branches — the sphenopalatine and descending palatine arteries. They are isolated by blunt dissection and ligated with clips (see text).

the maxillary artery as near to the nose as possible. No postoperative antral pack should be needed.

It may also be necessary to ligate the anterior ethmoidal artery when the nasal bleeding appears to come from the upper part of the nasal cavity. This should be done before the transantral attack on the maxillary artery. A skin incision is made equidistant from the medial canthus and the nasal dorsum, and curved slightly inferiorly. The periosteum is exposed and the lacrimal sac is freed from the lacrimal fossa with a blunt dissector. The periosteum is then elevated until the anterior ethmoidal artery is exposed. This artery penetrates the fronto-ethmoidal suture at the posterior limit of the anterior ethmoid cells, and it is usually found ~2.5 cm from the anterior lacrimal crest. The artery is identified and clipped.

In cases where bleeding persists, we have rarely had to perform ligation of one or both external carotid arteries, which can be exposed above or below the anterior belly of the digastric artery. However, embolization offers a good alternative, especially in cases of avulsive facial injury.

In CMF missile wounds, the carotid arteries and their branches may be severed. Surgical exploration and arterial ligation may be dangerous or impossible if the arterial wound is deeply sited. When the trajectory of the missile makes this likely, arterial embolization offers an alternative means of arresting bleeding. Dolin et al (1992) used angiography in 38 of 100 facial gunshot wounds, and coil embolization of bleeding arteries was employed in six cases. We have not yet had to employ this method of arresting bleeding in the CMF region, though it has been useful in other sites (Fig. 20.5).

It seems likely that interventional radiological measures to arrest deep bleeding will be used increasingly. Frerich et al (1991) review the options for intractable bleeding in midface fractures, and report success from selective embolization of the maxillary artery in three cases, one an 88-year-old man.

Laboratory investigations

Haemoglobin estimation, a full blood picture, serum electrolyte screen, protein screen and liver enzyme estimation are requested at once. A coagulation screen is carried out if any operation is contemplated (Table 20.2), or if bleeding has been copious. The blood group is determined, and blood matching is done if transfusion is likely to be needed. HIV and hepatitis antibody screening are requested in all cases where nursing or operative intervention will involve a risk of contamination by body fluids; in many countries, these tests require consent by the patient. In unconscious patients, the blood ethanol level is measured urgently; in our community, this is legally obligatory in all road crash victims over the age of 14.

Blood volume replacement

Estimation of blood loss is always difficult. Blood may have been lost at the accident site, or on the way to hospital. There may be much blood in the stomach, or lost from injuries elsewhere in the body. In children and young adults, intense peripheral vasoconstriction may maintain a normal pulse and systolic blood pressure until one-third of the blood volume has been lost. This does not happen in old people, who suffer marked falls in blood pressure after relatively small losses of blood; however, the elderly cardiovascular system may fail to respond by increasing the heart rate, especially if β-adrenergic blocking drugs have been prescribed. Acceleration of the heart rate may interfere with myocardial perfusion: as the rate increases, there is an increase in the time of systole relative to diastole, and during the period of systole the myocardial perfusion virtually ceases — indeed the flow in the coronary arteries is reversed.

The central venous pressure (CVP) is most useful as a guide in giving blood replacement, which should aim to keep the CVP at 5–10 cm above the midaxillary line in young people, 10–15 cm in the old. A central venous line is therefore inserted as soon as possible. Care should be taken not to prick the pleural cavity, and a chest radiograph should be obtained after the line is inserted. A urinary catheter is also inserted to monitor urinary output. An arterial line is also inserted when the circulatory state is very unstable. The choice of replacement fluid has been discussed: for reasons given above, we prefer to replace losses initially with colloid solutions and to transfuse blood to keep the haemoglobin level at ~10 g/dl.

The risk of wash-out coagulopathy arises when large volumes of blood have been replaced (p. 532). Wash-out coagulopathy does not occur until clotting factors have been reduced to 30% of the normal values; this is likely to happen after blood loss and replacement of about one blood volume.

Two units of fresh frozen plasma are therefore given when blood replacement approaches one blood volume. Blood coagulation studies are repeated, and also the platelet count, to see if specific haematological therapy, such as Prothrombinex or cryoprecipitate, is needed; platelet infusions are given if the count falls to < 60 000/ml. Consultation with the clinical haematologist is desirable in such situations, and the possibility of pre-existing blood dyscrasia or aspirin ingestion should be kept in mind.

Control of raised intracranial pressure

Raised intracranial pressure is a surgical emergency, and progressive signs of raised pressure may call for very rapid intervention. This aspect of emergency management is discussed in Chapter 13, and here it is only necessary to note that the emergency treatment of a deteriorating head injury sometimes entails endotracheal intubation, hyperventilation and/or infusion of mannitol (0.5–1.0 g/kg body weight as a bolus dose). Decisions on the management of such cases should be made jointly by the physician providing emergency management and the consultant neurosurgeon (Simpson et al 1988). We do not favour giving mannitol or other hyperosmolar agents as a routine measure. Steroid medication is no longer considered appropriate in the primary management of head injuries.

When a patient with CMF injury comes to the emergency room in status epilepticus, the fits should be controlled at once by intravenous diazepam (2 mg/min to total 10 mg). If there is no response, thiopentone and possibly intubation and ventilation will be needed.

Eye protection

In any eye injury, and especially in penetrating injury, the prevention of further ocular damage is essential. This can be caused by the patient, the first aid attendant, the casualty staff, the anaesthetist, the radiographer, the nursing staff, or the surgeon. The nature of the injury should be explained to the patient; all staff members must understand the risks of the injury and how these can be prevented.

We urge that cases of suspected or verified penetrating eye injury should be transported flat with the head and neck supported. To avoid elevation of intraocular pressure, vomiting or coughing should be prevented. The eye should be protected by a lightly applied pad or shield, or by plastic film (Fig. 9.8); pressure on the globe should be avoided. If the eye has been injured by a chemical agent, the conjunctiva should be irrigated thoroughly with normal saline and repeatedly from the time of injury until the patient can be assessed by an ophthalmologist.

Failure of vision is a surgical emergency, and should be discussed at once with an ophthalmologist. When caused by an increasingly tense orbital haematoma, there may be need for an emergency orbital decompression (p. 422); there are other remediable causes of visual failure, and in all of them delay may be disastrous.

Implanted objects

In some cases of penetrating injury, a knife or other sharp object is left projecting out of the orbit or the skull vault. To minimize the risk of further damage to the eye or brain, it is best to leave the object in situ until the patient is anaesthetized; after appropriate radiological investigation, which may include angiography, the object can be carefully withdrawn. The possibility of bleeding after withdrawal should be kept in mind.

Pain relief

This requires care and experience; relief of pain is essential, but excessive doses of narcotics are dangerous, especially if there is a cerebral injury. In patients with severe pain, we give initially small repeated intravenous bolus doses of morphine until the patient is reasonably comfortable. The appropriate bolus dose becomes the guide to further intravenous dosage by continuous infusion. Large intramuscular doses of narcotic analgesics are to be avoided if possible. In the injured person, absorption may be delayed and variable (Mather et al 1975); the peak level may be higher than is necessary for analgesia, and the trough level may be inadequate. The result may be respiratory depression, vomiting and impaired conscious level. Where close medical supervision is not possible, as in an ambulance, self-administration of Entonox (50% nitrous oxide in oxygen) or Penthrane (methoxyflurane) have been recommended. These gases are potentially hazardous in patients with impaired consciousness; however, such persons rarely need analgesia.

Antibiotic prophylaxis

This is a contentious subject (p. 236). It is our practice to give prophylactic chemotherapy as soon as possible, for the following conditions:

Compound facial fractures
— intravenous flucloxacillin (usual adult dose 1 g 6 hourly; maximum 100 mg/kg body weight/day)
— intravenous metronidazole (usual adult dose 500 mg 12 hourly infused over 20 min; maximum 20 mg/kg body weight/day in 3 doses)

Compound calvarial fractures
— intravenous flucloxacillin only

Fractures of the skull base
— intravenous amoxycillin or ampicillin (usual adult dose 1 g 6 hourly; maximum 100 mg/kg body weight/day)
— intravenous or oral trimethoprim–sulphamethoxazole (usual adult dose two tablets or 10 ml by infusion 12 hourly; maximum 8 mg trimethoprim/kg body weight/day in 2 doses)

Penetrating eye wounds
— intravenous gentamicin (usual adult dose 120–160 mg 12 hourly)
— a third-generation cephalosporin, e.g. ceftriaxone, 1–2 g daily (maximum 50 mg/kg/day as single dose).

Our arguments for this policy of prophylaxis, and for these choices of antibiotics, are set out in Chapter 9 and elsewhere in relation to injuries of organs with specific drug barriers, such as the brain (p. 371) and the eye (p. 409); doses should be modified in cases of hepatic or renal dysfunction, and in children. These doses express our own practice, but we urge that each trauma unit should form its own policies in collaboration with a clinical pharmacologist, and our doses are not necessarily appropriate in all settings.

Special care is needed in patients with a history of drug sensitivity, especially sensitivity to the penicillins and the sulphonamides; in such cases, it may be wise to withhold prophylactic medication of any kind, since the arguments for prophylactic antibiotic medication are not unchallenged. The risk of cross hypersensitivity should be remembered; in perhaps as many as 9% of persons hypersensitive to penicillin, there is also hypersensitivity to cephalosporins (Garrod et al 1981).

Tetanus prophylaxis

This is needed unless the injured person is known to have been fully immunized within the last 10 years. If the record suggests that immunization was > 10 years ago, or if the wound seems especially prone to tetanus and immunization was 5–10 years ago, 0.5 ml adsorbed tetanus toxoid is injected. This is also given when the immunization status is unknown but the wound looks clean and not especially prone to tetanus. When the patient is not known to have been properly immunized, and the wound is associated with contamination or tissue damage, toxoid is given, and also passive immunization by human tetanus immune globulin (250 units). Full immunization by toxoid can be given later. Wounds in the CMF region are not as a rule prone to tetanus, since *Clostridium tetani* requires an anaerobic environment, but immunization is nevertheless essential. Facial burns should be regarded as prone to tetanus, since there is likely to be necrosis and ischaemia.

There is only one contraindication to tetanus immunization and that is a history of neurological or severe systemic reaction to a previous dose; a history of a local reaction need not preclude another dose (American College of Surgeons Committee on Trauma 1984).

Emergency operative intervention

In many cases of CMF trauma, definitive treatment should not be undertaken immediately: the best results are obtained by elective operation done after careful investigation and team planning. Moreover, injuries elsewhere in the body may take precedence. However, some forms of CMF injury have high priority and should be dealt with as soon as possible (Weaver 1988). These include:

1. Jaw fractures causing airway obstruction
2. Inhaled tooth fragments and dental plates
3. Open wounds of the eye
4. Open wounds, especially wounds of the lips, eyelids and face generally, and especially if bleeding (see above)
5. Incised wounds of the facial nerve
6. Open wounds involving the parotid or nasolacrimal duct
7. Craniocerebral injuries complicated by raised intracranial pressure, e.g. acute intracranial haemorrhage, intracranial aerocele
8. Open brain wounds.

These injuries are discussed in Chapters 11–15. It is necessary to emphasize that during the process of emergency assessment and resuscitation, the various injuries are identified, and their priorities are determined (Mektubjian, 1982). In cases of multiple injuries, this process of triage is best done by a multidisciplinary team with a designated team leader.

ASSESSMENT OF VIABILITY

The team members may have to decide on the viability of the injured person, either in the emergency room or at a later stage in management. Some cases of CMF trauma are moribund when admitted; others become moribund from cardiac failure due to exsanguination, despite vigorous resuscitation; the decision to cease supportive treatment may have to be taken. More often, however, the cause of death after CMF trauma is failure of the brainstem centres as a result of irreversible cerebral swelling and/or intracranial bleeding. When brainstem death is established, further supportive therapy is not indicated.

When the apparently moribund person is young (< 50 years) and previously in good health, then it is usually right to continue cardiopulmonary resuscitation and to look for a remediable condition, such as a ruptured intrathoracic or intra-abdominal viscus, or an intracranial haemorrhage. In comatose patients the possibility of a non-traumatic cause of coma (e.g. drug ingestion) should be considered. Even in older persons, efforts to restore cerebral perfusion may be justifiable, though the likelihood of a good response is much less, and the decision to cease supportive measures may be reached sooner. The previously expressed views of the victim may be helpful in this often difficult decision.

Brainstem death

The diagnosis of irreversible brainstem failure should be based on well defined criteria. In the UK, these were laid down by a joint conference representing medical surgical and anaesthetic authorities (Royal Colleges and Faculties in the United Kingdom, 1976). It is first necessary to exclude brainstem depression by drugs, metabolic abnormalities or hypothermia. A diagnosis of irremediable structural brain damage must be made. The following tests of reflex function should be made and should show no response:

— pupillary light reflexes
— corneal reflexes
— vestibulo-ocular reflexes, in response to head movement and to irrigation of the external auditory canals with ice-cold water
— responses to pain in the cranial nerve territory
— gag reflex
— respiration in response to elevation of arterial carbon dioxide tension.

In our practice, the last test is given particular importance. The pCO_2 is allowed to rise to 50 mmHg while 100% oxygen is administered by catheter into the trachea and ventilation is ceased; apnoea is seen as evidence of brainstem failure if there is no evidence of a high cervical cord lesion. The tests are usually repeated independently after 30 min or more; this is always done if organ donation is intended. Reflex activity below the brainstem level need not negate the diagnosis of brain death; the term 'Lazarus sign' has been applied to such activity when seemingly integrated limb movements appear in a brain-dead patient.

The professional and legal criteria of brainstem death vary considerably in different parts of the world (Walker 1985); in some countries, the criteria include specific procedures such as cerebral angiography, to show absence of cerebral perfusion, and electroencephalograpy, to show absence of cortical electical activity. We have not used these procedures routinely, but have occasionally employed cerebral angiography in doubtful cases; it has a place when there are confounding factors, such as a high cervical lesion or a high serum level of therapeutic barbiturate. We have also made use of nuclear scanning (Fig. 8.5). This has received greater acceptance with the advent of Ceretec ([^{99m}Tc]HMPAO), a lipophilic perfusion tracer that readily crosses the blood–brain barrier; with the aid of a bedside SPECT scan, it is easy to visualize the presence or absence of blood flow in the brain within

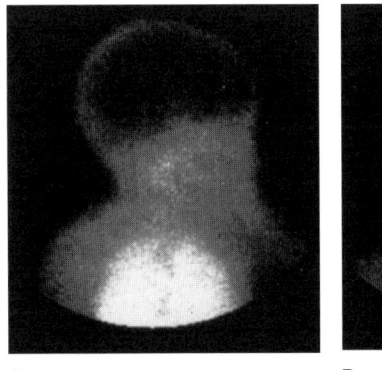 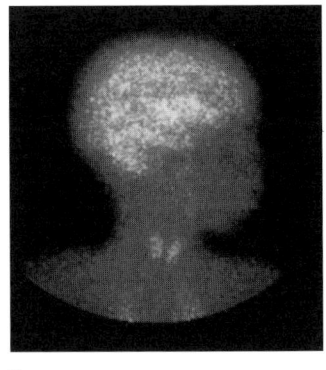

A   B

Fig. 8.5 Ceretec radioisotope angiogram: brain death. A 2-year-old child swallowed an insecticide and was admitted in coma. There was no recovery after a period of intensive care, and the criteria of brain death were evident. **A** The Ceretec angiogram shows no cerebral circulation; there is a good circulation in the lungs. **B** By comparison, an older child with normal cerebral circulation.

5–10 min after injection (Wieler et al 1993). It has however been found that in infants and young children, evidence of normal cerebral perfusion and active glucose metabolism does not exclude brain death (Medlock et al 1993). Doppler sonography has also been used but we have no personal experience of this method of verifying cerebral circulatory arrest.

REFERENCES

Alexander J 1989 Oral and maxillofacial trauma: triage to definitive care. In: Becker D P, Gudeman S K (eds) Textbook of head injury. Saunders, Philadelphia, Ch 17

American College of Surgeons Committee on Trauma 1984 Prophylaxis against tetanus in wound management. Bull Am Coll Surg 69: 22–23

Advanced Trauma Life Support 1993 American College of Surgeons, Chicago

Arajärvi E, Linqvist C, Santavirta S, Tolonen J, Kiviluoto O 1986 Maxillofacial trauma in fatally injured victims of motor vehicle accidents. Br J Oral Maxillofac Surg 24: 251–257

Colvin J 1981 Effective management of penetrating eye injuries in remote Australia. Med J Aust 1: 329–334

Dieckert J P, O'Connor P S, Schacklett D E et al 1986 Air travel and intraocular gas. Ophthalmology 93: 642–645

Dolin J, Scalea T, Manner L, Sclafani S, Trooskin S 1992 The management of gunshot wounds to the face. J Trauma 33: 508–515

Fischer M M 1989 The crystalloid versus colloid controversy: bias, logic and toss-up. Thor Surg 4: 205–211

Frerich B, Ehrenfeld M, Schwenzer N, Bien S, Riediger D 1991 Notfallmassnahmen bei akuten Blutungen infolge Mittelgesichtsfrakturen. Fortschr Kiefer Gesichtschir 39: 45–48

Friedman W H 1985 Surgery of the pterygopalatine fossa. In: Blitzer A, Lawson W, Friedman W H (eds) Surgery of the paranasal sinuses. Saunders, Philadelphia, Ch 13

Garrod L P, Lambert H P, O'Grady F, Waterworth P M 1981 Antibiotic and chemotherapy. Churchill Livingstone, Edinburgh, Ch 3

Gilligan J E 1990 Transport of the critically ill. In: Oh T E (ed) Intensive care manual, 3rd edn. Butterworth, London

Hoffman E 1982 Road accidents: resuscitation on site. Injury 14: 245–249

Holcroft R W, Vassar M J, Turner J E, Derlet R W, Kramer G C 1987 3% NaCl and 7.5% NaCl/dextran 70 in resuscitation of severely injured patients. Ann Surg 206: 279–287

Hossack D W 1972 The pattern of injuries received by 500 drivers and passengers killed in road accidents. Med J Aust 2: 193–195

Hunt R N 1977 Peace River Region FACTS project — final statistical report (including overview). The Workers Compensation Board of Alberta, Alberta

Ivatury R, Siegel J II, Stahl W M, Simon R, Scorpio R, Gens D R 1992 Percutaneous tracheostomy after trauma and critical illness. J Trauma 32: 133–140

Kox W J, Gamble J (eds) 1988 Fluid resuscitation. Baillière's clinical anaesthesiology. Baillière Tindall, London, Vol. 2: 443–760

Lamke L O, Liljedah I S O 1978 Plasma volume changes after infusion of various plasma volume expanders. Resuscitation 5: 93–102

Liskiewicz W J 1992 An evaluation of the Royal Air Force helicopter search and rescue service in Britain with reference to Royal Air Force Valley, 1980–1989. J R Soc Med 85: 727–729

Mather L E, Lindop M J, Tucker F T, Pflug A E 1975 Pethidine revisited: plasma concentrations and effects after intramuscular injections. Br J Anaesth 47: 1269–1275

Medlock M D, Hanigan W C, Cruse R P 1993 Dissociation of cerebral blood flow, glucose metabolism, and electrical activity in pediatric brain death. J Neurosurg 79: 752–755

Mektubjian S R 1982 Operative policy in severe facial trauma in combination with other severe injuries. J Maxillofac Surg 10: 14–17

Nahum A M 1969 Immediate care of acute blunt laryngeal trauma. J Trauma 9: 112–125

Nordström C-H, Messeter K, Sundbärg G, Wåhlander S 1989 Severe traumatic brain lesions in Sweden. Part I: aspects of management in non-neurosurgical clinics. Brain Injury 3: 247–265

Ottoson A 1985 Aspiration and obstructed airways as a cause of death in 158 consecutive fatalities. J Trauma 25: 538–540

Reines H D, Bartlett R L, Chudy N E, Kiragu K R, McKnew M A 1988 Is advanced life support appropriate for victims of motor vehicle accidents: the South Carolina Highway Trauma project. J Trauma 28: 563–570

Ross S E, O'Malley K F, De Long W G, Born C T, Schwab C W 1992 Clinical predictors of unstable cervical spinal injury in multiply injured patients. Injury 23: 217–319

Royal Colleges and Faculties in the United Kingdom 1976 Br Med J 2: 1069–1070

Schaefer S D 1991 The treatment of acute laryngeal injuries. Arch Otolaryngol Head Neck Surg 117: 35–39

Schmidt U, Frame S B, Nerlich M L, Rowe D W et al 1992 On-scene helicopter transfer of patients with multiple injuries — comparison of a German and an American system. J Trauma 33: 548–555

Schneider M, Schneider G H 1987 Erste-Hilfe-Ausbildung für Fuhrerscheinanwarter. Unzureichendes "Muss"? Rettungsdienst 10: 524

Selecki B R, Ring I T, Simpson D A, Vanderfield G K, Sewell M F 1981 Injuries to the head, spine and peripheral nerves. Report on a study. New South Wales Government Printer, Sydney

Shoemaker W C 1976 Comparison of the relative effectiveness of whole blood transfusions and various types of fluid therapy in resuscitation. Crit Care Med 4: 71–78

Simpson D, North B, Gilligan J et al 1984 Neurological injuries in South Australia: the influence of distance on management and outcome. Aust NZ J Surg 54: 29–35

Simpson D A, Heyworth J S, McLean A J, Gilligan J E, North J B 1988 Extradural haemorrhage: strategies for management in remote places. Injury 19: 307–312

Spiessl B 1990 Resuscitation with massive oropharyngeal and facial bleeding. In: Border J R, Allgöwer M, Hansen S T, Rüedi T P (eds) Blunt multiple trauma. Dekker, New York & Basel, Ch 22

Spittal M J, Hunter S J, Spencer I, Blake D, McLaren C A B 1992 Secondary patient transfer by air: an audit of 3 years' experience of the Royal Air Force in the world-wide transport of critically ill patients. J R Soc Med 85: 730–732

Takaori M, Safar P 1966 Adaptation to acute haemorrhage to acute severe haemodilution with dextran 75 in dogs. Arch Surg 92: 743–746

Tscherne H, Kalbe P M, Wisner D H 1990 Pre-hospital care of the polytrauma patient: the role of the physician. In: Border J R, Allgöwer M, Hansen S T, Rüedi T P (eds) Blunt multiple trauma. Dekker, New York & Basel, Ch 16.

Walker A E 1985 Cerebral death, 3rd edn. Urban & Schwarzenberg, Baltimore

Weaver T 1988 Anaesthetic management of facio-maxillary trauma. In: Kerr D R (ed) Australasian anaesthesia. Faculty of Anaesthetists, Royal Australasian College of Surgeons, Melbourne, pp 62–66

Wieler H, Marohl K, Kaiser K P, Klawki P, Frössler H 1993 Tc-99m HMPAO cerebral scintigraphy. A reliable, noninvasive method for determination of brain death. Clin Nucl Med 18: 104–109

Woodring J H, Lee C 1993 Limitations of cervical radiography in the evaluation of acute cervical trauma. J Trauma 34: 32–39

Definitive management: principles, priorities and basic techniques

J. Trott   D. J. David
Contributing authors: M. Hammerton   D. A. Simpson
R. Edwards

INTRODUCTION

This chapter considers the organizational structure of a craniofacial unit, and how it can be employed in the prioritization and definitive management of craniomaxillo-facial (CMF) injuries. Also considered are some of the basic policies and techniques used in combined operations for repair of complex injuries.

ORGANIZATION

Facility and personnel

In the management of CMF injuries, an organizational structure should be established to allow the best use of resources and to provide appropriate levels of care. This structure is composed of two basic elements: the facility and the personnel. The term 'facility' comprehends the wards, operating theatres, diagnostic services, clinics and other hospital systems essential in the modern management of trauma. The personnel comprise not only the committed core members of the multidisciplinary trauma team, but also the numerous less directly committed colleagues who contribute in the surgical treatment, nursing and rehabilitation of the injured patient.

Ideally, the facility should be established in a single location; if this is not possible then the locations must be geographically close to allow ease of access and inter-communication (Fig. 9.1). The facility should have a central location in relation to the main mass of the population to be served. Patients must be able to reach the facility with a minimum of delay and if possible there should be a nearby heliport or airport to enable rapid transfer of

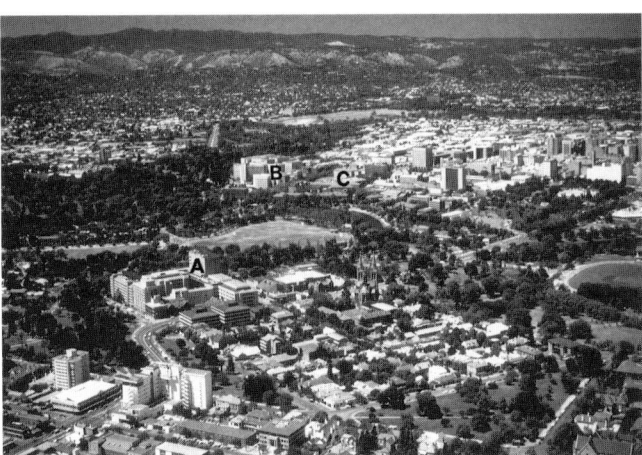

Fig. 9.1 Adelaide, South Australia. Aerial view of the Women's and Children's Hospital (**A**), the Royal Adelaide Hospital (**B**), and the University of Adelaide (**C**). Their close proximity to each other and to the city centre facilitates the management of major trauma. The sports field between the hospitals has been used for helicopter landings; direct landing on a hospital building is preferable.

critically injured patients from outlying areas. The facility must have an adequately staffed emergency or casualty area with emergency operating rooms available 24 h a day. An intensive care unit will be needed to manage the critically injured patient. Relevant specialist services must be available immediately. These include diagnostic imaging services, medical laboratory and haematology services, and blood transfusion services, as well as the relevant clinical departments. The ideal facility for managing CMF injuries should have geographical proximity to a university campus. This will allow the very important activities of teaching and research to be undertaken with appropriate academic support and rigor. These are further discussed in Chapter 23.

Personnel with a special interest in CMF trauma bond together as a team dedicated to managing these injuries. They may be part of an extended craniofacial team already in existence. The trauma subsection of the extended craniofacial team has the following members: craniofacial surgeons (p. 683), neurosurgeons, ophthalmologists, specialist anaesthetists, ENT surgeons, and dental specialists including dentists, orthodontists, and restorative dental experts. Psychosocial workers and specialist nurses are further important members of such a team. Working as a dedicated team, the group constitutes a structure which provides ease of communication and referral within its membership, and also an ability to collect data both for research and for regular peer reviews of all aspects of CMF injury management. Peer review is an intrinsic component of the team concept, and this presupposes an efficient record system and a good library service.

Admission policies

After the emergency assessment and resuscitation (see Chs 6 and 8) come the allocation of immediate priorities and the decision on admission to specialized departments (Fig. 9.2). In our system of management, the patient with multiple injuries is admitted under the care of the hospital department appropriate for the most serious injury. A severe brain injury is admitted under the neurosurgery department, a proven or suspect ruptured abdominal viscus is admitted under the general surgery department and a case of spinal injury under the orthopaedic department. Facial fractures occurring in isolation or in the presence of less severe injuries are admitted to the plastic surgery department under the care of the on-call craniofacial specialist; in many trauma services, the oral surgical department has this role. Isolated eye injuries are admitted to the ophthalmological department. After admission, baseline investigations and consultations within the CMF trauma team are carried out. Data from the clinical, laboratory and radiological investigations described in

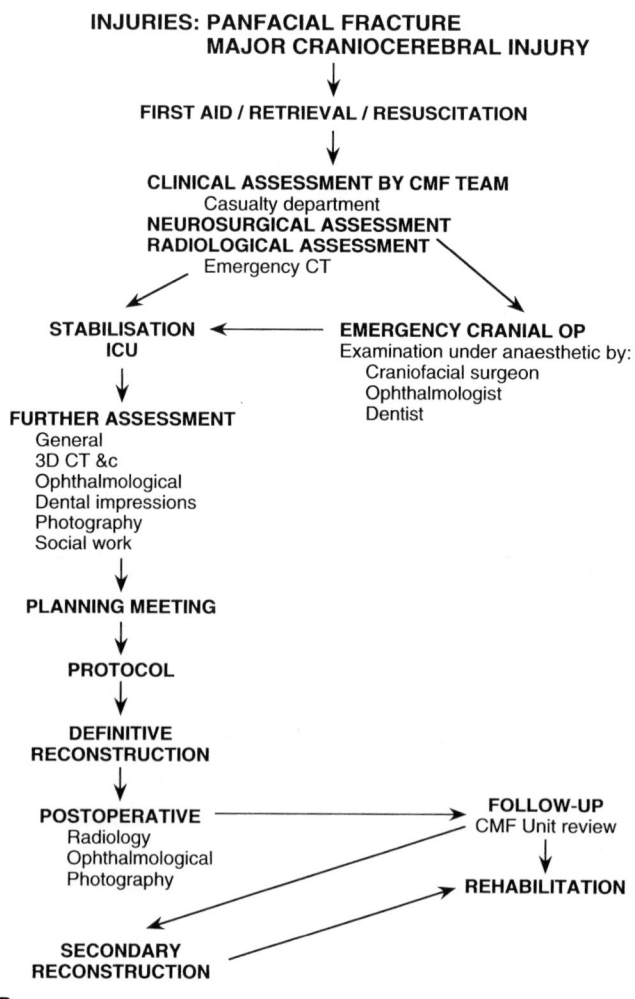

Fig. 9.2 Trauma management by a CMF unit. The skills of a multidisciplinary unit can be deployed in trauma management in response to the pattern and severity of the injuries. **A** A unidisciplinary problem, such as a possible depressed fracture of zygoma, engages the attention of one specialist, in this case a craniofacial surgeon. Investigation, diagnosis, treatment and follow-up are coordinated by the same unit. A similar scheme is applied in the management of an isolated corneal wound, or depressed skull fracture. **B** A multidisciplinary problem, such as a panfacial fracture with a major craniocerebral injury, engages the attention of a number of specialists. In this case, the neurosurgeon initiates urgent treatment, but the craniofacial, ophthalmological and dental specialists are consulted as soon as possible, and the further management of the case is coordinated by the multidisciplinary team.

Chapters 6–8 are combined in a work-up which allows the formulation of a plan of management appropriate to the unique needs of the individual patient.

Specialist clinical assessment and consultations

The craniofacial surgeon examines the patient and the X-ray pictures shortly after admission. Diagnosis of the bony and soft-tissue injury is then confirmed and recorded. All proven or suspected craniocerebral injuries are assessed by a neurosurgeon if this has not been already done in the emergency department. All eye injuries and all orbital fractures require an ophthalmological consultation. All jaw fractures affecting the occlusion are seen by the team dental consultant, who inspects teeth for traumatic damage and takes dental impressions of both upper and lower jaws (p. 355). These impressions are used to cast plaster study models for planning surgical reduction and fixation. All consultants record their findings, diagnoses and recommended management plans in the case records.

The anaesthetist or intensivist reviews the progress of the case in the light of the serial clinical records (p. 160) and laboratory tests to confirm that the pathophysiological effects of trauma, especially hypovolaemia, anaemia and electrolyte disorders, have been corrected. The definitive anaesthetic assessment may be deferred until the operative management plan is prepared. This assessment is of great and sometimes decisive importance, especially in the elderly and where there is some significant pre-existing disease (see Chs 19 and 20).

Prevention of infection

While the multidisciplinary assessments are being made, measures are instituted to minimize the risk of infection.

Microbial infection is a threat after any open wound or any surgical operation, whether done electively or as an emergency. In the CMF region, infection may be disastrous. Cerebral infection may cause death or severe disability (p. 387). Ocular infection may cause blindness (p. 416); postoperative facial infection may lead to rejection of bone grafts and prolonged morbidity. Craniofacial reconstructions entail substantial risks of infection: they are often long, they may expose cavities that cannot readily be sterilized, and there may be postoperative dead space, especially in the anterior cranial fossa. In early reports on craniofacial surgery, high infection rates were recorded: in our own initial experiences, we had an overall incidence of 6.5% infection in 170 transcranial procedures of all kinds, and the incidence was especially high in adults with pre-existing tracheostomies (David & Cooter 1987).

Given the nature of CMF trauma and the orofacial microbial environment (p. 119), it seems unlikely that any surgical routine will wholly eliminate post-traumatic infection, but every effort must be made to reduce the incidence and the severity. Experience and theoretical considerations support:

1. Early wound toilet, appropriate debridement, and early primary wound closure
2. Operative planning to reduce wound exposure time, and to avoid procedures known to increase the risk of serious infection, such as tracheostomy and prolonged ventricular drainage
3. Elimination of local sources of microbial infection
4. Pre- and peroperative prophylactic antibiotics
5. Nutritional support.

It is not difficult to justify these ideals as generalizations, but in reality, many compromises must be made. Wound closure may have to be deferred because of other more urgent problems. Debridement of cerebral wounds and the removal of deeply placed foreign bodies may conflict with the paramount need to conserve cerebral function (p. 373). Bactericidal skin cleansing and prophylactic chemotherapy must be used with discrimination and at the right time.

Skin wounds must be cleaned and dressed; in our service, gauze packs moistened with saline and changed every 2 h are considered to be the most effective; the techniques used in skin lacerations and abrasions are discussed in Chapter 15.

With jaw fractures, the care of the mouth is important. Nursing staff may have to pick away dried blood from inside the mouth; moistened probes and forceps are useful in this. An appropriate diet is prescribed with the help of the hospital dietician; this will usually need to be in a non-chew or liquid form. Oral hygiene is maintained with mouth washes of chlorhexidine or other antiseptic; attention to this after each meal is mandatory. Where eyelids are swollen, eye toilets may be needed as the poorly draining tears rapidly become mucopurulent. Eye ointments may also need to be used where eyelid closure is compromised (p. 246).

Theatre aseptic routine must be meticulous, especially where two or more disciplines are joined in a combined procedure: often, each has its own different rituals, and it is necessary to combine these, even if the resultant procedure appears cumbersome, to avoid a perception by staff members that their standards have been lowered. Preoperative 'disinfection' of the skin and the various facial cavities has limited value. Complete sterility is unattainable in the mouth, and in the skin, it is impossible to sterilize the hair follicles and skin glands (Lowbury 1981). However, it is possible to reduce the bacterial count very substantially by an appropriate bactericide; we favour povidone–iodine (Betadine®) applied with sponges a few minutes before incision. Scalp wounds are covered with Ioban®, a polymeric plastic film coated with a bactericidal iodophor.

The value of prophylactic antibiotics has been disputed, both for facial fractures and for craniocerebral wounds. It has been shown that prolonged use of antibiotics promotes the growth of resistant organisms in the pharynx (Ignelzi & Van der Ark 1975) and elsewhere. However, there is now much evidence to support the routine use of peroperative chemotherapy in elective orthopaedic and vascular surgery (Strachan 1993) and in elective neurosurgical operations (Young & Lawner 1987); we believe that this experience supports a similar policy with CMF trauma. The choice of antibiotic depends partly on the local microbiota and the likely pathogens, and partly on the capacity of the chosen antibiotic to cross the blood–brain and blood–eye barriers, and to penetrate bone.

With the exception of isolated fractures of the zygomatic arch and condylar fractures, facial fractures are usually compound through mucosal surfaces. Some authorities, relying on very early rigid fixation, do not give prophylactic antibiotics. Our plan of management does not require such early intervention as a routine, and we give prophylactic antibiotics to all patients with compound facial fractures, usually intravenously (David & Cooter 1987); in our present management plan, flucloxacillin and metronidazole as a combination are used (p. 229). This regime is continued peroperatively and for 48 h thereafter; in some cases, oral antibiotics may be continued for a further 5 days. The roles of prophylactic antibiotics in craniocerebral wounds and cerebrospinal fistulas are discussed in Chapter 13. In our practice, flucloxacillin has been given for compound skull fractures and for penetrating wounds of the brain, while patients having CSF leakage receive in addition co-trimoxazole (a sulphonamide–trimethoprim combination); this drug penetrates the blood–brain barrier. For calvarial compound fractures, metronidazole is omitted unless there is special reason to fear infection by a gram-negative organism. Hitherto, we have not given cephalosporins prophylactically from fear of promoting resistance; however, in view of its good penetration across the blood–brain barrier, ceftriaxone may prove to be a justifiable choice (Demetriades et al 1992). For open wounds of the eye, we favour a third generation cephalosporin and an aminoglycoside (p. 409).

Great care is needed in respect to antibiotic dosages, both for prophylactic and for therapeutic purposes. In this book, the dosages suggested for the various antibiotics are those recommended in our hospitals (p. 229); opinions on the choice and the dosages of many antibiotics vary, and it is wise to formulate general policies in consultation with a clinical pharmacologist and a clinical microbiologist. Similar consultations are also desirable in individual patients with unusual or life-threatening infections in any site, or when there is evidence of drug sensitivity.

Topical antibiotics, in powders, sprays, or irrigations, remain a controversial subject; Haines (1982) found no evidence to support their use in clean neurosurgical procedures, though he saw applications in treating heavily contaminated wounds. We routinely immerse bone grafts in a solution of 0.2% flucloxacillin during facial reconstructions, and some use is made of this solution in irrigating the extradural space. All the penicillins are epileptogenic, and although small doses (e.g. 10 mg penicillin G or methicillin in 5 ml Ringer's solution) have often been used by intrathecal or intraventricular injection, we do not advise this for prophylactic purposes.

Topical antibiotic ointments and eyedrops are often used in ophthalmological injuries, but should be chosen and used with some care, especially in the presence of a penetrating eye wound. In the treatment of some eye infections, intravitreous chemotherapy may be necessary, and this should be given in precisely calculated doses and concentrations known to be within tolerated limits. Chloramphenicol eye ointments and drops have been incriminated as possible causes of blood dyscrasias, and should not be used unless there is no effective alternative (Fraunfelder et al 1993).

Multidisciplinary planning

Once all necessary assessments are completed an operative plan is produced. If other specialists are to be involved in the surgery then discussions will be held at an interdisciplinary planning meeting (Fig. 9.2B). As a result of this meeting a protocol is produced discussing the proposed airway management, the order of exposure, the method of fixation and any ancillary procedures. This protocol is circulated to operating theatre, anaesthetic and ward nursing staff, as well as to the members of the relevant departments.

PRINCIPLES OF MANAGEMENT OF FACIAL FRACTURES

Priorities

When a facial injury obstructs the airway or causes massive bleeding, immediate action is needed, but the definitive treatment of facial fractures is rarely urgent and can be carried out as one or more elective procedures. In recent years, there has been a trend towards earlier intervention and to the use of combined procedures in an attempt to minimize morbidity and shorten time in hospital (p. 267). Arguments for early surgery of facial fractures include the belief that reconstruction of the bony framework should be done before the formation of contractile scar tissue (p. 123) which may prevent the correct placement of soft tissues, particularly those within the orbit (Gruss 1990). Our experience with secondary surgery indicates that this argument is not always valid. We prefer to delay surgery until the patient's general condition has stabilized, the swelling has largely settled and the dental and ophthalmological work-ups are complete. We also feel that surgery should be performed on elective operating lists and not in emergency suites at odd hours of the night. We argue that this allows the development of better operative techniques and better teaching, without detriment to the final result. There are some exceptions to this timing policy. Early bony reduction and stabilization are carried out in massive open wounds where there has been significant soft-tissue disruption or loss (p. 450). Even in these cases, however, the bony reduction and stabilization may be only a temporary splintage done at the time of soft-tissue repair with a view to redoing the bony reconstruction once the full work-up is completed. Minor, uncomplicated, undisplaced or minimally displaced fractures will go on the next elective operating list following completion of work-up.

Operative procedures

Reduction and fixation

The principles of surgical treatment of facial fractures have evolved rapidly over the last 30 years (p. 27). At the beginning of this period mandibular fractures were immobilized by using the teeth as external fixateurs with various types of intermaxillary splints; they were reduced in a closed fashion and stabilized with these splints. Maxillary fractures were also reduced by closed methods and stabilized with an external frame (Fig. 1.16) or internal suspension wiring (Fig. 1.21). Orbital fractures were also reduced by closed methods, often without attempt to provide stabilization. These methods were often satisfactory, but sometimes led to secondary deformities such as enophthalmos and foreshortening of the midface. Following the advent of craniofacial surgery in the late 1950s, emphasis moved from closed reduction to wide exposure and open reduction of all facial fractures and stabilization by interosseous wiring (Gruss et al 1985), now virtually replaced by the use of plates and screws. At the occlusal level the teeth are now of secondary importance in fracture fixation, while at the midface and orbital levels, primary bone grafting has significantly reduced problems of enophthalmos and midfacial shortening (Luce 1992).

Craniofacial instruments

It is important to have appropriate instrumentation to carry out the exposure required to visualize the facial fracture pattern and to provide stabilization. Soft-tissue dissection is done with fine sharp craniofacial surgery instruments. A range of periosteal elevators is essential;

we use the Obwegeser type. The smaller periosteal elevator is used within the orbit and in areas of sharply changing contour while the large instruments are used over broad flat surfaces. Malleable metal brain retractors of various sizes are used to retract orbital and cranial contents. Rigid blade retractors are used to retract the lips and cheeks over the jaws and face. Metal cheek retractors and metal tongue depressors are used in wiring dental arch bars to the teeth. We prefer the soft metal dental arch bars if possible as these are less damaging to the gingiva. In adults, 26 gauge stainless steel wire is used to locate the arch bars to the teeth; in children, 28 or 30 gauge stainless steel wire may be used. Where wiring is to be used for interosseous stabilization then similar gauges of wire are used. A power drill is used to drill holes in the bone for passage of the wire; we use the Hall drill powered by compressed nitrogen. Electric drills have the advantage of being more portable.

Plates

While intraosseous wiring is used successfully in many centres the advent of miniplating systems with their ability to provide three dimensional stability has been a great advance in fracture management. Plates secured by small self-tapping screws give rigid bone fixation and rapid union. Among the miniplating systems available are the Luhr Vitallium® plates, the Würzburg titanium system, and the plates designed by Champy and by the AO group (Hobar 1992) (p. 270). At our institution we use AusSystem® plates devised and produced in Adelaide (Fig. 9.3).* These plates are made of titanium and unlike the Vitallium plates of the Luhr system they do not scatter radiation which may affect postoperative computed tomography (CT) scans adversely. Furthermore the AusSystem plates have an advantage over the Würzburg system in that they are much more malleable and easily moulded to the contour of the bone, thereby facilitating stabilization of midface fractures and positioning of bone grafts; they can be moulded by screw pressure, and do not show 'memory' — that is, they do not tend to recoil when other forms of fixation have been released.

Miniplates may cause noticeable deformity when placed on prominent parts of the facial skeleton, in sites such as the orbital rims and the bridge of the nose, where there is relatively little subcutaneous tissue. The plate and screw heads usually become palpable and even visible through the skin. This may be prevented by countersinking the miniplate and screws, or by the use of interosseous wires. Alternatively, one may use the microplate systems, developed in titanium by Leibinger and in Vitallium by Howmedica. The components of these systems are no

---

* AusSystems Pty Ltd, 116 Melbourne Street, Adelaide, SA 5006, Australia.

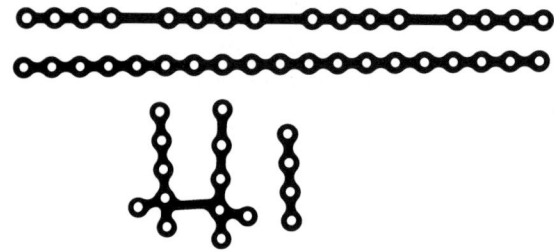

A

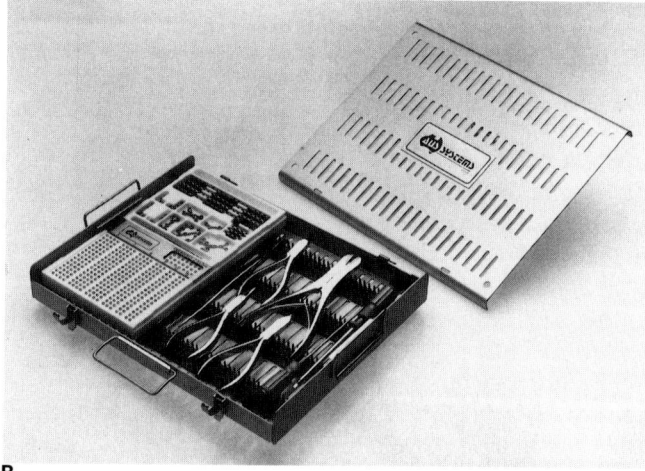

B

Fig. 9.3 Titanium miniplates. The AusSystem® plating set. **A** A range of AusSystem plates, comprising low profile screws and plates for frontal bone and orbital rim use as well as heavier but malleable plates, suitable for mandible and maxillary reconstruction. **B** Instrument kit for AusSystem plates.

higher in profile than 28 gauge wire, and unlike wire they confer three-dimensional stability. It remains to be proved that microplates will stabilize fractures under high load stress, but their use in frontal and orbital rim fractures has helped to solve the problem of miniplate prominence. Special mesh-like microplates can also be used for orbital wall reconstruction, in conjunction with bone grafts; however, these are still under trial.

Craniofacial exposures

As far as possible, surgical exposure of the facial skeleton is carried out without leaving visible scars. In the upper facial skeleton this has been made possible by the use of the extended bicoronal scalp incision. The exact line of this incision may be dictated by the need to deal with cranial components of the fracture or by the site of the patient's hairline. The bicoronal flap is raised in a subgaleal plane to a horizontal level 2–4 cm above the supraorbital rim or to the site of any fractures of the frontal bone. From this level dissection proceeds subpericranially over the orbital rim and into the orbit. The supraorbital neurovascular bundle is carefully preserved; it is usually necessary to free it in the supraorbital notch

by cuts with a fine chisel. Over the temporalis muscle it is important to dissect strictly against the temporal fascia or to incise through the superficial layer of the temporal fascia and dissect in the subfascial fat down to the zygomatic arch (Fig. 9.4). At the level of the zygomatic arch the periosteum must be stripped with great care particularly on the middle and posterior thirds. This may not be easy where fractures are present. Only by careful attention to these details will damage to the frontal branch of the facial nerve be avoided. Within the orbit the periorbita is dissected well back to the apex of the orbit. Where orbital fractures are present the orbital soft tissue may be trapped between the bony fragments and these must be separated to release the soft tissue. This is mandatory for fractures of the orbital roof and medial orbital wall as well as for complicated lateral orbital wall fractures. The temporomandibular joint and neck of the condyle can be approached by extending the bicoronal flap incision in the natural contours down to the lobule of the ear. Careful dissection of the soft tissue from the lateral ligaments of the temporomandibular joint capsule visualizes the neck of the condyle and the sigmoid notch. Further access can be gained by dividing the most posterior fibres of the masseter muscle, and a subperiosteal dissection can be taken down to the angle of the mandible. Again, care should be taken to avoid excessive traction on soft tissues which may produce a temporary palsy of the frontal branch of the facial nerve (Fig. 9.4C).

A subciliary lower eyelid incision or transconjunctival incision (David 1974), with or without lateral canthotomy, produces excellent exposure of the orbital floor (Manson et al 1987; Fig. 9.5). When the lateral canthotomy is performed it can be extended up to provide exposure not only of the floor and inferior rim of the orbit, but also of the lateral orbital wall and rim as far as the frontozygomatic suture. Combined with a bicoronal approach this will allow visualization of the entire orbit and any fractures in its vicinity.

Intraoral incisions in the upper or lower buccal sulcus provide exposures of the remaining facial skeleton with the exception of the pterygoid plate (Fig. 9.6). Care must be taken to avoid damage to branches of the infraorbital nerve in the upper buccal sulcus incision and to the inferior dental nerve in the lower buccal sulcus incision. Because of the risk of damage to the inferior dental nerve in fractures of the edentulous mandible, we prefer an external submandibular incision in such cases; this incision can also be used in the reduction and fixation of difficult mandibular angle fractures (Fig. 9.4C). When lacerations are located immediately over a fracture, they can be used in exposure.

Bone grafts

The practice of wide exposure and open reduction of

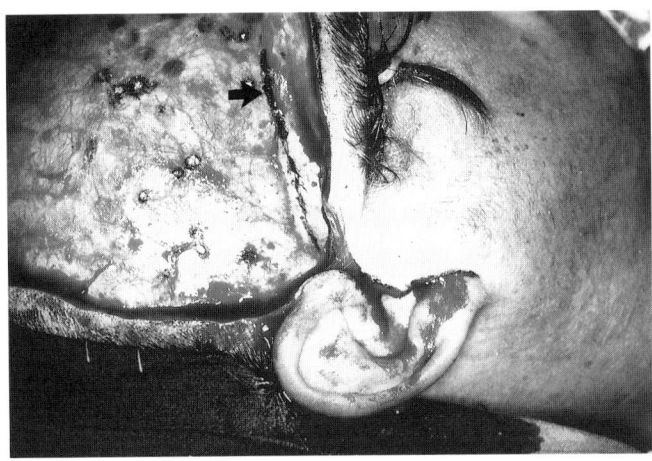

A

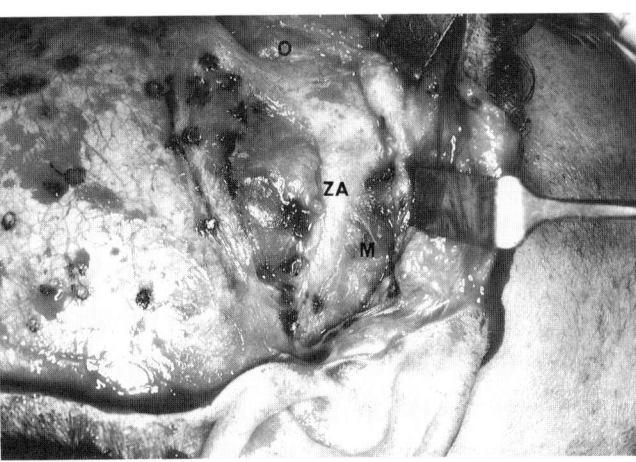

B

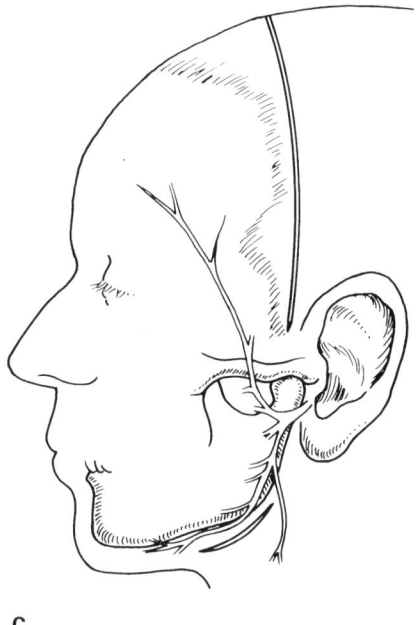

C

Fig. 9.4 Exposure through coronal scalp incision. A The bicoronal scalp flap is elevated over the superficial temporal fascia. On the level of the superior orbital rim (line indicated by an arrow), the fascia is incised and dissection then proceeds in a plane deep to the superficial temporal fascia down to the zygomatic body and arch. This dissection protects the frontal branch of the facial nerve. **B** The zygomatic arch (ZA) and the upper part of the masseter muscle (M) are then exposed. The orbital contents (O) are also exposed. Dissection is subperiosteal over the bone and deep to fascia over the masseter. **C** The diagram shows the incision in relation to the frontal branch of the facial nerve. Also shown is the relation of the submandibular incision to the mandibular branches of the facial nerve.

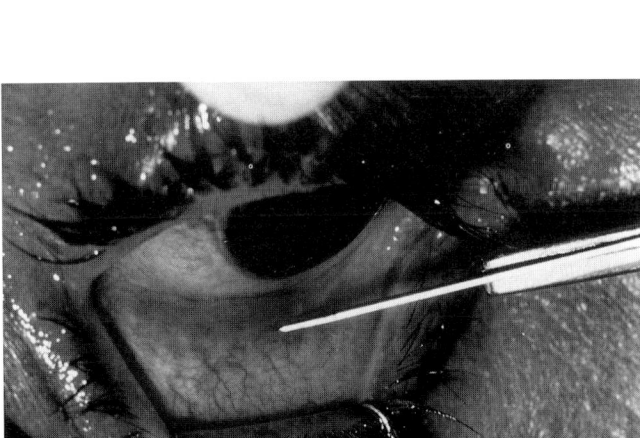

A

Fig. 9.5 Conjunctival incision. A When extended through the lateral canthus, wide exposure of the inferior and lateral orbit is obtained through this approach. The incision is taken across the conjunctiva just inferior to the tarsal plate. **B** Dissection (broken line) is carried deep to the orbicularis oculi muscle to the orbital rim, where the periosteum is incised. Subperiosteal incision then exposes the inferior orbital rim, the orbital floor and the lateral orbital wall and rim. Diagram by S. Cantrell.

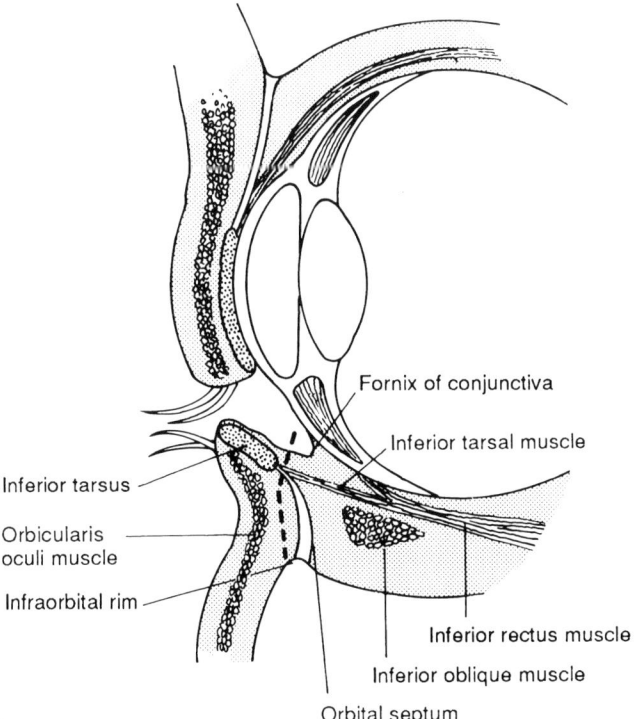

B

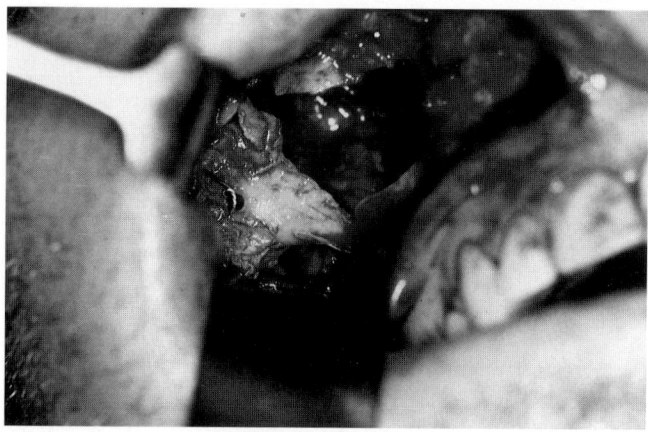

Fig. 9.6 Upper buccal sulcus incision. This is used to expose the anterior maxilla. Care should be taken to avoid damaging branches of the inferior orbital nerve. In this illustration, a comminuted fracture of the zygomatic buttress is seen, associated with a fractured zygoma. A large fragment of the buttress has been temporarily stabilized with an interosseous wire. Part of the anterior maxilla is missing, exposing the maxillary antrum.

facial fractures has highlighted the need for bone grafting in many situations. This is particularly so when bone is found to be missing from the vertical bony pillars of the midface in association with jaw fractures involving the occlusion (Gruss & Phillips 1989). The pillars must be reconstructed to allow the correct vertical height of the midface to be restored and also to stabilize the upper alveolus during the action of chewing. The egg-shell bone of the floor and medial wall of the orbit is often lost in orbital fractures (p. 327) and for adequate reconstruction bone grafting is commonly required. Primary bone grafting is sometimes needed to reconstruct deficits in the orbital rim, or to correct the nasal bridge line where there has been severe comminution of the nasal bone and bony nasal septum resulting in total loss of support to the nasal pyramid.

Gunshot wounds may result in a significant loss of bone, especially in the mandible; when this loss is > 3 cm in length we prefer to use vascularized bone to give more certain healing. This may be a free graft of iliac bone taken on the deep circumflex iliac arterial system, or may be some other appropriate free flap (p. 622). The most commonly used sites for harvesting bone graft are the iliac crest, the rib cage and the skull vault (calvaria); Salyer & Taylor (1987) have reviewed their merits. Many factors are important in increasing the chances of survival of bone grafts, but perhaps the most important is rigid fixation followed by good soft tissue coverage preferably with a periosteal surface (Rahn 1989). Other factors promoting graft survival are discussed in Chapter 5; these include a well vascularized bed in the host tissues and prevention of haematoma formation.

Hip grafts

The wing of the ilium is perhaps the most versatile of

all bone graft sites. Large pieces can be harvested, and the structure of the ilium offers a range of cortical and cancellous grafts. Cortical bone plates taken from the ilium are strong yet malleable, and are far less brittle than calvarial bone; they provide excellent reconstructive material for the orbital walls and also for mandibular reconstruction both as vascularized and non-vascularized grafts. The inner table can be harvested separately. After removal of a small amount of inner table, cancellous bone may be scooped out and used alone or with cortical bone. For strong grafts, both tables can be taken. It is important not to take the crest itself, both in adults and in children. Preservation of the crest with its attached muscles preserves the contour of the hip. If the scar is well placed even the skimpiest of undergarments will conceal it. In children the iliac crest is still in part cartilaginous up to 12–13 years of age; depending on the developmental state of the child, the crest may be cartilaginous even at somewhat later ages.

Technique. In the older child or adult the hip can be harvested by a second team working while the major craniofacial dissection is under way, thus saving time. A sandbag is placed under the hip. The skin incision is made 2 cm below the crest on the lateral side; if the skin is rolled medially the cut can then be made straight down to the bone. The dissection of the ilium proceeds according to the size of the graft to be taken. Often, only a small amount of bone is required, such as a disk for a 'bath-plug' reconstruction of the frontal region or when a small medial cortical window is opened for the harvesting of some cancellous bone. In such cases, all the muscular attachments of the crest are preserved and a cut is made down to the medial side of the periosteum which is stripped exposing the blade of the ilium directly. Alternatively the medial and lateral lips of the crest may be split free with an osteotome leaving the muscle and periosteal attachments on the mobilized segments of bone, thus exposing the ilium on one or both sides (see Fig. 9.7). At the end of the procedure, the bone segments can be reattached with very strong nylon sutures or occasionally wires. It is important to step the bone at the point of severance with the adjacent anterior spine or posteriorly so that the reconstructed segments do not collapse after the wound is closed. If the cut is made a little more medially then the lid can be lifted off and hinged on the lateral periosteal attachments. This lid may then be replaced quite easily on the pre-cut steps. It is our custom to drain the space carefully with suction drains and we use the reciprocating power saw or the sagittal power saw to facilitate the taking of the graft.

Rib grafts

Rib grafts can be readily harvested by a submammary incision and large lengths are available. Rib has the advantage of being malleable. It is useful within the orbit,

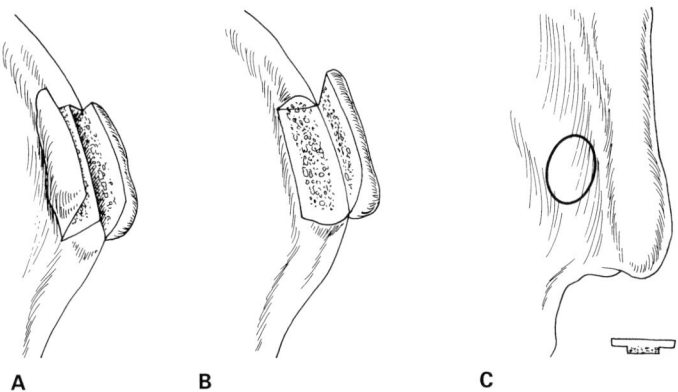

Fig. 9.7 Bone graft from the iliac crest. A Incision over the iliac crest, down to the periosteum; lids of bone and periosteum are hinged medially and/or laterally to expose the bone which can then be harvested. The crest is then reconstructed by wiring or stitching the lids back. **B** Incision is made down through the periosteum over the crest and a segment of bone is lifted to medial or lateral side. The segment can be wired back into position after harvesting. **C** A circular trephine graft is taken with cortex and attached cancellous bone like a bath plug (see inset).

for reconstruction of the calvaria (Fig. 17.20), and as a costochondral graft in the nose or temporomandibular joint. In our practice, rib is most often used for reconstruction of the cheek bone, often as an onlay graft, and for the costochondral grafting techniques.

Technique (Fig. 21.6). The incision should be at the level of the submammary fold in women and at the equivalent in men. It is possible to harvest ribs through relatively short (5–6 cm) incisions, and great cuts should not be made across the chest. It is important to have a good assistant and proper instruments. The initial cut is made onto the preselected rib after injection of a solution containing 0.5% adrenaline. The periosteum can be raised quite easily, and using a sharp elevator the superficial surface of the rib can be exposed. The initial dissection on the deep side of the rib may cause trouble; damage to the neurovascular bundle may occur, and occasionally damage to the pleura. Pleural damage is an unusual event and is easily repaired with a few sutures providing that the lung has not been damaged. A Doyen's rib raspatory or a similar curved elevator is then inserted in the small tunnel under the rib, and the deep periosteum stripped. One end of the rib is divided by lifting it and dividing it with rib shears; by holding it, delivering it further into the wound, and retracting firmly, a large segment can be obtained. If more than two ribs are needed, it is important to harvest two, leave one and then harvest a third, to prevent a flail chest. It is important not to leave jagged cut ends of the rib — they may cause damage to the lung and pleura — and to secure bleeding carefully. It is also important to resuture the periosteum very carefully as ribs reconstitute and may be reharvested if necessary. The quality of rib graft is variable. Sometimes the rib is so soft that it is hardly usable; in other subjects, it provides stout and useful material with good cancellous content. The rib is split on a separated table. It is held by an assistant with a bone-holding forceps. A sharp osteotome, usually without the use of a mallet, is worked from one end of the rib along its edge in a rocking motion to split the rib. In poorer quality ribs which are brittle and without much cancellous content one may have to use a mallet or even a saw.

Calvarial bone

This is a popular source of bone grafts because of a lack of donor site morbidity; there is also a widespread but unsubstantiated view that calvarial bone is better because it is developed in membrane and hence more suitable for reconstruction of the facial bones. It does have the drawback of being more rigid than either iliac bone or rib. The services of a neurosurgeon on the craniofacial team are occasionally needed. A secondary contour defect may result if the edges are not smoothed as much as possible. It should not be necessary to point out that in harvesting calvarial bone, the sagittal sinus and its parasagittal venous tributaries should be avoided, and great care should be taken to preserve the dura mater; anecdotal accounts of dural damage abound.

It has been said that the parieto-occipital area over the nondominant hemisphere is the donor site of choice. This seems to imply that there is a significant potential for cerebral complications. This implication should be dismissed: there should be no cerebral complications, and brain injury in this site is as reprehensible as in any other.

Technique. When a craniotomy is being performed, the inner table can be split from the bony flap raised by the neurosurgeon. In other situations, the outer table can be safely split from the skull where there is a reasonably well formed diploic space as is usual in the parietal area. It is important to view the X-ray pictures before operation as there is a wide variety of diploic anatomy and some patients have thin skulls. Where the coronal incision is being used, the posterior flap can be dissected backwards and an area of pericranium exposed. When one wishes to take only the outer table, for example to repair the orbital floor, an area of bone is defined by cutting through the pericranium around it. The pericranium is then dissected away from the proposed bone graft site, leaving a patch of pericranium overlying the bone to be taken. A trench is then cut with a large flame-shaped burr through the outer table into the cancellous bone. A thin curved osteotome is then worked around the periphery of the graft until it is freed. Sometimes the outer table is very brittle and by maintaining the pericranial cover, the bone fragments will be held together. Where calvarial bone is needed for a large cranioplasty then almost all the parietal bone should be harvested by the neurosurgeon and very carefully split using fine osteotomes and power saws. The inner table is usually replaced in the donor (parietal) region, the outer table being used in the cranioplasty. For an isolated harvesting not done through a bicoronal scalp flap, a transverse or oblique scalp incision above the ear can be used (p. 557).

Done by a proficient surgeon, this is a very safe procedure; damage to the sagittal sinus or to the brain has nevertheless been recorded, and postoperative intracranial haemorrhage is also a possible complication. Calvarial grafts should not be harvested by operators unfamiliar with the technique (Kline & Wolfe 1994), and if there are any signs of neurological impairment after such an operation, full evaluation, including CT scanning, should be done at once.

Other bone donor sites

The anterior surface of the tibia has been used in the past, but we have no experience of its use in CMF repairs.

Vascularized bone grafts have been taken from the humerus, radius, scapula, and clavicle, as well as from the ilium and the calvaria; our preferred techniques of revascularized free grafts are discussed on p. 626.

Cartilage grafts

Costal cartilage can be harvested as described above and used in small orbital floor defects which can also be repaired with cartilage harvested from the nasal septum or the concha of the ear.

Alloplastic materials

Synthetic materials, including Silastic® and Teflon® sheeting and hydroxyapatite, have all been used in attempts to reconstruct the fractured orbital floor, and as onlays in restoring facial contours. They are easy to use, do not absorb, and have no donor site morbidity, but the risk of delayed infection and movement or extrusion make them a second choice when compared to the advantages of autogenous materials. Alloplastic materials (titanium, acrylic etc.) are widely used to cover calvarial bone defects and are often very satisfactory, although delayed infection and exposure sometimes occur. In Adelaide we favour the use of titanium plates, either shaped by hydraulic pressure (Blair et al 1980) or cast in a mould modelled from CT scan data by the CAD/CAM (computer-aided design and computer-aided manufacture).

Fixation techniques

There are certain sites where secure fixation should be achieved; these include the horizontal and vertical buttresses of the face. These buttresses are the framework or structural pillars of the face and stabilization of properly reduced fractures in these areas will re-establish normal skeletal anatomy. Miniplating systems have greatly enhanced the ability to provide three-dimensional stabilization of bony fragments in these buttress areas.

Interosseous steel wires still have many applications in CMF fracture fixation. Wires may be used to locate bone temporarily before the application of plates and screws; this strategy is useful where all fixation points of the bone cannot be visualized at once. Fine wire may be used to stabilize the inferior orbital rim where the overlying subcutaneous tissue is very thin and where plates and screws may be palpable percutaneously. And in many parts of the world, wires may be employed because miniplate systems are unobtainable or prohibitively costly. Pre-stretched wire should be used, inserted through holes drilled with a fine burr and twisted clockwise to tighten and to achieve firm apposition of bone ends. The twisted end is cut long enough to be buried in an adjacent burr hole, yet not so long as to be palpable through the skin. Wire has been a great surgical standby, and skill in the use of wire remains essential.

Plates must be used with caution in childhood; there is ample evidence from animal experiments that plates and screws placed across sutures in a growing animal will reduce growth at that suture site (Lin et al 1991). It therefore seems reasonable to remove plates and screws in a planned fashion when the plates and screws have been placed across a growth centre, for example the mandibular condyle (p. 504).

PRINCIPLES OF SOFT-TISSUE REPAIR

Priorities

Primary repair of soft tissues of the face and scalp should, if possible, be carried out within 12 h of injury. But in practice, delay up to 48 h has not led to detrimental consequences, and can be accepted where there are more urgent priorities.

Management of skin wounds

Debridement

Accurate conservative debridement is the key to early primary closure. The cheeks and scalp are the only areas of the face where there is some redundancy of tissue; elsewhere, debridement must conserve vital structures such as eyelids, lip, nose and ears. Therefore an accurate repair of these structures is essential with matching of landmarks, and this should not be delayed unless there are compelling reasons. The techniques of skin closure are discussed in Chapter 15.

Plastic procedures

Where there is such loss of skin that direct closure is not possible without distortion of a key anatomical structure, then skin grafting may be the preferred primary option. In different situations, we have used split-skin grafts, full-thickness grafts and virtually all the flaps devised by plastic surgeons (p. 451). These procedures also find many applications in the management of burns (Ch. 17).

Microsurgical procedures

Microvascular tissue transfers are now routinely used in repairing avulsive soft-tissue injuries (pp. 437 and 454) and in reconstructing defects in the facial skeleton by vascularized bone grafts (p. 623). The success of these depends on microvascular anastomoses by a skilled operator with appropriate equipment. In our service, the Wild M691 microscope has been chiefly used; the anastomoses are normally performed with 10/0 nylon sutures on 70 μm tapered needles. In the replantation of avulsed structures, staff and facilities for microvascular repair must be available at short notice.

In the management of CMF trauma, there are other applications for microsurgery, especially in ophthalmic and neurosurgical procedures. Each discipline has its own preferences in choice of microscope, and this can cause difficulties in combined operations.

Muscles, nerves and ducts

Careful alignment and suture of these deeper structures should also be carried out early. In most cases, use of the microscope will be required to effect accurate repairs. Where major branches of the facial nerve have been divided posterolateral to the line of the lateral canthus, careful microscopic repair is mandatory. If there is a laceration of the supraorbital nerve at the superior orbital rim then this too should be repaired to prevent troublesome numbness of the forehead. Lacerations of the inferior dental nerve where it issues from the mental foramen should also be primarily repaired. The microscope should be used for early repair of ductal structures; these include Stensen's duct and the canaliculi of the nasolacrimal drainage apparatus (pp. 429 and 439).

PRINCIPLES OF DENTAL MANAGEMENT

Priorities

Injuries of the teeth are not high in the list of priorities in cases of multiple trauma. Ideally, replantation of an avulsed tooth should be done within 30 min of the avulsion (p. 353), but this is rarely possible in cases of serious CMF injury. Fractures exposing the dental pulp may result in loss of an otherwise salvageable tooth and the chances of survival are increased by application of calcium hydroxide paste and appropriate endodontal therapy. Other dental injuries can be treated less urgently.

Nevertheless, the dental assessment is often of great importance, and should not be delayed in injuries involving the oral cavity. This is especially so when fractures of the facial skeleton disrupt the dental occlusion.

Dental techniques

These are discussed in Chapter 12. The skills of the prosthodontist are indispensible in the treatment and rehabilitation of fractures of the jaws. In our unit, dental specialists have led in designing and manufacturing oral and extraoral prostheses, in the use of osseointegrated implants (p. 637) and in the application of CAD/CAM techniques for fabrication of titanium and other implants. The prosthodontist has been involved increasingly in preparing ears, noses and ocular prostheses, and the role of this important discipline is likely to expand.

PRINCIPLES OF BRAIN INJURY MANAGEMENT

Priorities

Brain injury management has some imperative priorities, which express the need to protect the brain from the secondary complications of head injury. These include:

1. Prevention of hypoxia and hypotension, especially in comatose patients
2. Control of raised intracranial pressure (ICP) and prevention or treatment of cerebral compression
3. Prevention of craniocerebral infection.

Coma management

Coma with depression of the protective reflexes is an immediate threat to life; the threat is increased when fractures of the facial skeleton compromise the airway. Coma management is discussed on p. 381; it is important here to emphasize that persisting coma may delay the definitive management of other CMF injuries. In patients remaining in coma (Glasgow Coma Scale ≤ 8) after resuscitation, we routinely institute endotracheal intubation, ventilation and respiratory paralysis as soon as possible — usually in the emergency room, sometimes at the roadside or in the retrieval ambulance. This entails many neurosurgical and metabolic dangers, and to avoid these, close 24 h collaboration with the team of intensivists is essential. CMF injuries in coma are managed in this way until the physiological state is stable and the risk of serious intracranial complications is acceptably low.

Raised intracranial pressure and cerebral compression

The patient with a craniocerebral injury complicated by raised ICP is in danger of irreversible impairments of neuronal physiology, and modern neurosurgical intensive care is planned to keep the ICP at a tolerable level: 20 mmHg is usually given as the maximum acceptable pressure, though patients have survived much higher pressures for periods of days. The need to monitor and control ICP has a high priority in victims of CMF trauma who are in coma; our methods are set out in Chapter 13.

When ICP is elevated by a mass lesion, especially an expanding intracranial clot, other considerations become dominant. The danger is not only the effect of a general elevation in ICP: there is the more immediate threat of transtentorial herniation, brainstem compression, and irreversible damage to the vital brainstem nuclei (Fig. 2.28). Modern head injury management aims to detect intracranial clots and areas of brain swelling by early and repeated CT scanning, and to a lesser extent by ICP manometry; detection by observation of the conscious level is still an essential part of the management of minor head injuries, but is excluded in comatose patients by the use of respiratory paralysis and ventilation. An extradural or subdural clot causing cerebral displacement is an imperative surgical emergency; when there is evidence of rapid deterioration or severe displacement, the patient must be rushed to the theatre. Although small haematomas may be treated conservatively, it is wise to evacuate all except the most trivial extracerebral haematomas at once by an adequate craniotomy if there is any impairment of the conscious level. Intracerebral haemorrhage, if large, may also require craniotomy, and there is sometimes justification for operating on haemorrhagic contusions constituting a mass lesion; Gudeman et al (1989) have been able to do this without increasing the eventual neurological deficit. In our experience of CMF trauma, an operation for haemorrhagic contusion is likely to end with a frontal or temporal lobectomy as an 'internal decompression', and we have avoided such mutilating operations if at all possible. External decompression, by removal of a large bone flap and enlarging the dural capacity by a fascial graft, is less detrimental, but is often ineffective. Operation for intracranial haemorrhage will usually take priority over any other procedure for CMF injury. However, in doing these urgent operations, the neurosurgeon should keep the needs of facial fracture repair in mind, especially when planning the exposure (see below); in such cases, it is helpful if a craniofacial colleague can be in the theatre to advise on this, to examine the fracture under anaesthesia, and to view the radiological images.

Intracranial infection

Prevention of intracranial infection is an important part of management of CMF trauma. Ideally, open craniocerebral wounds should be closed as soon as possible, with watertight reconstitution of the dura mater and good scalp closure. However, these injuries do not carry the highest priority. Compound depressed calvarial fractures can be left for 24 h, or even longer, if covered with a sterile dressing and treated with systemic antibiotics. Both in peace and war, closures of penetrating missile wounds have been similarly delayed without adverse effects, though it is certainly not advisable to do so. Persisting cerebrospinal fluid leaks through the nose and other cranionasal fistulas should also be closed before infection can supervene. However, it is highly inadvisable to attempt to close a cranionasal fistula until ICP has returned to normal. Moreover, cranionasal fistulas may heal spontaneously, and cerebrospinal rhinorrhoea is usually treated expectantly for 7–10 days in the hope of spontaneous cessation of the leak. During the waiting period, we give prophylactic antibiotics in such cases, though their value is disputed. Since fistula repair is not seen as urgent, it can be combined with elective repair of complex facial fractures (Simpson et al 1990).

Neurosurgical techniques

Instruments

For craniocerebral injuries, standard neurosurgical instruments are appropriate; microsurgical instruments, though rarely essential, are very helpful in difficult dissections in the region of the optic nerves and chiasm. Adjustable self-retaining retractors are useful, especially when used in conjunction with the rigid skull fixation given by the Mayfield head rest. When exploring war-time missile wounds of the brain without a skilled assistant, the Scoville brain spatula forceps is a most helpful substitute for a self-retaining retractor; no doubt the simple wire double retractor devised by Miyake & Ohta (1993) could be used in the same way. The operative microscope is routinely used in subfrontal explorations, especially in the vicinity of the optic chiasm; in our service, the Contraves microscope has been favoured. However, if a microscope is not available, binocular loupes and a strong headlight are usually satisfactory. Powered drills (see above) have become part of standard neurosurgical operative technique; diamond burrs are essential in opening the optic canal (see p. 425). The neurosurgeon who has to manage gunshot wounds of the head without plastic surgical assistance should be prepared to close scalp defects by split-skin grafting when the use of a rotation flap alone is insufficient to effect watertight closure without tension — always assuming that the pericranium in the secondary defect will accept a graft.

Neurosurgical exposures

The use of the standard bifrontal scalp flap is strongly advocated for frontal mass lesions and for exploration of the anterior cranial fossa, whether by a bifrontal or unifrontal bone flap (Fig. 13.11). If a lateral craniotomy is needed, the skin incision should be planned to permit a frontal flap at a later date. Occasionally, we have been able to combine operation for intracranial clot with repair of a fracture of the facial skeleton, but there are dangers in prolonged one-stage operations in severely injured patients.

Wound closure

The dura mater is always closed; at present, 4/0 braided Neurolon is used, but fine absorbable sutures have been found satisfactory. If necessary, a graft of temporalis fascia, pericranium or fascia lata is inserted. Bone flaps are replaced; in the past, these have been secured with silk or steel wire, but titanium wires or miniplates are preferable. The scalp is closed in two layers; for the galea, we use a continuous absorbable suture (e.g. Vicryl: polyglactin 910), the skin edges being apposed with staples or a continuous monofilament Prolene (polypropylene) stitch. Drainage is used as little as possible, since suction may aspirate excessive volumes of cerebrospinal fluid if there is a breach in the dura (McCulloch & Pattison 1981). But where there appears to be a risk of postoperative bleeding, low-pressure suction drainage is used.

Postoperative monitoring

All craniotomies carry the risk of postoperative bleeding, especially in the extradural space; neurosurgical nursing observations are planned to detect such complications. However, changes in the conscious level may be masked if narcotic analgesics must be given because of painful procedures such as thoracotomy for rib grafts or exposure of the iliac crest; in such cases, small bolus doses of intravenous morphine are a reasonably safe means of giving analgesia without greatly impairing consciousness. Likewise, after exposure of the facial skeleton, the pupillary light reflexes may be masked by orbital swelling. The neurosurgeon must then rely on ICP monitoring (p. 369) and on repeated CT scanning; monitoring of vision and other cerebral functions by computer-averaged records of evoked potentials has not played a large part in our practice (p. 248) but may be used as an additional safeguard.

PRINCIPLES OF MANAGEMENT OF EYE INJURIES

Priorities

Penetrating eye injuries should take priority over all other CMF injuries save those that are immediately life-threatening. In children, there is special urgency, since a child may aggravate the eye damage by rubbing or picking at the wounded eye. In adults with such injuries, it may be justifiable to delay the definitive repair overnight, or for whatever time is needed to transfer the injured person to a centre that can offer more expert treatment. If this is done, precautions should be taken to prevent expulsion of the contents of the eye or infection.

Remediable conditions imperilling the blood supply of the retina or optic nerve also deserve high priority. These include:

1. Optic nerve compression
2. Intraorbital haematoma
3. Occlusion of the central retinal artery
4. Acute glaucoma.

These conditions are discussed in Chapter 14; in practice, urgent surgical treatment of these conditions is rarely indicated and still less often is it successful.

The timing of secondary eye surgery is important. Vitrectomy may be needed in wounds involving the posterior segment of the eye (p. 405); this operation is best done 7–10 days after injury, and no later than 2 weeks. Lens extraction may also be needed, and this is best delayed until anterior chamber haemorrhage has resorbed, and any corneal wound has healed, so that there is a good operative view of the intraocular structures. Moreover, if an intraocular lens is to be implanted, preoperative measurements by keratometry and A-scan ultrasound will be needed; these need careful and unhurried measurement. The timing of lens implantation depends on the patient's age: in a child in the age where there is a risk of amblyopia, operation is done at 2–6 weeks, in an adult at 2–12 weeks.

Organization

Some eye injuries, especially those in the posterior segment of the eye, demand much diagnostic and operative skill. In planning a trauma service, it is important to ensure that an ophthalmologist with these skills is always available at short notice. It is equally important to ensure that all members of the trauma team are alert to detect eye injuries, and sufficiently familiar with the management of ocular trauma to participate in assigning priorities in cases of multiple injury with eye involvement. It is also important that medical and nursing staff should be trained to detect delayed visual failure.

It is not always easy to combine ophthalmological procedures in a single-stage multidisciplinary operation, as is often done with conditions requiring plastic surgery, neurosurgery, or oral surgery. Eye surgeons are accustomed to use dedicated theatres, special equipment and nursing staff with special skills. However, many less demanding ophthalmological procedures can and should be done as part of a definitive multidisciplinary procedure.

This is often true of enucleation or evisceration of a severely damaged eye; it is also true of tarsorrhaphy, which has many applications in CMF trauma.

Ophthalmological techniques

These are discussed in Chapter 14, in relation to the various types of eye injury. Penetrating eye wounds may require vitrectomy. Simple removal (abscission) of prolapsed vitreous can be done with scissors and cellulose sponges at the time of the primary operation, and any ophthalmologist involved in traumatic eye surgery is competent to do this. But more complex vitrectomies may be necessary for injuries involving the posterior segment of the eye, to remove vitreous haemorrhage, to deal with vitreous traction bands, to remove deeply sited foreign bodies, and for retinal detachments. These exacting procedures need special instruments and the special skills of an ophthalmologist who is dedicated to this field of surgery. The techniques of vitrectomy are beyond the scope of this book, but a general account is given in Chapter 14. Optic nerve decompression is another procedure requiring specialized instruments and skills, and the craniofacial unit should be able to provide these at short notice: the swing away from transfrontal neurosurgical decompression to transethmoid decompression may enlist the ENT surgeon in these still debatable procedures (p. 426).

Protection of vision

In the course of the management of CMF trauma, vision may be imperilled in many ways, and it is necessary to adopt routine measures designed to minimize the known risks. Morax (1984) has given an interesting review of peroperative visual dangers, and there are also risks in the intensive care unit and in the ward.

There are many situations in which a previously normal cornea may be injured, or a recoverable corneal injury may become irreversible. These include:

1. Accidents in emergency management or in the operating theatre, resulting in mechanical or chemical trauma
2. Later injury from impaired lid closure, proptosis, exposure, impaired tear production or a combination of these.

The prevention of corneal injury is an immediate responsibility for many members of the CMF team. Measures for eye protection in emergency management are discussed on p. 229. In the operating theatre, great care is needed to avoid accidental contact with the exposed eye. If possible, the eye is protected by the anaesthetist after induction, by covering the cornea with a suitable ointment

(e.g. white paraffin ointment) and sealing the eyelids with a waterproof adhesive film or strapping. However, this is often impossible; in many operations in the orbital region, the eye is necessarily part of the sterile field. Strong antiseptic solutions should be avoided: we have seen permanent blindness when a skin preparation of 70% alcohol was inadvertently placed in contact with the cornea. A half-strength aqueous solution of povidone–iodine is well tolerated; some surgeons prefer to use 0.2% aqueous chlorhexidine. Throughout the operation, care is taken to avoid mechanical contact or desiccation. We place discs of absorbent material covered with plastic (e.g. Telfa® dressings) over the eye, irrigating them from time to time; Morax (1984) mentions the use of coloured contact lenses to cover the cornea during surgery.

The cornea is endangered if there is impaired lid closure. Initially, it is usually appropriate to employ temporary measures to close the lids and to prevent desiccation. These include:

1. Copious use of lubricants, artificial tears and lid massage
2. Application of clear plastic film (Fig. 9.8A); this has largely replace the use of a watch glass taped to the face (Fig. 9.8B)
3. Taping the lids together, or sealing them with tissue adhesive
4. Inserting a 4/0 silk suture through the upper (or lower) lid, and taping this to the cheek (or eye brow); a version of this procedure is shown in Fig. 9.8C.

Tarsorrhaphy

These measures may fail, and are of course unsuitable for long-term protection; a tarsorrhaphy may then be necessary. In some situations, tarsorrhaphy may indeed be indicated forthwith. The chief of these is a combination of facial and trigeminal paralysis, with abolition of both the motor and sensory arcs of the corneal reflex. This is unusual as a consequence of an impact in the CMF region, but we have seen it after a crushing injury of the skull, and it is very likely to lead to severe keratitis.

Temporary tarsorrhaphy is appropriate when the need for eye closure is expected to be over in 3–6 weeks at most; this is so when the cause is postoperative orbital swelling and proptosis. The lids are sutured together without removal of any lid tissue; when the sutures are removed, the eye will open. We use 4/0 silk or 3/0 Nylon sutures, passed through the upper tarsal plate to emerge in the line between the orifices of the Meibomian glands and the line of the lashes, and then through the lower plate in the reverse direction; on each side of the palpebral fissure and the line of eyelashes, the stitch is passed through a short (5–10 mm) length of rubber tubing to

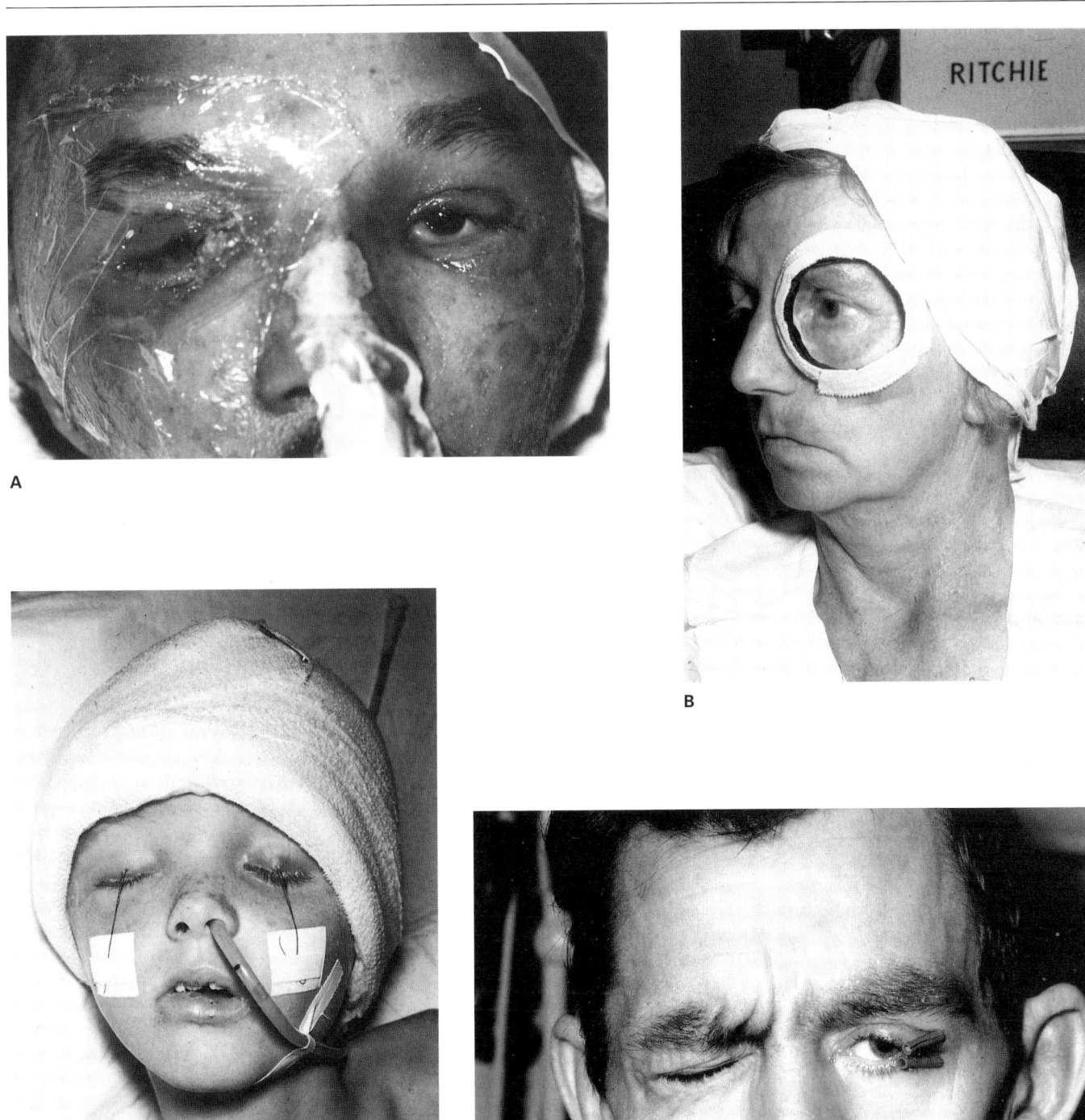

Fig. 9.8 Protection of the cornea. A The eye can be covered with clear polyethylene film (Glad®-wrap). This is now in routine use as an initial protective measure. **B** A watch glass or plastic cover can be taped to the skin; this allows use of the eye. Little use is made of this now, but it has a place when the cornea is anaesthetic, as it makes it difficult for the patient to rub or scratch the eye. **C** A suture can be passed through the eyelid and taped to the cheek: the suture is used to open the eye when the pupils are tested. In practice, this method is often unsuccessful because attachment of the taped suture soon becomes loose. We no longer advise this, but it has its advocates. **D** Tarsorrhaphy is a versatile and usually safe method of securing eye closure. The figure shows a permanent partial tarsorrhaphy done for facial paralysis; rubber tubing is used to prevent sutures from cutting through the lid margins.

act as a bolster. Usually two of these mattress sutures will suffice.

In a permanent tarsorrhaphy, a strip of tissue is removed to allow the lids to fuse together by tissue union. To effect this, a strip of lid may be excised between the lashes and the orifices of the Meibomian glands on both the upper and lower lids; alternatively the whole of the inner lid margin may be excised. The lids are then sutured together with 4/0 silk or 5/0 Nylon stitches passed into the lid and out again as mattress sutures: they are tied on rubber bolsters, as described above. If bolsters are not used, then it is likely that the stitches will cut through the delicate lid tissue, especially in a young patient. This may lead to scarring, distortion of the lid margins and impairment of the lid function of tear spreading. In temporary tarsorrhaphy, it is important to preserve the lid margins, and in permanent tarsorrhaphy it is important to ensure that the direction of the lashes is not disturbed. If a permanent tarsorrhaphy leaves lashes misdirected inwards, the cornea and the conjunctiva may be irritated.

Tarsorrhaphy is a simple procedure, but it should be done carefully by a capable surgeon to ensure a satisfactory outcome. If a partial tarsorrhaphy is required (Fig. 9.8D), and this is often appropriate in cases of facial paralysis, then it is wise to make the tarsorrhaphy more extensive than seems necessary, since it is easier to open an over-large tarsorrhaphy than to resuture one that is too small.

Optic nerve protection: visual evoked responses

The optic nerve may be injured during operation, by manipulation or by the injection of an agent able to cause ischaemia or nerve damage. It may be injured after operation from compression by haematoma formation. In all orbital procedures and especially in craniofacial operations requiring correction of orbital dystopias (p. 573), it is necessary to avoid any manoeuvre likely to cause traction or compression of the optic nerves. At the close of any operation of this type, the pupils must be inspected and the light reflexes must be tested. If vision is lost, under circumstances suggesting optic nerve compression, the area of possible compression should be explored immediately.

Harding (1991) and others have used the elicitation of visual evoked responses (VER) to monitor optic nerve function during and after craniofacial surgery, and we have made some use of this diagnostic procedure. We employ a 44 mm hand-held flash stimulator which easily penetrates a closed eyelid; the stimulator contains an array of 19 light-emitting diodes. Recordings are taken from an electroencephalographic scalp electrode placed over the midoccipital cortex and about 3 cm above the inion, with a reference electrode on the ear or forehead. The evoked potentials are filtered in the range 1.6–3000 Hz,

and averaged until a stable and reproducible response is recognized. Usually 25–100 averages, repeated 1–3 times, are sufficient either to confirm optic nerve transmission or to raise concern about the possibility of damage. However, this is not a sensitive test of optic nerve function, and is used only to detect gross failure of vision.

Our use of VER monitoring in practice has been limited, chiefly to cases where there is already visual impairment. In elective operations known to place the optic nerve in some jeopardy, such as extensive orbital dissections, we have routinely performed a baseline VER measurement before operation. We do not perform the investigation during operation, because the VER is affected by anaesthetic agents, especially halothane, but if there is postoperative orbital swelling preventing tests of the pupillary light reflex, then a normal recording is very reassuring. Our chief use for VER recording has been in traumatic optic neuropathy, especially where the patient is uncooperative or where there is orbital swelling (p. 424).

PRIORITIES AND STAGING OF PROCEDURES

In isolated injuries, there are usually no difficulties from conflicting priorities. Multiple injuries always present the need to put first things first. In several possible scenarios, it may necessary to plan a staged sequence of operations on the basis of the clinical priorities. The high priority of the major neurosurgical and ophthalmological emergencies is indisputable. Soft-tissue lacerations, both of the skin and the oral mucosa, should be closed as soon as possible; this will lessen the risk of infection and further tissue loss. At the same time, repair of vital structures such as eyelids, nerves and ducts can be undertaken; these procedures are discussed in Chapters 14–16. Urgent operative intervention may be needed for life-threatening injuries of other body symptoms within the first 24 h after injury, e.g. ruptured thoracic or abdominal viscera.

On the other hand, decision on the management of facial skeletal injury should usually wait until completion of the full work-up. When the definitive plan of management of facial injury is prepared, less urgent treatment of injuries in other systems may be scheduled to be done at the same time as the operative reduction and fixation of the facial fractures. An example would be the simultaneous management of the facial and craniocerebral components of a CMF injury (e.g. a facial fracture and a closed depressed frontal bone fracture or dural repair of the anterior cranial fossa) + enucleation of a ruptured eye + some elective extracranial orthopaedic procedures.

PRINCIPLES OF COUNSELLING

When the management plan is completed, it must be explained to the patient, and usually also to the relatives.

This is essential in helping the patient to make a wise choice, whether between operative and non-operative management, or between a range of operative procedures. The explanation is the responsibility, often onerous, of the surgeon(s) chiefly involved; it is easier if there are already good communications between the team members, the patient and the family. Mutual confidence is always desirable, and never more so than when the initial injury assessment points to the likelihood of some permanent deformity or loss of function. When the patient is a child, the legal guardian must give informed consent to surgery; however, it is important to explain to children, in whatever depth is possible, what has to be done and why. For elective procedures, time can usefully be spent in games that illustrate the management plan in ways that are reassuring to the child.

Informed consent

Possible complications must be explained by the surgical specialist who will conduct, or at least supervise, the recommended operative procedure(s); the risks of anaesthesia are explained by or on behalf of the anaesthetist who will give the anaesthetic. It is well when counselling can be done in an unhurried way, giving the patient time to think and take advice, or to request a second opinion in doubtful cases. In explaining possible adverse outcomes, the counsellor has to be frank yet should avoid frightening the patient unduly.

The explanation has medicolegal implications. Throughout the world, but especially in jurisdictions based on some variant of English Common Law (the UK, the USA and many countries formerly in the British Empire), surgeons are increasingly being sued by patients disappointed by the results of treatment. Among the grounds for such legal actions has been alleged failure to explain the possible complications, both those which are relatively frequent and those which are known to be very rare. It has been our practice to explain the obvious risks inherent in the treatment of a particular pattern of CMF injuries, which almost always include death and often include blindness, and to offer to list the rarer risks, while stressing their rarity. This can be done in a reassuring way. In our experience, few patients wish to know more than the major risks, and many indeed are satisfied by the statement: 'I would want this operation if I was in your position'. Nevertheless, it is the duty of the counselling surgeon to make sure that the anxieties of the individual patient are fully brought out, and that he or she is given an explanation of the extent to which these are well grounded. In the USA, some surgeons provide a lengthy printed list of possible complications; we believe that this could become a perfunctory ritual, and might actually hinder a proper explanation. It is agreed that the surgeon has a duty to give an explanation of the risks in a proposed course of action, but different jurisdictions have given different opinions on what standards should be used in deciding whether this has been done to a reasonable extent. In the case of Sidaway v The Bethlem Royal Hospital (1985), the highest British appellate court held that the adequacy of the explanation should be judged by the standard of medical practice at the time, presented as expert testimony. Nevertheless, the same court emphasized that there could be exceptions to this rule, and in a recent judgement, the full Australian High Court held that the standard must be the general concept of reasonable behaviour (Rogers v Whittaker 1992). This case is of particular interest to surgeons working with CMF injuries because it related to postoperative sympathetic ophthalmitis resulting in bilateral blindness. Medical opinion confirmed that the risk of this devastating complication was very low, but the court held that in the context of a largely cosmetic operation, it would have been reasonable to mention this possibility. In our practice, few difficulties have arisen in the early counselling of the victims of CMF trauma, and in particular the giving of informed consent has rarely caused distress or delay. Written forms of consent, signed by the surgeon and the patient, are routinely used, though such forms would not be a valid defence if the explanation given were held to be inadequate.

REFERENCES

Blair G A S, Gordon D S, Simpson D A 1980 Cranioplasty in children. Child's Brain 6: 82–91
David D J 1974 Exploration of the orbital floor through a conjunctival approach. Aust NZ J Surg 44: 25–27
David D J, Cooter R D 1987 Craniofacial infection in 10 years of transcranial surgery. Plast Reconstr Surg 80: 213–225
Demetriades D, Charalambides D, Lakhoo M, Pantanowitz D 1992 Role of prophylactic antibiotics in open and basilar fractures of the skull: a randomized study. Injury 23: 377–380
Frauenfelder F T, Morgan R L, Yunis A A 1993 Blood dyscrasias and topical ophthalmic chloramphenicol (Letter). Am J Ophthalmol 115: 812–813
Gruss J, Phillips J 1989 Complex facial trauma: The evolving role of rigid fixation and immediate bone graft reconstruction. Clin Plast Surg 16: 93–104
Gruss J, Mackinnon S, Kassel E, Cooper D 1985 The role of primary bone grafting in complex craniomaxillofacial trauma. Plast Reconstr Surg 75: 17–24
Gruss J Discussion on Derdyn C, Persing J, Broaddus W et al 1990 Craniofacial trauma: an assessment of risk related to timing of surgery. Plast Reconstr Surg 86: 246–247
Gudeman S K, Young H F, Miller J D, Ward J D, Becker D P 1989 Indications for operative treatment and operative technique in closed head injury. In: Becker C P, Gudeman S K (eds) Textbook of head injury. Saunders, Philadelphia, Ch 6
Haines S J 1982 Topical antibiotic prophylaxis in neurosurgery. Neurosurgery 11: 250–253
Harding G F A 1991 Intraoperative and intensive care unit monitoring with visual evoked potentials and electroretinography. In: Heckenlively J R, Arden G B (eds) Principles and practice of clinical electrophysiology of vision. Mosby, St Louis
Hobar P 1992 Methods of rigid fixation. Clin Plast Surg 19: 31–39

Ignelzi R J, Van der Ark G D 1975 Analysis of the treatment of basilar skull fractures with and without antibiotics. J Neurosurg 43: 721–726

Kline R M, Wolfe S A 1994 Complications associated with the harvesting of cranial bone grafts. Plast Reconstr Surg (in press)

Lin K, Bartlett S, Yaremchuk M, Grossman R, Udupa J, Whitaker L 1991 An experimental study on the effect of rigid fixation on the developing craniofacial skeleton. Plast Reconstr Surg 87: 229–235

Lowbury E J L 1981 Topical antimicrobials: perspectives and issues. In: Maibach H I, Aly R (eds) Skin microbiology. Relevance to clinical infection. Springer, New York, Ch 19

Luce E 1992 Developing concepts and treatment of complex maxillary fractures. Clin Plast Surg 19: 125–131

Manson P, Ruas E, Iliff N 1987 Deep orbital reconstruction for correction of posttraumatic enophthalmos. Clin Plast Surg 14: 113–121

McCulloch G A, Pattison W J 1981 Circulatory changes caused by a closed, negative pressure drainage system after craniotomy. Neurosurgery 9: 380–382

Miyake H, Ohta T 1993 A new brain retractor. Technical note. J Neurosurg 79: 462–463

Morax S 1984 Surveillance de l'appareil visuel au cours de la chirurgie plastique orbito-palpébrale. Ann Chir Plast Esthét 29: 311–317

Rahn B 1989 Theoretical considerations in rigid fixation of facial bones. Clin Plast Surg 16: 21–27

Rogers v Whittaker 1992 Full Court of the High Court of Australia 109 ALR 625

Salyer K, Taylor D 1987 Bone grafts in craniofacial surgery. Clin Plast Surg 14: 27–35

Sidaway v Governors the Bethlem Royal Hospital and others 1985 1 All ER 643–666 (HL)

Simpson D A, David D J, Reilly P L 1990 Fractures of the anterior cranial fossa: the craniofacial approach. Asian J Surg 13: 23–31

Strachan C J 1993 Antibiotic prophylaxis in peripheral vascular and orthopaedic surgery. J Antimicrob Chemother 31 Suppl B 65–78

Young R F, Lawner P M 1987 Perioperative antibiotic prophylaxis for prevention of postoperative neurosurgical infections. J Neurosurg 66: 701–705

Anaesthesia and postoperative care

R. Edwards   J. Barritt   R. Walter
Contributing authors: J. Abbott   J. Trott

INTRODUCTION

In general the definitive management of craniomaxillo-facial (CMF) trauma is not urgent, the exceptions being those life-threatening conditions described in Chapter 8. CMF trauma surgery is therefore usually performed when the patient is stable and after completion of any surgery necessary for other injuries causing systemic instability. However, the operations are often challenging for the anaesthetist (Bahr & Stoll 1992; Schulz 1992). Many are long and some entail severe blood loss. In operations for intracranial injuries, and in transcranial procedures done to correct injuries or deformities involving the skull base, the control of intracranial pressure (ICP) is an additional requirement. In operations on the jaws, encroachments on the airway may present further difficulties for the anaesthetist.

At the conclusion of the operative repair of any CMF injury there is much to be done to ensure the patient's well-being, both physical and psychological. In cases of severe injury or deformity, the team of multidisciplinary trauma specialists is still required to care for the patient and its members must consult with one another closely, especially in the provision of psychosocial support.

ANAESTHESIA

The airway

Nasotracheal intubation provides a convenient and secure airway during and after surgery and allows the jaws to be wired together with teeth in occlusion. We prefer to use armoured tubes and secure them with a stitch through the ala of the nose (Fig. 10.1). There are, however, two instances described in the literature where nasal tubes

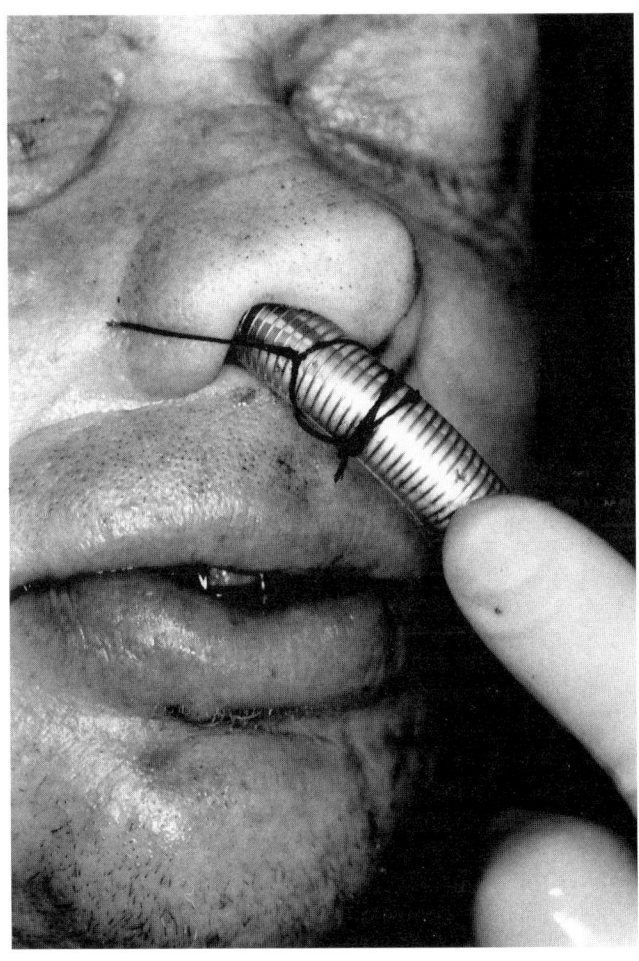

Fig. 10.1 Anchoring a nasal endotracheal tube. A 56-year-old man suffered fractures of the maxilla and mandible when a plane made a crash landing. The tube is sutured to the nose: the stitch (2/0 silk) is passed through the alar cartilage.

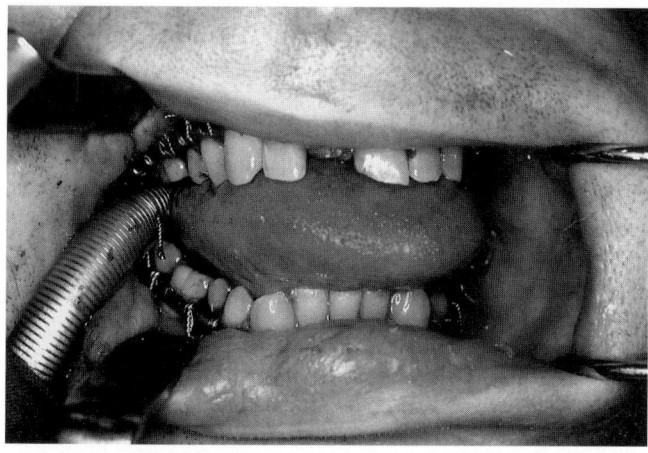

Fig. 10.2 Anchoring an oral endotracheal tube. The tube is wired to the third molar tooth; it can be led out through the corner of the mouth when intermaxillary fixation is needed.

have penetrated the cranial cavity through a fracture of the cribriform plate (Horellou et al 1978, Patrick 1987). The skilled anaesthetist who passes the endotracheal tube directly along the floor of the nasal cavity is unlikely to produce this appalling injury; nevertheless it is our practice to use an oral endotracheal tube for those patients whose anterior cranial fossa floor is not intact. The orally placed armoured tube can be secured to an eyelet wire attached to a third molar tooth (Fig. 10.2). The tube exits from the mouth behind this tooth allowing the teeth to be placed in occlusion. There are many more reports of nasogastric tubes entering the cranial cavity in cases of anterior fossa fracture; the nasogastric tube is smaller and more flexible than an endotracheal tube and therefore more likely to be misplaced (Seebacher et al 1975, Wyler & Reynolds 1977, Fremstadt & Martin 1978, Galloway & Grudis 1979, Borovich et al 1981, Moustoukas & Litwin 1983).

Care must be taken not to cause an intracranial aerocele by forcing gas into the cranium with positive pressure ventilation from a face mask. In those patients requiring urgent surgery to repair a penetrating eye injury there is a conflict between the risk of expelling more intraocular contents during induction of anaesthesia and the risks of vomiting from a stomach often loaded with alcohol and food (Bruce et al 1982, Libonarti et al 1985). The safest compromise is to pre-oxygenate prior to a rapid sequence induction with sodium thiopentone and suxamethonium; fasciculation is prevented by pretreatment with a non-depolarizing agent such as vecuronium 0.6 mg.

Maintenance of anaesthesia

After anaesthesia has been induced the following measures will help to give optimal operating conditions:

1. The head is placed so that the great veins draining the brain are unobstructed, by putting the head and neck in as neutral a position as possible
2. Cerebral venous drainage is assisted by means of a 10–15° head up tilt and by ensuring that wet heavy drapes or other equipment do not lie across the neck
3. Ventilation is aimed so to avoid hypoxia and to induce a modest hypocarbia (pCO$_2$ 30 mmHg)
4. Ventilator settings are chosen to impede the circulation as little as possible.

Circulatory impediments include obstruction of venous return, constriction of alveolar capillaries and 'tamponade' of the heart by distended lungs which reduce filling during diastole. These are likely to occur while positive pressure is applied by the ventilator. The tendency for cardiac output to fall is mitigated by active intact vascular reflexes mediated through the baroreceptors; it is reported that these may be inadequate in cases of severe diabetic neuropathy (p. 538). It is of particular importance to ensure that the inspiratory time is between 0.5 and 1.5 s and that positive pressure should not be held after inspiratory flow has ceased. Respiratory rate and tidal volume are determined according to the age and weight of the patient; the standard figure for tidal volume (7–10 ml/kg) should be reduced for the obese. The obese patient should be regarded as a normal-sized person surrounded by a fatty overcoat whose mass must be disregarded in calculating the tidal volume; an estimate must be made from the ideal weight for the height. If the tidal volume is overestimated by reference to the actual weight of an obese patient, the lungs will be overdistended and the cardiac output will fall.

These principles are especially relevant in neurosurgical anaesthesia. Properly applied, they will provide the surgeon with a quiet field in which to operate unless there is already post-traumatic brain swelling, when osmotic diuretics may be needed to ensure safe exposure. For this, we favour 20% mannitol, to a maximum dose of 1 g/kg; some prefer to add frusemide (up to 1 mg/kg) as a loop diuretic. Elective neurosurgery should not be carried out when there is reason to expect that the brain is still swollen.

Anaesthetic agents

The choice of anaesthetic agents depends largely on the anaesthetist's experience and skills; economic considerations may also require consideration. Three volatile agents have been widely used in neurosurgical and other major CMF procedures, either alone or as an adjunct to nitrous oxide anaesthesia. Halothane is a potent vasodilator. One minimal anaesthetic concentration (MAC) trebles the cerebral blood flow (CBF) and abolishes autoregulation (Michenfelder 1988). This marked increase in CBF causes an elevation in ICP, by altering arteriolar resistance and promoting cerebral venous dilatation; the experimental evidence for this is reviewed by Campkin & Turner (1986). However, in spite of these disadvantages, halothane was widely used in neurosurgery before the advent of more modern inhalational anaesthetics, and is still in common use in developing countries because of its lower cost. If halothane is to be used, a period of some 10 min of hyperventilation should precede the introduction of halothane, to lower the pCO_2 to 25–35 mmHg; provided that the preoperative ICP was not raised, this should give good operative conditions.

Isoflurane is a mild cerebral vasodilator. There is no rise in CBF at < 1–1.5 MAC, and there is no need to induce hyperventilation before using isoflurane.

Enflurane is midway between halothane and isoflurane in its effects on CBF, and may cause an elevation in ICP. Moreover, enflurane may cause convulsions at $\geqslant 1.5$ MAC, especially if the pCO_2 is low. Although isoflurane may also cause convulsions, it is considered to be the best of the volatile agents for neurosurgery because of the small effect on CBF and ICP. If enflurane is chosen, the concentration must be kept to < 1 MAC.

If there is elevation in ICP before an operative procedure, a small increase in CBF may cause an alarming increase in ICP. An intravenous infusion of propofol will lower ICP by reducing CBF and this may offer advantages over the volatile agents (Moss 1989).

In the islands north of Australia, and no doubt elsewhere in the developing world, many millions of people depend on diethyl ether for necessary anaesthesia, often administered through an EMO (Epstein–Macintosh Oxford) inhaler, and we have been impressed by the skill of colleagues in these parts in using this historic mode of anaesthesia. Other volatile inhalational agents are too expensive, and the logistics of transporting heavy gas cylinders often prevents the use of nitrous oxide. Ether–air mixtures from the EMO inhaler are unlikely to detonate, though deflagration may cause burns (Macintosh et al 1963); in CMF surgery, diathermy is often very useful, and the use of halothane in oxygen-enriched air is a compromise solution.

Maintenance of blood volume

During prolonged surgery it becomes difficult to estimate the blood loss. There may be hundreds of partially soaked gauze swabs and many packs. Much saline is used for irrigation and cooling of saws and drills. Blood may be spilt on the floor and on drapes, or may lie under the patient. We have found large quantities of blood in the stomach at the end of surgery in spite of a throat pack. We therefore use the central venous pressure (CVP) as the chief guide to transfusion and transfuse so as to maintain a normal CVP. If whole blood is not available, transfusion with packed cells and normal serum albumin (5% albumin: see p. 221) is satisfactory.

Transfusion with large volumes of blood is sometimes necessary, especially for large ablative wounds of the face, but has well-known dangers. These include hyperkalaemia and wash-out coagulopathy (p. 228).

Blood stored by refrigeration at the usual temperature (4°C) has undesirable biochemical characteristics. The serum contains excessive potassium, because the potassium pump fails at low temperatures; the potassium level may be up to 30 mmol/l. The pCO_2 is high, as is the blood sugar, and the pH is very low. If cold blood is given without preliminary warming, then moderate or even severe hypothermia may be induced; if there is hyperkalaemia > 7 mmol/l and the patient is cold, there may be cardiac arrhythmias or even ventricular fibrillation. To correct the dangerous combination of hypothermia and hyperkalaemia, it is usual to warm the patient and to give by intravenous injection:

1. 10% $CaCl_2$ (10 ml)
2. Soluble insulin (20 units)
3. 50% glucose (50 ml).

These measures should restore physiological stability and normothermia, with reduction of the potassium level to an acceptable value. If this does not happen, ion exchange may be needed.

Coagulation defects may be expected when coagulation factors are reduced in concentration to about 30% of their normal value. This is likely after the replacement of one blood volume (70–90 ml/kg) and when blood loss approaches that amount, coagulation factor levels and a platelet count should be measured at once. Specific deficiencies should be corrected by appropriate therapy; even if coagulation investigations are normal it is reasonable to give fresh frozen plasma prophylactically after loss of one blood volume. Consultation with a haematologist is essential (p. 532): clotting factors and platelets should only be administered to correct proven coagulation factor deficiencies. Extravascular space fluid losses should be estimated and replaced when large areas of open tissue are exposed to the air for long periods of time.

Suppression of vascular reflexes

Bradycardia and peripheral vasoconstriction are commonly seen during dissection of the face. If bradycardia is abolished with atropine, tachycardia and hypertension result, showing that the reflex has a sympathetic as well as a parasympathetic component. This causes increased bleeding. Vascular reflexes can be suppressed by deepening anaesthesia with narcotics and an inhalation agent. Transient bradycardia is best ignored.

Deliberate hypotension

Other writers have reported marked reductions in

operation time and bleeding following the institution of deliberate hypotension as a routine procedure (Davies & Munro 1975). We have halved the operative time and the amount of blood loss for transcranial operations during 15 years of craniofacial surgical experience without resorting to deliberate hypotension. This has been due to improvements in surgical technique and teamwork. We do not allow reflex hypertension, but deliberate hypotension is used only in those parts of a procedure where real advantages can be demonstrated for the surgeon, such as dissection of the facial nerve. We have also found that facial nerve surgery is facilitated by the absence of non-depolarizing muscle relaxants. This allows surgeons to use a nerve stimulator as an aid in locating the nerve (p. 440). Liberal doses of narcotic analgesics such as phenoperidine in short cases, or morphine in longer cases, combined with a volatile inhalational agent such as isoflurane, allow the use of mechanical ventilation and control of blood pressure. Good operating conditions for the surgeon are achieved by these simple measures. The control of blood volume is much more difficult when deliberate hypotension is used, and there is also a greater risk of postoperative bleeding. We believe these added risks are seldom justified.

Hypothermia

It is desirable that normothermia should be maintained, and precautions should be taken to avoid hypothermia, especially in children. Prolonged surgery and exposure of large areas of body surface during multiple operations lower the body temperature, in spite of warming blankets, heated humidification of inspired gas and warming of blood, intravenous fluids and operative irrigations.

A rise in temperature is sometimes noted when the face is osteotomized or fractured, due to embolization of marrow, bone fragments and saliva. Broad spectrum antibiotics should be administered well in advance of such manipulations to prevent septicaemia.

Monitoring

Patient safety requirements demand full monitoring for prolonged surgery involving the risk of airway compromise. The following are required:

— direct arterial blood pressure or frequent dynamap blood pressure recording
— electrocardiogram (ECG)
— core temperature
— CVP
— respiratory rate
— oesophageal or chest stethography
— circuit oxygen concentration
— arterial blood gas analysis
— circuit pressure alarms to detect ventilation disconnection
— chest X-ray picture to confirm position of endotracheal tube and central venous catheter
— CO_2 capnography
— pulse oximetry.

Capnography and pulse oximetry improve patient safety and allow less reliance on invasive monitoring procedures such as direct arterial blood pressure estimations and arterial blood gas analysis. Capnography, combined with oesophageal stethography and the ECG, are sensitive indicators of a significant entry of air into the heart; air embolism is not a frequent complication of CMF trauma, but could occur when a wound of the large cranial venous sinuses is being repaired (p. 372). Meirowsky (1965) described a wartime death from air embolism occurring under such circumstances and warned against elevating the head when a sinus is open. If air embolism does occur, the head is lowered and the surgeon floods the operative field with irrigation fluid. The anaesthetist turns off the supply of nitrous oxide, because this gas is much more soluble than nitrogen, and diffuses more rapidly into a bubble of embolized air, thus increasing its volume. Cardiac massage may be necessary. Campkin & Turner (1986) recommend initial precautionary placing of a catheter in the right atrium to aspirate a large air embolism; we have not had a need for this in CMF surgery, though it was usual to take this precaution when neurosurgical operations were done in the sitting position.

Arterial blood pressure may be measured by the usual pneumatic cuff in short operations with little bleeding, though Dynamap recording is convenient. For long operations, and where much bleeding is expected, we use direct arterial monitoring with a pressure transducer, and if deliberate hypotension is to be employed, this is essential.

Cannulation of the radial artery should be performed only after an Allen test has confirmed that the ulnar system is patent: in this test, the radial artery is occluded by finger pressure, and finger perfusion is checked (Allen 1929, Brown et al 1969). We often prefer to cannulate the dorsalis pedis artery, which is more accessible when a large surgical team surrounds the patient's head.

We have not used Swan–Ganz manometry during surgery for CMF trauma. An indication might be found in a case of left ventricular malfunction, as a sequel of myocardial ischaemia (p. 540). This may be suspected when a falling systemic arterial pressure, in the absence of drug-induced myocardial depression, does not respond to blood volume expansion though the central venous pressure rises. Pulmonary wedge pressure measurement with a Swan–Ganz catheter will also be helpful to monitor the effects of inotropic agents, or drugs such as nitroglycerine and sodium nitroprusside.

Local anaesthesia

Operations on the soft tissues of the face may be done under local anaesthesia; a solution of 2% lignocaine and 1:80 000 adrenaline is usually effective both for anaesthesia and for control of bleeding. The dose of lignocaine should not exceed 7 mg/kg; for an adult weighing 70 kg, the maximum dose is therefore ~25 ml 2% lignocaine, or 100 ml of the 0.5% solution used by neurosurgeons in scalp infiltration. Below the age of 2 years, the risk of exceeding the safe dose justifies the use of 0.25% lignocaine; indeed, it may be wiser to dispense with local anaesthesia, since all operations are done under general anaesthesia and the infiltration is chiefly used for haemostasis. The total dose of adrenaline is also important, especially in children: the maximum dose for an adult of average size is 0.5 mg, or for children 0.01 mg/kg. In practice, plastic surgeons who perform facial surgery under local anaesthesia rarely use more than a few millilitres of 2% lignocaine and 1:80 000 adrenaline, and do not approach toxic levels. However, there is a risk of causing vasovagal syncope in susceptible individuals by inadvertent intravenous injection of a small bolus of local anaesthetic, especially when pain and fear may predispose to syncope. Under general anaesthesia, this is unlikely to occur, though the adrenaline may cause transient hypertension and other undesirable cardiovascular effects, especially when halothane is used; this is a further argument for isoflurane (Campkin & Turner 1986).

Local infiltration of the scalp with 0.5% lignocaine and 1:200 000 adrenaline is a standard neurosurgical adjunct to general anaesthesia, and has been used by us routinely for its haemostatic effect and to facilitate dissection.

POSTOPERATIVE CARE

Recovery from anaesthesia

Recovery from anaesthesia may be allowed to occur in recovery, special care or intensive care wards. No patient should be extubated at the conclusion of surgery unless haemostasis is assured, there is free movement of the lower jaw and minimal swelling of the mouth, tongue and pharynx. There should be no possibility of significant swelling developing later. The patient must have adequate sensory and motor control of the airway to cope with breathing, swallowing, coughing and vomiting.

Airway management

Except in those minor cases where the airway is and will remain secure, arrangements should be made to leave the endotracheal tube in position until the need for it can be assessed the next morning. However, it often becomes apparent an hour or two after surgery that the patient is awake, that the amount of swelling is acceptable and that the patient is in no danger; the decision may then be made to remove the tube. But it must be stressed that there should be no pressure on staff to extubate the patient as no harm will come from leaving a tube overnight in a well-run intensive care unit (ICU). If after having removed the tube the staff have any concerns about the airway then the decision to remove the tube was unequivocally wrong and a hazardous situation was created unnecessarily. Airway decisions are best made after consultation between the anaesthetist (who has had the opportunity to inspect the airway), the surgeon and the intensivist.

Swelling of injured orofacial tissues may increase for some days, threatening the airway. When the protective reflexes are compromised, airway obstruction or the inhalation of blood or vomitus is possible, and the airway should be left secure. The nasotracheal tube or tracheostomy tube through which anaesthesia was administered can generally be left in place. Nasal endotracheal tubes are generally more comfortable for the awake patient than oral endotracheal tubes. However, an oral tube wired to a lower molar tooth (see above) may be needed to give a suitable airway for a patient whose jaws must remain fixed together post operatively. Staff caring for patients must be familiar with the type of airway and the mechanisms fixing tubes and teeth. They must know how to open the jaws and wire cutters should be available for that purpose. But the anaesthetist, in consultation with the surgeon, should be able to secure the airway safely so that this does not happen. The length of time that our patients remain intubated has been reduced by miniplating systems which allow the jaws to be unwired at the conclusion of surgery, giving a mobile mandible and good access to the airway.

Endotracheal intubation and tracheostomy

The indications for tracheostomy are basically the same as for endotracheal intubation:

— to bypass upper airway obstruction
— to prevent the inhalation of blood or gastric contents
— to allow tracheobronchial toilet
— to permit mechanical ventilation.

Tracheostomy is preferred when it is expected that the need for these measures will continue for several weeks, or where it is thought that there may be special difficulties with an oral or nasal endotracheal tube, as in cases with massive avulsive facial injuries. Tracheostomy is also indicated when there is a laryngeal injury (see above). Though similar in purpose, tracheostomy and prolonged oral or nasal intubation have different complications. Prolonged intubation may be complicated by:

— displacement, kinking or blockage
— subglottic stenosis

—laryngeal granuloma
—trauma to the nasal cavity
—postextubation croup.

Tracheostomy may also be complicated by displacement of the tube. In addition, tracheostomy may lead to:

—erosion into surrounding structures, such as the oesophagus or the innominate artery
—infection both local and pulmonary
—tracheal granuloma
—tracheal dilatation
—tracheal stenosis.

It should also be said that tracheostomy is somewhat more distressing for relatives: it looks very unnatural, and local purulent infection is often noted.

Staff must be familiar with the likely complications of tracheostomy and their likely timing. During the first 24 h, before the tissues around the stoma have become fixed, accidental decannulation may occur, though with careful technique, this can be avoided; we have often found it useful to suture the tube to the skin until the stoma is established. If the tube does come out, the stoma in the trachea may be separated from the stoma in the skin. Attempts to recannulate the trachea may be unsuccessful especially in the hands of inexperienced staff. Therefore, nursing in ICU for the first 24 h is essential.

When tracheostomy is performed by the open technique, a small flap of trachea, hinged on the caudal side of the stoma (Björk flap) is sutured to the deep cervical fascia to prevent this dangerous complication. We accept that the Björk flap is sometimes complicated by tethering of the stoma to the skin or by a persistent cutaneous fistula. But these complications are easily rectified by a small operation under local infiltration anaesthesia. In infants and children the trachea should be opened by a vertical slit, secured by a stay suture on each side. When the percutaneous technique of tracheostomy is used (p. 382), this safeguard cannot be employed, and even greater care is needed.

During the last 20 years, the number of tracheostomies performed has fallen markedly. Most patients can be safely managed with an endotracheal tube to secure the airway. However, unless intensive care facilities are of a high standard the use of tracheostomy has to be more liberal.

Fluid and electrolyte replacement

There are many formulae devised to estimate fluid requirements at all ages. Very simply, mature infants require 100 ml/kg/day, up to 1000 ml for a 10 kg infant; adults require 40 ml/kg/day; in old age, the requirement may be reduced to 30 ml/kg/day. Wallace's formula bridges the period between infancy and adult life:

Fluid requirement (ml/kg/day) = $100 - (3 \times$ age in years)

The daily requirements of sodium and potassium are of the order 1–3 mmol/kg/day (1 g NaCl = 13.5 mmol Na; 1 g KCl = 17 mmol K). In children and young adults, the sodium need is met if the maintenance fluid is equivalent to 1/3 normal saline. Potassium should not be added postoperatively until it is known that renal function is adequate to excrete excess potassium. In cases of cerebral injury, the fluid and electrolyte requirements must be monitored carefully, as derangements are often seen, some resulting from hypothalamic damage and some from the use of osmolar diuretics. After major injury, there is retention of fluid, and it has been usual to restrict fluid intake after cerebral injury to two thirds of the normal requirement; it is hoped that this will prevent or minimize cerebral swelling. Current thinking emphasizes the importance of maintaining normal cerebral blood flow, and if there is any suggestion of hypovolaemia, fluid replacement should be more liberal; however, Luerssen & Marshall (1990) have reported severe brain swelling as a sequel of rapid resuscitation with large volumes of saline. CVP monitoring is recommended when rapid fluid replacement is needed.

In planning fluid replacement, it is important to take into account fluid withheld during fasting and fluid lost into the tissues ('third space' fluid loss). The blood loss during surgery may have been underestimated and bleeding may continue. This can be underestimated because blood may be wiped away on tissues and swabs or may fill the stomach. If there is concern about raised ICP, the serum electrolytes and osmolality must be monitored, to avoid both dehydration and hyponatraemia.

Neurological management

When there has been a cerebral injury, the postoperative observation of conscious level, pupillary light reflexes and vital functions should be especially careful. As a rule, the preoperative CT scan will have excluded any serious intracranial complication; however, the scan should be repeated if there is any suspicion of impaired consciousness or failure to wake up. If the patient was unconscious before operation, then ICP monitoring is usually necessary (p. 369), and a sustained rise (> 20 mmHg) should arouse suspicion.

Ophthalmological management

During anaesthesia, the cornea is protected by instillation of white paraffin ointment in each conjunctival sac and the lids are closed with clear adhesive tape, unless the eye is necessarily part of the surgical field.

After operation, the cornea must be protected along the lines described in Chapter 9; if necessary, eye toilet is performed by irrigation with artificial tears (e.g. methyl cellulose eye drops).

Sedation and analgesia

Patients require sedation and analgesia to allow them to tolerate endotracheal tubes. This may be accomplished by narcotics and benzodiazepine drugs. The dose must be determined on an individual basis as the range from patient to patient is quite wide. A suggested regime is midazolam 1–2 mg hourly (20–40 μg/kg) and phenoperidine 1–2 mg hourly (20–40 mg/kg). Fentanyl or phenoperidine should be used for those patients with cranial injury who might subsequently develop subdural or extradural haematoma.

Morphine may be used when the danger of postoperative intracranial haematoma has passed; even before this, morphine is not absolutely contraindicated if dosage control is good. Infusion of narcotics by the intravenous route enables pain relief on a longer term basis with the lowest possible blood level. Large bolus intravenous doses or intramuscular injections of narcotics may give initial blood levels much higher than is required to relieve pain and may produce nausea, vomiting and excessive drowsiness. Blood levels may then rapidly fall and inadequate analgesia is the result.

In cases of CMF injury, patient-controlled analgesia is usually contraindicated because the effects of trauma, alcoholism and head injury may make the patient unable to judge his or her needs.

Postoperative bleeding

Persistent oozing of blood into the pharynx may, if swallowed, cause unpleasant vomiting or be of sufficient amount to contribute to hypovolaemic shock. Patients should be encouraged to spit out blood rather than swallow it; a 14 gauge catheter or a Yankauer sucker can be given to the patient to aid in removal of oral blood. A gastric tube of reasonable bore (16–22 french gauge) placed during surgery may be useful in removing some fluid blood after surgery, though it will not remove thick clots. Care must be taken in placing the tube to ensure that recently sutured tissues are not disrupted and that the tube cannot gain access to the anterior cranial fossa through a fracture. Surgeon and anaesthetist must discuss these possibilities before placement. During this period the maintenance of blood volume may require attention because blood may continue to be lost or because the amount of loss was initially underestimated. Coagulation status should be checked if bleeding continues on after a loss of one blood volume. The haematologist will provide advice as to specific therapy.

Antibiotics

The role of prophylactic antibiotic therapy is discussed on p. 236. In our routine management of fractures compound into the mouth, peroperative intravenous chemotherapy is continued for 48 h and then ceased, though oral antibiotics may be given for a further 5 days if there is very poor oral hygiene. It is important to ensure that clear orders are given on the duration of the course: prolonged administration of broad spectrum antibiotics is a sure way of promoting resistant strains, and in the environment of an ICU, this may be disastrous. However, antibiotic therapy for an established infection, such as osteomyelitis, may have to be maintained until the infection is controlled.

Steroid medication

Glucocorticoids are often given postoperatively, in the hope of alleviating post-traumatic swelling in the facial tissues. We do not favour this, on the theoretical ground that this medication may impair wound healing (p. 122), and on the practical ground that swelling usually subsides with acceptable speed if the patient is encouraged to sit up early. In cases of severe facial swelling, ice packs are sometimes useful.

Steroids, in the form of dexamethasone, are often prescribed for cerebral swelling, and in certain forms of cerebral oedema the response is sometimes dramatic: this is especially so when the swelling surrounds a cerebral abscess. In general, however, the evidence that steroid medication promotes survival after severe head injury is unconvincing (North & Reilly 1990).

Oral hygiene

This must be maintained, especially if there is an intra-oral injury. If the patient is unable to use a tooth brush, nursing care must include careful oral cleansing. In the early stages after operation, blood clots are gently removed from suture lines and wound surfaces by the nursing staff; as mentioned above, the patient is encouraged to use oral suction to help in this, and the use of the sucker is explained before operation. A mouth wash, such as 0.2% chlorhexidine gluconate, is used 2 hourly. If arch bars and wires have been used, the patient is shown how to use wax to smooth over any sharp protrusions.

Diet

In conscious patients, oral feeding is begun as soon as possible. Initially sterile water is given in small amounts, to test the capacity to swallow and to be sure that there is no vomiting; when amounts totalling 100 ml/h are being drunk without incident, an appropriate diet is begun. This will depend on the nature of the injury and its surgical treatment. After operation for a fracture of the upper or lower jaw, there are three possible situations:

1. The fracture(s) have been stabilized by miniplates, with no intermaxillary fixation of any kind.

2. The fracture(s) have been stabilized by miniplates, with light elastic band traction between upper and lower jaw: jaw opening is possible but is restricted. There may be an occlusal bite wafer secured to the teeth of the upper jaw into which the lower teeth will function.
3. There is intermaxillary fixation with arch bars and wires, and no jaw movement is possible.

In the first two situations, the patient is given a non-chew diet; when the jaws are wired, a full fluid diet is necessary. The diet is designed by the hospital dietitian in collaboration with the nursing staff; patients are given booklets detailing the variety of foods to be eaten daily, the frequency and volume of the meals needed for adequate nutrition, and the implements needed to prepare and to ingest the food. The non-chew diet is designed to supply food which is soft to stiff in consistency, as well as being smooth and relatively moist. The non-chew diet can be eaten without producing stress or compression forces at recently stabilized fracture sites, and the food will not tend to collect in areas of the mouth which are insensitive. Patients on a full liquid diet are warned that the large volume needed to maintain nutrition will induce feelings of gastric fullness; small feeds given up to six times daily are advised. Weight loss may result when the amount of food does not meet the patient's energy needs. Should this happen, the calorie intake must be increased by enriching the diet with high calorie foods such as cream, grated cheese, full cream milk powder, butter or margarine. Constipation may be avoided by adding whole grain cereals, vegetables and fruit.

The dietary management of the unconscious patient is discussed on p. 383.

Wound care

External facial wounds are inspected after 48 h; the suture lines are then cleaned twice daily if necessary, with dressed probes and saline or dilute hydrogen peroxide, and the wound is then left exposed. Sutures are removed after 7 days. Scalp wounds are usually left covered until the stitches or staples are removed, though attention is given to the possibility of haematoma formation under the incision; this can usually be felt through the dressing. Scalp drains are removed as soon as there is no increase in the volume of aspirated fluid; this is usually on the first day after operation. The tip of the drainage tube is sent for bacterial culture.

Mobilization

Patients are encouraged to sit up as soon as possible after recovery from anaesthesia, and to walk when their injuries make this possible. Early mobility helps to minimize facial swelling, and facilitates clearing oral, nasal and chest secretions; it also encourages a sense of independence and promotes early discharge. Depending on the nature of the injury, physiotherapy may be needed to help the patient to become mobile.

Psychosocial rehabilitation

This begins as soon as the injured person has been admitted to hospital, and may involve team members from many disciplines. Social workers are engaged in almost every case of CMF injury, but the depth of involvement varies. The hospital chaplain or other minister of religion may be of great value.

Special needs may arise from the cause of the injury. Thus, injuries from attempted suicide or criminal assault may need psychiatric management, whereas sporting injuries commonly entail less stress. Injuries from burns and some motor vehicle accidents may cause great emotional trauma, as do injuries causing blindness, deformity or brain damage. Whatever the cause and nature, the injury is usually unexpected and deeply distressing for the victim and the family. Support is urgently needed (Goodstein 1985, Roberts & Appleton 1989).

Management can be conceptualized in four stages.

First stage

In a multidisciplinary team such as a craniofacial unit or a burns unit, the social worker is notified by the medical or nursing staff as soon as possible after the patient's admission. If the patient is conscious and accessible, the social worker takes a brief history, focused on immediate practical issues, such as the urgent care of young children. The timing of visits by children to the injured parent is discussed; visits are encouraged, and advice is given on preparing the child for the visual and emotional impact of the visit. An interview with the family is held as soon as possible, to engage them as partners in treatment and to assess the impact of the crisis on both patient and family. Information is collected regarding the circumstances of the accident; the social consequences are assessed and discussed, and enquiry is made into the premorbid personality, lifestyle and reaction to stress, all essential in planning the overall treatment program (Bailey et al 1988, Shepherd et al 1988). Other practical issues are then raised, such as legal needs, employment, finance, and accommodation, and these are acted on when the time is appropriate. Contact with community agencies may be needed: urgent liaison may be necessary with an agency for the victims of violent crime, or with an insurance company, or on request with the police, to report an alleged assault or to trace property (Shepherd 1989). The obligation to notify the police of a criminal assault varies in different jurisdictions: in many communities, it is mandatory to do so in cases of suspected child abuse. The information gathered by all members of the treatment team is communicated and formulated in the treatment plan, which may be periodically revised in ward-based planning meetings.

Second stage

This comes when a programme of surgical management has been planned and explained to the patient and the family by the surgeon responsible (p. 248). Team members must also explain what can be expected, such as pain, facial swelling, dressing procedures, possible impairments of vision or speech, and dietary restrictions. The social worker's role at this stage includes frequent clarification with the patient regarding the information given: there is always difficulty in absorbing medical information when one is still in shock from trauma, and where there has been no opportunity, as there is in elective surgery, for intensive preoperative preparation. Reassurance from the staff is essential in supporting the patient, but team members must be conscious of what expectations on the outcome are realistic.

At this point, the social worker takes a more detailed psychosocial history, focused on the likely disruption in lifestyle and the emotional reactions to the trauma. The patient is assisted in coping with early grieving and anger, and with altered body image (Bernstein 1982, Williams & Griffiths 1991).

Case example. Mr X, an active self-employed young farmer, was married with two small children. He was experiencing severe marital difficulties which contributed to attempted suicide by gunshot. Management included multiple surgical reconstructions. Tracheostomy was needed and this affected communication. Disfigurement and other losses from the injuries required psychiatric intervention, the social worker and other allied health professionals working with medical and nursing staff. Interventions centred around supportive therapy, grief and marital counselling, the effects on the children, and in particular the losses in self-esteem and body image. Despite her decision for marital separation, Mrs X agreed to stay at home to assist in the early stages of home care. Support from the local community was mobilized to run the farm and to give emotional support to both husband and wife.

Third stage

This follows definitive surgery. The patient begins to face the reality of the injury, with prolonged hospitalization, perhaps further reconstruction for facial deformity, often pain and scarring in donor sites and sensory loss. (Patients with frontal lobe damage may, however, have little insight into these problems.) Team members should be aware that the patient will be experiencing grief and a range

of options in counselling should be prepared. Discussion of the realities of the injury must be carefully timed. Even when full recovery can be expected, careful counselling is needed (Mathog et al 1988). This is especially important in cases of minor brain injury, since long-term disabilities may sometimes be seen in such cases. In a seminal neuropsychological study, Gronwall & Wrightson (1974) showed that impaired concentration may follow a head injury with brief loss of consciousness, and often this persists for a month or more; they demonstrated a reduction in the rate of information processing. It is wise to reassure patients who have had a minor head injury that impaired concentration is to be expected, that it should improve, and that return to work should be done in planned stages. When there is likely to be permanent facial deformity, the patient and the family must be prepared for, and assisted in, the adaptation to changes in body image, with positive emphasis on management of the loss. Advice is given on prostheses and cosmetics. The long-term emotional and physical adjustments are discussed. Psychiatric assessment may be recommended — sometimes urgently.

When disability from brain damage is likely, the patient and the family must be prepared for a long period of rehabilitation, and the neurological rehabilitation plan must be explained. The degree of recovery after brain injury is usually unpredictable in the first few months, and the support and information given to both patient and family must be sensitive but realistic. The neurosurgeon and/or the neuropsychologist have important roles in assessment, and in giving information and advice. It should be emphasized to the patient that recovery from brain damage is a slow process, taking several years to reach a plateau level. It may be necessary to give the patient's partner or parent a somewhat bleaker forecast, but experience has shown that it is unwise to be wholly pessimistic, except in the rare case of persistent vegetative state.

In this third stage, the support services needed after discharge are discussed with the patient and the family and action is taken where requested. Community social services and legal agencies may be notified; care supervised by the general medical practitioner may be organized, or transfer to a unit offering specialist rehabilitation for brain damage or blindness (p. 649), or for drug or alcohol abuse (p. 531). If the injury was inflicted in a domestic or public assault, there may be need for shelter accommodation. Patients who are already using social support services are encouraged to reactivate them. The social worker is ideally placed to be the link with these diverse services.

Before discharge, a family meeting is advisable to review the treatment, to coordinate ongoing rehabilitation and to address anxieties and uncertainties. There should be a discussion with the responsible surgeon, or his/her deputy, at this stage, to be sure that the patient and the immediate family understand the medical situation: it is common experience that explanations given earlier are forgotten or misunderstood. Problems such as loss of the sense of smell should be explained, also any need for long-term medication, such as anti-epileptic drugs.

Fourth stage

This begins before discharge and involves both the medical and social team members in planning coordinated outpatient clinic appointments; an interdisciplinary case conference is often needed. Liaison with the various agencies listed above is coordinated by the social worker in conjunction with other allied health professionals. There may be need for housing relocation, domiciliary services, vocational retraining, and legal advice on accident compensation or disability pensions. Injured children are referred to the paediatric team psychologist, who will usually have seen the child in hospital and can coordinate the educational assistance needed to get the child back to school.

Psychiatric support

In some instances, psychiatric referral is imperative. A number of pathological reactions may be observed after severe injury. Post-traumatic stress disorder (PTSD) is common and can be the cause of considerable psychological disability and impaired physical recovery; Mayou et al (1993) have found acute mood disorders and horrific memories of the accident in 31/171 (18%) of a series of road crash victims studied prospectively. PTSD may have an acute or delayed onset, and is easily overlooked; the victim may re-experience the trauma in a variety of ways, or may show disorders of attention and arousal, or emotional lability. Depression and anxiety are common. The aetiology and the management of PTSD are discussed by Ettedgui & Bridges (1985) and McFarlane (1989).

Long-term support

Patients frequently return for ongoing reconstructive surgery. Team members must be aware that the patient may need to experience all four phases of treatment and support again, though usually for briefer periods of time.

Encouragement and the building of confidence are important in the continuing psychological management of changed appearance and altered body image. While families may accept and support, the victims often shun social contacts, fearing rejection because of visible aesthetic and functional changes. In some cases, there is need for a major career change, and patients will need support and encouragement in coming to terms with this. Referral to a support group for the burned, the visually impaired or the victims of brain injury may be useful for particular social and psychological needs. Concepts and organizational bases for the management of permanent impairments are discussed in Chapter 22.

REFERENCES

Allen E V 1929 Thromboangiitis obliterans; methods of diagnosis of chronic occlusive arterial lesions distal to wrist with illustrative cases. Am J Med Sci 179: 237–244

Bahr W, Stoll P 1992 Nasal intubation in the presence of frontobasal fractures: J Oral Maxillofac Surg 50: 445–447

Bailey B M, Carr R J, Bermingham D F, Shepherd R G 1988 A comparative study of psycho-social data on patients with maxillofacial injuries in an urban population – a preliminary study. Br J Oral Maxillofac Surg 26: 199–204

Bernstein N R 1982 Psychosocial results of burns. The damaged self-image. Clin Plast Surg 9: 337–346

Borovich B, Braun J, Yosefovich T, Guilbird J N, Grushkiewicz J, Peyser E. 1981 Intracranial penetration of nasogastric tube. Neurosurgery 8: 245–247

Brown A E, Sweeney D B, Lumley J 1969 Percutaneous radial artery cannulation. Anaesthesia 24: 532–536

Bruce R A, McGoldrick E, Oppenheimer P. 1982 Anaesthesia for ophthalmology. Aesculapius, Birmingham, pp 75–76

Campkin T V, Turner J M 1986 Neurosurgical anaesthesia and intensive care, 2nd edn. Butterworth, London, Ch 3, p 8

Davies D W, Munro I R 1975 The anesthetic management and intraoperative care of patients undergoing major facial osteotomies. Plast Reconstr Surg 55: 50–56

Ettedgui E, Bridges M 1985 Post-traumatic stress disorder. Psychiatr Clin North Am 8: 89–103

Fremstadt J D, Martin S H 1978 Lethal complication from insertion of nasogastric tube after severe basilar skull fracture. J Trauma 18: 820–822

Galloway D S, Grudis J 1979 Inadvertent intracranial placement of a nasogastric tube through a skull base fracture. South Med J 72: 240–241

Goodstein R K 1985 Burns: an overview of clinical consequences affecting patient, staff and family. Comp Psychiatr 26: 43–57

Gronwall D, Wrightson P 1974 Delayed recovery of intellectual function after minor head injury. Lancet 2: 605–609

Horellou M F, Mathe D, Feiss P 1978 A hazard of nasotracheal intubation (letter). Anaesthesia 33: 73–74

Libonarti M M, Leahy J J, Ellison N 1985 The use of succinylcholine in open eye surgery. Anaesthiology 62: 637–40

Luerssen T G, Marshall L F 1990 The medical management of head injury. In: Vinken P J, Bruyn G W, Klawans H L (eds) Handbook of clinical neurology, revised series 13. Elsevier, Amsterdam, Vol 57, Ch 9

Mathog R H, Nelson R J, Petrilli A, Humphreys B 1988 Self-inflicted shotgun wounds of the face: surgical and psychiatric considerations. Otolaryngol Head Neck Surg 98: 568–574

McFarlane A C 1989 The treament of post-traumatic stress disorder. Br J Med Psychol 62: 81–90

Macintosh R, Mushin W W, Epstein H G 1963 Physics for the anaesthetist, 3rd edn. Blackwell, London, pp 284–415

Mayou R, Bryant B, Duthie R 1993 Psychiatric consequences of road accidents. Br Med J 307: 647–651

Meirowsky A M 1965 Wounds of dural sinuses. In: Meirowsky A M (ed) Neurological surgery of trauma. Office of the Surgeon General, Department of the Army Washington D C, Ch 16

Michenfelder J P 1988 Anaesthesia and the brain. Churchill Livingstone, New York

Moss E 1989 Editorial II. Volatile anaesthetic agents in neurosurgery. Br J Anaesth 63: 4–6

Moustoukas N, Litwin M S 1983 Intracranial placement of nasogastric tube: an unusual complication. Southern Med J 1983 76: 816–817

North J B, Reilly P L 1990 Raised intracranial pressure. A clinical guide. Heinemann, Oxford

Patrick M R 1987 Airway manipulations. In: Taylor T H, Major E (eds) Hazards and complications of anaesthesia. Churchill Livingstone, Edinburgh, p 341

Roberts D, Appleton V 1989 Psychosocial care of burn-injured patients. Plastic Surg Nurs 9: 62–65

Schulz R C 1992 Nasotracheal intubation in the presence of facial fractures. Plast Reconstr Surg 89: 165–166

Seebacher J, Nozik D, Mathieu A 1975 Inadvertent intracranial introduction of a nasogastric tube, a complication of severe maxillofacial trauma. Anaesthesia 42: 100–102

Shepherd J P 1989 Surgical, socio-economic and forensic aspects of assault: a review. Br J Oral Maxillofac Surg 27: 89–98

Shepherd J P, Gayford J J, Leslie I J, Scully C 1988 Female victims of assault. A study of hospital attenders, J Craniomaxillofac Surg 16: 233–237

Williams E E, Griffiths T A 1991 Psychosocial consequences of burn injury. Burns 17: 478–480

Wyler A R, Reynolds A F 1977 An intracranial complication of nasogastric intubation. Case report. J Neurosurg 47: 297–298

Facial fractures

J. A. Trott   M. H. Moore   D. J. David
Contributing author: M. Jay

INTRODUCTION

Facial fractures vary greatly in severity and significance. Some are fractures of a single bone or small bony complex, caused by a relatively low level of force impacting on a salient part of the face. Fractures of the nose, the commonest facial fracture, are usually the result of such impacts: as a rule, a broken nose is an aesthetic problem, with only minor functional inconveniences. At the other end of the spectrum of severity, panfacial fractures are the result of very severe force impacting on the entire face and causing gross deformity and functional impairment, sometimes even a threat to life (p. 219). Facial fractures are very common, and their causes reflect the social environment in which the face is struck. The aetiology of facial injuries is discussed in Chapter 3, and our own recent experience is set out in Table 3.1

This chapter deals with the management of fractures and dislocations of the adult facial skeleton caused by blunt impacts or relatively low velocity missiles; in Chapter 16, the massive facial injuries caused by high velocity missiles and other avulsive agents are discussed, and the modifying effects of immaturity and senescence are considered in Chapter 19.

General classification of facial fractures

Facial fracture patterns express the complex anatomy of the facial skeleton, and especially the lines of strength and weakness described in Chapter 2. Some fractures are named after their discoverers (p. 18) or by the causative mechanism (p. 104). However, an anatomical nomenclature is more specific. Cooter & David (1989) have devised an alphanumeric system in which major and minor components of the entire cranium are identified by letters (see Tables 2.1 and 2.2), while bony injury is assessed on a scale of 0–3 (see Table 2.3):

0 = no fracture
1 = undisplaced fracture
2 = obviously displaced fracture
3 = comminuted and/or compound fracture.

A numerical value for the severity of injury is given for each major anatomical zone; this is derived from the sum of the injury scores for each minor zone in that major zone, to a maximum score of 5. Since there are 10 major anatomical zones, and each of these is bilateral, the summation of the scores for the 20 zones gives a value of 100 for maximal craniomaxillofacial (CMF) disruption, lesser degrees of injury being expressed as percentages. The percentage for a given case is termed the Craniofacial Disruption Score. Standard charts are used for recording the fractures as located by X-ray and/or operation. The system is designed for easy coding and computer storage, rather than for verbal description of a clinical case.

For the present purposes (Fig. 11.1), facial fractures are considered in functional groupings:

1. Fractures primarily affecting occlusion — fractures of the jaws and dento-alveolar fractures
2. Fractures primarily affecting the orbit — fractures of the naso-ethmoid region, zygoma, orbital walls and orbital roof
3. Fractures primarily affecting the nasal airway — fractures of the nasal bones and cartilages
4. Fractures primarily affecting the skull base; fractures

FUNCTIONAL ZONES OF FACE

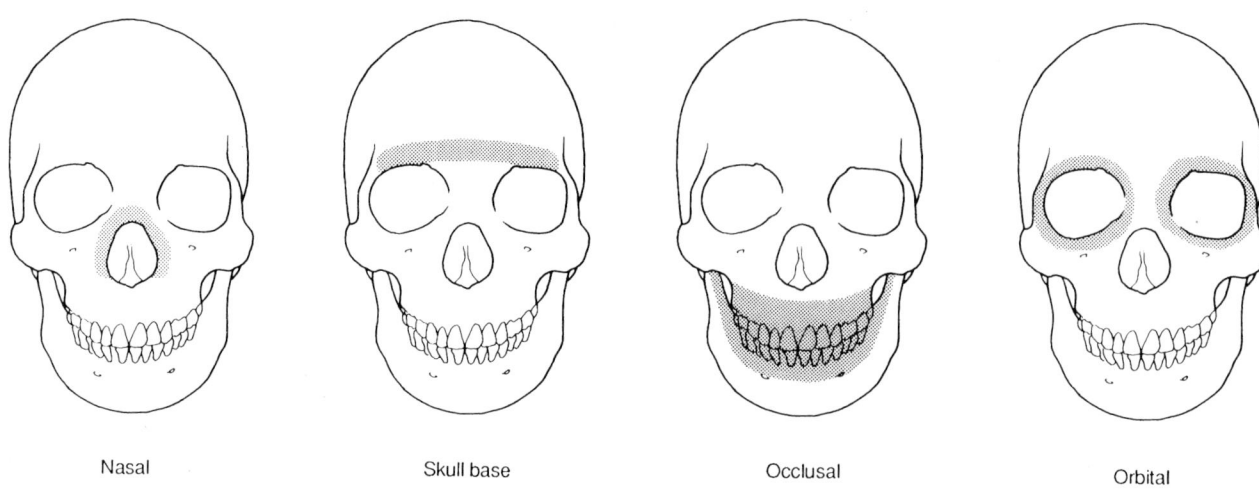

Nasal   Skull base   Occlusal   Orbital

Fig. 11.1 Functional groupings of facial fractures. Shaded areas represent the functional zones of the face. Restoration of these areas in three dimensions following fractures is mandatory for return of normal function and form.

of the anterior cranial fossa are especially important and these are considered in Chapter 13

5. Fractures affecting more than one of the above functional areas — panfacial fractures, fractures involving both the orbit and the occlusion etc.

FRACTURES AFFECTING OCCLUSION

FRACTURES OF THE RAMUS, ANGLE AND BODY OF THE MANDIBLE

Surgical pathology

The anatomy of the mandible has been discussed in Chapter 2. It is a very strong bone (p. 105), designed to withstand the forces applied in mastication, but it has areas of weakness. These include the condylar process, the angle, and the anterior body in relation to the deep root of the canine tooth; the angle is especially weak if there is an unerupted third molar tooth. Fig. 11.2 shows the common fracture sites relating to these points of weakness; these fractures may be unilateral, bilateral or combined in any permutation.

Classification

Mandibular fractures may be classified simply on the anatomical site of the fracture. They may be linear or comminuted; comminution may be slight or very extensive. Fragment size is important: large fragments may lose soft-tissue attachments and then behave as a free graft. The fracture may be displaced or undisplaced, and this is relevant in selecting a treatment strategy: almost always a displaced fracture of angle or body in an adult requires reduction and stabilization for 6 weeks, whereas

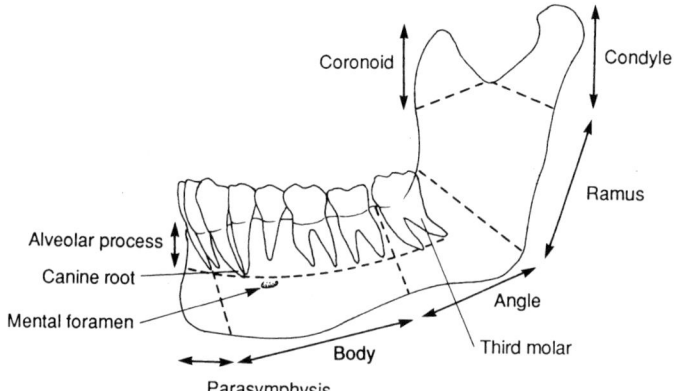

Fig. 11.2 Common fracture sites of mandible. Commonly used descriptive terms for the anatomy of the mandible and the anatomical classification of fractures are also given.

undisplaced fractures of the ramus or condyle are treated conservatively.

The distinction between compound and non-compound mandibular fractures is important. Any displaced fracture through a tooth root is inevitably compound; fractures of the ramus and condylar region are non-compound unless caused by a penetrating agent, e.g. gunshot. The presence or absence of teeth on either side of the fracture line is also important from the viewpoint of treatment by intermaxillary fixation, and this has justified a classification:

Class I: teeth on either side of the fracture line
Class II: teeth on one side only
Class III: edentulous.

Fractures of the young child's mandible and of the edentulous mandible are discussed in Chapter 19. Special problems arise when mandibular fractures are associated with avulsive tissue loss: these are discussed in Chapter 16 and the resultant deformities in Chapter 21. Pathological fractures of the mandible, expressing local or general weakening of the bone by disease, are discussed in Chapter 20.

Clinical assessment

The history points to the likely site of the fracture. Ellis et al (1985) found that the incidence of angle fractures was higher in victims of assault (30.6%) than in those hurt in falls (17.2%) or in road crashes (10.9%); conversely, condylar fractures were less often due to assault: 24.3% as compared with 36.3% in the victims of falls and 34.1% after road crashes. This may reflect a higher incidence of assaults causing lateral jaw impacts, rather than impact on the point of the chin. Interrogation should also establish whether dentures were worn at the time of the accident, and whether there had been any relevant previous disease.

In cases of severe multiple trauma, resuscitation will have priority. But it is of vital importance, even in cases with life-threatening injuries, to make a preliminary assessment by palpating the facial skeleton and to examine the interior of the mouth, with a good light, using cheek retractors where necessary.

When circumstances allow, a more systematic examination of the mandible is carried out (p. 163). The patient and the examiner sit comfortably facing each other. The patient is asked to point to any areas of pain or tenderness, and to run the tongue along the teeth to detect dental irregularities, chipping, loss of a crown; the tongue is very sensitive to these and also to loss of oral sensation. The patient is asked to map out any area of numbness. Swelling and/or bruising are noted and the patient is asked to open the mouth (Fig. 11.3). Chin lacerations may give a clue to a condylar fracture (Fig. 11.4). Intraoral inspection may then be carried out, with special attention to irregularities in the teeth and steps in the dental arch: these may indicate a fracture, as may local swelling, bruising of gingival tissues or laceration of the mucosa (Fig. 11.5).

The patient is next asked to bite the teeth together, and to say whether the occlusion feels normal; the nature of the occlusion is noted. If the patient is edentulous, the dentures are inspected for signs of injury (p. 520).

Finally the mandible is palpated through the overlying soft tissues. Initially the examiner stands behind the seated patient. Bilateral palpation begins over the condylar heads and moves down to the angle and forward along the lower border to the symphysis (Fig. 6.5). Tenderness, swelling and deformity support the diagnosis of a fracture; compression on both angles will usually cause pain in an otherwise occult fracture. Neurological examination may show sensory loss in the lower lip, from damage to

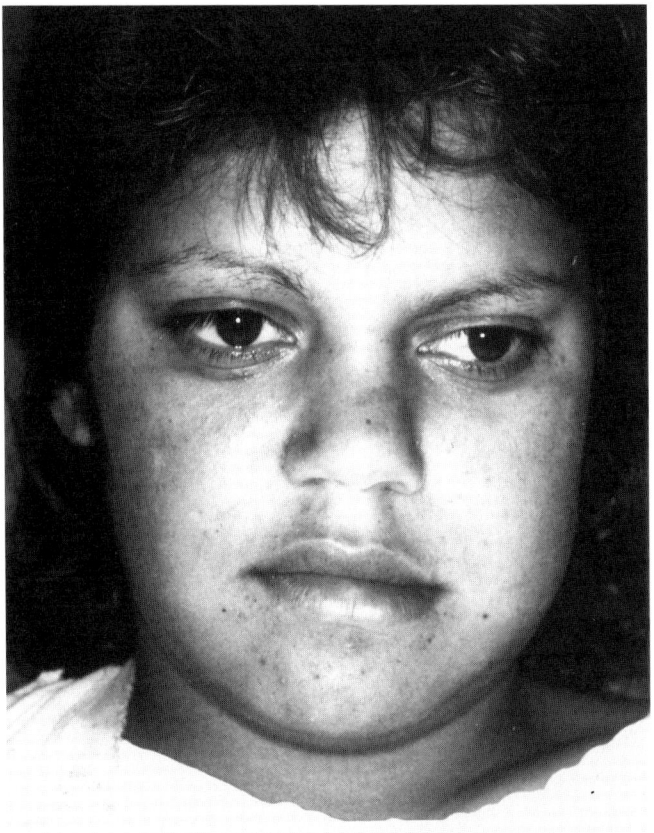

A

B

Fig. 11.3 Clinical signs of mandibular fractures: the angle.
A Minimal swelling of the right cheek seen in a young woman with an undisplaced right angle fracture of the mandible. **B** Bruising of the right masseter and medial pterygoid muscles result in restricted mouth opening on the affected side.

the inferior dental nerve, even in the absence of a complaint of numbness. Finally, intraoral palpation with a gloved finger may be revealing.

Radiological assessment

If the clinical findings suggest that the mandible alone

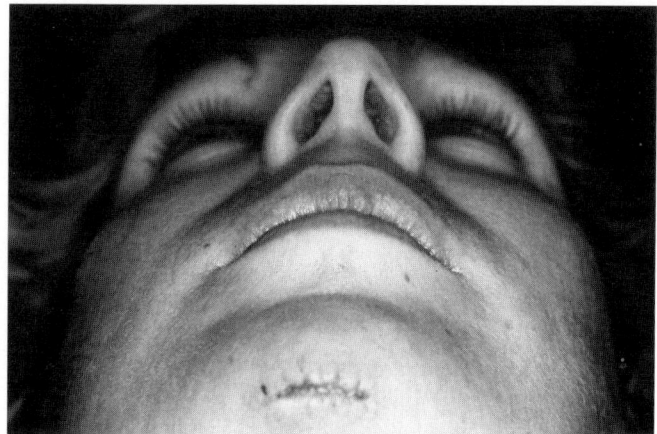

A

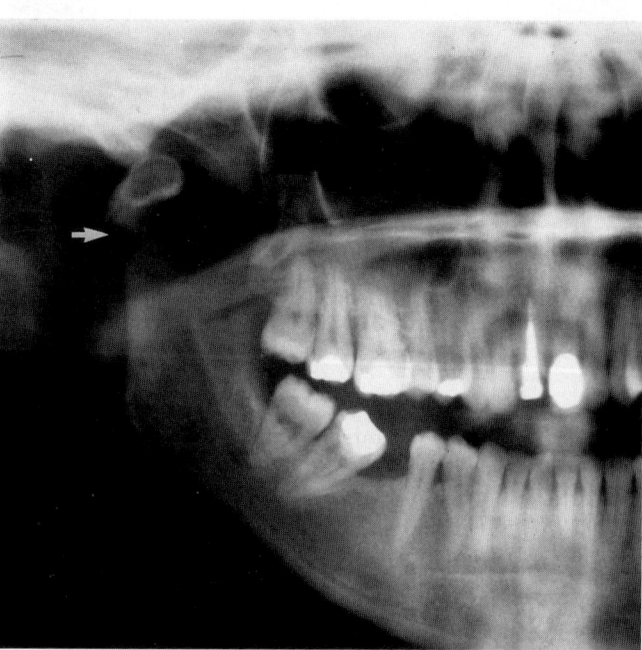

B

Fig. 11.4 Clinical signs of mandibular fractures: the condyle.
A This patient fell from a bicycle onto the point of her chin. The accompanying chin laceration has been sutured. **B** The right condyle fracture associated with this injury (arrow).

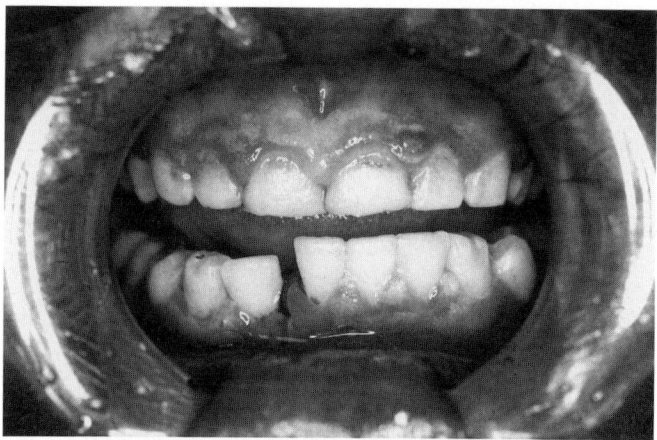

Fig. 11.5 Clinical signs of mandibular fractures: the body.
Separation between right lower central and right lower lateral incisors with a step in the occlusal plane associated with a parasymphyseal fracture of the mandible.

is injured, the X-ray examinations of choice are the orthopantomogram (OPG) and the Towne's anteroposterior view (p. 176). The OPG allows inspection of the entire mandible and mandibular dentition on a single film, being a composite of two lateral views. However, the tomographic process entails blurring in the symphyseal region and fractures here may be missed; moreover, lateral displacement at the angle may not be evident (Fig. 11.6A,B). The Towne's view is a useful complementary examination to demonstrate lateral displacement and fractures at the symphysis.

To obtain an OPG, the patient must sit and this is impossible in severely injured or uncooperative patients.

It may then be necessary to obtain lateral oblique views on each side (Fig. 11.7). A computed tomographic (CT) scan may give useful information on the integrity of the buccal and lingual plates, which are sometimes separated or fractured in isolation (Fig. 11.8).

Early management

Patients with compound mandibular fractures are admitted to hospital and intravenous antibiotics are given: we favour flucloxacillin and metronidazole. The rationale for this choice and the dosages are discussed on p. 236. Pain relief may be needed, but narcotics are if possible withheld, especially if there is a cerebral injury. Clear fluids are allowed and later a liquid diet is given. Oral hygiene is maintained by cleansing the mouth with dressed probes, soft toothbrushes and irrigation with 0.2% chlorhexidine solution.

Dental assessment

This is described in Chapter 12. In dentate patients with a displaced fracture, dental impressions are taken to provide plaster casts of the occlusion in the position resulting from the injury. These casts are then cut at the fracture site and mounted on an articulator in the predicted pretraumatic position so that they can be used as models in planning how to restore the pretraumatic occlusion as accurately as possible. An acrylic wafer is made from the articulated dental model for use in the surgical reduction and fixation of the fracture.

Timing of definitive treatment

This is decided as soon as the clinical priorities of other injuries have been established. Soft-tissue lacerations, if

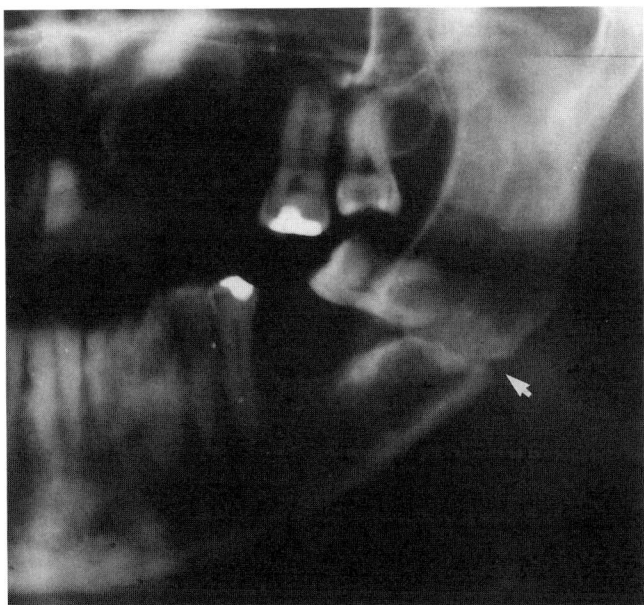

A

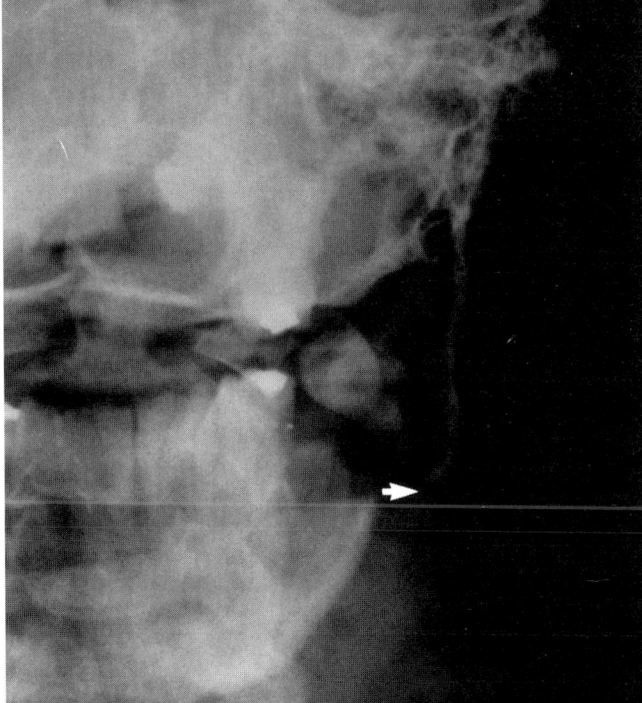

B

Fig. 11.6 Radiology of mandibular fractures: the angle.
A Fracture of the left angle of mandible seen in orthopantomogram
(arrow). Anteroposterior and some superior displacement is seen in this
view. **B** Anteroposterior Townes view of the same fracture demonstrating
more significant lateral displacement not visible in the orthopantomogram.

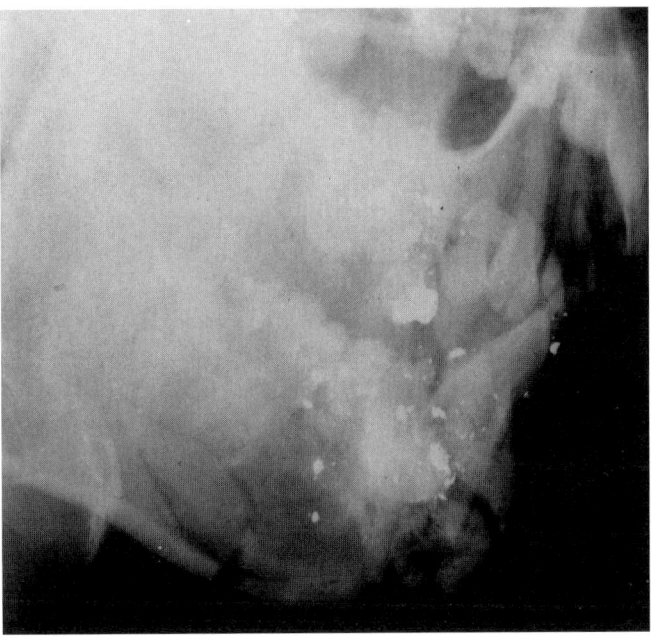

Fig. 11.7 Radiology of mandibular fractures: the body.
Comminuted fracture of the left body of mandible demonstrated on an
oblique lateral X-ray.

significant, are debrided and sutured within 12 h of the
injury (p. 433).

Many authorities favour early surgical reduction and
immobilization of compound fractures of the mandible.
Maloney et al (1991) state that this policy has reduced
postoperative infection from 4% to <1%, and Champy
et al (1986) suggest that fractures should be plated within
12 h of injury for the same reason. We emphasize the
importance of a detailed dental assessment and stabilization of the general condition before operation, and
therefore our procedures are usually done electively rather
than as emergencies, though at times a definitive mandibular operation is done early under a general anaesthetic
needed for some urgent procedure, such as fixation of a
limb fracture. We believe that results are better if operations are done with the best available instruments and
with experienced theatre staff; these may not be provided
by an emergency operating service. In a series of 50 cases
of angle fractures of the mandible treated by delayed
fixation, at an average time of 4 days after injury, we
found only one case of infection (Moore et al 1990).
However, this policy of elective operation after full dental
evaluation requires cost-benefit analysis, and we do not
deny that good results have been achieved by early
intervention.

Conservative management

Stable fractures without displacement are best treated
conservatively, by a liquid non-chew diet and analgesics;
a soft padded neck collar may be worn to support the

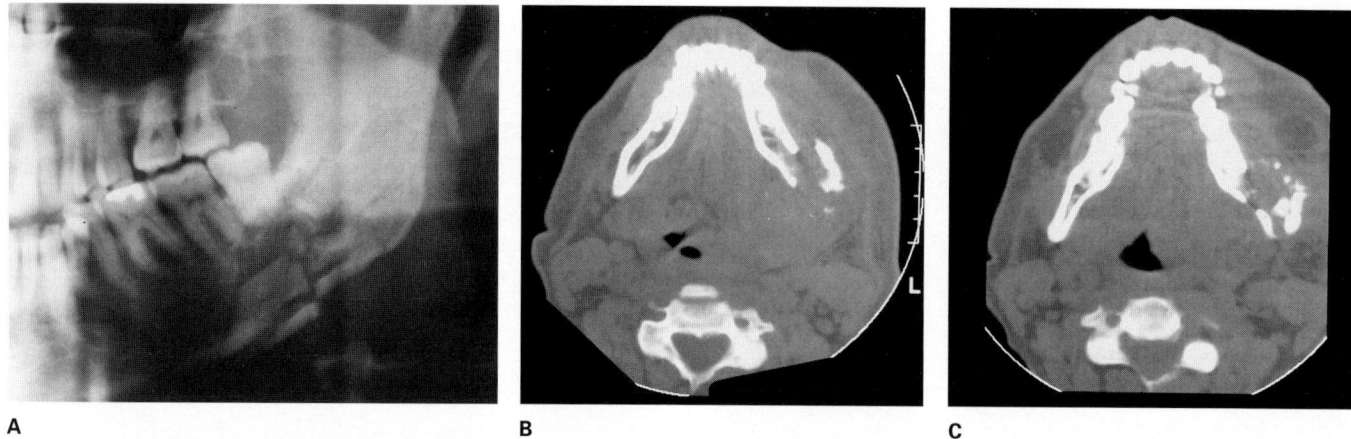

A   B   C

Fig. 11.8 Radiology of mandibular fractures. A Orthopantomogram of a comminuted fracture of the left angle of mandible. In this view it was not possible to tell whether the lingual cortex was intact. **B** CT scan of this patient revealed a displaced fracture of the lingual cortex at the lower border of the mandible. **C** CT scan of the upper border of the mandible in this patient also revealed a fracture of the lingual plate, confirming the need for surgical stabilization of the fracture.

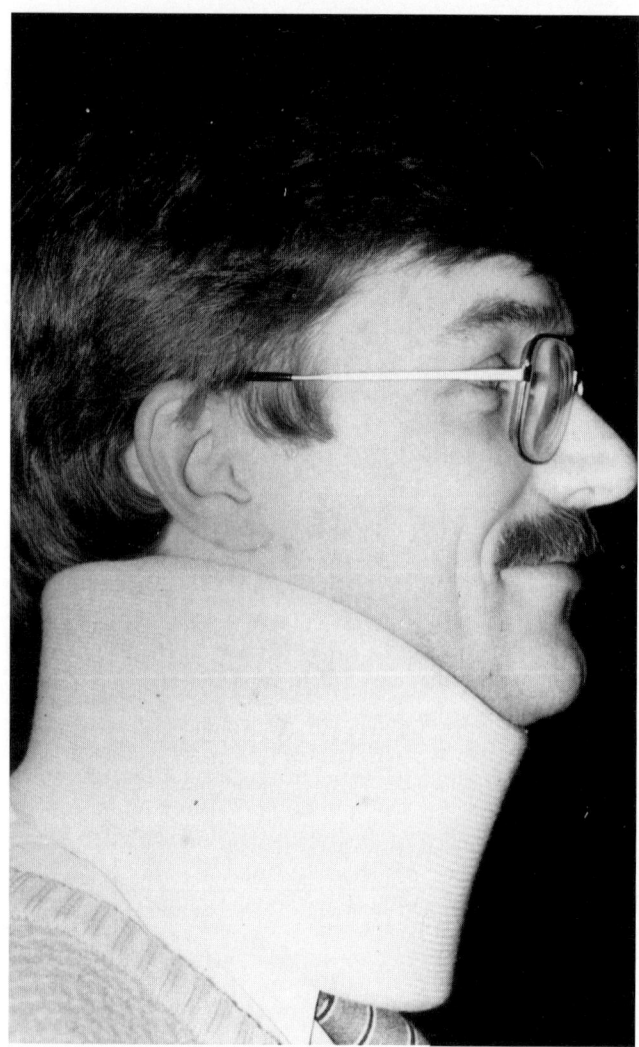

Fig. 11.9 Conservative treatment. A soft, padded (e.g. polyurethane foam) neck collar may be worn to provide symptomatic relief via chin support.

chin (Fig. 11.9). This conservative regimen is appropriate for many unilateral fractures of the angle and body, especially in the elderly edentulous patient, and for the greenstick fractures of children (p. 503). Most ramus fractures are securely splinted by the masseter muscle laterally and the medial pterygoid muscle medially; displacement is rare and these fractures can usually be treated conservatively. In a young adult with an undisplaced hairline fracture of the body or angle which extends to a dental root, decision may be more difficult. If the patient is judged to be sensible and likely to comply with the programme, then conservative treatment should have a good chance of success. If there is doubt about compliance, then operative treatment should be considered.

Principles of operative fixation

Until the advent of internal osteosynthesis with miniplates (pp. 26 and 237), external intermaxillary fixation was the main surgical strategy in the management of mandibular fractures — a strategy of some antiquity (p. 16). But the arguments against closed reduction and intermaxillary fixation are numerous and cogent (Thaller et al 1990).

Closed reduction demands a correct evaluation of the pretraumatic occlusion, and it may be impossible to achieve this if the dentition was incomplete or grossly diseased. Intermaxillary fixation must usually be maintained for 6 weeks, to allow callus to establish a stable secondary union (p. 129), and this is an ordeal for the patient. Hygiene and feeding present problems. There is often buccal and labial irritation and even ulceration of the mucosal surfaces. It is impossible for the tongue to be used to clean the teeth and gums; manual cleaning is made difficult by the presence of wires and the wax often used to reduce their irritative effects. Plaque may build up on the teeth, causing gingivitis with potential long-term dental problems. Liquid diets delivered by syringe are tedious and unappetizing; weight loss is common and sometimes serious. For all these reasons, some patients will not endure intermaxillary fixation: they remove the wires, sometimes with disastrous results. Moreover, the teeth may move or even loosen. When arch bars are applied to premolars and molars, this is unlikely, but it is a real danger if canine or incisor teeth are ligated; if possible, these teeth should not be ligated, and if an arch bar must be supported in the central region, then this should be done by circummandibular and/or transpalatal wiring. Intermaxillary fixation is also a potential airway hazard, especially if there is a risk of sudden loss of consciousness, as in epileptics and diabetics.

Finally, there is experimental evidence to show that prolonged mandibular immobilization causes atrophy of the muscles of mastication, fibrosis of the periarticular connective tissues and degenerative changes in the cartilage of the mandibular condyle; these changes can reduce the range of passive bite opening (Ellis & Carlson 1989). J. O. Andreasen (personal communication) has warned that teeth involved in fractures can be devitalized when ligated to the commonly used Erich bar. Brown et al (1991) compared the costs of managing isolated fractures of the mandible by miniplate osteosynthesis and by intermaxillary fixation. Miniplate fixation was considerably cheaper when account was taken of the duration of hospital stay and the service charges incurred in feeding, dental hygiene and nursing; the complication rates were similar in both series.

We are therefore strong advocates for internal fixation. There is, however, one situation in which intermaxillary fixation is still the treatment of choice. This is in the child with mixed dentition, where a fracture line runs through multiple unerupted tooth buds, with thin bone plates unsuitable for screw fixation. The management of such fractures is discussed in Chapter 19 (p. 504).

Teeth in fracture line

When the fracture goes into a dental root, it has been argued whether it is necessary to extract the tooth to lessen the risk of subsequent infection. This issue was particularly important when the teeth were used in intermaxillary fixation. When miniplate fixation is the primary treatment of choice, the teeth have virtually no role in stabilizing the fracture, but are important as indicators to guide accurate reduction. Our policy has been to retain teeth in the fracture line where these teeth have potential function either in the occlusion or as fixation posts for subsequent prosthodontic work — always assuming that the teeth appear likely to survive. Should the tooth lose vitality, then early restorative dentistry is undertaken

(p. 358). When the tooth root is fractured, with comminution of the alveolar bone around it, then infection is almost certain and the tooth should be extracted, with removal of loose bone fragments. When an impacted third molar is involved in an angle fracture, we extract it because this tooth is rarely a functional part of the occlusion, and because we have seen chronic pain, with or without infection, develop when the tooth is not extracted. However, clinical studies by Rubin et al (1990) have shown that incompletely erupted molars may be left in the fracture line without increasing the risk of complications.

Interosseous wiring

This is indicated when intermaxillary fixation is used as the mainstay of treatment, in fractures with displacement or when there is a tooth on only one side of the fracture (type II fracture: see above). Wiring is used in conjunction with arch bars, interdental eyelet wires and/or dental splints (see below). We see this mode of treatment as inferior to miniplate fixation, but it should be remembered since miniplates may not always be available.

Where a fracture at the angle is to be stabilized, the upper border of the external oblique ridge is the obvious site to insert the wire. Exposure is transoral, allowing extraction of the third molar if it is impacted and not part of the occlusion. Placing a transosseous wire at the upper border of the ridge provides a one-dimensional stabilization against the tensile forces exerted by the muscles of mastication (Fig. 11.10). In other areas of the body of

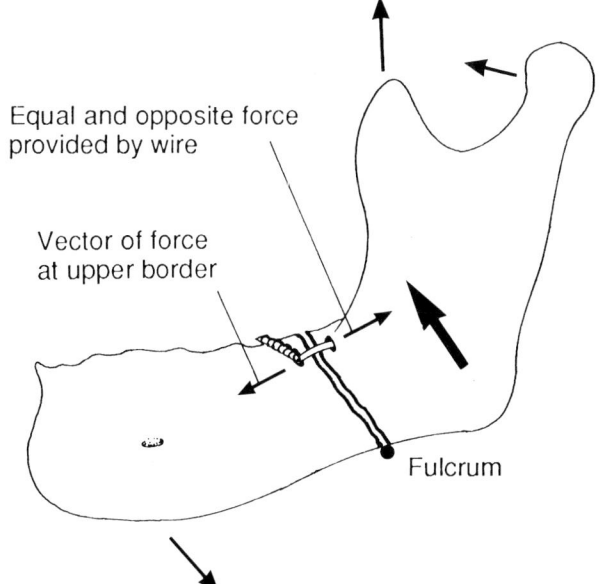

Equal and opposite force provided by wire

Vector of force at upper border

Fulcrum

Fig. 11.10 Interosseous wiring. Placing an interosseous wire at the upper border of an angle fracture counteracts the tensile forces produced by the muscles of mastication (arrows) around the lower border of the fracture which are acting as a fulcrum. In addition to the wire, intermaxillary fixation is required.

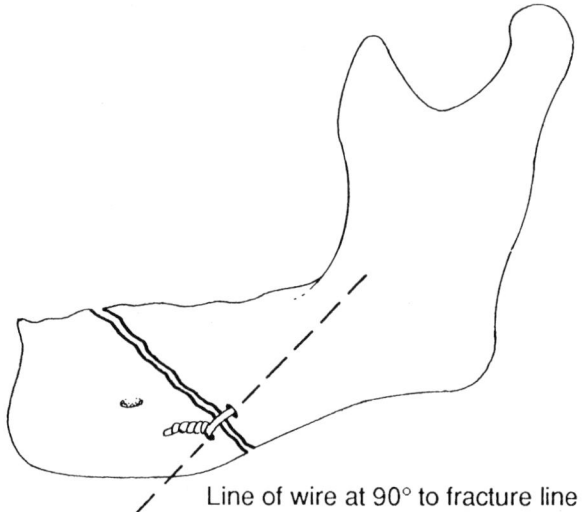

Line of wire at 90° to fracture line

Fig. 11.11 Interosseous wiring. Interosseous wire is placed at 90° to the line of fracture to avoid displacing the fracture along its length as the wire is tightened. In the body area of a dentate mandible, wires must be placed inferiorly to avoid damage to dental roots and the inferior dental nerve.

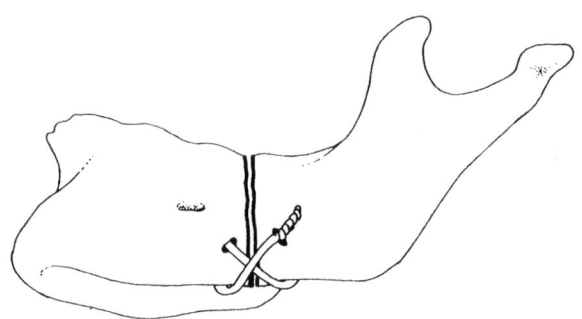

Fig. 11.12 Interosseous wiring. Figure-of-8 technique may provide additional vertical stability at the lower border of the mandible.

the mandible, transosseous wires are placed at the lower border or midbody region. Stabilization is best when the wire crosses the line of the fracture at 90° (Fig. 11.11). When the lower border is exposed, figure-of-eight wiring may be used for greater stability (Fig. 11.12). Alternatively, when the fracture splits the body in the sagittal plane, the wire may be passed through the two plates of bone and then around the lower border of the mandible (Fig. 11.13). After wiring, intermaxillary fixation is maintained for 4–6 weeks.

In edentulous cases, the approach is extraoral, as dental splints will be needed for intermaxillary fixation, again for up to 6 weeks, and the presence of a sutured mucosal incision and the subsequent scar line may impede both the splints and the later use of dentures.

Dental splints

Moulded acrylic dental splints can be stabilized by cir-

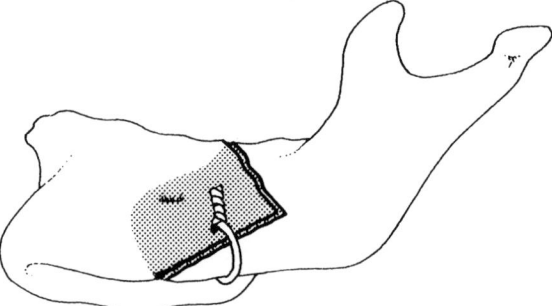

Fig. 11.13 Interosseous wiring. Where the plane of fracture is parasagittal there may be considerable overlap of the lingual and buccal cortical bone plates (shaded area). A 'lag' wire passed across the fracture and across the bony plates will provide a compressive force between the plates, further enhancing stabilization.

cumosseous wires and have been advocated for many purposes. We see two specific clinical indications. The first is in the management of dento-alveolar injuries and extruded teeth. Various types of splints can be etched on to the crowns of teeth and connected to adjacent sound teeth by rods or bars: these are purpose-made appliances, and will promote survival of endangered teeth. The other use for dental splints is in the management of the fractured mandible in very young children: this is discussed on p. 504.

Miniplate osteosynthesis

In 1958, the Swiss Arbeitsgemeinschaft für Osteosynthesefragen formed a study group to consider the principles of internal fixation. This now famous body, the AO/ASIF, showed the value of rigid immobilization and coaption of bone ends in securing primary bone union (p. 129); compression was seen as advantageous, and compression miniplates were designed for use in the craniofacial area. Initially, stainless steel was used, but this metal has some disadvantages, being radio-opaque and also more liable to corrosion than titanium. Luhr of Würzburg developed miniplates and microplates for use in all parts of the CMF region: for the mandible, his system employed compression by bicortical screws, which had to be inserted in the lower border to avoid damage to the inferior dental nerve and to the tooth roots. Luhr used Vitallium, but more recently titanium has been preferred because of its malleability, radiolucency and high biocompatibility (p. 155).

Success in plating fractures of the mandible depends on an understanding of the mechanical forces acting through the mandible in mastication. The mandible is normally subjected to tension forces at its upper border and to compression forces at its lower border. Unless the fracture is inherently self-stabilizing, there will therefore be distraction of the upper or alveolar end of the fracture line. The plating system must counteract this distraction.

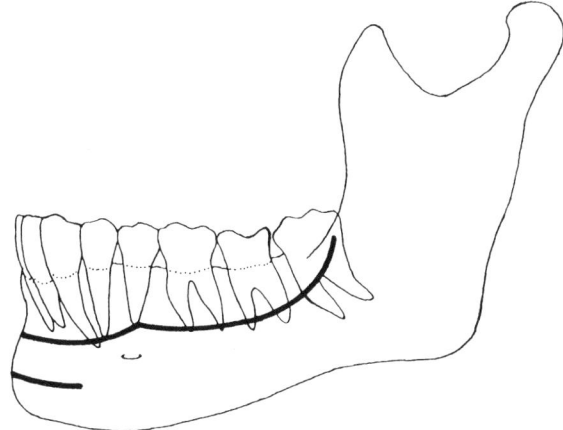

Fig. 11.14 Mandibular tension line. The mandibular tension line is the junction of dento-alveolar and body bone (after Champy).

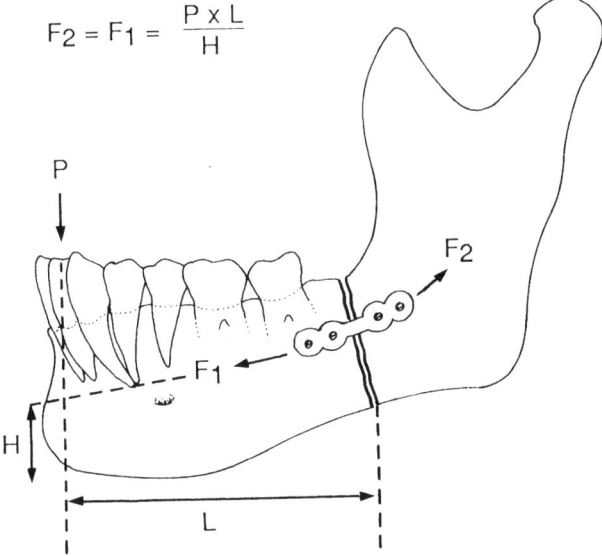

$$F_2 = F_1 = \frac{P \times L}{H}$$

CALCULATION OF MOMENT OF FORCE

P = Applied force

L = Horizontal distance from applied force to fracture

H = Distance from line of plate to lower border

Fig. 11.15 The equation of forces of a mandibular angle fracture (after Champy).

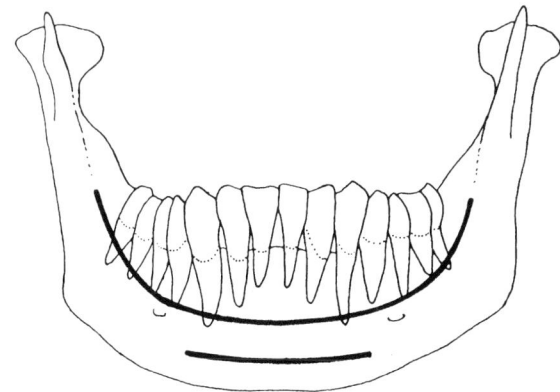

Fig. 11.16 Anterior body reverse-tension line. The anterior lower borderline is the site for lower-border plates in conjunction with upper-border plates when fractures transgress this area (after Champy).

Champy et al (1986), following Michelet et al (1973) of Strasbourg, described an ideal line for the siting of the plate (Fig. 11.14). Where a force F_2 is needed to counteract the distracting force F_1, it will be equal to the downward force in the symphyseal region multiplied by the distance L between the downward force and the fracture itself, and divided by the height H between the point of tension banding and the fulcrum or lower border of the mandible. It can be seen that the greater the value of H, the less force will be needed to control the fracture. It is also clear that the distance L will be greatest in fractures of the angle, and stronger plating will be needed for fractures in this area (Fig. 11.15). Champy also demonstrated the presence of rotational torsion forces in the anterior mandible, which is a three dimensional structure upon which bilateral muscular groups act. He recommended lower border plates as well as upper border plates to give better control of these torsional forces (Fig. 11.16.) In the tooth-bearing alveolar area, the thickness of bone is variable, and unsuitable for screw fixation; the upper border of the mandible is therefore the ideal site. Champy showed that the average thickness of the outer cortex of the mandible is 5 mm, but in some areas the cortex is < 3 mm thick: there is therefore some danger of injuring the inferior dental nerve (Fig. 2.6). Care should therefore be taken to drill only through the outer cortex, and to use only 5 mm screws.

In certain situations, the usual tension–compression relations can be reversed. This may be the case when a bite load is placed just anterior to an angle fracture, and the contralateral muscle sling is functioning normally but the ipsilateral sling is ineffective from traumatic oedema and bruising (Rudderman & Mullen 1992). In addition to this theoretical concept of intermittent reversal of the normal tension–compression zones, there is also some clinical evidence of unfavourable results with angle fractures treated by a single plate sited in Champy's ideal osteosynthesis line. Levy et al (1991) recently reported on 61 patients with 63 angle fractures, treated according to Champy's principle of monocortical non-compression. When only one plate was used for osteosynthesis at the mandibular angle, complications were seen in 5/19 patients; when two miniplates were used, only one of 32 patients experienced complications. Although Levy and co-authors do not state exactly where the second plate was placed, one of their illustrations shows the second plate to be close to the lower border of the mandible and

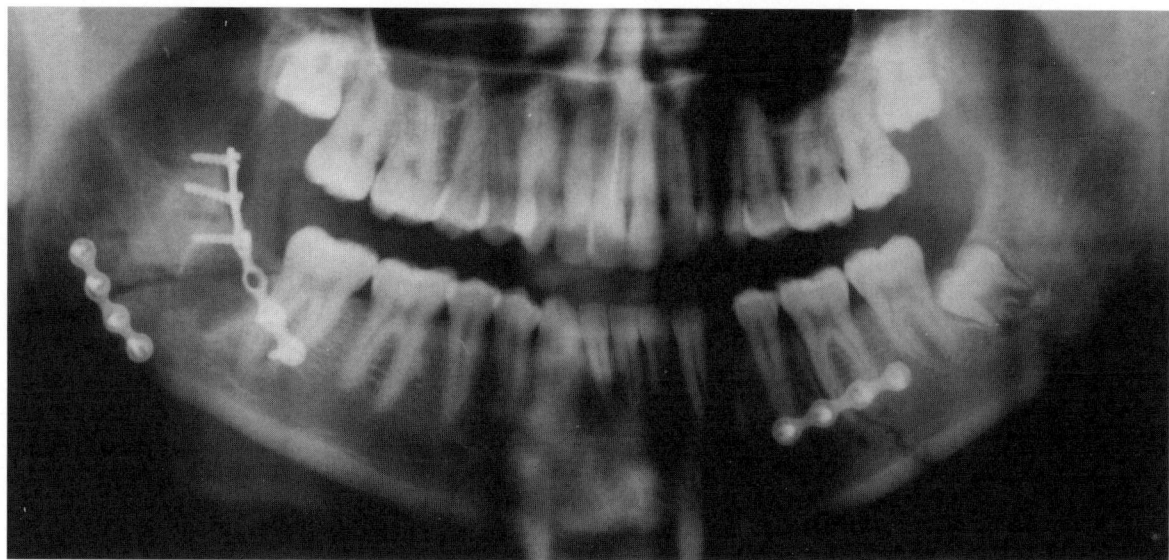

Fig. 11.17 Miniplating mandibular fractures. Orthopantomogram following miniplate stabilization of fractured left body and right angle of mandible. Difficulty was found in obtaining accurate reduction of the inferior part of the fracture at the angle via an intraoral exposure. Accordingly an external submandibular approach was made following application of the upper-border miniplate and screws. The lower border was reduced under direct vision and stabilized with a 4-hole miniplate and screws as shown.

therefore able to act as a compression band against the intermittent reversal of tension–compression zones (see above).

Our experience with 50 cases of mandibular angle fractures treated according to Champy's principles with single upper-border non-compression plates has been satisfactory, with only one adverse result due to infection (Moore et al 1990). However, there are two clinical situations in which an additional lower-border plate is needed. First, the accuracy of reduction of an angle fracture by the intraoral route may be uncertain, because the lower border of the mandible cannot be seen. It may then be necessary to expose this area by an external incision and to achieve accurate reduction and fixation with a second miniplate to reinforce the plate inserted by the intraoral route (Fig. 11.17). Second, if it is uncertain whether the patient will obey the injunction not to chew, it may be wise to insert a second plate.

In summary, the Champy technique of upper-border single-plate osteosynthesis will be successful in most cases of angle fractures, provided that the patient does not chew and the reduction is accurate. Failure in these respects may lead to an unusual bite force, reversal of the normal tension–compression zones, and movement at the fracture site, with greater risk of infection. In muscular male adults with angle fractures, the mechanical considerations summarized above mean that a greater banding force may be needed: this may justify the use of 6-hole plates rather than the usual 4-hole plates, and longer screws may be inserted in the proximal fragment (Fig. 11.18).

Supplementary intermaxillary fixation remains as a resort when internal fixation seems likely to be insufficient alone.

Compression plates

As stated, these require bicortical screws, and must therefore be inserted into the lower border of the mandible; to control the upper-border tension zone, the plates must be strong and rigid, and the screws must be large. A modified form of compression plate has been designed for mandibular fractures, in which the outer plate holes provide compression at the inferior border, while the inner holes of the plate provide a downward movement of the fracture to counteract the distracting tension at the upper border (Hobar 1992).

The merits of compression and non-compression plates remain under debate. Compression plates increase bone contact at the fracture site, and provide rigid stabilization; this promotes primary bone union with no callus formation. However, in practice it appears that healing is equally good with non-compression systems, despite the transient appearance of callus. Compression plating systems have one potential drawback: as compression is applied across the buccal plate of bone, there is a potential risk that the fracture line may be opened on the lingual side. A small difference in reduction between lingual and buccal or labial bone can lead to a significant crossbite and potentially to a post-traumatic malocclusion. To prevent this, the flexible miniplates must be shaped to conform to the bone surface accurately: if anything, they

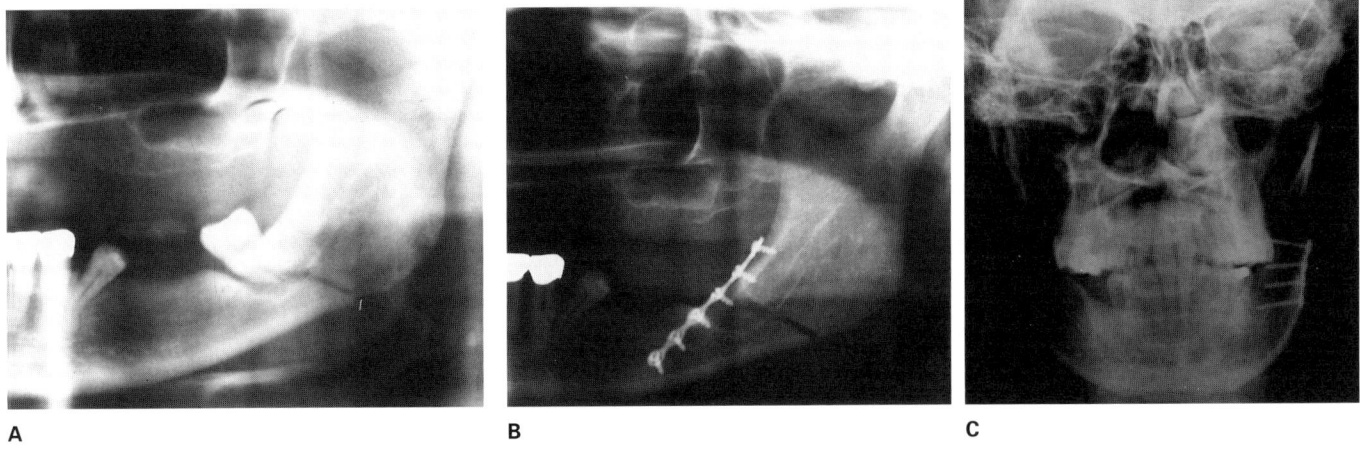

Fig. 11.18 Miniplating mandibular fractures. A Left angle fracture in a patient who was believed to be unreliable in complying with dietary restrictions. **B** Stabilization of fracture with 6-hole plate and screws for greater banding force. **C** 13 mm screws may give greater purchase via bicortical fixation.

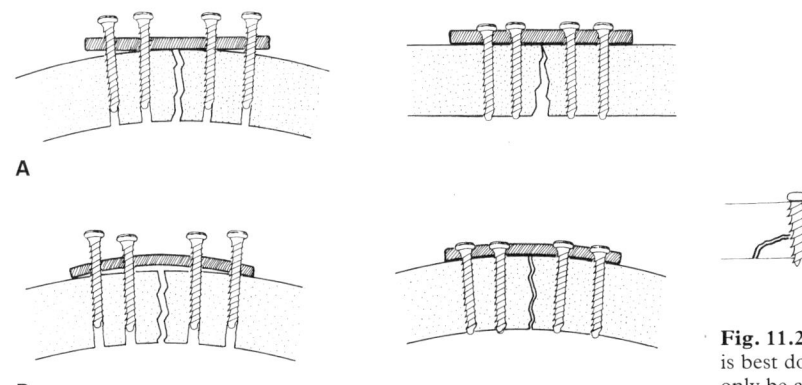

Fig. 11.19 Compression plating mandibular fractures. A Where compression plate does not exactly conform to the curvature of the underlying bone, compression will result in opening of the lingual cortex fracture line. **B** To prevent this, the plate must be exactly shaped to the curve of the underlying buccal cortex or even slightly overcurved.

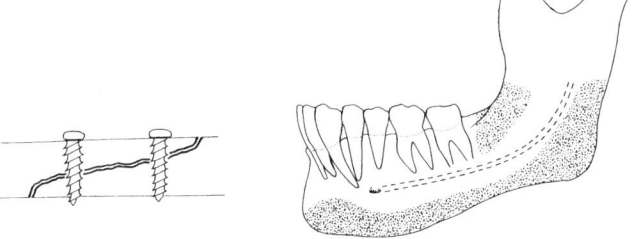

Fig. 11.20 Lag screwing mandibular fractures. Lag screw fixation is best done where there is overlap of cortical bone plates. Screws can only be applied in areas where damage to dental roots or the inferior dental nerve will not ensue (shaded).

should be overcurved, so that compression will affect both buccal and lingual surfaces equally (Fig. 11.19; Calloway et al 1992).

Lag screws

The principle of lag screwing is to overdrill the hole made in the outer plate of bone, so that the screw will engage only in the smaller hole in the inner cortex; when the screw is tightened, there will be compression between the outer and inner plates. For maximum compression, the axis of the screw must be close to 90° to the plane of the fracture, without displacing or distracting the fragments.

When a fracture shears between the lingual and buccal plates, the wide surfaces of opposed cortical bone offer ideal conditions for lag screw fixation, though this must be done where there is no risk of injuring the inferior dental nerve or dental roots (Fig. 11.20). The fragments to be screwed must not be comminuted.

When the fracture is behind the last tooth, screws can be inserted in the upper border. Niederdellman & Shetty (1987) have proposed a method of lag screw fixation of angle fractures, and report good results; Ellis & Ghali (1991) also report favourably on lag screw fixation for anterior mandibular fractures. This method may be technically demanding, and requires a good deal of practice and competence to give consistent results.

Operative management (Champy technique)

Operation is done under general anaesthesia; a nasotracheal tube is passed and sutured to the base of the nostril (Fig. 10.1). The incision sites are infiltrated with 2% lignocaine and 1/80 000 adrenaline. Schuchardt or Erich arch bars are ligated to the premolar and first molar teeth with 26 gauge stainless steel wire; if a centre of support is needed for the arch bars in the incisor–canine region, the bars are anchored with circummandibular or transpalatal wires as described above. The teeth are cleaned with a toothbrush and dilute (half-strength) Betadine solution. Irreparably damaged teeth or dental roots are extracted.

The operator may use a headlight to give good illumination when working in the angle area. The incision to explore an angle fracture is placed just lateral to the anterior border of the ramus, and runs down beyond the third molar just lateral to the inferior buccal sulcus. With scalpel or cutting diathermy, the incision is deepened to the bone and the fracture line is then exposed by subperiosteal dissection down to the inferior border of the mandible. A posterior border retractor, combined with a notched anterior border retractor, will give good retraction of the soft tissues. If the third molar is to be extracted, this is now done, care being taken not to fracture the external oblique ridge of bone. The socket is cleaned and irrigated; care is taken not to injure the inferior dental nerve, which is sometimes exposed by the fracture. The fracture edges are cleared of granulation tissue with a small sharp angled dissector, and the area is irrigated with weak antibiotic solution (e.g. 0.2 % flucloxacillin in saline) to wash away debris and reduce contamination. The fracture is now reduced manually into correct anatomical position.

The incision to explore a fracture of the body is placed to the buccal or the labial side of the inferior sulcus. To preserve the mental nerve, the scalpel is angled back sharply, under this sulcus, down to the bone. The periosteum is incised; the fracture is then exposed by subperiosteal dissection in the manner described above. If the fracture is laterally placed, the mental nerve and its foramen may also be exposed (Fig. 11.21).

When the fracture has been manually reduced, the occlusion is established and intermaxillary fixation is applied. The pretraumatic position of occlusion is established by the dental wafer and the plaster study models; however, on very rare occasions, even with the occlusion stabilised by the wafer, anatomical reduction is not achieved. When this is so, and assuming that there is no other fracture, then there must have been some error in model planning and wafer construction; the operative impression of anatomical reduction must therefore be accepted.

When the jaws are thus secured by intermaxillary wiring, and the fracture(s) reduced anatomically, it is relatively easy to achieve fixation with a miniplate applied in accord with Champy's principles. We apply a 4-hole AusSystem® plate to the upper border of the body, placing two monocortical 5 mm screws on either side of the fracture line; a similar plate is applied to the lower border in anterior body fractures. At the upper level of the body, where it joins with the alveolar bone, care is taken to

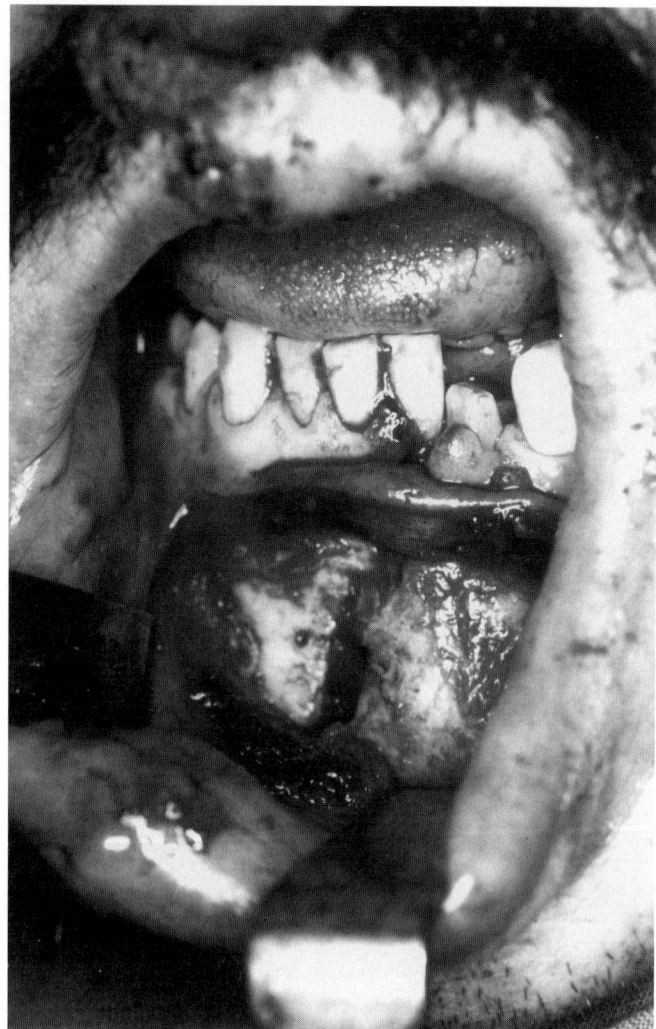

Fig. 11.21 Intraoral exposure. Inferior labial sulcus incision to expose a parasymphyseal fracture of the mandible. Care is taken to protect the fibres of the mental nerve as they traverse the muscle of the lower lip.

drill only the outer cortex, the drill being kept at 90° to the surface; copious irrigation is used. The plates are bent as accurately as possible to conform with the contours of the mandible; however, this is less important when using these malleable titanium plates than when steel or vitallium compression systems are employed (Figs 11.22 and 21.23).

Modifications in this standard method may be appropriate in fractures in the angle area, on the external oblique ridge. A 6-hole plate may be preferred, and longer screws may be used in the ramus, to give better purchase in the bone (Fig. 11.18). If a second lower-border plate is needed for an angle fracture, it may be attached by an intraoral approach combined with percutaneous drilling and screwing through a cannula. But if there is doubt about the reduction of the inferior border, there need be no reluctance to expose the area by an external incision. This is made about 1 cm below the inferior border of the

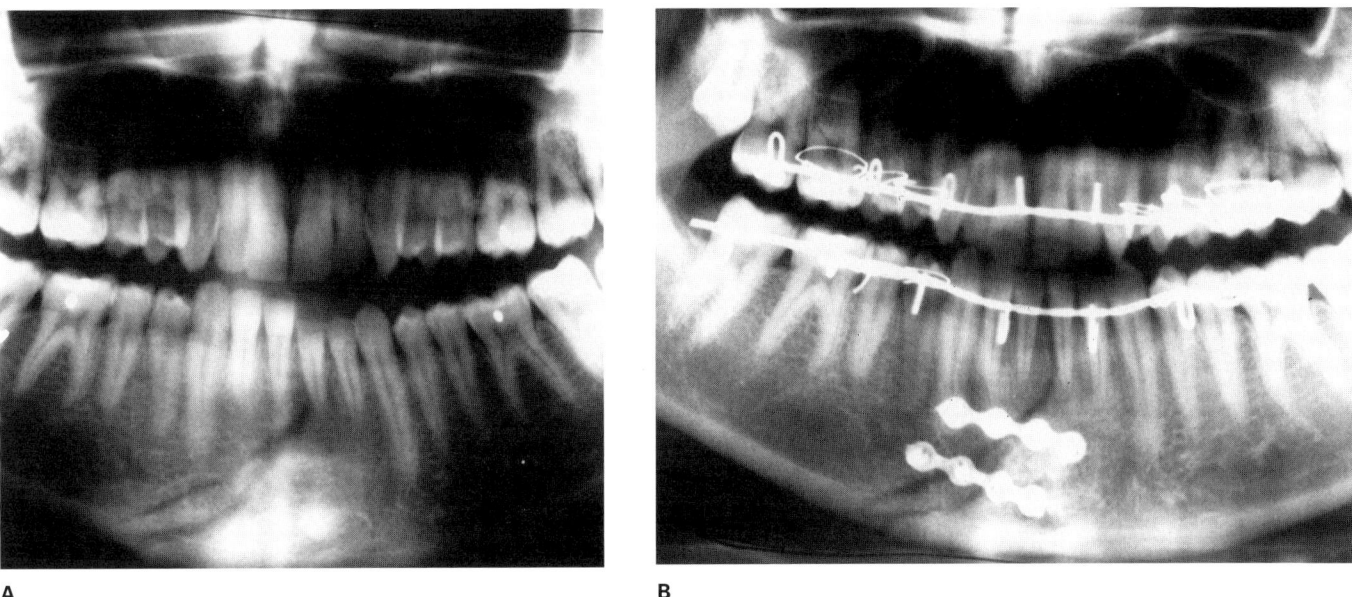

A   B

Fig. 11.22 Miniplating mandibular fractures: parasymphyseal. A and **B** X-rays pre- and post-surgical treatment of a parasymphyseal mandibular fracture using 4-hole miniplates applied in accordance with Champy's principles.

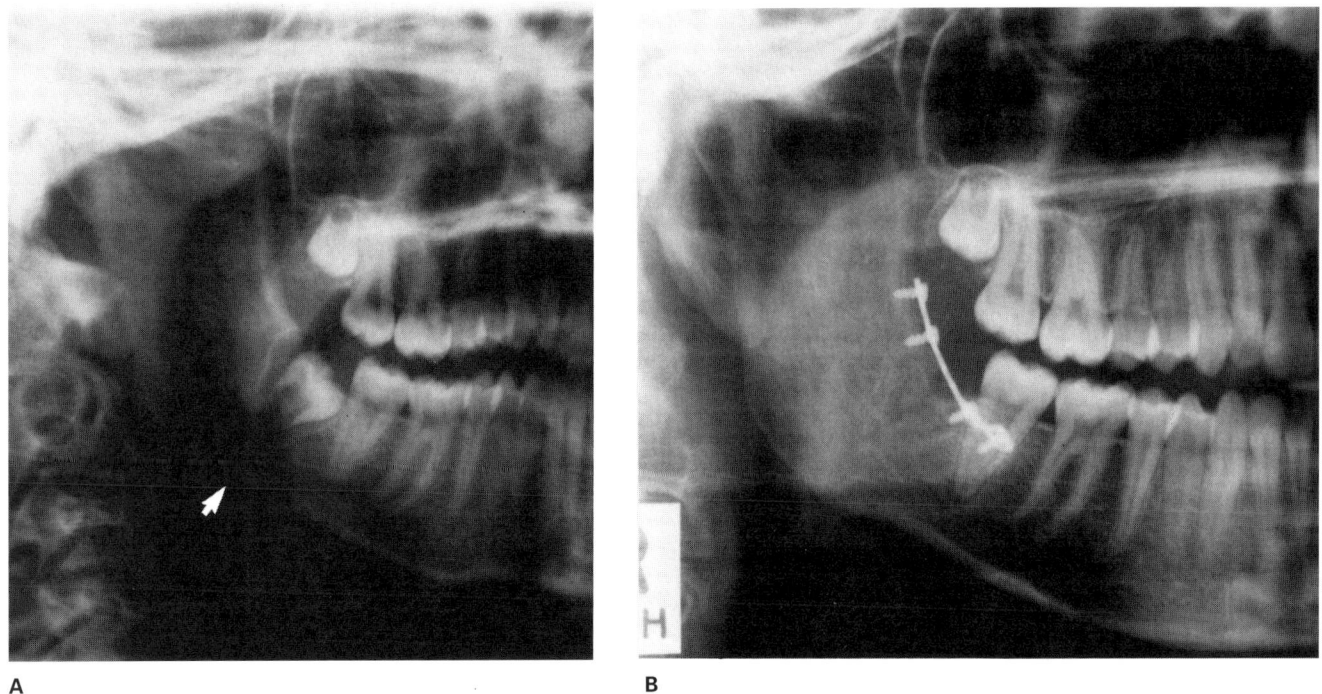

A   B

Fig. 11.23 Miniplating mandibular fractures: angle. A and **B.** X-rays pre- and post-treatment of a mandibular angle fracture using a contoured miniplate with four screws in accordance with Champy's principles. In this case the post-treatment X-ray was taken after 6 months and no sign of fracture was seen.

mandible, below the course of the mandibular ramus of the facial nerve (Fig. 2.30). The incision is usually about 3–5 cm long, and is deepened through fat and platysma to the fascia of the submandibular gland (Fig. 9.4C). This is incised, and the dissection is then taken upwards, so that the mandibular branch of the facial nerve remains in a superficial plane and need not be identified. Large branches of the facial artery and vein will be encountered running over the top of the submandibular gland, and these should be ligated and cut. Sharp dissection through the masseter and the periosteum will then expose the fracture site. Since there is already stabilization by a miniplate at the upper border, the fracture edges can easily be manipulated into anatomical reduction and fixed by a 4-hole non-compression plate (Fig. 11.17). The skin wound is then irrigated with antibiotic solution and closed in two layers, drainage being used only if there is much oozing. When it is not necessary to visualize the lower border of the mandible, the plate can be fixed to the lower border percutaneously by drilling and screwing through a cannula.

Intraoral wounds are closed with a running 3/0 chromicized catgut stitch, taking bites of mucosa and muscle. The temporary intermaxillary fixation is then removed and the excursions of the mandible are checked, with special attention to its ability to bite into occlusion. The arch bars are usually left in situ; if the patient readily settles into normal occlusion, the bars are removed on the second or third day, but if this does not happen then the bars can be used to allow light rubber elastic traction to help to overcome the imbalance in the masticatory muscles caused by injury and swelling. This elastic traction may be maintained for 7 days, being removed when the patient settles into normal occlusion.

Postoperative management includes intravenous antibiotics for 48 h. Clear fluids are given for 12–24 h, then a liquid or non-chew diet. Oral hygiene is maintained with mouth washes and small tooth brushes; this becomes easier when the arch bars are removed. Pain relief is rarely needed after 48 h. X-ray pictures (OPG and Towne's view) are obtained on the first day after operation. If these are satisfactory, and if mandibular mobilization is going well, the patient is discharged, usually after 2 or 3 days. External stitches are removed 1 week after operation, when oral hygiene and mobilization of the jaw are checked. There are normally further reviews at 3 and 6 weeks, after which there should be a 4 cm opening between the incisor teeth and little local swelling. A dental assessment is then made, with special attention to oral hygiene and occlusion, as well as estimation of the viability of teeth in the fracture line. A non-chew diet is taken for 6 weeks; thereafter a normal diet is allowed. Between 6 weeks and 12 months, the patient is seen if there are clinical reasons; the healing of scars, the recovery of any areas of sensory loss and the return of normal mastication are verified. Restorative dentistry is sometimes needed.

COMMINUTED MANDIBULAR BODY FRACTURES

Management

When there is a moderate degree of comminution and little or no bone loss, as is sometimes seen after wounds from small bore weapons, the fractures may be treated by the regimen just described, with some modifications.

Debridement is performed first, small fragments of

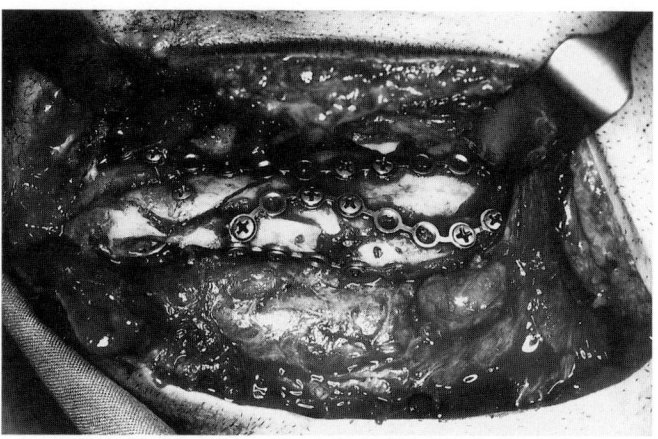

Fig. 11.24 Miniplating and lag screwing mandibular fractures. Use of multiple plates and screws to stabilize the comminuted left body fracture seen in Fig. 11.7. This was combined with intermaxillary fixation for 6 weeks.

bone being removed. If the alveolus is comminuted, the shattered bone and associated teeth, and any blood clot, are removed, and the injured area is irrigated with weak antibiotic solution.

The mandible is then stabilized. After manual reduction, the teeth are held in occlusion by intermaxillary fixation with arch bars and the wafer. It may then be appropriate to stabilize the bone fragments by inserting upper and lower border plates, with at least two screws gripping the chief proximal and distal bone fragments. If there is insufficient bone to hold an upper-border plate, then it may be best to use a Luhr type of compression plate, with bicortical screws on the lower border. Where there is doubt about the reduction of the lower border, it may be wise to expose the area by an extraoral approach. If the stability of the fixation given by the miniplates is in doubt, the intermaxillary fixation should be maintained for 4–6 weeks (Fig. 11.24).

Complications of fractures of the body and angle of the mandible

These include:

- Infection
- Non-union
- Malocclusion and malunion
- Plate exposure
- Nerve injury and/or dental injury due to drilling the body of the mandible.

Infection

The incidence varies in different reports and the causes are disputed. Bochlogyrus (1985) reported abscess, cellulitis or osteomyelitis in 61 of 853 patients (7%); various methods of reduction and fixation were used, but it

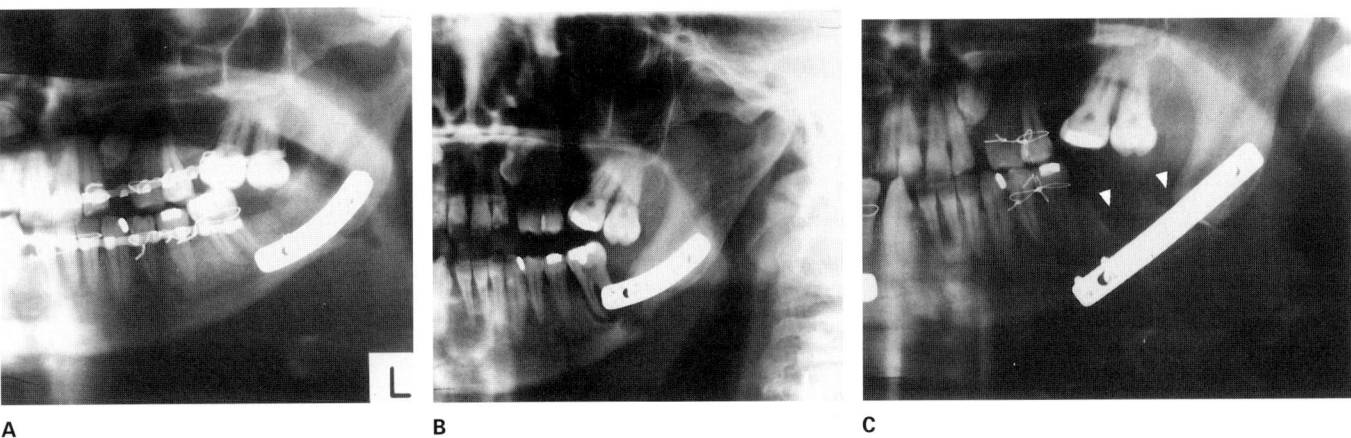

Fig. 11.25 Management of an infected angle fracture. A A fracture of the left angle of mandible following an assault to a 29-year-old male. The fracture was treated using a heavy lower-border compression plate and bicortical screws. **B** After 18 months lost to follow-up, the patient returned with clinical signs of infection and non-union. The orthopantomogram showed non-union and loss of bone around first molar. **C** Following debridement of necrotic bone and the first molar tooth, intermaxillary fixation, iliac bone grafting to the gap and stabilization with heavy lower border compression plate using eight bicortical screws, he went on to uneventful healing. The bone graft is located between the arrow heads.

appeared that the incidence of infection was not significantly greater after open operations. Moore et al (1985) found an incidence of 16% in a study of 100 fractures in 56 patients, with osteomyelitis in 3%. Maloney et al (1991) found no infections at all when the fractures were reduced by the closed technique and immobilized within 72 h of injury; open reduction within 72 h had an infection rate of 2%. Iizuka et al (1991a) reported infections in 6% of patients stabilized with compression plates, all save one being fractures at the angle. Champy et al (1986) reported an incidence of 3% in cases treated by his principles; he urged treatment within 12 h of injury. Anderson & Alpert (1992) reported the high incidence of 16% infection in 75 plated fractures; however, there was only one case of frank osteomyelitis, and the authors believed that preventable errors in technique were often responsible. Levy et al (1991) gave special attention to fractures of the mandibular angle: when only one miniplate was used, without intermaxillary fixation, the infection rate was 22%, but when two miniplates were used, no infections were seen. In our report on 50 fractures at the angle (Moore et al 1990) only one infection was seen.

When infection is diagnosed, a wound culture is taken and intravenous flucloxacillin and metronidazole are at once given. X-ray pictures of the mandible are taken, to exclude fracture displacement, bone sequestrum or any complication relating to the plate, such as fracture or dislodgement. If there is non-union and/or osteomyelitis, the fracture is explored and necrotic material is excised, together with loose fragments of bone. Teeth in the fracture line are extracted and all plates and screws are removed. The occlusion is then established and intermaxillary fixation is reinstituted. If there is bony contact at the fracture site, a heavy mandibular compression plate is immediately inserted on the lower border of the man-

dible, with 4–6 bicortical screws. If there is discontinuity of bone, a bone graft is inserted; intermaxillary fixation is maintained for 6 weeks (Fig. 11.25A–C). With rigid fixation and adequate drainage, osteomyelitis usually subsides (Koury & Ellis 1992).

Non-union

This is clinically indistinguishable from infection, and in principle the treatment is the same.

Malocclusion and malunion

These can result from inadequate or inappropriate reduction of the fracture, but may also be the consequence of orthodontic movement of teeth which have been wired to arch bars, or the result of imbalance of masticatory muscles. Unilateral muscle injury forces the mandible into the position of greatest comfort, which may entail crossbite or overbite even when the reduction is anatomically correct. If this is the case, the malocclusion can be managed by appropriate dental methods — or more simply by rest and patience, since the complaint usually subsides with time. If the cause of malocclusion is shown by X-ray to be due to inadequate reduction of the fracture, two possibilities arise. First, the operative procedure may have been at fault: malunion from this cause should be detected by postoperative X-ray examination (Fig. 11.26A,B). Second, the patient may have been at fault, in failing to comply with the dietary programme: chewing on solid food may have fractured the plate itself, or fractured the bone around the screws. Reoperation is necessary in either case, to reduce the fracture again and to fix it more strongly. If the bone has already united — malunion in the true sense — an osteotomy will be

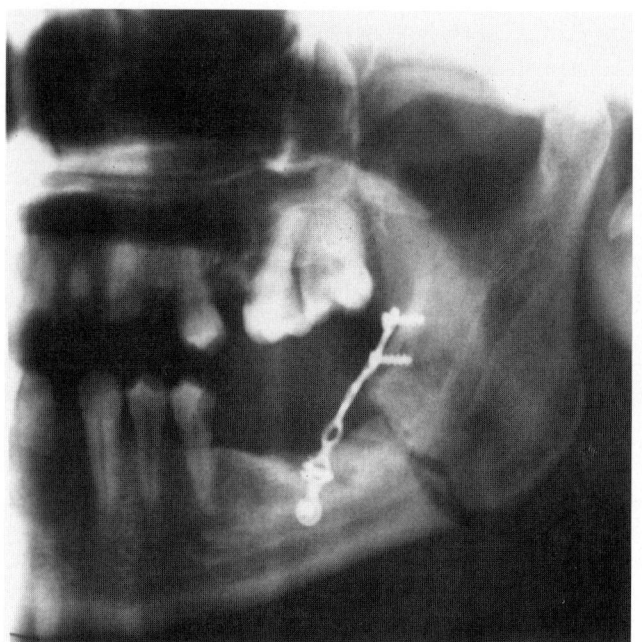
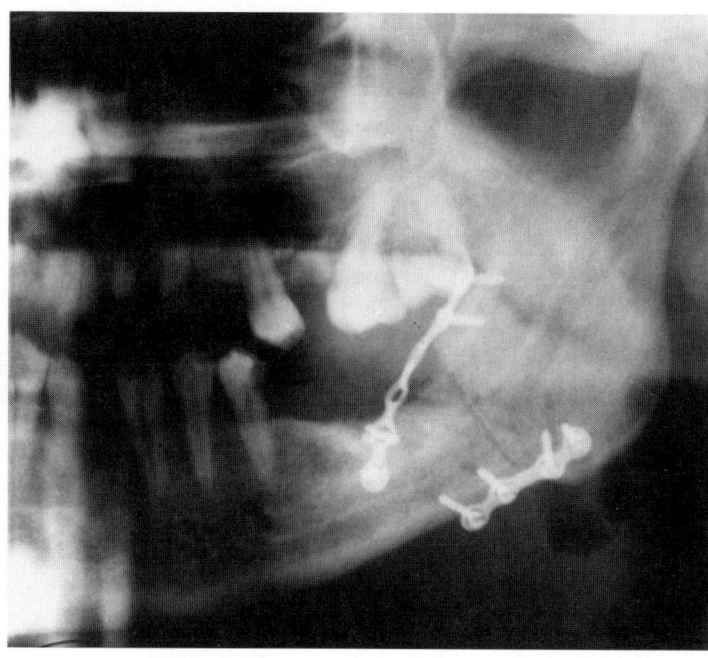

A   **B**

Fig. 11.26 Faulty operative reduction. A A left angle fracture of the mandible, inadequately reduced. This mistake was revealed in the X-ray pictures taken immediately after surgery. **B** The fracture was re-explored via an external submandibular incision. This enabled satisfactory reduction with added stabilization using a lower border miniplate.

needed to give correct occlusion; this is usually done at the level of the angle or through the body with preservation of the neurovascular bundle. The corrected occlusion is maintained by intermaxillary fixation, with either lag screws or plates to stabilize the reduction.

Plate exposure

Miniplate exposure may be due to poor operative technique in suturing the mucosa or to postoperative trauma, as from excessive zeal in using a tooth brush before the mucosa is fully healed. If there are no other problems, it is safe to leave the plate exposed until healing is complete, in 6 weeks, after which the plate can be removed without compromising the result.

Nerve injury and/or dental injury due to drilling the body of the mandible

Injuries of the inferior dental nerve, dental roots and/or tooth buds may occur when an inexperienced operator drills the outer cortex, or from the use of unduly long screws. If there is clinical and X-ray evidence that a screw is impinging on any of the listed structures, then the screw, or screws, should come out at once. It will then be necessary to follow the patient's progress for signs of loss of tooth vitality, failure of teeth to erupt, or sensory loss in the mental nerve territory. Sensory recovery, or failure of recovery, should be watched for over 12–18 months.

DENTOALVEOLAR FRACTURES

Surgical pathology

These may occur in isolation, either when a segment of two or more teeth is displaced en bloc, or as an area of gross comminution.

Management

When the displaced fragment of bone and teeth retains a good mucosal attachment on the lingual side, it can be preserved. The displacement is reduced, the mucosal laceration is repaired if necessary, and the reduction is stabilized: this is done by etching pillars on to the crowns of both the involved and the adjacent unaffected teeth, to which an acrylic rod or bar is then fixed (Fig. 11.27). But when there is gross comminution, it is best to remove the teeth and shattered bone and to suture the mucosa over the area of denuded bone.

FRACTURES OF THE CORONOID PROCESS

Surgical pathology

The coronoid process is a thin plate of bone, serving as the insertion of the temporalis muscle onto the ramus: as such, it is stressed to withstand vertical tension but not force applied to its lateral aspect. The process is therefore most vulnerable to a lateral impact when the mouth is open; it may also be injured by sudden contraction of

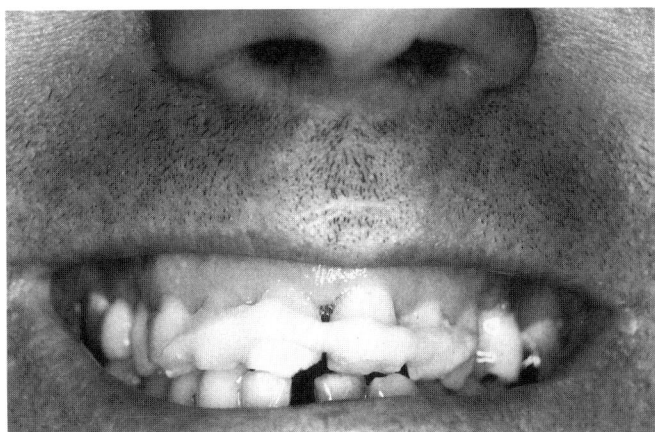

Fig. 11.27 Stabilization of dento-aleolar fractures. An acrylic rod is etched onto the crowns of upper central teeth to stabilize a dento-alveolar fracture.

the temporalis muscle at the time of an impact, or by a penetrating agent. Nevertheless, solitary fractures of the coronoid process are unusual, because the process is well protected by the temporalis and masseter muscles and by the zygomatic arch. In our retrospective review of facial fractures treated over a 3 year period (p. 87), there was only one coronoid fracture among 324 cases of mandibular fracture — an incidence of 0.3%. Rapidis et al (1985) found that coronoid process fractures accounted for 0.6–4.7% of all facial fractures in several reported series reviewed by them. In an analysis of 52 cases of coronoid fractures, they found fractures in other parts of the facial skeleton in 77%; in 44% there were fractures elsewhere in the mandible, these being evenly distributed between symphysis, body, angle and condyle, and in 19% there was an associated fracture of the zygoma, while in only 4% were there fractures of the maxilla.

Clinical assessment

The signs may include trismus and crossbite due to injury of the ipsilateral masticatory muscles; there may be intraoral swelling and bruising in the upper retromolar region. However, these signs may be masked by the effects of associated injuries.

Radiological assessment

The fracture may be seen in the standard OPG and Towne's views; if not, it will be readily demonstrated by CT, which will also show the proximity of a depressed fracture of the zygomatic arch and hence the potential for bony fusion between coronoid and zygoma (Fig. 11.28).

Management

This is essentially the treatment of the associated injuries,

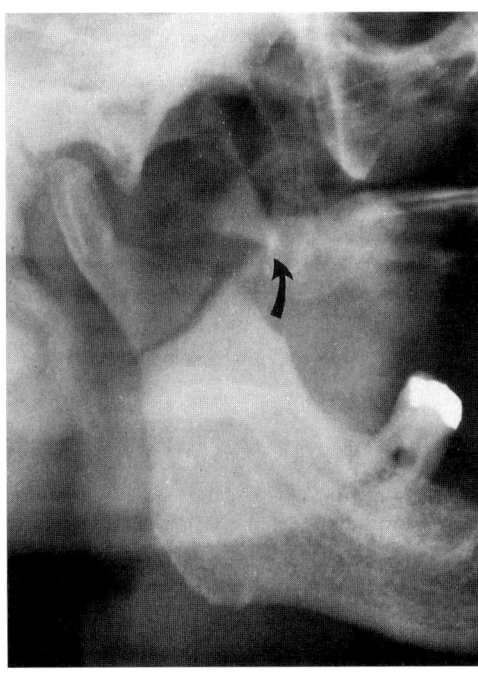

Fig. 11.28 Radiology of coronoid fractures. X-ray demonstrating a coronoid fracture associated with a condylar fracture. The coronoid process is displaced superiorly and posteriorly.

followed by early mandibular mobilization. There is no indication for open reduction and fixation of the fractured coronoid process, provided that the normal transverse space between the squamous temporal bone and the zygomatic arch has been restored.

FRACTURES AND DISLOCATIONS OF THE CONDYLE

Surgical pathology

The condyle is that part of the mandible which passes vertically up from the posterior border above the sigmoid notch to the glenoid fossa of the temporal bone. Fractures may occur at any level in the sigmoid notch, thus including a variable amount of the ramus in the condylar fragment (Figs 11.29 and 11.30). Rarely, there may be a sagittal fracture of the condylar head without involvement of the sigmoid notch (Fig. 11.31). There may be dislocation of the fractured condyle, either posterior, anterior, medial or lateral; rarely there is vertical dislocation into the middle cranial fossa (p. 289).

Classification

There are many classifications of condylar fractures, based on the level, the degree of obliquity, the presence of comminution or compound injury, the displacement, and the presence or absence of dislocation of the head from

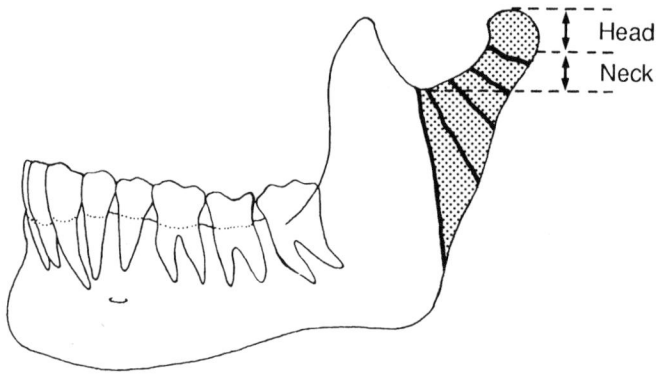

Head
Neck

Fig. 11.29 Anatomy of condylar fractures. A condylar fracture is any fracture which separates the condylar head from the corpus of the mandible but excludes the coronoid (see shaded area). All pass through the sigmoid notch and, depending on the level, are high or low.

the glenoid fossa. Lund's (1974) classification has merit because of its simplicity (Fig. 11.32):

- Type I: enlocated head with or without displacement at the fracture site, and with no more than 60° angulation
- Type II: dislocated head, with 90° or more angulation.

Lund also described these fractures as high, involving the head or neck, and low, at the base of the condylar process.

Clinical assessment

Pain in the region of the temporomandibular joint (TMJ) may be a symptom, and trismus is a common sign. When the patient attempts to open the mouth, there will be pain and restriction of movement: this may be bilateral, but if unilateral, there may be deviation of the chin point towards the affected side. This sign is not specific: it may express any injury causing unilateral contusion of the masticatory muscles, e.g. fracture of the zygomatic arch, coronoid process, pterygoid plates or temporal bone. Indeed, a sprain of the TMJ may produce this sign. Other clinical findings may help to differentiate these types of injury, but in a severe panfacial fracture only radiology will determine the state of the condylar region. Otoscopic examination of the external auditory meatus may show bleeding from a tear in the lining of the canal: posterior displacement of the condylar head may indeed split the cartilaginous part of the canal or fracture the tympanic plate, and hearing should be tested.

Bimanual palpation of the condyles during opening and closing of the mouth may detect swelling, tenderness and perhaps absence of the normal condylar head. This can be done either by placing the fingers over the TMJ just in front of the tragus, or by inserting the finger tip gently into the external auditory canal on each side. Systematic palpation of the rest of the mandible may reveal another coexisting fracture or fractures.

Neurological examination is usually unremarkable: injury to branches of the mandibular division of the trigeminal nerve is very rare in condylar fractures. Damage to the facial nerve is also unusual, but may occur, especially if there is lateral dislocation of the condylar head.

The mouth is then inspected and the occlusion is examined. Typically, bilateral condylar fractures cause an anterior open bite not present before injury, while a

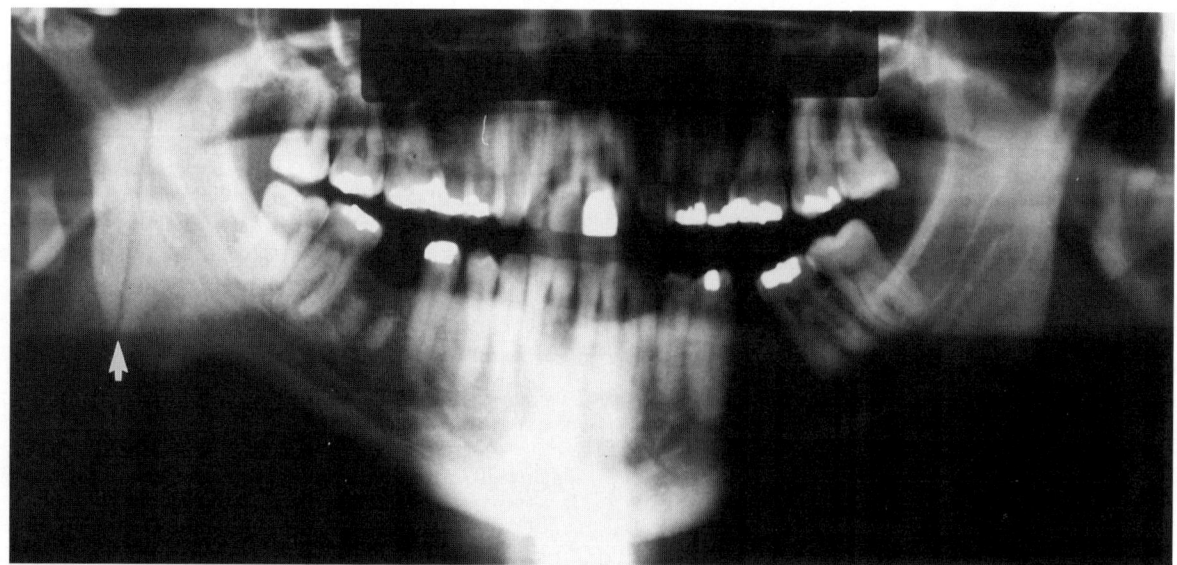

Fig. 11.30 Anatomy of condylar fractures. A low condylar fracture extending to inferior border of ramus. To be compared with higher level in Fig. 11.28.

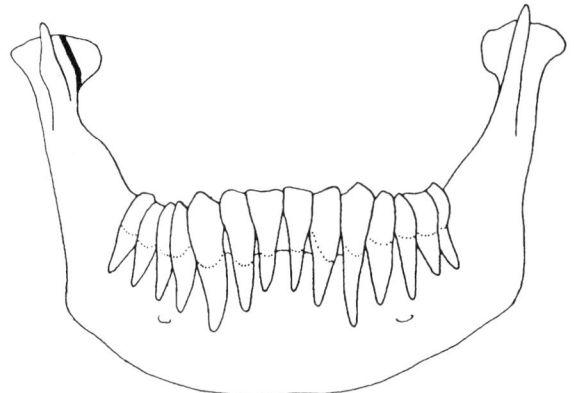

Fig. 11.31 Anatomy of condylar fractures. A sagittal fracture of the head of the condyle may be associated with an intact sigmoid notch. Such fracture may occur in isolation or as a part of a comminuted pattern of condylar fracture.

unilateral fracture causes a lateral crossbite. The teeth and alveoli must be examined: there is a significant association between injuries in these structures and condylar fractures. Indeed, Lindahl (1977a) found injured teeth in 46(37.4%) of 123 cases of condylar fracture, the association being most frequent in bilateral fractures and when the condylar head was involved.

Radiological assessment

The standard OPG and Towne's views will usually show fractures of the condyle. The OPG is especially helpful in showing the site of the fracture; for surgical planning, it is important to know whether the condylar fragment is large enough to allow fixation by a miniplate (Fig. 11.33).

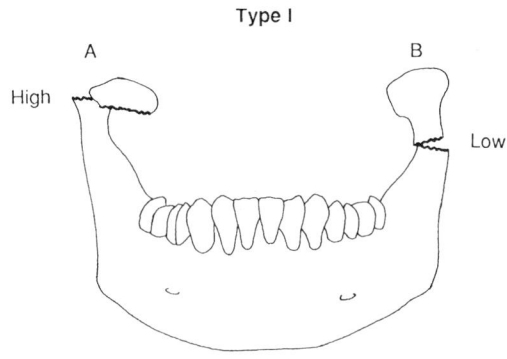

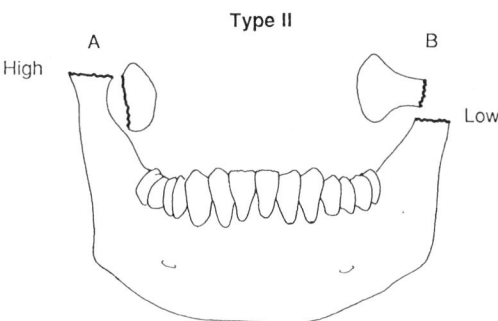

Fig. 11.32 Classification of condylar fractures. Lund's 1974 classification of condylar fractures. Subtypes A and B denote high or low fractures respectively.

This view also shows anteroposterior or vertical displacement of the condylar head as well as anteroposterior displacement and/or overriding at the fracture site. The Towne's view is complementary in showing medial or lateral displacement of the head or the fracture fragments

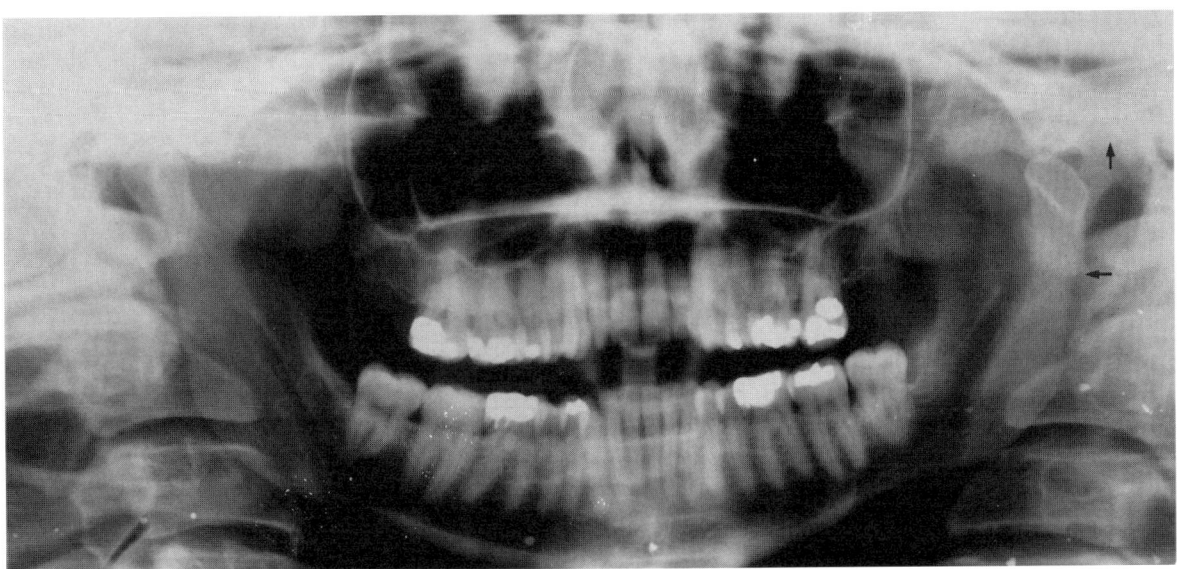

Fig. 11.33 Radiology of condylar fractures. Orthopantomogram demonstrating medium to low level fracture of left condyle in a 14-year-old. The level of the fracture is placed above the lowest point of the sigmoid notch and below the head of the condyle.

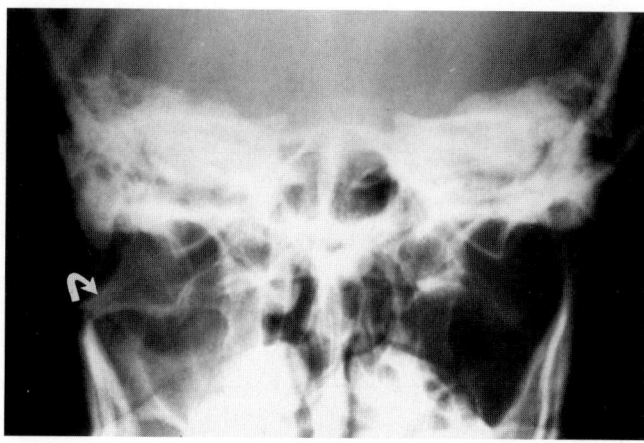

Fig. 11.34 Radiology of condylar fractures. A Townes view demonstrating medial dislocation of the condylar head from the glenoid fossa. Angulation at the fracture site is approximately 90°.

(Fig. 11.34). CT scan may be helpful in showing a sagittal split, or even comminution, of the condylar head: such fractures may lead to ankylosis and need early recognition and treatment (Fig. 11.35).

Dental assessment

This is done along the lines described above; the preparation of plaster study models showing the desired final occlusion, and also an acrylic dental wafer, are necessary

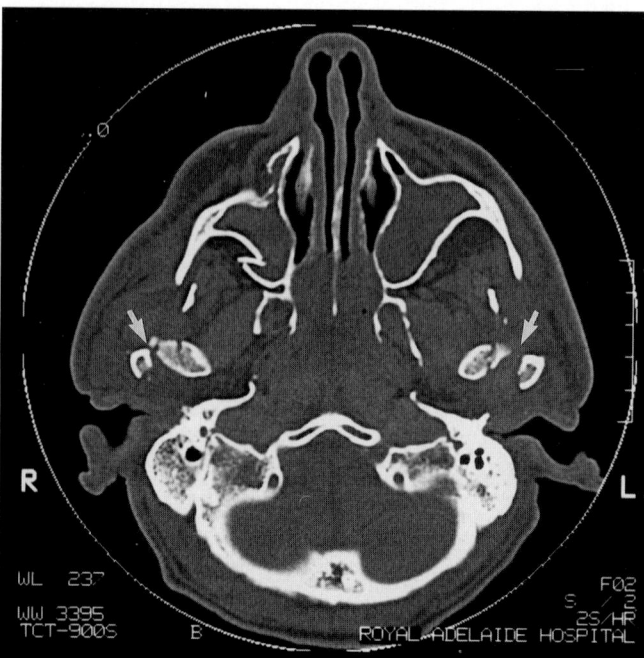

Fig. 11.35 Radiology of condylar fracture. CT scan demonstrating bilateral sagittal fractures of the condylar heads in association with a midface fracture.

preludes to surgical treatment. The dentist will also plan treatment of any dental injuries. The dental findings are then discussed, together with the clinical and radiological findings, and treatment is then planned according to a formal protocol which is discussed below.

Principles of treatment

The management of these injuries is controversial, chiefly because there is uncertainty over the natural history of the unreduced fracture in children and in adults.

Lund (1974), Lindahl (1977a–c) and Lindahl & Hollender (1977) published studies on restitutional re-modelling of the displaced condylar fracture in childhood, and the associated compensatory growth, which tend to support a conservative plan of management; indeed, Lund found that remodelling could result in a normal condyle. However, this process was significantly less effective when growth was nearing completion or completed. Remodelling was also incomplete when the condylar head was dislocated from the glenoid fossa, and when the fracture was low on the condylar neck. Compensatory growth of the mandible on the affected side was observed only if body growth was still occurring. In unilateral cases, compensatory growth was evident in 78% of the studied cases; in 30% this compensatory growth was excessive, causing deviation of the chin point to the unaffected side. Compensatory growth was found to be most pronounced when fractures occurred at puberty, and when the condylar head was not dislocated. Lund found no relationship between the degree of compensatory growth and the height of the fracture.

Lindahl treated 123 patients in the Maxillofacial Unit School of Dentistry in Gothenburg over a 4 year period. He noted that all the children in the series developed a satisfactory occlusion. He did not say whether this was spontaneous or the result of orthodontic treatment, nor did he relate any need for orthodontic treatment to the type of fracture, the degree of remodelling and compensatory growth or the patient age. Nor was a time-cost analysis of the achievement of satisfactory occlusion given for the various fracture types. However, Lindahl did look at the long-term effects of conservative management on mastication. He found that in children, the asymmetry of mandibular movements usually disappeared in 2 years. But in adults, the signs of asymmetrical movement persisted or became worse. Moreover, symptoms such as clicking tenderness or pain, rare in children, were frequent in adults (Lindahl 1977a,b).

Other authors have questioned whether conservative treatment will give a satisfactory, albeit adjusted, occlusion (Hinds & Parnes 1966, Robinson & Rowe 1971). It seems clear that while the results of conservative treatment may be acceptable, they are far from perfect in respect to chin deviation and to TMJ function in adults.

Moreover, the so-called satisfactory results may require protracted and expensive orthodontic treatment.

In some centres, aggressive strategies of treatment have been proposed. Schettler & Rehrmann (1975) in Düsseldorf employed elastic traction from a long bridle attached to a plaster head cap: this was applied to the mandible through a bone hook inserted into the chin. They reported complete restoration of articular function in all treated cases; however, patients had to wear this elaborate appliance for an average period of 3.5 weeks. Open anatomical reduction of the condylar fracture has been also been favoured (Brown & Obeid 1984), but hitherto this has not gained universal acceptance and there are several reasons for this. First, methods of stabilization have been imperfect, and have allowed malunion in one or other plane, or even complete relapse (Fig. 11.36A,B). Second, methods of exposure have not always been safe, or even effective in all types of fracture. Some reports have given no emphasis on the importance of preserving muscle attachments, such as that of the lateral pterygoid to the proximal fragment, or to the maintenance of the capsular attachments to the condyle (Takenoshita et al 1989). Moreover, operative techniques have often been reported without long-term results. For all these reasons, operative intervention has been suspect. Several criteria should be fulfilled for operative procedures to be acceptable:

1. The operative procedure must provide for restoration of normal function and occlusion within 6–12 weeks

2. The fracture must be reduced so that the muscles which act on the condyle regain normal tension and position
3. The displaced fragment must be large enough to be reduced and stabilized in three dimensions
4. The stabilization must be maintainable until bone union occurs
5. The operation must not damage the attachments of the lateral pterygoid muscle to the condylar head
6. There must be no operative morbidity from injury to nerves or other important structures, or to mandibular growth.

If these criteria can be met, operation offers the prospect of rapid restoration of function and of occlusion, by achieving an anatomical reduction of the fracture and of the TMJ joint, followed by early mobilization.

Conservative management

In most cases this is principally the encouragement of early mobilization by active jaw movement. With adequate pain relief and a liquid diet, the patient will usually bite into the pretraumatic occlusion within a couple of days. Active encouragement continues until an opening close to 40 mm between the upper and lower incisors is achieved. If the patient cannot regain the pretraumatic occlusion, arch bars are applied and occlusion is established and maintained for 2 weeks by intermaxillary wire fixation.

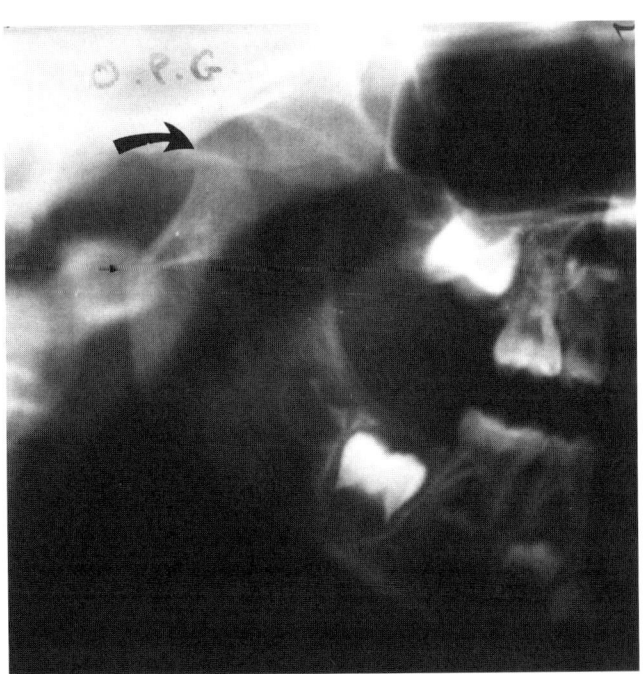
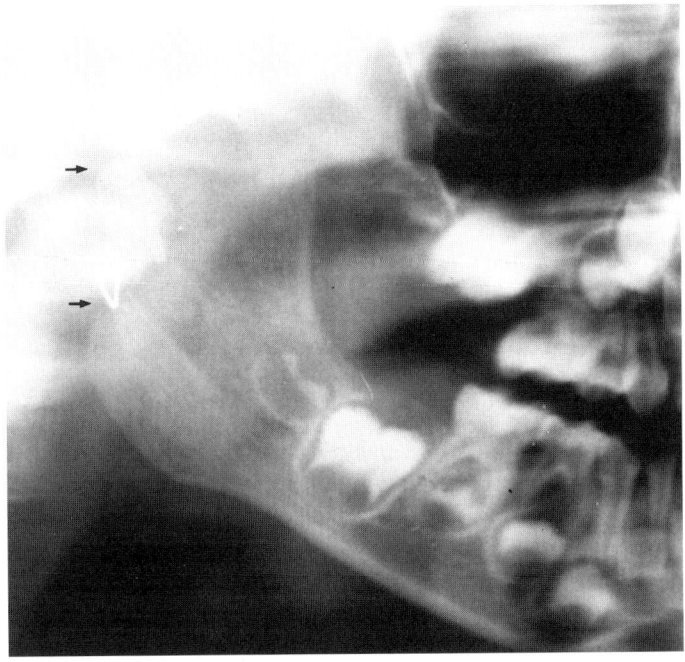

A   B

Fig. 11.36 Attempted wire stabilization of condylar fracture. A Displaced and dislocated condylar fracture in a 7-year-old. The large arrow indicates the dislocation of the condylar head, and the small arrow indicates the angulation at the fracture site. **B** 1 year following reduction and stabilisation with an interosseous wire, there has been relapse followed by malunion. Remodelling did not take place, probably because of the invasive nature of the surgery (all muscle was stripped from the condyle) and inadequate stabilisation (wire only). Arrows point to condylar remnant.

By this time, the pain should have ceased and the inter-maxillary wires can be replaced by elastic bands — light by day, heavy by night. The bands are intended to counteract the usual tendency to deviation of the chin to the affected side (in unilateral injuries) or to anterior open bite (in bilateral injuries); the light bands allow active movement, which is encouraged. This regimen is continued for another 6–8 weeks and is ceased only when the patient can maintain the pretraumatic occlusion. It may then be necessary to encourage wider opening of the mouth by an exercise programme. After eating, the patient spends 5 min three times a day before a mirror, opening – protruding – retracting – and laterally deviating the lower jaw. The patient, after these exercises, is given a stack of wooden spatulae and inserts each day an increasing number of these between the incisor teeth, until a 40 mm interincisal opening is achieved. Pain is to be expected, and the patient is reassured that this is a necessary result of stretching scarred tissues.

The best reported results from conservative management are those of Lindahl, discussed above, and they are far from perfect. In adults with fracture-dislocation of the condyle, conservative management may lead to malocclusion, loss of teeth, and pain in the TMJ (Robinson & Rowe 1971). Nevertheless, conservative treatment is indicated if there is little or no displacement, or if the fracture line is so high that surgical stabilization is impossible.

Operative management

Zide & Kent (1983) have given as absolute indications for operation:

1. Fracture dislocation of the head into the middle fossa, or into the temporal fossa if associated with clinical disability
2. Intra-articular foreign body
3. Lateral extracapsular dislocation of the condyle
4. Inability to open the mouth or to bring the mandible into occlusion after 1 week with evidence of a bony block
5. Compound injuries, e.g. gunshot wounds.

Zide's relative indications include:

6. Displaced condylar fracture, where the fracture line is near the lower border of the sigmoid notch and the head is dislocated from the glenoid fossa
7. Condylar fracture, where vertical displacement is associated with displaced fracture(s) of the upper jaw.

We endorse these indications, and believe that in adults, when there is displacement of the fracture and where the proximal fragment has sufficient length to accept two screws to hold a plate, then anatomical reduction and rigid plate fixation will allow immediate mobilization and good prospects of a satisfactory functional and aesthetic outcome. The scope of operative intervention in children is considered in Chapter 19.

The condyle may be approached through an intraoral incision, or through various skin incisions discussed by Ellis & Dean (1993). Whichever route is chosen, the approach must give good exposure of the fracture site, must allow reduction without damage to the joint capsule or disk, and must not interfere with the attachment of the lateral pterygoid muscle. It must enable the surgeon to establish three-dimensional stability after reduction.

We have found these aims achievable through the bicoronal scalp incision described on p. 238, but extended in front of the ear to the level of the ear lobe. It is often unnecessary to make the full coronal incision: one may spare the contralateral side. The incision is run along the natural contour of the helix and the tragus to be inconspicuous when healed; the temporal part of the incision is likewise designed to be hidden by the fall of the hair. The scalp flap is turned down in the subgaleal plane to a level 1–2 cm above the superior orbital margin, and thereafter is taken subperiosteally to the orbital rim on the affected side. The superficial temporal fascia is then incised, and the dissection proceeds through the fat to expose the zygomatic arch. This method of dissection spares the frontal branch of the facial nerve. The masseter is next exposed a distance at least 2 cm below the zygomatic arch, and the capsule of the TMJ is seen (Fig. 11.37). The parotid gland is separated from the cartilaginous external auditory canal, but no further, and the facial nerve is kept covered by soft tissue. The masseter is then divided 1–2 cm below the arch of the zygoma, the cut being taken from the posterior border forward, care being

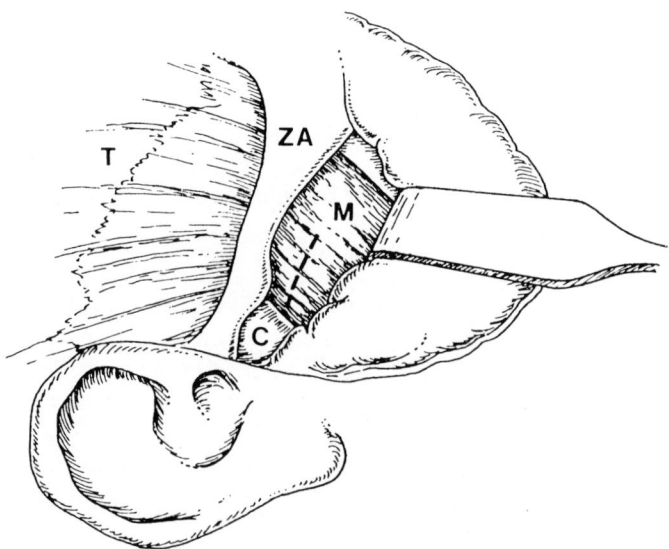

Fig. 11.37 Surgical exposure of condylar fractures. Anatomy on display after turning down the bicoronal flap. T, temporalis muscle; M, masseter muscle; C, capsule of temporomandibular joint; ZA, zygomatic arch.

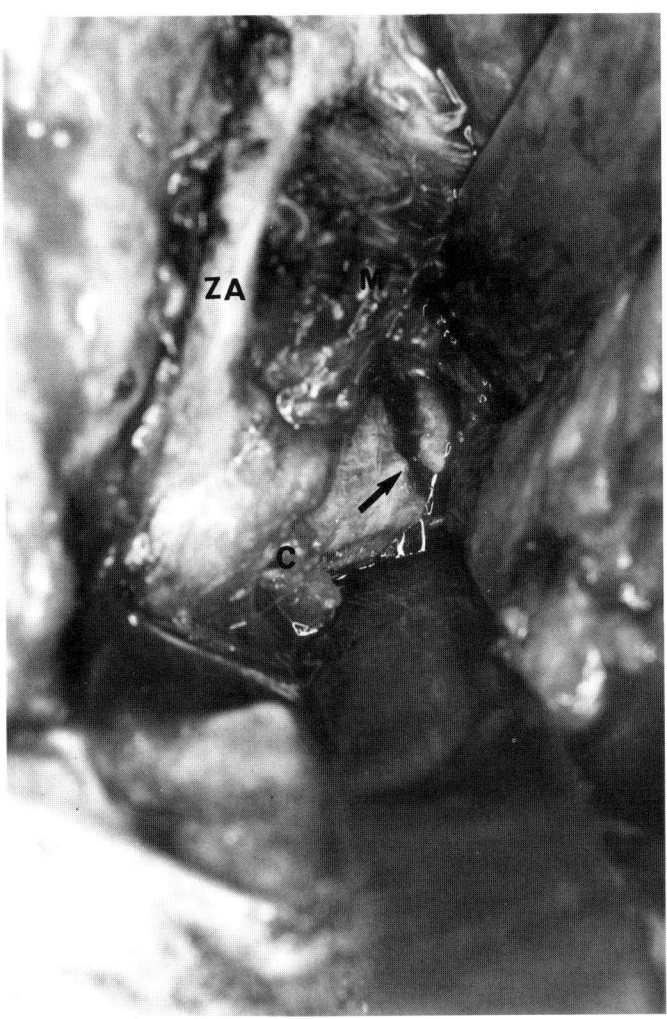

Fig. 11.38 Surgical exposure of condylar fractures. Operative view of condylar fracture (arrowed). The posterior masseter has been cut to expose the fracture. M, masseter muscle; C, capsule of temporomandibular joint; ZA, zygomatic arch.

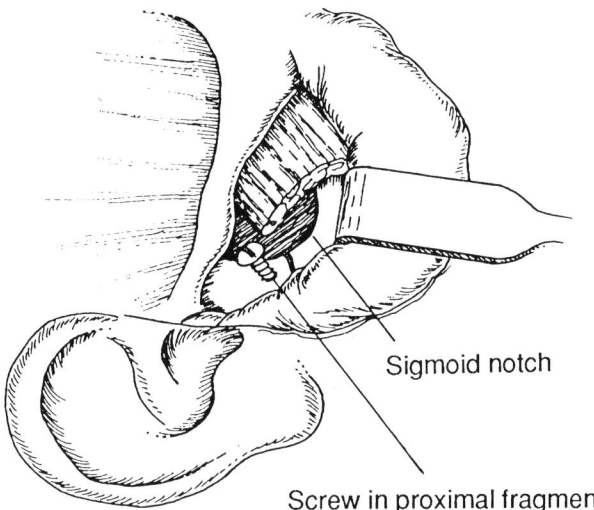

Fig. 11.39 Surgical exposure of condylar fractures. Via a myotomy of the posterior masseter muscle, a hole has been drilled in the accessible proximal fragment and a screw inserted. The latter acts as a 'handle' on the proximal fragment, allowing its reduction without further trauma to its capsular or muscular attachments.

taken to avoid injury to the nerves and vessels passing through the sigmoid notch. It is now possible to expose the neck of the condyle, the upper ramus, and the sigmoid notch: the fracture site is on view and can be fully exposed with only light retraction (Fig. 11.38).

A drill hole is then placed in the proximal fragment, and a 13 mm screw is inserted a distance of 9 mm (Fig. 11.39). This screw is then used as a handle: it is grasped with strong artery forceps and the proximal fragment is manipulated into the position of anatomical reduction: this reduction is aided by downward pressure on the ramus via the sigmoid notch. At no time is the joint capsule or the lateral pterygoid muscle injured or dissected. When reduction is effected, a 4-hole miniplate is bent to conform with the lateral concavity of the bone and fitted with four screws (Figs. 11.40 and 11.41). The screw used in manipulation is then removed. The masseter and superficial temporal fascia are repaired with 3/0 Vicryl

sutures. The scalp wound is closed in two layers, 6/0 Vicryl being used in the pre-auricular area. Drainage is rarely needed. Arch bars and intermaxillary fixation are not used, except when there is a concurrent fracture elsewhere in the mandible or the upper jaw: in such cases, intermaxillary fixation is left until the scalp is healed. Postoperative care is as described for fractures of the mandibular body. The jaw is mobilized in the manner described as conservative management. At 6 weeks, mobilization is usually complete and the patient may take a normal diet.

Steinhäuser (1964) described an intraoral approach to the fractured condyle and Lachner et al (1991) have used this exposure for miniplate fixation in 14 cases, with satisfactory results; they did not indicate what degree of displacement was an indication for open reduction. We see this exposure as adequate in very low oblique condylar fractures, but not in more horizontal higher fractures (Fig. 11.42A,B). Indeed, Habel et al (1990) found it necessary to osteotomize the coronoid process to gain access to the proximal fragment when using an intraoral incision. Other external approaches to the condyle have been proposed: in the pre-auricular area (Al-Kayat & Bramley 1980), through the postauricular area (Hoopes et al 1970) and through various submandibular incisions (Fig. 11.43). But we favour the extended coronal scalp incision described here, because it gives the surgeon direct exposure of the fracture without heavy soft tissue retraction and risks of damage to the facial nerve (Fig. 11.44).

Brown & Obeid (1984) have reviewed the methods of stabilizing the fracture when it has been exposed and reduced. Surgeons have used various types of interosseous

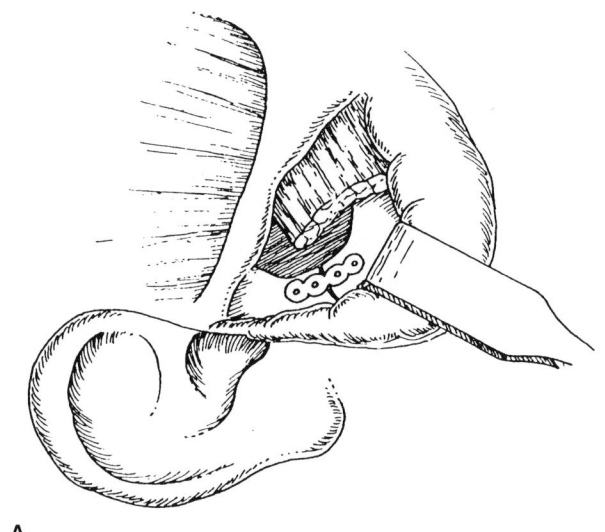

A

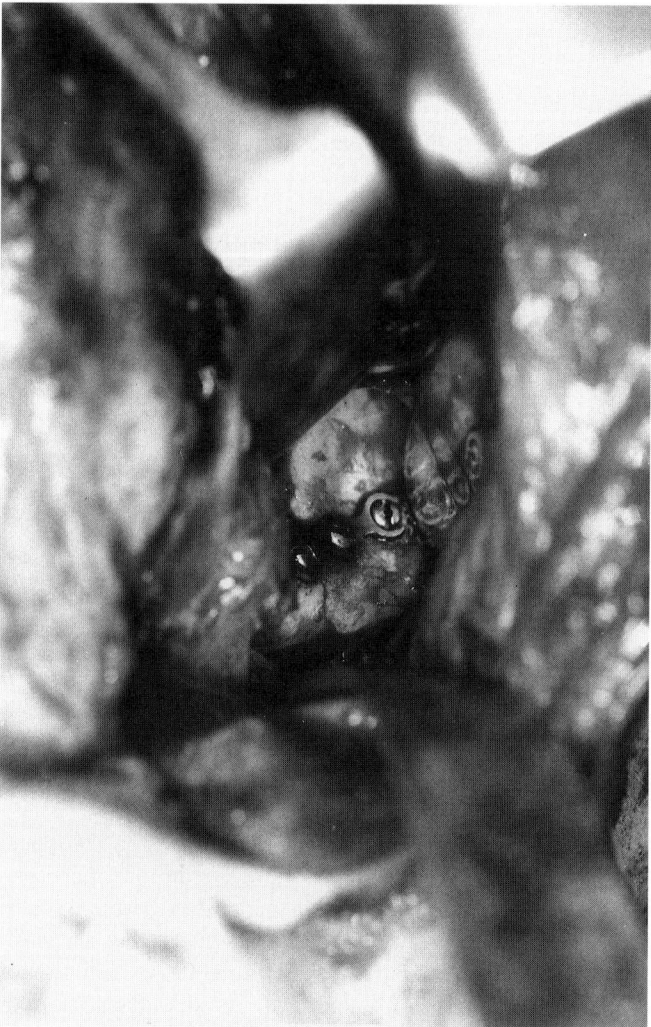

B

Fig. 11.40 Surgical exposure of condylar fractures. A At least two screws through holes in a plate on each side of the fracture line provides three-dimensional stabilization, allowing early return of function. **B** Operative view.

wiring, Steinmann's pins with or without wiring, external fixateurs, and miniplates. Miniplates have the great advantage of giving three-dimensional stabilization while allowing mobilization and early return to normal function. With the exception of external fixateurs, the other methods listed do not give stability, and the jaws must be immobilized by intermaxillary fixation, which is detrimental to early functional recovery. External fixateurs, by their nature, must totally prevent mobilization.

Complications of condylar fractures

The condyle is isolated from the teeth by vascular soft tissues, and condylar fractures usually heal well. However, complications can occur. These include:

- Growth disturbance
- Avascular necrosis
- Ankylosis of the TMJ
- Malunion
- Other TMJ dysfunctions.

Growth disturbance

This problem is peculiar to childhood and is discussed in Chapters 19 and 21.

Avascular necrosis

This is sometimes seen when an intracapsular fracture detaches a fragment of the head of the condyle which is denuded of its blood supply; the cortical surface of the condylar head is eroded and the surface becomes rough and flattened. This complication is well described by Sanders et al (1977). The patient complains of pain and limitation of movement; changes in the condylar surface may be demonstrated by X-ray. Sanders advised removal of the avascular fragment of the head of the condyle and smoothing of the remaining bone. Avascular necrosis can also result from damage to the blood supply in the course of an open operation on the TMJ (Iizuka et al 1991b). When it is necessary to stabilize the condyle by open surgery, we believe that it is important to retain all residual capsular attachments of the proximal fragment, and also the insertion of the lateral pterygoid muscle. Some surgeons indeed have completely isolated the proximal fragment by dividing all soft tissue attachments prior to reduction and fixation, and have reported no problems from this (Takenoshita 1989), but we believe that avascular necrosis can occur under these circumstances, and we have seen an example of this (Fig. 11.36).

Ankylosis of the TMJ

TMJ ankylosis is more likely to develop when there has been tearing or disruption of the articular disk, associated

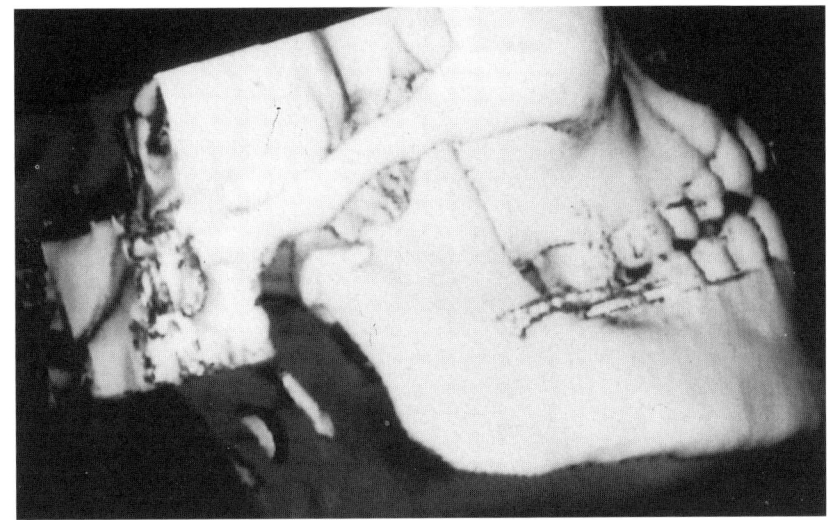

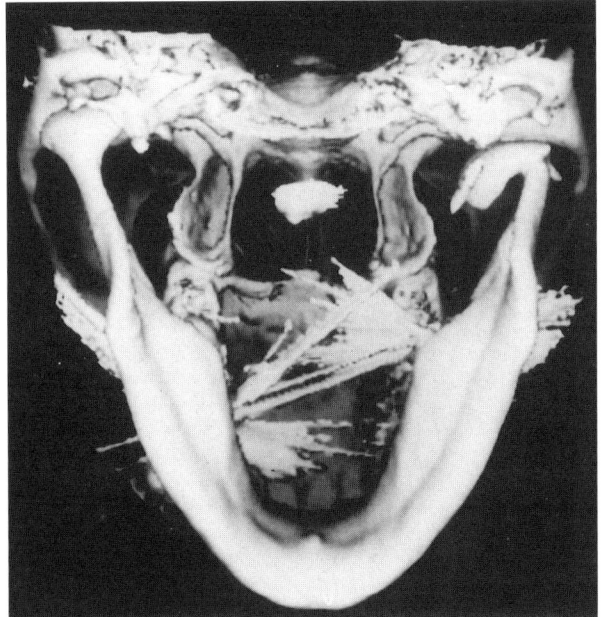

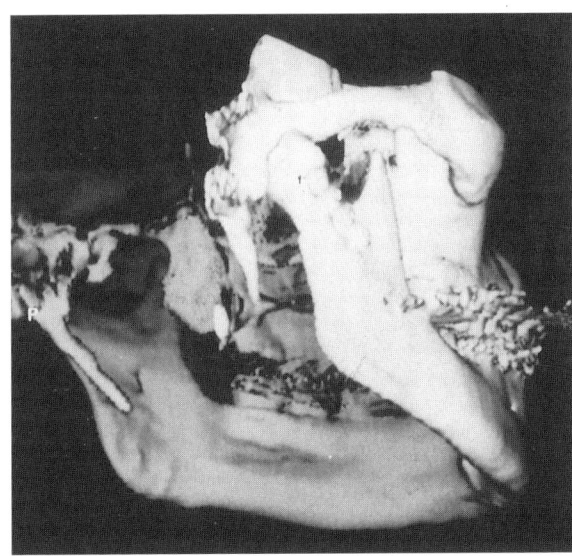

Fig. 11.41 Surgical exposure of condylar fractures. A Three-dimensional CT scan of a condylar fracture with medial dislocation of the head.
B Three-dimensional CT scan from below, showing the head displaced into the medial pterygoid region. **C** CT scan after reduction and
stabilization via an extended bi-coronal approach with myotomy of the posterior fibres of the masseter muscle. The four-hole plate and screw heads
can be readily seen.

with comminution of the condylar articular surface, as in intracapsular fractures. In such cases, early zealous mobilization of the jaw is mandatory, with close supervision and careful follow-up. If there are associated fractures of other parts of the mandible, it is important to avoid treating these by intermaxillary fixation: miniplate osteosynthesis is the treatment of choice, followed by early progressive mobilization. This regimen requires patient compliance, and this will as a rule be lacking in patients who are in coma or disturbed consciousness from head injuries, or who are demented, psychotic, addicted to drugs, or intellectually disabled.

TMJ ankylosis has many implications: it causes difficulties in feeding, and may result in poor dental hygiene and consequent oral sepsis. The condition may also be a potentially dangerous factor in inducing anaesthesia; the anaesthetist should always be warned of possible difficulty in intubation and a flexible fibroscope may be useful.

In an established case, treatment can be offered. If compliance is assured, an arthroplasty is possible. The scope of the arthroplasty to be undertaken ranges from simple freeing of soft tissues and interposition of cartilage or muscle, through to total joint reconstruction, which is indicated when there is a significant bony ankylosis. Various reconstructive materials have been recommended (p. 602). Our experience is chiefly with costochondral grafts: we have used onlay rib grafts, secured to the ramus with lag screws or plates, at least 1.5–2 cm of the attached cartilage being inserted into the glenoid fossa. Our operative techniques are discussed in Chapter 21 (p. 601).

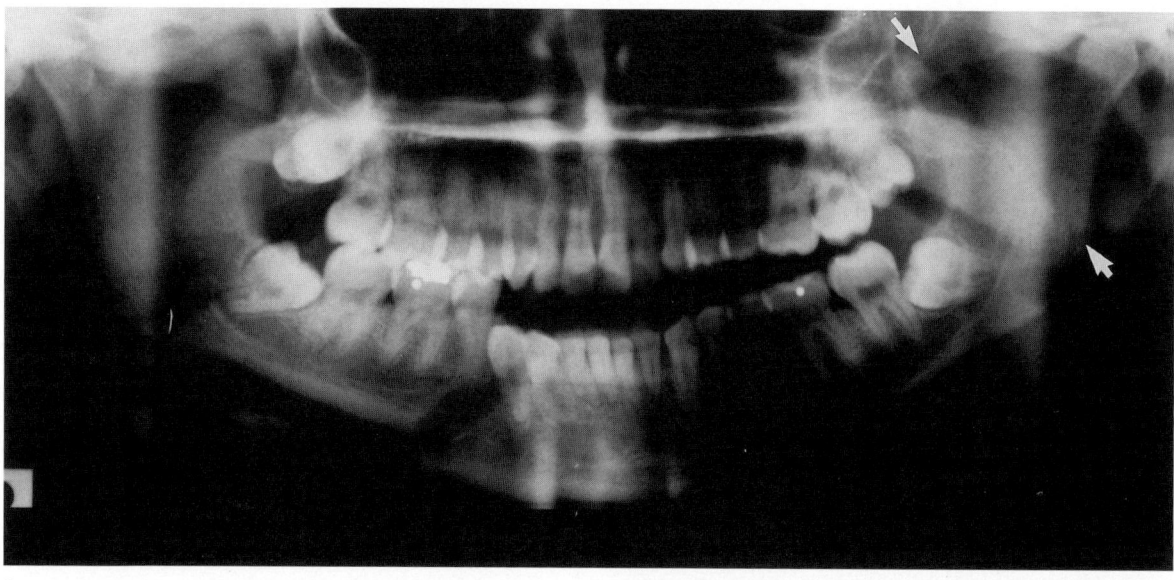

A

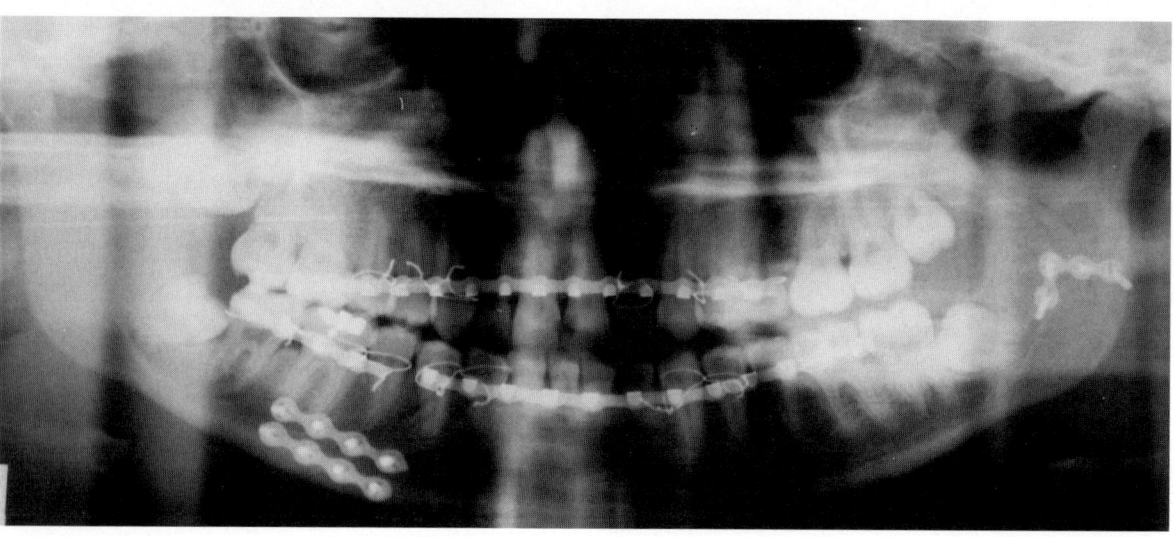

B

Fig. 11.42 Surgical exposure of condylar fractures. A Orthopantomogram of condylar fracture low enough for intraoral reduction (arrow). **B** After reduction and stabilization using an intraoral approach.

Malunion; other TMJ dysfunctions

Malunion can be tolerated unless occlusion is deranged. If after 12 weeks of conservative therapy and dental occlusal adjustment, there is still a significant open bite, with or without an occlusion likely to cause impairment of the vitality of the teeth, then there is a strong case for surgical correction of the malocclusion forthwith (Hinds & Parnes 1966). Failure to do so may result in tooth loss and/or TMJ dysfunction. Standard osteotomies through the ramus will easily correct buccal anterior crossbites. Vertical subsigmoid osteotomy with plate fixation (p. 612) and sagittal split osteotomy with lag screw fixation (p. 609) will allow early mobilization; these procedures should be done after intensive physiotherapy has given the fullest possible range of jaw opening.

DISLOCATIONS OF THE CONDYLE

Classification and surgical pathology

While dislocation of the condyle from the glenoid fossa is often associated with a fracture of the condylar process, simple dislocations of the condyle do occur in the absence of such a fracture. They can be classified as:

1. Anteromedial or anterior — the common form
2. Posterior — relatively uncommon

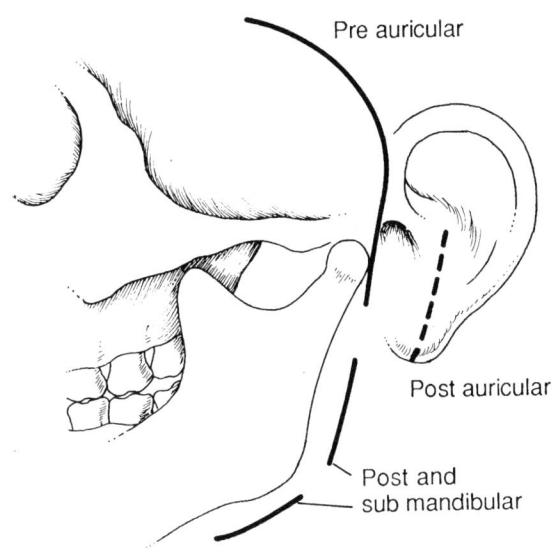

Fig. 11.43 External incisions for exposure of condylar fractures. External skin incisions described for access to condylar fractures.

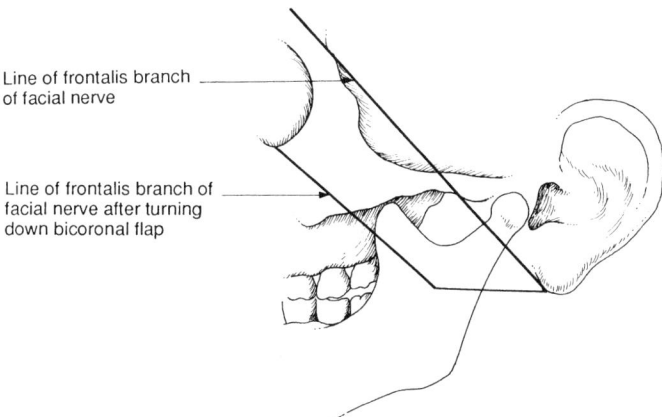

Fig. 11.44 Bicoronal flap 'relocation' of the frontalis nerve. The act of turning down the bicoronal flap including frontalis muscle locates the frontalis branch of the facial nerve below the sigmoid notch of the mandible. Retraction on the nerve is extremely light as a result.

3. Medial — relatively uncommon
4. Lateral — relatively uncommon
5. Vertical (upward) or central dislocation through a fracture in the glenoid fossa — rare (Pieritz & Schmidseder 1981, Worthington 1982).

Clinical assessment

In the common anteromedial dislocation, which is likely to be bilateral, there is usually pain in the region of the affected joint(s), prognathism, an open mouth and an inability to close into normal occlusion. It is said that this dislocation is typically caused by a blow to the chin, especially when the mouth is open. There may be a history of previous dislocation.

The less common dislocations are likely to be associated with fracture of the body of the mandible. In lateral dislocation, there will be obvious deformity and often an ipsilateral facial paralysis, a rare finding in other mandibular dislocations and fractures. In posterior dislocation, the external auditory canal is likely to be bruised or even obstructed by the dislocated condyle.

Radiological assessment

It is necessary to exclude other fractures as well as to locate the position of the condyle in relation to the glenoid fossa; CT is especially useful in this.

Management

The treatment of anterior dislocation, whether unilateral or bilateral, has not changed much since the time of Hippocrates (p. 9). Pain relief is given, and under either intravenous sedation or general anaesthesia, the dislocation is reduced. To do this, a downward pull is applied with the thumbs on the retromolar area; when the muscular resistance is overcome the ramus comes down and the condylar head can be levered back over the articular eminence into the glenoid fossa. It may be appropriate to rest the jaws by intermaxillary fixation, using light elastic band traction, for several days at least, and then to mobilize the jaw slowly. Recurrent anterior and anteromedial dislocation may require a surgical procedure to block excessive forward movement over the articular eminence. To do this we have used the procedure reported by Dautrey & Pepersack (1982). In this, a posterior osteotomy of the zygomatic arch is performed, allowing downward fracture of the arch to form a block against dislocation of the condylar head (Fig. 11.45).

Medial and lateral dislocations are more difficult to reduce (Ferguson et al 1989, Worthington 1982). The induction of anaesthesia can be dangerous: the condyle can be tightly wedged in the temporal fossa, and the displacement of the jaw may prevent the anaesthetist from visualizing the larynx. The anaesthetist must know of this hazard, and the surgeon must be ready to perform an emergency tracheotomy.

Medial dislocation has been reduced by cutting and temporarily displacing a segment of the zygomatic arch to permit strong downward traction of the ramus. Lateral dislocation has been reduced by traction exerted through a wire passed through the ramus. Exposure through the extended coronal scalp flap described above allows visualization of these difficult dislocations, which can then be reduced with or without osteotomy of the zygomatic arch (Fig. 11.46A,B). Because these dislocations entail damage to the capsule, disc and muscle attachments, early mobilization after a short period of rest is desirable: to allow this, any associated mandibular fractures should be plated.

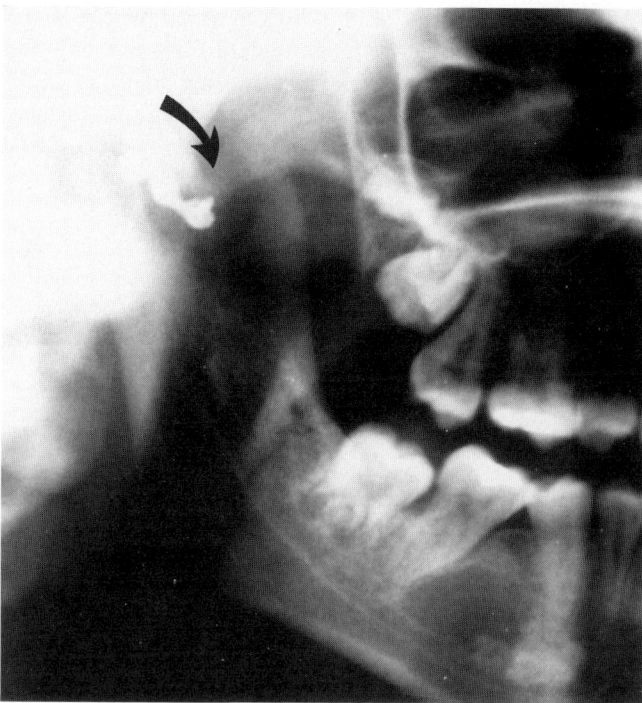

Fig. 11.45 Surgical 'blocking' of anterior dislocation. OPG of Dautrey procedure. The zygomatic arch has been down fractured in the region of the articular eminence (arrow) and stabilised with a miniplate. This acts to block excessive forward translation of the condylar head.

Patterns of mandibular fracture

In our retrospective study of adults with facial fractures treated in a 3-year period (p. 87), there were 324 patients with 491 fractures of mandible. Table 11.1 shows the anatomical distribution of these fractures, in comparison with some other reported series. It is noteworthy that in nearly half of our cases, the mandible was broken in more than one place: in 152 (46.9%) there were two fractures, and in eight (2.5%) there were three.

Of the cases with double fractures, the commonest combination was angle + body (23.5%). In descending order of frequency came condyle + body (14.5%), bilateral body (3.5%), bilateral angle (3%), and condyle + angle (2.4%). Of the small group with triple fractures, all had combined fractures of condyle + body + angle, and in three of these, both condyles were fractured. Examples of patterns of multiple mandibular fracture are shown in Figs 11.47–11.51.

MAXILLARY FRACTURES

Surgical pathology

An understanding of the blood and nerve supply to the

Table 11.1 Classification of mandibular fractures, with percentage incidences in series from South Australia (Australian Craniomaxillofacial Unit: ACFU), Western Scotland (Ellis et al 1985) and Iowa, USA (Olson et al 1982)

	ACFU (%)	Ellis et al 1985 (%)	Olson et al 1982 (%)
Condyle	20.2	29.3	29.1
Coronoid process	0.3	2.2	1.3
Ramus	3.05	2.6	1.7
Angle	36.46	23.1	24.5
Body	16.50	33.0	16.0
Symphyseal	23.82	8.4	22.0

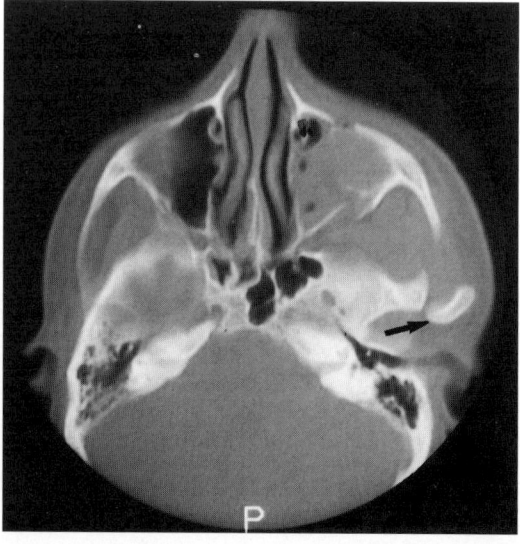

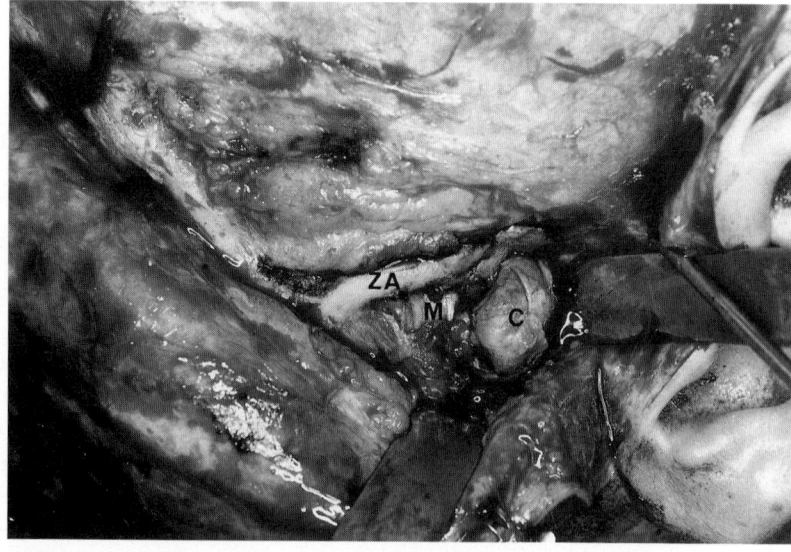

A   B

Fig. 11.46 Management of lateral dislocation of condyle. A CT scan of lateral dislocation of left condyle (arrow). This was associated with a left body of mandible fracture, right condylar fracture and upper jaw fractures. **B** Operative appearance via extended bicoronal flap exposure and myotomy of masseter. The condylar head can be seen lateral to the zygomatic arch. C, condylar head; M, masseter muscle; ZA, zygomatic arch.

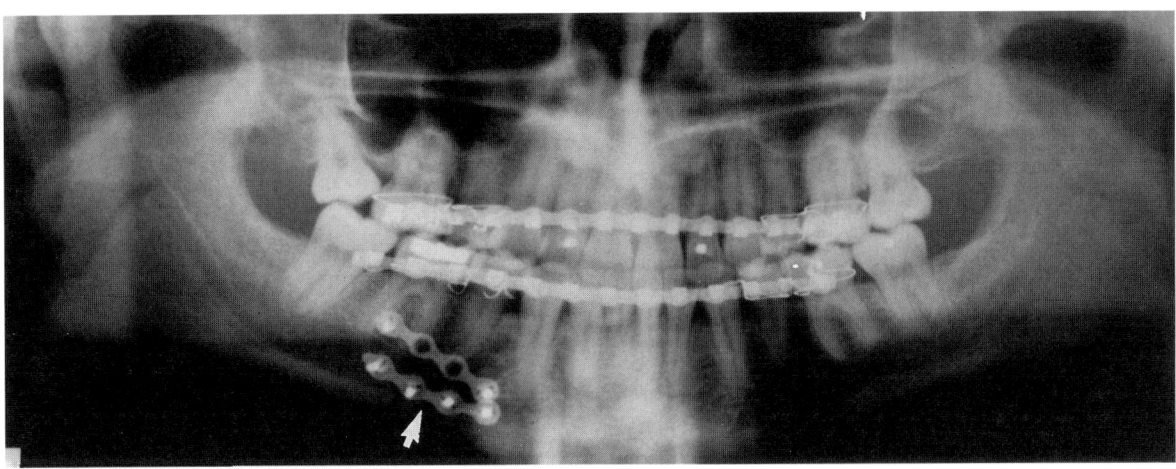

Fig. 11.47 Mandibular fracture patterns. Post-fixation orthopantomogram of body fracture through the bicuspid/first molar area (arrow). This is relatively rare.

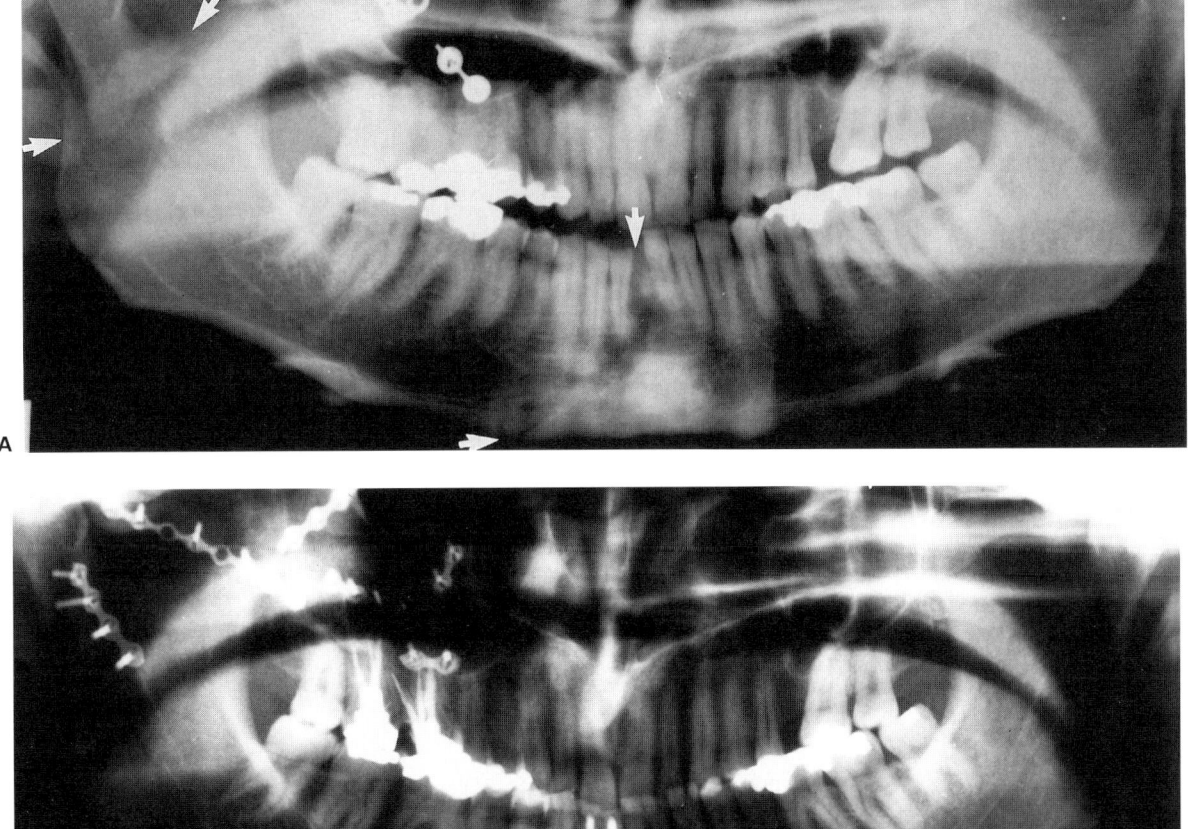

Fig. 11.48 Mandibular fracture patterns. A Pre-operative orthopantomogram of right condylar fracture associated with symphyseal fracture (arrows). This is a relatively common problem. However, this case also included fractured zygoma and maxillary dento-alveolar fracture. **B** Post-surgical reduction and plating of mandibular and midface fractures.

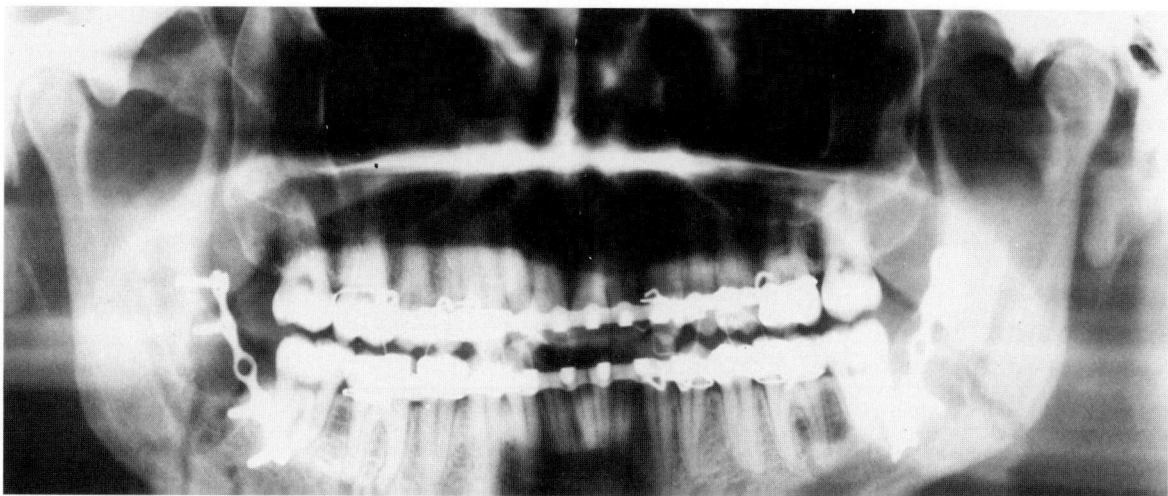

Fig. 11.49 Mandibular fracture patterns. Bilateral angle fractures stabilised with miniplates. This method allows immediate movement of the mandible and rapid return to function.

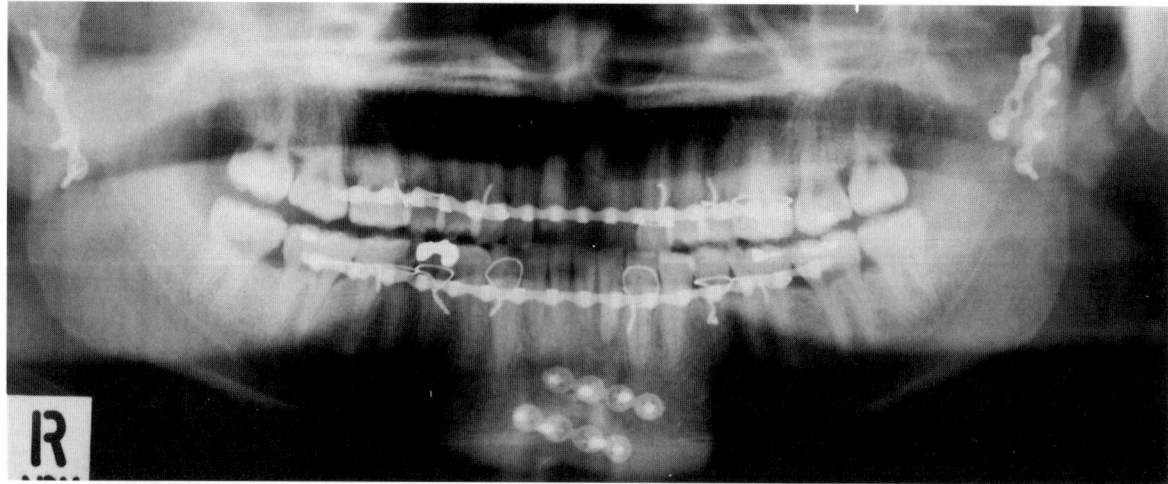

Fig. 11.50 Mandibular fracture patterns. Post-surgical orthopantomogram of bilateral condylar fractures associated with symphyseal fracture. Miniplate stabilization of these fractures provides rapid return to function.

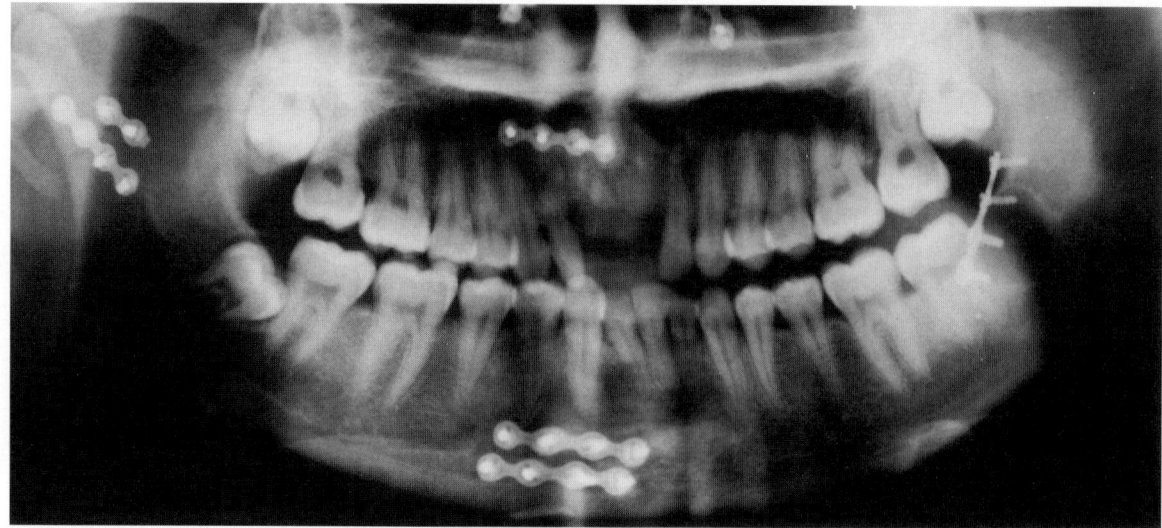

Fig. 11.51 Mandibular fracture patterns. Post-surgical orthopantomogram of condyle, body and angle fracture pattern associated with upper jaw fracture. Miniplate stabilization leads to rapid return of function.

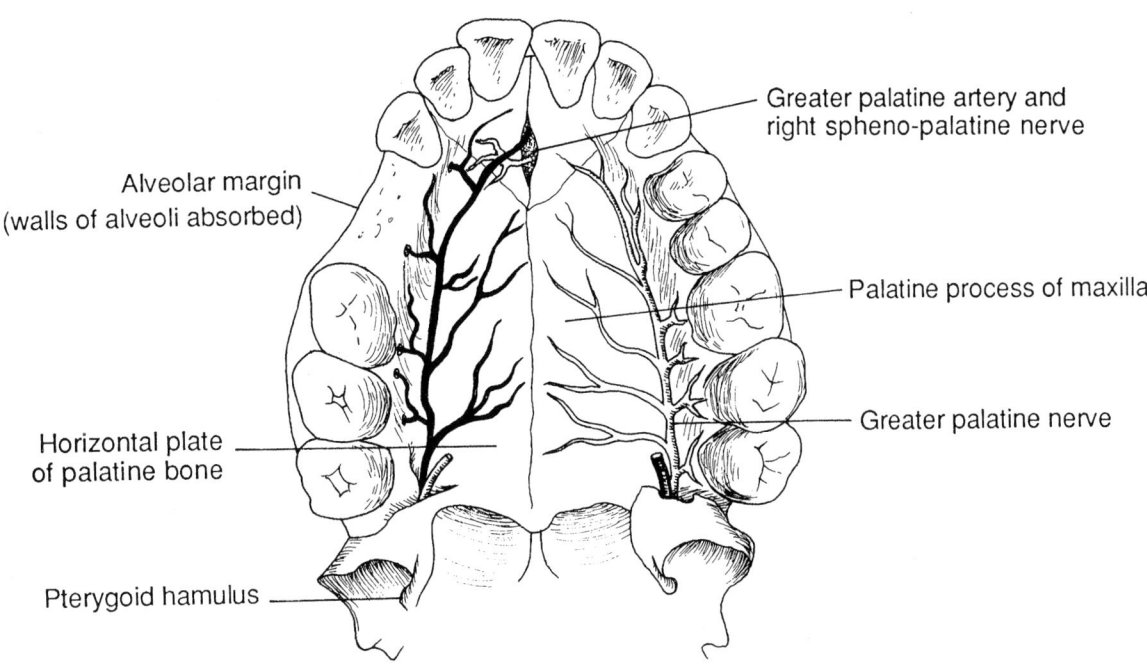

Greater palatine artery and
right spheno-palatine nerve

Alveolar margin
(walls of alveoli absorbed)

Palatine process of maxilla

Greater palatine nerve

Horizontal plate
of palatine bone

Pterygoid hamulus

Fig. 11.52 Maxillary anatomy. Nerve and artery supply of the hard palate, alveolar bone and mucosa.

maxilla and upper dental arch is essential both in planning safe incisions for exposure of an already damaged maxilla and in understanding the patterns of numbness associated with maxillary fractures (pp. 48 and 61). On each side, the greater palatine canal transmits the greater palatine artery and nerve which supply all of the bone and mucosa of the hard palate (Fig. 11.52). Branches of the maxillary artery and maxillary nerve enter the posterior maxilla through small foramina to become the posterior superior alveolar (or dental) artery and nerve; the nerve supplies the molar teeth through the dental plexus. Branches from the infraorbital artery and nerve enter the anterior maxillary bone from the orbital floor and supply the anterior teeth (Fig. 11.53A,B) It can be seen that fractures of the orbital floor and/or the anterior maxilla may result in numbness of anterior teeth while fractures extending low in the maxilla posterior to the first molar region may result in numbness of the posterior teeth. Apart from the above-named arteries the maxilla gains blood supply from gingival attachments to the alveolar bone and through its attachments to the soft palate from the pharyngeal and palatine branches of the facial artery and the ascending pharyngeal branches of the external carotid artery. Where this profuse blood supply is interfered with by a significant degloving of soft tissue, and particularly if there is associated detachment of the soft palate from the posterior hard palate, then care must be taken in surgical exposure of the maxilla lest dissection detaches the remaining blood supply from the maxillary bone and the associated teeth.

The skeleton of the midfacial region appears designed to transmit the powerful forces of mastication through to the base of skull. The strong horizontal elements in the maxillae, alveoli and hard palate make up a foundation to support the three paired vertical bony condensations or buttresses (Fig. 2.15). The most anterior of these extends from the dento-alveolar arch in the lateral incisor/canine region superiorly along the piriform margin to the medial orbital rim and frontomaxillary suture. The middle buttress extends from the region of the first molar tooth to the body of the zygoma and through this bone as the lateral orbital wall to the frontozygomatic suture. The posterior buttress is represented by the attachment of the maxillary tuberosity to the pterygoid plates and hence to the sphenoid (Fig. 11.54) (Manson et al 1980).

The biomechanical stresses in the midface have been harder to assess than those in the mandible. However, the load paths for distribution of force appear to be the buttresses described above and analysed in more detail in Chapter 2 (p. 44). Ideally, surgical plates screwed in place along the buttresses should stabilize and reconstruct the load paths, and the more screws that are used on each side of a fracture line, the more evenly the distribution of force will be applied along these paths (Fig. 11.55) (Rudderman & Mullen 1992).

Classification

In classifying occlusal fractures of the maxilla, little can be added to Le Fort's original description (p. 18). The common denominator in each of the Le Fort types of maxillary fracture is the status of the upper jaw and the occlusion. In the Le Fort I pattern the upper jaw is detached from the cranial skeleton at a horizontal fracture

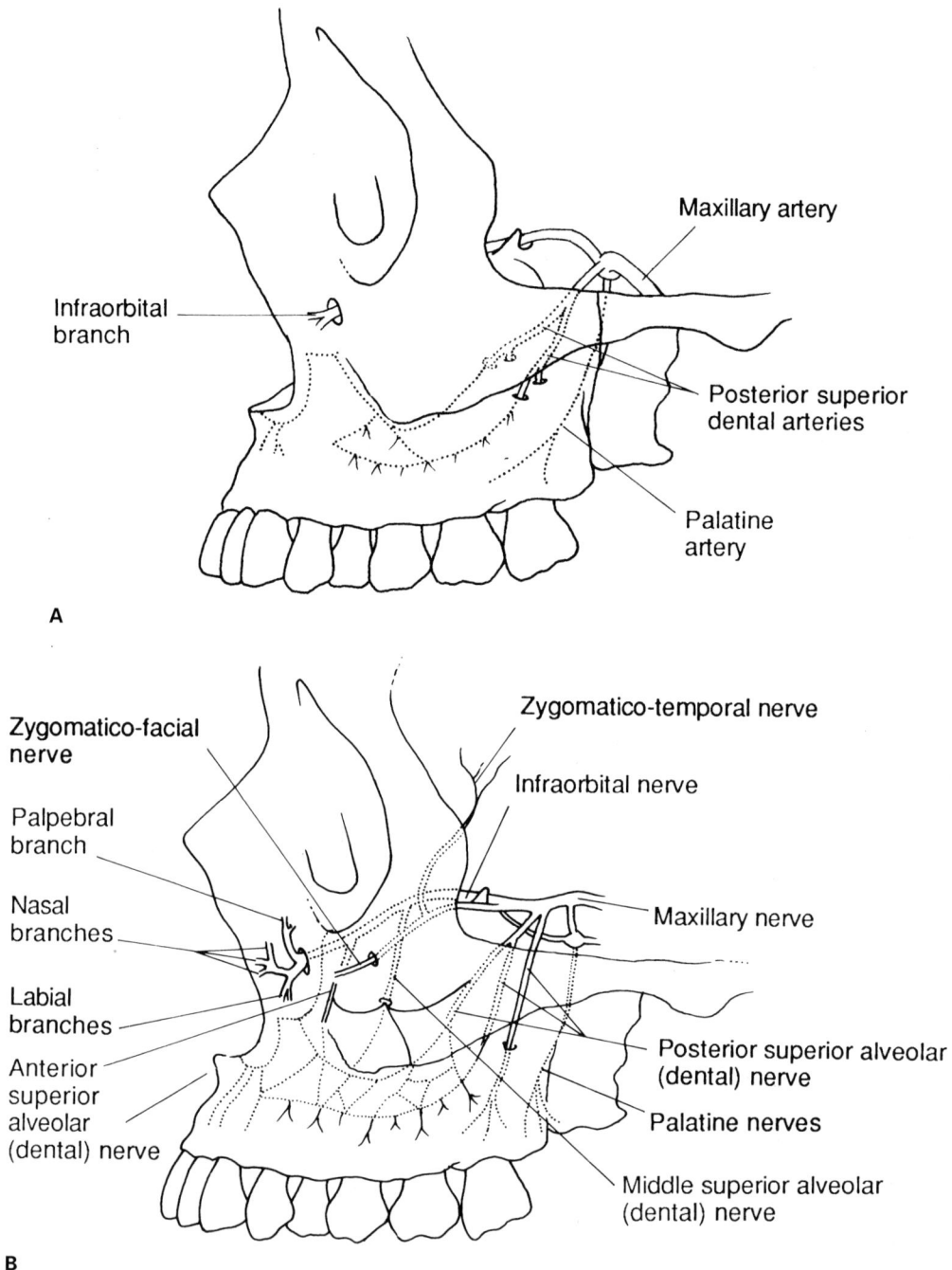

Fig. 11.53 Maxillary anatomy. A Arterial supply to the anterolateral maxilla. **B** Nerve supply to the anterolateral maxilla.

through the piriform aperture, the zygomatic buttresses and the pterygoid plates. In the Le Fort II fracture pattern, the upper jaw is detached at a fracture line running across the nasal bones through the inferior orbital rims and through the zygomatic buttresses and pterygoid plates. In the Le Fort III pattern the upper jaw is detached from the base of skull at a fracture line running through the nasofrontal suture, the ethmoid bone, the frontozygomatic sutures, the arches of the zygomas and the pterygoid

plates (Fig. 11.56). However, this time-honoured classification does not provide a full description of the degrees of comminution and displacement, nor does it mention two common associated and very important lesions — the parasagittal fracture of the hard palate and the smaller dento-alveolar segment fractures of the upper jaw. Furthermore the Le Fort classification does not relate the severity of the maxillary fracture to other areas of the craniofacial skeleton. These deficiencies are redressed

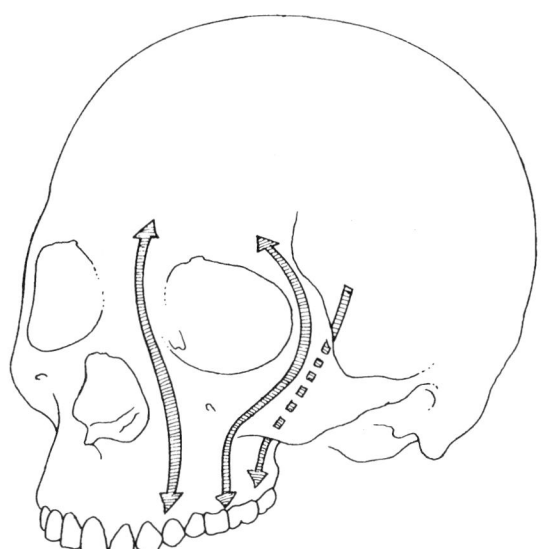

Fig. 11.54 Maxillary anatomy. The load-bearing vertical bony buttresses of the midface.

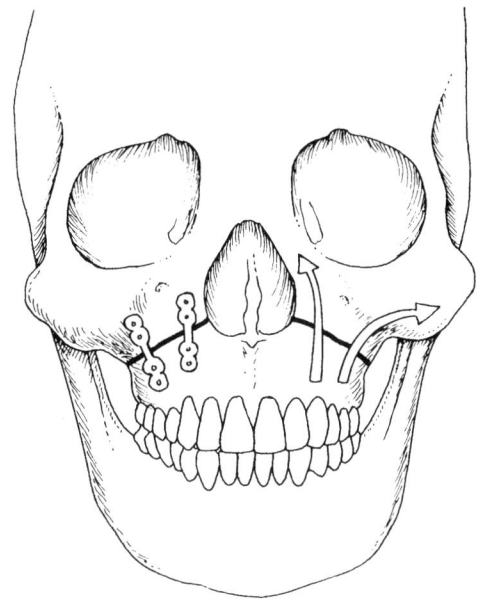

Fig. 11.55 Maxillary anatomy. If possible, plates should be placed longitudinally along the line of the load-bearing buttresses.

in the alphanumeric classification system proposed by Cooter & David (p. 35).

Clinical assessment

The signs depend on the degree of displacement and comminution, and on whether the fracture extends to the orbits and skull base. Intraoral inspection may show the upper alveolar arch to be intact, or split into two fragments by a longitudinal (parasagittal) fracture, or mobile dental alveolar segments may be seen. Gross loss of bone

and oral mucosa can occur in high velocity missile injuries (p. 445). Malocclusion may be evident: it may be complained of by the patient, or be obvious on inspection. However, the examiner must keep in mind the common occurrence of pretraumatic occlusal disharmony, especially anterior open bite and crossbites. In the typical fracture of the upper jaw with an intact alveolar arch, posterior and inferior displacement of the occlusal surface will result in an anterior open bite (Fig. 11.57). This backward and downward movement is in part due to the inclination of

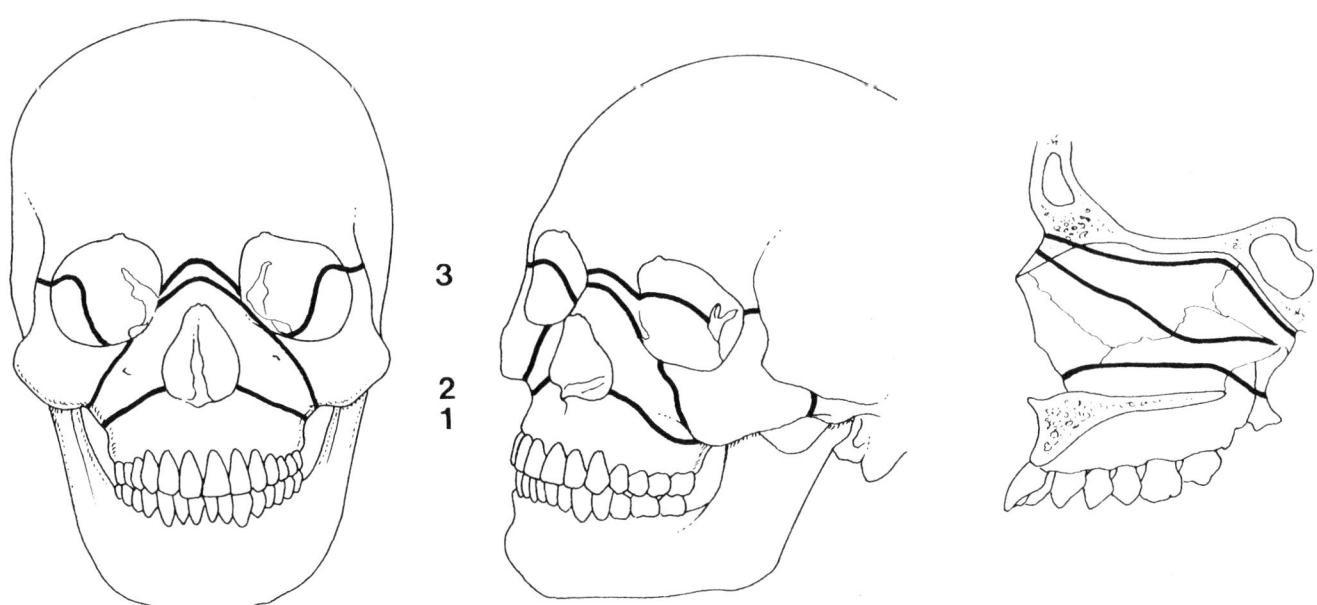

Fig. 11.56 Maxillary fracture classification. The classical fracture lines of Le Fort.

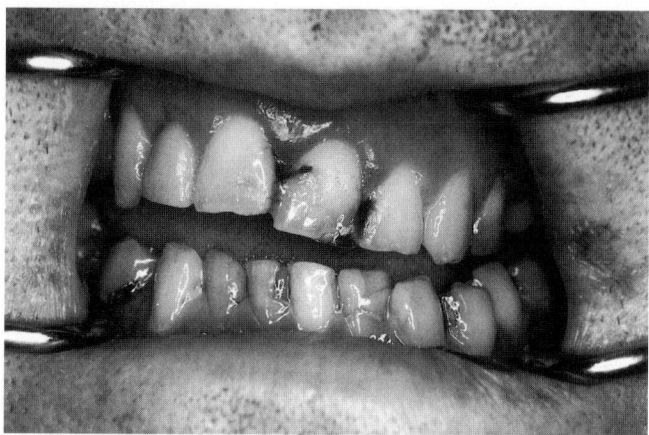

Fig. 11.57 Clinical signs of maxillary fractures. Anterior open bite associated with posterior displacement of an upper jaw fracture and gagging of the posterior dentition.

the base of the skull, and in part to the vectors of pull by the medial pterygoid muscles. The movement forces the mandible open producing the appearance of elongation of the midface.

On external inspection the cheeks are typically swollen by post-traumatic oedema, bleeding and bruising, or by emphysema from air forced out of the paranasal sinuses. If the fracture of the upper jaw extends into the orbit, then swelling and bruising of the eyelids may be apparent (Fig. 11.58). The clinical methods of examination described in Chapter 6 may be diagnostic. A gloved finger on the hard palate exerting an upward and rocking force may elicit pain, crepitus and abnormal mobility (Fig. 6.5). It may be possible to locate the site or sites of abnormal mobility by performing bimanual palpation at the piriform base and the nasofrontal and frontozygomatic suture areas in turn while applying the upward and rocking force to the hard palate. In some cases gross midface instability can be demonstrated by asking the patient to bite upward with his mandible, resulting in upward movement of the upper jaw. Careful examination along these lines will often enable the examiner to deduce the most likely pattern and level of a fracture of the maxilla.

Radiological assessment

The radiological findings provide back-up evidence for the clinical diagnosis. Plain anteroposterior and occipitomental X-ray pictures may demonstrate fluid in the maxillary sinuses (Fig. 11.59), or displaced fracture lines in the zygomatic buttress, inferior orbital rim or piriform margin. Parasagittal fractures of the hard palate can sometimes be visualized in plain X-ray pictures. However, the most useful radiological investigation is the CT scan with axial, coronal and three-dimensional (3D) reformatting. This is our standard radiological examination for fractures

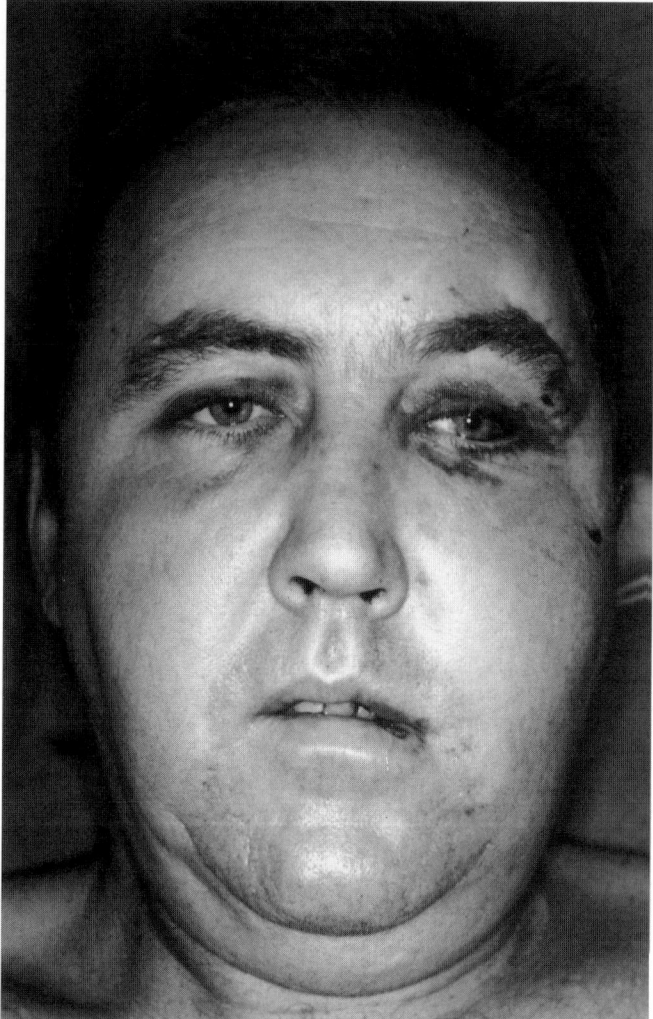

Fig. 11.58 Clinical signs of maxillary fractures. Elongation of the midface, bruising and swelling of the cheeks and eyelids accompany a midface fracture involving upper jaw and orbits.

of the upper jaw (p. 190). Axial cuts show fractures of the posterior wall of the maxillary antrum and of the pterygoid plates (Fig. 11.60). Splits of the hard palate and alveolus, as well as dento-alveolar segmental fractures, are readily seen (Fig. 11.61A,B). Coronal CT scans of the midface give detailed information on fractures of the anterior maxilla, especially those in which the fractures transgress the piriform buttress and/or the inferior orbital rim (Fig. 11.62). The coronal scan also visualizes parasagittal fractures of the palate (Fig. 11.63). Axial CT scans must be studied to detect fractures in the region of the pterygoid plates, a confirmatory sign of a fracture of the upper jaw; in the absence of this, the anterior maxillary fracture may be part of an upper midface/naso-orbital fracture with an intact upper jaw (Fig. 11.64). 3D reformatting may add little when displacements are slight, but when displacements and comminution are

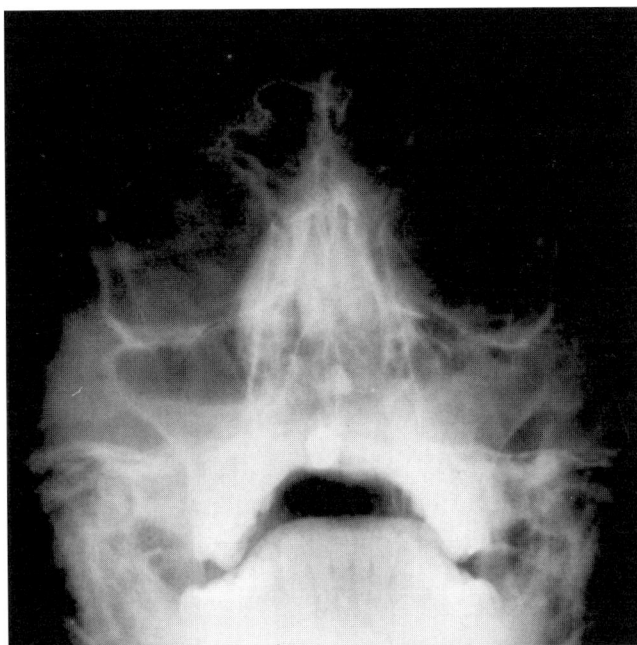

Fig. 11.59 Radiology of maxillary fractures. Occipitomental view demonstrating fluid levels in both maxillary antra and fractured nose, but little else.

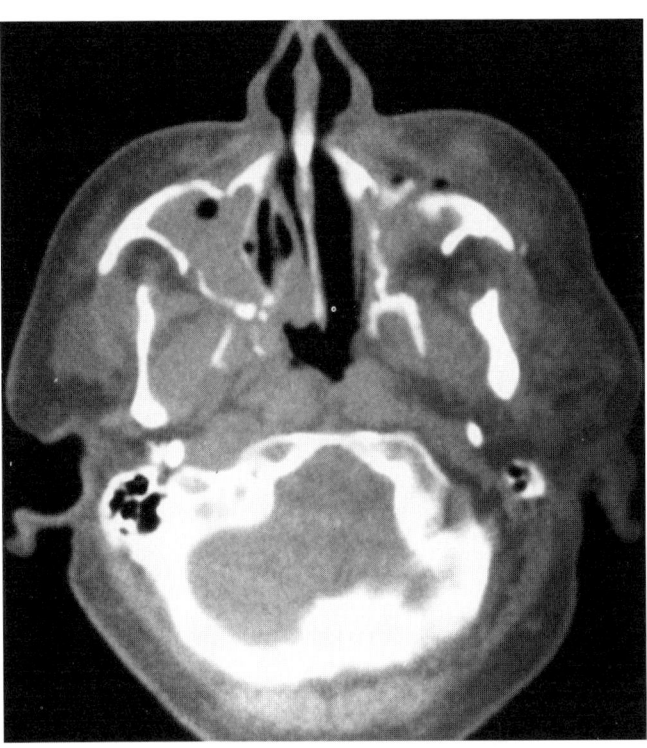

Fig. 11.60 Radiology of maxillary fractures. Axial CT scan of midmaxilla, demonstrating fractures of the anterior, posterior and medial walls of both maxillae and the right side pterygoid plates.

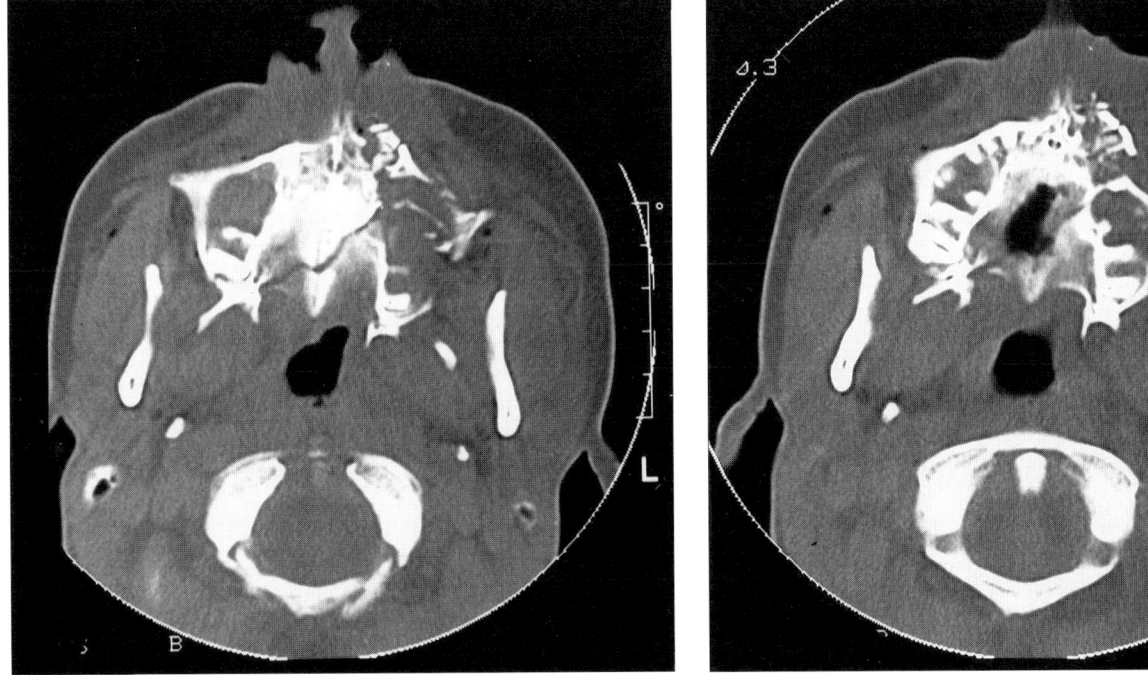

A   B

Fig. 11.61 Radiology of maxillary fractures. A A diagonal fracture of the hard palate and associated dento-alveolar area. **B** A higher cut through the same fracture.

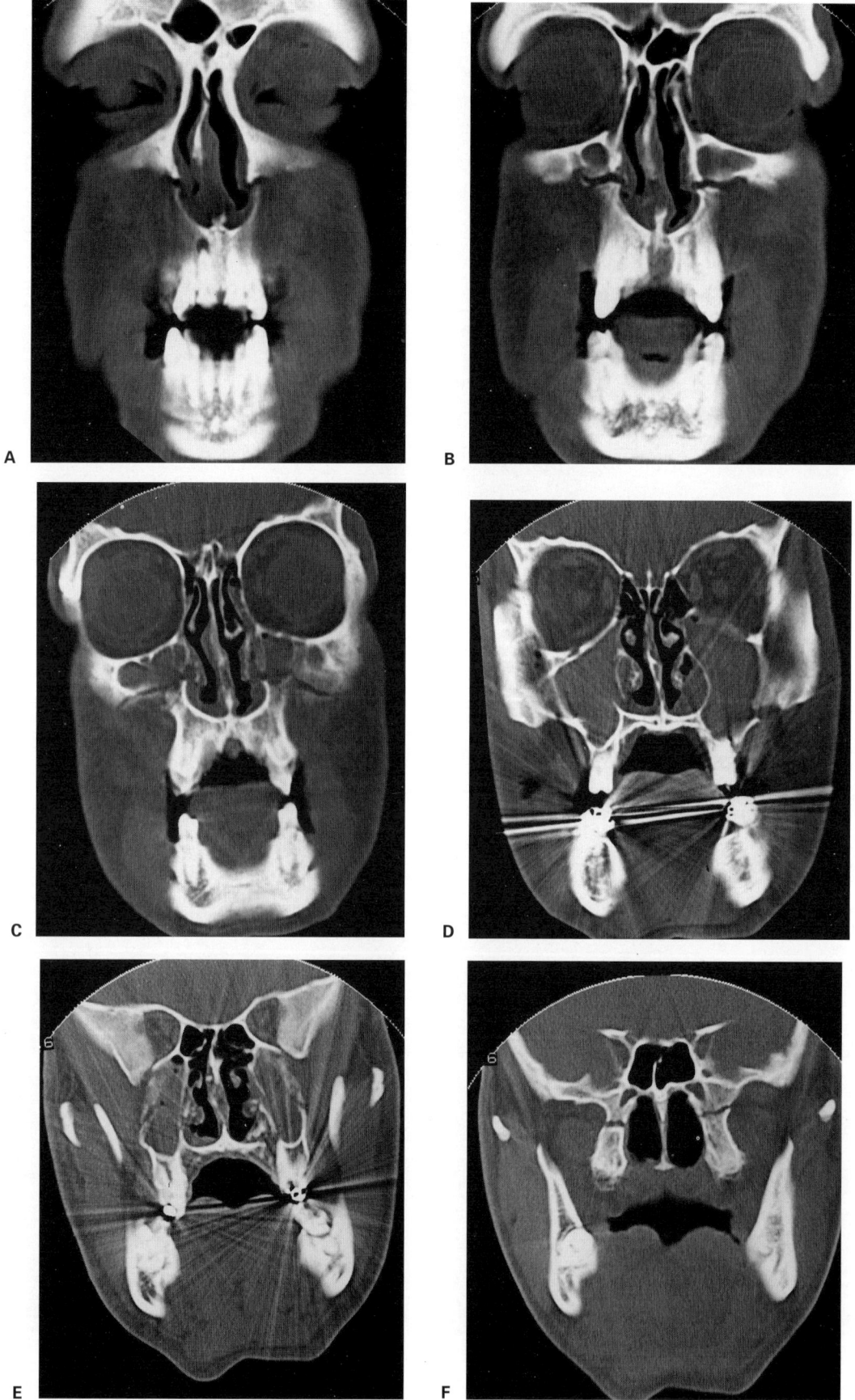

Fig. 11.62 Radiology of maxillary fractures. Series of coronal scans anterior to posterior maxilla demonstrating the progression of horizontal maxillary fracture lines from the piriform margins (**A** and **B**) through the mid anterior maxilla (**C**) to the zygomatic buttress areas (**D**) and thence to the posterior maxillae (**E**) and finally the pterygoid plates (**F**).

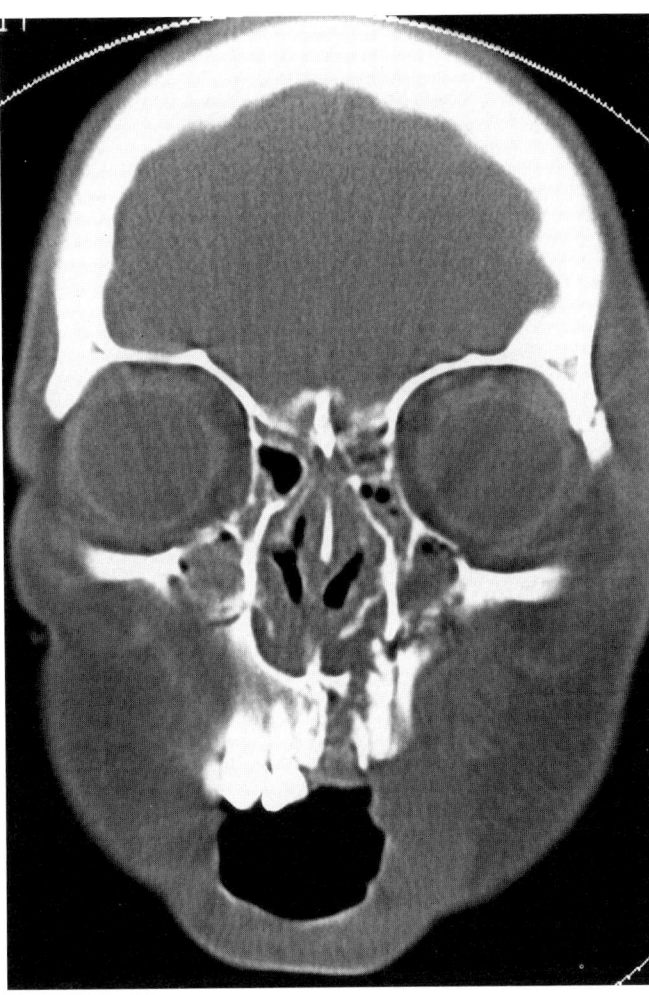

Fig. 11.63 Radiology of maxillary fractures. Coronal views of fractures through both piriform margins, the left side of the palate and fractures into both orbital floors.

extensive, the graphic visualization given by the 3D scan is valuable and may indicate a need for bone grafting.

Principles of management

Management of these fractures depends in the first place on whether the fracture is thought to be in need of surgical reduction and stabilization. There are several clinical situations where surgical reduction would be contraindicated:

1. Where clinical and radiological examination confirms an undisplaced fracture. In both edentulous and immature patients, an undisplaced fracture is invariably stable to masticatory forces.
2. In the edentulous patient where there is only minor radiological evidence of displacement, and where the fracture appears to be stable to masticatory forces. Bony union of these fractures can be confidently expected (Thaller & Kawamoto 1990). In these cases, prosthodontic adjustment will be sufficient. Patients

are given a soft non-chew diet for 6 weeks and then allowed a graduated return to normal eating.
3. Patients with associated severe brain injuries who are not expected to survive.

When none of the above contraindications exist and where there is displacement and instability, then consideration must be given to anatomical reduction and stabilization of upper jaw fractures.

Preoperative dental assessment

In addition to full clinical and radiological examination, patients will require assessment by a dental specialist (p. 355). Impressions of the dental arch and teeth will be used to cast a plaster model. An expert in dental occlusion will study the model, cutting it at sites of vertical fractures through the occlusion and then mounting the fragments on an articulator in the exact position of pretraumatic occlusion. An acrylic bite wafer will then be constructed which will be used peroperatively and often postoperatively to maintain correct occlusal relationship. Close dental collaboration is even more important with upper jaw fractures than with lower jaw fractures. In the latter, the strength and solid form of the mandible ensure that anatomical reduction of the fracture site is relatively easy and the occlusion is used as a secondary check on the correctness of the reduction. In fractures of the upper jaw the complex structure of the maxillary bone makes certainty about anatomical reduction of a fracture more difficult and the dental relationships assume a high degree of importance in establishing that reduction is achieved. This is especially important where there are vertical fractures of the upper jaw, e.g. parasagittal fractures and dento-alveolar segmental fractures. In these fractures, the acrylic bite wafer can be used to control rotational forces on the teeth during the period of healing.

Where open reduction and miniplate fixation are indicated in the edentulous patient then Gunning or modified denture splints may be used temporarily. But where intermaxillary fixation and suspension wiring or interfragment wiring are the only option for fracture stabilization, then appropriate dental splints must be maintained for 6–8 weeks. Similarly, where external frames are the only stabilization method available for an upper jaw fracture, cast metal cap splints must be bonded to the teeth before surgery: a rod is then attached to the cap splints, and in turn fixed to the external frame. The dental specialist will also manage any acute dental injuries along the lines described in Chapter 12.

Timing of definitive treatment

Much has been written on the desirability of performing surgical correction of the midface fracture as early as

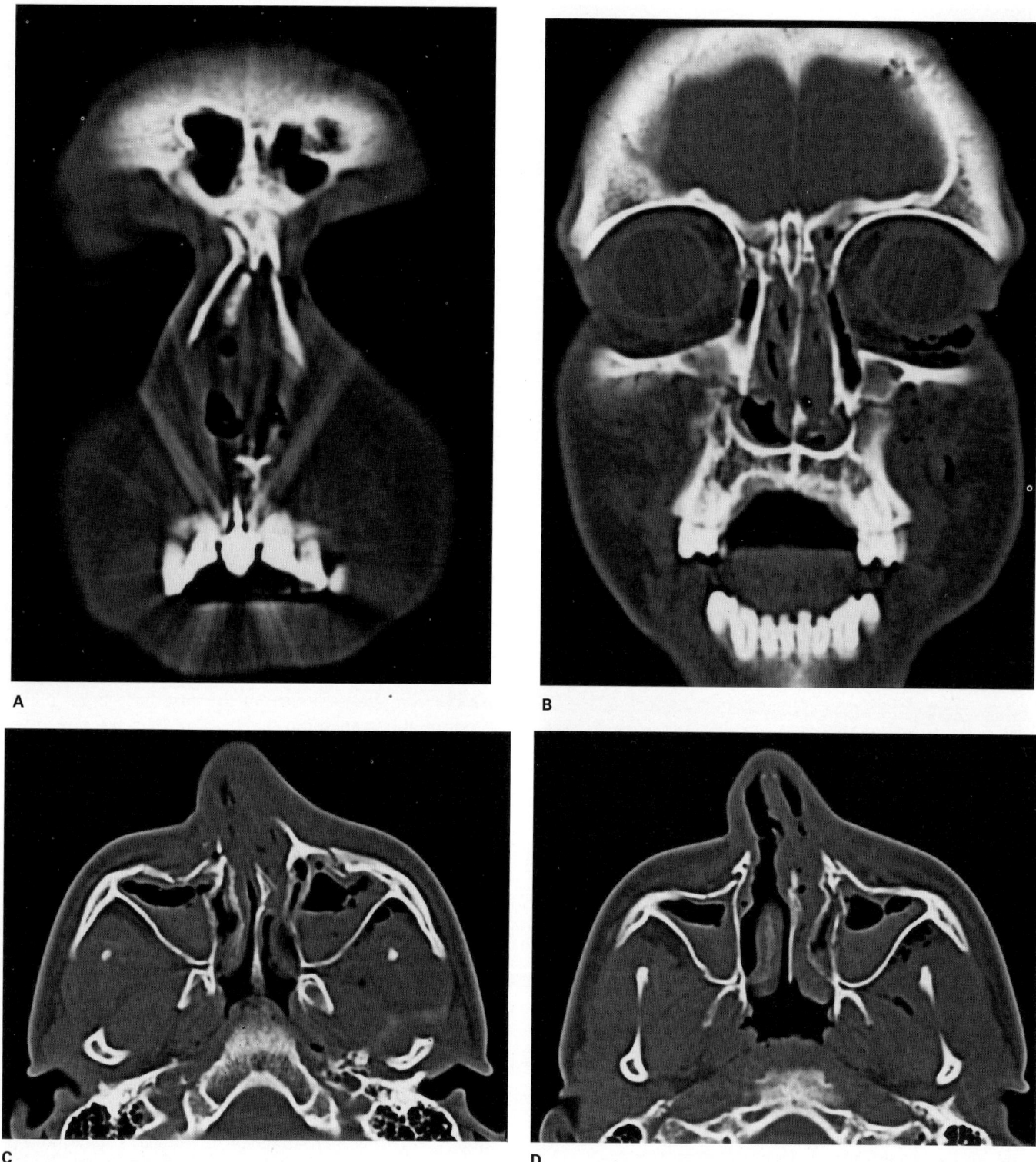

A

B

C

D

Fig. 11.64 Radiology of maxillary fractures. Coronal views of anterior maxillary fracture associated with naso-orbital fracture (**A** and **B**). The upper jaw was intact as evidenced by the intact pterygoid plates on axial cuts (**C** and **D**).

possible after injury (Gruss & McKinnon 1986; Manson et al 1985b). The chief argument is the belief that early accurate bony reconstruction will prevent the development of soft-tissue contractures which in turn will lead

to post-traumatic deformity. Gruss (1990) has stated that he believes such an outcome will be unavoidable if repair of midface fractures is not accomplished within 10–14 days after the injury. However, there are other factors which must be considered when deciding on the timing of surgery for upper jaw fracture reduction. Perhaps the foremost of these is the consideration of priorities of management of other injuries. Brain injury is often associated with facial fractures and disturbances of cerebral physiology may take some time to stabilize. Derdyn et al (1990) studied patients with combined facial fractures and cerebral injuries and identified factors which they felt were contraindications to early surgical reduction of facial fractures. These included a Glasgow Coma Score of five or less, CT evidence of intracranial haemorrhage with midline cranial shift and/or basal cistern effacement, and intracranial pressure > 15 mmHg (p. 369). Brandt et al (1991) in a similar study were unable to identify any neurological complications directly attributable to craniofacial repair in the first 24 h after injury. However, they stated that craniofacial repairs should be delayed in patients with documented intracranial pressure > 25 mmHg. Other systemic injuries that may demand delay in facial fracture treatment include unstable cervical spine injuries, cardiovascular instability and severe intrathoracic injuries; ocular injuries that represent an immediate threat to vision (p. 245) may also impose delay if a combined operation is undesirable. Moreover, a certain amount of time will be required to perform a radiological and dental work-up necessary to allow adequate fracture management. In our unit, this usually takes 2 or 3 days. Finally, consideration will need to be given to the practical requirements of co-ordinating surgery with other specialties. This may involve collaboration with a neurosurgeon in management of intracranial injuries or with an orthopaedic surgeon in management of distal skeletal injuries. David (1984) has shown the cost-effectiveness of a combined approach in craniofacial injuries. Where there are no contraindications, our unit policy is to repair midfacial fractures as soon as possible, which is usually 2 or 3 days after injury, but may be any time up to 10 days.

It used to be argued that early reduction and immobilization of Le Fort III fractures will reduce the risk of meningitis. Experience and study of the pathology of anterior fossa fractures give little evidence to support this view. Nevertheless, this consideration suggests that if there are no contraindications, unstable fractures of this type should be fixed as soon as the appropriate preparations have been completed.

Airway management

Upper jaw fractures may compromise both the oral cavity and the nasal cavity, and placement of an endotracheal tube requires careful consideration and discussion with the anaesthetist. When the nasal bones are not significantly displaced or comminuted a nasotracheal tube will allow the necessary surgical procedures to be carried out without special difficulty (Fig. 10.1). If a nasal fracture requires reduction then there are only two alternatives: oral tracheal intubation or tracheostomy. It is often possible to place an armoured tube behind the mandibular molars. This tube is fixed with a wire to the posterior dentition, allowing intermaxillary fixation to be applied during the operation (Fig. 10.2). This avoids the need for tracheostomy. But should the eruption of the posterior molars be such that there is not enough room for even a small tube, then there will be no choice but tracheostomy. Zachariades et al (1983) have listed several other indications for tracheostomy. These include severe gunshot injuries, severe crush injuries, bilateral mandibular and maxillary fractures, gross maxillary fracture with profuse bleeding and midface fractures associated with cranial, thoracic or spinal injuries. We agree that combined cerebral, facial and chest injuries are best managed by early tracheostomy to lessen the risk of cerebral oedema due to hypoxia or increased venous pressure (p. 381): in such cases, tracheostomy should be done as soon as possible. Also we accept tracheostomy as part of the management of profuse facial bleeding from midface fractures, to secure the airway while the facial cavities are packed to control bleeding. However, since the advent of miniplate fixation we have not routinely used tracheostomy in bilateral maxillary and mandibular fractures, preferring nasotracheal or orotracheal intubation as described above.

Disimpaction

Where closed methods of fixation are used, reduction may be carried out using the specially designed forceps described by Rowe & Killey (1955). One blade of each forcep is inserted along each nostril floor while the other blade is placed via the mouth over the hard palate mucosa. When both forceps are in position the surgeon is able to exert powerful leverage on the upper jaw via the hard palate which is securely gripped between the blades of the forceps (Fig. 11.65). It is important to exercise care to avoid tearing the soft palate attachment to the hard palate, which may result in loss of vascularity to the jaw and teeth (see above). While these instruments may also be used in methods employing open exposure of maxillary fractures, disimpaction and mobilization of the upper jaw may be obtained by tapping an osteotome into some part of the fracture and then exerting digital pressure over the alveolus anteriorly in a downward direction. This method avoids the risk of damage to the junction of soft and hard palate with forceps. Minimally displaced non-comminuted fractures of the upper jaw may be difficult to disimpact but this can be achieved in all cases by using one or other or a combination of the above methods.

Fracture stabilization

Until the last decade, stabilization of upper jaw fractures

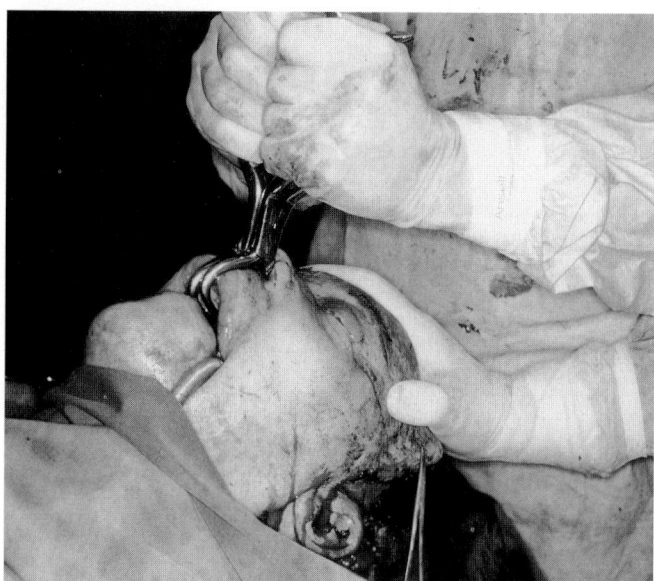

Fig. 11.65 Mobilizing upper jaw fractures. Two forceps have been applied to grasp the hard palate and mobilize the upper jaw fracture. This manoeuvre must be done with the head stabilized to avoid injury to the neck and will usually be accompanied by brisk bleeding.

was carried out either by external frame fixation or by internal suspension wiring depending on the clinical indications. In both techniques the upper jaw was fixed to the lower jaw in the position of pretraumatic occlusion by intermaxillary wiring or cap splints, or in the case of edentulous patients by Gunning splints; the conjoined upper and lower jaw complex was then secured to the intact upper midface or to the skull base. With fractures having minimal comminution and good vertical stability, stabilization was achieved by internal suspension wires passed to the intact zygomatic arches. Where there was gross comminution and vertical instability, the jaws were stabilized with an external frame. This frame was removed 6–8 weeks after surgery, as were the suspension wires. As recently as 1985, Wallace described a new frame for craniomaxillary fixation (p. 24). In the past, we have used external frames styled after Le Vant, fixed to the frontal skull by pins in the outer table (Le Vant et al 1969). Halo frames have also been used when frontal bone fractures have dictated the need to use pins inserted more laterally; this frame provides a very rigid platform for stabilizing bars. However, no matter how mechanically refined the external frame may be, there are practical problems. For the patient, the halo frame has a major disadvantage: lying with the framed head on a pillow is uncomfortable. For the surgeon, judgment as to the exact vertical position of the jaw complex in relation to the skull base is more an educated guess than an exact judgment based on anatomical bony landmarks. Finally, the cumbersome linkage of rods and universal joints cannot provide rigid stability. In 1942 Adams (Fig. 1.22) described a method of internal stabilization of upper jaw fractures.

After reduction, as described above, the upper and lower jaws were stabilized in the pretraumatic occlusion using arch bars and intermaxillary wiring. By this means the intact lower jaw provided anteroposterior stability to the upper jaw. Where the zygomas were also fractured, these were first reduced and stabilized with interosseous wires inserted through incisions over the frontozygomatic and inferior orbital rim fractures sites. The central jaw complex was then stabilized against the now stable lateral midface complex using a heavy wire loop inserted through a drill hole in the frontozygomatic area and passed immediately behind the body of the zygoma through an upper buccal incision to the intermaxillary wiring. The wire was secured to the arch bar in the region of the mandibular first molar on each side and tightened to provide an upward and backward compressive force and hence stabilization. When the lateral midface did not require reduction and stabilization, the suspension wire was passed around the most anterior part of the zygomatic arch via a small cutaneous stab incision; the wire was then secured to the mandibular arch bar and tightening was then carried out. This technique has had wide application and modifications have been described as recently as 1986 (Farole 1986). But for suspension wiring to be successful, there must be effective integrity of the upper jaw buttresses. Clinical experience and high resolution CT scan imaging have shown that this integrity is often lacking: it is far more common to see significant comminution in one or more of these buttresses. When this is so, suspension wires and intermaxillary fixation will not prevent upward movement of the jaw complex along an arc centred at the TMJs (Fig. 11.66). While external frames could be used to greater effect in such cases, they do not provide absolutely rigid stabilization. Moreover, the problem of correct judgment of midfacial height remains when the midfacial buttresses are not directly visualized.

In the early 1980s, many surgeons were dissatisfied with these methods of upper jaw reduction stabilization and began looking for new approaches. This movement was stimulated by the new technology of CT scanning which allowed preoperative imaging of the degree of comminution and displacement in midfacial fractures. Stoll et al (1983) in Germany described a method of stabilization of the midface by an internal metal frame. Two stainless steel rods were passed subcutaneously through an incision over the glabella, one on each side of the nose, down to the anterior maxillae. After the jaws were secured in intermaxillary fixation, two screws were placed at each end of the rods providing stability in both the vertical and sagittal planes (Fig. 11.67). These rods were removed under local anaesthesia 6–8 weeks later. The authors recommended this method in cases with associated cerebral injury as fixation could be carried out quickly. On the other side of the Atlantic, Gruss and Manson extolled the

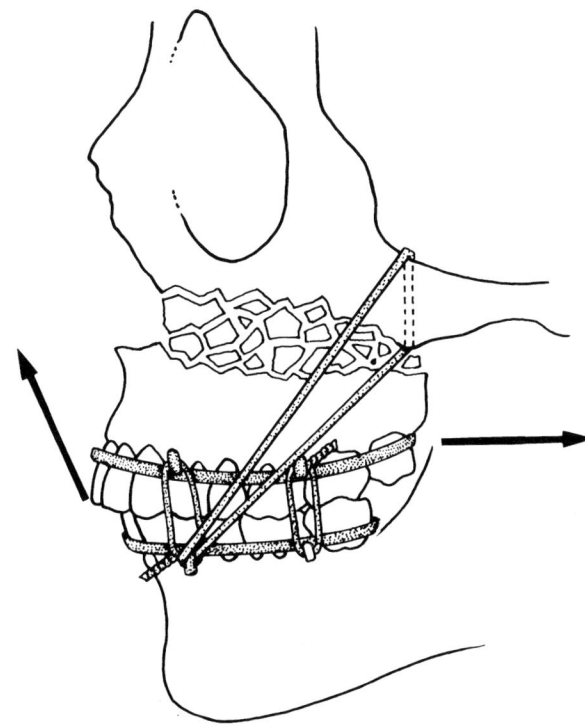

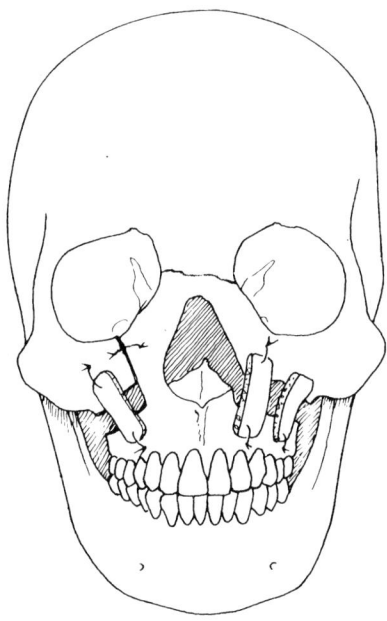

Fig. 11.68 Upper jaw stabilization. Interfragmentary wiring and primary bone grafting as popularized by Gruss and Manson.

Fig. 11.66 Vectors of force following suspension wiring. Adams circumzygomatic compression wiring results in upward movement of the midface when there is comminution of the midface vertical buttresses. Posterior displacement is prevented by the mandibular condyle remaining seated in the glenoid fossa.

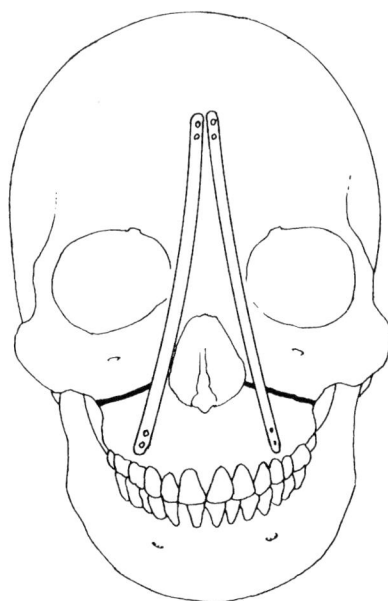

Fig. 11.67 Upper jaw stabilization. Temporary midface stabilizing rods as used by Stoll et al.

virtues of extended open reduction of midface fractures and immediate reconstruction of buttresses with direct fragment wiring and bone grafting if necessary. Only the accessible nasofrontal and zygomaticofrontal buttresses

were reconstructed but the combination of interfragmentary wiring and bone grafts produced good stability and avoided the need for suspension wiring or internal frames (Fig. 11.68) (Manson et al 1985b, Gruss et al 1985b). Schilli et al (1981) pointed out the benefits of extended open reduction followed by stabilization by miniplates and screws to give three-dimensional stability and less need for bone grafting. In a recent review of midface stabilization, Gruss & Phillips (1989) confirmed that miniplate fixation of the midface had almost totally replaced interosseous wires and primary bone grafts in their practice. However, when there were bony buttress defects > 0.5 cm in length they felt that interposition bone grafting was indicated, the bone graft being stabilized to the miniplate. The advent of malleable titanium miniplates has been an important part of the evolution of treatment.

Miniplate technique

Since 1987 open reduction with stabilization by miniplates has been our treatment of choice for displaced upper jaw fractures. Originally we used the titanium miniplates of the Würzburg System, but latterly we have moved to locally manufactured titanium plates and screws (see above). We find these more malleable, conforming better to the underlying bone and reducing the risk of plate spring with subsequent movement and malunion.

Operative management

As stated above, operation is done under endotracheal

anaesthesia, tracheostomy being rarely required. Arch bars are located to teeth of upper and lower jaws. Exposure of the upper jaw fracture lines is performed through an incision in the mucosa of the upper buccal sulcus, taking care not to injure branches of the inferior orbital nerves. When a midface fracture involves the orbit(s), subciliary lower eyelid incisions (p. 238), with or without a coronal scalp flap, may be needed to complete the exposure. The soft tissues are dissected from the maxillae on each side to expose the nasomaxillary and the zygomaticomaxillary buttresses and the related fractures. Often there is significant comminution and small fragments of bone are removed. Larger fragments will be preserved in a weak antibiotic solution — usually 0.2% flucloxacillin in normal saline. This solution is used copiously to irrigate the maxillary sinuses. Disimpaction of the fracture and mobilization of the upper jaw are carefully carried out as described above. An acrylic occlusal wafer is wired to the upper jaw and the jaw is placed into occlusion and stabilized with intermaxillary wires. We are aware that in some centres, interocclusal acrylic wafers are not considered necessary when there is a good dentition, an accurately determined pretraumatic occlusion, and no dento-alveolar fracturing. However, we find the use of wafers invaluable in fractures with more complicated impairments of occlusion. The relationship of the upper jaw to the midface buttresses is then established; an assistant maintains the seating of the mandibular condyles in the glenoid fossae. Usually at least one of the four anterior vertical midface buttresses will not be severely comminuted, providing a guide to the correct vertical relationships between the upper jaw and the remaining midface. Once the relationship is established an AusSystem miniplate is used to stabilize the reduced fracture, with adherence to the principle of reconstructing the vertical load lines and using at least two screws on either side of the fracture line. Accurate shaping of the plate to the bone contours is also important. Care must be taken to avoid damaging dental roots when fractures extend inferiorly in the zygomaticomaxillary buttress. When all four anterior vertical midface buttresses are severely comminuted, it will be necessary to judge the correct vertical positioning of the upper jaws by eye, using the line of contour of the buttresses as a guide; in such cases, bone grafts may be required. Depending on the operator's preference, either outer table of calvaria or split rib graft will be suitable: we prefer calvarial bone, because it is more rigid and holds screws very well and because donor site morbidity is less (p. 241). All four buttresses are stabilized with miniplates and screws before intermaxillary fixation is released. The success of the reduction is then finally confirmed. All surgical fields are copiously irrigated with weak antibiotic solution. Oral mucosal wounds are closed with 3/0 chromicized cat gut or 4/0 Vicryl, depending on individual

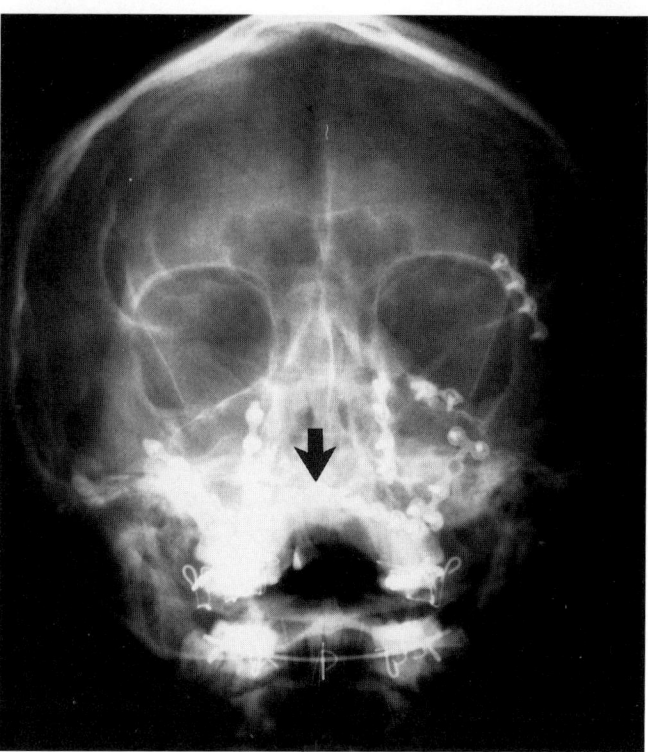

Fig. 11.69 Miniplating of upper jaw fractures. Post-surgical reduction anteroposterior radiograph showing stabilization of fractures seen in Fig. 11.61. The fracture of the alveolus and hard palate has been controlled by locating the teeth in an acrylic bite wafer and interosseous stabilization with a horizontal miniplate and screws (arrow). Four vertical buttress miniplates and screws can be seen stabilizing the occlusal complex to the upper midface.

preference. Finally the mandible is manipulated back and forth into the bite facets of the wafer: the surgeon then confirms that the reduction is satisfactory and that the lower teeth engage cleanly into the wafer and all at the same time (Fig. 11.69).

Management of complex midfacial fractures

The above discussion relates to fractures of the upper jaw at the Le Fort I level. Different treatment sequences must be considered when other bones of the midface are also fractured, and when there is a simultaneous mandibular fracture. Our policy is based on the principles outlined by Markowitz & Manson (1989).

Vertical fractures through the alveolar process of the upper jaw and associated palate can occur with any type of Le Fort fractures. Antoniades et al (1990) found an incidence of 24% of parasagittal fractures of the alveolus and hard palate associated with Le Fort fractures; in this group, there was a 78% incidence of associated mandibular fractures. Manson et al (1990a) described difficulty in preventing rotation of the minor dento-alveolar segment in parasagittal fractures of the upper jaw and recommended open reduction of the posterior aspects of the

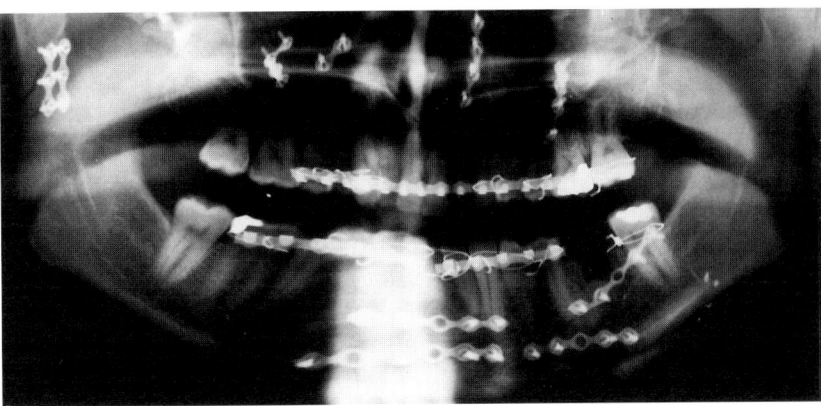

Fig. 11.70 Miniplating of upper and lower jaw fractures.
Orthopantomogram (**A**) and lateral plain film (**B**) demonstrating
miniplate stabilization of a complex mandibular fracture including right
condylar fracture. Doing this first allowed accurate localization and
plating of the upper jaw fracture and associated midface complex
fracture.

hard palate fracture with stabilization by miniplate and
screws under direct vision; miniplate fixation was also
used across the fracture in the vicinity of the piriform
margin. Acrylic occlusal wafers were needed to stabilize
the occlusion in 15% of patients. With this technique,
there was a 10% incidence of plate exposure in the roof
of the mouth.

Where the mandible is also fractured, it is stabilized
with miniplates (see above). This is particularly important
when there is a displaced condylar fracture in association
with an upper jaw fracture; only by open reduction and
miniplate stabilization of the condylar fracture can the
correct anatomical height of the posterior facial skeleton
be established (Fig. 11.70A,B).

More than in any other constellation of CMF fractures, the combined maxillary and mandibular fractures
with comminution and detached dento-alveolar segments
demand expert presurgical dental model planning. We
routinely use an acrylic wafer to locate the teeth on both
upper and lower jaws. The mandibular arch is stabilized
first and checked against the wafer. The maxillary arch
is then reduced by an extended open approach through
the upper buccal sulcus incision. Arch bars are ligated
to the teeth either segmentally or along the whole upper
arch and the teeth are then fixed into the wafer which is
stabilized to the arch bars with wires. Miniplate fixation
across the alveolar fracture, at the level of the piriform
margin or further posteriorly, is carried out and then the
lower jaw is again brought into the wafer to complete
intermaxillary fixation (Fig. 11.69). The patient must
wear the acrylic splint and arch bars on the upper teeth
for a minimum of 6 weeks. With this approach we have
only infrequently found it to be necessary to expose the

hard palate and apply miniplate fixation. But when there
has been loss of alveolar bone and teeth, with significant
comminution, then exposure and miniplate stabilization
of the hard palate component of the fracture may be the
only way of establishing the correct transverse posterior
maxillary relationships.

Where the upper jaw fracture is associated with displaced orbital fractures then these are stabilized in the
manner described below. The occlusal complex, consisting
of the upper and lower jaws united by intermaxillary
fixation, is then brought to the stabilized upper midface
and final stabilization (with or without bone grafting) is
carried out at the Le Fort I level using miniplates according to the principles already described (Fig. 11.71).
Particular care is taken at the close of the reduction to
ensure that the occlusion is satisfactory.

Edentulous upper or lower jaws

In all cases, it is necessary to establish the pretraumatic
anteroposterior jaw relationships; in the edentulous patient it is also important that the correct vertical posterior
facial height be established so that dentures can be fitted.
If possible a Gunning-type splint is made from the
patient's denture. If this is not available then a splint or
splints made from models cast from dental impressions
of the edentulous jaw should be used. These splints are
wired to the upper and lower jaws and then to each
other during the surgery to allow correct reduction of the
fractures in both the anteroposterior and vertical planes
(Fig. 11.72A,B). The management of fractures of the
edentulous jaws is further discussed in Chapter 19
(p. 520).

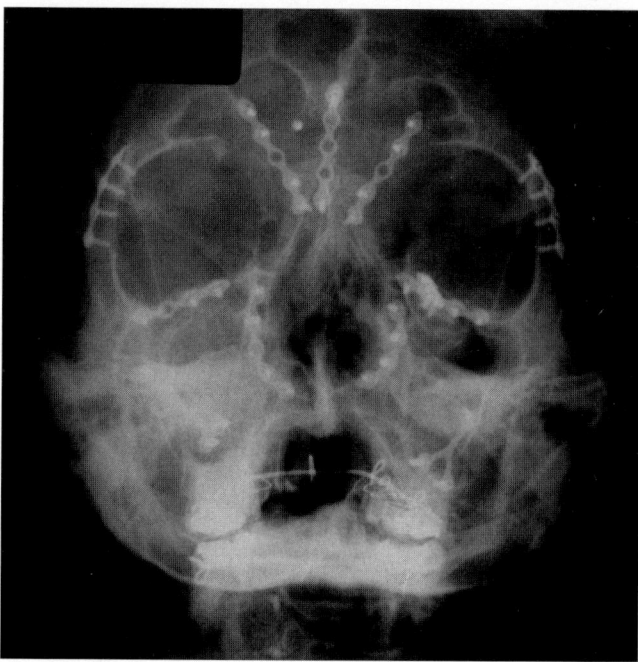

Fig. 11.71 Miniplating of combined upper jaw and orbital fractures. Post-surgical reduction X-ray of upper jaw fractures combined with orbital fractures (Le Fort I, II and III). The reduced occlusal complex has been stabilized to the reduced and stabilized orbital complex using vertical buttress miniplates and screws.

Postoperative management

This is virtually as for mandibular fractures, and can be divided into the same temporal sequences. We release the intermaxillary fixation during the first 24 h to allow safe recovery of the airway (p. 255). The acrylic occlusal wafer may be left on the upper jaw and the mandible permitted to engage in the dental facets on the inferior aspects of the wafer. Light rubber band traction may be placed between upper and lower jaws in the premolar region after the first 24 h to inhibit contraction of the medial pterygoid muscles during the early stages of mobilization. These muscles may cause posterior and caudal displacement of the upper jaw if used strenuously; by providing a closing force, the rubber band effectively inhibits the muscle action. Depending on the severity of the injury, this elastic traction is maintained for 7–14 days before removal. At that time the acrylic bite wafer will also be removed unless it is needed to stabilize the upper jaw arch form as in parasagittal and dento-alveolar fractures, when the acrylic bite wafer will be left in situ for 6–8 weeks. During the first 24 h the patient is allowed to sip water by mouth and oral hygiene is attended to by nursing staff using suction, dressed probes or more sophisticated water picks or air guns. A small-headed soft toothbrush is useful for cleaning around arch bars and wires while mouthwashes will give the patient a sense of comfort and improved hygiene.

The intraoperative antibiotics are continued intravenously for 48 h; we use flucloxacillin and metronidazole (p. 236).

The patient is nursed sitting up as soon as possible to reduce facial swelling. Jaw mobilization is commenced

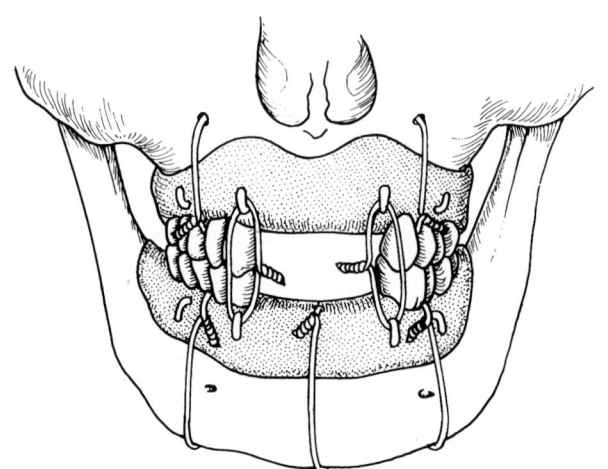

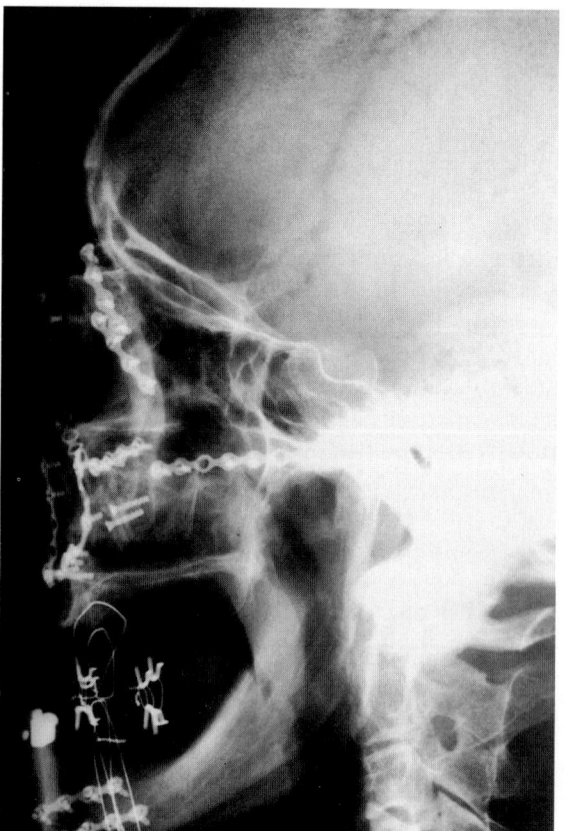

Fig. 11.72 Denture splintage of upper jaw fractures. A Diagram of denture type splints wired to the upper and lower jaws and then to each other. **B** Lateral radiograph of an edentulous patient with upper and lower jaw fractures where the dentures were modified to enable intermaxillary fixation of the jaws and aid in reduction of the upper jaw fracture.

as soon as possible, unless other injuries cause delay. Pain relief is given as required (p. 257). Over the first week a non-chew diet is instituted with appropriate caloric and nutritional content. Once the patient is managing this diet and maintaining good oral hygiene, and depending on the demands of other injuries, then he/she is discharged from hospital, often as early as 2–5 days after surgery. Before discharge, the position of plates and screws and the relationships of the condyles in the glenoid fossae are checked by OPG of the mandible, and antero-posterior and lateral views of the skull and facial bones as well as appropriately tilted occipitomental views. Between 2 and 6 weeks, outpatient follow-up is maintained on a fortnightly basis. Hygiene and nutritional status are checked as well as mouth opening and occlusion. Dental arch bars and bite wafer are removed between 6 and 8 weeks in cases where these had been judged to be necessary. Patients are then referred for dental assessment of tooth vitality, occlusion and hygiene (p. 360). Further reviews are carried out over 1 year to establish the restoration of oral function as well as recovery of soft-tissue scarring and cutaneous nerve function. The success of dental restorative measures is also confirmed and recorded.

Complications

These include:

- Malunion and malocclusion
- Non-union
- Facial deformity, especially soft-tissue sagging
- Infection
- Nasal obstruction
- Lacrimal duct obstruction.

Malunion and malocclusion

Malunion with associated malocclusion and loss of normal facial form are the most significant complications of upper jaw fractures. Severe comminution of midfacial buttresses with or without bone loss may make stabilization of upper jaw fractures difficult. Poor fixation of screws in thin maxillary bone may lead to movement after operation; to prevent this, it may be worth using a piece of bone graft behind the maxillary bone to act as a nut for the screw, which thus acts as a bolt. Failure to seat the condyles in the glenoid fossae during the time that the plates are being applied is another cause of relapse and malocclusion, commonly resulting in anterior open bite. Failure to produce good conformation of plates to the underlying bony shapes may result in additive displacing forces and again malunion is the result; this is less likely to occur with the more malleable plates favoured by us. The finding of malunion will require full dental and radiological reassessment. If deformity is mild, spot grinding of

tooth facets may provide sufficient adjustment to allow normal function. Where malunion is gross, then osteotomy may be required with or without preliminary bone grafting of the anterior maxilla and appropriate buttress stabilization with miniplates.

Non-union

Today this is a rare event in maxillary fractures, though occasionally seen when severely comminuted fractures were treated by closed suspension wiring.

Facial deformity

While the positioning of the posterior maxilla, in any plane, probably has little or no effect on the facial contour, the anterior maxilla is critical for proper balance. Inadvertent impaction of the maxilla, a significant problem in the days of wire fixation, creates the impression of an aged face by eliminating maxillary incisor display and foreshortening the face. Inferior malpositioning, much less common, creates an anterior open bite (due to posterior interference) and displays excessive gingiva. Obviously, improper positioning in the anteroposterior direction creates similar problems. Furthermore a discrepancy in midline position is readily apparent to the casual observer.

Where fracture exposure has required dissection of soft tissues from the zygomatic body, careful attention must be given to adequate suspension of soft tissue in this area. Failure to appreciate this point may lead to loss of pretraumatic cheek prominence through soft-tissue sagging.

Infection

We have seen several cases of chronic maxillary sinusitis some years after a fracture of the upper jaw. Management includes removal of buttress plates and screws, after which the infection will usually subside.

Nasal obstruction

Nasal obstructive symptoms may follow upper jaw fractures through fracture dislocations of nasal septal cartilage and bone. Once the nasal mucosa has soundly healed then appropriate septoplasty may solve this problem.

Lacrimal duct obstruction

Lacrimal obstruction is an uncommon complication of upper jaw fractures. Balle et al (1989) found eight cases of lacrimal obstruction in 104 maxillary fractures of Le Fort types II and III. Obstruction presents as epiphora, with or without recurrent dacryocystitis. Diagnosis of the level of lacrimal obstruction is confirmed on dacryocystography; if confirmed the condition may be treated by dacryocystorhinostomy (p. 429).

FRACTURES AFFECTING THE ORBIT

NASO-ORBITO-ETHMOID FRACTURES

Surgical pathology

Naso-orbito-ethmoid fractures are relatively uncommon injuries. The result of direct trauma to the midface, the fractures may be confined to the naso-orbito-ethmoid region, or more frequently occur in association with other midfacial injuries. While the primary point of injury is the nasal bone complex, a high energy impact often produces radiation posteriorly in the underlying delicate ethmoid framework, superiorly into the frontal sinus, laterally to the orbital floor and inferiorly into the nasal septum and maxillae (Fig. 11.73). Consequently the nomenclature to describe these injuries has varied according to the particular area of interest to individual authors. McCoy (1959) coined the term 'naso-ethmoid-orbital', more frequently phrased as naso-orbito-ethmoid, which best delineates these injuries. Management is challenging because of the intricate and complex three-dimensional skeletal anatomy of the region, the frequent coexisting soft-tissue injuries (especially of the medial canthal ligament and nasolacrimal duct) and the difficulties in achieving and maintaining fracture reduction.

As with most facial fractures there has been a move from techniques of closed reduction and splinting, often with poor outcomes, to a more invasive strategy of open reduction and stable internal fixation. The challenge in the treatment of naso-orbito-ethmoid fractures remains the restoration of bony nasal projection and the restitution of nasal and orbital soft tissues, in particular the medial canthal ligament. Only by understanding the anatomy of this region is optimal management possible.

These fractures are characterized by disruption of the naso-orbito-ethmoid region with isolation of a central unstable bone fragment to which the medial canthal ligament remains attached, exerting a laterally displacing force. The resultant deformity is a depressed nasal root, telecanthus and shortening of the palpebral fissure (Fig. 11.74).

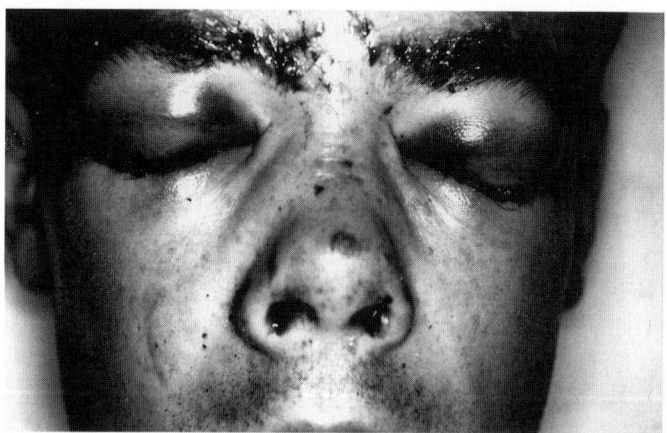

A

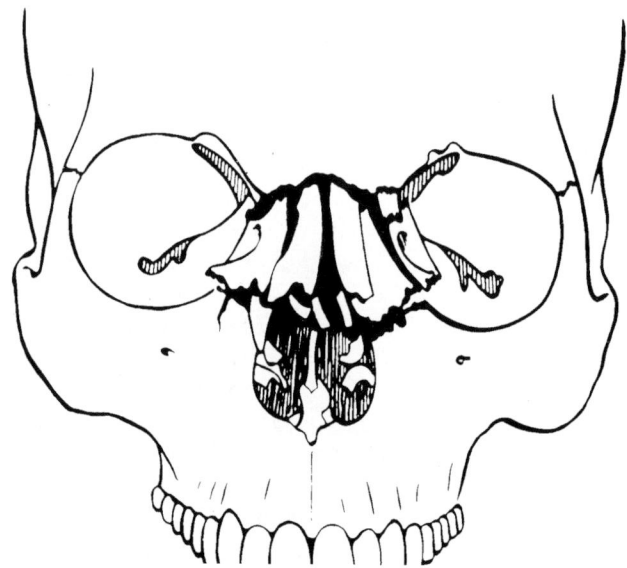

Fig. 11.73 Anatomy of naso-orbito-ethmoid fractures.
Conventional pattern of naso-orbito-ethmoid fracturing with comminution.

B

Fig. 11.74 Clinical signs of naso-orbito-ethmoid fractures.
A and **B** Frontal and right lateral views reveal depression of nasal root, mild telecanthus and foreshortening of the nasal dorsum.

The naso-orbito-ethmoid region lies at the confluence of the cranium, orbit, nose and maxilla and the reconstruction of all these regions is required for an acceptable outcome.

The frontal process of the maxilla, the maxillary process of the frontal bone and the proximal segment of the nasal bones constitute the upper portion of the central midfacial buttress or pillar. Protected posteriorly is the thin medial orbital wall composed largely of the lacrimal bone, and the orbital plate of the ethmoid bone (lamina papyracea). Dissipation of the impacting force as it proceeds posteriorly usually prevents the fracture displacement from extending to the optic canal. Above and laterally, the medial orbital wall becomes the thin orbital roof, the anterior portion of which is the floor of the frontal sinus. Medial to, and lying behind, the naso-ethmoid buttress, and below the anterior cranial fossa, the interorbital space is composed of the ethmoid sinuses. The posterior boundary is the sphenoid bone. With the application of significant force to the naso-orbito-ethmoid region, disruption and buckling of the interorbital space occurs, with potential for displacement posteriorly. Radiation of fracture lines superiorly will involve the anterior cranial fossa floor with attendant risks of a cranionasal fistula (p. 376) and olfactory tract disruption. In our experience, the association of a naso-orbito-ethmoid fracture with extensive disruption of the anterior cranial fossa is not very common (Table 13.2); however, when this association does occur, it may have serious implications.

The frontal sinus lies above the anterior interorbital space, with variable lateral extensions. The anterior wall is thick, providing structural support from side to side. Bony septa, the patterns of which vary, traverse the sinus, attaching the anterior wall to the thin posterior wall. The floor of the frontal sinus is the medial roof of the orbit. Centrally the frontal sinus drains into the nose; the drainage of the sinus into the ethmoid infundibulum or middle meatus (Fig. 2.8) is at risk when the anterior ethmoidal labyrinth is severely comminuted. The nasal bones complete the bony pyramid anteriorly. The medial canthal ligament and lacrimal drainage system comprise the soft-tissue elements likely to be injured in this region. The three limbs of the medial canthal ligament — superior, anterior and posterior — envelope the lacrimal sac. The ligament maintains eyelid position in relation to the globe and forms the medial component of the suspensory sling of the eyelids (Fig. 11.75). Disruption by laceration, or through mobilization of the bony attachment, allows an unopposed lateral pull in the suspensory sling, causing telecanthus and shortened palpebral fissure.

Lacrimal drainage occurs via both lacrimal canaliculi which run in a fibrous sheath, the palpebral extensions of the medial canthal ligament. Uniting, they enter the posterolateral aspect of the lacrimal sac located in the lacrimal fossa and overlaid in its upper portion by the me-

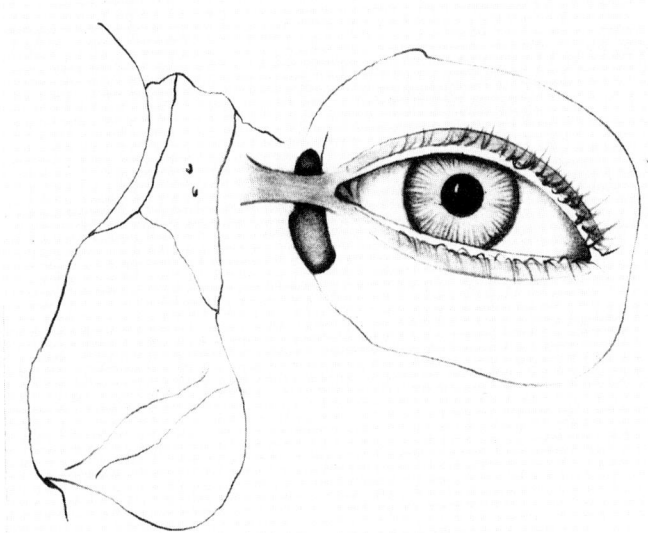

Fig. 11.75 Anatomy of medial canthal region. Diagrammatic representation of the medial canthal ligament as the medial component of the eyelid suspensory sling overlying the lacrimal sac.

dial canthal ligament (Robinson & Stranc 1970). The sac is continuous with the nasolacrimal duct (Fig. 2.38) as it passes inferiorly, posteriorly and slightly laterally through a distance of approximately 12 mm in the bone to enter the nose below the inferior turbinate (Gruss et al 1985a).

Classification

The fractures may be unilateral or bilateral, simple or comminuted, closed or compound; they may occur in isolation or in association with more extensive fracturing of the forehead, orbit or maxilla. Fractures are bilateral in two-thirds of cases; while in > 90% there are other associated facial fractures (Cruse et al 1980). These authors reported 33 cases in 182 patients, an incidence of 18%. With improved imaging techniques and wide exposures, the true incidence of these injuries should be better understood.

Several classifications of naso-orbito-ethmoid fractures have been proposed. Markowitz et al (1991) group them into Types I–III, within each subdivision an ascending scale of severity of comminution. Gruss (1982) extends his classification in accord with the almost uniform extension of these fractures into the adjacent bony skeleton (Table 11.2).

Our system of scoring by the craniofacial disruption index quantifies the extent and pattern of bony damage in a global fashion.

Clinical assessment

A history of significant blunt trauma to the central midface, especially the glabella and nasal root region, should evoke suspicion of a naso-orbito-ethmoid fracture.

Table 11.2 Classification of naso-orbito-ethmoid fractures

A. Markowitz et al (1991)

Type I Single central fragment bearing medial canthus
      — unilateral
      — bilateral
Type II Comminution of bony central fragment without extension beneath area of canthal insertion
      — unilateral
      — bilateral
Type III Comminution of bony central segment with extension beneath area of canthal insertion
      — unilateral
      — bilateral

B. Gruss (1982)

1. Naso-orbital alone
2. Naso-orbital and central maxillary
3. Naso-orbital and Le Fort II and III
4. Naso-orbital and orbital dystopia
5. Naso-orbital and loss of bone

In the past, extreme soft-tissue swelling and the absence of significant early localizing functional deficits often led to late diagnosis or misdiagnosis. The resulting cosmetic and functional deformities were significant and almost impossible to correct by secondary means.

The advent of axial and coronal CT scan delineation of the central midface has allowed detailed display of the anatomy of the fracture patterns. Specific clinical examination confirms or refutes the CT diagnosis and establishes whether there is a need for intervention, while the radiological assessment determines the operative approach and the patterns of fixation.

Inspection reveals localized bruising and ecchymoses, sometimes burst open lacerations over the nasal root, and periorbital swelling. Where the fractures spread more widely, diffuse facial oedema is usually seen and obscures the clinical findings. Medially located subconjunctival and periorbital haemorrhages are common. The presence of a laceration in the region of the medial canthal ligament raises the possibility of injury to the nasolacrimal drainage (p. 428).

The characteristic skeletal disruption is best seen in the lateral profile (Figs 11.74 and 11.76). Collapse of the entire bony nasal pyramid results in gross posterior displacement of the nasal dorsum, with tilting superiorly of the nasal tip and creation of an abnormally obtuse nasolabial angle. In frontal view, there is an increase in nasal width superiorly, with obvious upward rotation of the nasal tip. The caudal end of the nasal septum is usually buckled laterally beneath the collapsed nasal dorsum.

Palpation of the naso-orbito-ethmoid region confirms the loss of nasal bony support. Backward pressure on the nasal dorsum accentuates the collapse of nasal contour; there may be bony crepitus. Transverse compression of this region between thumb and index finger over the region of the medial canthal ligaments will elicit painful bony movement. Under anaesthesia, bimanual examination is performed by placing a blunt-tipped clamp intranasally against the portion of the medial orbital wall to which the medial canthal ligament attaches; this produces movement in the unstable fracture. Paskert & Manson (1989) advocate this as a test of need for surgical repair.

A complete ophthalmological assessment is mandatory to exclude associated injuries and as a baseline for follow-up after surgical repair. Neurosurgical evaluation is also needed because of the proximity to the anterior cranial fossa and the potential for fracture extension into this area, often with a dural tear, pneumocephalus, CSF rhinorrhoea and olfactory tract injury. Olfaction should be tested if possible (p. 166), though nasal obstruction often prevents this.

Radiological assessment

Plain radiographs have usually been performed in the emergency room as part of the screening assessment. These seldom contribute significantly to the diagnosis of the fracture pattern and planning management, except when there is pneumocephalus or other sign of anterior fossa involvement.

Direct axial and coronal CT scan evaluation of the naso-orbito-ethmoid region is essential to document the pattern and extent of the bony injury (Fig. 11.76). Extensions of the fracture into the adjacent frontal sinus above, and midface below, are identified; these may modify treatment.

Principles of treatment

In the past these injuries were treated by closed reduction, with fixation by external splintage. A number of authors, including Adams (1942) and Converse & Smith (1966), employed external lead plates or buttons held by transnasal wires to restore nasal form. The inevitable result, in anything but a minimally displaced fracture, was a characteristic nasal root flattening and collapse. Where comminution was marked the compression plates indeed accentuated the posterior recession of the nasal dorsum. The associated shrinkage and contracture of the overlying soft-tissue envelope produced a state almost insoluble by secondary reconstructive means.

Mustardé (1963), Dingman & Natvig (1964) and Stranc (1970) identified and advocated the importance of direct open reduction, direct fixation with wire and reattachment of the medial canthal ligament (Fig. 11.77). When performed through restricted incisions, and where the extent and severity of comminution of the fractures were not accurately defined, the results remained suboptimal.

Modern management identifies in detail the pattern of skeletal injury, to permit planned early wide exposure,

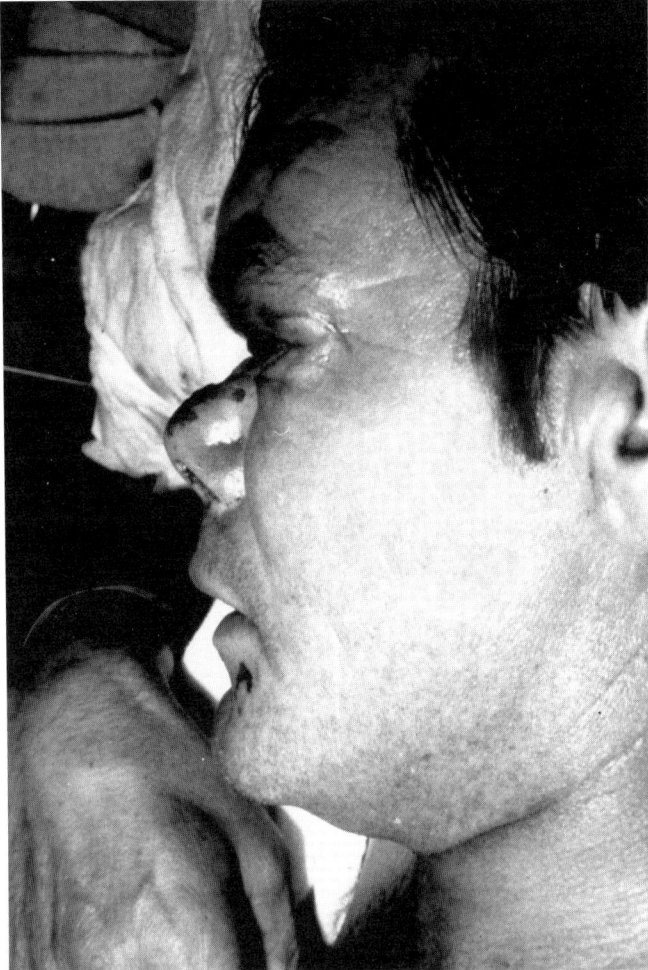

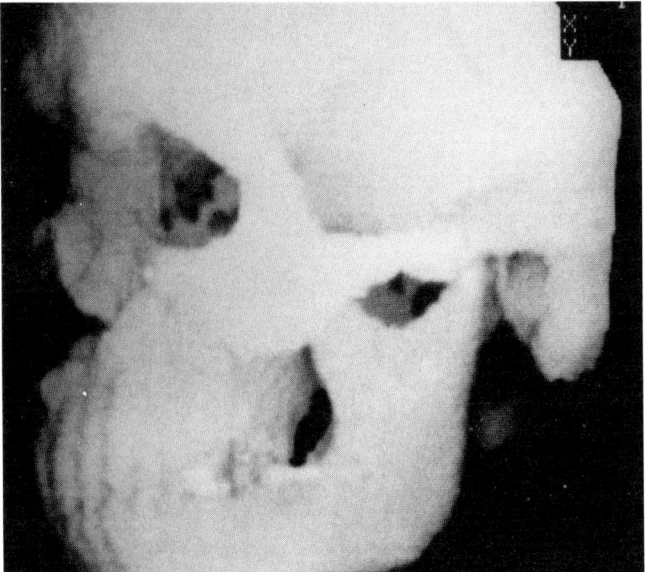

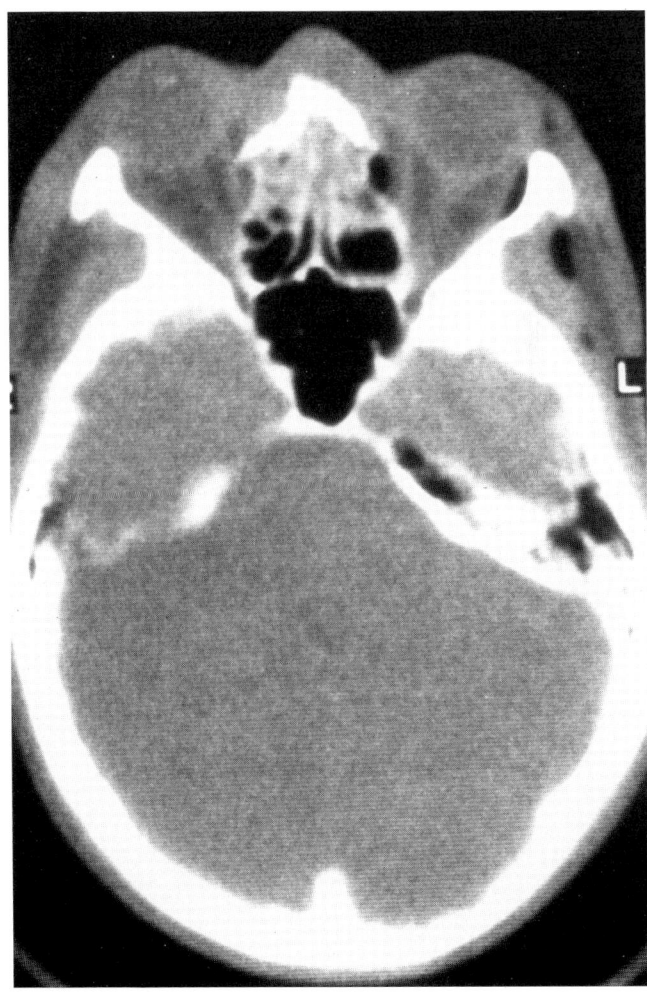

Fig. 11.76 Naso-orbito-ethmoid fractures. A Collapse of bony nasal pyramid with superior tilting of the nasal tip. **B** 3D CT reconstruction confirms the clinical findings. **C** 2D axial CT scans identifies medial orbital comminution posterior to the collapsed nasal dorsum.

accurate anatomical reduction with stable internal fixation and primary bone grafting where bone loss or comminution is extreme (Leipziger & Manson 1992). Just as the complex facial fracture demands accurate reconstruction of facial skeletal width and projection, with precise redraping of the soft-tissue cover, so injury to the naso-orbito-ethmoid region requires restoration in three dimensions in a discrete fashion, correction of the intercanthal distance and anteroposterior positioning being of critical importance. Maintenance of the close bond of the soft tissues to the underlying skeleton, particularly in the medial canthal region, will permit ideal reconstruction in both transverse and anteroposterior directions. Finally the functional and aesthetic reconstruction is completed by appropriate redraping of the soft-tissue envelope, with repositioning of the medial canthal ligament and repair of the nasolacrimal drainage system where necessary.

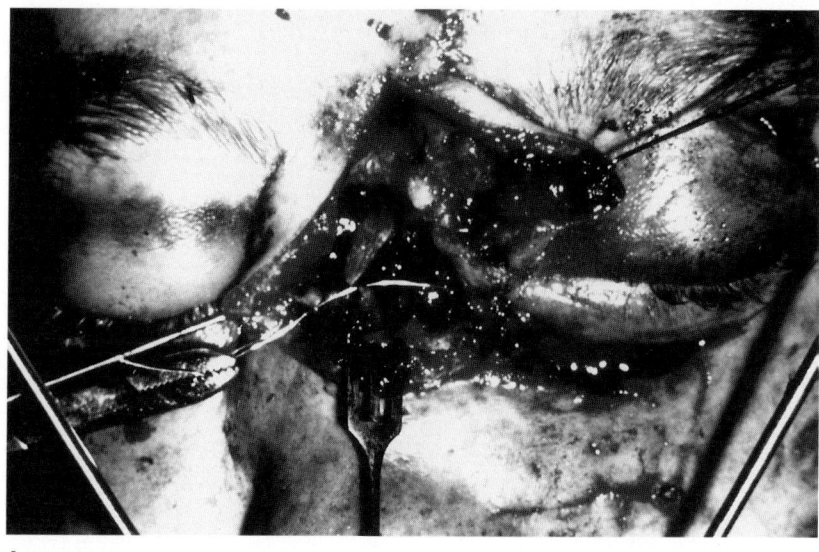

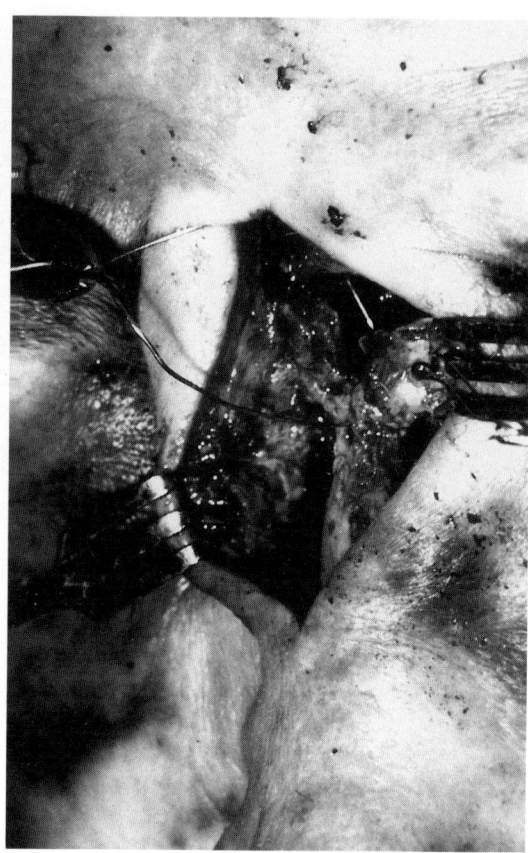

Fig. 11.77 Interosseous wiring. A and **B** Older techniques of direct exposure of fractures with wire fixation performed via existing lacerations and vertical nasal incisions.

Operative management

A coronal scalp incision gives the best exposure. Subperiosteal dissection of the entire lateral orbital wall and orbital roof allows wide, tension-free exposure of the medial orbital walls, nasal bones and frontal process of the maxilla. The trochlea is elevated, but care is taken to preserve the bony insertion of the medial canthal ligament.

A conjunctival incision with lateral canthotomy or lower eyelid subciliary incision exposes the inferior medial orbital wall and orbital floor (Fig. 9.5).

An upper vestibular (buccal sulcus) incision will identify and enable fixation of fracture extension to the nasomaxillary buttress and margin of the piriform aperture.

Local nasofrontal lacerations may provide midline exposure, but open incisions in this region have a place only in the elderly or bald patient where there is a localized fracture and where the coronal approach is aesthetically undesirable; except in such circumstances, the 'open-sky' incision of Converse & Hogan (1970) is now largely of historical interest.

Previously, multiple interosseous wires were employed to reassemble the bony jigsaw, but these suffered from the same inability to maintain nasal projection and width that had been experienced with external frames and splints. The demand for precise stable anatomic reduction in this area has seen the rapid implementation of miniplate, microplate and screw fixation.

Where the naso-orbito-ethmoid region is fractured as a single segment, either on one side or bilaterally, the deformity can be controlled by miniplate or microplate and screw fixation at two points: in some cases, a single plate on the piriform aperture or medial inferior orbital rim may be sufficient. In these cases the canthal attachment is in continuity with the major bony fragment and hence canthal position is restored by the skeletal reduction.

In injuries where bony comminution is more severe, adequate exposure is necessary to identify the nature of the bony attachment of the medial canthal ligament. Where this is intact, and the segment of bone of sufficient size, the segment itself may be used to maintain the correct intercanthal distance. Either by 28 gauge transnasal wires placed posterior and superior to the lacrimal fossa and tightened, or by an appropriately contoured microplate or miniplate, the central segment is reduced to minimize the bony distance between bony medial orbital margins. This is most frequently undercorrected, with inappropriately anterior placement of the medial canthus so that over correction should be attempted. The central segment is then fixed above and below to the stable bony elements by plates and screws.

Reconstruction of the medial orbital wall with rib or calvarial graft is usually necessary. In extreme comminution with avulsion of the medial canthal ligament, transnasal canthopexy with wires is required; this is done through a hole in the bone graft of sufficient size (~3 mm) to allow anchoring of the soft tissue. Use of a primary bony graft as a cantilever restores the nasal bridge projection, and maintains the soft tissues in correct length, by tissue expansion, which both minimizes and aids later secondary reconstruction. The nasal dorsum is reconstructed by an appropriately contoured costochondral graft or calvarial bone graft fixed superiorly at the nasofrontal region by miniplate and screws. The distal portion of the graft is inserted under the lower lateral cartilages to preserve normal tip anatomy. A columella strut is seldom required at the time of primary reconstruction if cantilever nasal support is adequate (Figs 11.78 and 11.79).

The nasal septum, which is invariably grossly buckled and oedematous, may be centred by a closed manipulation. A later definitive correction may be necessary. Primary septal reconstruction has so far not been widely attempted; the risks and difficulties are discussed below (p. 335).

Associated frontal sinus and cranial fractures are repaired at the same time with stabilizing miniplates or microplates and screws. The presence of such fractures demands care in ensuring that the support for cantilevering the nasal dorsum is stable; this may require extension of plates further superiorly on the forehead. Compromise of the frontonasal drainage is only seen where both anterior and posterior walls of the lower portion of the frontal sinus are grossly fractured, and only then is exenteration and obliteration of the sinus necessary.

Management of nasolacrimal injuries

Despite its proximity, damage to the nasolacrimal system in naso-orbito-ethmoid fractures is not very frequent even in severe injuries; Cruse et al (1980) recorded laceration of the nasolacrimal duct system in 7 (21%) of 33 cases. Early exploration is not indicated except where there is an obvious lacrimal system transection in an external laceration, when standard repair over a silicone tube or nylon suture produces satisfactory results. Late obstructive symptoms requiring dacryocystorhinostomy are seen in only 5–10% of patients treated by open acute fracture reduction. When obstruction is noted it is usually in the bony nasolacrimal canal; this can be confirmed by dacryocystography (p. 178). Definitive dacryocystorhinostomy is best performed at least 3 months after the primary fracture repair. By contrast, closed reduction and external splinting of naso-orbito-ethmoid fractures was associated with a higher rate of obstruction by malpositioned bones and more frequent need for later dacryocystorhinostomy (Gruss et al 1985a).

Complications

These include:

- Uncorrected deformity
- Nasal obstruction
- Enophthalmos
- Soft-tissue thickening and contractures
- Prominent plates and screws.

Uncorrected deformity

This is the chief complication. Diagnosis of the naso-orbito-ethmoid fracture in the severely comminuted case is seldom difficult, even when diffuse soft-tissue swelling is evident. But where displacement is not so marked, oedema and swelling may result in misdiagnosis and a later presentation with deformity. Loss of nasal projection and increased nasal width produce a contracted, distorted soft-tissue envelope in which osteotomy and bone grafting is likely to produce a result inferior to what can be achieved by early correction.

Following early open reduction and fixation of naso-orbito-ethmoid fractures, telecanthus and inappropriately anterior placement of the medial canthus remain a common problem. This reinforces the importance of maintaining the central bony attachment of the medial canthus, as exposing and reducing this structure is technically difficult and seldom recreates the pretraumatic state. Late reconstruction then demands osteotomy to reduce bony intercanthal distance together with a repeated medial canthopexy.

Collapse of the bony nasal dorsum is usually satisfactorily reconstructed by augmentation with a bone graft. Resorption and late irregularity may be corrected by further grafting, using standard rhinoplasty incisions and approaches (p. 577).

Nasal obstruction

Nasal airway obstruction is not infrequent following these injuries. Appropriate evaluation and septoplasty are commonly required.

Enophthalmos

Post-traumatic enophthalmos may result from failure to restore the position and continuity of the medial orbital walls where the injuries extend significantly into the orbit. Careful stable orbital wall reconstruction will prevent or mitigate this deformity; the late treatment of enophthalmos is difficult and often unsatisfactory (p. 559).

Soft-tissue thickening and contractures

Soft-tissue thickening and scar contracture with webbing may follow open lacerations and the surgical correction of the underlying fractures. The soft tissues in the medial canthal region are normally thin and pliable; trauma in

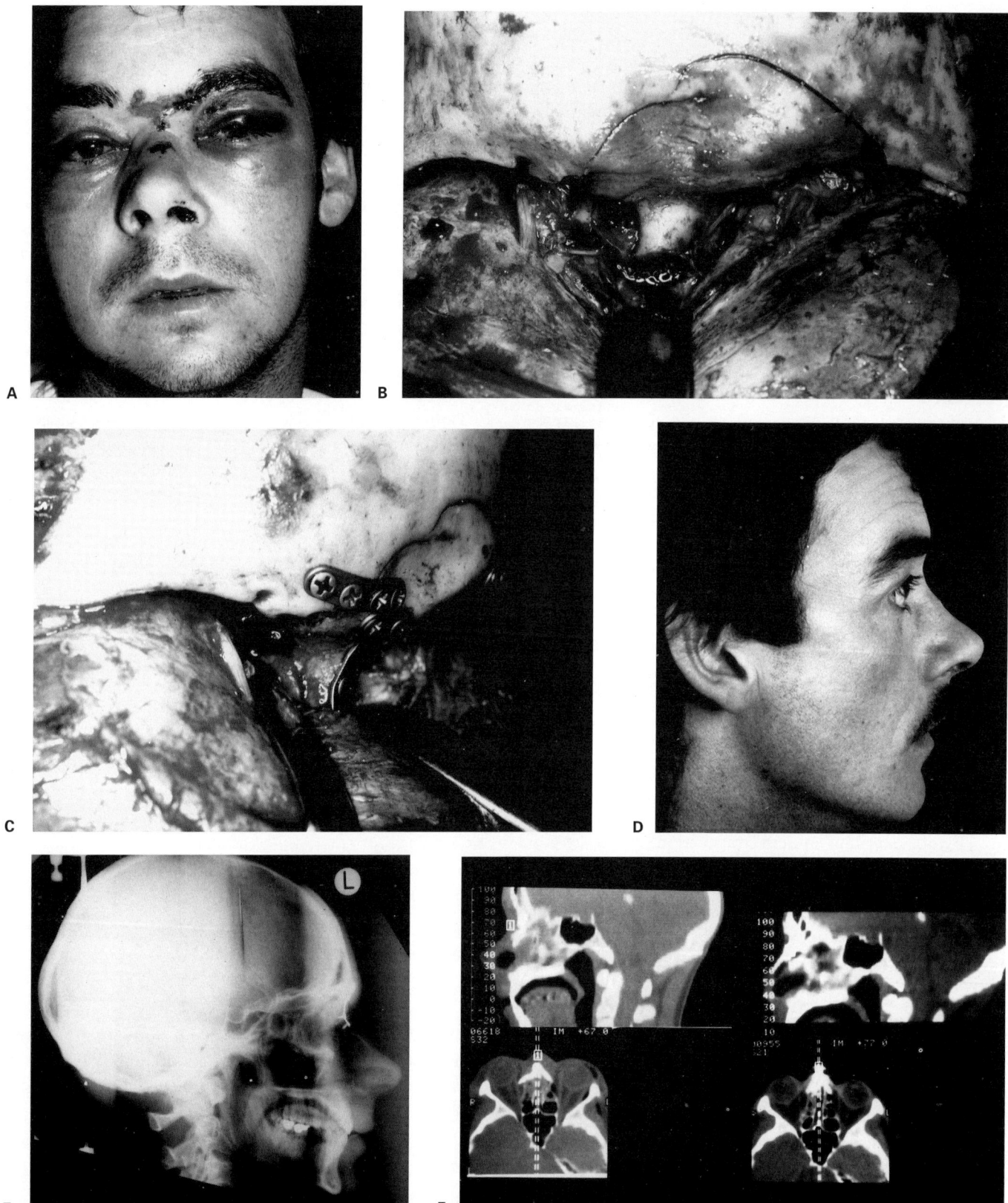

Fig. 11.78 Management of naso-orbito-ethmoid fracture with a nasal graft. A Significantly depressed naso-orbito-ethmoid fracture with frontal extension following assault with baseball bat. **B** Operative exposure via bicoronal flap confirms extension into anterior wall of the frontal sinus. **C** Operative view following reduction and internal fixation with miniplates. **D** Postoperative clinical appearance with restoration of nasal dorsum including primary bone graft. **E** Postoperative plain lateral radiograph. **F** Pre- and postoperative midsagittal 2D CT reformats detail restoration of profile.

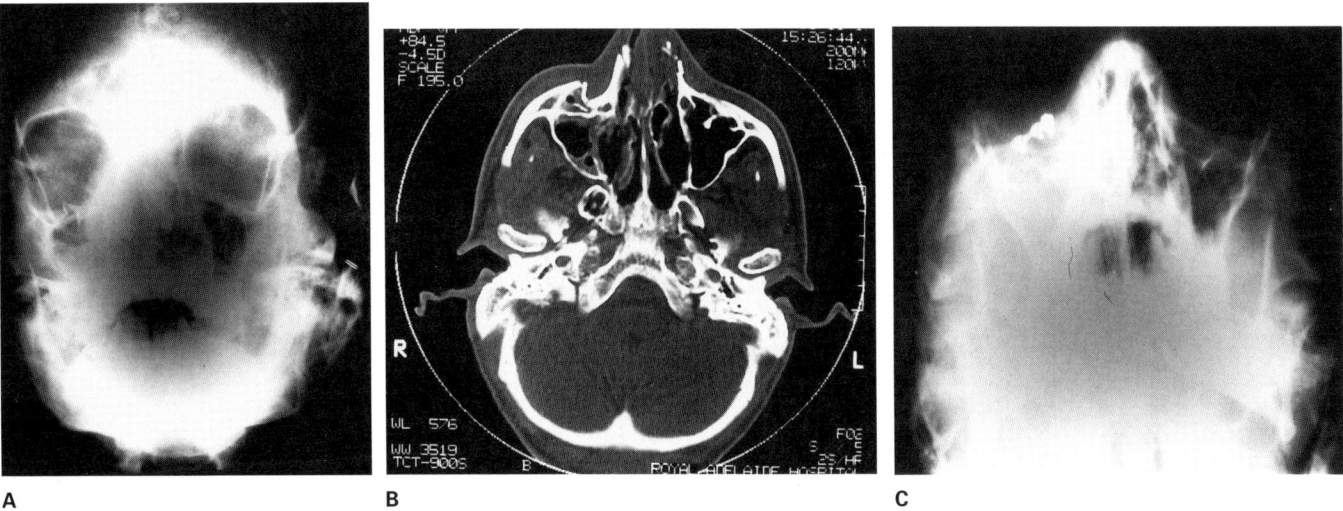

Fig. 11.79 Management of naso-orbito-ethmoid fracture. A Plain radiograph of isolated right naso-orbito-ethmoid fracture. **B** Axial 2D CT scan details posterior displacement at right nasomaxillary region. **C** Postoperative plain radiograph confirms reduction and fixation at the medial end of infraorbital rim and the piriform margin.

dissection of this area must be minimal to avoid intractable problems with the soft tissues.

Prominent plates and screws

Miniplate fixation has greatly improved fragment stability. However, prominent plates and screws in this region may become visible or palpable and the soft tissues around them may be thickened. Microplates and small screws will minimize this problem; alternatively, fine interosseous wires may be used.

FRACTURES OF THE ZYGOMA

Surgical pathology

The description and management of fractures of the orbit and zygoma have often suffered from imprecision and inaccuracy. A superficial consideration of these injuries frequently fails to elucidate the complexities of the extent and pattern of the bony disruption and of the soft-tissue elements which act to displace the skeleton or are themselves disrupted by the fracture. Inadequate understanding leads to inadequate treatment, and the resulting orbitozygomatic depression, enophthalmos and ocular dystopia are among the more difficult facial deformities to treat.

Advanced imaging techniques and wide exposure of the orbitozygomatic region have revealed the true extent of these injuries and provided an impetus to prevention of the frequent complications which used to attend operative treatment in this region.

Zygomatic fractures are among the most frequent facial injuries. They have frequently been described as '*tripod*' fractures: this term focuses attention on the resilient bony extensions of the zygoma that locally relate to adjacent bones, without due recognition of the almost inevitable involvement of the orbital wall and of the fourth bony process — the zygomatic arch. In fact, the zygomatic bone is truly a '*quadripod*' which borders the inferolateral margin of the orbit. Displaced fractures of the zygoma therefore involve the boundaries and walls of the orbit, though to a variable degree (Fig. 11.80).

For many years, there was a belief that restoration of the solid bony contours of the cheek was sufficient, and this favoured the use of simple techniques of fracture reduction. But when older techniques of reduction were seen to produce a high incidence of residual displacement, and with the increasing frequency of high velocity severely comminuted fractures, there arose a demand for techniques of stable fixation in three dimensions and accurate restoration of all bony orbital contours both external and internal.

The zygomatic bone makes a key contribution to orbital contour, facial width and projection (Figs 11.80 and 11.81). Comprising the inferolateral orbital rim, the zygoma articulates with the frontal bone superiorly, the maxilla inferiorly and medially, and with both the sphenoid and temporal bones posteriorly and laterally. Four bony processes radiate from the zygomatic body providing strong articulations with the frontal, maxillary and temporal bones. The bony junction between the temporal process of the zygoma and the zygomatic process of the temporal bone constitutes the zygomatic arch. Attached to the arch are the temporalis fascia and masseter muscle, this muscle being usually considered to be the major deforming force in maintaining displacement of a depressed zygomatic fracture, though this is in debate (Dal Santo et al 1992). Immediately superficial to the arch are the superficial temporal vessels and frontal branch of the

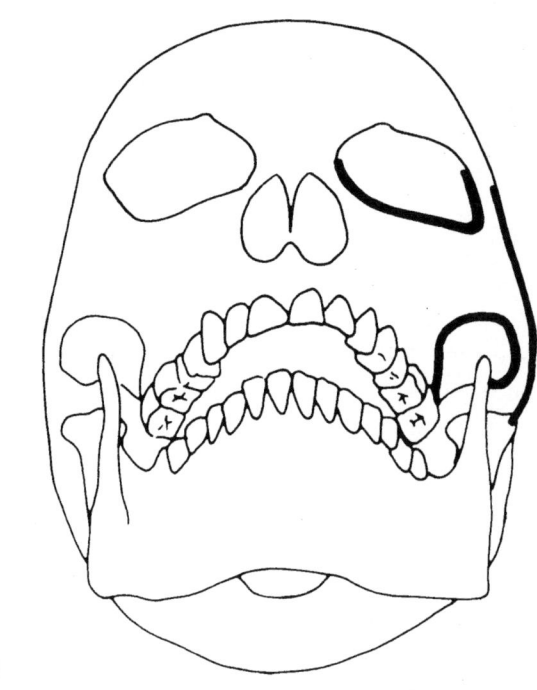
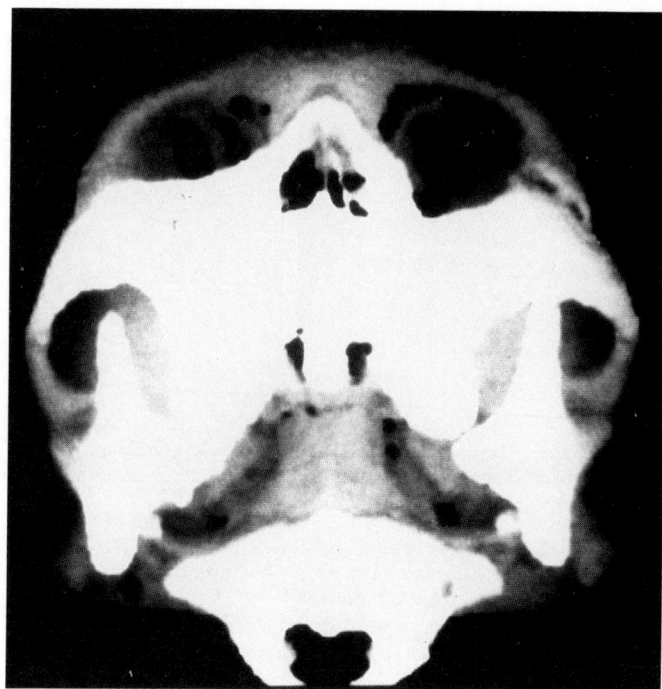

A   **B**

Fig. 11.80 Anatomy of zygomatic fractures. A and **B** Diagram and 3D CT reconstruction identify the contribution of the zygoma to the orbital contour and facial width and projection.

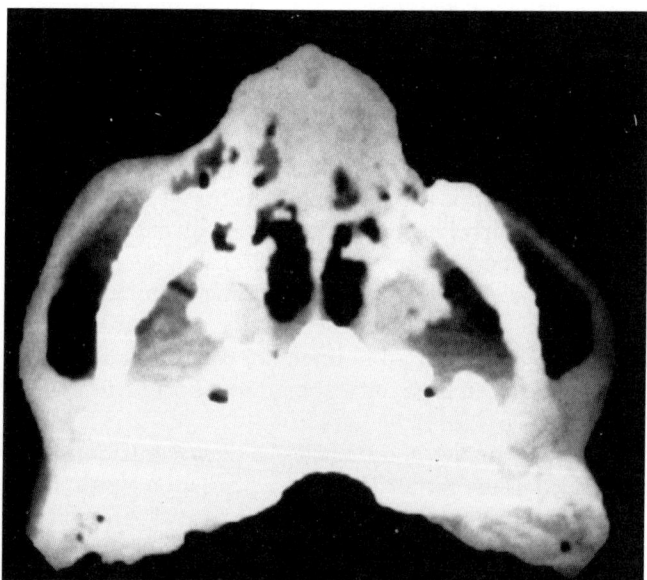

Fig. 11.81 Radiology of zygomatic fractures. Basal 3D CT reconstruction of untreated displaced left zygomatic fracture. Lateral bowing of the zygomatic arch accompanies posterior displacement of the zygomatic body.

facial nerve, while deeply pass the internal maxillary vessels, temporalis muscle and coronoid process.

Gruss et al (1990) emphasize the importance of the position of the zygomatic arch to locate the zygoma appropriately in relation to the skull base in anteroposterior, vertical and transverse dimensions (Fig. 11.81); more

recently Gruss has also stressed that the arch is actually a flattened arciform structure, and that this shape should be reconstructed as accurately as possible. Perhaps equally important, the orbital portion of the zygoma, where it meets the greater wing of the sphenoid along the lateral orbital wall, provides similar information regarding the relationship to the cranial base. Relocation of the displaced zygoma cannot be anatomically guaranteed without recourse to exposure of a number of these articulations.

Classification

Various classifications have been proposed for fractures of the zygoma. The system of Knight and North (1961) achieved early widespread use. These authors detailed patterns of zygomatic fracturing according to direction of displacement and rotation of the zygoma as viewed on plain radiographs. This was a simplification of the pattern of injury, implying dislocation in two dimensions about a single axis or point of rotation; the classification was consistent with the imaging techniques and level of open surgical exposure available at that time. With the advent of CT scanning, and with improved methods of operative exposure and fixation of the orbitozygomatic region, the extent rather than the pattern of fracturing was seen to be of greater significance. Where low velocity impacts produce linear fractures with lesser degrees of displacement, high velocity impacts result in comminution, displacement and extension into the adjacent facial skeleton. Jackson (1989) evolved a simplified general classification

Table 11.3 Classifications of zygomatic fractures*

A. Jackson (1989)

Group I	Undisplaced fractures — no treatment
Group II	Localized segmental fractures — exposure and fixation
Group III	Displaced 'tripod' fractures (low velocity) — simple elevations, or elevations, exposure and fixation
Group IV	Displaced comminuted fractures (high velocity) wide exposure and multiple point fixation

B. Gruss et al (1990)

1. Zygomatic body	2. Zygomatic arch
(a) Intact	(a) Intact
(b) Undisplaced	(b) Undisplaced
(c) Segmental	(c) Segmental
(d) Displaced	(d) Displaced — inferiorly with depression — laterally
(e) Comminuted	(e) Comminuted

* These simple systems of classification provide a grading of severity which can be related to management protocols.

of zygomatic fractures relating pattern and displacement to treatment (Table 11.3). Gruss et al (1990) recognized the role of the zygomatic arch injury in accurate reduction and classified these injuries according to the level of bony damage to the zygomatic body and the zygomatic arch. We (Cooter & David 1989) quantify the degree of bony comminution in each element of the zygoma as well as the level of displacement of the skeletal articulations. This system, although complex, permits more accurate comparison of treatment results between different series (p. 35).

Clinical assessment

A history of local trauma to the cheek should arouse suspicion of orbitozygomatic fracture. Recording the mechanism, direction and particularly the velocity of impact is essential; and the observer should maintain a high index of suspicion for associated ocular, midfacial, craniocerebral and cervical spine injuries. The association of zygomatic fractures with other midfacial injuries and with fractures of the adjacent segments of the mandible (condylar process, ramus, coronoid and angle) has to be kept in mind; mandibular injury is especially likely where a localized high velocity impact is sustained.

The symptomatology typically relates to the effect of the displaced zygomatic bone on the surrounding soft tissues. The orbital soft tissues manifest swelling, ecchymoses and subconjunctival haemorrhages, particularly laterally (Figs 11.82–85). Diplopia or blurred vision may be a complaint due to orbital soft-tissue swelling, ocular dystopia or primary ocular injury. Numbness or altered sensation in the distribution of the infraorbital nerve (cheek, lateral portion of nose and upper lip) indicates infraorbital rim fracturing. Trismus and complaints of malocclusion are recorded where arch fractures impinge on the underlying temporalis muscle. A sense of an altered occlusion may also follow injury to the infraorbital and superior alveolar nerves. In both situations a true occlusal disturbance by extension of the zygomatic fracture into the maxillary alveolar process must be excluded by careful intraoral examination (Fig. 11.83).

As the zygoma is largely superficial, physical examination and especially palpation will readily identify displacement. Observation from above (bird's eye view) provides an impression of loss of the zygomatic prominence (Fig. 11.84). This is confirmed by placing examining fingers on the most prominent part of the zygomatic body and comparing with the non-injured side. When there is displacement in the inferior orbital rim, there may be a palpable step-down as one feels from medial to lateral

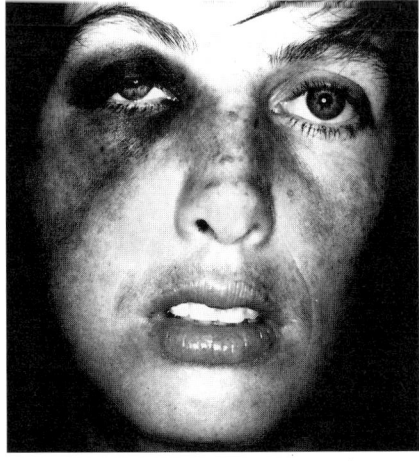 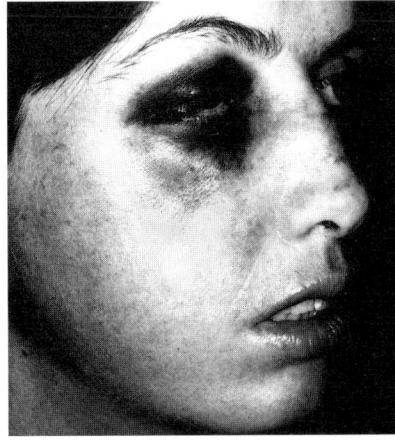 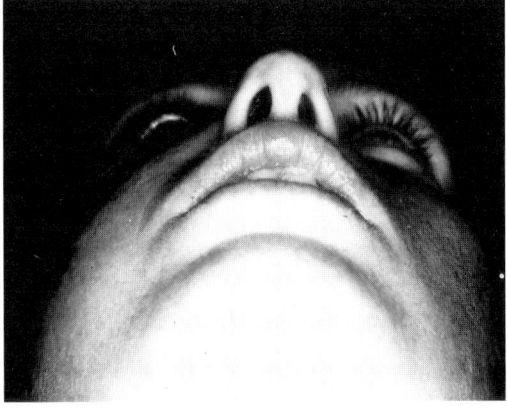

A   B   C

Fig. 11.82 Clinical signs of zygomatic fractures. A Frontal, **B** right oblique and **C** worm's-eye views of a woman with depressed right zygoma after horse riding accident. Marked periorbital bruising does not disguise the flattening of the right cheek. Enophthalmos on the right produces a pseudoptosis.

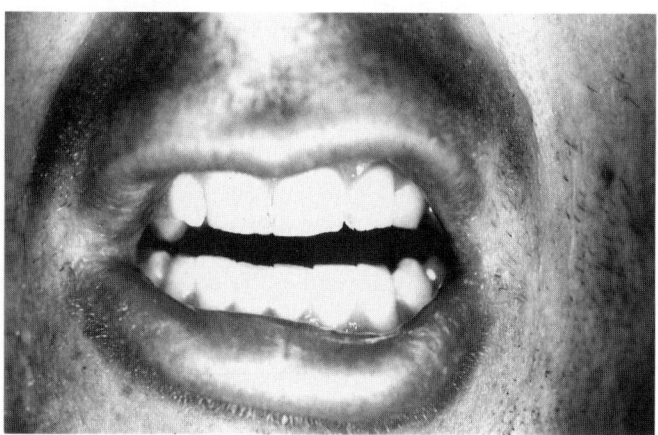

Fig. 11.83 Clinical signs of zygomatic fractures with maxillary extension. Open-bite occlusal disturbance in patient with a depressed zygomatic fracture with extension into the maxillary alveolus.

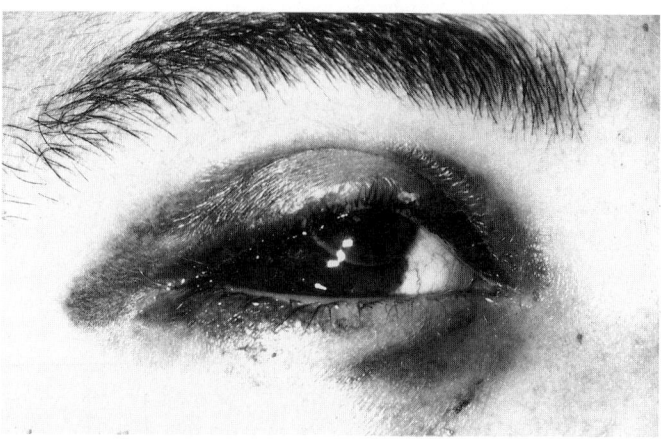

Fig. 11.85 Clinical signs of zygomatic fractures. Laterally based subconjunctival haemorrhage in a fracture of the right zygoma.

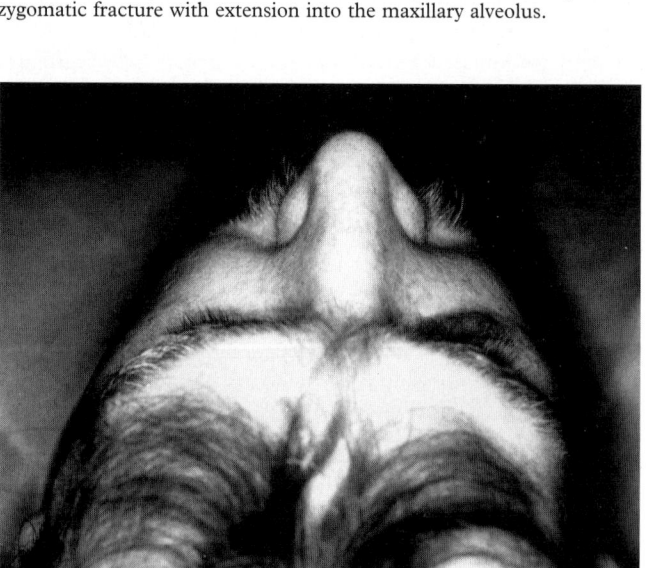

Fig. 11.84 Clinical signs of zygomatic fractures. Bird's-eye view identifies flattening of the left zygoma.

at the infraorbital rim, with associated tenderness. More laterally a tender palpable depression in the zygomatic arch is present, often the only abnormality in isolated arch fractures. In contrast, where the zygomatic fracture accompanies extensive midfacial fracturing the zygomatic arch is bowed outward and the anteroposterior projection of the zygomatic prominence is diminished.

Intraoral examination will identify bruising in the upper vestibule where fractures of the maxillary buttress may also be palpable. Alveolar extensions of the fracture or malocclusions caused by trismus or associated midfacial and mandibular fractures may also be noted.

Detailed ophthalmological examination (p. 167) includes assessment of visual acuity, extraocular muscle function and degree of enophthalmos. Enophthalmos may

be masked by early severe facial and periorbital swelling, and indeed exophthalmos is not uncommonly the early finding. Unusual zygomatic fractures with medial impaction may be associated with a reduction in the bony orbital volume and hence a tendency to exophthalmos. Ophthalmoscopic examination will disclose any retinal injury or hyphema, the presence of which sometimes requires further investigation and perhaps delay in the operative repair of the skeletal injuries.

Radiological assessment

Plain radiological assessment of the zygoma consists of the Waters, reverse Waters, Caldwell, submentovertical and lateral views (p. 199). The Waters view records displacement at the inferior orbital rim, maxillary buttress and zygomatic body; the Caldwell view shows the frontozygomatic region and zygomatic arch; the submentovertical view shows the zygomatic arch. For isolated zygomatic arch fractures, no further radiological assessment is really necessary, though we commonly perform CT scanning to amplify the anatomical diagnosis and as a baseline for postoperative verification of reduction.

For more complex patterns of fracturing requiring accurate assessment of orbital wall involvement, degree of zygomatic body and arch displacement, and degree of comminution, axial and coronal two-dimensional (2D) CT scanning of the orbitozygomatic region is certainly indicated (Fig. 11.86). Coronal scans visualize the orbital walls and the orbital floor; the axial views show accurately any deformation of the zygomatic body, arch and lateral and medial orbital walls. Both views, by identifying the appropriate stable skeletal elements, assist in planning the surgical exposures necessary for reduction and stable fixation (Fig. 11.87). 3D CT scan reconstructions provide graphic pictorial assistance but add nothing to surgical decision-making which relies much more on the baseline 2D CT scan data.

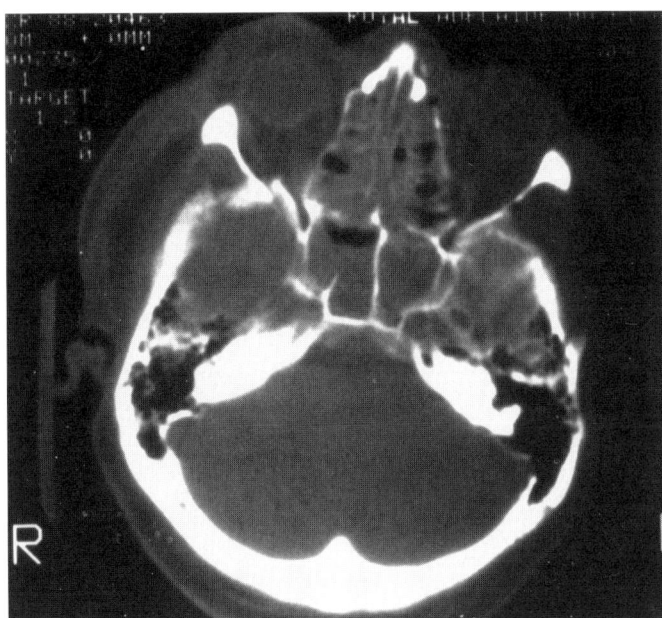

Fig. 11.86 Radiology of zygomatic fractures. Axial 2D CT scan shows very posterior fracturing of the lateral orbital wall, medial impaction of the orbital rim and marked exophthalmos.

Principles of management

The evolution of treatment of zygomatic fractures has seen continuing debate with regard to the indications for reduction and the techniques and patterns of fixation of zygomatic fractures.

The mainstay of reduction alone has been Gillies' technique of percutaneous elevation by leverage from an incision in the temporal hair-bearing scalp (Gillies et al 1927), or Dingman's variation (Dingman & Natvig 1964) of elevation from the eyebrow, or even from an intraoral approach. Few studies have detailed objective results regarding outcome after simple Gillies reduction. Melmed

(1972) studied a group of low velocity, minimally displaced body and depressed arch fractures and reported a 30% rate of results considered to be less than acceptable. This report also detailed an improved aesthetic outcome and fewer poor results when fixation was added, with further increments of benefit when reduction was performed under direct vision. An opposing view has been presented by Schubert (1991), with excellent anatomical restoration in 73% of cases treated by percutaneous reduction alone, but in this study the comminuted or significantly displaced fractures were treated by some form of fixation while the more stable, minimally displaced, low velocity fractures were treated by reduction alone.

The progression through techniques of antral packing, interosseous wiring and transfixion with Kirschner wire to the use of miniplate fixation has seen more consistent restoration of symmetry. Rohrich et al (1992) reported fewer problems with infraorbital nerve complications, malpositions of the globe and inaccurate cheek positioning when miniplate fixation was compared with fixation by interosseous wires. It is now standard practice to employ miniplate fixation and wide operative exposure of the orbitozygomatic skeleton, thus allowing anatomical restoration of the zygomatic prominence with fewer positional disturbances of the globe, such as enophthalmos and vertical dystopia.

Locating the required points of fixation demands an understanding of which articulations are most easily displaced. Fracturing and comminution begin in the zygomaticomaxillary buttress and inferior orbital rim, with extension to and involvement of the greater sphenoid wing (lateral orbital wall); disruptions of the zygomatic arch and zygomaticofrontal suture are seen in the more severe injuries. Since the masseter muscle is the major displacing force acting on the zygoma, miniplate fixation of the zygomaticomaxillary buttress and the zygomatico-

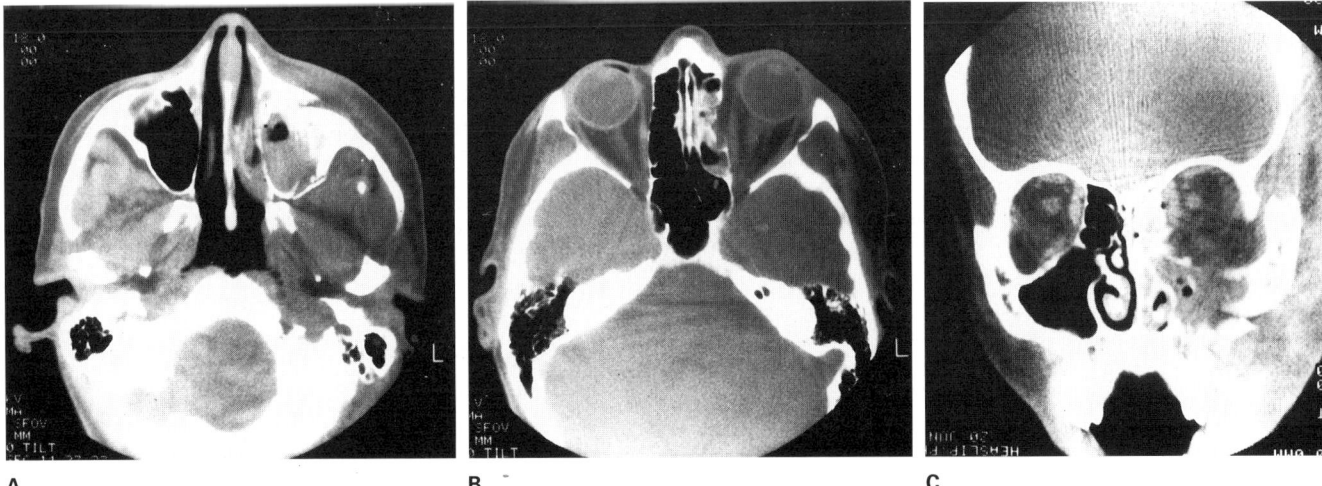

A   B   C

Fig. 11.87 Radiology of zygomatic fractures. A Axial 2D CT scan identifies posterior displacement of the zygomatic body, fracturing through the infraorbital rim and lateral bowing of the zygomatic arch. **B** Medial orbital wall blow-out in association with displaced zygomatic fracture. **C** Coronal 2D CT scan displays zygomatic body displacement, medial and lateral wall, and orbital floor damage in a high-velocity impact.

frontal articulation should orientate the vectors of fixation in the optimal axis. The techniques of exposure, reduction and miniplate fixation are now well described, but surgeons differ on how these principles are applied in each pattern of fracture.

In discussing treatment approaches, it is logical to subdivide fractures of the zygoma into those where there is no orbital wall involvement (isolated zygomatic arch fracture) and the more common orbitozygomatic fracture, where the fracture lines involve at least one wall of the orbital cavity.

Isolated zygomatic arch fracture

The isolated zygomatic arch fracture is usually a low velocity injury, with characteristic symptoms of trismus and clinical signs of localized arch contour depression. Treatment is by the closed reduction technique of Gillies et al (1927). A short oblique incision in the hair-bearing temple allows passage of an elevator deep to the temporalis fascia behind the depressed arch. This achieves stable reduction in the majority of cases (Fig. 11.88). In rare cases, isolated arch fractures may be unstable after reduction. While it is possible to fix arch fractures internally via a bicoronal approach, the degree of contour abnormality seldom justifies an open operation of such magnitude. The less invasive technique of stenting of the arch with a percutaneous needle or tubing sutured over the arch may have a role. Alternatively, the swelling and oedema in the temporalis muscle after the performance of the Gillies manoeuvre may provide a degree of internal

splintage sufficient for contour maintenance in these cases.

When untreated or neglected, zygomatic fractures manifest a cosmetic deformity — the localized depression of the lateral cheek. Only in extreme cases where the depression is marked is there a long-term disturbance of jaw opening and closing. There are no significant complications of the percutaneous surgical correction.

Orbitozygomatic fractures

Undisplaced fractures require no operative treatment. Advice is provided to avoid local pressure on the zygomatic prominence during the initial weeks, with follow-up maintained until healing at about 6 weeks. The incidence of late displacement of initially conservatively managed undisplaced zygomatic fractures is unknown, but appears to be very low. Early recognition will permit appropriate operative intervention.

Displaced orbitozygomatic fractures demand careful open reduction and internal fixation on an individualized basis. Most fractures fall within the category of mild to moderate displacement, in association with a variable degree of comminution. Fracture separation in these cases is invariably more marked at the zygomaticomaxillary buttress and the inferior orbital rim, with lesser injuries at the superior articulations. Exposure via a lower eyelid subciliary skin-muscle flap or transconjunctival incision with lateral canthotomy reveals the zygomaticofrontal suture, lateral orbital wall, inferior orbital rim, orbital floor and anterior zygomatic arch (Fig. 11.89). An upper

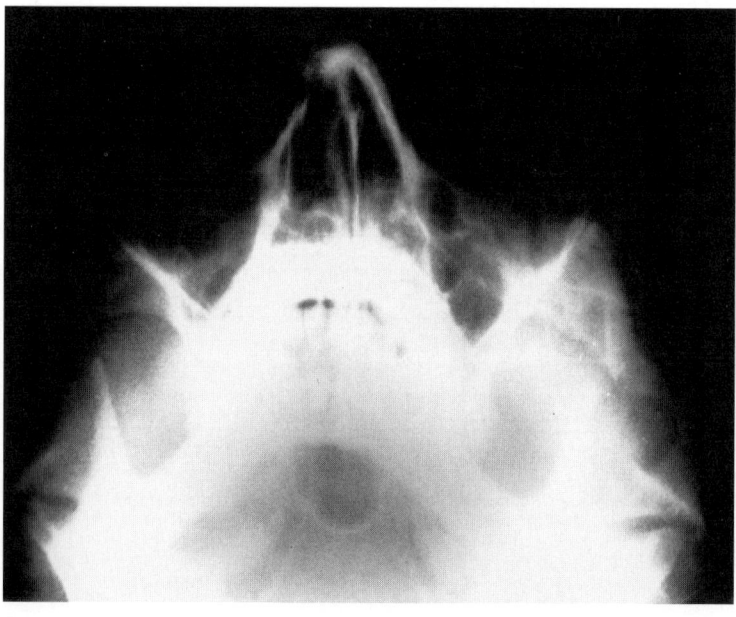
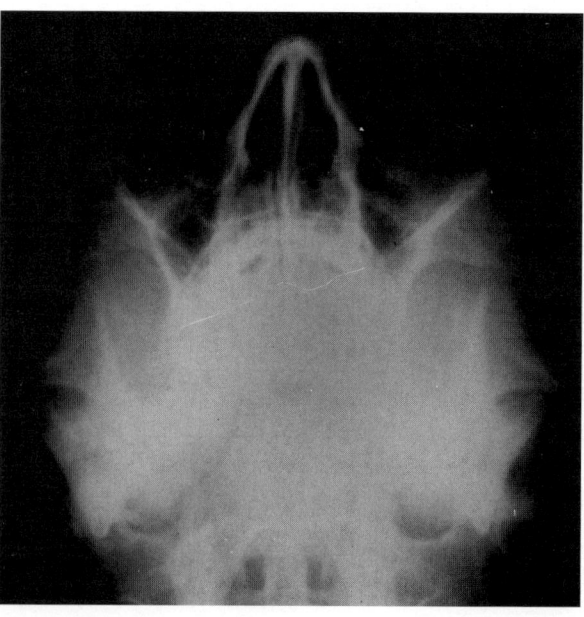

A

B

Fig. 11.88 Radiology of zygomatic arch fractures. A and **B** Plain radiographs confirm reduction of an isolated left zygomatic arch fracture following a Gillies elevation.

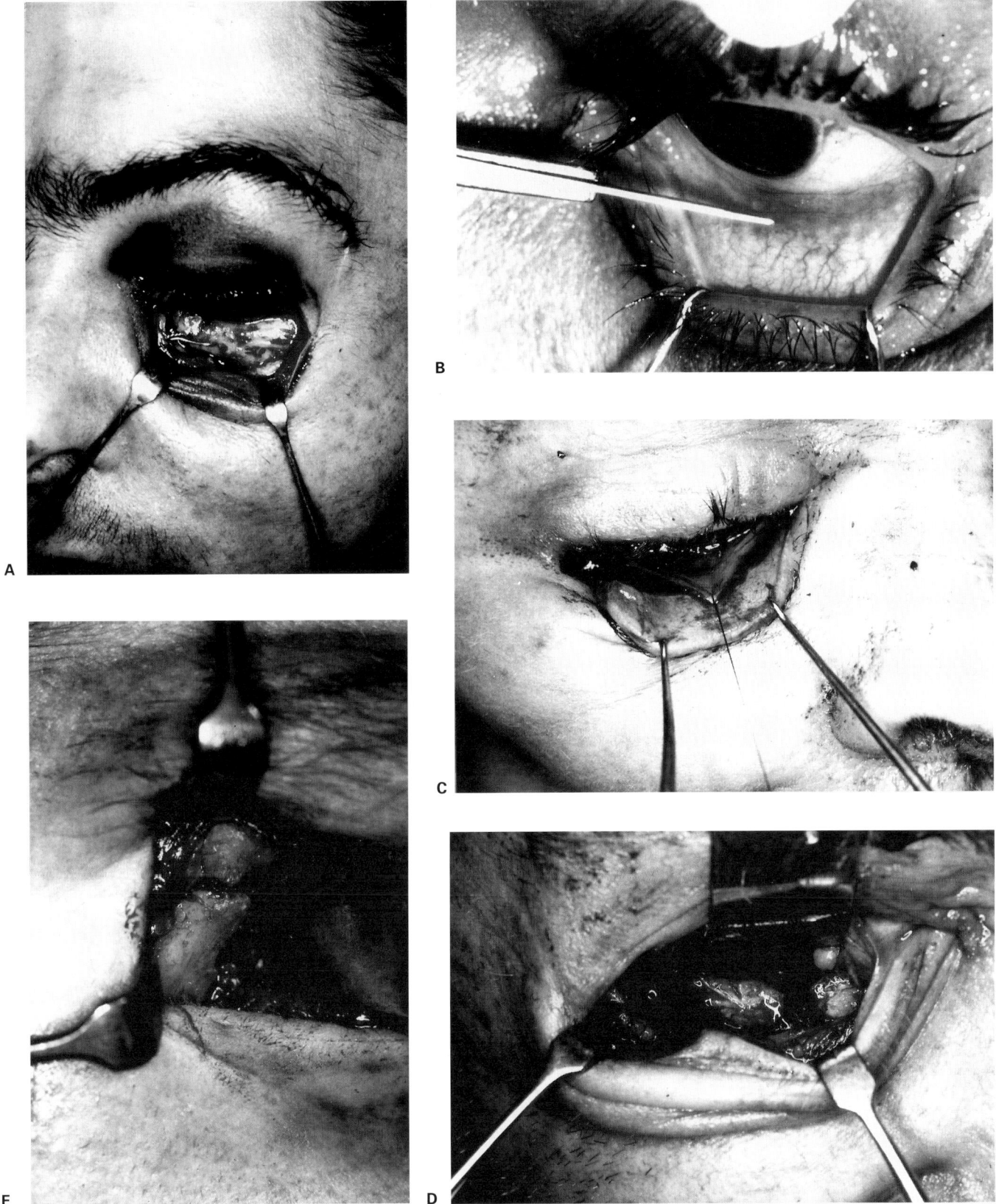

Fig. 11.89 Surgical exposure of orbital rim. A Subciliary skin–muscle flap approach to the inferior orbital rim and floor. **B** Transconjunctival approach begins inferior to the tarsal plate of the lower eyelid. **C** Extension with a lateral canthotomy improves width of exposure. **D** Displaced fracture of the inferior orbital rim easily exposed. **E** Lateral and superior dissection allows exposure and plating of the frontozygomatic fracture via conjunctival incision and lateral canthotomy.

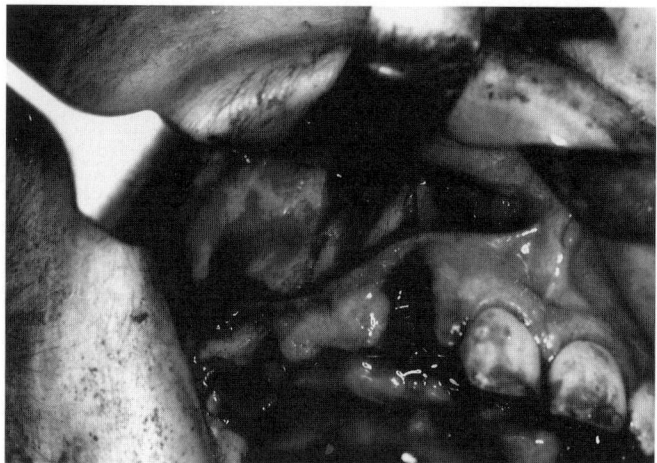

Fig. 11.90 Surgical exposure of zygomaticomaxillary region.
Upper vestibular incision exposes the anterior maxilla, piriform margin and zygomaticomaxillary fracture.

buccal vestibular incision permits exposure of the zygomaticomaxillary articulation and anterior attachment of the masseter muscle to the zygoma (Fig. 11.90). Following fracture mobilization and elevation either by the intraoral approach or by Gillies' procedure, anatomical restoration is achieved by visualizing the anterior zygomatic articulations, and comparing the anteroposterior projection of the zygoma and inferior orbital rim with the contralateral side. The addition of lateral orbital wall exposure reveals the alignment of the zygoma with the greater wing of sphenoid and confirms accurate reduction.

Miniplate fixation in the zygomaticomaxillary buttress has a vector of action which opposes the displacing influence of the masseter, albeit in bone which is thin and has little strength. The zygomaticofrontal suture, while a poor single indicator of reduction, provides the strongest bone for miniplate fixation. This two-site fixation will provide sufficient stability in the majority of fractures of this type. An additional third point of fixation at the inferior orbital rim with miniplates, or preferably a microplate or fine wire, will counteract the remote possibility of lateral rotation. Where significant comminution is present in the zygomaticomaxillary buttress, inferior orbital rim fixation will contribute significantly to stability in this level of injury; this may be unnecessary if bone grafting is employed (see below). Operative treatment is completed by careful reattachment of the midfacial and periorbital soft tissues to the zygomatic skeleton to minimize subsequent soft-tissue sagging under gravity, causing scleral show, lower lid ectropion, lateral canthal distortion and depression of the zygomatic soft-tissue prominence.

In many zygomatic fractures where displacement is significant, but where comminution is not marked, single miniplate fixation at the zygomaticofrontal suture is adequate (Figs 11.91 and 11.92). Visualization of the orbital rim, lateral orbital wall and zygomaticomaxillary region is also required to confirm the accuracy of the reduction.

In thinly built individuals and females the zygomaticofrontal miniplate is often palpable and sometimes visible, requiring later removal. This is accentuated where there is dissection, displacement or atrophy of the temporalis muscle. Countersinking the miniplate by burring or contouring the bone prior to plate placement, or by locating the plate on the posterior, rather than lateral aspect of suture may obviate this problem. Microplate fixation causes fewer cosmetic problems (Fig. 11.93). Yaremchuk et al (1993) recommend miniplate fixation of the zygomaticomaxillary suture, with microplates at the zygomaticofrontal suture and the infraorbital rim. This fixation appears to be at least as stable as the more conventional pattern of two- or three-point miniplate fixation, and has less likelihood of aesthetic complications.

Comminuted and grossly displaced orbitozygomatic

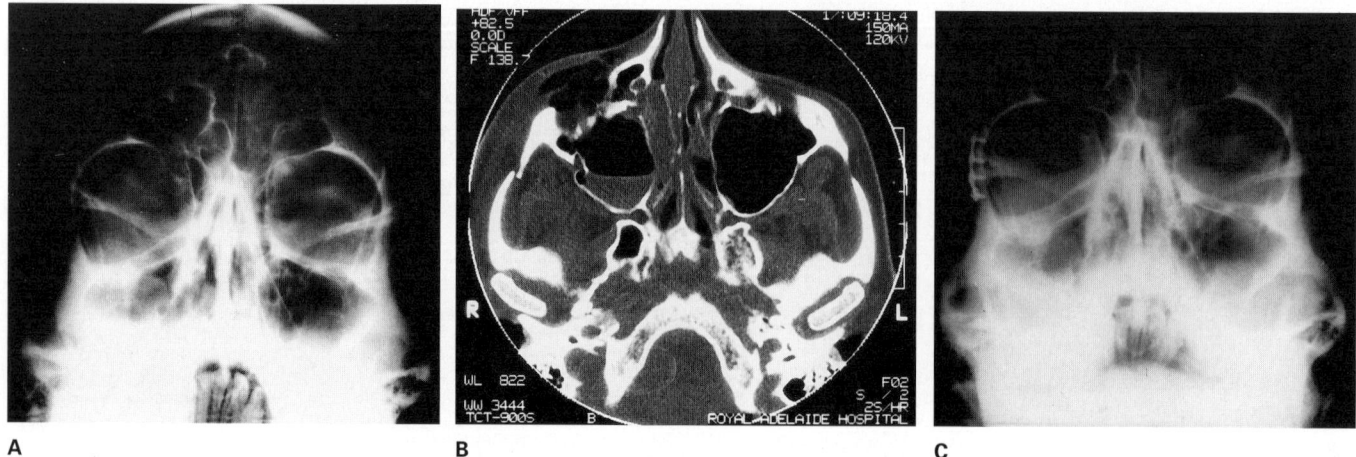

A   B   C

Fig. 11.91 Radiology of zygomatic fracture management. A Displaced but minimally comminuted fracture of the right zygoma. **B** Axial 2D CT scan confirms displacement. **C** Postoperative plain radiograph displays satisfactory reduction with single frontozygomatic miniplate fixation.

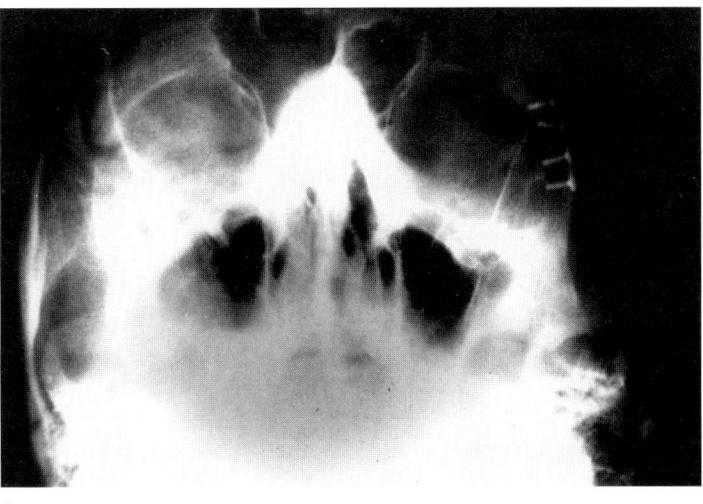
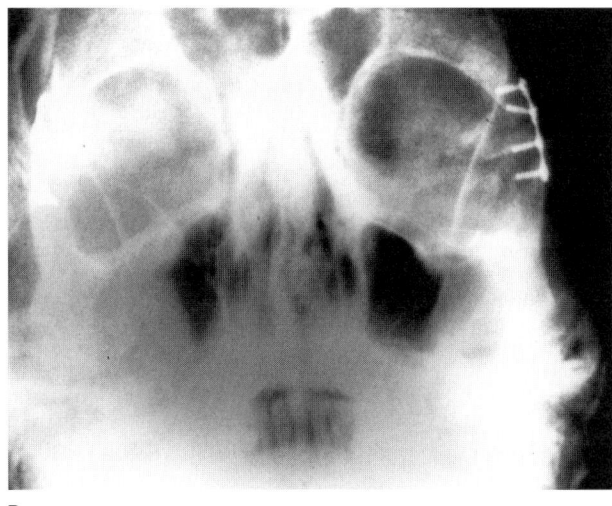

A   B

Fig. 11.92 Radiology of zygomatic fracture management. A Displaced right zygomatic fracture in patient with previously treated old fracture of the left zygoma. **B** Postoperative radiograph with single frontozygomatic plate fixation.

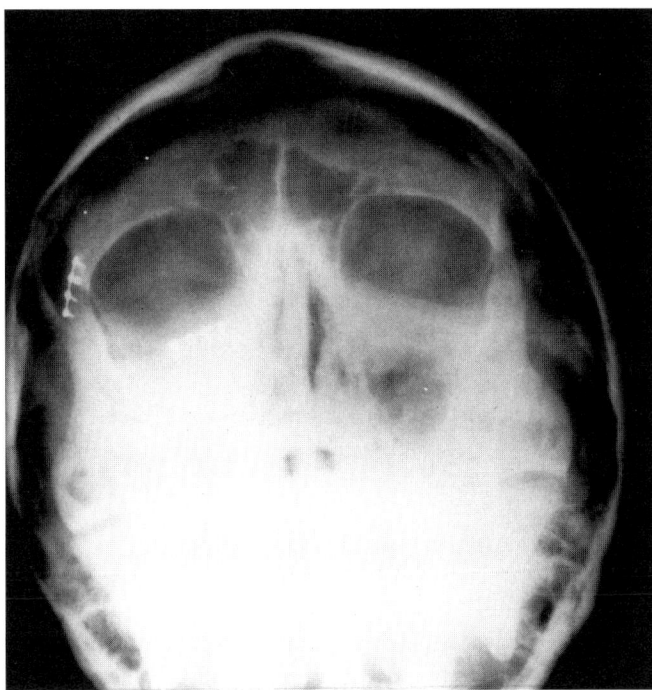

Fig. 11.93 Microplate fixation of zygomatic fractures.
Significantly displaced right orbitozygomatic fracture with microplate fixation at frontozygomatic fracture and micromesh at inferior rim to restore orbital floor position.

fractures seldom occur in isolation. Almost always these fractures occur in high velocity impacts producing major midfacial or panfacial fractures, of which the zygomatic injury forms one portion. Superimposed on the pattern of the moderately displaced fracture group, and reflecting more violent distortion, are comminution of the lateral orbital wall, including the greater wing of the sphenoid, and disruption of the zygomatic arch. Recognizing the disruption and restoring the arch, as advised by Gruss

et al (1990), is the key to restoration of the zygomatic projection, the midfacial width and the anteroposterior projection (Fig. 11.94). Axial CT scan images identify the arch fractures, usually anteriorly at the junction with the zygomatic body and posteriorly passing obliquely close to the glenoid fossa, with intervening lateral bowing of the arch. A bicoronal approach facilitates exposure, mobilization and reduction of the arch fractures. Disinsertion of the masseter muscle may be required for reduction; correct anatomical positioning is achieved by comparison with the contralateral side.

Fixation in these cases follows the 'best fit' principle, comparison with the normal contralateral side being readily available. Temporary stabilization at the zygomatico-frontal suture with an interosseous wire or miniplate allows the surgeon to verify that there is correct rotational and projectional alignment at the zygomaticomaxillary buttress, inferior orbital rim and lateral orbital wall, before proceeding to definitive miniplate and screw fixation of the zygomatic arch. Formal miniplate fixation of the re-maining sites is then performed to position the zygoma rigidly between the fronto-orbital borders above and the midface below.

The role of microplate fixation in these high energy injuries has not been clearly defined. Yaremchuk et al (1993) believe these to be inadequate on their own in situations where extreme soft-tissue swelling may exert considerable deforming forces. We have had no experiences to support or disprove this view.

Comminution and loss of bone at the major articula-tions, the anterior maxillary wall, the orbital floor and the lateral orbital wall demand careful operative display, reduction and reconstruction by primary bone grafting if the major complications of enophthalmos and orbito-ocular dystopia are to be avoided (Fig. 11.95). High

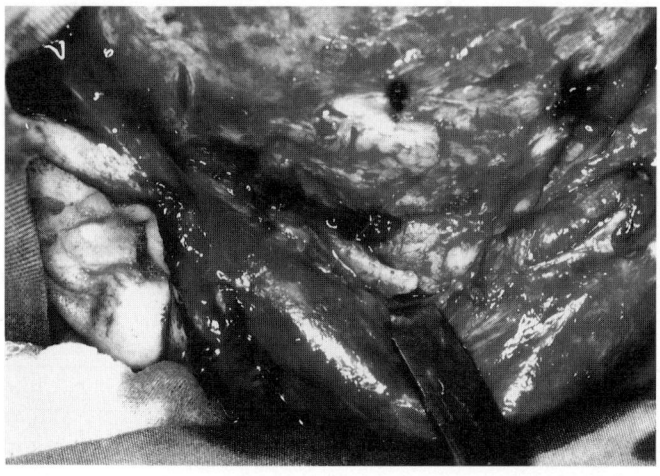

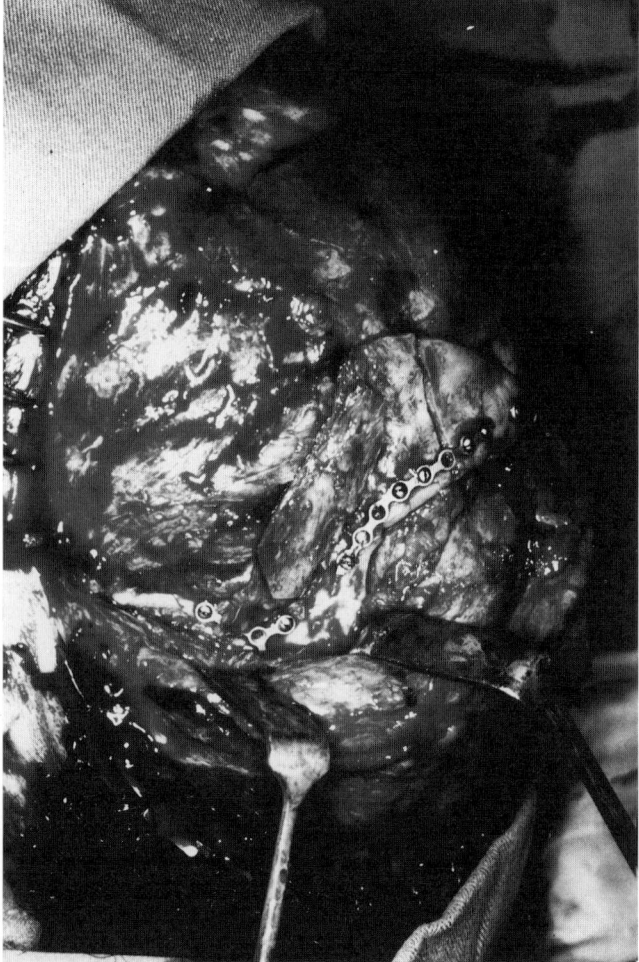

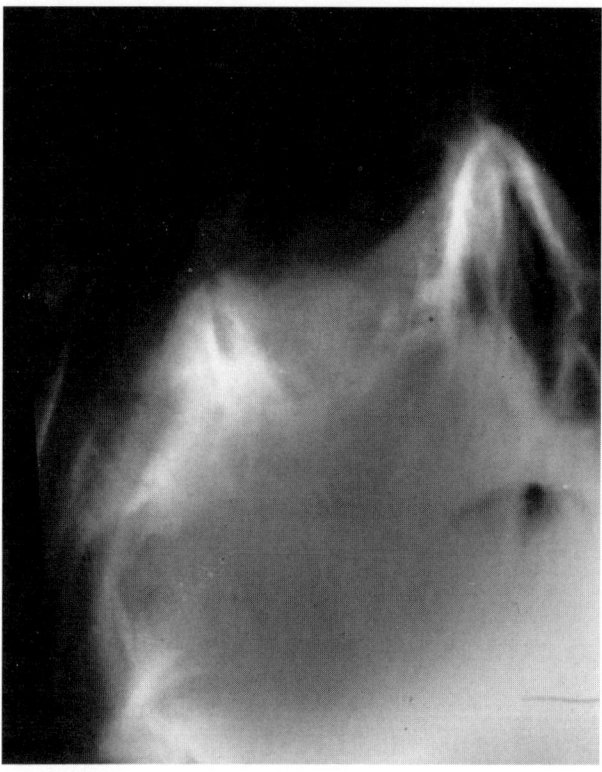

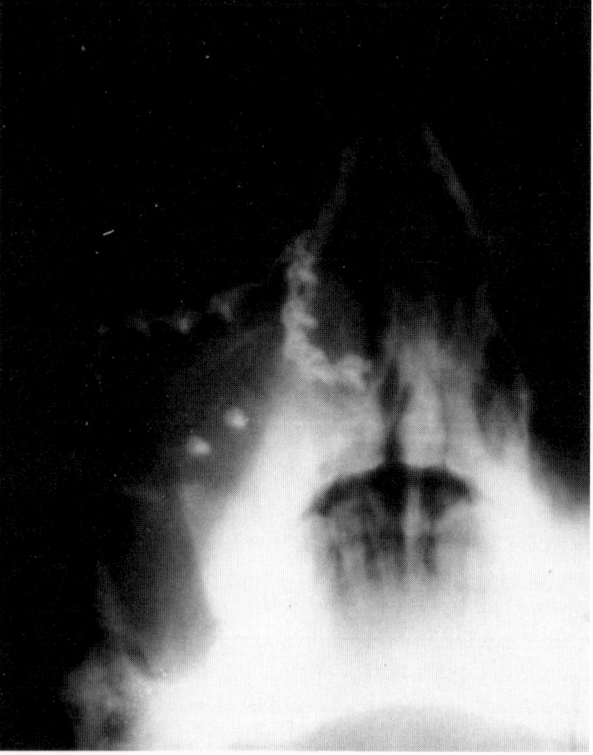

Fig. 11.94 Management of zygomatic arch fractures. A Zygomatic fracture occurring in association with midfacial fractures. Displaced arch fragments at tip of retractor. **B** Stabilization at the frontozygomatic region and zygomatic arch restores facial projection and width.

Fig. 11.95 Management of comminuted zygomatic fractures. A Severely comminuted right zygomatic fracture. **B** Plain radiograph after wide exposure, reduction, internal fixation and primary bone grafting.

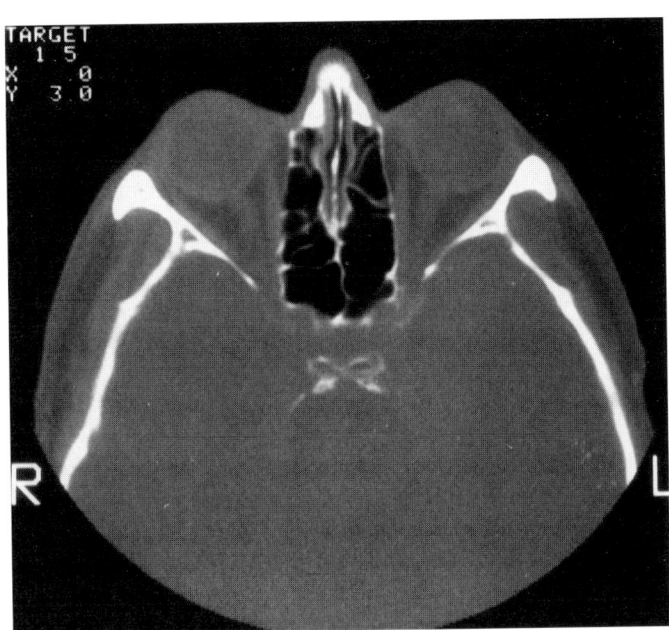

Fig. 11.96 Radiology of orbital margins. Axial 2D CT scan of uninjured orbits. *The lateral wall lies entirely behind the equator of the globe.*

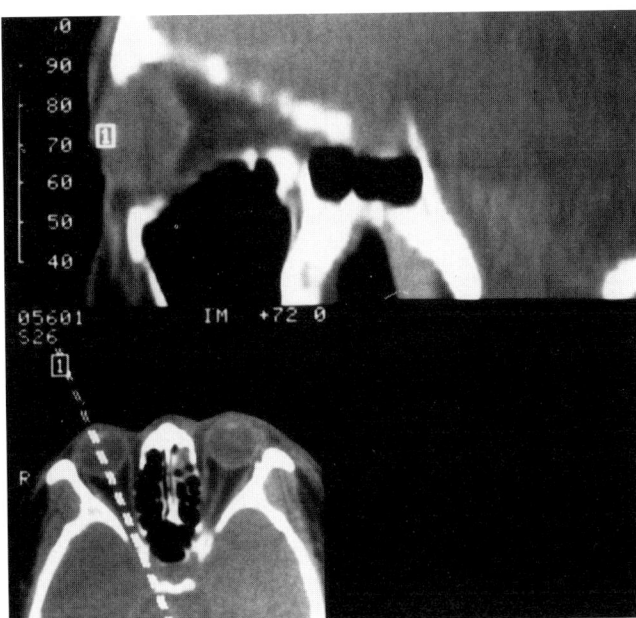

Fig. 11.97 Radiology of orbital floor. Oblique sagittal 2D CT reformat identifies the upward bulge of the orbital floor in its posterior portion.

velocity injuries with their characteristic comminution all require exploration of at least the orbital floor and lateral orbital wall. The lateral orbital wall is situated entirely posterior to the axis of the globe, and non-anatomical reduction produces an increase in bony orbital volume with resulting enophthalmos (Fig. 11.96). Comminution in this region invariably requires the addition of bone grafts from calvarial, rib or iliac donor sites. Grafts are easily placed into any wall of the orbit, particularly where the posterior 'ledges' are used as guides to alignment and stability, but bone graft displacement is too often seen. Stabilizing these grafts by miniscrew, miniplate, microplate or titanium mesh should improve predictability of outcome and reduce the incidence of resistant enophthalmos.

The orbital floor characteristically bulges upward in its most posterior extent, 35–38 mm behind the inferior orbital rim where the intact bony ledges are located (Fig. 11.97). Failure to expose this area and to employ it for bone grafting may lead to inadequate initial bony orbital wall reconstruction and also to subsequent graft displacement and orbital volume expansion.

The case for routine wide orbital exploration in medium velocity orbitozygomatic fractures is not so well defined. Orbital wall components of the zygomatic fracture do not require exploration if CT scanning shows no displacement: in such cases the periorbita is intact and maintains the soft-tissue orbital volume. Unnecessary exploration risks disruption of the periorbita and may cause orbital volume changes secondary to the surgery.

Complications

These include:

- Deformity
- Prominent plates
- Disturbance of globe position
- Ocular injury
- Nerve injury.

Deformity

The chief complication of the older techniques of management was inadequately or uncorrected deformity. Osseous deformity has been much reduced by wide exposure, open reduction, internal fixation and primary bone grafting; these techniques carry with them certain side-effects which demand finesse in surgical technique. Soft-tissue deformities include sagging of eyelid and cheek after zygomatic dissections (Phillips et al 1991); meticulous redraping of the dissected soft tissues should lessen the risk of this deformity.

Prominent plates

Plate prominence is common: plate placement must minimize palpability and visibility.

Disturbance of globe position

Disturbance of globe position in both the anteroposterior

and vertical dimension remains the major long-term complication. Enophthalmos and vertical ocular dystopia as late post-traumatic manifestations are cosmetically and often functionally disturbing, and almost impossible to correct perfectly when well established. These deformities constitute the major complication in high velocity, severely comminuted zygomatic fractures (Fig. 11.98).

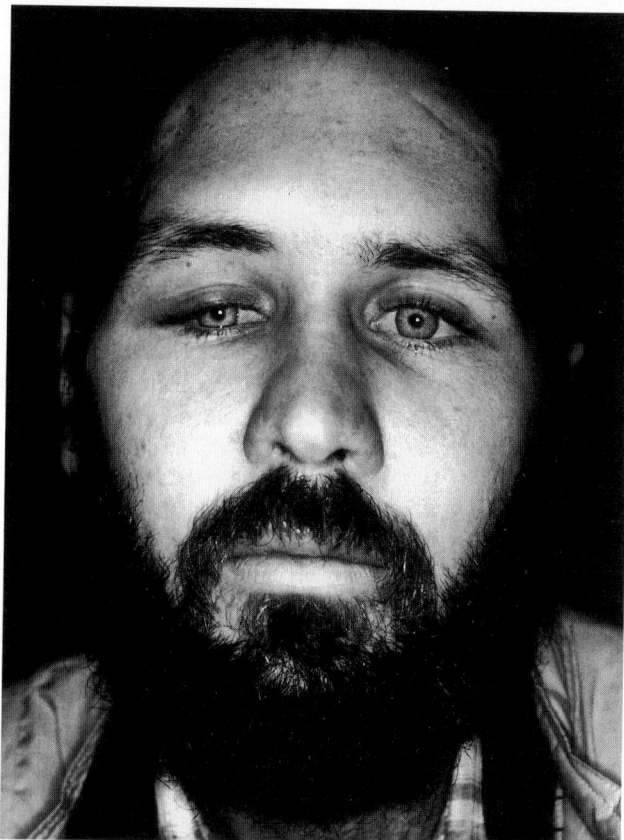

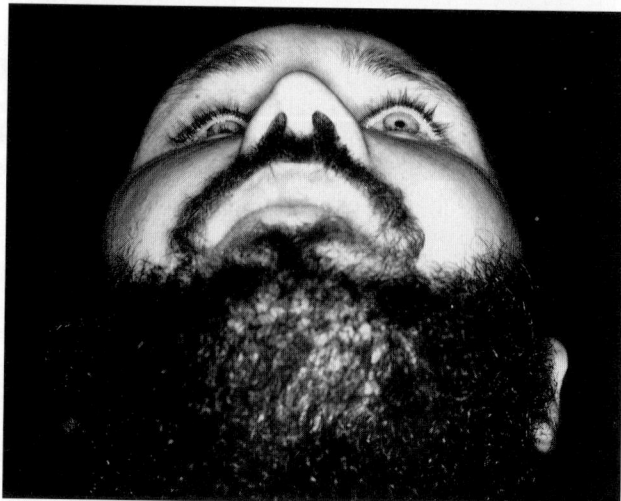

Fig. 11.98 Post-traumatic enophthalmos. A Frontal and **B** worm's-eye view of marked enophthalmos on right side following severe right frontozygomatic fracture. Note the supratarsal hollowing and pseudoptosis.

Ocular injury

Direct globe injuries are common in association with these fractures, but most are not serious and without long-term sequelae. These injuries are discussed in detail in Chapter 14.

Nerve injury

Infraorbital nerve injuries causing persistent numbness, paraesthesia or hyperaesthesia in the distribution of the nerve may occur; Dielert & Jais (1992) reviewed 176 cases of zygomatic fractures, and found disturbed sensation in the face in as many as 28.5%. Most patients experience significant recovery of function early, but occasional patients experience progressive improvement as late as 18 months after injury.

ORBITAL FRACTURES

Surgical pathology

The position of the orbit at the interface between the cranium above and the midface below, in intimate relation to the thin-walled paranasal sinuses, demands that this region be carefully evaluated in the assessment of facial trauma.

Advances in the management of orbital injuries have resulted from better understanding of the bony and soft-tissue anatomy (Pearl 1987), and have improved awareness of how each component relates to the other to produce the final position of the globe in three dimensions. Advances in the imaging of these injuries now permit preoperative planning, appropriate operative exposure, and reconstruction of both skeletal and soft tissues to minimize the major long-term sequelae of enophthalmos and attendant soft-tissue contractures. A high and predictable level of anatomical skeletal restoration by rigidly fixed bone grafts now appears possible, and the only remaining unpredictable variable for outcome is the periorbital soft tissue and how this changes after the initial injury and the subsequent surgery. Good primary correction is essential; late correction will not reverse the soft-tissue disorganization and muscle shortening resulting from prolonged posterior displacement of the globe.

Simplistically a quadrilateral pyramid composed of seven bones, the orbit has a strong anterior rim or base and four thin walls which converge on a strong bony apex. The thick protective outer rim is formed by the frontal, zygomatic and maxillary bones; at the rim, the orbit is ovoid in coronal section, becoming more rectangular as one proceeds posteriorly to the apex, where the cavity is almost triangular (Fig. 2.7). The orbit has four walls — superior (roof), medial, inferior (floor) and lateral — all thin and delicate and each unique in the manner in which it responds to trauma. Lang (1983) quoted measurements

Table 11.4 Classification of orbital fractures

1. Intrinsic — orbital rim intact
   (a) Blow-out
   (b) Blow-in
2. Extrinsic — orbital rim fractured
   (a) Blow-out
   (b) Blow-in

of the orbital walls in adults; these are given on p. 37. The portion of the orbit in front of the transverse axis of the globe — the anterior segment — has little effect on bony orbital volume and hence on the projection of the globe of the eye, and relatively more influence on its vertical and transverse ocular position (Fig. 11.97). Alterations to the size and shape of the posterior segment, the portion of the orbital cavity behind the axis of the globe, determine the orbital skeletal volume and therefore the ocular projection.

Disruption of the orbit may result from fracture of the orbital rim and walls by extension of *extrinsic* (= external) fractures, which are classified according to their major anatomical component, or from indirect forces transmitted via the globe and periorbital soft tissues to produce an *intrinsic* blow-out fracture of the floor or medial wall (Table 11.4).

The superior orbital rim, formed by the frontal bone, is thick. The orbital roof is arched in both anteroposterior and transverse directions, and relatively resistant to fracturing. 'Blow-in' fractures (inferior displacement) of the roof occur as frequently as blow-out fractures in this area and in most cases are associated with orbital rim disruption. Orbital roof fractures, usually occurring in high energy impact injuries with extension into the face, are more frequently seen in children (p. 511); such fractures often result from direct impacts on the frontal bone (p. 102).

The orbital floor is the classic site of 'blow-out' fractures. The anterior orbital floor medial to the infraorbital canal is concave in an anteroposterior direction. Posterior to the axis of the globe it becomes convex upwards, the underlying maxillary antrum bulging superiorly and obliterating the angle between the floor and the medial wall (Fig. 11.97). Restoration of this orbital floor convexity after injury significantly influences forward positioning of the globe.

The medial walls are approximately vertical and run parallel with each other. The most inferior portion diverges laterally and runs into the floor. The lacrimal bone and the lamina papyracea (orbital plate) of the ethmoid comprise the thin, vulnerable portion of the medial wall. Supported by the bony septae of the ethmoidal air sinuses, the medial wall, although often thinner than the floor, does not fracture as frequently as the orbital floor in pure 'blow-out' injuries. Isolated medial wall defects in the middle third of the orbit produce increases in orbital

volume posterior to the ocular axis and may cause enophthalmos. Medial rectus entrapment in such injuries is possible but infrequent. At the anterior extent of the medial wall lie the lacrimal drainage system and medial canthal ligament; injuries of these structures are most frequently seen in association with naso-orbito-ethmoid and complex midfacial injuries.

The lateral orbital wall (greater wing of the sphenoid and orbital process of the zygoma) diverges from the medial wall at 45° (Fig. 11.96), and lies entirely posterior to the transverse ocular axis. Infrequently fractured in isolation, a fracture in this site is an almost invariable accompaniment of zygomatic fractures. Any disturbance in orientation or positioning of the lateral wall, lying as it does posterior to the globe axis, produces orbital volume change and alteration in globe projection (Fig. 11.99). Muscle incarceration in these injuries is rare, but muscle contusion may occur.

The posterior third of the orbit and orbital apex is composed of thicker, more resilient bone, surrounding the inferior and superior orbital fissure and optic foramen. Comminution of the thinner, more anteriorly placed orbital bones minimizes transmission of displacement forces to the posterior orbit.

Extraocular muscles in the anterior half of the orbit are separated from the bony walls by small fatty cushions, in contrast to the posterior orbit where they are close to the walls and more vulnerable to injury from the fracture or from the trauma of surgical dissection. The orbital fat of the anterior orbit is extraconal. Of special interest is a sausage-shaped orbital fat compartment which separates the levator palpebrae superioris, superior rectus and superior oblique muscles from the orbital roof. Where dystopia of the globe occurs with orbital fracture this superior fat pad prolapses away from the upper eyelid producing

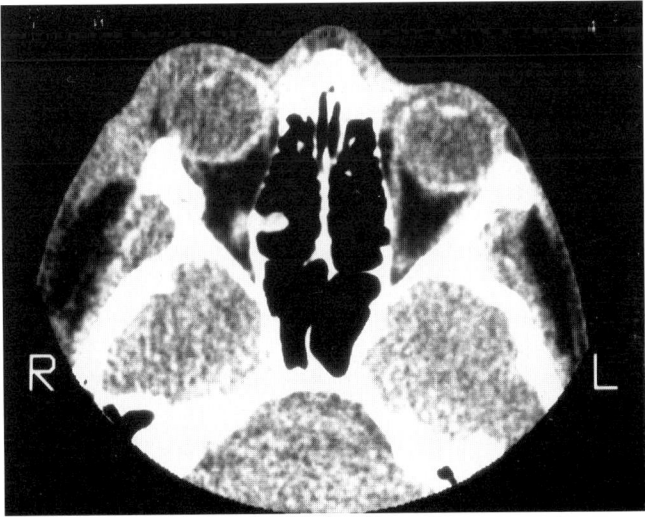

Fig. 11.99 Radiology of blow-in fractures. Axial 2D CT scan of lateral orbital wall 'blow-in' fracture (impure) with resultant exophthalmos.

'supratarsal hollowing' — corrected by repositioning and elevation of the globe behind the equator. In the posterior orbit most fat is intraconal and it is the volume of this fat that is the most important determinant of globe position. Most authors believe that loss of extraconal fat produces no significant change in globe position, but fat displacement from the intraconal to the extraconal compartment in the posterior orbit reduces globe support, with possible resultant enophthalmos (Manson et al 1985a).

Classification and mechanisms

Fractures of the orbit may be simply grouped as those which are intrinsic to the orbital walls and those fractures of the orbital walls which occur in association with extrinsic (extraorbital) fractures involving the frontal, zygomatic, midfacial or naso-ethmoid regions (Table 11.4). Intrinsic fractures of the orbital walls are categorized as blow-out and blow-in fractures. The pure blow-out or blow-in fracture is distinguished by an intact orbital rim, while what are often inaccurately referred to as 'impure' blow-out or blow-in fractures are characterised by extension of an orbital wall fracture to involve the orbital rim.

The application of sudden blunt trauma to the periorbital soft tissues is transmitted as a hydraulic pressure wave to the orbital walls, resulting in a characteristic pattern of fracturing of these walls. Because of its thin, fragile and comparatively unsupported position the orbital floor gives way medial to the infraorbital nerve and medial orbital wall. The sequelae of this disturbance include enophthalmos, muscle entrapment and diplopia: these are direct consequences of the suddenly increased orbital volume and the displacement of the globe and its related muscles and periorbital fibrous septae. Pure blow-out fractures usually result from a low energy impact: the typical cause is a ball striking the orbit from in front (Fig. 4.5). Controversies on the mechanisms producing blow-out fractures are discussed in Chapter 4 (p. 104). The blow-in fracture, described more recently (Antonyshyn et al 1989), and much rarer, is characterized by inward displacement of bony fragments of the walls and/or rim (pure and impure) with resultant decreased orbital volume and increased globe projection (Fig. 11.99).

Low velocity impacts from assaults or falls most commonly produce simple, isolated linear, or 'blow-out' type fractures, with minimal comminution involving one or two orbital walls. Medium velocity impacts produce similar injuries, but usually with associated orbital rim disturbance and involvement of at least two orbital walls. The extrinsic fractures which extend to involve the orbital walls invariably result from medium and high energy impacts.

High velocity impacts result in complex orbital fractures, involving three or four walls, with associated panfacial fractures and increased incidence of orbital soft tissue and globe injuries; such fractures exhibit much less well defined patterns of fracturing, and more comminution and bone loss.

Clinical assessment

Clinical examination of the orbit in trauma is often of limited value, but a history of the velocity of impact, and the presence or absence of associated craniofacial and multisystem injuries will alert the observer to the likelihood of simple or complex orbital injuries. Periorbital bruising and swelling is inevitable, and in major injuries is at first so severe as to obscure the globe (Fig. 11.100). Eversion of the eyelids with Desmarre retractors in these severe cases is mandatory and should be done early to avoid missing primary globe injuries, which occur with increased frequency as the impact energy rises.

Visual disturbance, blurring or diplopia may be complained of, and these symptoms require full ophthalmological assessment. Holt & Holt (1983) reported on a large series of patients with facial trauma and identified ocular and/or periorbital soft tissue injury in 65%; 18% had severe injuries and 3% blinding injuries. Our experience suggests a much lower incidence (4.9%) of significant ocular injuries, predominantly in association with pure orbital, zygomatic or mid- or pan facial fractures (p. 397). Altered sensation and numbness in the distribution of the infraorbital nerve and the anterior and middle superior alveolar nerves are frequent accompaniments of orbital floor fractures (Fig. 2.29).

Clinical examination follows the sequence detailed for zygomatic fractures. Assessment of alterations in the anteroposterior projection of the globe is frequently difficult during the acute phase when swelling is marked. The enophthalmos associated with a significant orbital wall

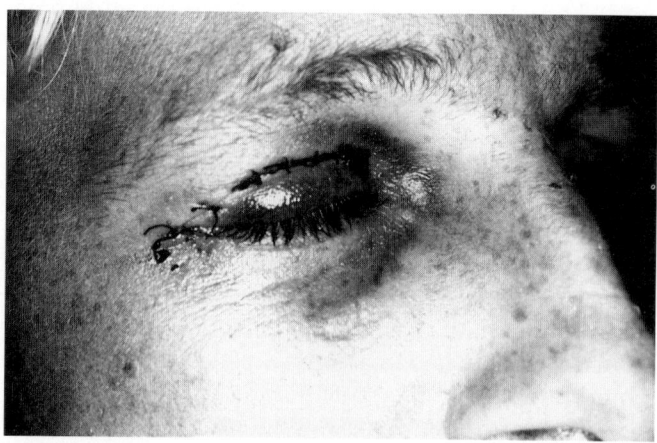

Fig. 11.100 Clinical signs of orbital blow-out fractures. Right orbital blow-out fracture following blunt trauma. Moderate periorbital bruising closes the eye acutely.

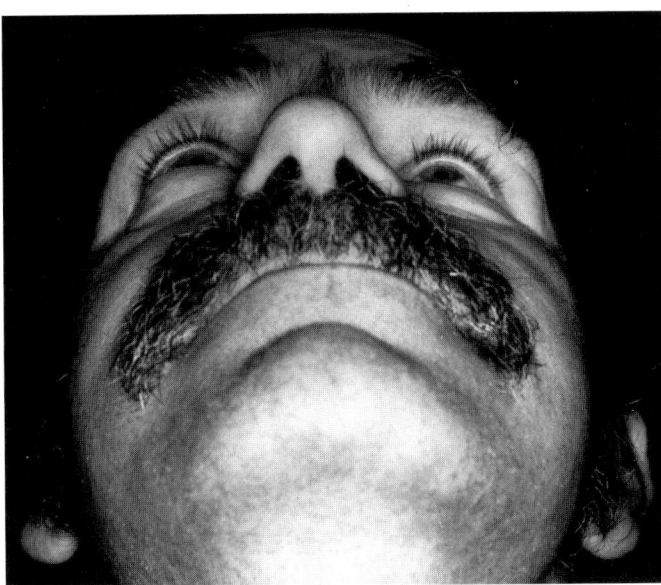

Fig. 11.101 **Clinical signs of orbital blow-out fractures.** Worm's-eye view identifies significant enophthalmos in blow-out fracture after resolution of oedema.

injury may only become overt after the oedema has subsided (Fig. 11.101). Early marked exophthalmos suggests a significant reduction in bony orbital volume and requires urgent and complete ophthalmological and radiological examination to exclude an orbital injury which may be directly injurious to the globe or contents of the orbital apex. The ophthalmological assessment of the globe and the ocular motility is especially important; Antonyshyn et al (1989) reported a 12% incidence of

globe rupture and 10% incidence of superior orbital fissure syndrome in patients with blow-in fractures.

Radiological assessment

CT examination is now the diagnostic investigation of choice in orbital trauma. Plain radiographic studies are often employed as screening tests, but CT scan assessment is mandatory for accurate diagnosis and in planning appropriate reconstruction (Fig. 11.102).

High resolution axial CT scan examination with films of both bone and soft-tissue windows show damage to the medial and lateral walls and extension of fractures into the cranial base, zygoma and midface. Direct coronal views, or those produced by reformatting the data obtained from the axial scans, visualize the status of the orbital roof, medial wall and orbital floor (Fig. 11.103). When a pure blow-out fracture is suspected, direct coronal scans of the orbit will accurately identify both the extent of the floor and medial wall involvement and the nature of the soft-tissue abnormality (p. 193). Fatty prolapse into the area of the blowout fracture without muscle entrapment is identified by the presence of the muscles in the orbit above the orbital wall fracture (Fig. 11.104). Muscle displacement into the sinus or muscle impinging on the bony fragments may mean muscle entrapment. Submucosal haematomas or mucosal polyps of the maxillary sinus roof, which on conventional radiology may resemble herniated soft tissues, can be differentiated on coronal CT scan. Sagittal oblique reformats of CT image data in the line of the inferior rectus muscle will similarly relate

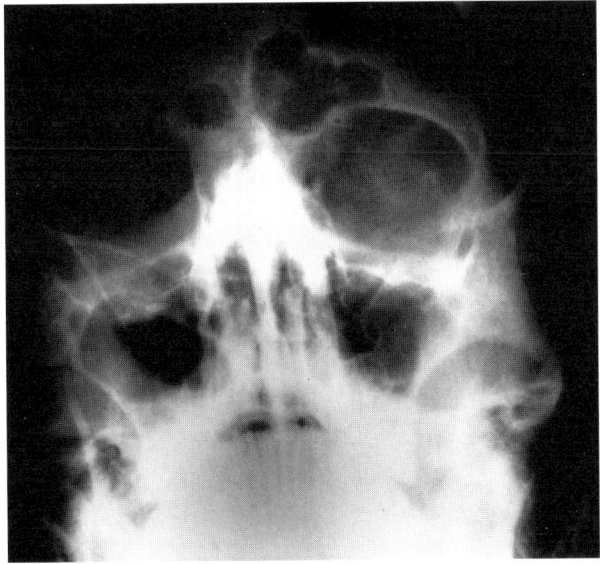

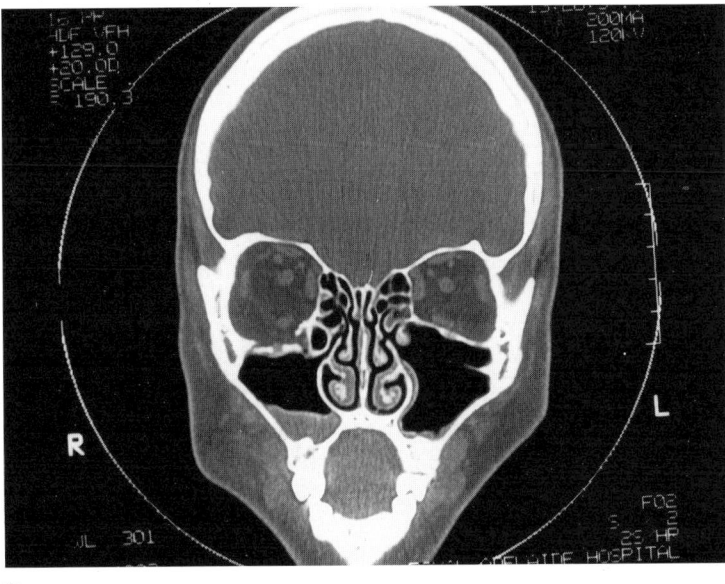

A   B

Fig. 11.102 **Radiology of orbital blow-out fractures. A** Plain radiograph shows 'tear-drop' deformity of right orbital floor, with inferiorly displaced orbital floor bony fragments. **B** Coronal 2D CT scan details the isolated right orbital floor fracture with no involvement of the medial orbital wall.

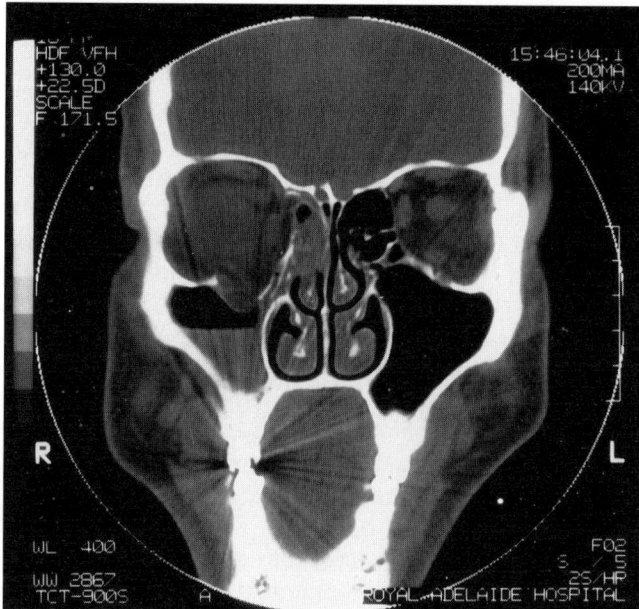

Fig. 11.103 Radiology of orbital blow-out fractures. Coronal 2D CT scan pictures the trap-door like depression of the right orbital floor with concomitant blow-out of the medial orbital wall. Note the transverse narrowing of the ethmoid air cells on the right.

this muscle and the adjacent orbital soft tissues to bony damage to the orbital floor. Comparison with the contralateral orbit provides a qualitative assessment of the degree of enophthalmos; quantification of post-traumatic enophthalmos and the changes produced by surgical correction is also possible (Marsh & Gado 1983).

Management

Closed methods of managing fractures which involve the orbital walls risk non-anatomical reconstruction of the bony orbit, post-traumatic enophthalmos, ocular dystopia and motility disturbances. Some authors have advocated conservative management of blow-out fractures on the basis that the soft-tissue ligamentous supports of the globe remain undamaged and able to maintain eye position (Korneef 1982). These views have been largely rejected because of the incidence of unacceptable late post-traumatic enophthalmos, which is very difficult to treat. Non-operative management is considered only in those cases where bony displacement is negligible and there are no other clinical signs of note; there is no evidence to support infraorbital nerve numbness alone as an indicator for operative intervention.

Management now aims at accurate restoration of the orbital rim and walls, thus minimizing the troublesome secondary soft tissue disturbances. The orbital rim is reduced and fixed internally with a combination of mini-plates and microplates, while the orbital walls are reconstructed with primary bone autografts if comminution or bone loss is extensive (Figs 11.93 and 11.95).

Operative repair is performed as early as possible to minimize the development of soft tissue fibrotic changes. Acute periorbital swelling prevents exploration and repair within the first 24–48 h except in such exceptional circumstances as the presence of a bony fragment impinging on the globe or optic nerve in a 'blow-in' fracture. This demands immediate exploration.

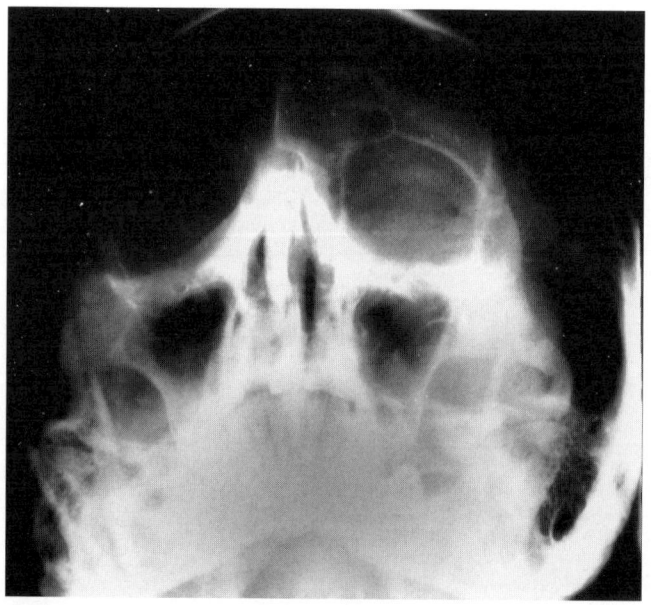

A

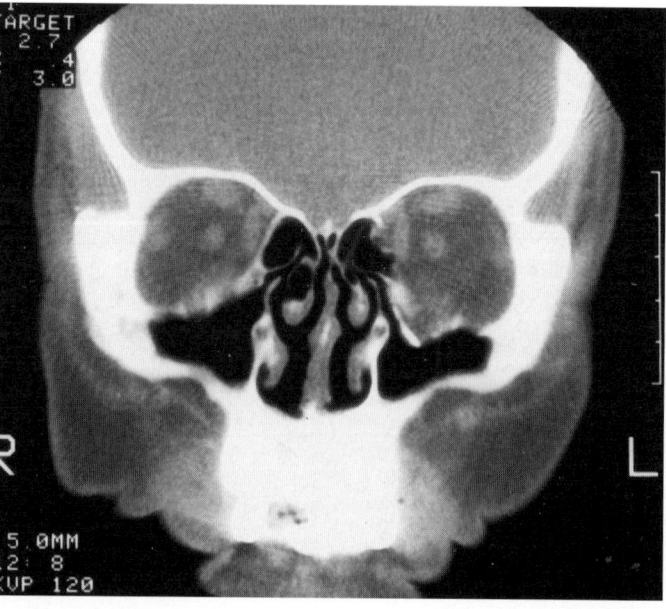

B

Fig. 11.104 Radiology of orbital blow-out fractures. A Plain radiograph identifies relatively minor irregularity and depression of left orbital floor bony fragments. **B** Coronal 2D CT scan denotes irregularity of the left orbital floor and apparent inferior displacement of the inferior rectus muscle into the region of the fracture.

The exposure, exploration, reduction and fixation of the orbital rim are described in the section on orbito-zygomatic fractures (p. 320).

Reconstruction of the orbital cavity, together with orbital rim restoration, returns the globe to its pre-injury position with full maintenance of ocular motility. Subperiosteal dissection of the orbital walls delineates the site and pattern of the fracture, identifying the areas of bony deficiency and the surrounding stable, intact bony margins. All the herniated soft tissues are retrieved from the bony defect, minimizing fibrosis or loss of soft tissues.

In small isolated blow-out fractures, the displaced bony fragment may be elevated and allowed to override, producing a stable restoration of the orbital wall anatomy. For most defects this is inadequate, and correction requires the introduction of an orbital wall substitute.

The choice of materials for orbital reconstruction lies between autogenous bone or cartilage grafts and alloplastic implants, either resorbable or non-resorbable. Supposedly resorbable alloplastic materials such as Gelfilm® and Vicryl® mesh have little strength and are of use only where orbital wall defects are minimal, or where the surgeon feels that a small smooth space filler will improve a localized contour irregularity in the restored orbital cavity. Being resorbable, they are well tolerated and are not associated with late infective or extrusion problems. Various non-resorbable alloplastic implants have been employed for small and large orbital defects (Maas et al 1990). The easy availability of compounds such as Silastic® sheeting, Marlex® mesh, Prolene®, Teflon® and titanium or Vitallium® mesh, and the wish to avoid secondary donor site problems, have continued to promote the widespread use of these compounds in the orbit despite significant graft extrusion rates. As with similar grafts utilized elsewhere in the body the orbital tissues respond to the foreign body with the production of a fibrous avascular capsule. Situated in close proximity to the paranasal sinuses and often immediately subcutaneous, alloplastic implants remain at long-term risk of infection and extrusion. The biocompatibility of titanium has encouraged its use as a mesh to restore orbital cavity contours, especially in complex orbital and extensive panfacial fractures where all normal orbital supporting structures are lost. Able to be bent and shaped very accurately, titanium mesh is best utilized as a framework on which autogenous bone may be placed. Some of the bone will resorb, but experimental studies by Sullivan et al (1993) suggest that enough remains to constitute a smooth orbital floor. The use of mesh in isolation allows extensive soft-tissue ingrowth, making removal of the mesh at a later date for infective or other complications a possibly insurmountable technical challenge. In addition the porosity of the mesh does not prevent soft-tissue loss from the orbit and hence the development of enophthalmos. We believe that autogenous bone is usually the best material for orbital repair, provided that the grafts are properly shaped, placed anatomically, rigidly fixed, and with substantial volumetric overcorrection to allow for future resorption. Autogenous grafts have indeed been utilized in this way for many years, being favoured because of the lack of infective and extrusion problems. Nevertheless, autogenous grafts are attended by variable degrees of disadvantage relating to donor site morbidity and graft resorption. These relate to the choice of bone or cartilage, and to the site from which the graft is obtained.

Calvarial bone enjoys widespread popularity for use as onlay and inlay grafts in the craniofacial region. The need for a further incision may be avoided if bone is harvested from the inner table when a formal craniotomy has been performed, or split from the outer table of the temporoparietal skull when a coronal flap is used; with a sharp osteotome, calvarial bone can be cut with preservation of the overlying pericranium. The brittle nature of calvarial bone makes contouring of the graft to the appropriate orbital wall shape rather difficult. Calvarial bone appears most useful where it can accurately reconstruct a single orbital wall, or as an autogenous onlay overlying titanium mesh restoring two or more orbital walls.

Split-rib graft is available in large quantities and is most readily contoured to the correct curvature of the orbital walls. It is the graft material of choice in those cases where several orbital walls require reconstruction. Resorption of onlay rib or iliac grafts is said to be higher than when calvarial bone is employed (Zins & Whitaker 1983). Stacking bone graft from anterior to posterior, making use of the stable posterior ledge, gives the correct convex upslope of the orbital floor and minimizes the risk of displacement of the graft. Rigid internal fixation by lag screws or contoured microplates or miniplates improves graft retention and gives ideal orbital wall reconstruction. These additional techniques are seldom necessary in the isolated blow-out fracture, but increase the predictability of a good outcome in complex injuries.

Autogenous cartilage graft, either costal or auricular, can be valuable in correcting small orbital wall defects. While not prone to significant resorption, cartilage grafts have a tendency to warp; if placed in the orbit, difficulties with fixation may lead to displacement of the cartilage into the adjacent maxillary sinus. Few studies have detailed significant experience with the use of cartilage graft in the orbit.

In uncomplicated blow-out fractures, after anatomical correction of the orbital bony anatomy with or without a graft, the orbital soft tissues are simply allowed to redrape. A forced duction test is performed by grasping the rectus muscle insertion with forceps to ensure that all muscle entrapment has been relieved. The lower lid incision or conjunctival incision is then closed in a single layer. In complex orbital injuries where the exposure requires extensive subperiosteal dissection of the facial soft tissues, the final act in operative treatment is careful fixation of the periorbital soft tissues.

Complications

Complications of orbital fractures are still seen despite open reduction and primary bone grafting. Residual problems may result from the initial injurious process, or from failure to correct the disordered anatomy, or from changes induced by the operative exposure (Wolfe 1988). Common complications include:

- Ocular problems
- Enophthalmos
- Ocular dystopia
- Canthal dystopia.

Ocular problems

These relate primarily to the initial injury and are not affected by the bony reconstruction. Persistent diplopia in the initial postoperative period is not infrequent but is seldom noted on long-term follow-up. Some patients do continue to have subjective complaints of double vision on extremes of gaze. It is sometimes suggested that these complaints are not supported by objective evidence of ocular disturbance; nevertheless a careful test of ocular motility will usually show muscle weakness or restriction of gaze and some of these patients need ocular muscle surgery (p. 420).

Where significant bony displacement occurs in the region of the orbital apex and superior fissure with associated optic nerve injury and/or ophthalmoplegia, the outcome after bony reduction is often unhappy. In most cases of blindness following high energy impacts the optic nerve is irreversibly damaged in the optic canal (p. 422). By contrast Antonyshyn et al (1989) were able to show a significant improvement after immediate orbital decompression in orbital blow-in fractures complicated by ophthalmoplegia.

Enophthalmos

The commonest complication remains persistent enophthalmos. This relates principally to inadequate exposure of the extent of the bony defect, and particularly the medial orbital wall extension. Inadequate or inaccurate orbital wall reconstructions by graft, or graft displacement and resorption, contribute significantly to this problem. In complex orbital injuries a degree of bony overcorrection is needed to achieve an acceptable long-term outcome with respect to globe position; the unpredictable factors of oedema, fibrosis and fat loss make it impossible to get a perfect result.

Ocular dystopia

Transverse and vertical dystopia of the globe may follow inaccurate reduction of the zygoma, and hence the portion of the orbital walls anterior to the axis of the globe, or from incorrect graft placement in the same region.

Canthal dystopia

The main complications relating to the surgical exposure and subperiosteal dissection of the orbit are degrees of medial and lateral canthal dystopia. Careful maintenance of the bony attachment of the medial canthus in isolated orbital injuries should prevent the development of telecanthus or medial canthal dystopia. Medial canthal abnormalities are more frequent and are difficult to correct where bony orbital injury is accompanied by local soft-tissue lacerations in this region. In addition to telecanthus an inappropriately anterior positioning of the medial canthal ligament is a frequent complication. Lateral canthal dystopia, with poor apposition of the lower lid to the globe, is a common finding soon after a lateral canthotomy performed to expose the orbit but settles with time. Careful attention to wound closure and reattachment of the lateral canthus will prevent the development of this eyelid abnormality.

FRACTURES PRIMARILY AFFECTING THE NASAL AIRWAY

NASAL FRACTURES

Surgical pathology

Whether alone or in combination with more complex injuries, fractures of the nose are the commonest facial fracture in most published series. The prominent position of the nose makes it often injured in isolation when struck by a low energy impact (Fig. 11.105); the nasal bones are the most fragile element in the facial skeleton, and break under forces well below those needed to fracture the other components of the middle third of the face (p. 103). With high energy impacts, nasal fractures are often seen as one element of a more complex facial injury. The exposed position of the nose makes it liable to injury in assaults, accidents and falls. An understanding of the mechanisms and patterns of injury and their variation according to the force and direction of the blow is of importance both for individual patient management and prognosis and also in the prediction of outcome and resolution of litigation arising from assault.

While the visible injury of the nose demands immediate attention, most nasal fractures have posterior extensions which produce bending or displacement of the bony and cartilaginous nasal septum. The management of these is a great long-term challenge.

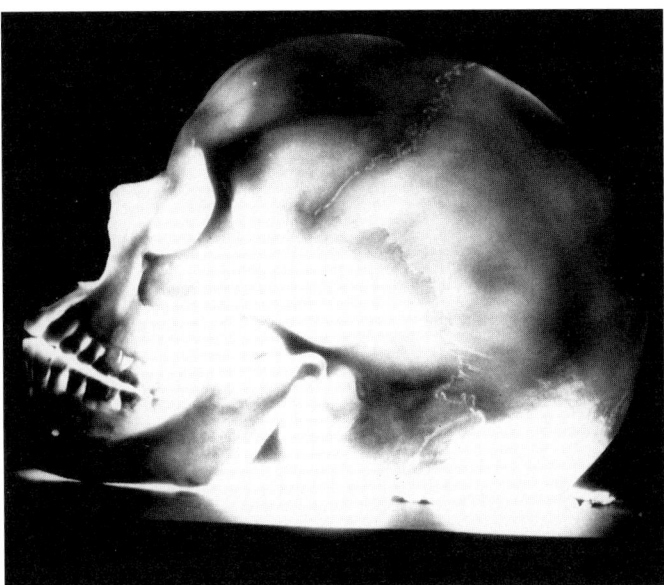

Fig. 11.105 Nasal skeleton. Lateral profile of adult skull confirms the prominent position of the nose, exposed to frontal and oblique lateral impacts.

The patterns of nasal injury relate to the complex anatomy of the nose (p. 37) and to the velocity, mass, direction and site of impact. High energy impacts, by objects with high velocity and/or large mass, cause increased comminution, loss of nasal dorsal support and likely extension into adjacent facial regions; the nasal bones and anterior nasal spine are likely to collapse under an impact force able to create a Le Fort type of fracture (p. 103). The spread of bony–cartilaginous disruption widens as the effective force of impact increases (Pollock 1992). Direct frontal impact usually displaces and comminutes both the nasal skeleton and septum. Laterally directed forces produce deformation ranging from minor unilateral medial displacement of a single nasal bone through to significant lateral displacement of the entire nasal complex; with the latter, septal involvement may be complex in several dimensions. Inferior impacts damage initially the anterior nasal spine with extension more posteriorly to involve the septum and lateral nasal structures, injuring both soft tissues and bony elements.

Stranc and Robertson (1979) analysed nasal fractures according to lateral and posterior displacement and by the unilateral or bilateral extent of the injury. They noted that lateral force fractures were most common, and because there is seldom serious disruption between the bony and cartilaginous elements, the aesthetic and functional result after reduction is usually good. By contrast injury from a frontal impact is less common and less well defined and the results are less often acceptable. Generally the degree of posterior displacement correlates closely with the amount of comminution of the nasal bony–cartilaginous complex.

As with other regions of the facial skeleton, identical fracture patterns are seldom seen in the nose, yet a degree of predictability is evident. The cartilaginous elements are the most forward-projecting portions of the nose and are thus the first components to deform on impact. The dissipation of energy then proceeds through the next most vulnerable structures, the nasal bones and septum, and so on into the skeletal base until dissipated. The fractures due to high energy impacts are invariably bilateral with extensions proximally toward the glabella, inferiorly to the piriform margin, with involvement of the supporting facial skeleton.

Clinical assessment

The history of injury usually identifies the probable energy of impact and the likely extent of injury. Details of the nature of the traumatic force, and its direction, will aid in predicting fracture patterns. A record of pre-existing nasal deformity and previous operations on the nose should be sought.

Examination early after injury is ideal, but is seldom possible before the onset of oedema obscures the definition of the nasal bones and cartilages. Local injury to the region of the anterior nasal spine produces swelling and pain in the upper lip with marked tenderness on palpation of the columella. Where the injury is localized to the nasal bones and frontal processes of the maxilla periorbital bruising and paranasal oedema are evident (Fig. 11.106). With further extension of the injury into the naso-ethmoid and midfacial regions the deformity associated with these injuries predominates and the clinical indications of displacement of the nasal bones are correspondingly less evident. In general, the more extensive the injuries, the greater the oedema and bruising.

A systematic examination and palpation of the nose, with attention both to intra- and extranasal structures, is done along routine lines (Fig. 6.5). This must be gentle, and may rarely require local or general anaesthesia, especially in children. Palpation of the nasal bones and frontal processes of the maxilla is performed to elicit mobility, bony deformity and crepitus. Oedema often limits the detailed assessment of the displacement of the thin nasal bones.

Intranasal examination allows assessment of nasal obstruction from blood clot, or bleeding from mucosal lacerations which may require control to allow complete evaluation. Displacement of the septal cartilage, bony deviation, mucosal tears and septal haematoma are all assessable by intranasal examination (Fig. 11.107).

Reassessment may be indicated when the initial examination occurs at a time of maximal swelling, in order to avoid missing a fracture. The final and often most effective clinical evaluation for surgical planning may be performed intraoperatively. A periosteal elevator placed high

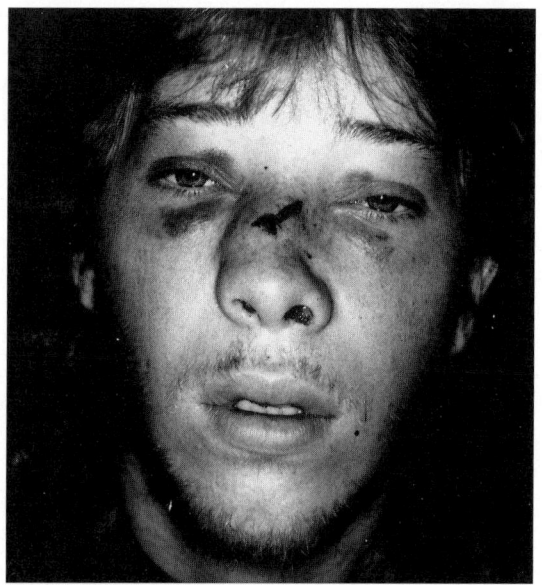

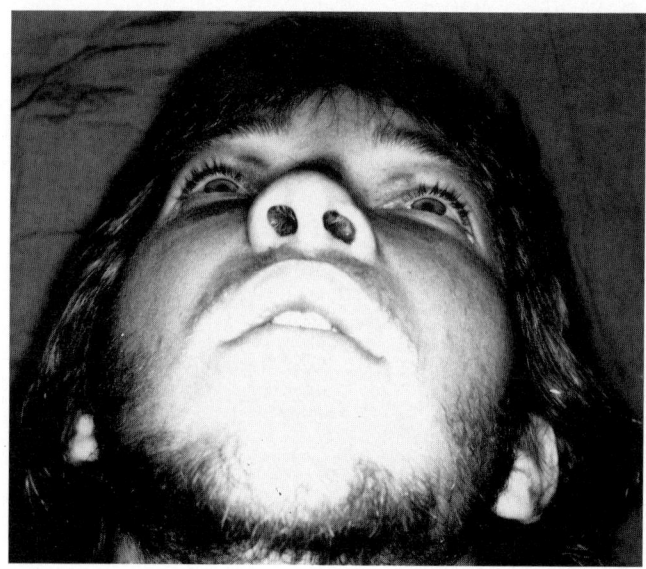

Fig. 11.106 Clinical signs of nasal fractures. A and **B** Clinical appearance where gross deviation of the nasal bony skeleton to the right with attendant tilting of the cartilaginous septum.

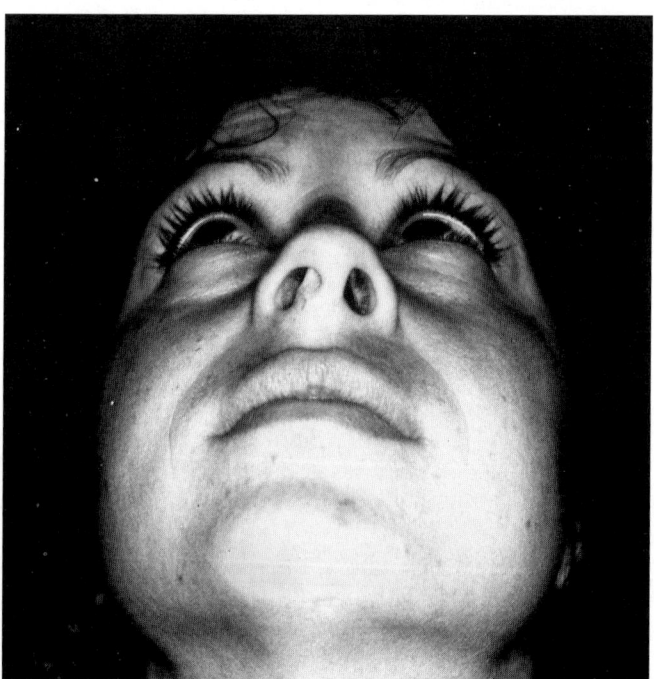

Fig. 11.107 Nasal septal injury. Worm's-eye view identifies characteristic caudal septal dislocation.

in the nasal vault will help in bimanual palpation of individual nasal bones and the nasal bone complex as a whole. Intraoperative pressure over the nasal dorsum is helpful in assessing collapse of the underlying bony–cartilaginous structure (Gruss 1982). Although this procedure was originally used in the assessment of naso-orbito-ethmoid fractures, Pollock (1992) has utilized it selectively at dif-

ferent levels of the nose to identify collapse of the upper, middle or lower vault. When applied to the upper nose in complex injuries, the nasal bridge is found to disappear back between the eyes.

Radiological assessment

Routine radiographical examination of the facial bones may not always reveal the nasal fracture. A lateral view coned on the nose and occipitomental views with additional backward projection may improve the visualization of bony injury. These views are frequently requested in the casualty department, particularly if the mechanism is an assault and litigation is likely; however, the radiographs seldom influence the decision on operative repair. Coronal or axial CT scans, with the addition of 3D CT reconstruction, will elegantly visualize a nasal fracture superimposed on a major midfacial or naso-orbito-ethmoid fracture (p. 198), but CT investigation is certainly not indicated for isolated simple nasal fractures.

Management

Treatment aims at restoration of appearance and re-establishment of nasal airway function bilaterally. As a rule, the nasal fracture must be reduced. Convention has it that reduction is ideally undertaken either immediately following injury, prior to the development of oedema, or up to 14 days later when the oedema has subsided. Most cases fall within the latter category, whether simple or complex. Where there are other extensive facial fractures reduction may be further delayed while the patient is resuscitated and appropriately investigated. In fact, the timing of operative treatment must be individualized. While immediate centralization of the nasal pyramid in a laterally deviated nose is possible, an inadequately treated nasal septum or inaccurately reduced nasal bones will necessitate more complex secondary surgery. Most nasal fractures are reduced within the first 7–10 days although it is possible to accomplish an appropriate reduction after a delay of 3–4 weeks.

Because simple techniques of reduction will not suffice in all cases, nasal fractures should as a rule be treated in an operating theatre, so that more complex forms of treatment can be undertaken at once if necessary.

Simple closed reduction is the standard treatment for nasal injuries due to low and middle levels of impact energy. In the acute period, the application of local thumb pressure may successfully reduce the displaced nasal complex to its normal position, sometimes without the need for an anaesthetic. Delayed reduction may be possible in the same fashion, using local anaesthetic and sedation or general anaesthesia. General anaesthesia permits detailed examination, and is particularly useful in the younger patient where cooperation might otherwise be difficult. Intranasal packing and external tapes and splints minimize subsequent swelling and bleeding, and may aid in positioning unstable fragments.

In middle level energy impacts where displacement of the nasal complex may be both posterior and lateral, closed reduction is similarly employed, but requires the use of elevating instruments. Upward and outward manipulation of the nasal bone fragments with a Howarth elevator or similar blunt edged tool permits realignment whilst minimizing damage to the nasal lining. Nasal compression forceps (e.g. Walsham's forceps) are widely employed but may cause additional soft-tissue crush injury. Sharper instruments such as a large curved haemostat have been used, but risk tearing the nasal mucosa.

Treatment of low and middle energy nasal injuries by simple closed reduction has been generally accepted, despite studies which indicate that this method has potential for a poor outcome. Mayell (1973) in a retrospective report showed that only 30% of cases had restoration of normal appearance, though 50% had normal nasal airway function. Similarly Harrison (1979) identified only 33% of his patients as having both adequate airway and ideal cosmesis.

Closed reduction is ideal for the unilateral, depressed nasal bone fracture where septal injury is absent; inadequately treated septal displacement is the chief cause of the poor results of closed reduction. In the middle energy impacts the nasal complex displacement is both posterior and lateral with resultant increased septal injury, and more elaborate procedures may be needed.

Nevertheless, nasal septal dislocation is routinely man-aged in the first instance by closed reduction (Fig. 11.107). As the septal position will often influence nasal bone position, the reduction must be rechecked and occasionally repositioned. Asch septal forceps will correct both superior and inferior septal deviations. The superior portion of the cartilaginous septum, being contiguous with the bony septum, is reduced first before dealing with the inferior septum. Adequate reduction of the superior portion can usually be achieved; inferior septal deviations are not so often successfully reduced with closed techniques.

Where closed reduction has failed, the choice lies between acute open reduction or a late secondary procedure. Early open reduction is difficult because of the soft-tissue swelling and the increased risk of lacerations when elevating the mucoperichondrium of the septum. Harrison (1979) suggested early limited submucosal resection of the bony–cartilaginous junction for those cases where septal deviation is marked: after lower horizontal and posterior vertical submucous septal resection, the cosmetic and functional results were improved. There has been only limited acceptance of this management, because it could result in mucosal injury and septal perforation. Pollock (1992) has advocated early cartilage repositioning and fixation where significant septal deviation adversely affects nasal bone positioning, using techniques of cartilage preservation. This has not been our policy: rather, we have advocated secondary correction.

Lacerations of the overlying skin are frequent in cases of nasal fracture, and may permit open reduction and fixation with interosseous wires, miniplates or microplates. When bicoronal and upper vestibular incisions are used for exposure of associated complex fractures, ideal exposure of the nasal region is given.

Complex nasal fractures demand careful reconstruction proceeding from a stable proximal base. The nasal bony anatomy must be restored and the bones must be re-attached at the frontal articulation to recreate the naso-frontal angle. Interosseous wires, micro- and miniplates and screws will provide anatomical reconstruction where the bony fragments are sufficiently large. The middle and lower thirds of the nose are then reconstituted using the techniques of closed reduction and limited open septal reduction described above. In all cases nasal packing is employed for 1–2 days in concert with a moulded nasal splint or plaster for the first 5–7 days. Where bony comminution is extreme and proximal skeletal support inadequate this approach is insufficient to expand the nasal soft-tissue envelope. If uncorrected, severe comminution may result in a variable combination of saddle deformity, loss of nasal tip projection and nasal foreshortening in the vertical dimension. There is a need for bone or cartilage grafts to augment the skeleton and to splint the nasal soft tissue.

Cantilever bone grafts overlying the existing nasal

bone and interposed into the nasal tip will satisfy this reconstructive need. Introduced via a bicoronal approach if this is already available, or through a local intranasal incision or an external rhinoplasty approach, the graft is fixed to the stable proximal elements of the nasal bones with miniscrews or by a contoured miniplate anchored to the central forehead. In the less complex fractures where no bicoronal incision has been used the anchoring screws can be inserted through a small skin incision in the glabella. Attention to nasal tip aesthetics is essential when using these grafts to ensure accurate positioning and attachment of the alar cartilages, and to minimize the need for secondary revision. Underlay grafts have been described as a variation with miniplate fixation of the graft below at the anterior nasal spine. No significant advantage over onlay cantilever grafting has been noted, especially in operations performed soon after injury. Cartilage grafts may be of value in the middle section of the nasal dorsum overlying the upper lateral cartilages where isolated collapse in this region is noted; they are usually inadequate to maintain forward nasal projection in severe complex injuries.

Complications

These may be broadly classified as either aesthetic or functional, interplay between both being common.

Facial aesthetics

In terms of facial aesthetics, persistent lateral deviation of the nose, and loss of nasal projection and saddle deformity, are the most significant common residual problems.

In the common low and middle energy nasal fractures persistent lateral deviation and irregularities of the nasal bridgeline, particularly a nasal hump, are the commonest aesthetic problems requiring secondary surgery. Corrective rhinoplasty with hump reduction and infracture together with septoplasty may be required (p. 575), the timing being variable; usually the rhinoplasty is performed some months following the initial injury.

Loss of nasal dorsum projection is managed in the same fashion, with an autograft for augmentation. Contracture of the soft-tissue envelope is the major limitation on what can be achieved to restore the nasal dorsum; as a rule, less projection can be achieved than with primary surgery and attempts at over-projection risk graft exposure at the nasal tip.

Function

Nasal obstructive symptoms from inadequate correction of the nasal septal cartilage represent the chief functional disturbance. Obstructive symptoms are managed by de-finitive septoplasty in conjunction with any external nasal surgery that may be required; this is done when the nasal mucosa is soundly healed from the initial injury.

MULTIPLE AND PANFACIAL FRACTURES

Clinical significance

Modern retrieval and resuscitation services result in the survival of many very severely injured patients, some of whom present for management of panfacial and craniofacial fractures. These victims of high velocity impacts with multi-system injuries which include craniofacial fractures need initial intensive care and treatment of life-threatening injuries; they then require acute stable fixation of their cranial and facial fractures to maximize the restoration of form and function.

Each injury is unique, demanding a flexibility of management that is not conveyed in any cookbook recipe approach. The confusion and poor outcome that follow rigid application of such approaches can be overcome by correct understanding of the aims and principles of reconstruction and proper sequencing of repair. In essence repair proceeds from knowledge of the stable, uninjured bony buttresses, determined preoperatively by detailed radiology and intraoperatively by wide exposure. The aim of treatment is correct restoration of midfacial projection and width in relation to the cranial base above and the mandible below. The twin requirements of form and function can then be realized. Management of these injuries involves the application of all the principles and approaches to individual subregions with a specific focus on timing and sequence of repair.

Surgical pathology

The patterns of fracture in these injuries are not defined by any conventional classification system applicable to individual facial subregions. However, in the majority of cases there are three important anatomical sites of injury, and an understanding of the fracture patterns and exposure of each of these is necessary for effective repair.

1. Cranio-orbital interface. This is the junction between the anterior cranial fossa and frontal sinus above and the orbits and naso-ethmoid region below. Anteriorly the sinus and its nasal drainage conduit (p. 37) demand consideration in the repair process, to minimize the risk of secondary sinusitis, mucocele and other infective problems. More posteriorly, maintenance or restoration of the normal interface between the contents of the anterior cranial fossa and the nasal cavity is essential in avoiding cerebral infection ascending from the nasal air passages; a dural tear makes cerebral infection a threatening possibility in both the short and the long term (p. 147). At the posterior limits of the craniofacial junction, extension of cranial base fractures through the sphenoid bone risks injury to the neurovascular structures at the orbital apex, superior orbital fissure and cavernous sinus. Away from the midline, damage to the orbital roof and lateral orbital walls may affect the projection and/or motility of the eye, or may cause orbital pulsation. Injuries in this area are often complicated by frontal lobe damage.

2. Zygomaticomaxillary junction. The zygomatic arch and the lateral orbital wall most accurately relate the orbit and midface to the cranial base above. Correct stable arch position determines lateral midface projection and midfacial width. Reconstruction of the maxilla in its correct place between the zygomas will complete the midfacial arch and central midfacial projection, with a proper relation to the mandible.

3. Mandibular condyles. These demarcate the posterior lateral limit of the craniofacial interface. The mandibular condyles and the rami establish posterior facial height. The condyles are frequently injured in panfacial fractures and demand careful restoration to re-establish the vertical dimension of the face. It is the intact mandibular arch to which the midface must be related at the occlusal level, and the mandibular arch determines facial height and to a lesser extent central facial projection.

Classification

The extent and range of bony injury in high velocity impacts frustrate any attempt to produce a detailed and precise system of classification. However, groupings have been formulated in relation to the direction and point of impact on the craniofacial region, and related to areas of skeletal strength, the facial buttresses, and adjacent zones of relative bony weakness — the sinuses and the nasal, orbital and oral cavities.

Gruss et al (1989) have grouped these injuries into three broad anatomical divisions:

1. Central craniofacial fractures
2. Lateral craniofacial fractures
3. Combined central and lateral fractures

Centrally directed impacts over the frontonasal region cleave the central facial buttresses from the anterior cranial base. Variable extensions into the frontal bone and orbital roof occur around and through the impact-absorbing frontal sinus. In the paediatric group where frontal sinus development is not complete (Fig. 2.10), impacted oblique linear and segmental fractures of the frontal bone and orbital roof occur more frequently. More extensive and/or high velocity impacts produce vertical extension of the fracture pattern through the midface and central mandible.

Laterally situated impacts damage the frontozygo-maticomaxillary (lateral facial) buttress with posterior extension to the greater wing of the sphenoid, temporal and parietal bones. Intracranial complications are less common, but extension into the lower face is often seen.

Extremely violent impacts produce gross comminution of both the central and lateral facial elements with frequent sagittal fracturing of both the midface and mandible, mandibular condylar fractures and an increased incidence of intracranial injury. Although collapse of the facial skeleton has protective value (p. 106), the brain may suffer both local and diffuse damage, and the floor of the anterior cranial fossa is often disrupted.

Clinical assessment

This begins with evaluation of airway, breathing, circulation and conscious level. The immediate concern in the management of these severely injured cases is the institution of appropriate life-support measures and the assessment of life-threatening intracranial and extracranial complications.

The hallmark clinical features are deformation of extreme aesthetic and functional significance, and marked skeletal instability. Clinical observation reveals extensive diffuse facial swelling and bruising, often with lacerations over the bony prominences — the forehead, the supraorbital ridges and the root of the nose. Visible bony deformation is often evident with loss of nasal projection and disturbances in midfacial projection, symmetry and height.

Palpation of the facial skeleton may reveal contour irregularities of the orbital margins and widespread bony instability involving both orbital and occlusal skeletal elements (Fig. 6.5). Irregularities of the supraorbital rim may identify cranial extensions of the fracture patterns whilst flattening of the zygomatic region may be accompanied by marked proptosis, raising suspicion of a blow-in displacement of the lateral orbital wall, including the greater wing of the sphenoid with involvement of the orbital apex. Compressive force applied to the nasal root in both anteroposterior and transverse dimensions may demonstrate massive comminution and mobility of the naso-ethmoid region on the anterior cranial base.

Intraoral examination identifies bruising, soft-tissue lacerations or even tissue loss, and may show segmental and sagittal maxillary and mandibular fractures often involving dento-alveolar segments. The extreme mobility of a flail midfacial segment is often easily demonstrable. Detection of condylar fractures is especially easy in patients who are already intubated and ventilated when the first detailed clinical examination is carried out. By grasping and moving the mandible in the region of the mandibular angle with a gloved hand while the index finger of the opposite hand palpates the anterior wall of the external auditory canal, it is possible to appreciate crepitus, abnormal mobility and/or displacement of the mandibular condylar process.

In most though not all cases of panfacial fractures, there are impairments of neurological function, and a neurological assessment should be carried out as soon as possible (p. 159), though often this is limited by the need to institute endotracheal intubation and ventilation. It is also desirable to assess visual function as soon as possible and especially to exclude a penetrating injury of the globe; this may be impeded by orbital swelling.

Radiological assessment

Definitive description of the fracture pattern in these cases is possible only with high resolution CT scans. Ideally axial scan data from the vertex to chin point should be provided on bony settings. Soft-tissue window hard copy images should be provided in the cranial slices to identify the nature of any intracranial involvement and to visualize the globes and the optic nerves. The creation of 3D CT images from the axial data provides a qualitative ready reference image pre- and intraoperatively to assist in planning treatment (Broumand et al 1993). However, these images do not provide an accurate guide to fracture patterns and displacement in all areas of the facial skeleton.

Management

The treatment of these complex injuries is the sum of the repair of all the fractures of individual facial and cranial structures. It is desirable to minimize reoperation and prolonged hospitalization. In the past, difficulties often arose in the timing of facial repair in relation to neurosurgical or less often ophthalmological interventions; the modern craniofacial unit allows interdisciplinary coordination of effort and the development of a coherent, logical sequence of repair which is applicable to all eventualities. In particular, the combined craniofacial and neurosurgical operation permits repair of multiple facial fractures and closure of cranionasal fistulas in a single procedure (David 1984).

Preoperative care

The patient's cardiorespiratory condition must first be fully stabilized. Tracheostomy is no longer required solely for airway management of complex facial fractures, but where prolonged intubation is necessary for coma or other injuries then tracheostomy may be employed (p. 382).

It may be necessary to monitor the intracranial pressure (ICP), since the clinical signs of a fall in the conscious level may be masked by orbital swelling or by the use of artificial ventilation (p. 369). The initial CT scan gives warning of the likelihood of delayed cerebral swelling and other complications, and it is our policy to institute ICP monitoring if there is CT evidence of intracerebral haemorrhage, obliteration of basal cisterns or midline shift. Even if the CT scan is within normal limits, it may be wise to monitor the ICP, at least during the first 48 h.

Timing of repair

The severely injured patient with complex craniofacial/panfacial fractures ideally requires definitive correction of the bony injuries within the first 5–7 days. Some have suggested primary fixation within 12–48 h of injury (Gruss 1990), but such a time frame may be incompatible with adequate preoperative radiological, ophthalmological and dental assessment — especially when the patient is comatose or poorly cooperative. This is also the period when soft-tissue swelling peaks and operative exposure and assessments of facial projection and symmetry are at their most difficult. Cerebrospinal rhinorrhoea or intracranial aerocele may provide an additional reason for delay: for reasons set out in Chapter 13, we believe that these signs of a cranionasal fistula do not invariably demand an anterior cranial fossa dural repair, and delay of a few days will often clarify the need for this procedure, besides allowing raised ICP to subside.

Where early acute neurosurgical intervention is necessary for intracranial bleeding or compound depressed calvarial fractures the collaboration of the craniofacial surgeon is mandatory. If scalp incisions are made and cranial bone flaps elevated, it is important that they be designed so as not to complicate the exposure and stabilization of cranio-orbital fractures. For example, where fixation of the mobile face below demands an intact fronto-orbital bar above, any frontal bone flap elevated for exposure of the anterior cranial fossa must be positioned so as to maintain these stable superior points. Loss of the fronto-orbital bar complicates superior localization and predisposes to inaccurate fracture reduction. Where depressed fractures of the temporal region have extensions to involve the lateral orbital wall and greater wing of the sphenoid, the opportunity exists to correct and stabilize the orbital component as well as elevating the cranial element of the fracture. Leaving the orbital fracture element till a later definitive facial repair risks displacing the already corrected cranial component and may cause intracranial bleeding or dural injury.

Occasionally, patients with panfacial or complex facial fractures present late, more than 3 weeks after injury, having undergone extensive life-saving procedures for extracranial injuries. In such cases bone union is often well advanced, and soft-tissue contracture may already be evident. Soft-tissue dissection for exposure must then be extensive and the fractures must be disimpacted to permit stable reduction and anatomical fixation; fracture mobilization will often require formal osteotomy of the fracture lines.

Sequence of repair

There are several possible approaches to the complex panfacial fracture, relating to the status of the stable boundaries of the injured face — the calvarial vault above and the mandible below.

Where the frontal cranium is intact, or where there is fracture but no loss of bone in the anterior cranial fossa or fronto-orbital bar, or where these structures have already been rigidly reconstituted, the orbito-zygomatic and midfacial regions can be built *from above downward*. Projection and symmetry of the orbitozygomatic façade sets the facial width and lateral facial projection, between which the midfacial arch can be positioned to recreate midline facial projection and pretraumatic occlusion.

There are situations where repair proceeds *from below upward*. When the mandibular arch is disrupted, it should be repaired as the first part of the procedure. If the mandibular condyles are fractured either unilaterally or bilaterally, they require early reduction and internal fixation by miniplate, to re-establish posterior facial height. In the presence of comminuted intracapsular condylar fractures this may not be possible and intermaxillary fixation must be maintained; primary costochondral graft reconstruction of the mandibular condyle can be contemplated (p. 604). Once the mandible is rigidly restored the midface may be disimpacted and placed into the predicted occlusion; intermaxillary fixation is then instituted. Repair then proceeds *from above down* to meet the already fixed maxillomandibular segment.

Sagittal fractures of the midface introduce another dimension in reconstruction. Where the mandibular arch is intact an occlusal reference point exists below to restore lower midfacial width and maxillary dental arch form. The upper midfacial width is set by correct positioning of the zygomas and this determines the transverse dimension of the split midface at its upper border. Fixation of the sagittal fracture may be possible with transversely placed miniplates anteriorly on the maxilla, or may rarely require posterior microplate fixation of the hard palate. Where sagittal midfacial and complex mandibular fractures occur concomitantly, both upper and lower dental arches appear splayed open and there are no immediately available reference points. Gruss et al (1990) stress the importance in such cases of using the zygomatic arches to set the facial width. The maxillary arch width is then set between these boundaries with miniplate fixation of the midface to produce stability both transversely and vertically in relation to the orbitozygomatic region above. The mandibular arch can then be rebuilt on the above structure, producing ideally a stable functional result and (most importantly) a symmetrical aesthetic result. In these cases, the danger

in the reverse approach, proceeding from below upwards, is that reconstruction commences at a distance from the only stable symmetrical element — the cranial base. The inaccuracies inherent in condylar fracture repair and repositioning are great and introduce variables of asymmetry much beyond what can be achieved by starting at the zygomas and zygomatic arches, which are a direct extension of the cranial base.

The only other situation of note where a repair involves rebuilding *from below upward* is in the presence of cranial bone loss and disruption of the floor of the anterior cranial fossa. There the reference points are lost or distorted. To repair the frontal cranial base and then secure on it the midface may risk damaging or displacing the already repaired anterior cranial fossa. The mandible and midface are therefore first repaired and this reconstituted complex is reattached to the cranium above once its form has been restored and the appropriate barriers between nose and intradural space have been repaired if this is considered necessary. The indications and technique of transcranial repair of the anterior cranial fossa are detailed in Chapter 13 (p. 376); when this is done as part of a combined procedure, great care is needed to maintain appropriate asepsis. We have not employed subcranial extradural repair of the shattered anterior fossa when there is likelihood of a cranionasal fistula. If extradural repair can be shown to be reliable, the procedure has attractions both with respect to simplicity and because it need not be contraindicated by the presence of brain swelling (p. 381). At present, we are sceptical of the reliability of this method of closing a cranionasal dural fistula except under very favourable conditions.

At all levels, an acceptable outcome demands repositioning of existing bone, with primary autogenous bone grafting where there is severe bony comminution or bone loss and replacement or expansion of the craniofacial soft tissues to the pretraumatic state.

A predictably good outcome for the skeletal elements in these complex injuries is now achievable. But further attention to the soft tissues is required. The older semi-closed management of these injuries by suspension wiring and external frames was followed by contracture of the soft tissues because of failure to restore normal bony contours, whether orbital with post-traumatic enophthalmos, or paranasal with loss of nasal projection. Modern subperiosteal dissection of the facial soft tissues permits anatomical skeletal repositioning, primary bone graft augmentation and anterior re-expansion of the facial soft tissues to approximately the pre-injury situation. Such exposures, however, risk sagging of the facial soft tissues especially the cheeks, under the influence of gravity, if resuspension of the soft-tissues to the underlying bone has been inadequate. The resulting soft-tissue alterations may produce a perception of asymmetry and a disappointing aesthetic outcome, attributable to unsatisfactory soft-tissue cover and not to skeletal deformity. Reattachment of the periosteum to the zygoma and zygomatic arch has been advocated (Gruss et al 1990) but no long-term results have been reported on maintenance of the soft-tissue position.

Atrophy of the temporal soft tissues (the temporalis muscle and the temporal fat pad) may also follow these wide exposures. Secondary correction with bone grafts placed deep to temporalis is then necessary to augment the contour of the region and to restore symmetry.

Complications

The complications attending these injuries are those seen in each individual craniofacial subregion. The potential for asymmetry of appearance and disturbance of function is extreme. The continued evolution of exposure, rigid fixation and primary bone grafting should ensure increasing accuracy of reconstruction and reduction in rates of post-traumatic deformities and other complications in the facial region.

The complications of concurrent transcranial anterior fossa repair include frontal lobe oedema and early or late cerebral infection (p. 380); we believe that the risks of these complications are acceptably low if our criteria for transdural exploration are respected and if operation is withheld until cerebral swelling has subsided.

REFERENCES

Adams W M 1942 Internal wiring fixation of facial fractures. Surgery 12: 523–540

Al-Kayat A, Bramley P 1980 A modified preauricular approach to the temporomandibular joint and malar arch. Br J Oral Surg. 17: 91–103

Anderson T, Alpert B 1992 Experience with rigid fixation of mandibular fractures and immediate function. J Oral Maxillofac Surg 50: 555–560

Antoniades K, Dimitriou C, Triaridis C, Karabouta I, Layaridis N, Karakasis D 1990 Sagittal fracture of the maxilla. J Craniomaxillofac Surg 18: 260–262

Antonyshyn O, Gruss J S, Kassel E E 1989 Blow-in fractures of the orbit. Plast Reconstr Surg 84: 10–20

Balle V H, Andersen R, Siim C 1989 Incidence of lacrimal obstruction following trauma to the facial skeleton. Ear Nose Throat J 67: 66, 68, 70

Bochlogyros P N 1985 A retrospective study of 1521 mandibular fractures. J Oral Maxillofac Surg 43: 597–599

Brandt K E, Burruss G L, Hickerson W L, White C E, DeLozier J B 1991 The management of mid-face fractures with intracranial injury. J Trauma 31: 15–19

Broumand S R, Labs J D, Novelline R A, Markowitz B L, Yaremchuk M J 1993 The role of three-dimensional computed tomography in the evaluation of acute craniofacial trauma. Ann Plast Surg 30: 488–494

Brown A E, Obeid G 1984 A simplified method for the internal fixation of fractures of the mandibular condyle. Br J Oral Maxillofac Surg 22: 145–150

Brown J S, Grew N, Taylor C, Millar B G 1991 Intermaxillary fixation compared to miniplate osteosynthesis in the management of the fractured mandible: an audit. Br J Oral Maxillofac Surg 29: 308–311

Calloway D M, Anton M A, Jacobs J S 1992 Changing concepts and controversies in the management of mandibular fractures. Clin Plast Surg 19: 59–69

Champy M, Pape H D, Gerlach K L et al 1986 Mandibular fractures. The Strasbourg miniplate osteosynthesis. In: Kruger E and Schilli W (eds) Oral and maxillofacial traumatology. Quintessence Publishing, Chicago, Vol 2

Converse J M, Hogan V M 1970 Open-sky approach for reduction of naso-orbital fractures. Case report. Plast Reconstr Surg 46: 396–398

Converse J M, Smith B 1966 Naso-orbital fractures and traumatic deformities of the medial canthus. Plast Reconstr Surg 38: 147–162

Cooter R D, David D J 1989 Computer-based coding of fractures in the craniofacial region. Br J Plast Surg 42: 17–26

Cruse C W, Blevins P K, Luce E A 1980 Naso-ethmoid-orbital fractures. J Trauma 20: 551–556

Dal Santo F, Ellis E, Throckmorton C S 1992 The effects of zygomatic complex fractures on masseteric muscle force. J Oral Maxillofac Surg 50: 791–799

Dautrey J, Pepersack W 1982 Functional surgery of the temporomandibular joint. Clin Plast Surg 9: 591–601

David D J 1984 New perspectives in the management of severe cranio-facial deformity. Ann R Coll Surg Engl 66: 270–279

Derdyn C, Persing J A, Broaddus W C et al 1990 Craniofacial trauma: an assessment of risk related to timing of surgery. Plast Reconstr Surg 86: 238–245

Dielert E, Jais M 1991 Methoden und Ergebnisse der chirurgischen Versorgung lateraler Mittelgesichtsfrakturen. Fortschr Kiefer Gesichtschir 36: 105–108

Dingman R O, Natvig P 1964 Surgery of facial fractures. Saunders, Philadelphia

Ellis E, Carlson D S 1989 The effects of mandibular immobilization on the masticatory system. A review. Clin Plast Surg 16: 133–146

Ellis E, Dean J 1993 Rigid fixation of condylar fractures. Oral Surg Oral Med Oral Pathol 76: 6–15

Ellis E, Ghali C E 1991 Lag screw fixation of anterior mandibular fractures. J Oral Maxillofac Surg 49: 13–21

Ellis E, Moos K F, El Attar A 1985 Ten years of mandibular fractures: an analysis of 2137 cases. Oral Surg Oral Med Oral Pathol 59: 120–129

Farole A 1986 Temporal screw suspension for complicated midface fractures. J Oral Maxillofac Surg 44: 491–492

Ferguson J W, Stewart I A, Whitley B D 1989 Lateral displacement of the intact mandibular condyle. Review of literature and report of case with associated facial nerve palsy. J Craniomaxillofac Surg 17: 125–127

Gillies H D, Kilner T P, Stone D 1927 Fractures of the malar-zygomatic compound, with description of a new x-ray position. Br J Surg 14: 651–656

Gruss J S 1982 Fronto-naso-orbital trauma. Clin Plast Surg 9: 577–589

Gruss J S 1990 Craniofacial trauma: an assessment of risk related to timing of surgery [Discussion]. Plast Reconstr Surg 86: 246–247

Gruss J S, Hurwitz J J, Nik N A, Kassel E E 1985a The pattern and incidence of nasolacrimal injury in naso-orbital-ethmoid fractures: the role of delayed assessment and dacryocystorhinostomy. Br J Plast Surg 38: 116–121

Gruss J S, Mackinnon S E, Kassell E E, Cooper P W 1985b The role of primary bone grafting in complex craniomaxillofacial trauma. Plast Reconstr Surg 75: 17–23

Gruss J S, Mackinnon S E 1986 Complex maxillary fractures: role of buttress reconstruction and immediate bone grafts. Plast Reconstr Surg 78: 9–24

Gruss J S, Phillips J H 1989 Complex facial trauma: the evolving role of rigid fixation and immediate bone graft reconstruction. Clin Plast Surg 16: 93–104

Gruss J S, Pollock R A, Phillips J H Antonyshyn O 1989 Combined injuries of the cranium and face. Br J Plast Surg 42: 385–398

Gruss J S, Van Wyck L, Phillips J H Antonyshyn O 1990 The importance of the zygomatic arch in complex midfacial fracture repair and correction of post traumatic orbitozygomatic deformities. Plast Reconstr Surg 85: 878–890

Habel G, O'Regan B, Hidding J, Eissing A 1990 A transcoronoidal approach of fractures of the condylar neck. J Craniomaxillofac Surg 18: 348–351

Harrison D H 1979 Nasal injuries: their pathegenesis and treatment. Br J Plast Surg 32: 57–64

Hinds E C, Parnes E I 1966 Late management of condylar fractures by means of subcondylar osteotomy: reports of cases. J Oral Surg 24: 54–59

Hobar P C 1992 Methods of rigid fixation. Clin Plast Surg 19: 31–39

Holt G R, Holt J E 1983 Incidence of eye injuries in facial fractures: an analysis of 727 cases. Otolaryngol Head Neck Surg 91: 276–279

Hoopes J E, Wolfort F G, Jabaley M E 1970 Operative treatment of fractures of the mandibular condyle in children. Using the post-auricular approach. Plast Reconstr Surg 46: 357–362

Iizuka T, Lindqvist C, Hallikainen D, Paukku P 1991a Infection after rigid internal fixation of mandibular fractures: a clinical and radiologic study. J Oral Maxillofac Surg 49: 585–593

Iizuka T, Lindqvist C, Hallikainen D, Mikkonen P, Paukku P 1991b Severe bone resorption and osteoarthrosis after miniplate fixation of high condylar fracture. A clinical and radiologic study of thirteen patients. Oral Surg Oral Med Oral Pathol 72: 400–407

Jackson I T 1989 Classification and treatment of orbitozygomatic and orbitoethmoid fractures. The place of bone grafting and plate fixation. Clin Plast Surg 16: 77–91

Knight J S, North J F 1961 The classification of malar fractures: an analysis of displacement as a guide to treatment. Br J Plast Surg 13: 325–339

Korneef L 1982 Current concepts on the management of orbital blow-out fractures. Ann Plast Surg 9: 185–200

Koury M, Ellis E 1992 Rigid internal fixation for the treatment of infected mandibular fractures. J Oral Maxillofac Surg 50: 434–443

Lachner J, Clanton J T, Waite P D 1991 Open reduction and internal rigid fixation of subcondylar fractures via an intraoral approach. Oral Surg Oral Med Oral Pathol 71: 257–261

Lang J 1983 Clinical anatomy of the head. Neurocranium, orbit, craniocervical regions. Springer, Berlin

Leipziger L S, Manson P N 1992 Naso-ethmoid-orbital fractures. Current concepts and management principles. Clin Plast Surg 19: 167–193

LeVant B A, Gardner-Berry D, Snow R S 1969 An improved cranio-maxillary fixation. Br J Plast Surg 22: 288–290

Levy F E, Smith R W, Odland R M et al 1991 Monocortical miniplate fixation of mandibular angle fractures. Arch Otolaryngol Head Neck Surg 117: 149–154

Lindahl L 1977a Condylar fractures of the mandible. I. Classification and relation to age, occlusion and concomitant injuries of teeth and teeth supporting structures, and fractures of the mandibular body. Int J Oral Surg 6: 12–21

Lindahl L 1977b Condylar fractures of the mandible. III. Positional changes of the chin. Int J Oral Surg 6: 166–172

Lindahl L 1977c Condylar fractures of the mandible. IV. Function of the masticatory system. Int J Oral Surg 6: 195–203

Lindahl L, Hollender L 1977 Condylar fractures of the mandible. II. A radiographic study of remodeling processes in the temporomandibular joint. Int J Oral Surg 6: 153–165

Lund K 1974 Mandibular growth and remodelling processes after condylar fracture. A longitudinal roentgencephalometric study. Acta Odontol Scand 32: 3–117

Maas C S, Merwin G E, Wilson J, Frey M D, Manes M D 1990 Comparison of biomaterials for facial bone augmentation. Arch Otolaryngol Head Neck Surg 116: 551–556

Maloney P L, Welch T B, Doku H C 1991 Early immobilization of mandibular fractures: a retrospective study. J Oral Maxillofac Surg 49: 698–702

Manson P N, Clifford C M, Su C T, Iliff N T, Morgan R 1985a Mechanisms of global support and post-traumatic enophthalmos: I. The anatomy of the ligament sling and its relation to intramuscular cone orbital fat. Plast Reconstr Surg 77: 193–202

Manson P N, Crawley W A, Yaremchuk M J, Rochman G M, Hoopes J E, French J H 1985b Midface fractures: advantages of immediate extended open reduction and bone grafting. Plast Reconstr Surg 76: 1–12

Manson P N, Hoopes J E, Su C T 1980 Structural pillars of the facial skeleton: an approach to the management of Le Fort fractures. Plast Reconstr Surg 66: 54–62

Manson P N, Glassman D, Vanderkolk C, Petty P, Crawley W A 1990a Rigid stabilization of sagittal fractures of the maxilla and palate. Plast Reconstr Surg 85: 711–717

Manson P N, Markowitz B, Mirvis S, Dunham M, Yaremchuk M 1990b Toward CT-based facial fracture treatment. Plast Reconstr Surg 85: 202–212

Markowitz B L, Manson P N 1989 Panfacial fractures: organization of treatment. Clin Plast Surg 16: 105–114

Markowitz B L. Manson P N, Sargent L, Vanderkolk C A, Yaremchuk M, Glassman O, Crawley W A 1991 Management of the medial canthal tendon in nasoethmoid orbital fractures: the importance of the central fragment in classification and treatment. Plast Reconstr Surg 87: 843–853

Marsh J L, Gado M 1983 The longitudinal orbital CT projection: a versatile image for orbital assessment. Plast Reconstr Surg 71: 308–317

Mayell 1973 Nasal fractures: their occurrence, management and some late results. J R Cell Surg Edinb 18: 31–36

McCoy F J 1959 Fractures of the naso-orbital ethmoidal complex. In: Georgiade N H (ed) Plastic and maxillo-facial trauma symposium. Mosby, St Louis, Ch 17

Melmed E P 1972 Fractures of the zygomatic-malar complex. S Afr Med J 46: 569–572

Michelet F X, Deymes J, Dessus B 1973 Osteosynthesis with miniaturized screwed plates in maxillo-facial surgery. J Maxillofac Surg 1: 79–84

Moore G F, Olson T S, Yonkers A J 1985 Complications of mandibular fracture: a retrospective review of 100 fractures in 56 patients. Nebr Med J 70: 120–123

Moore M H, Abbott J R, Abbott A H, Trott J A, David D J 1990 Monocortical non-compression miniplate osteosynthesis of mandibular angle fractures. Aust NZ J Surg 60: 805–809

Mustardé J C 1963 Epicanthus and telecanthus. Br J Plast Surg 16: 346–356

Niederdellmann H, Shetty V 1987 Solitary lag screw osteosynthesis in the treatment of fractures of the angle of the mandible: a retrospective study. Plast Reconstr Surg 80: 68–74

Olson R A, Fonseca R J, Zeitler D L, Osbon D B 1982 Fractures of the mandible: a review of 580 cases. J Oral Maxillofac Surg 40: 23–28

Paskert J P, Manson P N 1989 The bimanual examination for assessing instability in naso-orbito-ethmoidal injuries. Plast Reconstr Surg 83: 165–167

Pearl R M 1987 Surgical management of volumetric changes in the bony orbit. Ann Plast Surg 19: 349–358

Phillips J M, Gruss J S, Wells M D, Chollet A 1991 Periosteal suspension of the lower eyelid and cheek following subciliary exposure of facial fractures. Plast Reconstr Surg 88: 145–148

Pieritz U, Schmidseder R 1981 Central dislocation of the jaw-joint into the middle cranial fossa. Case report. J Maxillofac Surg 9: 61–63

Pollock R A 1992 Nasal trauma. Pathomechanics and surgical management of acute injuries. Clin Plast Surg 19: 133–147

Rapidis A D, Papavassiliou D, Papadimitriou J, Koundouris J, Zachariades N 1985 Fracture of the coronoid process of the mandible. An analysis of 52 cases. Int J Oral Surg 14: 126–130

Robinson M E, Rowe E 1971 Delayed surgical–occlusal treatment of malocclusion and pain from displaced subcondylar fracture: report of a case. J Am Dent Assoc 83: 639–642

Robinson T J, Stranc M F 1970 The anatomy of the medial canthal ligament. Br J Plast Surg 23: 1–7

Rohrich R J, Hollier L M, Watermull D 1992 Optimizing the management of orbitozygomatic fractures. Clin Plast Surg 19: 149–165

Rowe N L, Killey H C 1955 Fractures of the facial skeleton. Livingstone, Edinburgh

Rubin M M, Koll T J, Sadoff R S 1990 Morbidity associated with incompletely erupted third molars in the line of mandibular fractures. J Oral Maxillofac Surg 48: 1045–1047

Rudderman R H, Mullen R L 1992 Biomechanics of the facial skeleton. Clin Plast Surg 19: 11–29

Sanders B, McKelvy B, Adams D 1977 Aseptic osteomyelitis and necrosis of the mandibular condylar head after intracapsular fracture. Oral Surg Oral Med Oral Pathol 43: 665–670

Schettler D, Rehrmann A 1975 Long term results of functional treatment of condylar fractures with the long bridle according to A. Rehrmann. J Maxillofac Surg 3: 14–22

Schilli W, Ewers R, Niederdellmann H 1981 Bone fixation with screws and plates in the maxillofacial region. Int J Oral Surg 10 (Suppl 1): 329–342

Schubert J 1991 Stellenwert konservativ-chirurgischer Therapie von Frakturen des lateralen Mittelgesichts. Fortschr Kiefer Gesichtschir 36: 86–87

Steinhäuser E 1964 Eingriffe am processus articularis auf dem totalen Weg. Dtsch Zahn Mund Kieferheilkd Zentralbl 19: 694–700

Stoll P Schilli W, Joos U 1983 The stabilization of midface fractures in the vertical dimension. J Maxillofac Surg 11: 248–251

Stranc M F 1970 Primary treatment of naso-ethmoid injuries with increased intercanthal distance. Br J Plast Surg 23: 8–25

Stranc M F, Robertson G A 1979 A classification of injuries of the nasal skeleton. Ann Plast Surg 2: 468–474

Sullivan P K, Rosenstein D A, Holmes R E, Craig D, Manson P N 1993 Bone graft reconstruction of the monkey orbital floor with iliac grafts and titanium mesh plates: a histometric study. Plast Reconstr Surg 91: 769–775

Takenoshita Y, Oka M, Tashiro H 1989 Surgical treatment of fractures of the mandibular condylar neck. J Craniomaxillofac Surg 17: 119–124

Thaller S R, Kawamoto H K 1990 A histologic evaluation of fracture repair in the midface. Plast Reconstr Surg 85: 196–201

Thaller S R, Reavie D, Daniller A 1990 Rigid internal fixation with miniplates and screws: a cost-effective technique for treating mandible fractures? Ann Plast Surg 24: 469–474

Wallace J 1985 A new frame for cranio-maxillary fixation. Br J Oral Maxillofac Surg 23: 304–307

Wolfe S A 1988 Treatment of post-traumatic orbital deformities. Clin Plast Surg 15: 225–238

Worthington P 1982 Dislocation of the mandibular condyle into the temporal fossa. J Maxillofac Surg 10: 24–27

Yaremchuk M J, Del Vecchio D A, Fiala T G, Lee W P 1993 Microfixation of acute orbital fractures. Ann Plast Surg 30: 385–397

Zachariades N, Rapidis A D, Papademetriou J, Koundouris J, Papavassiliou D 1983 The significance of tracheostomy in the management of fractures of the facial skeleton. J Maxillofac Surg 11: 180–186

Zide M F, Kent J N 1983 Indications for open reduction of mandibular condyle fractures. J Oral Maxillofac Surg 41: 89–98

Zins J E, Whitaker L A 1983 Membranous versus endochondral bone: implications for craniofacial reconstruction. Plast Reconstr Surg 72: 778–785

CHAPTER 12 | Dental injuries

T. Brown   J. R. Abbott   L. L. Daenke

INTRODUCTION

Impacts to the middle and lower facial regions often injure the teeth. The number and type of teeth involved and the extent of the injuries depend on many factors including the nature, direction and magnitude of the external force and the velocity of impact (see Ch. 4). The majority of middle and lower facial injuries involving the teeth arise from vehicle accidents, where a solid object is impacted against the victim or vice versa; criminal assaults, gunshot wounds and sporting accidents may also be responsible. In many instances tissue damage and loss of function can be extensive.

For many patients with severe trauma, life-saving measures will take priority over dental procedures and it may not be possible to undertake a detailed oral examination until some time after the initial trauma. The delay may extend for a few days or as long as several weeks. Delay is also likely to happen after accidents in remote regions where facilities for the treatment of dentofacial disruption are limited. In Australia, for example, a great deal of trauma results from tourists overturning four-wheel drive vehicles while on safari; emergency treatment is performed at the nearest hospital or medical facility and the patient, when stabilized, is then air-lifted to a major trauma centre in a capital city (Ch. 8). Under such circumstances, dental injuries can easily be overlooked in preoccupation with other cranial or extracranial injuries.

SURGICAL PATHOLOGY

Trauma to the dentition may be relatively minor and confined to injuries of one or a few teeth (Fig. 12.1). The dental injury may include any of the following: enamel crazing or chipping, crown fracture with or without exposure of the dental pulp (Fig. 12.2), root fracture, loosening of a tooth within its socket with or without displacement from its normal alignment, partial or full intrusion of a tooth following apically directed impact, or complete avulsion of a tooth from its socket. The types of dental fractures and the pathological complications of these injuries are discussed in Chapter 5. More extensive trauma to the dental structures often follows severe impact injuries. Neighbouring structures including alveolar bone, soft tissues of the face and oral cavity, bones of the facial skeleton, sinuses, or nerves and vessels may also be damaged. These more extensive dentoalveolar injuries may affect the dental occlusion (Figs 12.3–12.6). Avulsive trauma, such as a gunshot wound, may result in partial or complete loss of a jaw and its teeth.

DENTAL ASSESSMENT

A thorough oral and dental examination of the patient must be undertaken as soon as possible to determine the extent of the trauma and to provide information for future treatment planning. It is important to record the number and types of teeth present, missing or damaged, though in the presence of severe swelling, mouth opening may be severely limited; in such cases it will be necessary to postpone examination of the posterior teeth for 48 h or until the swelling has subsided sufficiently.

Definitive dental examination will usually involve all of the standard procedures including visual inspection, palpation, dental models, occlusal records, pulp vitality tests, intraoral and extraoral radiography, computed

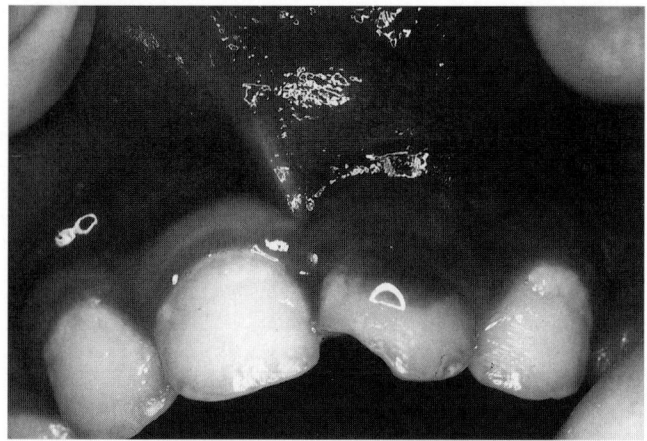

A

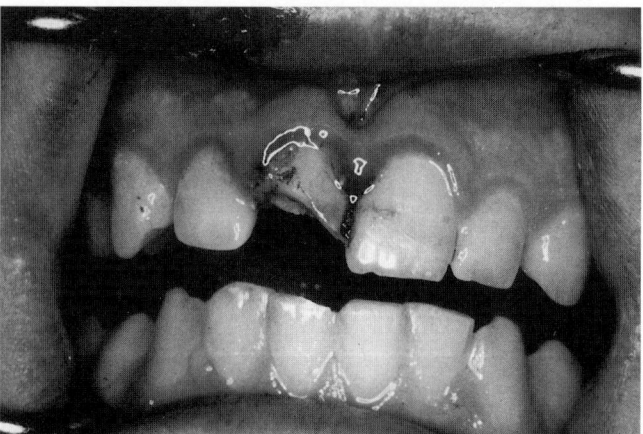

B

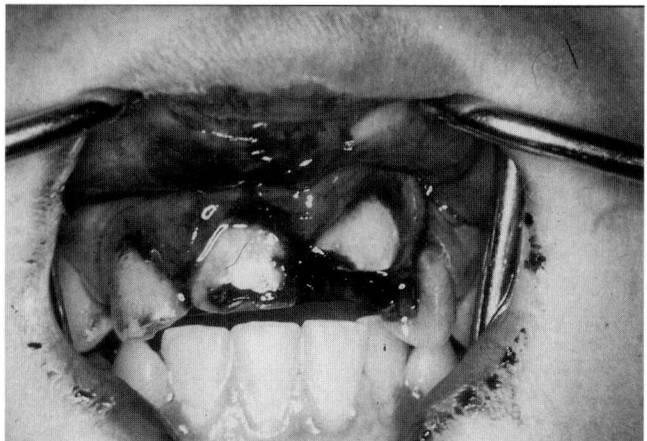

C

Fig. 12.1 Tooth fractures. Typical impact fractures of maxillary central incisors, showing various degrees of associated soft-tissue injury.

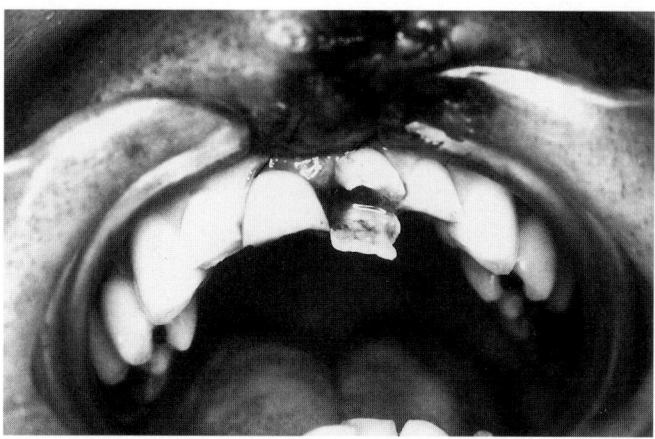

Fig. 12.2 Split tooth. Severe trauma to a maxillary left central incisor which is split vertically exposing the dental pulp.

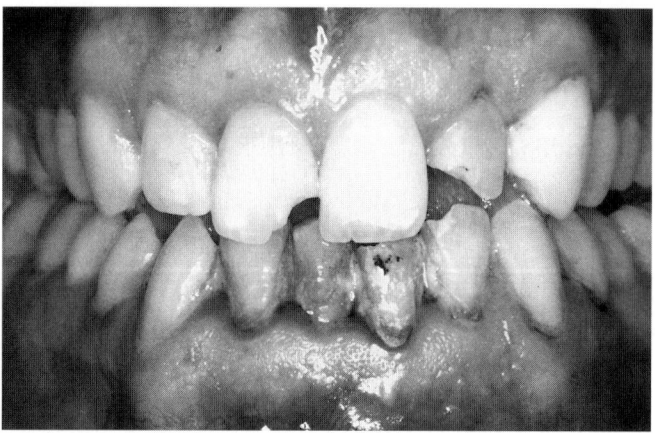

Fig. 12.3 Tooth fractures. A middle-aged woman fell from a bicycle and suffered a Le Fort I fracture. Fractures of maxillary incisors and open bite are shown.

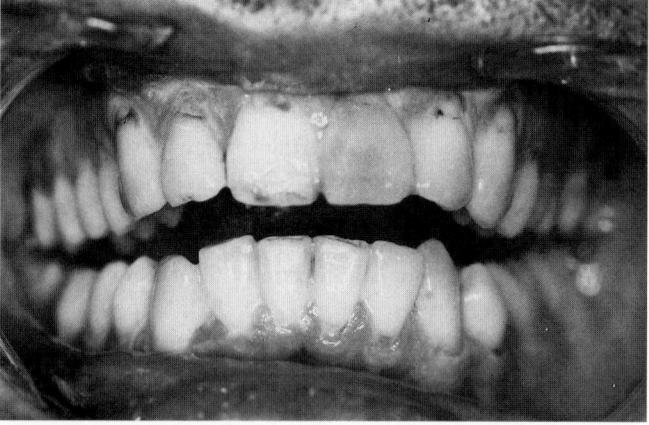

Fig. 12.4 Le Fort II fracture with anterior open bite. In this male patient the fracture has caused disruption of the occlusion with a pronounced anterior open bite.

tomographic (CT) scans and photography; these investigations are discussed in Chapters 6 and 7.

When patients are admitted to an intensive care ward, the use of oral intubation may limit a dental examination

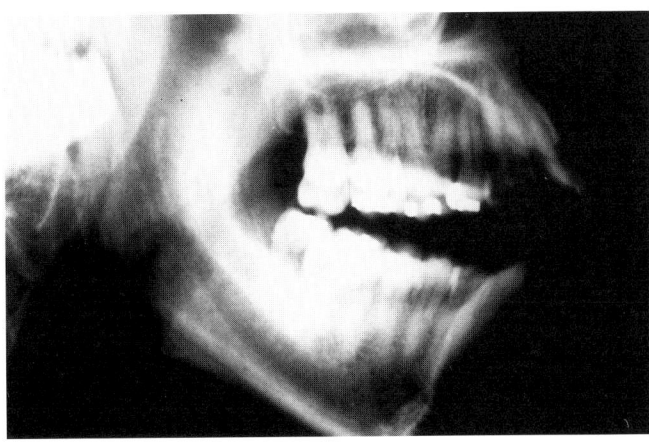

Fig. 12.5 Le Fort II fracture. Lateral radiograph of the patient showing tooth contact limited to the posterior region.

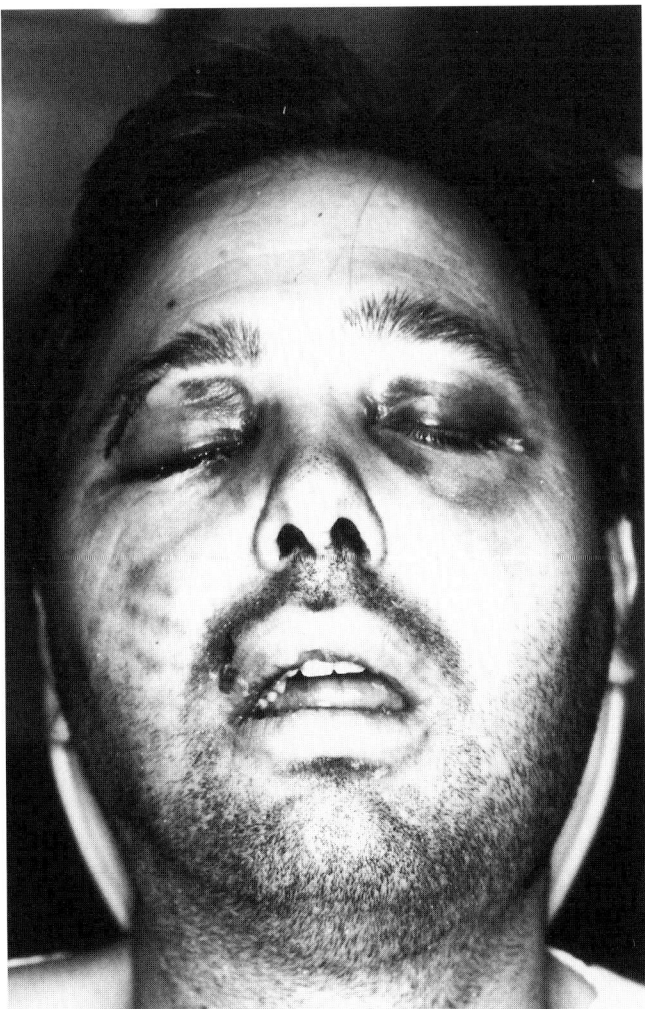

Fig. 12.6 Le Fort II fracture. Facial appearance of the patient showing the anterior open bite.

to the anterior teeth. Radiological visualization of the teeth may then be very helpful. CT examination of the head and neck will be performed if there is evidence of a craniocerebral or spinal injury, but plain radiographic films of the facial injuries may not be obtained initially. However, chest radiography is routinely performed, and this will detect inhaled foreign bodies, including teeth or fragments of teeth. Fortunately not all patients suffer severe trauma and in many cases definitive radiography need not be delayed. In cases of fracture of the facial skeleton, especially fractures of the maxilla or mandible, plain and orthopantomographic radiography are routinely used and give good visualization of the presence or absence of the teeth.

Major injuries of the brain, spine and trunk must take priority over the dental requirements. However, it may be possible to obtain preliminary dental alginate impressions and an occlusal wafer while the patient is under general anaesthesia for another procedure. Impression procedures will be hindered by oral intubation, for example in patients with severe nasal injury. While patients are receiving intensive care, good oral hygiene must be maintained and the regular use of a mouth wash such as chlorhexidine gluconate solution is recommended, particularly if the patient is unable to use a tooth brush or other mechanical aids effectively (p. 257).

The initial extraoral examination should determine the extent and sites of swelling, lacerations and any obvious deformities of the facial bones. Mandibular asymmetries and limitation in jaw movements must be noted as these may point to a mandibular fracture with displacement. Often the patient will be unable to close the anterior teeth together.

Intraoral examination of the soft tissues may reveal frank haematoma in the floor of the mouth, often accompanied by laceration of the lips and oedema. In such cases it may be impossible to palpate the soft tissues to detect forcign inclusions which can be best revealed on a small dental radiographic film of the type used for periapical images placed between the lips and given reduced exposure. The need for soft-tissue radiography is especially important when examining maxillary fractures as sharp, fractured incisal edges may have penetrated the upper lip, embedding chips of enamel in the tissue.

The dental examination includes an evaluation of the hard and soft tissues of the oral cavity including teeth present, absent or restored, periodontal health, pathological conditions such as soft tissue lesions, regions of bone resorption and dental caries. Lesions suggesting the possibility of acquired immune deficiency syndrome (p. 535) are noted (Greenspan et al 1990). Individual teeth should be checked for mobility and irregularities in position which may indicate luxation (dislocation) injuries or a fracture of the root. Edentulous regions require an assessment of the size, shape and resilience of residual ridges as well as any features that might hinder the taking of impressions. From a medicolegal point of view it is important to establish the status of the dentition and other oral tissues and to record this in the case notes. If possible this should be undertaken at the first examination.

All teeth should be examined for fractures which may range in severity from cracked or chipped enamel to loss of a major portion of the tooth crown and root. Frontal impact, for example, can shear off the crowns of teeth from their underlying roots. In some instances the tooth crown and small portions of the root will be loosely held in the gingival tissue. Palpation of the teeth between the fingers or gentle pressure with the handle of a dental mirror will reveal abnormal mobility. Subluxation, luxation or fractures of a tooth should be obvious to the examiner.

The finding of an avulsed tooth may call for immediate action. Teeth that have been avulsed can often be saved if they are replanted into the alveolus. However, the most critical factor in tooth replanting is time, since prolonged exposure causes drying and rapid death of the cells in the attached periodontal membrane: teeth that are not handled excessively and replanted within 30 min of avulsion have the best survival chance. The management of dental avulsion is discussed below.

With respect to the posterior teeth, facial impact causing mandibular or maxillary fractures can result in opposing teeth being forced hard against each other with consequent vertical enamel fractures or even split teeth. Blows to the chin, for example, are a common cause of crown or crown and root fracture of intact teeth. Cuspal fracture and dentine exposure with or without involvement of the dental pulp may also occur when indirect trauma applies a sudden load to the teeth (Madjar & Divon-Kuperschmidt 1992). Careful examination of the teeth may reveal loss of buccal or palatal cusps of the molar teeth. Vertically sheared enamel and root fragments may only be held in place by attachment to the gingival tissue. Patients may complain of pain when hot or cold fluids are ingested because of exposed dentine. In more severe cases, pin-point specks of blood on the dentine floor indicate a frank exposure of the dental pulp.

Jaw fractures are likely to disrupt the dental occlusion with a severity determined by the site of the injury. For example, a blow to the right side of the face can result in a posterior maxillary dento-alveolar fracture. Examination of the maxillary arch form and comparison with the unaffected side can give an indication of the degree of displacement. The palatal gingival tissue will also display evidence of haematoma and it is sometimes possible to trace the path of the fracture along the palatal surface. In some cases of major dento-alveolar fracture, the maxilla will be so damaged that subsequent procedures such as impression taking will be very difficult, as even the largest impression tray may be too small.

Tooth charting

The dental examination determines whether teeth are present, restored, missing, fractured, avulsed or subluxated and also establishes the state of each tooth including its vitality. Any occlusal or positional irregularities of individual teeth are also noted. Examination findings must be recorded legibly and unambiguously. Tooth notation is based on the appearance of the dentition when upper and lower dental arches are viewed from the occlusal aspect (Fig. 12.7). Any one of several systems of tooth notation may be used for dental examination; these are described in standard texts on dental anatomy (Berkovitz & Moxham 1982, Van Beek 1983). The notation described here is the Fédération Dentaire Internationale (FDI) system which assigns a two-digit code to each tooth. The first digit indicates the quadrant of the dental arch and the second digit indicates the tooth.

In the case of the permanent dentition, the first digit ranges from 1 for the maxillary right quadrant to 4 for the mandibular right quadrant, while the second digit ranges from 1 for central incisor to 8 for third molar:

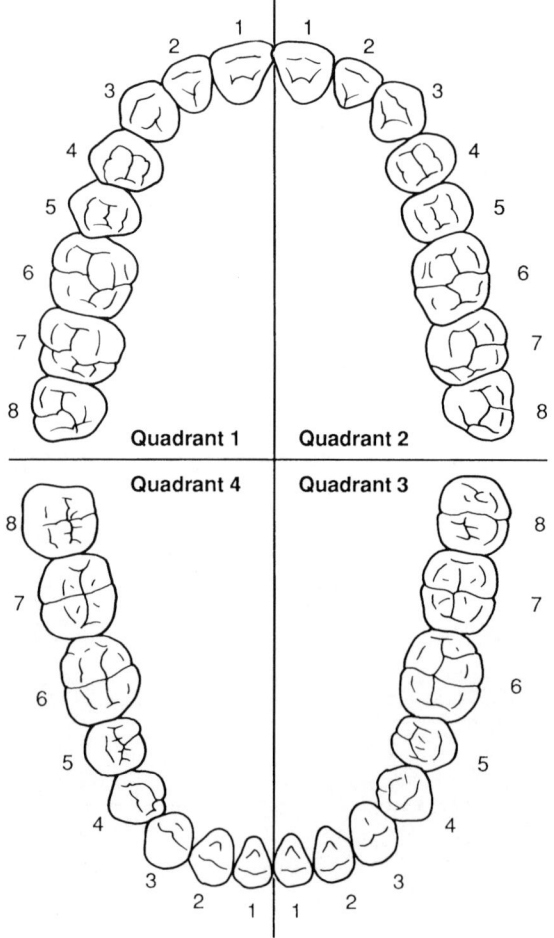

Fig. 12.7 Tooth notation. The permanent dentition is shown with division into arch quadrants with the number assigned to each tooth.

	Maxillary right							Maxillary left								
18	17	16	15	14	13	12	11	21	22	23	24	25	26	27	28
48	47	46	45	44	43	42	41	31	32	33	34	35	36	37	38

Mandibular right   Mandibular left

A similar notation applies to the deciduous dentition, the first digit ranging from 5 to 8 according to quadrant and the second digit from 1 for deciduous central incisor to 5 for deciduous second molar:

	Maxillary right				Maxillary left			
55	54	53	52	51	61	62	63	64	65
85	84	83	82	81	71	72	73	74	75

Mandibular right   Mandibular left

Thus each deciduous and permanent tooth has a two-digit code which is unique for that tooth; for example, 22 is the permanent left maxillary lateral incisor, 46 is the permanent right mandibular first molar, 74 is the deciduous left mandibular first molar and 81 is the deciduous right mandibular central incisor.

Classification of dental occlusion

The system commonly used to classify abnormalities in jaw relationships was developed by the orthodontist Edward H. Angle (p. 17). It is divided into three major categories termed Angle Class 1, 2 and 3 based on the anteroposterior relationships between maxillary and mandibular first molars (Fig. 12.8). Class 1 occlusion exists when the upper and lower first molars meet in a normal relationship: this occurs when the mesiobuccal cusp of the upper molar occludes with the mesiobuccal groove of the lower molar. In a Class 2 relationship, the lower molar occludes in a more posterior position than in Class 1 and this form of occlusion is sometimes termed post-normal. If the lower molar is more anteriorly located

in relationship to the upper molar than it is in Class 1 then the occlusion is referred to as Class 3 or pre-normal. Subdivisions are used by orthodontists to classify occlusal relationships further (Angle 1907, Proffit 1986, Foster 1990).

Dental radiographic assessment

Although the examiner of a patient with dental injuries associated with craniomaxillofacial (CMF) trauma will usually see the radiographs and CT scans obtained as part of the overall clinical assessment, special intraoral films and the extraoral panoramic view are especially important.

The most commonly used intraoral radiograph is the periapical view which provides good imaging of up to three or four teeth and their associated alveolar structures. Periapical films are often obtained by the relatively simple bisecting angle technique by which the operator positions the X-ray tube so that the central beam is directed towards a plane that bisects the angle between tooth and film (Fig. 12.9). The standard film, 40 mm × 30 mm in size, or slightly smaller for deciduous teeth, is held in position against tooth and palate or tooth and lower alveolus by the patient who must be instructed by the operator to take care not to bend the film. At times, because of a narrow dental arch or soft-tissue obstructions, the film and tube positions may need modification for patient comfort and to minimize distortion of the image.

As an alternative to the bisecting angle technique many clinicians prefer the paralleling or long cone technique. This method requires a special film holder which is attached to the cone of the X-ray equipment and positioned in the mouth so that the central beam passes perpendicular to both tooth and film (Fig. 12.10). A variety of film holders are available to facilitate radiography of

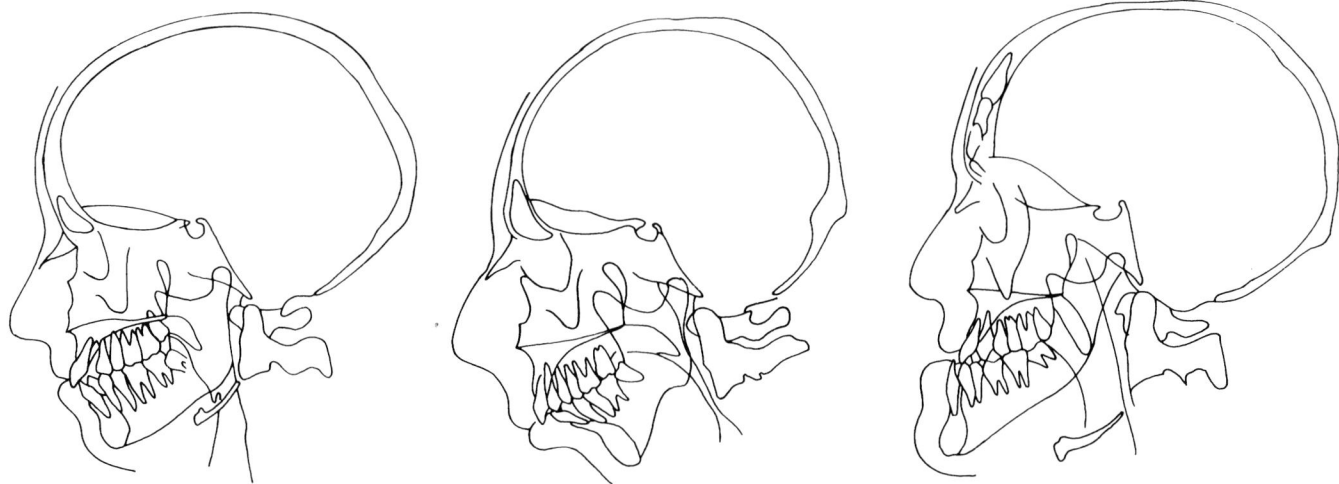

Fig. 12.8 Classification of occlusion. The characteristic profile appearances of subjects with dental occlusions corresponding to Angle Class 1 (left), 2 (centre) and 3 (right).

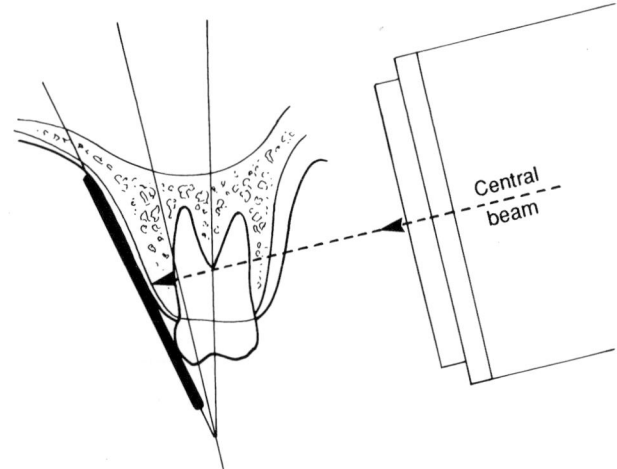

Fig. 12.9 Dental radiography: the bisecting angle technique. The central beam is directed at a line bisecting the planes of the film and the long axis of the tooth.

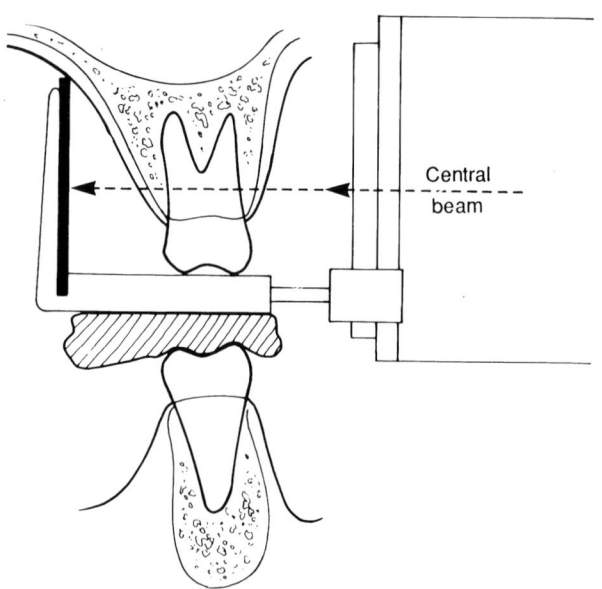

Fig. 12.10 Dental radiography: the long cone paralleling technique. The central beam passes perpendicular to the planes of the tooth and film.

different dental regions. The particular advantage of the paralleling technique lies in the relative freedom from distortion and the ability to determine tooth measurements and internal tooth morphology accurately, an important requirement of endodontic therapy.

Undistorted periapical films provide an excellent image of the dental hard tissues and the surrounding periodontium. They are essential when root fractures are suspected or when an accurate assessment of the periapical tissues is required.

As an adjunct to the periapical film, the bite-wing radiograph is used primarily for the diagnosis of dental caries. For this view, the film is held horizontally behind

the posterior teeth by the patient who closes on the horizontal arm of a special bite-wing holder. The film rests against the palate in the upper jaw and the lingual alveolus in the lower. Tooth crowns and the superior part of the alveolus are included in this view. As the view enables the examiner to visualize upper and lower posterior tooth crowns on the one film, the bite-wing is also important in a complete dental examination.

Occlusal view radiographs are useful to disclose unerupted or missing teeth and to assess the positions of any malaligned or displaced teeth relative to their neighbours within the dental arch. The occlusal film, which will adequately image the average dental arch, is held by the patient between the occlusal surfaces of upper and lower teeth. The central beam is directed through the bridge of the nose for a standard maxillary view and through the chin for the mandibular film. Occasionally, oblique occlusal films may be required for satisfactory imaging of some dental structures.

Panoramic dental radiographs are widely used for diagnostic purposes. By imaging all maxillary and mandibular teeth, the alveoli, mandibular ramus, temporomandibular joints, palate and part of the maxillary air spaces, a panoramic film provides an excellent aid for overall assessment of the dental region (Fig. 12.11). Fractured bones, missing, fractured or displaced teeth and other gross bony pathology can be readily detected. In spite of its general utility, this type of radiograph suffers from distortion and loss of clarity in some regions and must be supplemented by other views when finer detail is required.

The orthopantogram (OPG: p. 180) is obtained by exposure on an orbiting panoramic machine, and is the common form although views obtained with fixed machines are sometimes employed. The OPG is exposed in a special cassette that orbits around the patient's jaws, synchronously with the X-ray tube. To achieve a smooth transition from one region to the next, the tube and cassette move around three centres of rotation in succession. Even so, the OPG may provide rather poor imaging of the incisor region. Moreover, images of parts of the upper cervical column are usually superimposed upon other structures.

MEDICAL ASSESSMENT

The underlying purpose in the evaluation of the medical history and examination is to focus on any existing or previous medical conditions or medications that could interfere with desirable dental treatment options (Ch. 20). Such interference may take place early in management, or in the course of late restorative dentistry.

Apart from initial emergency dental treatment or treatment in the course of correcting a fracture involving the occlusion, the patient who has undergone surgery following CMF trauma may not be referred for reconstructive

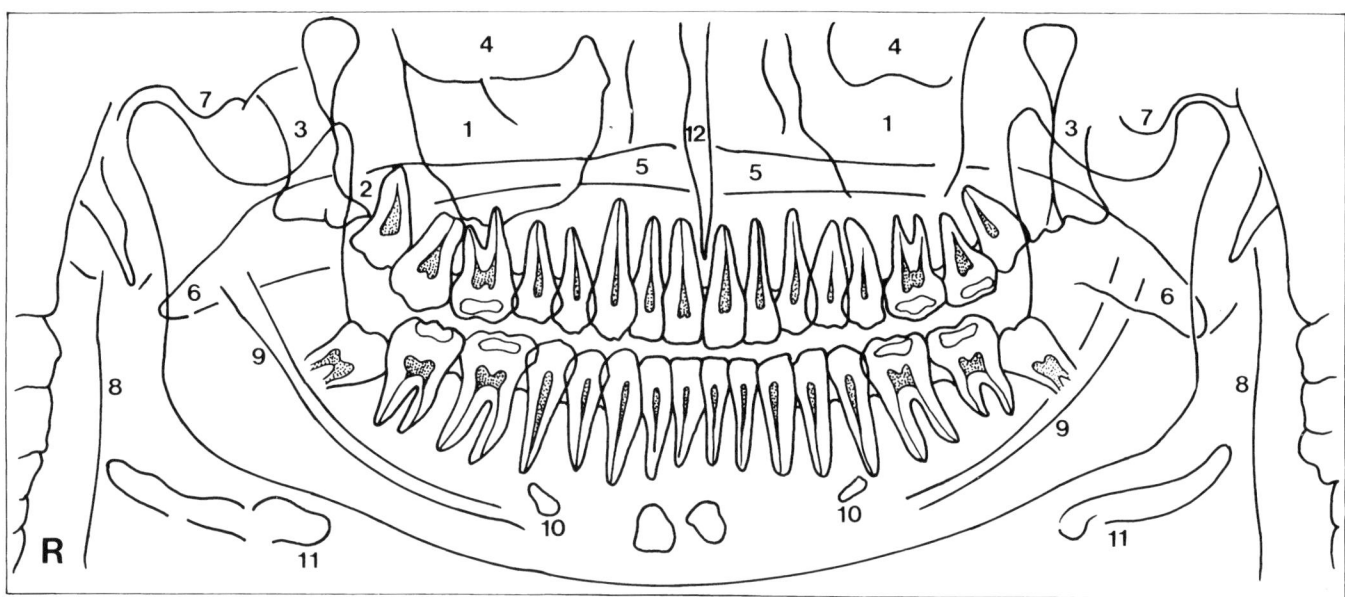

Fig. 12.11 Orthopantomogram of the permanent dentition. This provides images of both jaws, the teeth, alveoli and neighbouring structures: (1) maxillary sinus; (2) maxillary tuberosity; (3) lateral pterygoid plate; (4) orbital cavity; (5) hard palate; (6) soft palate; (7) articular eminence; (8) posterior pharyngeal wall; (9) inferior alveolar (mandibular) canal; (10) mental foramen; (11) hyoid bone; (12) nasal septum.

dental work for several months. During this healing phase, the patient may have visited a number of medical and paramedical specialists involved in treatment and rehabilitation. None the less, it should not be assumed that all relevant medical conditions have been properly investigated — or even diagnosed! At each appointment, the dental specialist should check the general health of the patient as well as the dental status. Preliminary data collection should include medical history, dental history, radiographs, dental study models, records of jaw relationships, facial and intraoral clinical photographs and a detailed oral examination. All of these data may interact in the development of a treatment plan. Some of the implications of concurrent medical diseases are discussed below.

INJURIES OF THE DENTAL PULP

Endodontic assessment

Endodontics is the dental speciality concerned with the sequelae of injuries to the dental pulp caused by trauma or the effects of untreated dental disease. Restorative procedures cannot be started on teeth with pulp injury until the endodontist has completed all necessary treatment. However, as noted above, considerable time may elapse before the patient's major injuries are sufficiently stabilized to allow the assessment of pulpal status of the teeth and the initiation of appropriate treatment regimes. By the time of referral for endodontic assessment and treatment, many patients who have suffered major craniofacial trauma involving the dental structures will have had teeth

with crown or crown–root fractures removed when the fractured facial bones were reduced and plated. Thus the number of teeth requiring endodontic intervention may be less than would otherwise be the case.

Pulp vitality tests

On presentation for endodontic evaluation all teeth, whether associated with fracture sites or not, must undergo pulp vitality tests as future treatment is dictated by the state of the dental pulp. Both thermal and electronic testing are mandatory.

In addition, the examiner must be alert for evidence of discoloration of the tooth crown, an indication of pulp pathology. To assist in the assessment of colour exchange it is helpful, where possible, to compare the colour of the suspect tooth with that of the contralateral tooth. A tooth crown exhibiting either pinkish or greyish colour change is a definite indication that pulpal damage has occurred.

The best method for testing the vitality of a tooth pulp is to induce rapid and positive thermal change by the application of a dry ice pencil to the tooth's gingival margin. The dry ice pencil used for pulp testing can be produced by a variety of instruments, most of which make a pencil 2–3 mm in diameter. However, we find that the extra thermal change produced by a thicker pencil of 4–5 mm diameter gives a significantly more reliable assessment of pulpal status. This is especially noticeable in fully crowned teeth. It is usually possible to establish a normal baseline reaction to the test by noting the reaction of obviously uninjured teeth. Electronic testing has limitations when applied to crowned or heavily restored teeth, conditions that tend to reduce pulpal response to electronic pulp testers. Sensitivity to percussion on the tooth crown can also indicate the presence of a compromised pulp, but thermal testing using the dry ice pencil is the most reliable. Any tooth that gives an abnormal response to pulp tests should be radiographed using standard intraoral periapical films. The finding of periapical rarefaction and/or thickened peridental ligaments gives further confirmation of pulpal pathology. Panoramic radiographs are not reliable for assessing periapical lesions.

A complete absence of reaction to the rapid cooling of a tooth indicates the presence of a totally necrotic pulp. An obviously enhanced reaction with an after-glow lasting for more than a minute indicates a pulp in a state of irreversible inflammation. In all instances of abnormal pulpal reaction endodontic intervention is mandatory if the affected tooth is to remain as a permanent entity in the dental arch.

However, pulp testing is not always a straightforward procedure in patients who have suffered craniofacial injuries. Pulp vitality depends on an intact and healthy vascular supply. If the neural connections have been severed by the trauma, or by subsequent treatment, but the vascular supply is still intact, the tooth may contain a perfectly healthy pulp but still respond negatively to pulp tests. Endodontic intervention in such instances is contraindicated. At present, techniques for assessing coronal blood flow such as laser Doppler flow metering and pulse oximetry are in their infancy but, in time, techniques such as these may well take all the subjectivity out of the determination of pulpal status (Schnettler & Wallace 1991, Gilbert et al 1992).

Management

Clinical endodontic therapy is well established and the methods are documented in standard texts as well as in specialized journals (Cohen & Burns 1984, Stock & Nehammer 1985, Messing & Stock 1988, Harty 1990). However, for those readers unfamiliar with endodontic procedures a brief description of endodontic therapy is in order. Unless a tooth that contains an injured pulp receives appropriate endodontic treatment, sooner or later periapical pathology will develop. If left untreated, the ultimate result is extraction of the tooth. Periapical pathology develops because toxins produced in the necrotic pulp tissue reach the vital periapical tissues via the apical foramina and initiate chronic or acute reactions in both the hard and soft tissues. Microorganisms are always involved in the pathological process. In order to prevent the establishment of such processes, endodontic intervention aims to remove all traces of diseased and traumatized pulp tissue from the tooth's pulp chamber and root canal system, render the subsequent empty root canals sterile and then hermetically seal them so that no further elements with the potential for producing toxic products can enter the root canal system.

Success depends on the three tenents of canal debridement (cleaning and preparation of the root canals), canal sterilization and canal obturation (root canal filling), all of which must be adhered to strictly. Debridement, the first phase of treatment, requires the removal of injured and necrotic pulp remnants from the coronal pulp chamber and the root canals. This is achieved by mechanically enlarging the root canal spaces laterally using special hand-operated instruments such as endodontic files and reamers together with copious irrigation of the canal spaces with a 2–5% solution of sodium hypochlorite. Mechanical and ultrasonically driven instruments for cleaning and preparing root canals are available but as yet these have not been developed to a stage where their use can be recommended.

Before treatment the diameter of the root canals can be as fine as 0.08 mm in adult teeth and well over 1 mm in younger teeth. The majority of teeth that are endodontically treated have canals at the finer end of the diameter range and during preparation of the canal an average diameter of 0.35–0.5 mm is achieved. The preparation and sterilization of the root canal spaces generally involve two to four treatments, the treatments ideally being several days apart. Between treatments, medicaments such as creams containing corticosteroids and calcium hydroxide are sealed into the canal spaces to assist in obtaining a sterile root canal environment.

Once a sterile canal system has been achieved, and this can be monitored by sampling cultures from the root canal, the canal space is totally obliterated with gutta percha cones and any one of a variety of suitable sealing cements. Various techniques for sealing the canals, all using gutta percha as the preferred filler, are available. Once canal obturation has been achieved the root system of a tooth, if treated correctly endodontically, remains perfectly healthy and provides an excellent foundation for an appropriate coronal restoration.

Endodontic therapy varies in complexity according to the state of the pulp and the anatomy of the root canals. A pulp which exhibits minimum infection may be treated in fewer sessions than a heavily infected root canal system. Teeth with multiple and twisted roots have correspondingly multiple and branching root canals. Furthermore, many teeth have lateral root canals that exit into the peridental space while others, usually older teeth, may present with exceedingly narrow root canals caused by calcific degeneration of the pulp tissue. Teeth such as these present a far greater treatment challenge than single-rooted anterior teeth.

Removal of the necrotic pulp tissue from the root canals is achieved via the coronal pulp chamber. Unless the pulp has been exposed by a fracture of the crown, pulp removal is achieved through access cavities which are usually prepared in the occlusal surfaces of posterior teeth and, for aesthetic reasons, the lingual surfaces of anterior teeth. This requires a detailed knowledge of the internal anatomy of each tooth, particularly the spatial relationship between the pulp chamber and the external surfaces of the tooth.

Knowledge of the correct root length is also essential in all phases of endodontic treatment. Insertion of instruments and subsequent placement of sealing material into the root canal spaces should terminate 0.5–1.0 mm short of the radiographic apex of the root. Instrumentation outside these limits only leads to unnecessary future complications and possible failure of treatment. Root length is usually determined accurately by means of a periapical radiograph of the tooth with a test instrument inserted into the root canal (Fig. 12.12). Such an instrument, usually a fine gauge reamer or endodontic file, is equipped with a moveable marker on its shank, such as a neoprene rubber disk, which can be positioned against a fixed and recordable point on the tooth crown. When the radiographs show that the tip of the instrument is correctly

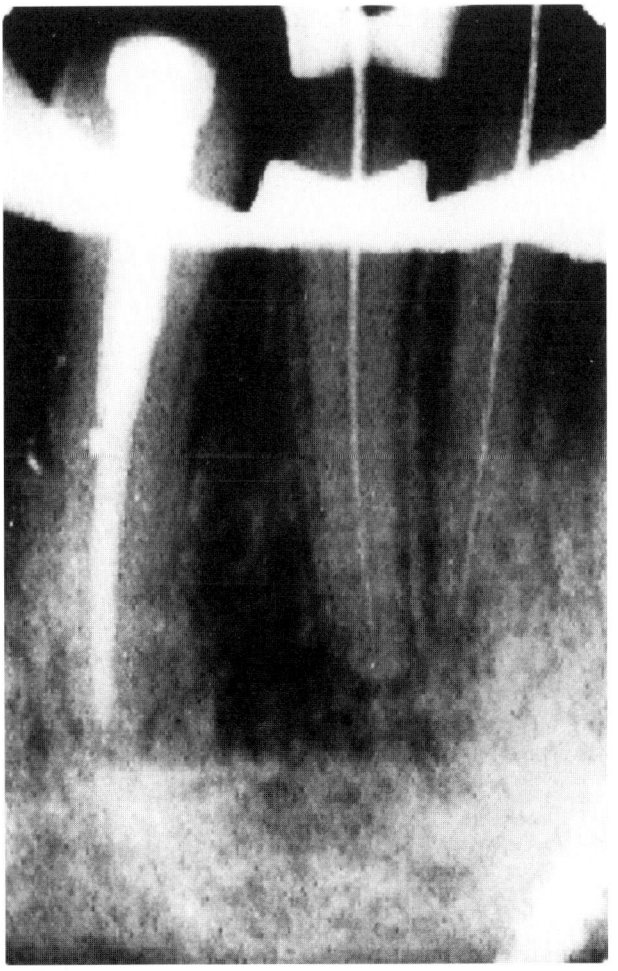

Fig. 12.12 Endodontics. Radiograph of mandibular incisors with instruments in place to indicate root canal length.

placed at the apical foramen the instrument is withdrawn and the distance between instrument tip and marker is measured. This measurement is then recorded as the working length for that particular root canal.

The length of a tooth's root can also be determined electronically by means of apex sensors but the accuracy of these devices is often suspect, except perhaps in teeth with straight root canals. However, these sensors, used in conjunction with other techniques, provide additional information to assist in determining a satisfactory root length measurement.

With treatment in the hands of a competent endodontist, the permanent retention rate for pulpally injured teeth is ~98%. However, the patient with CMF injury can present difficulties that are not encountered in the non-traumatized patient. Often, the patient may be unable to open the mouth widely enough for workable access to the posterior teeth and lower incisors. Generally with time and appropriate physiotherapy and jaw exercises the access difficulties will be overcome, but if acute pulp pathology with pain develops before access is possible, extraction of the offending tooth must be considered. In the case of lower anterior teeth where mouth opening is restricted it may sometimes be necessary to resort to labial access cavities rather than the conventional lingual approach.

A second and possibly more serious difficulty is the placement of fixation plates and screws in the jaws in positions that mask the radiographic images of root apices of teeth to be treated endodontically (Figs 12.13 and 12.14). This complicates the assessment of correct root length. The use of unusual radiographic projection angles can sometimes overcome this problem but in many cases the operator must rely on knowledge of the average lengths of teeth and tactile feedback through endodontic instruments inserted into the root canal. The use of local anaesthesia is contraindicated in these cases as the projection of a fine instrument through the apical foramen of a pulpless tooth will often elicit a reaction in the patient which helps in assessing the correct root length.

It should be noted that the endodontist is not responsible for the restoration of tooth crowns or the replacement of missing teeth. On completion of the endodontic treatment, the patient is referred to the dental practitioner responsible for further treatment. It is the responsibility of the endodontist to provide all other participating practitioners with information regarding the endodontically treated teeth together with radiographs of the completed canal seals. The administrative structure of an integrated craniofacial unit should facilitate this.

LUXATIONS AND ROOT FRACTURES

Surgical pathology

Luxation injuries arising from tooth impact are most

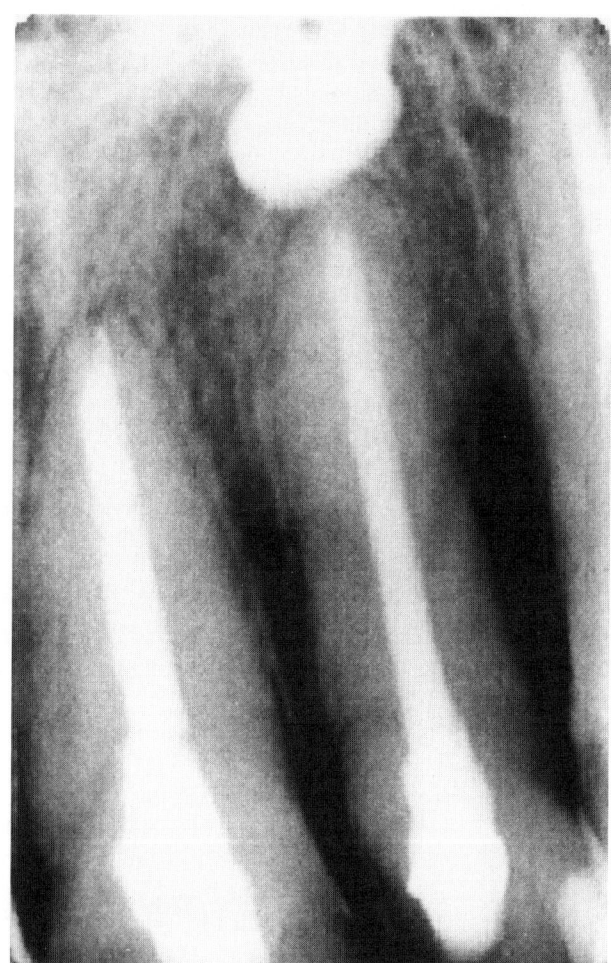

Fig. 12.13 Endodontics. Radiograph of maxillary teeth showing the proximity of a fixation device to the root apex of the lateral incisor.

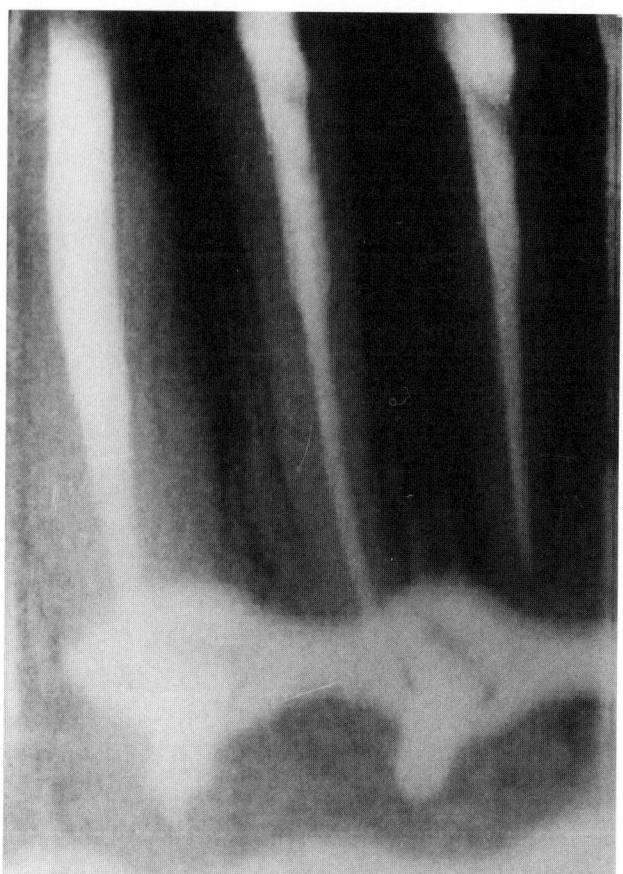

Fig. 12.14 Endodontics. Radiograph of mandibular teeth showing fixation devices obscuring images of the root apices of the lateral incisor and canine.

often seen in the anterior region of the dentition. Crona-Larsson & Norén (1989) found that maxillary central incisors represented ~70% of all teeth involved in impact injuries; the majority occurred in children aged 8–12 years. These authors found that the most frequent causes of anterior tooth trauma were falls, bicycle-riding, sports and assaults in that order. Boys suffered trauma more frequently than girls and tooth loosening without dislocation was the most common form of injury.

F. M. Andreasen (1989) used the following classification to describe luxation injuries:

1. Concussion: the tooth and periodontal tissues suffer minimal damage with tenderness to percussion being the predominant clinical symptom. Enamel crazing or chipping may occur as a result of concussion injuries.
2. Subluxation: the tooth is loosened within its socket but without displacement.
3. Extrusive luxation: the tooth is displaced from its socket in an occlusal direction so that it lies below the line of tooth occlusion.

4. Lateral luxation: the tooth suffers axial displacement in a lateral, labial or palatal direction. Damage to the alveolar bone occurs in this type of luxation.
5. Intrusive luxation: the tooth is impacted into the socket.

The three types of luxation injury all involve damage to the supporting tissues and furthermore are invariably accompanied by severance of the apical blood and nerve supply to the tooth with consequent pulpal necrosis.

Impact injuries to the teeth may cause fracture of the crown or root at any level (Fig. 5.11). In the case of root fracture, the unattached coronal portion of the tooth may be further displaced within the socket. F. M. Andreasen (1989) classified luxation injuries of the coronal portion of a root-fractured incisor in a manner similar to the luxation classification:

1. Concussion where there is no displacement of the fractured coronal portion
2. Subluxation with obvious mobility of the coronal portion
3. Extrusive luxation
4. Lateral luxation.

The latter two forms are characterized by displacement of the loose coronal portion of the tooth out of the socket.

In a detailed account of injuries to permanent teeth, F. M. Andreasen (1989) reviewed 637 luxated teeth and 95 root-fractured teeth over a period of up to 11 years. Behaviour of the dental pulp after injuries of these types determined the outcome of treatment and the long-term survival of the tooth. Pulpal healing patterns depended particularly on the nature and severity of the injury and the stage of root development. A passive form of splinting using acid-etched bonding with composite cements was found to be preferable to forceful cementation with orthodontic bands as less trauma to the injured tooth was involved.

With respect to luxation injuries, almost all teeth with the least severe injury, namely concussion, showed pulp survival with only a few suffering pulp necrosis or obliteration of the pulp canal by calcific deposit. Subluxation injuries were also followed by a high rate of pulp survival, particularly if the root apex was still open, as occurs when root formation is incomplete. A surprising finding of this study was that pulpal survival following luxation injuries could still occur even in the presence of classic signs of pulp necrosis such as coronal discoloration, loss of pulpal sensibility and periapical resorption as indicated by radiolucency. However, in the more severe extrusive, lateral and intrusive luxation injuries pulp survival occurred in relatively few cases, pulp necrosis, especially in teeth with closed apices, being the usual outcome.

Root fractures may heal by hard-tissue union, connective tissue union or the interposition of granulation tissue between the coronal and apical segments of the tooth. Almost all cases studied by F. M. Andreasen (1989) displayed resorption processes originating at the root fracture line or at the root apex. Hard-tissue union tended to occur commonly in root fractures following concussion or subluxation injuries to teeth with closed apices, but the other forms of fracture healing were more frequent following injuries involving extrusive and lateral luxation.

Management

The usual treatment of both luxated and root-fractured teeth is immobilization by splinting to adjacent teeth until healing of the damaged teeth has occurred. When obvious pulpal death has occurred, as in the more severe luxation injuries involving tooth displacement from the socket, endodontic treatment must be initiated. In other cases regular monitoring of pulpal status should be undertaken.

On the basis of the survey of pulpal healing quoted above, F. M. Andreasen (1989) recommended that luxation and root-fracture injuries should be treated with a relatively gentle splinting technique such as an acid-etched composite resin splint. Following the less traumatic luxation injuries, pulp survival may occur in spite of early signs of necrosis and therefore endodontic therapy should be delayed in these cases for up to 1 year so that pulpal status can be monitored regularly.

THE AVULSED TOOTH

Surgical pathology

More dramatic than the tooth luxation injuries caused by CMF trauma is the total avulsion of one or more teeth. As a rule, this type of injury is restricted to the anterior teeth: posterior teeth are rarely forced completely from their sockets.

Management

If the avulsed tooth can be found and replanted into its socket, regeneration of the periodontal ligament can occur with normal reattachment of the tooth to the bony socket after appropriate endodontic measures (J. O. Andreasen 1981, 1989). The long-term success of a replanted avulsed tooth depends on a number of factors, one of the most important being the time delay before replantation: after an extraoral time of 30 min the chances of a successful outcome are greatly reduced. However, the search for and replantation of avulsed teeth is not practicable when life saving procedures take priority.

Most documented avulsions and replantations have occurred as a result of relatively minor accidents such as occur on the sport field, at children's playgrounds and after minor bicycle mishaps. In these situations finding the missing tooth is rarely a problem. The case is very different when the tooth must be found in the wreckage of a crashed motor vehicle; in most vehicle accidents, the treatment priorities rarely allow for the finding and replantation of an avulsed tooth. The application of replantation techniques to the avulsed tooth depends on the seriousness of other injuries. Replantation is a viable option only in the absence of skeletal fractures and when swelling of the orofacial soft tissues does not make access to and manipulation of the dental structures too difficult.

The early management of the avulsed tooth is critical to a successful outcome and the following points should be noted:

1. If the tooth is clean it should be replaced immediately in the empty socket using gentle finger pressure, making sure that the tooth is correctly oriented with respect to its neighbours.
2. If debris is adhering to the tooth surface, the patient should suck the tooth clean or alternatively the tooth can be washed gently in milk.
3. If the primary aid provider is unable to replant the

tooth — and few can — the tooth should be stored in milk and the help of a dentist sought as soon as possible. It is essential to prevent the drying out of the root surface and if milk is not available the tooth should be wrapped in plastic film to retard dehydration of the cellular elements still adhering to the root surface.

4. When an avulsed tooth is handled, contact with the root surface should be kept to a minimum and the remnants of the peridental membrane adhering to the root surface must be protected as much as possible from further trauma.

5. At the time of replantation antibiotics and tetanus prophylaxis (p. 230) must be administered with the assumption that the avulsed tooth is likely to have been contaminated with microorganisms.

After the tooth has been replanted it must be stabilized as soon as possible by some form of temporary splinting by attachment to adjacent teeth. The splinting should be maintained for 1 week only, during which time endodontic therapy should be initiated and the debrided root canal dressed with a mixture of corticosteroid and calcium hydroxide paste. This procedure will give the greatest protection against redisplacement and inflammatory root resorption. The intracanal medication must be maintained for many months, and only when the stability of the root surface is reasonably assured should the root canal space be permanently sealed.

Factors affecting survival of replanted teeth

The chief cause of replantation failure is root resorption. This may be associated with an inflammatory response in the periodontal tissues which destroys cementum to open a pathway from the dental pulp. Root resorption may also be accompanied by bony ankylosis which follows the replantation of a tooth with a necrotic periodontal membrane (Hammarström et al 1986b). According to Andersson et al (1989), a tooth replanted with a necrotic periodontal membrane will be ankylosed with root resorption within 3–7 years in young patients but will remain in function for considerably longer in older patients. Hence the status of the pulp and periodontal membrane is the major determinant of successful replantation.

Several factors influence the healing processes following replantation. Damage to the periodontal membrane through excessive handling significantly increases the chances of post-replantation root resorption and ankylosis. Treatment of the tooth prior to replantation is also of critical importance in preserving the maximum vitality of the periodontal membrane. As stated above, the avulsed tooth must not be allowed to dry out as very few cells will remain vital after 1 h. If replantation must be delayed,

the tooth should be preserved in saliva or, preferably, milk until professional help is available (Blomlöf et al 1983).

In an experimental study, Andreasen & Schwartz (1986) found that avulsed teeth dried for 30 min and then stored in saline for 30 min before replantation suffered significantly more root resorption than teeth undergoing only 15 min drying. The extra period of drying apparently caused more necrosis of the periodontal membrane. These authors suggested that provided a tooth can be stored in saline after avulsion, a slight delay in replantation until a dentist or other qualified person is available is preferable to immediate replantation 'on-the-spot' by a person without dental knowledge.

Splinting of the replanted teeth should be minimal to permit physiological movements during mastication as this causes less root resorption than a tooth splinted with a rigid device. Moreover, endodontic treatment should be carried out within 14 days of replantation to minimize the passage of toxic material from an infected pulp to the periodontal ligament. An *in vivo* study of replanted lateral incisors in monkeys showed that systemic administration of antibiotics at the time of replantation prevented the development of rapid inflammatory root resorption (Hammarström et al 1986a).

FRACTURES LUXATIONS AND AVULSIONS IN CHILDHOOD

These are discussed in Chapter 19, and in more detail by Sowray (1985) and by Andreasen & Andreasen (1990). Apart from enamel chipping or crown fracture, a deciduous tooth may be completely avulsed, or displaced in any direction, or partially or completely intruded. The luxation injuries require special consideration because of the proximity of the permanent tooth and the possibility that it may be involved in the trauma. It is interesting that Garcia-Godoy et al (1989) found that very few parents of young children with primary tooth trauma were aware of the possible damage to underlying permanent teeth. The parents were more concerned with colour changes to their child's tooth and obvious pathological sequelae such as abscess formation. This study was conducted in private practice in the Dominican Republic; it is likely that similar views would be held in many other parts of the world, though public education in dental hygiene is more advanced in some countries.

Full clinical and radiographic examination is mandatory to determine whether the developing follicle is damaged; if this is the case, then as a rule the deciduous tooth should be carefully removed with the precautions described in Chapter 19. In many cases however, the follicle escapes injury and the deciduous tooth can be preserved. An avulsed deciduous tooth should never be reimplanted as damage to the developing permanent tooth is highly likely (Ch. 19).

FRACTURES OF THE JAWS

Management

CMF trauma involving teeth invariably disrupts the established dental occlusion and the disruption is most severe after jaw fractures. In such cases correct relationships between the teeth within the fractured segments and between these teeth and those of the opposite jaw must be re-established correctly. This is achieved by the use of various forms of splints and occlusal wafers which are fitted to the teeth when the fractures are reduced and definitive fixation is established by plates or intermaxillary wiring. This section reviews the dental principles and techniques involved in re-establishing the occlusion.

Dental impressions

The importance of these in the management of fractures of the jaws has been discussed in Chapter 11. In general, articulated models of the dentition are useful in ensuring that a correct occlusion is established. Very often it may be difficult to assess the true nature of the patient's occlusion, especially if there is an open bite or fractured bony segments. With modern dental alginate formulations it is possible for the dental technician to obtain at least two models from the impression so that one set can be articulated in the condition as presented while the other set is used as the master model for sectioning and construction of a bite wafer. Both sets of models are articulated. In this way the surgeon is given a meaningful guide as to the amount of bone reduction required to re-establish the occlusion.

Tray selection

Disposable impression trays are probably best for taking impressions, particularly if they are of the sectionable type. They are made in three sizes: small, medium and large; these are available for both the maxilla and mandible. The advantage of this type of tray is that the segments can be easily removed by a pair of wire-cutters to provide smaller trays for sectional impressions if required; moreover, when the patient's mouth cannot open fully, the lingual flange can be removed without destroying the rest of the tray. Once the tray has been cut, it is necessary to cover the ragged edges with a thin roll of the soft blue wax known as periphery wax. It is advisable to coat the inside surface of the tray with an alginate adhesive material to ensure that the impression material does not pull away from the tray with consequent distortion of the impression. A wafer constructed from a distorted model will not fit the patient's teeth accurately.

Alginate impression materials

The alginate or irreversible hydrocolloid is a very popular impression material in oral and maxillofacial surgery because of its relatively low cost and ease of mixing. If the plaster model is cast within 30 min after obtaining the impression, the reproduction will be accurate. Alginate impression material consists of sodium or potassium alginate, calcium sulphate, diatomaceous earth, trisodium phosphate, colouring material and a flavour. When the alginate reacts with water, insoluble calcium alginate forms very quickly, requiring the addition of trisodium phosphate as a retarding agent to provide sufficient working time for the operator to load the impression tray and seat it accurately in the patient's mouth.

There are two types of alginate powders available: type 1 (fast-set) and type 2 (slow-set). In most cases type 1 is preferred; at room temperature it allows ~1 min from mixing with water to setting. Type 2 alginate has a setting time of ~4 min. A fast setting time is important for some patients, for example those with a midface fracture which hinders nasal breathing, or those with a mandibular fracture limiting jaw opening. Traumatized patients often fear suffocation if bulky impression material remains in the mouth for an excessive length of time.

Mixing alginate can be done with a clean rubber bowl and a metal spatula. Mixing is carried out vigorously, the material being wiped against the side of the bowl for at least 45–60 s until the mix is smooth and creamy and does not fall off the spatula when raised from the bowl. The material is loaded into the impression tray and seated accurately in the patient's mouth.

Dental impressions are usually taken without the need of any anaesthetic as the small degree of pain can be tolerated. Removal of the impression when set may involve some pain, especially in patients with fractures, and if possible it is preferable to remove the impression with a quick snap action.

Following removal the impression is washed in water to remove traces of blood and saliva, wrapped in a moist towel and then placed in an air-tight container to avoid drying out. As a precaution against virus-contaminated blood or saliva remaining on the impression, it may be soaked in a 2% solution of glutaraldehyde for ~10 min without detriment to the impression. Some manufacturers now incorporate antiviral agents in the alginate powder. The impression should be poured using a high quality plaster or stone product 30 min after removal, this delay compensating for any distortion that may have occurred during removal from the mouth.

After setting, the dental models should be trimmed

and mounted on an articulator, a hinged device that enables upper and lower teeth to be brought together in correct occlusal relationship. In cases of major trauma the models are mounted on a plain line articulator avoiding the need to obtain records for the facebow record and jaw relations (see below). Disposal plastic articulators are available for this purpose. Although the plastic articulators are suitable for clinical presentation and study purposes, bite-wafers should be constructed from the master models mounted on a metal articulator.

Re-establishing the occlusion

The term dental occlusion, when used in its modern context, refers not only to the anatomical relationships between maxillary and mandibular teeth, but also includes consideration of the functional aspects of mandibular movements, temporomandibular joint physiology and the complex range of neuromuscular controls involved in jaw function. Dental occlusion is a very individual entity for each patient. The neuromuscular patterns controlling jaw movements and tooth-to-tooth contacts are developed early in life as the teeth emerge and they are constantly reinforced with every act of jaw closure involving tooth contact against opposing teeth, food or objects placed in the mouth (Thomson 1975, Ramfjord & Ash 1983).

Occlusal sense is a very refined sense involving perception of the shape, size, position and texture of objects placed between the teeth (Crum & Loiselle 1972). Even objects as small as grains of sand can be detected quite readily between occlusal surfaces. Therefore, any interference with the established form of dental occlusion by trauma or by restorative, orthodontic or surgical procedures will require a great deal of re-education by the patient as new neuromuscular patterns are learnt and then established. The success and comfort of any occlusal reconstruction, however small, will depend largely on the patient's ability to adjust to the changes in established functional patterns required by alterations to anatomical form and relationships within the dentition. While some patients display excellent adaptation to occlusal change, others, especially the elderly, have great difficulty and may never adapt satisfactorily to new occlusal sensation.

The majority of patients who have maxillary or mandibular fractures will have dental arch bars fitted by the surgeon. These bars can be adapted to the teeth in the operating theatre by the surgeon or to the dental cast by a technician using a wrought metal bar. Alternatively, they can be prefabricated with a silver alloy casting reproduced from a wax model of the arch bar prepared on the dental cast. The arch bar used in conjunction with an acrylic wafer provides the means for establishing and securing the patient's dental occlusion (Fig. 12.15).

When the dental models have set, they are sectioned

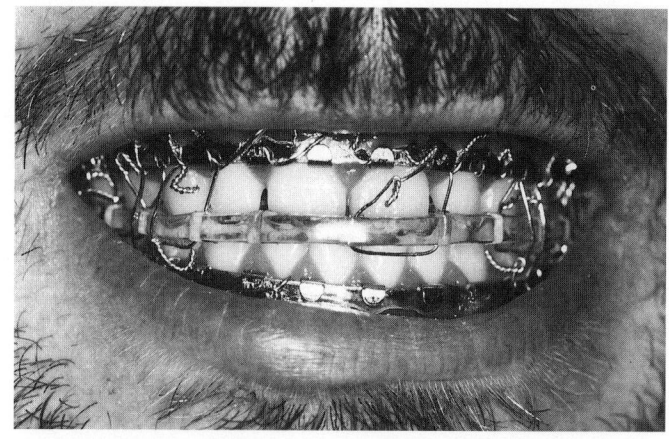

A

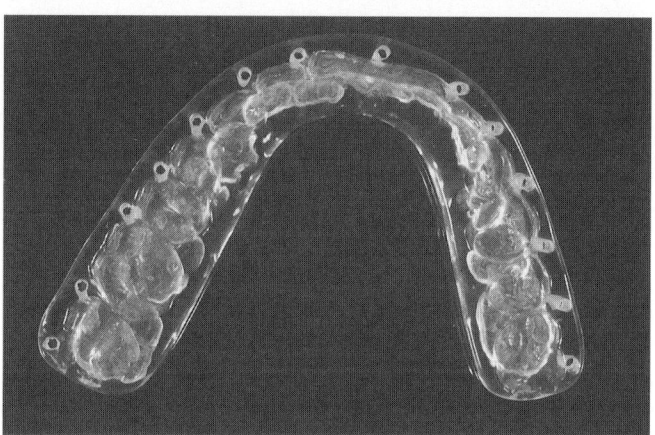

B

Fig. 12.15 Intermaxillary fixation. A Metal arch bars and occlusal wafer held in place by stainless steel ligature wire. **B** The occlusal wafer showing depressions for the opposing teeth and holes for the ligature wire.

with a round-bladed saw, examined carefully and aligned so that optimal occlusal relationships are established. The sections are then re-assembled using either sticky wax or quick-setting plaster to preserve the selected occlusion.

It may be difficult to determine an accurate occlusal relationship for a traumatized patient, particularly one without posterior teeth. In these cases it is necessary to examine wear facets on the remaining teeth to assess where the best interdigitation lies. This approach is not without difficulties as wear facets may have been produced when the patient was much younger or they may have been caused by non-functional movements of the mandible during bruxism or other habits. In these instances it is likely that the facets will represent arch relationships outside of the normal functional range. In some ethnic groups, for example Australian Aboriginals, the maxillary arch tends to be broad in relation to the mandible and in these subjects, maxillomandibular occlusal relationships as defined in conventional terms do not exist but are replaced by a form of alternate intercuspation which allows maximum interdigitation only on one side of the dental arch at a time (Brown et al 1987).

Another difficulty in establishing occlusion may arise in cross-bites when it is necessary to examine the wear facets carefully. When there is doubt about anterior tooth relationships, the patient can often remember whether the lower teeth closed in front of the upper teeth, edge-to-edge with them or behind them before the trauma. Dental records obtained on a previous occasion or even facial photographs can provide a valuable guide to re-establishing an accurate occlusion.

When the dentist is satisfied that correct occlusal relationships have been established, the model is now mounted on a dental articulator in the correct maxillomandibular relationship, and an acrylic bite wafer is made. First, a sheet of modelling wax is applied to the surface of the lower cast. Molten wax is then placed onto the top of the softened modelling wax along the line of tooth contacts and the articulator is closed to produce indentations of the tooth cusps as they approach the intercuspal position. The periphery of the wax is trimmed and smoothed and then the lower dental model complete with wax impression is invested in plaster within a special metal container termed a denture flask that opens into upper and lower sections. When the plaster is fully set the flask is opened and the wax boiled out with hot water. This leaves a space, previously occupied by the wax model, which is then packed with clear heat-cured resin which requires a 20 min curing cycle before it is safe to open the flask.

When the flask has cooled, the acrylic wafer is removed from the plaster and small holes are made around its periphery with a number 6 round burr. These holes enable the surgeon to place the interarch wires through the wafer in order to secure it firmly to the mandibular teeth. The wafer is then smoothed with pumice and polished with whiting (Fig. 12.16).

As a general rule acrylic dental wafers must be fairly thin, otherwise there may be difficulty in bringing the patient's teeth together. For example, in patients with an Angle Class II jaw relationship with deep overbite, a wafer constructed to position the anterior teeth correctly may cause disclusion of the posterior teeth to some extent.

Cast silver cap splints

Although these splints were once used extensively for intermaxillary fixation, it is now possible to achieve the same objective with acrylic occlusal wafers and titanium miniplates (p. 270). Construction of cap splints is very labour-intensive and expensive. The process requires an extensive wax-up on a dental model, investment and then casting in silver (Fig. 12.17). The cap splints are cemented into place in the operating theatre using either black copper cement or a polycarboxylate cement. Copper cement, however, can set prematurely if the critical manipulative procedures are not followed and it is very difficult to remove from teeth.

Gunning splints

In edentulous patients with jaw fractures, plastic Gunning splints (p. 16) may be constructed by the technician using impressions of the edentulous jaws and inserting metal cleats to allow intermaxillary wiring across maxillary and mandibular components of the splint. If the patient's dentures are available, these can be modified with the addition of the metal cleats to function in the same way as Gunning splints (Ch. 19).

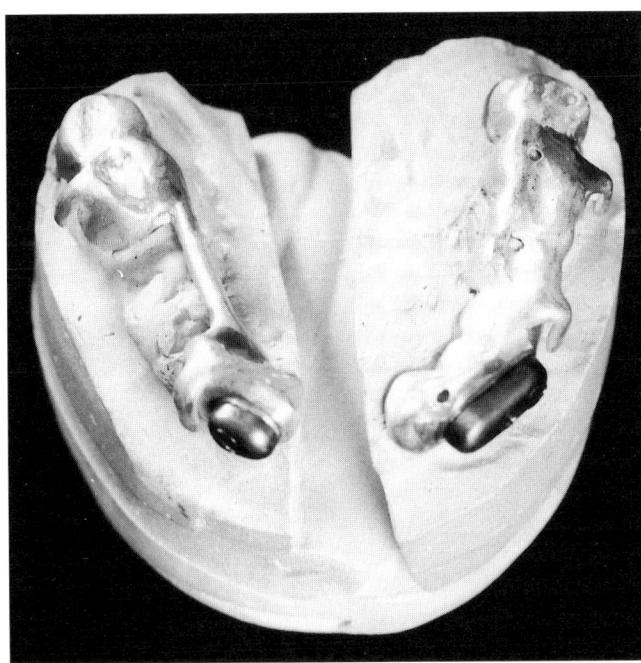

Fig. 12.17 Silver cap splint. A male patient aged 33 years suffered a Le Fort II fracture and a split palate in a motor cycle accident. Silver cap splints fitted to the maxillary arch were used to aid fixation.

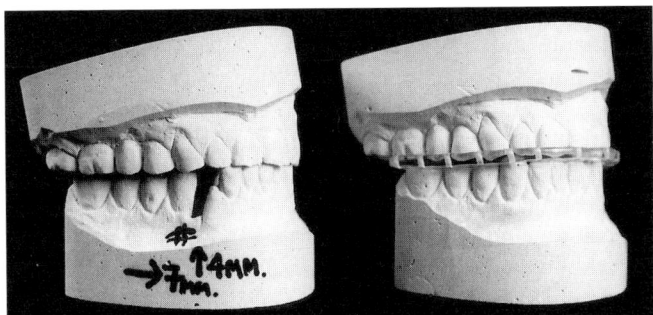

Fig. 12.16 Construction of an occlusal wafer. A mandibular fracture occurred in the region of the canine. Dental models were then reassembled to establish the occlusion by means of an occlusal wafer. The wafer is shown in place on the reassembled models.

MISSING OR DEFECTIVE TEETH

Dental restoration

The branch of dentistry concerned with the reconstruction of damaged, diseased or missing teeth is commonly referred to as restorative dentistry. It involves a wide spectrum of interests, knowledge and skills applied to diagnosis, prognosis, prevention and treatment planning. Teeth missing or damaged in CMF trauma can be restored or replaced with full function and aesthetics by use of modern restorative procedures. A dramatic improvement in the cosmetic appearance often greatly elevates the patient's self-esteem (Ch. 22).

As all dental treatment procedures involve the general health and welfare of patients, the dentist is bound to evaluate the individual totally. As a consequence, the optimal treatment for a particular patient may require referral to dental colleagues, medical specialists or other health care professionals. Although most procedures used in restorative dentistry are limited to the crowns of teeth and the supporting tissues, in many instances it will be essential to call upon the services of clinicians skilled in other dental specialties including oral surgery, endodontics, oral pathology, orthodontics, periodontics, paedodontics and both fixed and removable prosthodontics.

Many significant changes in the philosophy, methodologies and materials used in dental treatment have occurred, particularly over the past 20 years as evidenced by the vast body of information published in this period. As a result of the research and development being pursued throughout the world, concepts and treatments are subject to constant re-evaluation and many have become obsolete in a relatively short period of time. Over the past 10 years, for example, the practice of restorative dentistry has been significantly modified by new dental materials such as light-cured resins, glass-ionomer cements, dentine-bonding agents and titanium implants. Techniques, instruments and equipment have also changed. Restorative dentistry is a dynamic and ever-changing clinical discipline so that the types of treatment available today will, in all probability, be inadequate in a decade from now. The philosophies and methods of dental restoration as currently practised are outlined in general and specialized texts (Shillingburg et al 1981, Gettleman et al 1986, Solnit & Curnutte 1988, Wilson et al 1988, Mount 1991).

Dental assessment

First, a functional examination of the dental occlusion should be carried out with the teeth in the position of maximum interdigitation as well as in a range of protrusive and lateral contact positions. The degree of incisor overbite and overjet should be noted together with any discrepancies in posterior upper and lower tooth relationships in both the anteroposterior and transverse planes.

The use of articulating paper, carbon ribbon or occlusal wax during tooth closure will assist in identifying regions of occlusal interference, premature contacts and attrition, the latter sometimes being indicative of bruxism. The functional examination should also include palpation of the masticatory muscles to detect regions of tenderness or spasm and inspection of the temporomandibular joints by palpation during jaw movements and with the aid of a stethoscope to detect crepitus.

Models obtained from alginate impressions of the dental arches and mounted on an adjustable or semi-adjustable articulator (see above) by means of an occlusal registration and a facebow transfer are essential in complex restorative rehabilitation. The facebow record allows the upper dental model to be mounted in the same spatial relationship to the hinge axis of the articulator as the upper dental arch bears to the temporomandibular joints. The occlusal record is used to mount the lower dental cast on the articulator in the anatomically correct relation to the upper model. Further wax registrations taken with the jaws in protrusive or lateral contact positions are transferred to the articulator so that the mechanical condyle paths simulate the slope of the articular eminences. Depending on the degree of sophistication of the articulator, other adjustments can be made so that movements of the dental models made by the articulator produce tooth-to-tooth contacts that closely approximate those made by the patient during the same jaw movements. Thus important information on maxillomandibular relationships and other details of tooth contacts during excursions of the mandible, not readily apparent at the time of oral examination, can be obtained.

Duplicate models mounted on an adjustable articulator can also be used for diagnostic purposes involving the waxing up of regions to determine aesthetic tooth positioning for placement of retainers and titanium implants for prostheses if these are envisaged.

The type and extent of radiographic assessment necessary will be determined by the dental injuries: the examinations could range from a single periapical film to a full radiographic survey of the entire mouth. An OPG is a valuable diagnostic aid as it provides a survey of the entire maxillary and mandibular dentoalveolar region on a single film. If the treatment plan includes dental implants, lateral and antero-posterior head films may also be required. CT scans of the mandible may resolve doubt about the positioning of dental implants in relation to important anatomical structures such as the inferior dental nerve and the mental foramen.

Restorative procedures

Minor dental injuries, for example the fractured incisal edge of an anterior tooth, can usually be repaired with a composite resin restoration which is light-cured and

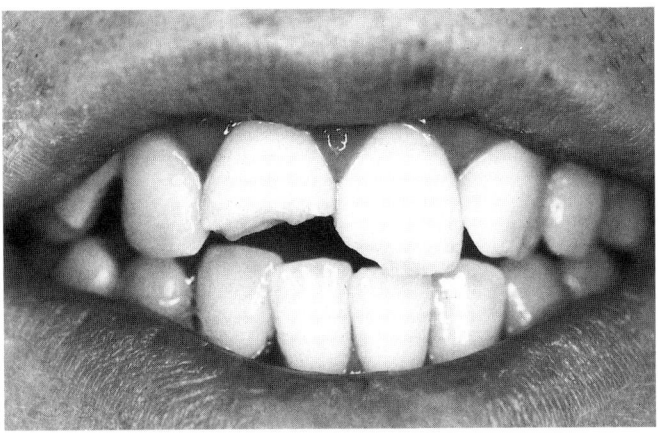

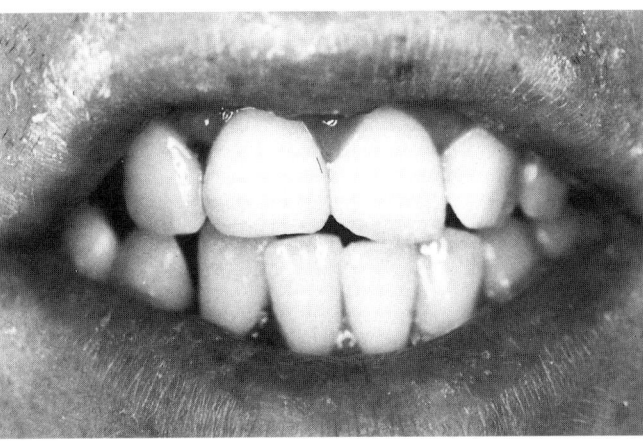

Fig. 12.18 Fractured incisor. A The maxillary central incisors were fractured in a bicycle accident. **B** Restoration of the right incisor was made with composite resin bonded to the acid-etched tooth surface.

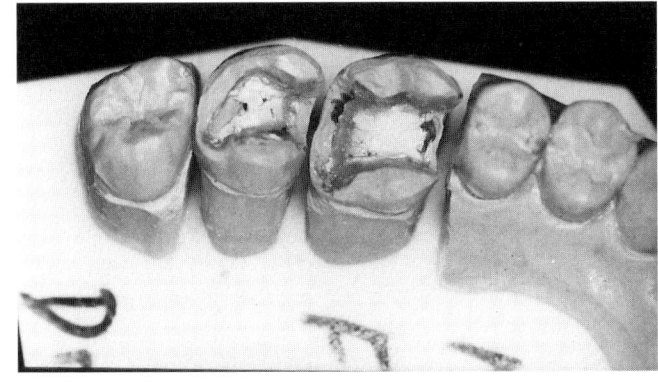

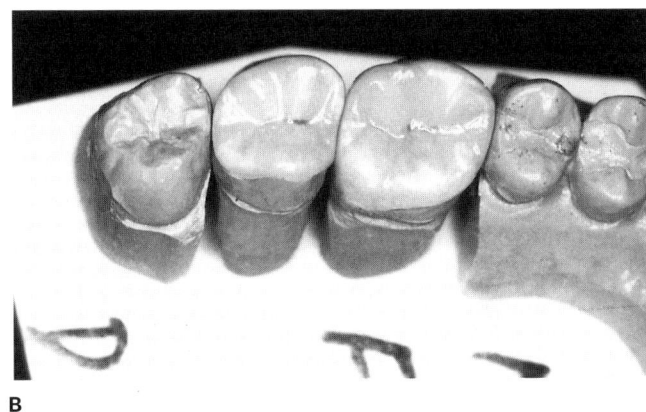

Fig. 12.19 Ceramic crowns. A Preparations for ceramic crowns on maxillary first and second molars. **B** The ceramic restorations in place on dies.

bonded onto an acid-etched tooth surface. This form of restoration provides a durable and excellent aesthetic result (Fig. 12.18). More extensive loss of tooth material requires more complex procedures including crowns, inlays and onlays, veneers, bridgework, partial dentures, or the use of osseo-integrated fixtures.

A *crown* is a cemented or adhesively bonded restoration that replaces the morphology, function and appearance of the damaged coronal portions of a tooth. A full crown covers the entire crown area whereas a partial crown covers only certain portions of the tooth. In the past, cast gold full crowns were used extensively in posterior teeth but the more aesthetic dental porcelain is now often preferred. Porcelain can be used by itself or fused to some other metal such as gold for greater strength. A crown is constructed upon a special model of the damaged tooth which has been prepared with cutting instruments according to well-defined principles (Fig. 12.19). When only the root of a tooth remains, a full crown can be constructed upon a dowel or core which is cemented into the already filled root canal.

An *inlay* is an intracoronal restoration with minimum extension whereas an *onlay* is used to restore more severely damaged teeth, particularly posterior teeth where it is necessary to protect cusps from potentially damaging occlusal forces. In modern dental practice adhesively bonded ceramic material is used for such restorations. Previously, wax patterns for inlays and onlays would often be prepared directly on the tooth in the patient's mouth but the current technique requires that the wax model be prepared indirectly on a special cast of the prepared tooth, especially when large restorations are required or where free access to the tooth is difficult.

A *veneer* can be either a composite resin or a porcelain ceramic restoration. As a rule, a porcelain veneer is < 0.5 mm thick; it is adhesively bonded to the remaining tooth structure by a thin layer of resin. These restorations are ideal for the aesthetic reconstruction of fractured anterior teeth as their preparation requires minimal removal of sound tooth structure (Fig. 12.20).

Single or multiple missing teeth can be replaced by implants, fixed bridgework or removable partial dentures. Conventional *fixed bridgework* involves the preparation of teeth on either side of the edentulous space. The artificial teeth suspended between the prepared teeth are

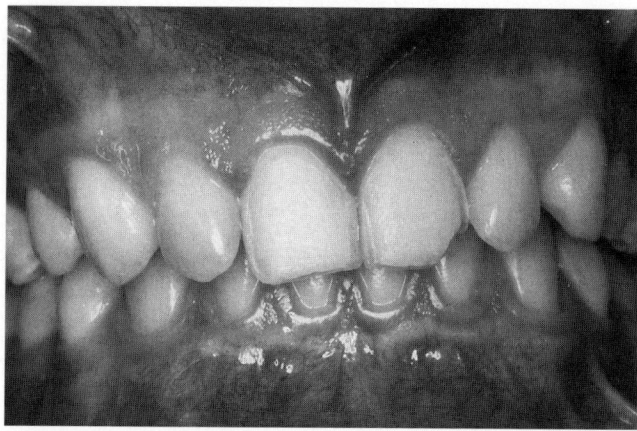

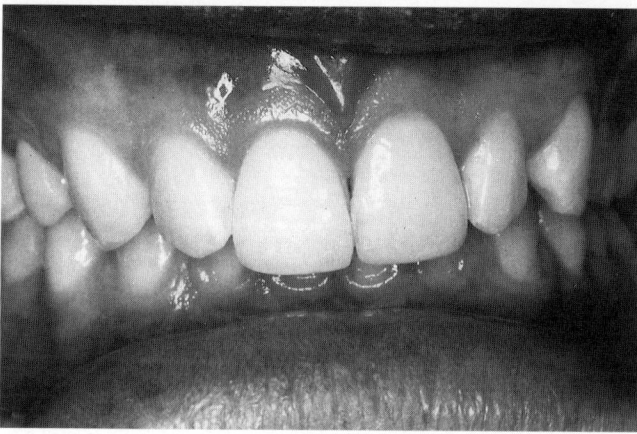

Fig. 12.20 Porcelain veneers. A Central incisors prepared for porcelain veneers. **B** Bonded porcelain veneers in place.

called pontics. These are connected to the bridge retainers which are cemented to the prepared abutment teeth (Fig. 12.21).

In the past decade, adhesively bonded bridgework has gained in popularity. The so-called *Maryland Bridge* was the first of a generation of bridgework; it utilizes a technique of surface etching of the tooth enamel on either side of the space before application of a thin layer of composite resin to cement the bridge. The advantage of this technique is that minimal tooth preparation avoids the loss of otherwise healthy tooth material required in preparation of conventional bridge abutments. It was widely used for the replacement of missing anterior teeth and generally limited to single teeth. The development of new porcelains with high strength has led to other bridgework designs, particularly the all-ceramic bonded bridge (Fig. 12.22).

Single and multiple tooth replacement by partial *dentures* and the construction of complete dentures to restore an edentulous jaw have been in vogue for over a hundred years. In the case of partial dentures, retention is effected by means of various attachments which are fitted to the existing natural teeth. While clasps built into the denture frame are still widely used, newer forms of precision attachments including magnets, clips and ball-joints offer a comprehensive choice for retainers of partial dentures. A dramatic example of complex restoration involving retaining devices is shown in Fig. 12.23, in a case requiring prosthetic replacement of the maxilla (Moore et al 1991).

Currently, the most exciting growth area in dentistry is the prosthetic application of *osseo-integrated fixtures* (Fig. 12.24). Originally implants were used in the symphysis region of the mandible to provide support for dentures resting on a severely resorbed alveolar ridge. They are now inserted in any partially edentulous segment of the arch providing that the underlying bone is adequate to provide the required support. Careful preoperative assessment and planning by the surgeon and the restorative dentist are critical to achieve the desired functional and aesthetic result. Mounted dental models prepared by the wax-up technique (see above, p. 358) are required in treatment planning. A surgical stent or template constructed on the models to indicate the site of implant placement is a valuable guide to the surgeon when the alveolar bone is prepared for implant insertion. With the implant in place, a period of healing will ensure that effective osseous integration takes place, after which the tooth or teeth can be constructed and fixed to the implants. Further details of the techniques involved in the use of osseo-integrated implants are given by Hobo et al (1989).

Postoperative dental care

As for any other form of dental treatment, the patient who has suffered dentofacial trauma followed by reconstruction requires regular postoperative care and evaluation. It is essential that adequate oral hygiene be maintained, particularly if bridgework, removable dentures or osseo-integrated implants have been provided. This is best achieved by instructing the patient on the use of oral hygiene aids such as tooth brushes, floss-silk, gum-massagers and mouth rinses.

At regular intervals the patient should attend for examination so that all restorative work can be checked for stability, integrity and correct function. These checks will include visual examination of the teeth, an occlusal analysis, photographs and, if necessary, radiographs. If endodontic treatment has been necessary, radiographic examination of the root apex and surrounding periapical bone must be undertaken at regular intervals.

Removable prosthetic appliances also need to be examined periodically to detect regions of alveolar bone resorption and to assess the need for relining or construction of a new appliance. The stability of the appliance and any retaining devices must also be checked.

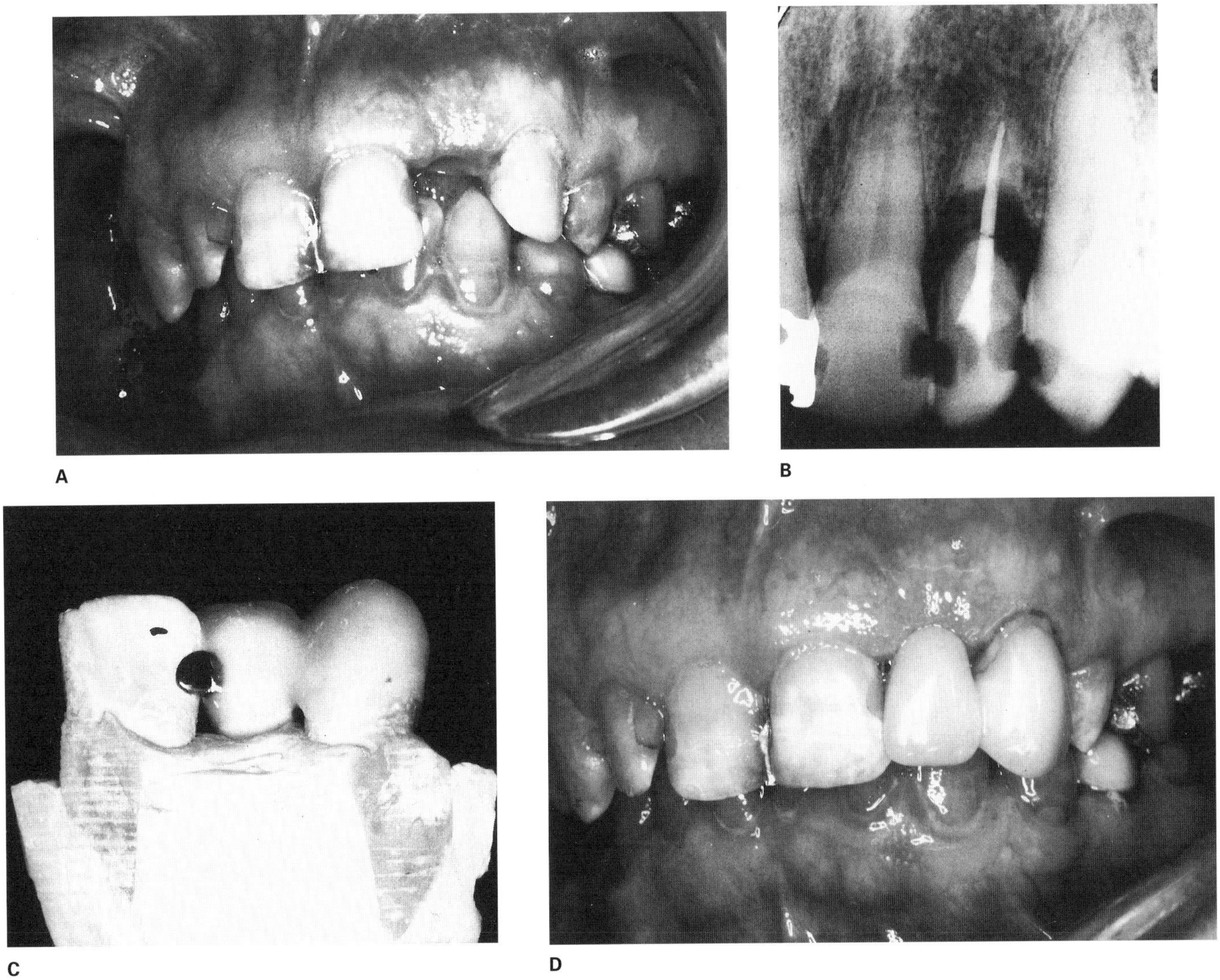

A

B

C

D

Fig. 12.21 Anterior porcelain bridge. A Intraoral view of a 60-year-old male who was involved in a motor vehicle accident 3 years previously. The maxillary left lateral incisor was severely concussed at the time and received endodontic treatment. However, after 3 years the tooth had undergone severe root resorption and it was extracted. **B** Periapical radiograph of the incisor taken before extraction demonstrates the advanced root resorption. **C** Porcelain bridge with a metal extension to replace the lateral incisor photographed from the palatal aspect. **D** The completed bridge bonded into position.

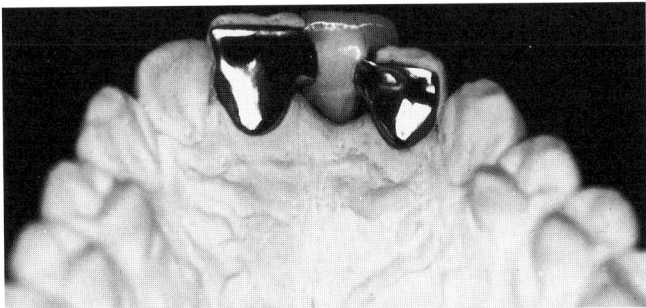

Fig. 12.22 A Maryland bridge viewed from the palatal aspect. This technique is useful for replacing single missing teeth as it requires minimal preparation to the abutment teeth. In the case illustrated, the maxillary left central incisor is bonded by acid-etching and composite resin to the teeth on either side of the space.

The patient should be informed that restorative procedures are not permanent but will require adjustments and repair and even replacement from time to time throughout the patient's life. The patient's own responsibility in maintaining good oral health and optimal oral function must also be stressed.

Longevity of restorative materials

In recent years there have been remarkable improvements in the dental materials and techniques used in the restoration of the human dentition. However, the procedures of restorative dentistry are not infallible and each patient presents a unique challenge, calling for treatment that

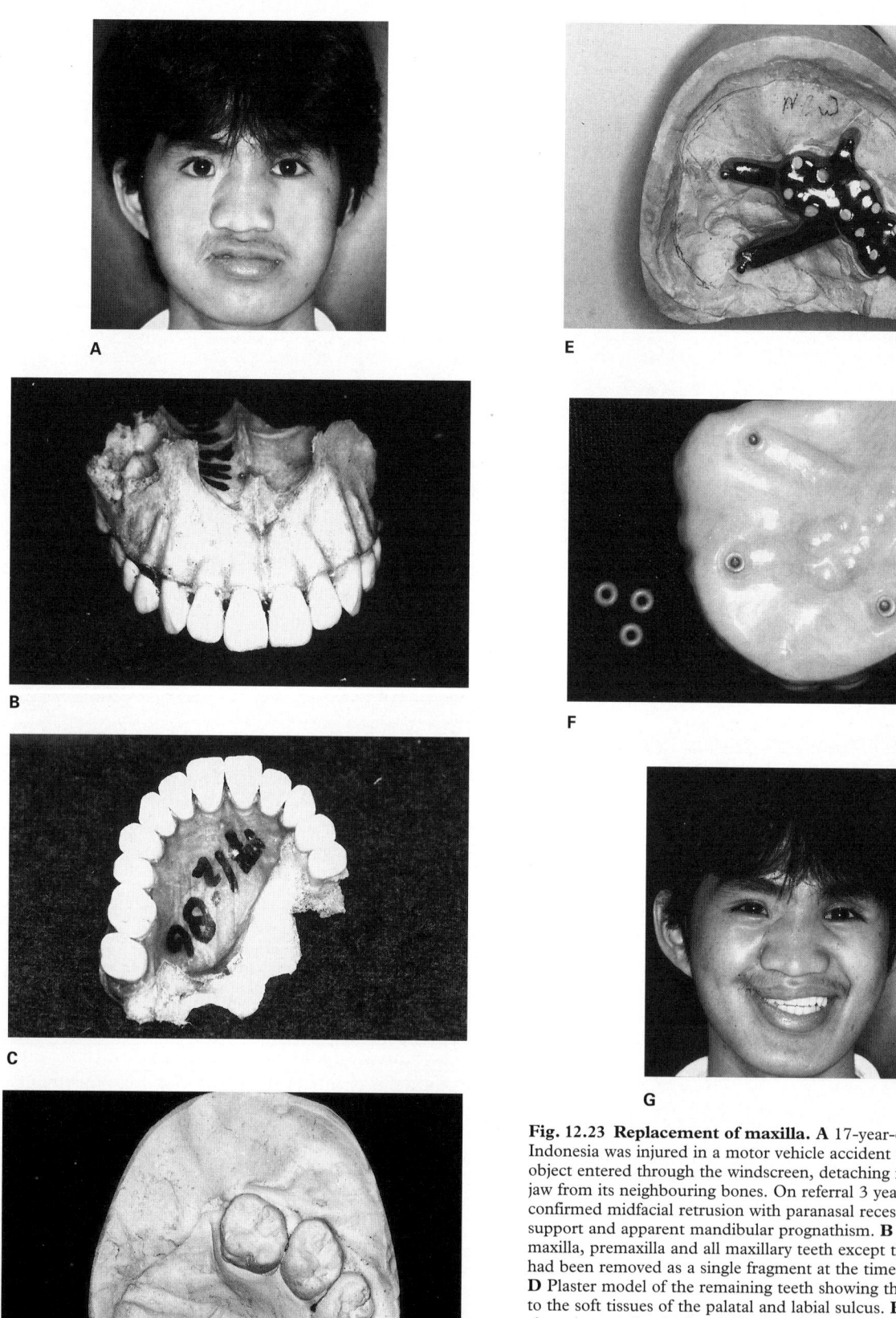

Fig. 12.23 Replacement of maxilla. A 17-year-old male from Indonesia was injured in a motor vehicle accident when a large metal object entered through the windscreen, detaching most of the upper jaw from its neighbouring bones. On referral 3 years later, examination confirmed midfacial retrusion with paranasal recession, loss of nasal tip support and apparent mandibular prognathism. **B** and **C** The bony maxilla, premaxilla and all maxillary teeth except the three left molars had been removed as a single fragment at the time of accident. **D** Plaster model of the remaining teeth showing their position relative to the soft tissues of the palatal and labial sulcus. **E** The nickel chromium casting is shown fitted to the dental model. The casting is etched on its fitting surface to assist the bond with tooth enamel using composite resin as the cementing medium. Note the metallic extensions which were designed to retain an acrylic upper denture. **F** The tissue surface of the acrylic denture illustrating small silicone rings used to clip over the metallic extensions shown in **E**. **G** The prosthesis in place.

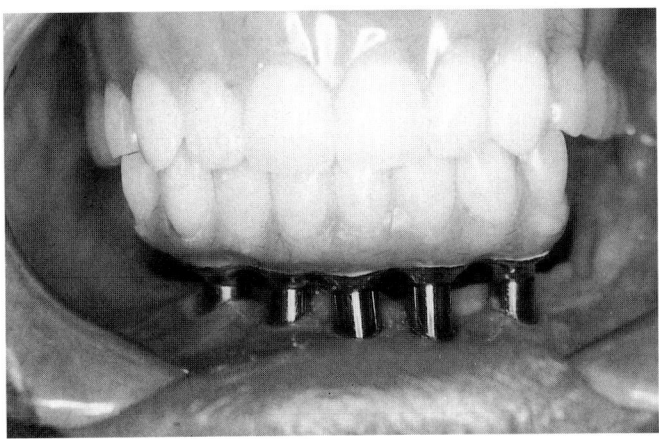

Fig. 12.24 Mandibular implant. A 52-year-old edentulous female was involved in a motor vehicle accident resulting in a Le Fort I and mandibular fractures. After fracture healing a lower denture could not be worn. A new maxillary denture was constructed together with a mandibular anterior bridge which is retained by a mandibular osseo-integrated implant. The lower teeth are screwed into the titanium transmucosal elements.

may range from routine and relatively simple procedures to procedures so complex that the knowledge and skills of a specialist restorative dentist are needed. Many patients with craniofacial trauma fall into the last category.

The survival of a dental restoration with continuing optimal function and appearance depends on a number of interacting factors including the material and its properties, the particular tooth restored and its preparation, the age of the patient, masticatory patterns and habits such as tooth grinding.

Without doubt amalgam has been the most widely used material for restoring posterior teeth. Recently the safety of amalgam has been questioned in some countries on the grounds of cumulative mercury toxicity. However, mercury release from amalgam restorations should be considered in relation to known environmental levels and toxicity. For example the exposure level from eight amalgam fillings has been measured at 1.2 µg per day, i.e. about 0.15 µg per day per amalgam. These levels represent only 5–10% of daily mercury intake from all sources and they are far below the published levels for toxicity (Jendresen et al 1992). Hypersensitivity to amalgam is very rare, affecting ~3% of the population, and even fewer show clinical symptoms which are invariably mild and short lived (Mackert 1991). Amalgam, therefore, remains an important and safe option for some forms of posterior tooth restoration.

Dental amalgam is often used to restore fractured cusps in posterior teeth where it may be rendered more durable by the cementation of threaded pins into the dentine for improved retention before the restoration is placed. Smales (1991a) assessed a large number of amalgam restorations with and without cusp coverage,

finding a high survival rate in both groups of ~72% after 15 years. Pin retention did not affect the survival rate significantly.

In further studies of amalgam survivals, Smales (1991b) and Smales et al (1991) reported high survival rates after 6–7 years of ~90% for high copper alloys, but only one low copper alloy matched this performance. Surprisingly, restorations of amalgam or composite resins placed in an Australian Defense Force Population had significantly better survival times than cast crowns (Dawson & Smales 1992).

Because of its excellent aesthetic qualities, composite resin has become the material of choice for many types of restoration in the anterior region of the mouth, particularly those concerned with the repair of enamel cracks or fractured incisors. For these restorations composite resins have replaced the earlier silicate cements and cast gold inlays. Composite resins are sometimes used for the restoration of posterior teeth, particularly if the patient objects to the appearance of amalgam. With improved compositions and methods of handling, the longevity of composite resins is increasing with respect to adherence to the tooth preparation and colour stability.

In the past, the major problems with composite resins have been occlusal wear and colour change. However, actual wear rates of the newer composites are very low (Leinfelder 1991). Several commercial products showed < 125 µm occlusal wear over a 5 year period (Tyas & Wassenaar 1991). Other researchers have reported similar results in clinical trials, e.g. 77% survival rates and only 253 µm wear after 8 years (Barnes et al 1991).

A median survival time of 8.9 years for several types of composite resins placed in the anterior teeth of patients in a dental teaching hospital was reported by Smales (1991c). For restorations involving the incisal angles, however, the median survival time reduced to 4 years. In a later study of three light-cured anterior composite resins survival rates after 4 years were reported (Smales & Gerke 1992). A skilled operator placed 700 light-cured resins in anterior teeth using a technique consisting of acid-etching of the enamel, placement of a cavity liner and application of a dentine adhesive. After 4 years, between 16% and 21% of the restorations were judged to have failed for various reasons but these were mainly placed in small cavities near the gingival margins where the dentine bonding was weak. In the case of fractured incisal angles, however, the failure rate was lower.

Tooth replacement by means of resin bonding to adjacent abutment teeth remains an important method of restorative dentistry as this technique requires very little destruction of healthy tooth material for retention purposes compared with conventional cemented fixed bridgework. A knowledge of failure rates in resin-bonded prostheses is obviously important but data from different studies are difficult to compare because of varying patient conditions, methods of preparation and observation times and, in some instances, lack of this information.

Of 49 resin-bonded fixed prostheses evaluated after 2–67 months, 35% had debonded, mandibular prostheses more frequently than maxillary (Chang et al 1991). In contrast to this high failure rate, other authors who used extracoronal precision attachments, air-abraded castings and cementation with a new effective adhesive reported an 80% success rate after 5 years for the resin-bonded retainers used to support removable partial prostheses (Marinello et al 1991).

In a study of 99 resin-bonded prostheses that were in place for up to 10 years, a debonding rate of 31% was found, 11% of the debonding being caused by trauma. The average age of debonding was 2.2 years with a range of 0.2–6.8 years (Williams et al 1989). Similar results were reported by Berekally & Smales (1993) who retrospectively evaluated resin-bonded bridges that had been inserted in a public teaching hospital. Over a period of 6 years, the failure rate from all causes including debonding for Rochette-type bridges (retention of composite by undercut holes in the metal retainers) was 75% with a median survival of 2.14 years. For Maryland bridges (retention of composite by acid-etching the metal retainers) the failure rate over 5 years was 42% with a median survival time of 2.6 years. Pontic fracture and debonding due to occlusal stress, non-retentive designs or resin failure were the main causes of the bridge failures.

With continuing improvement of luting cements and preparation techniques the high failure rates for resin-bonded fixed prostheses can be expected to reduce significantly. However, as Berekally & Smales (1993) conclude, the important factors for success in this type of restoration are patient selection, bridge design, technical and operative excellence and regular reviews.

This advice applies equally to all other restorative procedures and especially to the repair of traumatized dentitions.

DENTAL IMPLICATIONS OF MEDICAL DISEASE

For medically compromised patients requiring dental treatment arising from CMF trauma, appropriate precautions need to be taken and often special management procedures will be necessary. At all times the operator must be alert to the physical condition of the patient and prepared to record a detailed general and medical history before any dental treatment is commenced.

In almost all cases presenting with other than minor dental injuries, the overall management of the patient will be decided in consultation with a number of specialists, and any medical condition or other special circumstances should have been recorded and acted upon well before the dentist commences treatment. None the less, dental management of the medically compromised patient must always involve appropriate consultation with the patient's surgeon and physician.

Of special concern to those providing dental treatment is the management of patients who test positive for human immunodeficiency virus (HIV) or hepatitis B infections. Strict and well-rehearsed procedures must be followed when treating these patients as the risk of infection to the operator or assistant following injury from a needle-prick, burr, scalpel or other instrument is high in oral operations. The risk of cross-infection is much higher in the case of hepatitis B than HIV. In emergency cases when the HIV/hepatitis status is unknown, a wise precaution is to adopt the same procedures as in the presence of a known infected patient or carrier. The precautions adopted in a general operating theatre should be followed in the dental surgery by both the dentist and assistants when treating patients with HIV/hepatitis B infections. These are discussed in Chapter 20.

When superimposed upon CMF trauma, a number of other medical conditions require special attention on the part of an operator undertaking the dental phase of overall treatment. Particularly important are cardiac conditions such as rheumatic fever or congenital heart disease in which transient bacteraemias must be avoided, and coronary atherosclerosis in which the risk of cardiac infarction following stress is present (p. 540). Patients with hypertensive disease may be at risk from the vasopressor agents present in local anaesthetics if not adequately controlled by medication. Congenital, acquired and iatrogenic coagulation deficiencies present problems when surgical procedures are undertaken in the oral region (p. 532). When prescribing antibiotics the dentist must be alert to the possibility of allergic reactions which are often severe and can be fatal. Diabetes mellitus is another condition that may present difficulties in the management of dentofacial trauma in view of retarded wound healing and increased susceptibility to infection (p. 537).

Many other medical conditions of varying degrees of seriousness that have implications for dental treatment are described by Little & Falace (1980).

REFERENCES

Andersson L, Bodin I, Sörensen S 1989 Progression of root resorption following replantation of human teeth after extended extraoral storage. Endod Dent Traumatol 5: 38–47
Andreasen F M 1989 Pulpal healing after luxation injuries and root fracture in the permanent dentition. Endod Dent Traumatol 5: 111–131
Andreasen J O 1981 Traumatic injuries to the teeth, 2nd edn. Munksgaard, Copenhagen

Andreasen J O 1989 Atlas of reimplantation and transplantation of teeth. Mediglobe, Fribourg

Andreasen J O, Andreasen F M 1990 Essentials of traumatic injuries to the teeth. Munksgaard, Copenhagen, pp 141–154

Andreasen J O, Schwartz O 1986 The effect of saline storage before replantation upon dry damage of the periodontal ligament. Endod Dent Traumatol 2: 67–70

Angle E H 1907 Treatment of malocclusion of the teeth. Angle's system, 7th edn. S S White Dental Manufacturing, Philadelphia

Barnes D M, Blank L W, Thompson V P, Holston A M, Gingell J C 1991 A 5- and 8-year clinical evaluation of a posterior composite resin. Quintinence Int 22: 143–151

Berekally T L, Smales R J 1993 A retrospective clinical evaluation of resin-bonded bridges inserted at the Adelaide Dental Hospital. Aust Dent J 38: 85–96

Berkovitz B K B, Moxham B 1981 Tooth morphology. In: Osborn J W (ed) Dental anatomy and embryology. Blackwell, Oxford, pp 118–154

Blomlöf L, Lindskog S, Andersson L, Hedström K G, Hammarström L 1983 Storage of experimentally avulsed teeth in milk prior to replantation. J Dent Res 62: 912–916

Brown T, Abbott A H, Burgess V B 1987 Longitudinal study of dental arch relationships in Australian Aboriginals with reference to alternate intercuspation. Am J Phys Anthropol 72: 49–57

Chang H-K, Zidan O, Lee I K, Gomez-Marin O 1991 Resin-bonded fixed partial dentures: a recall study. J Prosthet Dent 65: 778–781

Cohen S, Burns R C (eds) 1984 Pathways of the pulp, 3rd edn. Mosby, St Louis

Crona-Larsson G, Norén J G 1989 Luxation injuries to permanent teeth — a retrospective study of etiological factors. Endod Dent Traumatol 5: 176–179

Crum R J, Loiselle R J 1972 Oral perception and proprioception: a review of the literature and its significance to prosthodontics. J Prosthet Dent 28: 215–230

Dawson A S, Smales R J 1992 Restoration longevity in an Australian Defence Force population. Aust Dent J 37: 196–200

Foster T D 1990 A textbook of orthodontics, 3rd edn. Blackwell, Oxford

Garcia-Godoy F, Garcia-Godoy F, Garcia-Godoy F M 1989 Reasons for seeking treatment after traumatic dental injuries. Endod Dent Traumatol 5: 180–181

Gettleman L, Vrijhoef M M A, Uchiyama Y 1986 Adhesive prosthodontics: adhesive cements and techniques. Proceedings of the International Symposium on Adhesive Prosthodontics. Eurosound Drukkerij BV, Nijmegen

Gilbert T M, Pashley D H, Anderson R W 1992 Response of pulpal blood flow to intra-arterial infusion of endothelin. J Endond 18: 228–231

Greenspan D, Greenspan J S, Schmidt M, Pindborg J J 1990 AIDS and the mouth: diagnosis and management of oral lesions. Munksgaard, Copenhagen

Hammarström L, Blomlöf L, Feiglin B, Andersson L, Lindskog S 1986a Replantation of teeth and antibiotic treatment. Endod Dent Traumatol 2: 51–57

Hammarström L, Pierce A, Blomlöf L, Feiglin B, Lindskog S 1986b Tooth avulsion and replantation — a review. Endod Dent Traumatol 2: 1–8

Harty F J (ed) 1990 Endodontics in clinical practice, 3rd edn. Wright, London

Hobo S, Ichida E, Garcia L T 1989 Osseointegration and occlusal rehabilitation. Quintessence, Tokyo

Jendresen M D, Allen E P, Bayne S C, Hannson T L, Klooster J, Preston J D 1992 Report of the Committee on Scientific Investigation of the American Academy of Restorative Dentistry. J Prosthet Dent 68: 137–190

Leinfelder K F 1991 Using composite resin as a posterior restorative material. J Am Dent Assoc 122: 65–70

Little J W, Falace D A 1980 Dental management of the medically compromised patient. Mosby, St Louis

Mackert J R 1991 Dental amalgam and mercury. J Am Dent Assoc 122: 54–61

Madjar D, Divon-Kuperschmidt I 1992 Resin-bonded cast coverage for fractured posterior teeth. J Prosthet Dent 68: 15–18

Marinello C P, Scharer P, Meyenberg K 1991 Resin-bonded etched castings with extracoronal attachments for removable partial dentures. J Prosthet Dent 66: 52–55

Messing J J, Stock C J R 1988 A colour atlas of endodontics. Wolfe Medical, London

Moore M H, Abbott J R, David D J 1991 The missing maxilla: restoring aesthetic balance with mandibular surgery. J Craniofac Surg 2: 95–100

Mount G J 1991 An atlas of glass-ionomer cements: the clinician's guide. Martin Dunitz, London

Proffit W R 1986 Contemporary orthodontics. Mosby, St Louis

Ramfjord S, Ash M M 1983 Occlusion, 3rd edn. Saunders, Philadelphia

Schnettler J M, Wallace J A 1991 Pulse oximetry as a diagnostic tool of pulpal vitality. J Endod 17: 488–490

Shillingburg H T, Hobo S, Whitsett L D 1981 Fundamentals of fixed prosthodontics. Quintessence, Chicago

Smales R J 1991a Longevity of cusp-covered amalgams: survivals after 15 years. Oper Dent 16: 17–20

Smales R J 1991b Longevity of low- and high-copper amalgams analyzed by preparation class, tooth site, patient age, and operator. Oper Dent 16: 162–168

Smales R J 1991c Effects of enamel-bonding, type of restoration, patient age and operator on the longevity of an anterior composite resin. Am J Dent 4: 130–133

Smales R J, Gerke D C 1992 Clinical evaluation of light-cured anterior resin composites over periods of up to 4 years. Am J Dent 5: 208–212

Smales R J, Webster D A, Leppard P I 1991 Survival predictions of amalgam restorations. J Dent 19: 272–277

Solnit A, Curnutte D C 1988 Occlusal correction: principles and practice. Quintessence, Chicago

Sowray J H 1985 Localised injuries of the teeth and alveolar processes. In: Rowe N L, Williams J L (eds) Maxillofacial injuries. Churchill Livingstone, Edinburgh, pp 214–231

Stock C J R, Nehammer C F 1985 Endodontics in practice. British Dental Association, London

Thomson H 1975 Occlusion. Wright, Bristol, pp 33–46

Tyas M J, Wassenaar P 1991 Clinical evaluation of four composite resins in posterior teeth. Five year results. Aust Dent J 36: 369–73

Van Beek G C 1983 Dental morphology: an illustrated guide. Wright, Bristol

Williams V D, Thayer K E, Denehy G E, Boyer D B 1989 Cast metal, resin-bonded prostheses: a 10-year retrospective study. J Prosthet Dent 61: 436–441

Wilson H J, McLean J W, Brown D 1988 Dental materials and their clinical applications. British Dental Association, London

Craniocerebral injuries

P. L. Reilly   D. A. Simpson
Contributing author: A. Hanieh

INTRODUCTION

Injuries of the face are often accompanied by injuries of the brain and the cranial nerves. Forces impacting on the facial skeleton may be transmitted to the base of the skull; the effects on the brain may range from transient loss of consciousness to a lethal brainstem laceration (Simpson et al 1989). Alternatively, the forces causing injury may impact directly on the frontal bone, causing blunt or penetrating brain damage. The neuropathology of these injuries has been discussed (p. 138); in this chapter, the clinical features of injuries of the anterior cranial fossa and frontal lobes are set out and their neurosurgical management is discussed.

CLINICAL CLASSIFICATION

From the surgical viewpoint, the craniocerebral injuries resulting from impacts in the craniomaxillofacial (CMF) region fall into four main groups:

1. Externally compound frontal fractures and penetrating wounds, with varying degrees of local cerebral damage
2. Internally compound fractures of the anterior cranial fossa, often associated with some form of cranionasal fistula
3. Closed brain injuries resulting from impact-induced acceleration or deceleration (see Ch. 4)
4. Secondary complications, of which the chief are:
   — intracranial haemorrhage
   — cerebral oedema and other types of brain swelling
   — tissue hypoxia and metabolic disorders
   — cerebrospinal fluid (CSF) leakage and/or intracranial aerocele

— intracranial infection
— carotid-cavernous fistula
— post-traumatic epilepsy.

Each injury type causes specific problems in management, but two or more may be present simultaneously and neurosurgical strategy must be planned to detect and deal with any permutation of craniocerebral injuries. Injuries elsewhere in the CMF region often make team planning essential. This is especially so when a frontal impact has injured the facial skeleton, or some part of the visual apparatus. Anterior fossa fractures are often associated with injuries of the optic nerve and these may require combined ophthalmological and neurosurgical management; they are discussed in Chapter 14 (p. 422).

NEUROLOGICAL EVALUATION

Clinical assessment

The initial examination has been discussed in Chapter 6. The importance of an accurate and continuing evaluation of the conscious level must be reiterated; the Glasgow Coma Scale (GCS) has proven value both in assessing the severity of the initial impact and in detecting changes in cerebral status. The use of the paediatric variant (PGCS) of the Glasgow scale is discussed in Chapter 19.

External signs of injury should be carefully noted and recorded (Fig. 13.1). Lacerations are especially important, and the examiner should note the presence of brain tissue, pulsation, contamination or skin devitalization; in missile wounds, signs of powder tattooing (Fig. 6.2) are sought and an exit wound is looked for, though when the head has been hit by multiple fragments, the inter-

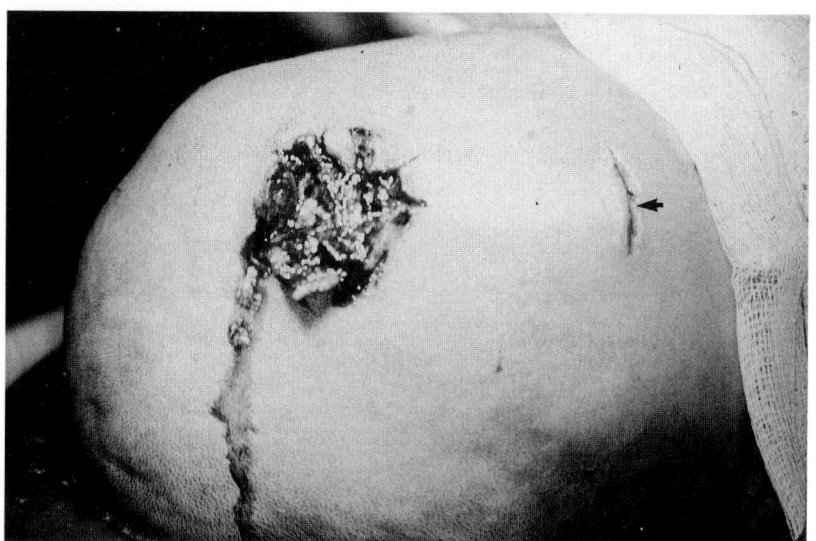 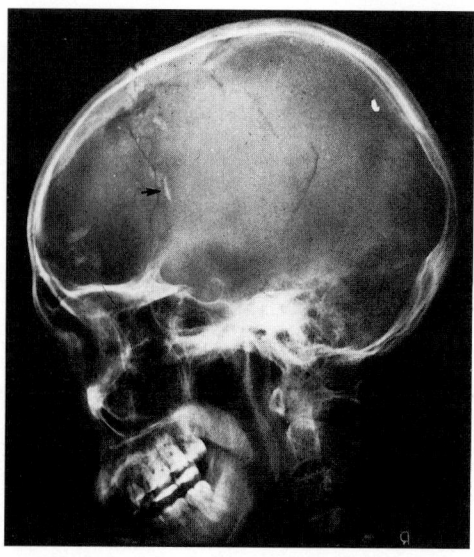

Fig. 13.1 Evaluation of a military missile wound. A young woman was wounded by a land mine; she was hit in the left forehead and became hemiplegic and aphasic. **A** Small entry wound (arrow) above the left eyebrow and large exit wound in the region of the coronal suture. **B** Plain radiographs showed bone chips low in the frontal lobe, a bone defect under the exit wound, a metallic fragment in the ipsilateral posterior parietal lobe, and a bone chip (arrow) in the region of the corpus callosum. At operation the entry wound was explored and the superficial bone chips were removed; the deeply placed bone chip could not be located. A re-exploration also failed to locate the chip which was in the vicinity of the anterior cerebral arteries. Modern opinion would criticize these attempts to remove the bone chip. The patient survived but was severely disabled when last seen.

pretation of the wounds may be difficult. Small wounds may be deceptive, concealing deeper penetration. A fracture of the skull base is suggested by periorbital haematomas, a sign known as raccoon eyes in North America, and as the spectacle/monocle sign in other parts of the world. Bruising about the mastoid process (Battle's sign) suggests a fracture of the temporal bone. The nose and ears must be examined for signs of a leakage of blood or cerebrospinal fluid (CSF) and a sample of any leakage fluid should be taken for immunochemical examination (see below).

The general neurological examination is done in whatever depth seems to be appropriate. It is always necessary to test the senses of smell and sight, and fundoscopy is always needed. Speech must be tested for signs of a dysphasic impairment, especially in cases with evidence of damage to the dominant cerebral hemisphere. A full examination may be difficult or impossible when the patient is first admitted: cooperation may be lacking, or facial damage may prevent a proper examination of the eyes and the sense of smell. When this is so, the examiner must ensure that these very important tests are done at a later time.

Continuing serial assessment is essential to detect changes in neurological status. The routine monitoring of conscious level, pupillary light reactions, pulse rate and blood pressure is especially necessary when the injured person is in a ward not accustomed to care for cerebral injuries: this is likely to happen when the chief injury is in the lower face and the cerebral injury has been seen as of minor significance.

Finally, the clinical assessment should take into account the possibility of extracranial injuries. These often complicate the neurosurgical management plan; they may demand urgent treatment, and they may also cause diagnostic confusion. The conscious level may be depressed by chest injuries causing hypoxia and hypercarbia or by impaired cerebral perfusion from blood loss and shock; the severity of the head injury should always be reassessed after resuscitation has been completed.

Tests for CSF leakage

If there is a nasal or aural discharge, a sample (> 0.1 ml) is taken for immunochemical estimation of the β_2-transferrin content (Oberascher 1988, Ryall et al 1992); this test replaces the often misleading tests for glucose content used in the past, since this transferrin isoform is almost specific for CSF and is detectable even in the presence of blood. It is also found in the serum in cases of hepatic cirrhosis and in a few persons with a genetically determined metabolic peculiarity, but these can be excluded by a concurrent assay of the serum level of β_2-transferrin.

Radiological assessment

Computed tomography (CT)

This is the primary radiological investigation and has largely replaced the routine plain X-ray examination of the head, though plain skull radiographs may be used as a screening examination when a CT scanner is not readily available. However, a lateral cervical X-ray picture of the neck should always be obtained in an unconscious patient who has had a head injury (p. 225).

The initial CT scan is done as soon as possible to assess the craniocerebral injury and to detect any life-threatening condition such as an intracranial clot or a tension aerocele. The CT scan also visualizes most fractures of the calvaria and skull base, though occasionally supplementary plain radiographs will be needed for this purpose. Intracranial air is well shown. Extradural air is seen as small bubbles, usually near a fracture into a paranasal or mastoid sinus (Fig. 7.25A); subdural, subarachnoid and intracerebral air collections are identifiable by their anatomical sites and shapes, and are unequivocal signs of a cranionasal or cranioaural fistula. Serial CT scans are used in monitoring the unconscious patient who is at risk of secondary complications.

Magnetic resonance imaging (MRI)

This gives better anatomical detail of the brain and other soft tissues, but currently available machines are less useful in the early management of craniocerebral injuries, both because of logistic problems in examining an unconscious patient requiring ventilation and because skull fractures are not well visualized. The superiority of MRI in demonstrating small brain lesions makes it the investigation of choice in assessing intrinsic brain damage at later stages of recovery. It is also superior to CT scanning in visualizing fragments of wood (Specht et al 1992). However, in our experience CT has proved satisfactory in showing large fragments of wood (Figs 13.6 and 14.1), which appear when dry as radiolucent lesions approximating to the density of air, but which may give different appearances when soaked in serum or other tissue fluid. MRI should not be used if there are ferromagnetic metal bodies, such as shell fragments, in the brain or eye (Teitelbaum et al 1990).

Cerebral angiography

Once the routine investigation to exclude an intracranial clot, angiography is now little used in the management of closed head injuries. Advances in MRI angiography are restricting the use of X-ray angiography still further. But at present carotid angiography, and sometimes vertebral angiography, have important roles in diagnosing vascular damage from penetrating wounds (p. 386) and in the diagnosis of carotid–cavernous fistulas (p. 392).

Intracranial pressure (ICP) manometry

ICP monitoring is routinely used in patients comatose from severe head injury, and more selectively when neurosurgical assessment is impaired by endotracheal intuba-tion and controlled ventilation in the management of a severe chest or faciomaxillary injury. ICP may be measured from a soft fluid-filled silastic catheter placed in a lateral ventricle; in some centres, this is done under X-ray or ultrasonic guidance. A ventricular catheter gives excellent recordings, and allows drainage of CSF to control raised ICP; however, catheterization is difficult when the ventricles are constricted by cerebral swelling. Subdural bolts, or catheters placed after a craniotomy, are easily inserted, and do not penetrate the brain. The quality of subdural recording is less good than that of a ventricular catheter (North & Reilly 1986).

Catheters such as the Camino catheter record from a sensor in the tip of the catheter (Ostrup et al 1987) and are now widely used. They provide records of high quality, and can be placed either in the ventricle, the subarachnoid or subdural space, or the brain parenchyma; they can be inserted in the emergency room or intensive care ward under local anaesthesia. The Camino sensors cannot be recalibrated in situ, but show minimal base line drift over several days (Fig. 13.2).

Complications of ICP monitoring include bleeding and clot formation, and infection. In a series of 340 cases, we (North & Reilly 1986) recorded two cases of frontal lobe haematoma, and eight infections; infections usually resulted from ventricular catheterization and the infection rate from this procedure was 3.6%. The complications of infection may be serious when a ventricular catheter is used. It is our practice to lead the ventricular catheter from the burrhole through a subcutaneous tunnel to a stab wound a few centimetres away, and to dress the egress point with povidone–iodine ointment; the catheter is usually removed after at most 3 days, and re-sited if drainage is still needed. Subdural sensors may be left somewhat longer. Fluid-filled catheters and bolts may leak, or become obstructed: this should be suspected when a previously normal pulsatile wave form becomes damped (North & Reilly 1990).

In CMF injuries, raised ICP may be due to intracranial bleeding, brain contusion and/or swelling, hydrocephalus, meningitis and various less common complications (Table 13.1). If the initial CT scan is entirely normal, the likelihood of clinically significant raised ICP is not great. However, intracranial haematomas do occasionally develop after an initially normal CT scan and unsatisfactory clinical progress always demands reassessment. If the initial scan shows intracranial haemorrhage of any type, or any mass lesion causing brain displacement, or obliteration of the third ventricle and/or perimesencephalic cisterns, then ICP is likely to be elevated and monitoring will be prudent — assuming that surgical treatment is not immediately needed. We advise routine ICP monitoring for:

- Patients with severe closed or open head injury, defined as a patient with a GCS ≤ 8 after resuscitation. In clinical terms, such a patient does not

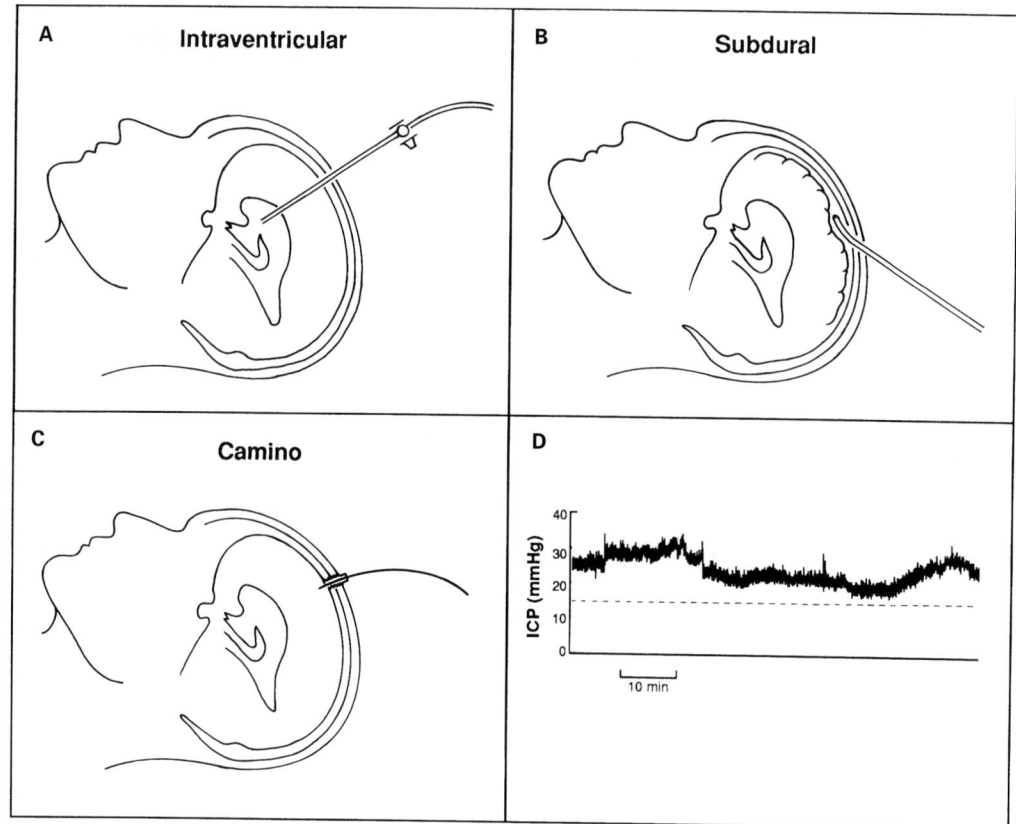

Fig. 13.2 Monitoring the intracranial pressure. Diagram showing standard techniques of recording intracranial pressure: **A** Ventricular catheter, inserted through a frontal burrhole. **B** Subdural catheter, inserted through a frontal burrhole; recordings may also be taken from a hollow screw (Richmond bolt) inserted through a smaller drill hole down to the subdural space. **C** Camino pressure transducer catheter inserted into the cerebral parenchyma through a hollow screw. **D** Intracranial pressure trace showing high pressure.

Table 13.1 Causes of raised intracranial pressure after CMF injury

Brain swelling
  Oedema
    Cytotoxic
    Vasogenic
  Vascular engorgement
Brain contusion
Intracranial clot
  Extradural
  Subdural
  Intracerebral
Hydrocephalus
Large skull depression
Pneumocephalus
Meningitis
Carotid–cavernous fistula

open the eyes, makes at best incomprehensible sounds, and responds to pain, if at all, by non-purposive flexor or extensor movements.

- Patients with brain swelling after surgery for clot removal.
- Patients who require prolonged ventilation after major

CMF surgery or chest injury, who cannot be assessed by regular neurological examination.

EXTERNALLY COMPOUND FRONTAL FRACTURES

Management

There is little controversy over the management of the compound depressed frontal fractures resulting from road crashes and other peacetime accidents. These are open wounds but as a rule there is no deep cerebral penetration (Fig. 13.3). Such wounds should be closed as soon as resuscitation is complete and an adequate assessment has been performed. Delay of up to 24 h does not appear to increase the risk of infection significantly, but delay in excess of 48 h is certainly hazardous, especially if the wound is grossly contaminated. Accidents involving a fall in 'fresh' water are especially likely to result in infection; unsurprisingly, Braakman (1972) reported cases of serious meningitis when open head wounds were immersed in

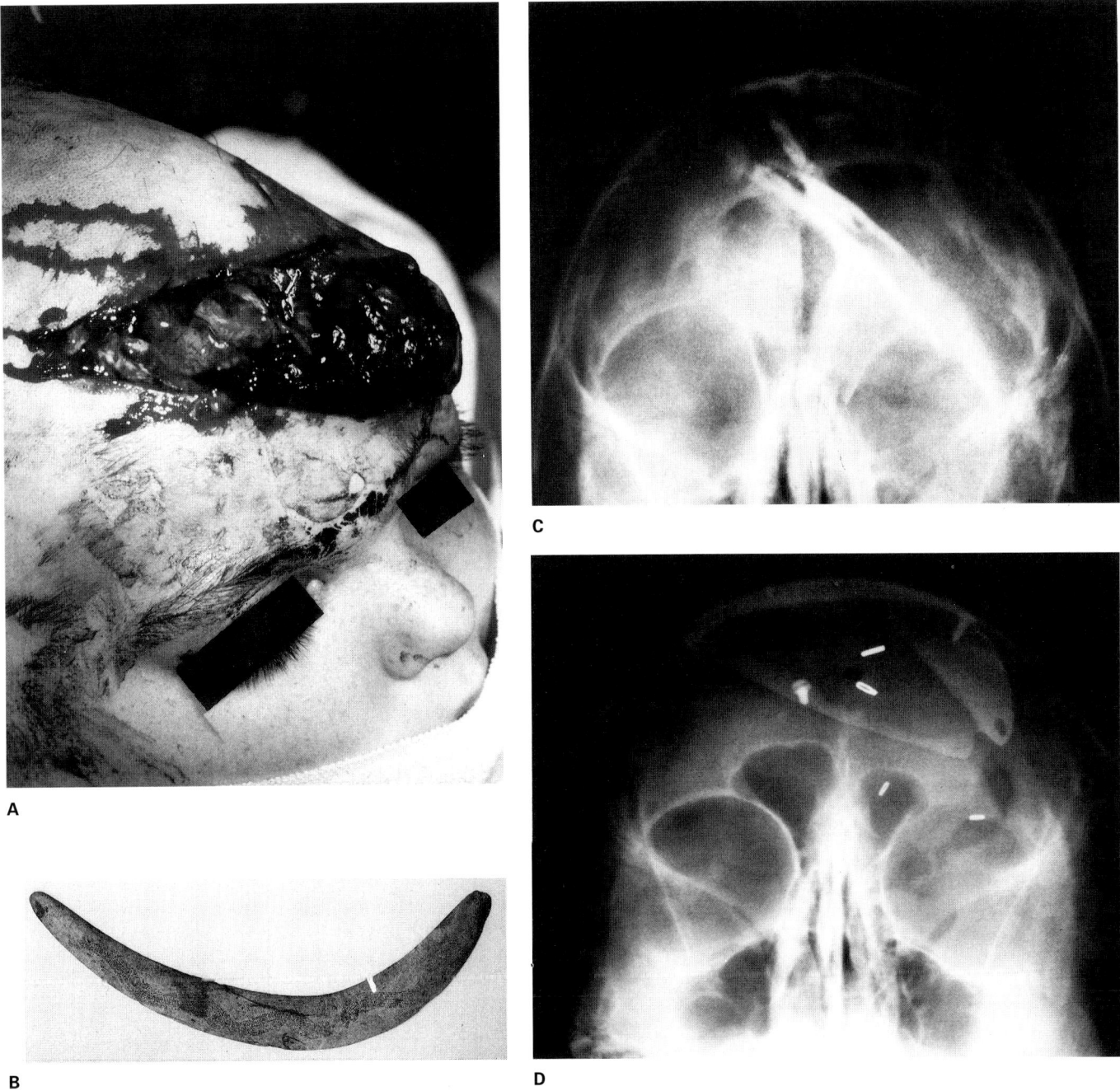

Fig. 13.3 Compound frontal wound from boomerang. An 8-year-old child was inadvertently struck in the right frontal region by a returning boomerang (Whittle 1980). **A** Compound depressed skull fracture with exposed brain. **B** The boomerang: traditional type, used in hunting. **C** Skull radiograph, showing a large frontal depressed fracture. **D** Skull radiograph after titanium cranioplasty. The child made a good recovery, with no detectable neurological deficit.

contaminated water in the vicinity of Rotterdam. It has been our practice to give an antibiotic from the time of admission, and to continue this for 5–7 days; a shorter period (e.g. 48 hours) may be preferable. For externally compound fractures, our prophylactic antibiotic of choice is intravenous flucloxacillin since the organism chiefly to be feared is *Staphylococcus aureus*; flucloxacillin is also effective against haemolytic streptococci. If there is a history of penicillin allergy, chloramphenicol or co-trimoxazole may be given. Some authorities oppose prophylactic chemotherapy, and certainly antibiotics are no substitute for early wound exploration and closure. However, Demetriades et al (1992) have reported on a randomized prospective trial of antibiotics in a series of 157 open and basilar skull fractures, the antibiotic being begun on admission and continued for 3 days. The incidence of infection was 8.7% in the control group, and 0.9% in the treated cases ($P < 0.05$). This study, though not based on a very large series, is in accord with other reports on the definite though modest benefits of prophylactic chemotherapy in high-risk cases.

Operative procedure

The operative repair of a compound skull fracture (Fig. 13.4) requires careful preparation, thorough cleaning of all layers down to the brain if the dura has been penetrated, and removal of all deep bone fragments and foreign matter. Haemostasis must be secured. In central frontal depressed fractures, the sagittal sinus is often injured. If at all possible, the sinus is preserved: there is considerable variation in the venous drainage of the frontal lobes, and sometimes occlusion of the anterior third of the sinus causes frontal venous infarction. It is usually possible to control bleeding from the sinus by tamponade with haemostatic agents (Oxycel, Gelfoam), or with pledgets of muscle or fascia, which can be sutured to the dura; control of venous bleeding is aided by elevating the head, with precautions against air embolism. The dura must be repaired; a fascial or pericranial graft is often needed. Bone fragments, if not grossly contaminated, are replaced. Large fragments are held in position by wires or miniplates to give a satisfactory frontal contour; this is important when the orbital margin is disrupted, and, in our service, this is done with neurosurgical–plastic surgical collaboration. This is especially appropriate when there is an associated fracture of the middle or lower face, which can be reduced and fixed under the same anaesthetic (p. 248).

If the skin wound is so large that the underlying fracture is well exposed, then the craniocerebral injury can be explored through the wound. Usually, however, it is better to explore through the standard bicoronal scalp flap, siting this to ensure that there is an adequate blood supply to the injured frontal skin. Scalp closure is usually not difficult.

COMPOUND DEPRESSED FRACTURES INVOLVING THE FRONTAL SINUS

Management

As a rule, these injuries do not present major operative problems. The depressed fracture is best approached through a bicoronal scalp flap. A small frontal craniotomy is made above the sinus area, to expose the posterior wall of the sinus and the depressed fracture extradurally. If the dura is torn, it is repaired in a water-tight manner (see below). The posterior wall of the frontal sinus is usually excised and the sinus mucosa is stripped away. The sinus ostia can be plugged with muscle. We have not inserted a drainage tube into the nose through the frontonasal duct or frontal recess, as advised by Raveh et al (1984). We believe that our method of management will usually result in obliteration of the sinus and have only once seen a mucocele develop some years later. Admittedly, cases of delayed sinusitis and even extradural infection have occurred after this type of management of the sinus (Simpson et al 1990), but in most of these there were other complicating factors. The anterior wall of the frontal sinus is preserved, and if it is shattered the frag-

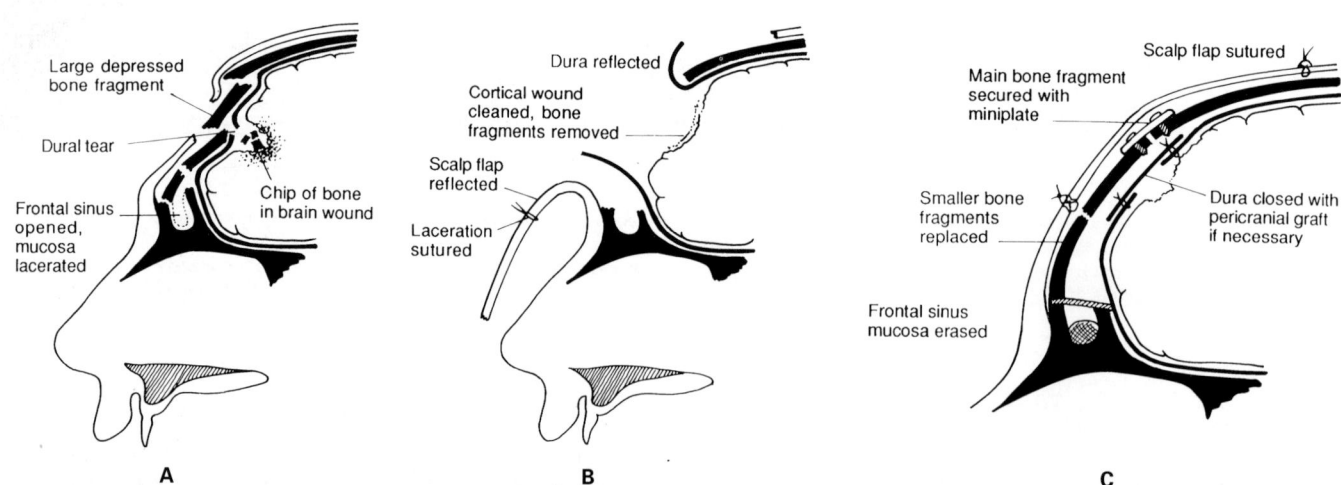

Fig. 13.4 Closure of frontal compound depressed fracture. A There is a wound in the forehead, with depression and comminution of the frontal bone; the dura and cerebral cortex are lacerated. **B** A standard coronal scalp flap is reflected and the depressed bone fragments are carefully removed; the dural tear is enlarged. The lacerated cortex is cleaned by irrigation and clot is removed by gentle suction. **C** The frontal sinus mucosa is removed and the posterior wall is resected (not shown). Sinus ostia may be closed with muscle and/or pericranial graft. The dura is closed, and the bone fragments are replaced, with miniplate or wire fixation. The scalp flap is sutured in two layers.

ments are wired or plated into good position; failure to do this may result in an ugly frontal concavity.

Central frontal depressed fractures may be associated with naso-orbito-ethmoid fractures (p. 310) and disruption of the anterior cranial fossa, often complicated by CSF rhinorrhoea. This constellation of injuries is best managed by a combined operation, in which all the fractures are elevated and fixed with miniplates. The anterior fossa may be explored intradurally and repaired at the same time if disruption is severe and the degree of brain swelling not prohibitive.

PENETRATING FRONTAL BRAIN WOUNDS

Management

This subset of compound frontal fractures needs separate consideration because there is some controversy over the surgical management.

When the penetrating agent is likely to be heavily contaminated or to have introduced foreign material, then the whole wound track should be explored under magnified vision. Clot and necrotic brain are gently sucked away; in doing this, care is taken not to remove viable brain and we do not share the belief that it is possible to reduce the risk of post-traumatic epilepsy by ablating brain up to the margin of a normal convolution (McDonald 1980); indeed there is reason to believe that smaller cerebral ablations carry a lower risk of seizures. Foreign material is meticulously removed; failure to remove fragments of clothing, dirt or wood may result in a brain abscess.

When the penetrating agent is a bullet or shell fragment, less aggressive management may be justifiable. Military experience in World War II laid stress on the risks of late infection if bone chips or missiles were left in the wound track, and bone chips were seen as especially dangerous since they are often contaminated by micro-organisms sucked into the brain in the wake of the missile. Standard military teaching enjoined meticulous search for bone chips; it was agreed that metallic missiles need not be removed if deeply placed or in a hazardous situation. Inexperienced military neurosurgeons often agonized over failure to locate a deeply placed bone chip, and re-exploration was often done when a postoperative X-ray picture showed a residual piece of bone (Fig. 13.1).

This policy has been called in question. Israeli wartime experience has favoured a much more conservative approach, intended to minimize operative brain damage. Brandvold et al (1990) did not attempt to remove deeply placed bone chips. Punctate wounds were not explored, larger wounds were debrided only when grossly contaminated and missile tracks were not opened with retractors. This conservative policy appeared justified by the good long-term results (see p. 376). Vietnamese military neurosurgeons have confirmed that the importance of im-

planted chips has been exaggerated; they have also emphasized that standard methods of management should be modified when brain wounds present late. Nguyen & Bui (1994) reported on 295 cases of wartime missile wounds, of which 58 came for neurosurgical treatment > 72 h after wounding. By using a limited wound debridement designed to avoid spreading infection, and with the use of antibiotics started at the battlefront, infection was avoided in nearly 70% of these.

Our own experience is chiefly of civilian bullet wounds, though some members of our team have had limited experience of wartime wounds. We have been at pains to remove bone chips; we have not been so concerned over metal fragments, except in the case of those known to contain copper (p. 153), such as pieces of cupronickel bullet jackets (Fig. 4.16).

It is possible that our policy of wound exploration has been unnecessarily radical. Nevertheless, experience from World War II should not be discarded until the safety of conservative management is confirmed. When the conscious level is reasonably well preserved, and especially when there has been delay in evacuation of the patient, we believe that at least a limited exploration of the missile track is warranted. In comatose patients, there is likely to be serious cerebral swelling, and conservative management is usually preferable. The entry wound is excised and closed, and ICP manometry is instituted; persisting coma is managed along standard lines (see below). CT scan is repeated later, with enhancement by contrast injection, to detect delayed abscess formation. Antibiotics (p. 236) have been routinely given; our usual choice is flucloxacillin.

Operative procedure

For penetration in the frontal convexity (Fig. 13.5), we have usually explored the wound as soon as resuscitation and assessment have been completed; the CT scan has been invaluable in showing the missile track and visualizing haematomas. A frontal craniotomy flap is reflected; exploration through an enlarged cranial entry wound may sometimes be appropriate in wartime operations, but will leave an unsightly frontal bone defect, necessitating later cranioplasty (p. 553). The dural wound is enlarged if necessary, and the missile track is gently irrigated and explored with the aid of Scoville's spatula forceps to allow removal of clot, necrotic brain and foreign material. The dura is closed, usually with a pericranial or fascial graft, absorbable sutures being used. The bone flap is replaced and the scalp is closed in standard fashion (p. 245) without tension. Missiles may avulse or otherwise destroy areas of scalp so extensive that normal closure is impossible; in such cases, the defect is closed by a large flap of scalp based on an artery such as the superficial temporal artery. This flap is advanced or

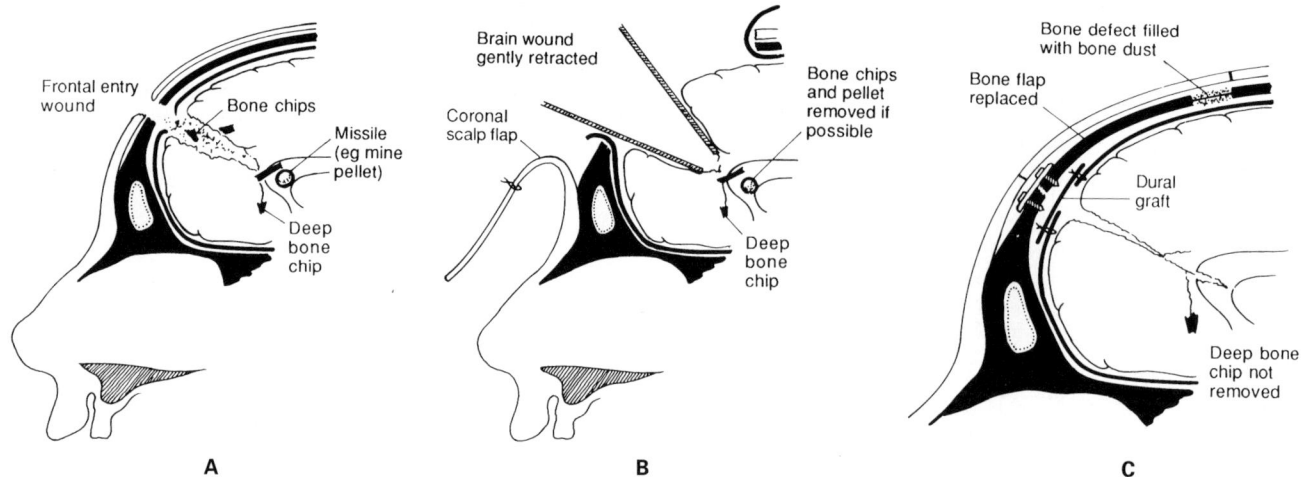

Fig. 13.5 Closure of frontal gunshot wound. A A missile has penetrated the frontal lobe and lodged near the lateral ventricle; the missile track contains bone chips and clot. **B** A standard coronal scalp flap is reflected and a frontal bone flap is used to expose the missile track. The brain wound is explored with gentle retraction; the accessible bone chips are removed, and if possible also the missile, since it may enter the ventricle. A deeply placed bone chip is not removed. **C** The dura is closed with a fascial graft, the bone flap is secured with miniplates to close the missile entry wound, and the small secondary bone defect is filled with bone dust.

rotated to cover the defect; the area exposed by the flap is covered with split-skin grafts. Postoperative ICP manometry is instituted.

ORBITOFRONTAL WOUNDS

Management

Penetrating orbitofrontal wounds, whether caused by a missile or by some other agent, deserve special consideration and very careful assessment. An ophthalmological consultation is always needed; in our practice, joint neurosurgical and ophthalmological management is usual. The clinical and radiological assessment should be rigorous, and the possibility of implanted foreign material must be kept in mind. Wood fragments in the orbit or cranial cavity are especially dangerous, and may not be seen in the preoperative CT scan. Miller et al (1977) reviewed the literature, and stressed the high incidence of infection, including tetanus, after implantation of wood. More recently, Mutlukan et al (1991) have reported a case of brain abscess and blindness from wood penetrating the orbit; we have seen a similar case (Fig. 13.6). The anatomical extent of the wound should be determined as fully as possible, since involvement of the paranasal air sinuses or the middle fossa may require more extensive surgical exposure.

Operative procedure

When investigation and team planning are complete, the orbit is explored from above, through a bicoronal scalp flap and fronto-orbital craniotomy (Fig. 13.7). The extent of the cerebral penetration is explored, and the dura is repaired with a fascial graft. The orbit is then explored by removing the superior orbital margin, and if necessary also the lateral orbital wall, as a free graft. The entry wound can be explored from the facial aspect, and the nature of the orbital injury can be assessed both from in front and from above. At the close, the orbital margin is reconstructed by plating or wiring the osteotomized bone in position.

Complications and results

Compound frontal fractures without deep cerebral injury have a low mortality when treated early and under favourable surgical conditions, unless there is severe impact-induced brain swelling. Unskilled operators occasionally meet severe bleeding from the anterior sagittal sinus. Delayed infection should be rare.

Mortality and morbidity are more formidable after penetrating frontal wounds, especially those caused by missiles. There is a large literature on wartime brain wounds but, in many reports, the site of the cerebral wound is not specified. The mortality in wartime wounds (p. 95) is of little relevance in considering methods of operative management, since it varies with the nature of the fighting and especially the battlefield triage. The incidence of infection is of greater interest, since this can relate to policies of management. Rish et al (1980) reported on 771 cases of penetrating craniocerebral wounds treated by craniectomy and wound debridement in Vietnam (1965–1970); epi- or subdural abscesses, cerebritis and brain abscesses were reported in 3.2%. However, this survey excluded wounds involving the anterior cranial

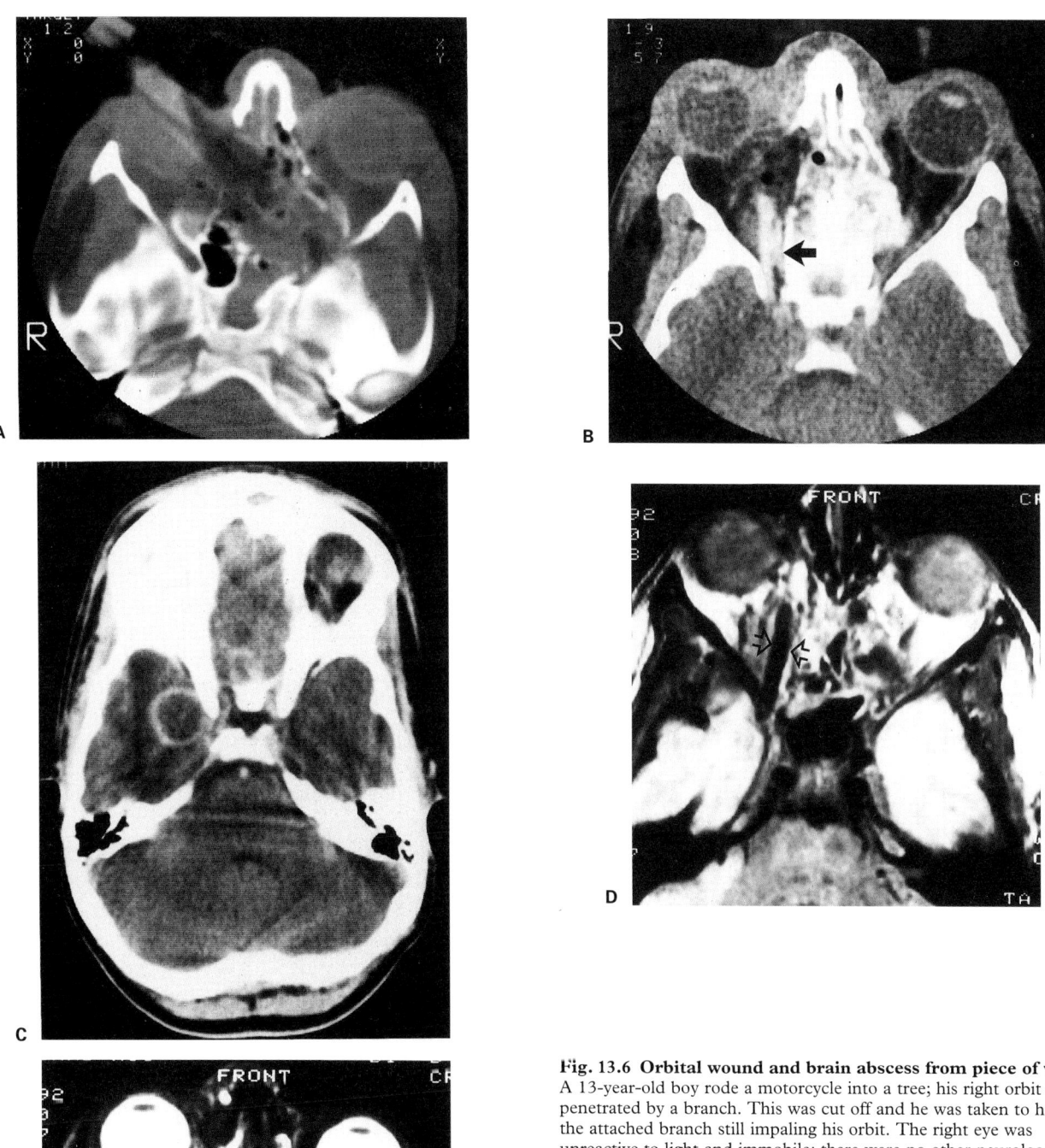

Fig. 13.6 Orbital wound and brain abscess from piece of wood.
A 13-year-old boy rode a motorcycle into a tree; his right orbit was
penetrated by a branch. This was cut off and he was taken to hospital,
the attached branch still impaling his orbit. The right eye was
unreactive to light and immobile; there were no other neurological
deficits. **A** CT scan on day 1 showed the branch in the right orbit,
ethmoid air cells and medial wall of left orbit. It was largely
radiolucent. The wood was removed and the wound was debrided and
closed. **B** CT scan on day 4 showed a piece of wood (arrow) in the
apex of the right orbit. Note that this was now radio-opaque, perhaps
from blood. **C** CT scan on day 11 showed a lesion with ring
enhancement in the right medial temporal lobe: an abscess was
diagnosed. **D** MRI scan (T1 image) showed the wood (arrows) as a
signal void. **E** MRI scan (T2 image) showed the abscess, with
surrounding high signal abnormality, presumably oedema. An anterior
temporal lobectomy was performed and the abscess was excised;
culture yielded *Enterobacter agglomerans*, an unusual organism which
had earlier been grown from the orbital wound. A piece of wood was
found penetrating the dura of the middle fossa. The boy made a good
recovery. A year later the right eye had no vision; there was a right
ptosis, with restricted ocular movement, especially upwards.

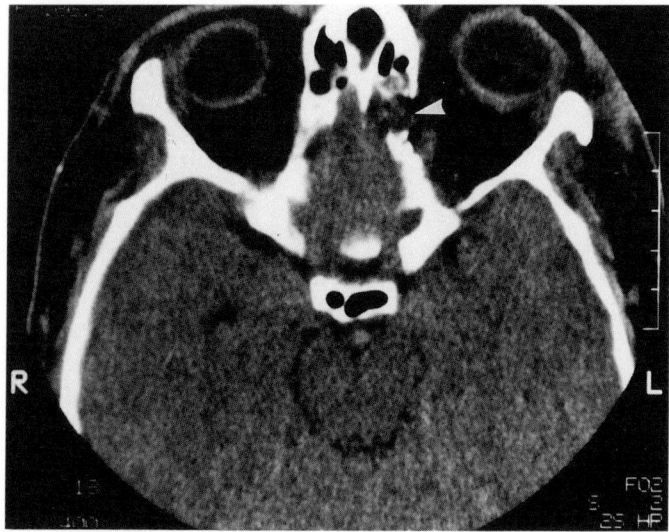

A

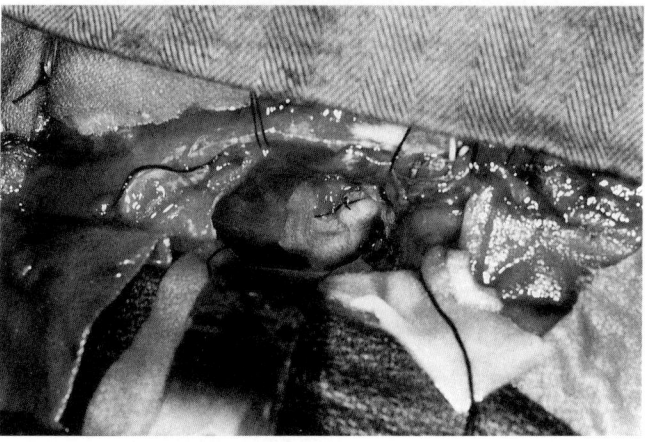

B

Fig. 13.7 Fronto-orbital wound from boat hook. A 45-year-old man was struck near the left inner canthus by a swinging boat hook. He did not lose consciousness. A small puncture wound was sutured. **A** CT scan showed a bony defect in the ethmoid–cribriform region. **B** At craniotomy, the falx was divided to give bilateral access; a puncture wound was seen in the right frontal lobe. The defect in the anterior fossa dura was covered with pericranium, sutured and sealed with autologous tissue glue.

fossa, which undoubtedly carry a much higher risk of infection (Rish et al 1981). The overall incidence of early infection in brain wounds treated in this war appears to have been low but the incidence of delayed meningitis and brain abscess was not insignificant. More recent wartime experience includes the Israeli report of Brandvold et al (1990) on 113 cases, including 18 with basal injuries, the cerebral wounds being treated by the conservative plan described above. The incidence of early meningitis was 8%, perhaps because the management of CSF leaks was also conservative (see below), but only one late brain abscess was reported despite residual bone chips in more than half the cases followed for 6 years or more. These cases were treated under very favourable logistic con-

ditions, the median time for arrival at a hospital with a neurosurgical service being 2.0 h after injury. By contrast, Nguyen & Bui (1944) reported on 295 cases wounded under conditions in which evacuation was often delayed. In 51, debridement was done within 24 h of wounding, when the infection rate was 13.7%. In 186, operation was done between 24 and 72 h, with an infection rate of 22.6%, rising to 31.0% in 58 cases treated at later times.

Peacetime missile wounds are likely to be treated under good conditions; however, they are usually due to bullets, often fired at short range, and the mortality is high. Since early operation is usually possible, the incidence of infection is likely to be low; Benzel et al (1991) described what they called aggressive management in 120 cases and reported only three superficial infections with no deep infections. In close range bullet wounds of the brain, it sometimes seems desirable to defer operation until brain swelling subsides, or until the likely quality of survival is clear, but this policy can be detrimental, because the victim may develop frontal lobe infection. Whether in war or peace, neurosurgeons planning the treatment of missile wounds in the frontal region should give careful attention to the factor of delay, as well as to the neurological state and the radiological anatomy.

Apart from the effects of delayed infection or rupture of a traumatic aneurysm (p. 146), the chief long-term complications of penetrating frontal wound are those relating to primary cerebral injury: post-traumatic epilepsy (pp. 295 and 659) and behavioural disorders (p. 653).

INTERNALLY COMPOUND FRACTURES OF THE ANTERIOR CRANIAL FOSSA

Management

There is controversy over the management of anterior fossa fractures involving the paranasal air sinuses and the nasal cavity. Long ago, Linell & Robinson (1941) showed that meningitis, both early and long delayed, may complicate these fractures, and these authors clearly showed that natural healing may be inadequate (p. 147). Intracranial aeroceles may develop after a skull base fracture (Fig. 13.8), and when there is a valvular mechanism, the aerocele may act as an expanding mass (North 1971). Awareness of these dangers became widespread during the decade after World War II. Hugh Cairns (p. 22) and his pupil Walpole Lewin (1954) reported experiences that appeared to justify routine antibiotic prophylaxis, surgical exploration and dural repair in all cases with a history of CSF leakage after anterior fossa fracture, even when the leakage had ceased spontaneously. This radical view was never accepted everywhere; it was argued that Lewin's control series was small and not representative of general experience. In the USA especially, much more conservative policies were advocated, and anterior fossa

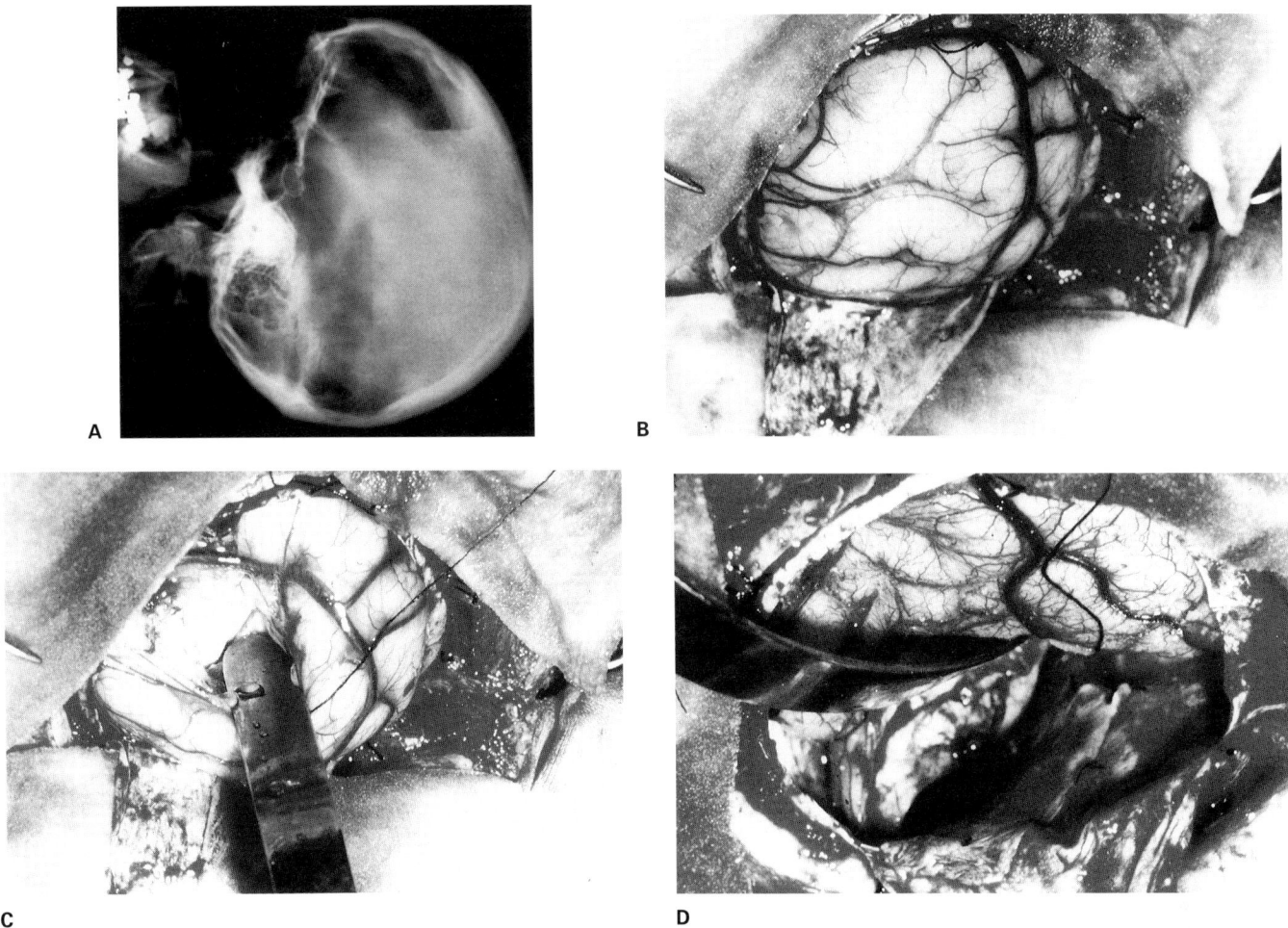

Fig. 13.8 Dural repair for intracranial aerocele. A 24-year-old woman was hurt in a car crash; her injuries included a left orbital blow-out fracture. 2 weeks later, she leaked CSF from her left nostril. A large frontal aerocele was found. **A** Lateral skull radiograph (brow-up), showing air and fluid level in the frontal lobe. **B** Tense brain at craniotomy, before aspiration of air. **C** Incision into the aerocele cavity — perhaps an unnecessary procedure? **D** Frontal lobe elevated to show traumatized orbital cortex, where a large spicule of the orbital roof was found opening the ethmoid air cells. A large sheet of fascia was sutured to cover the area of the cranionasal fistula.

repair was advocated only where CSF leakage persisted. It was widely believed that fixation of facial fractures would promote healing of a disrupted anterior cranial fossa.

An intermediate and very balanced view, based on both French and German experience, was presented by Loew et al (1984). These authors emphasized that anterior fossa exploration has a significant mortality and morbidity; Homburg – Saar, one of the two participating units, had indeed experienced a 25% mortality, though this was in severely injured cases undergoing early operation when the brain may still have been swollen. They argued that conservative treatment is appropriate when the leakage ceases within the first week, and were prepared to supplement the natural processes that arrest leakage by continuous external drainage of CSF by a lumbar spinal catheter. They saw continued CSF leakage, anosmia and a wide separation of fracture margins as indications for operative intervention.

More recently, Eljamel & Foy (1990a,b) have restated the case for preventive dural repair of fistulae These authors reviewed retrospectively a series of 160 cases of acute CSF leakage due to head injury, followed for a mean period of 6.5 years, and found a high incidence (30.6%) of meningitis. The risk was cumulative over time; without repair, some 85% had developed meningitis by 10 years. It was argued that operative dural repair is the only reliable long-term prophylaxis against meningitis after post-traumatic CSF rhinorrhoea. This series comprised cases referred to a neurosurgical service (the Mersey Regional Department of Neurosciences), and may have been in some way selected.

Our general indications for conservative or operative treatment of a cranionasal fistula have been evolved over a 40 year period (Dinning et al 1961, Caldicott et al 1973, Simpson et al 1990), and are based on an experience of 237 cases of anterior fossa fracture, of which 168 underwent formal dural repair.

We advise conservative treatment initially for CSF

rhinorrhoea and for subdural or subarachnoid intracranial air, if in small quantities. Our indications for operative repair are:

- CSF leakage persisting for 7 days, or 10 at most
- Recurrent CSF leakage after 7–10 days
- A large aerocele, especially if intracerebral, or if recurring after 7–10 days (Fig. 13.8)
- Escape of brain tissue through the nostrils
- Meningitis or brain abscess at any time after injury
- A basal fracture thought to communicate with one of the paranasal air sinuses and considered on X-ray evidence to be unlikely to heal, because of wide separation of bone edges, a tilted spicule of bone, or an appearance suggesting a cerebral herniation into the nasal cavity. We see this indication as valid even in the absence of any of the above indications.

Although we note carefully the presence or absence of olfaction, we do not give anosmia a great weight in deciding whether or not to advise operative repair, because this finding may be unreliable in the early period after CMF injury, and in any case anosmia may be misleading as a localizing sign (Leech 1974).

It has been said, and with some justification, that cranionasal fistulae associated with midface fractures of Le Fort type have a better prognosis than those resulting from severe frontal impacts (O'Brien & Reade 1984). It is often appropriate to treat CSF leakage complicating such fractures conservatively in the first instance. However, if the clinical and radiological findings suggest gross anterior fossa disruption, we advocate operative exploration and repair, and this can be very conveniently carried out in a combined operation when the midface fracture is repaired.

Chemoprophylaxis

When there is evidence, or suspicion, of a cranionasal fistula, prophylactic chemotherapy is given. The evidence that this is efficacious has been reviewed by Demetriades et al (1992) and earlier by Loew et al (1984), on the basis of several reported trials and comparisons of treated and untreated series. Loew et al concluded that there was no conclusive proof that antibiotics do prevent infection from a skull base fracture, and some suggestion that prophylactic chemotherapy encourages colonization of the nasal mucosa by more serious pathogens. Demetriades et al (1992) took a contrary view and although their own trial — cited above — was inconclusive with respect to meningitis, they found no convincing evidence that short courses of chemotherapy are detrimental. These authors did not cite the retrospective study by Leech & Paterson (1973), which showed a statistically significant benefit from prophylactic chemotherapy with penicillin and sulphadimidine, though this study is also open to

methodological criticism. Our views have been reported (Simpson et al 1990). We favour prophylaxis with intravenous co-trimoxazole (a trimethoprim–sulphonamide combination), aimed to give a bactericidal effect in the CSF, and ampicillin, aimed at a bactericidal effect in the nasal mucosa. These are given immediately when a skull base fracture is diagnosed, and continued for 7–10 days thereafter. This policy has been criticized, and certainly we cannot claim to have demonstrated that it has achieved a reduction in the incidence of meningitis. However, no detrimental consequences have been seen, either from serious toxicity or from the appearance of resistant microorganisms: when infections have developed in patients on these drugs, the organisms have responded well to other antibiotics. Apart from chemotherapy and warning against noseblowing, we do not advocate any special measures to promote spontaneous healing of a fistula; in particular, we do not favour spinal CSF drainage except as an adjunct to operative repair (see below).

Radiological assessment

The site of the fistula should be identified if possible. We have relied on fine-cut CT examination of the anterior fossa (p. 201); if there is a persisting CSF leak, intrathecal metrizamide may visualize the site, but this method is often disappointing when the leak is intermittent. Intrathecal injection of [^{99m}Tc]DTPA has been useful; cisternography is combined with the insertion of nasal pledgets to absorb the isotope, and this procedure has identified rhinorrhoea due to a petrous fracture (Williams et al 1977). But it is often difficult to demonstrate the site of the fistula, and where the clinical indications are strong the neurosurgeon must be prepared to explore the anterior cranial fossa bilaterally without a clear radiological diagnosis.

Timing of transcranial repair

In principle, operative repair of a cranionasal fistula should be done as soon as the indications are established. However, transcranial repair is best done as an elective procedure, when brain swelling has subsided, and if possible after the fistula site has been located. These requirements usually entail a few days delay, even when the need for repair is unquestioned.

In about one-third of our cases of anterior fossa fracture, there was an associated facial fracture or fractures, often needing operative reduction and fixation (Table 13.2). In the past, the need to immobilize fractures of the Le Fort type by external splints often complicated the neurosurgical programme of fistula repair: the advent of internal fixation has on the contrary made it simpler to plan an interdisciplinary operation at which both facial and anterior fossa repair is carried out through the

Table 13.2 Fractures of the mid and lower thirds of the face associated with anterior fossa fractures in a series of 238 cases

Principal facial fractures	No. of fractures	As % of series of anterior fossa fractures
Naso-orbito-ethmoid	4	1.7
Zygomatic	10	4.2
Orbital floor	6	2.5
Other orbital	13	5.5
LeFort I–III etc.	50	21.0
Mandibular	14	5.9
Other	7	2.9
Total mid and lower facial fractures	104	
Total cases with mid and lower fractures	89	37.4

In 15 cases, more than one fracture site was identified, hence the discrepancy between fracture and case numbers. From Simpson et al (1990).

bicoronal approach. The concept of one-stage total repair of panfacial fractures has been an important expression of the craniofacial philosophy (David 1984). Since our plan of management of panfacial fractures does not obligate very early operation (p. 338), it has been possible to stage combined operations of this type at about 5–7 days after injury, or even longer, when the indications for transcranial repair of the fistula have been appraised by the clinical and radiological criteria set out above. It has been argued that such delays predispose to infection (Brandt et al 1991), but this has not been our impression. Krafft et al (1991) reported a series of 70 cases of frontomaxillary fractures treated by combined one-stage neurosurgical and maxillofacial surgical procedures very similar in principle to those advocated here: in most of these, the operations were done between 5 and 10 days after injury and the authors saw no evidence of an increased infection rate. Nor were there any recurrent CSF leaks or postoperative meningitis.

Occasionally, a similar interdisciplinary combined operation is appropriate when it is necessary to repair the anterior cranial fossa as part of the correction of a post-traumatic deformity. However, many cases of cranionasal fistula present months or years after the causative injury has been treated, and then a neurosurgical repair may be done without a need for interdisciplinary collaboration. Even in such cases, it is often useful to review the patient's aesthetic status.

Operative techniques for transcranial repair

The standard bicoronal scalp flap is used (p. 238) wherever possible; neurosurgeons should keep in mind the requirements of craniofacial surgery, and place the incision well behind the hairline, even when no immediate craniofacial procedure is envisaged (Fig. 9.4). A unilateral or bilateral frontal craniotomy is performed, according to the need for a bilateral exploration: if olfaction is not lost, bilateral exploration should be avoided wherever possible, and this emphasizes the value of accurate preoperative radiographic localization of the site of the fistula. Extradural exploration may be sufficient when the fistula has been certainly located in the posterior wall of the frontal sinus. More often, the dura is opened; both for an adequate exploration, and because intradural grafts are more dependable, being firmly pressed into place by the brain which is not the case with an extradural graft (Fig. 13.9A). The frontal lobe is gently elevated, and the anterior fossa is explored systematically under magnified vision. If the fistula is located, the adherent brain, which often forms a hernia in the bone defect, is dissected away. The bone defect is then plugged with a piece of muscle soaked in an antibiotic solution, such as 2% flucloxacillin; large defects are closed with a small bone graft, which can be taken by splitting the bone flap (p. 241). We deprecate the use of alloplastic materials such as acrylic. Then, most

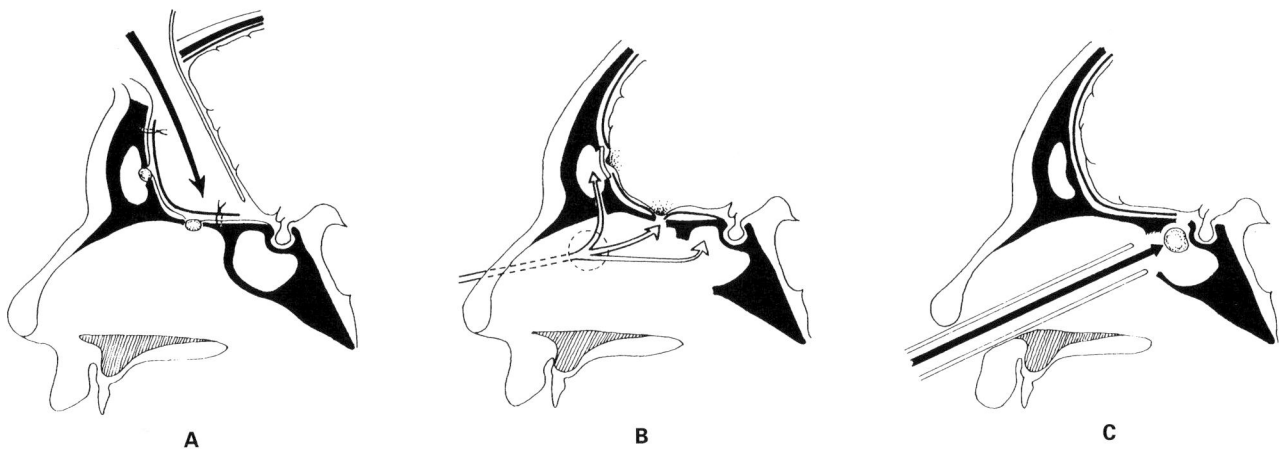

Fig. 13.9 Strategies for repair of a cranionasal fistula. A Frontal craniotomy and transdural application of a fascial graft, which is secured by sutures or fibrin glue. **B** Extradural fascial graft applied through an ethmoidectomy and secured with fibrin glue. **C** Trans-sphenoidal repair, a muscle or fascial graft being placed on the external aspect of the fistula; this may be combined with lumbar drainage.

importantly, the area of the fistula is carpeted with a large sheet of temporalis fascia, pericranium or fascia lata, sutured to the dura at four or more points around the site of the bone defect (Fig. 13.8) or secured with fibrin glue prepared from the patient's blood (Stechison 1992). When a bifrontal repair is needed, the fascial graft is given a median slit to take in the falx and crista galli; alternatively, the falx may be divided (Fig. 13.7). Watertight dural closure is desirable. The bone flap is replaced and secured. Postoperative spinal drainage is not used, unless the quality of the repair was in doubt.

Complications and results of transcranial repair

In our series of 168 cases, the operative mortality rate was 1.2%; the incidence of recurrent CSF leakage and/or meningitis was thought to be 5.4%, though follow-up was often incomplete. Probst (1990), in a larger series of 300 cases, reported a mortality rate of 9%, chiefly from associated severe brain injury, though in his earlier experience there were deaths directly due to operation, from 'local exacerbation of the brain oedema'. In his series, the incidence of fistula recurrence was 4%.

In general, we have been satisfied that anterior fossa repair by the transdural route will reliably obliterate most leaks. Nevertheless, the morbidity is not insignificant. There is a risk of imperilling olfaction when this is not already lost. Even more seriously, retraction of the frontal lobe can be detrimental if there is brain swelling. The exploration sometimes fails to locate the site of the fistula, especially when it is in the roof of the sphenoid air sinus; frontal and ethmoid fistulas are easier to locate and to repair. Furthermore, the repair sometimes fails. Our failure rate includes cases in which there were extenuating circumstances, but it must be recognized that recurrent CSF leakages and meningitis may occasionally occur after seemingly satisfactory intradural repair. It is therefore appropriate to consider alternatives to transcranial repair.

Lumbar drainage

Many authors have advocated continuous or intermittent spinal CSF drainage in the hope that this will promote natural healing of a cranionasal fistula. Findler et al (1977) reported on 14 cases of post-traumatic CSF leaks treated by this method: there were five failures, with one death from infection. Steimle et al (1990) see external CSF drainage as the treatment of first choice, but appear to accept extensive frontobasal comminution as an indication for primary surgical repair. Shapiro & Scully (1992) reported on five cases successfully treated by drainage, with no long-term relapses: however, Shapiro (personal communication) warns against relying on drainage if there is radiological evidence of a wide bone defect. It has been argued that external drainage increases the risk of retro-

grade spread of infection, but there is little support for this in the literature; however, there are reports of massive aerocele formation (Graf et al 1981) after low pressure drainage, and we have seen this alarming complication of excessive withdrawal of CSF after trans-sphenoidal surgery (Fig. 13.10). We feel that the evidence does not justify routine use of lumbar drainage in cases of post-traumatic CSF rhinorrhoea, since there is insufficient proof that the causative fistulas will heal permanently. Nevertheless, we are prepared to use this procedure

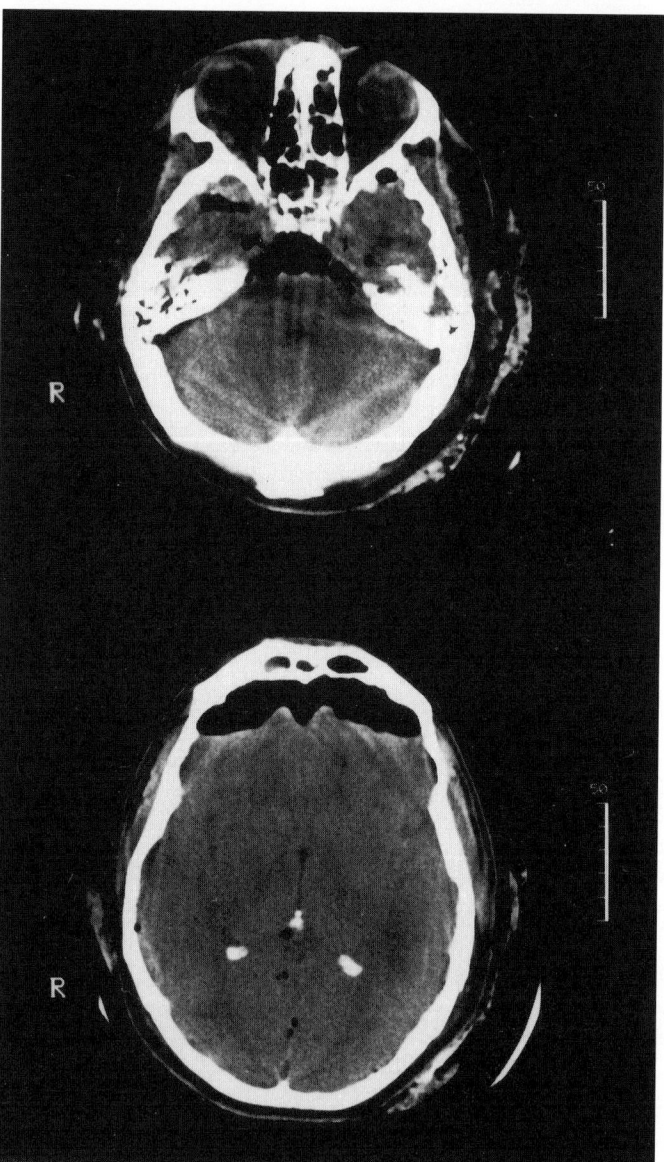

Fig. 13.10 Massive aerocele from excessive lumbar drainage.
A 33-year-old woman developed a CSF leakage after trans-sphenoidal surgery. Lumbar drainage was instituted to promote healing of the fistula, and the drainage pressure was inadvertently set too low. She became comatose. CT scan showed a large volume of intracranial air with posterior displacement of the brain and collapse of the ventricular system. She was placed head down and the drainage system was closed; she gradually improved.

when operative treatment has been unsatisfactory or is contraindicated.

Subcranial repair

Raveh et al (1984) reported on 153 cases of frontobasal skull fractures with rhinorrhoea; dural tears were exposed via an extended ethmoidectomy and repaired with extra-dural patches of fascia lata secured with fibrin glue (Fig. 13.9B). Transcranial repair was reserved for cases with 'vast frontal lobe lacerations'. This technique, com-bined with one-stage internal fixation and grafting of the associated facial fractures, was successful in most cases, though there were recurrent CSF leakages in 3.9%. The chief merits in this approach seem to be the capacity to operate early (2–4 days after injury), while the brain is still swollen and there is less risk of damage to the olfactory nerves; the chief demerit is the uncertainty of extradural graft fixation and the limited exposure. Other writers have also advocated extradural repair for frontal or ethmoid fistulas: we remain unconvinced, but the long-term results may justify these procedures.

Trans-sphenoid repair (Fig. 13.9C) is much easier to justify. Experience with fistulas occurring after pituitary surgery has shown that muscle packs and/or fascia may be an effective seal. Sphenoid leaks can be approached through the transnasal trans-septal route and we have used this for post-traumatic leaks; leaks which appear to involve both the sphenoid and ethmoid sinuses may be approached through an extended ethmoidectomy. The fracture and the dural defect must be identified carefully under the microscope; fluoroscein has been injected intrathecally to facilitate this (McCormack et al 1990), despite the reports of toxicity from this agent (Wallace et al 1972). The repair is done with fascia lata, secured with fibrin glue and supported by a muscle pack and struts of nasal septal bone or cartilage. However, the exposure given by this approach is limited, and we do not favour it if there is any doubt about the site or sites of the fistula.

CLOSED BRAIN INJURIES WITH PROLONGED LOSS OF CONSCIOUSNESS

Management

Blunt impacts in the CMF region often impair consciousness. The depth and duration of the loss of consciousness are good measures of the severity of the brain injury. Rimel et al (1982) ranked head injuries on the coma level 6 h after injury in three grades:

mild: GCS 13–15
moderate: GCS 9–12
severe: GCS $\leq$ 8

For the first two categories, management consists chiefly in watching for complications by serial reassessment and in organizing appropriate rehabilitation. Head injuries with persisting coma require supportive care and in most cases, planned team rehabilitation.

Management of the unconscious patient is aimed not only at detecting secondary complications, but also at providing optimum physiological conditions for neuronal survival. Prolonged unconsciousness, from whatever cause, is in itself a life-threatening condition; our management plan is applicable to coma resulting from open head inju-ries in the CMF region as well as to closed head injuries.

Controlled ventilation

In coma (GCS $\leq$ 8), the depression of the protective respiratory reflexes usually requires early endotracheal intubation and controlled ventilation. Other indications include upper airway obstruction from faciomaxillary injury, chest injury interfering with gas exchange, lung soiling by inhaled blood or vomit and severe pre-existing chronic pulmonary disease (p. 541). Severe head injuries are often complicated by pulmonary oedema, either as a neurogenic effect (Popp et al 1982) or from causes such as iatrogenic fluid overload or fat embolism. Pulmo-nary oedema is a dangerous cause of hypoxia, and may respond to controlled ventilation.

An oral or nasal endotracheal tube is inserted, with a soft cuff. In most trauma centres, controlled ventilation is then induced and maintained by various combinations of narcotics and pancuronium or other muscle relaxant. Narcotics (morphia or fentanyl) are used where the con-scious level is not profoundly depressed, to inhibit the reaction to tracheobronchial suction. Humidified oxygen (100%) is given until the arterial blood gases have been determined: ventilation is then regulated to give whatever levels are desired. Initially $pO_2 > 80$ mmHg and pCO_2 ~ 30–35 mmHg may be satisfactory; when ICP is stable, $pCO_2 = 40$ mmHg will be preferable, to give a margin for reduction by hyperventilation in emergency. Narcotics and relaxants are periodically withdrawn or reversed to allow testing of the conscious level.

There has been some controversy over the necessity for respiratory paralysis and prolonged controlled ventilation. Hypoxia and hypercapnia are unquestionably detrimental. Mechanical ventilation gives control of pulmonary gas exchange, unless there is very severe concurrent cardio-respiratory dysfunction, such as pulmonary oedema or lung injury; normal gas exchanges are of special impor-tance in cases of head injury with cerebral ischaemia. Controlled ventilation avoids the transient peaks of intra-cranial pressure seen in struggling or coughing patients, and allows hyperventilation when temporary hypocapnia is desired. But controlled ventilation deprives the clinician of the power to monitor conscious level and even the pupillary light reflexes may be abolished by narcotics.

Respiratory physiology is placed at the mercy of the neurosurgeon and the intensivist, and it is easy for errors and misjudgements to be made. Some years ago, Jennett & Teasdale (1981) reviewed the literature and argued in favour of a selective use of controlled ventilation. Our practice has been to use intubation and mechanical ventilation routinely in comatose patients with CMF injuries, and in some who are less deeply unconscious if there are chest or orofacial wounds; we accept that this policy has risks and we try to minimize these by meticulous supervision of the blood chemistry and by ICP manometry, with frequent CT scanning.

Endotracheal intubation can be continued for 10 days or more without great risk of laryngeal stenosis, but except in infants and young children, we prefer to use a tracheostomy when prolonged respiratory support is needed, or where the upper airway will be obstructed for some time by intermaxillary fixation. Percutaneous tracheal intubation, done in the ward, is a very convenient way of performing tracheostomy as an elective procedure (Ivatury et al 1992, Moore et al 1992).

Fluid balance

Hydration and cellular electrolyte status are monitored by serum analyses, the urinary output and the central venous pressure; changes in body weight may be noted, though this guide may be misleading if changes in equipment are overlooked. An accurate fluid balance is necessary. Initially, intravenous Hartmann's solution (compound Ringer–lactate solution) is given, and then as a rule 4% dextrose in $\frac{1}{5}$ normal saline. It is important to avoid overhydration in the early period after injury, since the physiological response to severe injury includes a phase of increased secretion of the antidiuretic hormone and hence fluid retention; although there is also increased production of aldosterone, the net effect is towards hyponatraemia. Therefore, when resuscitation is completed, we advocate restraint in fluid maintenance, with careful biochemical monitoring, especially of serum electrolytes and osmolality. For an adult of average weight, this usually means a daily administration of 1500–2000 ml. However, in cases of multiple trauma, continuing fluid loss into the tissues must be allowed for, and replaced with Hartmann's solution or normal saline.

The physiological antidiuretic response may be excessive or delayed, when it can truly be described as inappropriate; Born et al (1985) find this a frequent sequel of severe head injury. Hyponatraemia and even cerebral oedema may result. This potentially dangerous condition usually responds well to fluid restriction, sufficient to cause a negative fluid balance. If there are neurological complications, it is necessary to give intravenous saline in twice normal concentration in a volume calculated to return plasma sodium to near normal levels.

The converse condition of diabetes insipidus is in our experience by no means rare in cases of CMF injury: it was recorded in 15 (6.3%) of our series of fractures of the anterior fossa, presumably from damage to the hypothalamic nuclei or the pituitary stalk (p. 55). Diabetes insipidus usually becomes evident a few days after injury as an increased output of urine hypo-osmolar to the serum; the serum sodium is usually elevated. Diabetes insipidus must be distinguished from the polyuria due to mannitol therapy, in which there should be no difference between the osmolality of the serum and the urine, and the serum sodium is usually not elevated — indeed may be low. Sometimes diabetes insipidus may be transient or biphasic, remitting and returning; it is important not to over-react to the diagnosis, by giving immediate large doses of vasopressin, as this can cause a severe fluid retention. Fluid losses should be replaced exactly, with a sodium-free intravenous infusion; if the polyuria continues, small doses of synthetic vasopressin (desmopressin acetate) should be given intravenously, subcutaneously or intranasally. In our experience, most cases of post-traumatic diabetes insipidus subside spontaneously; if this does not happen, long-term medication with intranasal desmopressin acetate is needed.

Control of raised ICP

Factors increasing ICP are avoided. These include hyperpyrexia, fluid overload, hypertension, hypercarbia, hypoxia, and obstruction to venous drainage from the head. The patient is usually nursed 30° head up, with the neck in neutral rotation. Any neck ties must not constrict the veins. The body temperature is carefully controlled, if necessary by ice packs placed on the arteries of the groins, armpits and neck; chlorpromazine may be given to prevent shivering. Fluid balance is monitored. Blood gases are measured regularly and maintained in normoxia and normacarbia. Dexamethasone, formerly given routinely, is now in disfavour, though it remains possible that some forms of post-traumatic cerebral swelling will benefit from this drug (North & Reilly 1990).

If ICP remains high or rises, then the cause is sought: the factors listed above are checked, and as a rule a further CT scan is done. If no easily treated cause is found, a protocol of management is followed.

1. If a catheter has been inserted into the lateral ventricle, it is used to drain CSF at a constant pressure (e.g. 10 mmHg), to avoid ventricular collapse. If the ventricles are small, small quantities may be drained intermittently when ICP reaches a sustained high level.
2. Hyperventilation to reduce the pCO_2 to ~25 mmHg gives vasoconstriction and a reduction in cerebral blood volume, thus temporarily lowering ICP.

3. Cerebral dehydration can be next tried. Mannitol, an osmotic diuretic with a molecular weight of 180 and a configuration resembling glucose, crosses the blood–brain barrier slowly and reduces tissue water content. Frusemide (Lasix) is a diuretic acting powerfully on the distal loop of the nephron; it reduces ICP by overall dehydration, and perhaps also by specific reduction in CSF production by its action as an inhibitor of carbonic anhydrase. Together or singly, these drugs are the mainstay of medical management of raised ICP. Dosage is according to the severity of the elevation: usually we give small boluses of mannitol 0.5 g/kg and/or 20–40 mg frusemide. Osmolality must be carefully monitored, and kept below 305–310 mosmol/kg.

4. Hypnotic therapy is a last resort. Barbiturates in high dosage reduce metabolic activity and increase cerebrovascular resistance; the resulting reduction in cerebral blood flow lowers ICP. Care is needed to maintain blood pressure so that cerebral perfusion is not impaired.

5. Surgical decompression, other than in the form of removing intracranial clots, plays only a small part. When brain swelling is associated with extensive contusion, there may be justification for a wide cranial decompression, with removal of the bone flap and expansion of the dural capacity by a fascial graft. It is important to avoid leaving a bone defect through which the brain herniates, nipping the cerebral veins at the margin and so promoting further swelling.

A sustained increase in ICP which does not respond to simple conservative treatment should be investigated by CT before more hazardous methods of control are used.

Nutrition

After injury, there is a period of catabolic hyperactivity: energy requirements are increased and a greater percentage of energy is derived from protein breakdown (Clifton et al 1984). In the presence of decerebrate or decorticate spasms, the concomitant increase in metabolic activity may result in a 50% increase in the basal energy expenditure (BEE); fever also increases the energy expenditure (9% per 0.5°C elevation). The hypermetabolic state may persist for a week or more; nutritional support will not prevent this catabolic process, but can slow it down and reduce its effects. There is an obligatory loss of weight, regardless of the nutritional programme; we aim to keep this below 10% of admission weight. In developed countries, young victims of CMF trauma are usually in good nutritional status before the injury, and will tolerate relative starvation for a few days. But there is a real risk of malnutrition if feeding is withheld for more than a week. In communities subject to dietary deficiencies, especially

protein deprivation, and in alcoholics, the margin of safety may be narrower.

Two routes of feeding the unconscious patient are on offer: enteral and parenteral. Both present problems. Enteral feeding is unlikely to be efficient until gastric emptying has returned; indeed, it may be dangerous, since the use of a cuffed endotracheal or tracheostomy tube does not always prevent regurgitation and inhalation of gastric contents. Brain injury usually precludes enteral feeding for a few days. The cerebral insult has an adverse effect on gastric emptying: this impedes gastrointestinal absorption and increases the risk of lung infection from inhaled gastric contents. This is particularly dangerous if the brain injury is associated with extensive facial fractures necessitating surgical reduction and fixation. Inhalation of gastric contents can be prevented by regular aspiration of the stomach; in our feeding routine, this is done every 5 h, with close observation for signs of abdominal distension. If the volume of gastric aspirate exceeds 150–250 ml, depending on the rate of feeding, then feeding is temporarily withheld. Nasoenteric feeding is contraindicated if there is a fracture in the anterior cranial fossa through which the tube could enter the cranial cavity; there are grisly reports of this (Fremstad & Martin 1978).

Parenteral nutrition must be given through a central venous catheter, with attendant risks of septicaemia, pneumothorax and other complications. These are not unacceptable risks, and some authors favour routine total parenteral feeding; Young et al (1987), reporting on a randomized comparison of enteral and parenteral feeding, found that the patients fed by the parenteral route made more rapid neurological recoveries, and suffered fewer septic complications. However, this work has been challenged by Hadley (1992), who stresses the value of enteral feeding in maintaining normal gut function and cites experimental evidence to suggest that parenteral nutrition promotes gut mucosal atrophy and bacterial translocation (p. 120). Grahm et al (1989) advocate early jejunal feeding.

We have chiefly relied on gastric feeding, begun as soon as gastric function has returned, usually after the fifth day. A naso-enteric tube is passed and its position is confirmed by X-ray; when facial fractures require operative fixation, the tube is passed in the theatre before the operation is terminated. In cases of central anterior fossa fracture, an oral tube is passed. After aspiration has confirmed that the volume of gastric residues is < 150 ml, infusion feeding with 5% dextrose is begun at a rate of 40–50 ml/h for 10 h. If this is tolerated, the volume and duration of infusion are increased. In cases under intensive care, we often begin formula feeds without this preliminary dextrose regime. The appropriate nutritive formula is determined by the dietitian, who calculates the energy requirement from the patient's weight, age and height, according to the Harris–Benedict equation for the BEE; a multiplication factor of 1.5 is used to give the actual energy requirement.

For males, BEE = 276 + $(57.3 \times W)$ + $(20.9 \times H)$ − $(28.5 \times A)$ kJ/day, where W is the weight in kg, H the height in cm and A the age in years. For females BEE = 2740 + $(40.2 \times W)$ + $(7.1 \times H)$ − $(19.7 \times A)$ kJ/day.

Many nutritional formulae are available. We prefer an iso-osmolar formula, at least initially. Additional protein is desirable. Osmolite HN® (Ross–Abbotts) and Isocal HN® (Mead–Johnson) contain 88 g protein and 8800 kJ energy in 2000 ml. Formulae containing more protein are available.

If gastric feeding is not tolerated, parenteral nutrition is given through a central venous catheter. An amino acid – 35% dextrose solution is given, with soya bean emulsion (Intralipid®) and vitamin supplements; electrolytes are added according to the biochemical status.

The nutritional state of the comatose patient must be monitored, by regular serial weighing. Though unreliable in patients with fluctuations in fluid balance, the body weight is invaluable as a guide in the longer term. Gadisseux & Ward (1989), in an excellent review of the problems of nutrition in head-injured patients, point out the limitations of evaluation by body weight. They advocate regular measurement of arm muscle circumference to monitor protein stores and triceps skin-fold thickness to monitor subcutaneous fat stores; however, in the early stages after injury, these may not give a meaningful impression of the nutritional status. Serum protein levels, especially serum albumin, are routinely measured; the albumin level falls initially but should rise within 2 weeks of injury, and if it does not, the management may be at fault. Gadisseux & Ward state that the serum transferrin level is a more sensitive indicator of nutritional inadequacy, but we have not found it very helpful.

For long-term feeding, percutaneous endoscopic gastrostomy (PEG) has been very satisfactory and it is our practice to employ this route of enteral feeding in patients who are unable to begin ordinary oral feeding after 4 weeks. The procedure may be used earlier if nasogastric feeding is unsafe. The procedure is done under general anaesthesia or under local anaesthesia with sedation; a gastroscopy is performed, the stomach is distended by inflation, and a cannula is inserted through a small incision in the anterior abdominal wall. A guide-wire is passed through the cannula and snared through the gastroscope; a feeding tube is then passed from the mouth over the guide-wire and drawn out through the abdominal wound (Hollands et al 1989). PEG has been very satisfactory in our practice; complications include infection of the anterior abdominal wall and dislodgement of the feeding tube, but these have not had serious consequences. Moore et al (1992) combine PEG with percutaneous tracheostomy; this has not been our practice.

Bladder and bowels

The unconscious patient may show urinary retention, but intermittent incontinence is more often seen. In males, this can be managed by a penile sheath drain. However, in the acute phase of recovery, a urinary catheter may be unavoidable, to measure urinary output. A silicone rubber catheter is used to minimize urethral irritation.

Recovery from coma

Many studies have shown a clear relationship between duration of coma and long-term neurological disability (Bricolo et al 1980). It is therefore understandable that endeavours have been made to arouse the comatose patient by intensive sensory stimulation as early as possible. The merits of this approach are still in dispute (Mitchell et al 1990, Pierce et al 1990).

As awareness returns, benign sensory stimulation is unquestionably desirable, and a reassuring environment should be provided: familiar faces, voices and music have seemed beneficial, especially in injured children. At this stage, and indeed earlier if possible, family members are enlisted as key workers in the rehabilitation team, which should now form a rehabilitation programme based on assessment of the likely physical, cognitive and behavioural impairments. In our management plan, the post-acute rehabilitation of patients with such impairments resulting from CMF injuries is undertaken in a separate unit (p. 649); if this is done, there must be close liaison with other members of the craniofacial team to ensure that facial, dental and visual problems are not overlooked.

Duration of unconsciousness

The daily nursing GCS records, if properly used, indicate when the patient began to respond to orders and to speak. This event is for the lay person the 'waking-up time' and it should always be noted, though a speech impairment may be a confounding factor.

Full restoration of consciousness is taken as the emergence from post-traumatic amnesia (PTA), and the duration of the PTA is a most valuable measure of the severity of a closed brain injury (Russell & Smith 1961). In the past, the PTA has been estimated retrospectively by asking the patient to give his first clear recollection, and to time this from records of some verifiable event. This simple measure is often unreliable in adults and is worthless in young children. The duration of unconsciousness is better defined by questions on orientation and memory, periodically administered to the patient during recovery; several suitable questionnaires are now available (Levin et al 1979, Shores et al 1986).

Complications and outcomes of traumatic coma

When coma persists after resuscitation, the victim is likely to have sustained significant brain injury, especially diffuse axonal and vascular lesions. The outcome of coma management therefore depends very largely on the severity of the primary cerebral injury, though the quality of management of secondary cerebral injuries is an important contributory factor. There have been many studies of the outcome of closed head injuries, and the GCS has been widely used to rank the severity of the brain injury; if a severe head injury is defined as a case with GCS ≤ 8 6 hours after the impact, the mortality of severe head injuries thus defined is ~40% and recovery is often incomplete. Gennarelli et al (1982), in an early study of an aggregated series of 1107 cases in coma after non-missile head injury, found that the overall mortality was 41%, and survival with severe disability, or vegetative survival, was recorded in 17%; 'acceptable' recovery was recorded in 42%. Cases in deep coma (GCS 3–5 after 24 h), and decerebrate, showed a mortality of 57%. The pathogenesis of the coma had obvious relevance: patients comatose after extradural haemorrhage showed a 20% mortality, against 61% for patients comatose after acute subdural haemorrhage. In all series known to us, older age has worsened the outlook for post-traumatic coma, except in the paediatric age group (pp. 522 and 512).

It has been suggested that in general the likelihood of recovery after impacts in the CMF area is better than after lateral or posterior head impacts (p. 108). Whether this is true of the outcome of post-traumatic coma from a CMF impact remains to be determined.

EXTRADURAL HAEMATOMA

Surgical pathology

Extradural haemorrhage (EDH) may result from comparatively minor frontal impacts. If the rate of bleeding is rapid, there will be progressive worsening of the conscious level and the classic signs of transtentorial herniation – ipsilateral pupillary dilatation, slowing pulse etc. Often, however, the presentation of a frontal EDH is less dramatic: the patient may never lose consciousness, and may only complain of severe persistent headache (Fig. 4.14).

Alternatively, the EDH may be found as an unsuspected lesion in the investigation of a more severe frontal impact causing CMFT fractures and persisting impairment of consciousness.

Management

In all presentations, CT scan is diagnostic (p. 204), and should only be omitted when rapid deterioration makes even a short delay undesirable. Hyperacute presentation of an EDH is unusual in CMF trauma, being more characteristically due to a lateral impact.

A frontal EDH should be evacuated through the standard coronal scalp flap and a craniotomy of appropriate size (Fig. 13.11). After haemostasis, the dura should be sutured to the margins of the craniotomy; suction drainage is often desirable (p. 245). Conservative treatment of EDH is warranted only if the patient is conscious and the clot small and without evidence of cerebral displacement; in comatose patients, we evacuate even relatively small clots for fear of recurrent or continuing bleeding especially if ICP is elevated.

Complications and results

The overall mortality of uncomplicated EDH in our hands has improved since the advent of CT scanning to 8.5% during the period 1986–1990 (Jones et al 1993) — not too far from the enviable figure of 5% achieved in Verona by Bricolo & Pasut (1984). It has been our impression that the frontal extradural haematomas likely to result from impacts in the CMF region are especially favourable. In 209 cases of EDH treated during the years 1976–1990, the mortality in 29 cases of frontal EDH was 10.3%, compared with 12.8% in 180 cases of EDH in other sites; the proportion of good recoveries was 82.8% and 66.1% respectively. This is suggestive, but the difference in good recoveries does not achieve significance.

ACUTE SUBDURAL HAEMATOMA

Surgical pathology

Acute subdural haemorrhage (ASDH) is seen after more severe impacts, usually in the frontolateral or lateral area. Consciousness is usually impaired from the time of the impact, and often there are already signs of transtentorial herniation when the diagnosis is made. CT scan is essential, not only to visualize the ASDH (see p. 207), but also to assess signs of brain swelling and contusion.

Management

If the ASDH is > 5–10 mm thick, and especially if there is > 5 mm displacement of the midline structures, then operation should be done with all possible urgency — always assuming that the patient is not already moribund. The operation usually begins with a large frontotemporal scalp flap and an osteoplastic flap of similar size; the dura is widely opened, the clot is evacuated and any active bleeding is dealt with. It is desirable to avoid a bony decompression; if the brain swelling at operation seems to make replacing the bone flap impossible, then the dural opening is enlarged by inserting a fascial or pericranial graft. The graft is sutured to the dural margins, to avoid

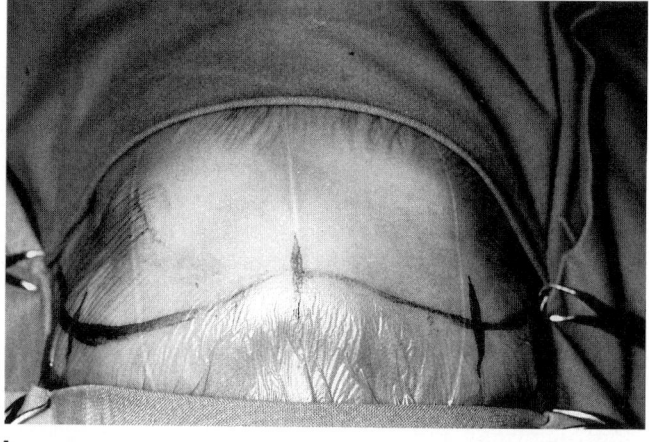

A

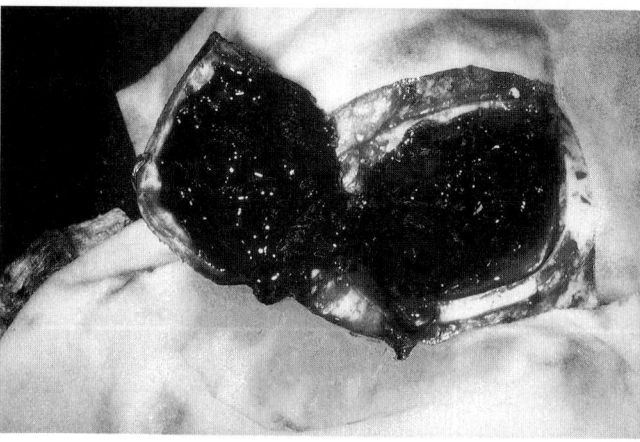

B

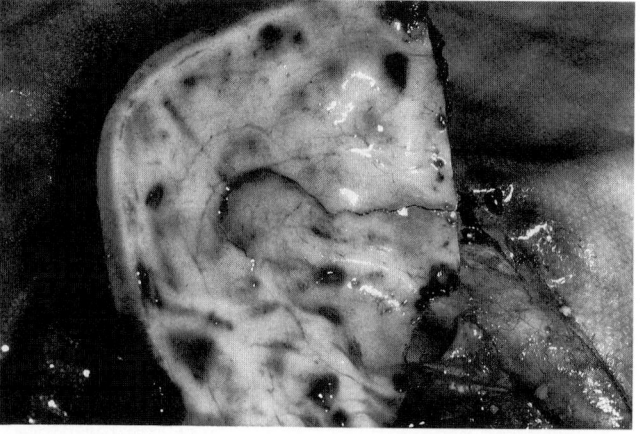

C

Fig. 13.11 Removal of a frontal extradural clot by osteoplastic craniotomy. An 8-year-old girl was struck in the left frontal region with a baseball club. She complained of intermittent headache, but retained consciousness. CT scan 13 days after injury showed a large left frontal extradural clot. **A** The standard coronal scalp flap gave good exposure without a visible scar. **B** Unilateral frontal craniotomy showed a large mass of solid clot. **C** There was a large fracture in the centre of the bone flap, with some depression at the point of impact.

venous nipping when the brain swells, as it usually does, in the postoperative period.

Complications and results

The general mortality of ASDH is high and permanent severe disability is unhappily common. In the series reported by Stening et al (1986), the mortality was 76%, with good recovery in only 8% and moderate disability in 11%. This was a population-based study and included many cases not treated by neurosurgeons; nevertheless, the mortality was 68% even when the initial treatment was under neurosurgical supervision. More recently, Wilberger et al (1991) reported a very similar mortality (66%) and 'functional recovery' (19%), with somewhat better results when operation was done within 4 h of injury.

INTRACEREBRAL HAEMATOMAS

Surgical pathology

Intracerebral haemorrhage (ICH) of surgical significance is not very common after blunt impact in the CMF area, but may occur from rupture of one of the striate arteries or in association with a frontal skull fracture. Sometimes a significant ICH presents at an interval of a day or more after the causative impact (Bullock & Teasdale 1990); this underlines the need to repeat the CT scan if progress is unsatisfactory.

ICH is a common sequel of penetrating frontal wounds due to missiles. Delayed ICH from traumatic aneurysms due to missile wounding has been reported, and if the track of the missile raises this possibility, angiography should be performed (Haddad et al 1991), especially when the missile is a small fragment.

Management

Many intracerebral haematomas are best treated conservatively in the expectation that the clot will liquefy and slowly resorb. However, if there is clinical or CT evidence of cerebral compression, operative intervention is usually necessary. Careful judgement is needed here: in the presence of severe brain swelling, an operation planned to evacuate an ICH may end as a frontal or temporal lobectomy, and the resulting disabilities may be very severe.

Solid haematomas are evacuated through a frontal craniotomy, though burrhole aspiration has been successful in some cases of chronic type. When an ICH results from rupture of a traumatic false aneurysm, recurrent bleeding is likely and it is usually necessary to clip the injured artery; the aneurysm is commonly not amenable to repair.

BRAIN SWELLING

Surgical pathology

CT may show diffuse or localized brain swelling. Brain swelling may be due to an increase in brain water from vasogenic or cytotoxic oedema, or to an increase in cerebral blood volume (p. 145). Underlying both forms of oedema is a disorder of fluid exchange across semipermeable membranes. This may be due to mechanical disruption, failure of energy dependent mechanisms or increase in transmembrane fluid pressure.

Brain swelling is a dynamic process and after head injury several types of brain swelling may coexist. For example, raised ICP due to vascular engorgement, or due to vasogenic oedema, may lead to ischaemia and hence to cytotoxic oedema.

Management

Because it is at present impossible to identify the dominant cause of brain swelling in a particular patient, treatment is the same for all types; it is predominantly effected by medical therapy (see above).

INTRACRANIAL INFECTION

Management

Early diagnosis is imperative. Fulminating meningitis rapidly becomes irreversible, and an undiagnosed brain abscess may cause death from brainstem compression or rupture into the ventricle. Treatment requires intimate collaboration with an experienced microbiologist, both in the choice of antibiotic (Table 13.3) and in the monitoring of progress.

MENINGITIS

Clinical and radiological assessment

Diagnosis is easy when the patient presents with the classical symptoms of headache, fever and neck stiffness, after recovery from a head injury known to have involved the paranasal air sinuses. Diagnosis may be much harder when the patient is still in coma, or otherwise suffering from the effects of a massive CMF injury. In our series of 31 patients who suffered one or more attacks of meningitis complicating a cranionasal fistula (see Table 5.2),

Table 13.3 Antibiotics recommended for organisms causing serious infections of the central nervous system

Organisms	Treatment Standard	Alternative
Penicillin/amoxycillin-sensitive organisms		
Haemophilus influenzae (β-lactamase negative)	Amoxycillin	Third-generation cephalosporin★ Chloramphenicol
Neisseria meningitidis	Penicillin G	Third-generation cephalosporin★ Chloramphenicol
Streptococcus species including *Strep. pneumonia*	Penicillin G	Third-generation cephalosporin★ Chloramphenicol
Staph. aureus/Staph. epidermidis (β-lactamase negative)	Penicillin G	Chloramphenicol, Vancomycin
Anaerobic bacteria — *Clostridia fusobacteria*	Penicillin G	Metronidazole
Relatively resistant organisms		
Haemophilus influenzae (β-lactamase negative)	Third-generation cephalosporin★	Chloramphenicol
Strept. pneumoniae (moderately penicillin resistant)	Third-generation cephalosporin★	Chloramphenicol
Staph. aureus (β-lactamase positive)	Flucloxacillin	Vancomycin
Enterobacteriaceae (β-lactamase inducible negative)	Third-generation cephalosporin★	Imipenem
Bacteroides species (β-lactamase positive)	Metronidazole	Chloramphenicol
Resistant organisms		
Enterobacteriaceae (β-lactamase inducible positive)	Imipenem ± aminoglycoside	Consult microbiologist
Pseudomonas aeruginosa	Anti-pseudomonad penicillin and aminoglycoside	Ceftazidime and aminoglycoside Imipenem with aminoglycoside
Staph. aureus/Staph. epidermidis (methicillin resistant)	Vancomycin and Rifampicin	Consult microbiologist

★ Third-generation cephalosporins: ceftriaxone or ceftaxime.

there were only five examples of onset within the first week after injury. Six others occurred during the first year, and the remainder after periods of 1–19 years. Lumbar puncture establishes the diagnosis and usually identifies the organism and its antibiotic sensitivities. However, CT scan should be done first, to exclude severe brain swelling or abscess, when withdrawal of CSF might precipitate transtentorial herniation. If lumbar puncture is contraindicated, burrhole exploration may sometimes be warranted, to obtain a little CSF from a cortical subarachnoid cistern or from the lateral ventricle if this is not collapsed. A blood culture is taken: in our experience, bacteraemia is unusual in cases of delayed meningitis complicating a cranionasal fistula, but may occur when infection supervenes in a severely injured patient under intensive care.

Management

Intravenous chemotherapy is begun as soon as possible. Ideally, CSF is taken first, but in very fulminating meningitis, any delay may be disastrous, and it is often wise to begin therapy immediately the diagnosis is suspected. The choice of antibiotics is now difficult. The commonest organisms causing post-traumatic meningitis are *Streptococcus pneumoniae* and *Haemophilus influenzae*, in that order, and in the past these organisms were sensitive to penicillin and ampicillin respectively. It was therefore reasonable to give these antibiotics in high dosage at once, or after direct CSF smear had given the probable diagnosis. Unhappily, this is no longer wise, at least in our community. Ampicillin-resistant haemophilus organisms have been prevalent for a long time. Penicillin-resistant pneumococci were first encountered in Australasia (Hansman & Bullen 1967, Hansman et al 1971) and are now prevalent in many parts of America and Europe, though still rare in our community. It is therefore prudent to give initially a third-generation cephalosporin. At present, we favour cefotaxime (200 mg/kg/day) in 6 h doses, or ceftriaxone (100 mg/kg/day) in a single daily dose: in practice, the daily adult dose of cefotaxime is 2–12 g, and the daily dose of ceftriaxone only 1–6 g. When the sensitivities are known, more selective chemotherapy may be given.

Staphylococcal meningitis is not common as a sequel of CMF injury. Flucloxacillin or oxacillin is recommended; vancomycin is appropriate when the organism is resistant to these antibiotics, and in persons sensitive to penicillins. Multiply-resistant Gram-negative organisms may be seen when meningitis occurs in patients under intensive care, especially when broad spectrum antibiotics have been given prophylactically (see above). For such organisms, β-lactam antibiotics such as imipenem (Primaxin) may be given, or an aminoglycoside. Aminoglycosides penetrate the CSF poorly, even when there

is active infection, and may have to be given intrathecally (e.g. tobramycin or gentamicin 4–10 mg per dose). In the past, we used various intrathecal or intraventricular antibiotics (penicillin, methicillin, chloramphenicol, gentamicin) routinely for severe meningitis, and provided the doses were small, we saw no adverse effects. However, contemporary wisdom condemns this route of administration unless there is an overriding need.

In all cases of meningitis, antibiotic therapy is monitored by blood level assays; if the clinical response is poor, lumbar puncture is repeated to determine the CSF antibiotic level and to check that the organism is still sensitive to the antibiotic chosen.

CEREBRAL ABSCESS

Surgical pathology

We recorded only five cases of brain abscess as a complication of cranionasal fistula (Table 5.2), and we have seen even fewer from compound frontal skull fractures or penetrating wounds (Fig. 13.6). However, when adequate primary neurosurgical management is for whatever reason not available, brain abscesses are common. In a South African series of 641 brain abscesses, 142 (22%) were caused by implantation, chiefly in scalp wounds and compound fractures (Keet 1990). We have seen similar cases referred from outback Australian hospitals. Brain abscesses complicating military missile injuries used to be a common cause of death; Rish et al (1981) reported an incidence of only 3% in American Vietnamese experience, but in wars fought under circumstances less favourable for neurosurgical management, it seems likely that more cases will be seen.

Clinical and radiological assessment

In our small experience, frontal cerebral abscesses complicating cranionasal fistulas have presented between 5 weeks and 2 years after injury. Much longer latent periods have been reported, both after anterior fossa fractures (Rath & Knöring 1989) and from implanted fragments of glass (Gordon et al 1992). Frontal cerebral abscesses may present with few or no localizing signs; epilepsy may be an early manifestation. CT scan is diagnostic (Fig. 13.6).

Management

Intravenous antibiotic therapy should be given at once. Various initial regimens have been favoured. In the past, we gave flucloxacillin and ampicillin pending a bacteriological diagnosis; this was inadequate in one tragic case, and it may now be wise to give a third-generation cephalosporin at once, together with intravenous metronidazole in view of the frequent finding of bacteroides and other anaerobes. Glucocorticoids (dexamethasone) can be given to combat cerebral oedema, but we do not like to use this until it is known that the organism is sensitive to the antibiotic(s) selected, except in cases showing severe elevation in ICP not controllable by surgical means.

Although there is a place for non-surgical management in some haematogenous brain abscesses, there is no question whatsoever that post-traumatic frontal lobe abscesses require operative aspiration and as a rule later excision. A burrhole is first made, the incision being planned with later craniotomy in mind. The abscess is aspirated under X-ray or ultrasonic guidance; stereotaxic aspiration is indicated if the abscess is small or deeply placed, and many favour this as a routine. Pus is aspirated gently (Fig. 13.12), to decompress the brain, and for microbiological diagnosis; it has been our practice to lavage the abscess cavity gently with a dilute solution of ampicillin (2 mg/ml) or other antibiotic, though with modern antibiotics this may be superfluous. Progress is monitored by CT; further aspiration is usually needed, and will allow assay of the penetration of the antibiotic into the pus.

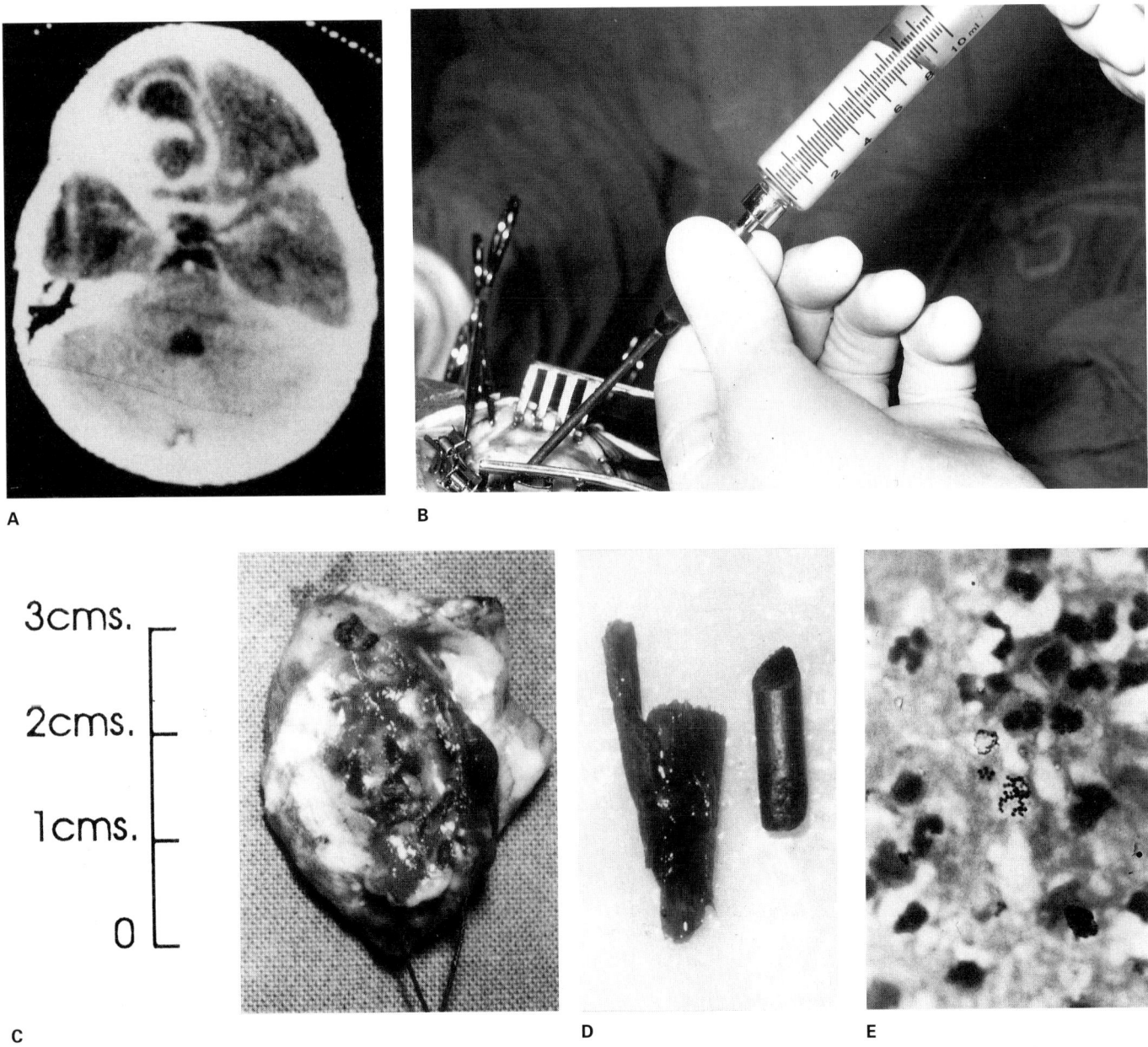

Fig. 13.12 Surgical management of a frontal brain abscess. A 6-year-old boy took a pencil to his teacher, and was tripped up by a schoolmate. He fell and drove the point of the pencil into his left orbit above the eye. The small wound was not explored. 5 weeks later, he was found to have a frontal brain abscess. Aspiration yielded pus containing a microaerophilic streptococcus and *Haemophilus aphrophilus*. 5 days later, the abscess was excised; the point of the pencil was found in the roof of the orbit. **A** CT scan, on an early scanner, showed a bilocular mass, with enhancement, in the right frontal lobe. **B** Aspiration through a frontal burrhole. **C** The frontal abscess, excised 5 days later. **D** Fragments of the pencil. **E** Gram stain showing streptococci in the abscess.

When the abscess has a firm capsule, it is excised (Fig. 13.12) en bloc. There is debate over the need for this, but in post-traumatic abscesses, there are often implanted bone chips or other foreign material (Figs 13.6 and 13.12) in relation to the abscess and this must be removed. If there is a cranionasal fistula, it must be repaired; this can be done as part of the same procedure.

SUBDURAL EMPYEMA

Surgical pathology

This is a rare complication of CMF trauma (Bannister et al 1981). We have seen two cases of devastating subdural empyema develop after minor frontal impacts (Fig. 13.13), perhaps due to pre-existing sinusitis, and cases have been reported where the subdural space has been infected from post-traumatic or postoperative osteomyelitis or from a scalp wound. Osgood et al (1975) reported an instructive case of frontal subdural empyema appearing 4 years after a craniofacial gunshot wound; the cause appeared to be a chronic frontal sinusitis.

Clinical and radiological assessment

Subdural empyema is usually an acute infection, with fever, impaired conscious level, and epileptic fits, which are often difficult to control. Loculation of pus in the parafalcine space may cause a leg monoplegia. CT with contrast enhancement should be diagnostic, though a thin film of subdural pus can be overlooked.

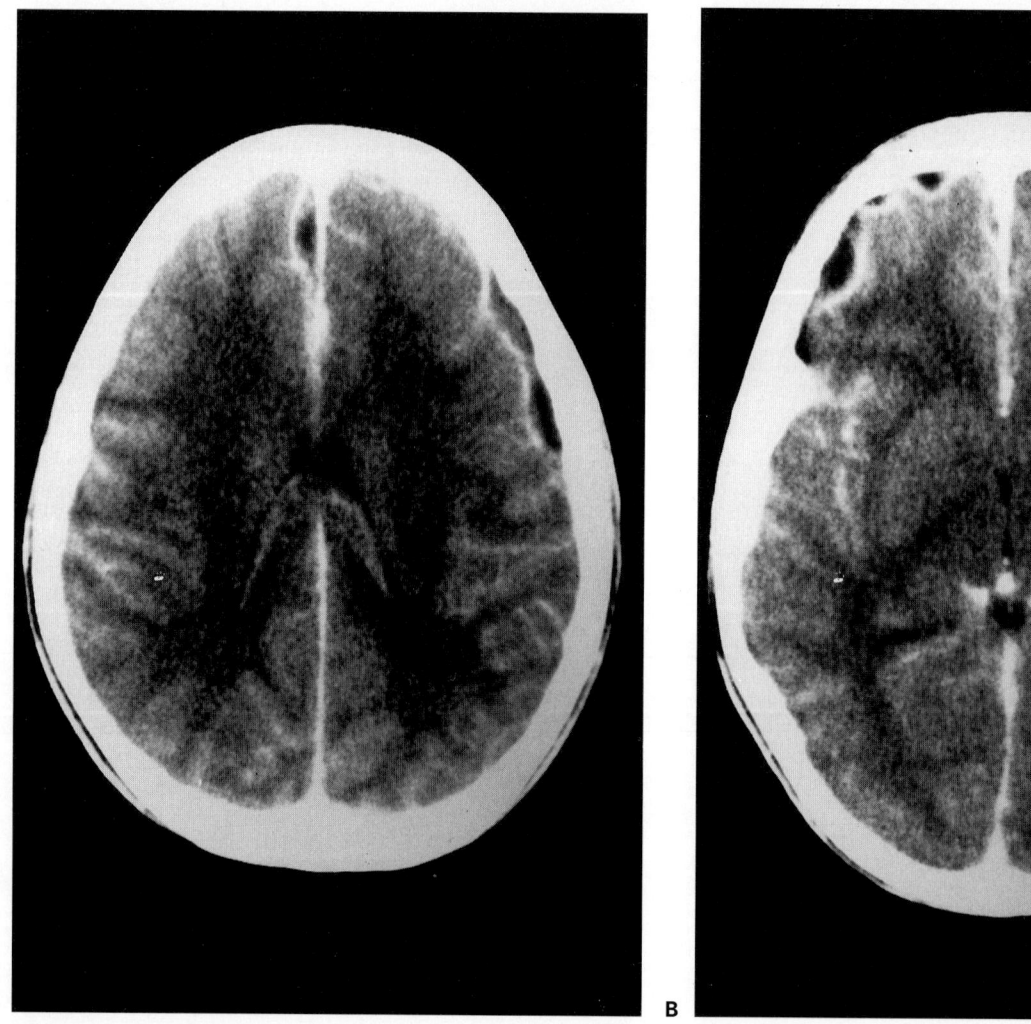

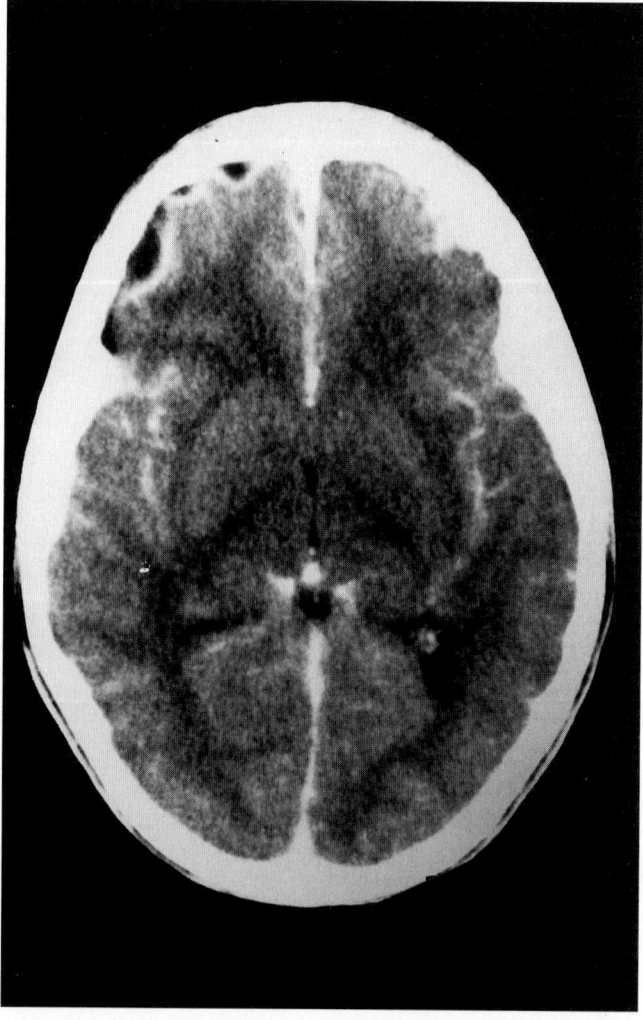

A B

Fig. 13.13 Surgical management of a subdural empyema. A 15-year-old aboriginal boy was kicked in the centre of the forehead. He developed a subcutaneous abscess which was drained in a local hospital; the pus yielded *Haemophilus influenzae*. He became febrile, drowsy and incontinent. He was flown to Adelaide where enhanced CT axial scan showed multiple loculi of subdural fluid. **A** Left frontal and interfalcine collections, with surrounding enhancement. **B** Right lower frontal collection. Three burrholes were sited over the chief loculi, and the diagnosis of subdural empyema was confirmed; in addition to *H. influenzae*, the pus yielded an anaerobic streptococcus. *Strept. milleri* was later identified. Amoxicillin and later ceftriaxone were given in large doses from the time of first microbiological diagnosis. The boy slowly made a good recovery. No frontal fracture was identified, but the microbiological findings suggested origin of the infection in a paranasal air sinus.

Management

Antibiotic therapy and immediate surgical drainage are indicated. Since subdural infection may be diffuse, or may form loculi in inaccessible places like the interhemispheric fissure, it has been usual to drain these dangerous infections through a wide craniotomy (Bannister et al 1981). This may no longer be appropriate when CT allows accurate localization of pockets of pus: Bok & Peter (1993) report excellent results in 77% of 90 patients mostly treated by burrhole evacuation, with craniectomies to expose parafalcine collections of pus. We have combined such operations with repeated antibiotic irrigation of the subdural space through catheters, but massive intravenous antibiotic therapy is probably much more important. Ingham et al (1991) have advocated an initial combination of ampicillin, gentamicin, and metronidazole or chloramphenicol. Glucocorticoids may be given, but again we prefer to withhold these until appropriate antibiotic therapy has been given. If there is evidence of sinusitis, drainage may be appropriate — in the case reported by Osgood et al (1975) the frontal sinus was exenterated and packed with fat.

OSTEOMYELITIS AND EXTRADURAL ABSCESS

These are much less serious complications of CMF trauma. Antibiotic therapy and surgical drainage, with removal of grossly infected bone, are usually effective. In modern craniofacial surgery, postoperative frontal infection and extradural abscess are troublesome complications, usually seen after procedures done for congenital deformities rather than for trauma (David & Cooter 1987). Infection gains entry during a prolonged operation, or through openings in the paranasal air sinuses; infections are usually by low-grade pathogens, and can be very prolonged. We found record of some kind of extradural infection in as many as 12 (5.1%) cases of anterior fossa fracture treated over a period of 35 years; in several of these, it was necessary to remove infected bone craniotomy flaps, but in general this complication was easily managed, as there is not a large dead space such as may follow a fronto-orbital advancement for deformity. We have also seen a large extradural abscess develop under an area of bone made necrotic by a severe burn; this required an extensive craniectomy, and greatly increased other difficulties in management (Fig. 17.20).

Cavernous thrombophlebitis

We have not seen this dangerous infection as a complication of trauma in the CMF region. However, Ingham et al (1991) mention the association, and cite cases in the literature where septic cavernous thrombophlebitis followed surgical procedures in the facial region. The possibility must therefore be kept in mind when proptosis, chemosis and limitation of eye movement appear with signs of sepsis after an injury or operation. The differential diagnosis will be from orbital cellulitis, a less uncommon complication, or from carotid–cavernous fistula; auscultation will usually rule out the latter condition. Diagnosis is by CT with strong contrast enhancement or by MRI angiography; Ingham et al (1991) describe the various changes seen in the cavernous sinuses. In the past, we have used cerebral angiography in non-traumatic cases, and have been impressed by the striking changes in the carotid artery, which may be narrowed and irregular. Treatment is by chemotherapy in high dosage; it appears that the risks of heparin therapy outweigh the advantages.

Complications and results of intracranial infection

In general, the results of treatment of post-traumatic meningitis are good. In our series of 31 cases of meningitis complicating a cranionasal fistula, there were two deaths, one after a seemingly trivial impact causing a crack fracture in the anterior fossa (Caldicott et al 1973: case 6). In at least one case, it seemed that there was an increased cerebral disability after a non-fatal attack of meningitis.

But this low mortality should not engender complacency. Patients still occasionally die from fulminating meningitis, or suffer irreversible cerebral damage from vasculitis, or develop postinfective hydrocephalus. The case for prevention is still valid.

The results of treatment of post-traumatic cerebral abscess are also not bad, and better than those with other types of brain abscess. But there is a high incidence of epilepsy, often permanent, and the case for preventive surgery is even stronger than with post-traumatic meningitis.

Earlier experience with non-traumatic subdural empyemas showed that these infections carried a high mortality, and permanent brain damage was recorded in a high proportion of survivors (Bannister et al 1981). In the series of Bok & Peter (1993) quoted above, the mortality was only 7.7%, with incapacitating sequelae in only 4%. This very gratifiying improvement was attributed largely to the use of CT scanning.

CAROTID CAVERNOUS FISTULA

Surgical pathology

The most common cause (75–90%) of carotid–cavernous fistula (CCF) is head trauma, and usually a blunt impact is responsible, though penetrating injuries account for a small percentage.

The internal carotid artery is strongly fixed by its dural attachment between the carotid canal and the cavernous sinus, and also where it leaves the sinus just below the anterior clinoid process. The artery is vulnerable to shearing forces acting between these fixed points of attachment. The pathology has been discussed; in most cases, there is a single tear in the artery, resulting in a high-flow fistula with massive arterialization of the cavernous sinus. The flow in the superior and inferior ophthalmic veins is often reversed, with engorgement and dilatation of these vessels. High venous pressure causes chemosis, proptosis and elevated intraocular pressure; venous distension may also cause paralysis of the third, fourth and sixth cranial nerves. There is often a latent interval between injury and the signs of fistula. In such cases, it is considered likely that the injury caused a minor tear in the carotid artery which subsequently gave rise to a traumatic aneurysm; rupture of the aneurysm leads to the fistula. A few patients suffer cerebral ischaemia from diversion of the arterial blood into the fistula (steal effect), especially if the circle of Willis is poorly developed.

Clinical assessment

An ophthalmological evaluation is needed to assess the threat to vision. The visual symptoms and signs are chiefly due to the elevated venous pressure, which may result in loss of vision from glaucoma. To prevent this, emergency treatment with appropriate medication (p. 417) should be instituted if the ocular pressure exceeds 25 mmHg; pressures > 40 mmHg represent a serious threat to vision.

The onset of symptoms is usually abrupt. Some days after injury the patient may become aware of a pulsatile bruit, and this is audible on auscultation. A pulsatile ex-ophthalmos develops and eventually there may be gross swelling of the orbital tissues, distended and arterialized conjunctival veins and venous engorgement of the retina.

In some (5–10%) cases, the fistula closes spontaneously; this is likely to happen with low-flow fistulas, and can be promoted by digital compression of the ipsilateral common carotid artery — a tedious and uncertain method of treatment. However, in about 70% of high-flow fistulas, the common post-traumatic variety, progressive ocular damage takes place. In these cases, blindness may result from the initial injury or from corneal ulceration due to exposure, but more commonly results from retinal ischaemia due to a combination of decreased arterial flow and venous hypertension (Harris & Barrow 1992). Patients also suffer from gross disfigurement and a persistent pulsatile bruit; there is a 3% mortality, chiefly from catastrophic epistaxis from arterialized nasal veins or from intracranial haemorrhage (Dohrmann et al 1985).

Radiological assessment

CT scan delineates the proptosis; contrast shows enlargement of the superior ophthalmic veins and the cavernous sinus (Fig. 13.14A). Cerebral angiography is needed to show the location of the CCF, and the pattern of drainage of the cavernous sinus. Ultrasonography has been used to demonstrate pulsatile veins, and to monitor the success of surgical measures.

Management

Various operations to trap and embolize the fistula have been described. These usually require permanent occlusion of the ipsilateral internal carotid artery and despite this have a high relapse rate. Incomplete obliteration of the fistula simply leads to enlarging of other venous channels. Better results were obtained by embolizing the artery with pieces of muscle introduced through a cervical arterotomy. This was procedure succeeded by the use of non-detachable balloons, and then by Serbinenko's (1974) elegant technique of embolization with a detachable balloon.

Today, there are two main approaches to treatment, both of which aim to preserve the internal carotid artery.

Intravascular radiology using intra-arterial or intravenous balloon embolization

This is now the treatment of choice (Higashida et al 1989). The intra-arterial approach is successful in ~90% of traumatic CCF. The uninflated latex or silicone balloon is directed by blood flow from the internal carotid artery, through the fistula into the cavernous sinus and then inflated. The inflation of the balloon results in occlusion of the cavernous sinus and the fistula; the balloon is then detached and the lumen of the carotid artery is maintained (Fig. 13.14B). In a large CCF, many balloons may be necessary. The balloons may be filled with a polymerizing solution (e.g. cyanoacrylate) so that the balloon is permanently inflated, to avoid premature deflation due to leakage of the radiological contrast medium.

The cavernous sinus may also be embolized through the internal jugular vein and inferior petrosal sinus or the superior ophthalmic vein. This approach is useful with low flow fistulas; it is indicated when the vein used has been dilated by arterialization for at least 3 months.

Exposure by craniotomy and repair of the intracavernous carotid artery

Techniques of transdural intracavernous surgery have been developed in recent years and this approach is gaining more support. The cavernous sinus can be obliterated with balloons injected into its lumen at operation (Debrun et al 1988), or with muscle fragments and/or fibrin sealant (Isamat et al 1986); under favourable circumstances, the rent in the internal carotid artery can be sutured under vision (Dolenc 1983).

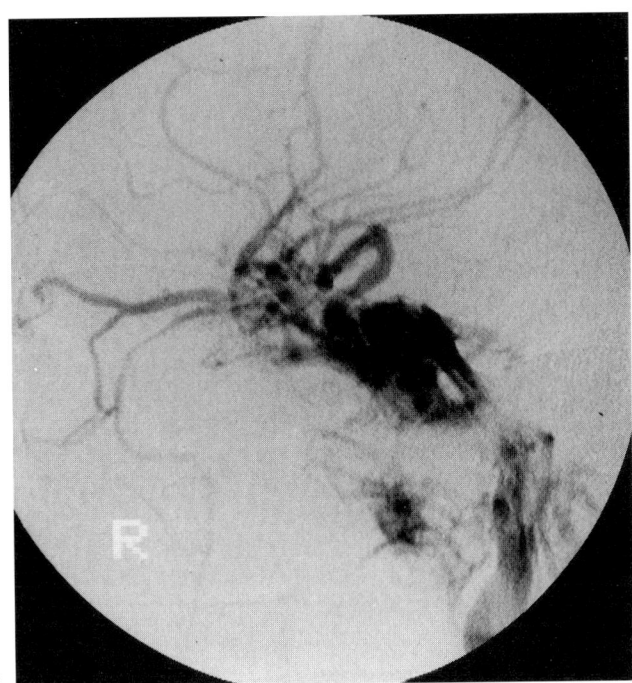 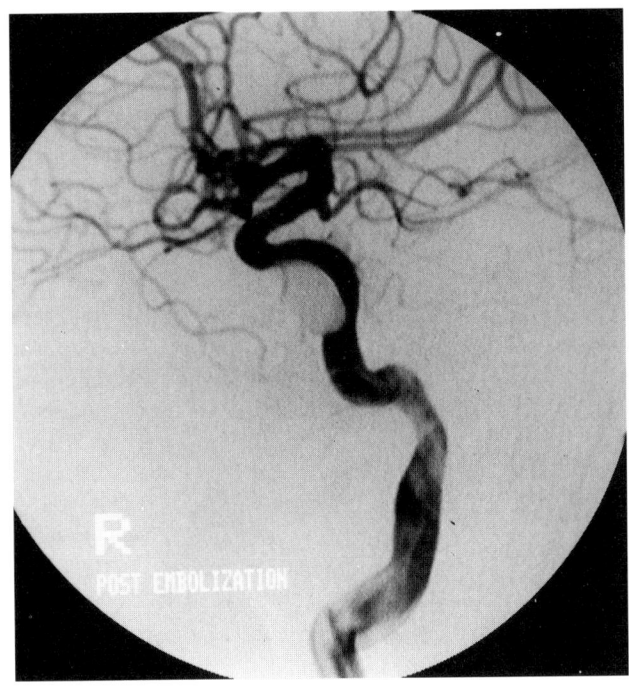

Fig. 13.14 Carotid-cavernous fistula obliterated by balloon embolization. A 60-year-old man fell from a ladder while pruning a tree. He struck his face and head on the right side. He suffered a fracture of the mandible, and exhibited right orbital swelling and paresis of the right sixth and third nerves. **A** Angiography showed a high flow carotid–cavernous fistula from the first part of the intracavernous internal carotid artery. **B** 12 days after the injury, the fistula was occluded with a flow-directed silicone balloon, initially filled with 0.8 ml of contrast medium, which was then exchanged for HEMA (hydroxyethylmethacrylate). The catheter was then detached. He required corrective surgery for a persisting sixth nerve weakness a year later; the fistula remained occluded.

Complications and results

Depending on the skill and experience of the radiologist, the intravascular therapy of traumatic CCF is successful in up to 95% of cases, or 100% if cases with loss of patency in the internal carotid artery are included (Debrun et al 1988); in most cases, the arterial approach is used. There is a possible risk of inadvertent embolization of a major cerebral artery, with resultant cerebral infarction; this form of treatment demands much experience in interventional radiology. Direct surgical repair is also a demanding operation, and we have not yet employed it.

POST-TRAUMATIC EPILEPSY

Incidence

Jennett (1975) studied a series of 300 depressed fractures of the skull, of which 118 (29%) were in the CMF region. The incidence of early epilepsy in the frontal group was 11%, not statistically different from other anatomical sites of injury. Late epilepsy occurred in 21% of these cases. The incidence of epilepsy after frontal missile wounds is even higher (Whitty 1961). Salazar et al (1985a) have correlated the incidence of seizures after missile wounds with the volume of loss of cerebral substance; the same study supported the impression that lesions in the temporal and frontal lobes are more likely to generate seizures than more posterior lesions (Salazar et al 1985b).

Prophylaxis

Post-traumatic epilepsy can be lethal and is often disabling. Status epilepticus may occur, with substantial risks and management problems. It has also been claimed that subclinical seizures in the unconscious patient may have detrimental effects on ICP (Marienne et al 1979). Early epileptic fits after head injury are associated with a four-fold risk of late epilepsy with its attendant social disabilities (p. 659). There are thus ample grounds for giving anticonvulsant medication to cases of head injury known to be at risk of seizures. Jennett's (1975) excellent data suggest that an intracranial haematoma, a history of early fits, focal signs of a brain wound, and a depressed skull fracture all raise the risk of late epilepsy above 20%. It seems likely that the intracranial haematomas at high risk of epilepsy are those with cerebral damage, and we do not regard extradural haematomas without CT evidence of intradural pathology as high-risk cases. We therefore give anticonvulsant medication as soon as possible after high-risk head injuries. An initial loading dose of phenytoin (adult loading dose 12 mg/kg) is given intravenously (rate 25 mg/min); thereafter, 5 mg/kg/day is given 6–8 hourly, either orally or intravenously; after discharge from hospital, carbamazepine (20 mg/kg/day in two divided doses) is progressively substituted, as it appears to have fewer side-effects than phenytoin (Smith & Collins 1987), though this is by no means proven to be the case. Medication is monitored by plasma level assays. Griebel et al (1990) monitor both free and total plasma phenytoin in paediatric cases of severe trauma, as the metabolism of the drug is disturbed and toxic effects may result; we have not routinely done this. Medication is continued for an arbitrary period of 2 years if no seizures occur; an EEG is usually done before medication is ceased.

As Janz (1994) has shown in a review of the copious literature, this policy rests on very uncertain foundations. The beneficial effects of giving phenytoin to suppress subclinical fits in cases of coma are yet to be confirmed. Our colleagues North et al (1983) showed convincingly that prophylactic phenytoin reduced the incidence of early postoperative fits in a controlled study of 281 cases (including 100 head injuries), and this was confirmed by Temkin et al (1990). But these studies showed no long-term protective benefit from phenytoin and it has yet to be proved that anticonvulsants reduce the risk of late post-traumatic epilepsy (McQueen et al 1983, Young et al 1983), nor is there any good evidence that the EEG has predictive value for the onset of late seizures. Nevertheless, the case for routine anticonvulsant therapy in high-risk head injuries is very persuasive, and despite these depressing reports we continue to give carbamazepine or phenytoin for up to 2 years in cases with an estimated risk of seizures in excess of 20%.

Management

If a seizure does occur in the early period after CMF injury, anticonvulsant control is essential; for established or threatening status epilepticus, intravenous diazepam (2 mg/min to 10–20 mg) or clonazepam is appropriate, and if the response is not immediate, endotracheal intubation and thiopentone anaesthesia should be instituted at once. Although it is unusual for a post-traumatic seizure to result from an intracranial haematoma of surgical significance (Jennett 1975), an urgent CT scan should be obtained, and the possibility of infection — especially subdural empyema — should be kept in mind.

REFERENCES

Bannister G, Williams B, Smith S 1981 Treatment of subdural empyema. J Neurosurg 55: 82–88

Benzel E C, Day W T, Kesterson L et al 1991 Civilian craniocerebral gunshot wounds. Neurosurgery 29: 67–72

Bok A P L, Peter J C 1993 Subdural empyema: burr holes or craniotomy? A retrospective computerized tomography—era analysis of treatment in 90 cases. J Neurosurg 78: 574–578

Born J D, Hans P, Smitz S, Legros J J, Kay S 1985 Syndrome of inappropriate secretion of antidiuretic hormone after severe head injury. Surg Neurol 23: 383–387

Braakman R 1972 Depressed skull fracture: data, treatment and follow-up in 225 consecutive cases. J Neurol Neurosurg Psychiat 35: 395–402

Brandt K E, Burruss G L, Hickerson W L, White C E 1991 The management of mid-face fractures with intracranial injury. J Trauma 31: 15–19

Brandvold B, Levi L, Feinsod M, George E D 1990 Penetrating craniocerebral injuries in the Israeli involvement in the Lebanese conflict, 1982–1985. Analysis of a less aggressive surgical approach. J Neurosurg 72: 15–21

Bricolo A P, Pasut L M 1984 Extradural hematoma: towards zero mortality: a prospective study. Neurosurgery 14: 8–12

Bricolo A, Turazzi S, Feriotti G 1980 Prolonged posttraumatic unconsciousness: therapeutic assets and liabilities. J Neurosurg 52: 625–634

Bullock R, Teasdale G 1990 Surgical management of traumatic intracranial haematomas. In: Vinken P J, Bruyn G W, Klawans H L (eds) Handbook of clinical neurology: revised series 13. Elsevier, Amsterdam, Vol 57, Ch 10

Caldicott W J H, North J B, Simpson D A 1973 Traumatic cerebrospinal fluid fistulas in children. J Neurosurg 38: 1–9

Clifton G L, Robertson C S, Grossman R G, Hodge S, Foltz R, Garza C 1984 The metabolic response to severe head injury. J Neurosurg 60: 687–696

David D J 1984 New perspectives in the management of severe craniofacial deformity. Ann R Coll Surg 66: 270–279

David D J, Cooter R D 1987 Craniofacial infection in 10 years of transcranial surgery. Plast Reconstr Surg 80: 213–225

Debrun G M, Viñuela F, Fox A J, Davis K R, Ahn H S 1988 Indications for treatment and classification of 132 carotid–cavernous fistulas. Neurosurgery 22: 285–289

Demetriades D, Charalambides D, Lakhoo M, Pantanowitz D 1992 Role of prophylactic antibiotics in open and basilar fractures of the skull: a randomized study. Injury 23: 377–380

Dinning T A R, Simpson D A, Tassie J A 1961 Infection complicating head injury. Aust NZ J Surg 30: 191–200

Dohrmann P J, Batjer H H, Samson D, Suss R A 1985 Recurrent subarachnoid hemorrhage complicating a traumatic carotid–cavernous fistula. Neurosurgery 17: 480–483

Dolenc V 1983 Direct microsurgical repair of intracavernous vascular lesions. J Neurosurg 58: 824–831

Eljamel M S, Foy P M 1990a Acute traumatic CSF fistulae: the risk of intracranial infection. Br J Neurosurg 4: 381–385

Eljamel M S, Foy P M 1990b Acute traumatic CSF fistulae: the case for surgical repair. Br J Neurosurg 4: 479–483

Findler G, Sahar A, Beller A J 1977 Continuous lumbar drainage of cerebrospinal fluid in neurosurgical patients. Surg Neurol 8: 455–457

Fremstad J D, Martin S H 1978 Lethal complication from insertion of nasogastric tube after severe basilar skull fracture. J Trauma 18: 820–822

Gadisseux P, Ward J D 1989 Nutritional support of head-injured patients. In: Becker D R, Gudeman S K (eds) Textbook of head injury. Saunders, Philadelphia, Ch 10

Gennarelli T A, Spielman G M, Langfitt T W et al 1982 Influence of the type of intracranial lesion on outcome from severe head injury. A multicenter study using a new classification system. J Neurosurg 56: 26–32

Gordon S B, Sharima B S, McKinstry C S, Fannin T F 1992 Brain abscess ten years after penetrating glass injury to skull. Ulster Med J 61: 116–118

Graf C J, Gross C E, Beck D W 1981 Complications of spinal drainage in the management of cerebrospinal fistula. J Neurosurg 54: 392–395

Grahm T W, Zadrozny D B, Harrington T 1989 The benefits of early jejunal hyperalimentation in the head-injured patient. Neurosurgery 25: 729–735

Griebel M L, Kearns G L, Fiser D H, Woody R C, Turley C D 1990 Phenytoin protein binding in pediatric patients with acute traumatic injury. Crit Care Med 18: 385–391

Haddad F S, Haddad G F, Taha J 1991 Traumatic intracranial aneurysms caused by missiles: their presentation and management. Neurosurgery 28: 1–7

Hadley M N 1992 Hypermetabolism following head trauma:

nutritional considerations. In: Barrow D L (ed) Complications and sequelae of head injury. American Association of Neurological Surgeons, Park Ridge, Illinois, Ch 11

Hansman D, Bullen M M 1967 A resistant pneumococcus. Lancet 2: 264–265

Hansman D, Glasgow H, Sturt J, Devitt L, Douglas R 1971 Increased resistance to penicillin of pneumococci isolated from man. N Engl J Med 284: 175–177

Harris M E, Barrow D L 1992 Traumatic carotid–cavernous fistula. In: Barrow D L (ed) Complications and sequelae of head injury. American Association of Neurological Surgeons, Park Ridge, Illinois, Ch 2

Higashida R T, Halbach V V, Tsai F Y et al 1989 Interventional neurovascular treatment of traumatic carotid and vertebral artery lesions: results in 234 cases. Am J Roentgenol 153: 577–582

Hollands M J, Fletcher J P, Young J 1989 Percutaneous feeding gastrostomy. Med J Aust 151: 328–331

Ingham H R, Sisson P R, Mendelow A D, Kalbag R M, McAllister V L 1991 Pyogenic neurosurgical infections. Edward Arnold, London

Isamat F, Ferrer E, Twose J 1986 Direct intracavernous obliteration of high-flow carotid–cavernous fistulas. J Neurosurg 65: 770–775

Ivatury R, Siegel J H, Stahl W M, Simon R, Scorpio R, Gens D R 1992 Percutaneous tracheostomy after trauma and critical illness. J Trauma 32: 133–140

Janz D 1994 Risiko und medicamentöse Prophylaxe von epileptischen Anfällen nach zerebralen Läsionen. Zentralbl Neurochir 55: 1–9

Jennett B 1975 Epilepsy after non-missile head injuries, 2nd edn. Heinemann, London

Jennett B, Teasdale G 1981 Management of head injuries. Davies, Philadelphia, pp 222–228

Jones N R, Molloy C J, Kloeden C N, North J B, Simpson D A 1993 Extradural haematoma: trends in outcome over 35 years. Br J Neurosurg 7: 465–471

Keet P C 1990 Cranial intradural abscess management of 641 patients during the 35 years from 1952 to 1986. Br J Neurosurg 4: 273–278

Krafft T, Spitzer W J, Farmand M, Laumer R, Seyer H 1991 Ergebnisse der kombinierten neurochirurgischen und mundkiefer-gesichtschirurgischen Behandlung von frontomaxillären Frakturen. Fortschr Kiefer Gesichtschir 36: 54–56

Leech P 1974 Cerebrospinal fluid leakage, dural fistulae and meningitis after basal skull fractures. Injury 6: 141–149

Leech P J, Paterson A 1973 Conservative and operative management for cerebrospinal leakage after closed head injury. Lancet 1: 1013–1015

Levin H S, O'Donnell V M, Grossman R G 1979 The Galveston Orientation and Amnesia Test: a practical scale to assess cognition after head injury. J Nerv Ment Dis 167: 675–684

Lewin W 1954 Cerebrospinal rhinorrhoea in closed head injuries. Br J Surg 42: 1–18

Linell E A, Robinson W L 1941 Head injuries and meningitis. J Neurol Neurosurg Psychiat 4: 23–31

Loew F, Pertuiset B, Chaumier E E, Jaksche H 1984 Traumatic, spontaneous and postoperative CSF rhinorrhoea. Adv Tech Stand Neurosurg 11: 169–207

McCormack B, Cooper P R, Persky M, Rothstein S 1990 Extracranial repair of cerebrospinal fluid fistulas: technique and results in 37 patients. Neurosurgery 27: 412–417

McDonald J V 1980 The surgical management of severe open brain injuries with consideration of the long-term results. J Trauma 20: 842–847

McQueen J K, Blackwood D H, Harris P, Kalbag R M, Johnson A L 1983 Low risk of late post-traumatic seizures following severe head injury: implications for clinical trials of prophylaxis. J Neurol Neurosurg Psychiat 46: 899–904

Marienne J P, Robert G, Bagnat E 1979 Post-traumatic acute rise of intracranial pressure related to subclinical epilepsy seizures. Acta Neurochir Suppl 28: 89–92

Miller C F, Brodkey J S, Colombi B J 1977 The danger of intracranial wood. Surg Neurol 7: 95–103

Mitchell S, Bradley V A, Welch J L, Britton P G 1990 Coma arousal procedure: a therapeutic intervention in the treatment of head injury. Brain Injury 4: 273–279

Moore F A, Haenel J B, Moore E E, Read R A 1992 Percutaneous tracheostomy/gastrostomy in brain-injured patients — a minimally invasive alternative. J Trauma 33: 435–439

Mutlukan E, Fleck B W, Cullen J F, Whittle I R 1991 Case of penetrating orbitocranial injury caused by wood. Br J Ophthalmol 75: 374–376

Nguyen T L, Bui N T 1994 Prevention of infective complications of cranio-cerebral wounds during the war on the south-west border of Vietnam (1978–9) J Clin Neurosci 1: 118–120

North J B 1971 On the importance of intracranial air. Br J Surg 58: 826–829

North B, Reilly P L 1986 Comparison among three methods of intracranial pressure recording. Neurosurgery 18: 730–732

North J B, Reilly P L 1990 Raised intracranial pressure. A clinical guide. Heinemann, Oxford

North J B, Penhall R K, Hanieh A, Frewin D B, Taylor W B 1983 Phenytoin and postoperative epilepsy. A double-blind study. J Neurosurg 58: 672–677

Oberascher G 1988 Cerebrospinal fluid otorrhoea — new trends in diagnosis. Am J Otol 9: 102–108

O'Brien M D, Reade P C 1984 The management of dural tear resulting from mid-facial fracture. Head Neck Surg 6: 810–818

Osgood C P, Dujovny M, Holm E, Postic B 1975 Delayed posttraumatic subdural empyema. J Trauma 15: 916–921

Ostrup R C, Luerssen T G, Marshall L F, Zornow M H 1987 Continuous monitoring of intracranial pressure with a miniaturized fiberoptic device. J Neurosurg 67: 206–209

Pierce J P, Lyle D M, Quine S, Evans N J, Morris J, Fearnside M 1990 The effectiveness of coma intervention. Brain Injury 4: 191–197

Popp A J, Shah D M, Berman R A et al 1982 Delayed pulmonary dysfunction in head-injured patients. J Neurosurg 57: 784–790

Probst C 1990 Neurosurgical treatment of traumatic frontobasal CSF fistulas in 300 patients (1967–1989). Acta Neurochir (Wien) 106: 37–47

Rath S A, Knöring P 1989 Late brain abscess after severe craniocerebral trauma with fronto-orbitobasal fracture. Childs Nerv Syst 5: 121–123

Raveh J, Redli M, Markwalder T M 1984 Operative management of 194 cases of combined maxillofacial frontobasal fractures: principles and surgical modifications. J Oral Maxillofac Surg 42: 555–564

Rimel R W, Giordani B, Barth J T, Jane J A 1982 Moderate head injury: completing the clinical spectrum of brain trauma. Neurosurgery 11: 344–351

Rish B L, Dillon J D, Caveness W F, Mohr J P, Kistler J, Weiss G H 1980 Evolution of craniotomy as a debridement technique for penetrating craniocerebral injuries. J Neurosurg 53: 772–775

Rish B L, Caveness W F, Dillon J D, Kistler J P, Mohr J P, Weiss G H 1981 Analysis of brain abscess after penetrating craniocerebral injuries in Vietnam. Neurosurgery 9: 535–541

Russell W R, Smith A 1961 Post-traumatic amnesia in closed head injury. Arch Neurol 5: 4–17

Ryall R G, Peacock M K, Simpson D A 1992 Usefulness of β$_2$-transferrin assay in the detection of cerebrospinal fluid leaks following head injury. J Neurosurg 77: 737–739

Salazar A M, Jabbari B, Vance S C, Grafman J, Amin D, Dillon J D 1985a Epilepsy after penetrating head injury. I. Clinical correlates: a report of the Vietnam Head Injury Study. Neurology 35: 1406–1414

Salazar A M, Amin D, Vance S C, Schlesselman S, Buck D, Grafman J 1985b Epilepsy after penetrating head injury: anatomic correlates. Neurology 35 Suppl 1: 230

Serbinenko F A 1974 Balloon catheterization and occlusion of major cerebral vessels. J Neurosurg 41: 125–145

Shapiro S A, Scully T 1992 Closed continuous drainage of cerebrospinal fluid via a lumbar subarachnoid catheter for treatment or prevention of cranial/spinal cerebrospinal fluid fistula. Neurosurgery 30: 241–245

Shores E A, Marosszeky J E, Sandanam J, Batchelor J 1986 Preliminary validation of a clinical scale for measuring the duration of post-traumatic amnesia. Med J Aust 144: 569–572

Simpson D A, Blumbergs P C, Cooter R D et al 1989 Pontomedullary tears and other gross brainstem injuries after vehicular accidents. J Trauma 29: 1519–1525

Simpson D A, David D J, Reilly P L 1990 Fractures of the anterior cranial fossa: the craniofacial approach. Asian J Surg 13: 23–31

Smith D B, Collins J B 1987 Behavioural effects of carbamazepine, phenobarbital, phenytoin, and primidone (abstract). Epilepsia 28: 598

Specht C S, Varga J H, Jalali M M, Edelstein J P 1992 Orbital cranial wooden foreign bodies diagnosed by magnetic resonance imaging. Dry wood can be isodense with air and orbital fat by computed tomography. Surv Ophthalmol 36: 341–344

Stechison M T 1992 Rapid polymerizing fibrin glue from autologous or single-donor blood: preparation and indications. J Neurosurg 76: 626–628

Steimle R, Jacquet G, Godard J, Chico F, Zaitouni A, Orabi M 1990 Die Liquorfistel — Indikationen zur Behandlung mit Lumbalpunktion und Drainage. Bericht über 66 Fälle. Zentralbl Neurochir 51: 140–144

Stening W A, Berry G, Dan N G et al 1986 Experience with acute subdural haematomas in New South Wales. Aust NZ J Surg 56: 549–556

Teitelbaum G P, Yee C A, Van Horn D D, Kim H S, Colletti P M 1990 Metallic ballistic fragments: MR imaging safety and artifacts. Radiology 175: 855–859

Temkin N R, Dikmen S S, Wilensky A J, Keihm J, Chabal S, Winn H R 1990 A randomized, double-blind study of phenytoin for the prevention of post-traumatic seizures. N Engl J Med 323: 497–502

Wallace J D, Weintraub M I, Mattson R H, Rosnagle R 1972 Status epilepticus as a complication of intrathecal fluorescein. J Neurosurg 36: 659–660

Whittle I R 1980 Beware of boomerangs and kangaroos! (Letter). Med J Aust 2: 347

Whitty C W 1961 Focal epilepsy and the study of cortical function. Med J Aust 1: 1–8

Wilberger J E, Harris M, Diamond D L 1991 Acute subdural haematoma: morbidity, mortality, and operative timing. J Neurosurg 74: 212–218

Williams D J, Simpson D A, Savage J P 1977 Cerebrospinal fluid otorhinorrhoea investigation and management. J Laryngol Otol 91: 433–436

Young B, Ott L, Twyman D et al 1987 The effect of nutritional support on outcome from severe head injury. J Neurosurg 67: 668–676

Young B, Rapp R P, Norton J A, Haack D, Tibbs P A, Bean J R 1983 Failure of prophylactically administered phenytoin to prevent late post-traumatic seizures. J Neurosurg 58: 236–241

CHAPTER 14

Ocular injuries

J. Crompton   M. Hammerton
Contributing author: E. Tan

INTRODUCTION

This chapter is not a comprehensive guide to the management of all types of ocular trauma. Such a guide would be a book in itself, and there are already several excellent texts written with this sole aim (Spoor & Nesi 1988, Shingleton et al 1991). Chapter 2 describes the anatomical and physiological basis of normal visual function, and Chapter 5 reviews the reactions of the eye to trauma. Chapter 6 sets out a system of routine ophthalmological examination, in which the minimum is a record of visual acuity: this is obligatory in virtually all craniomaxillofacial (CMF) injuries, and certainly in all ocular injuries. Our aim in this chapter is to provide building blocks on which one can found reliable management plans for the various ocular injuries commonly resulting from impacts in the CMF region. We highlight some specific measures and procedures, and offer practical tips learned from our own experience.

Classification of ocular injuries

The anatomy of the eye provides a simple basis for a clinical classification, and since the various ocular structures react to trauma in different ways, an anatomical classification is easily related to the diverse problems of management. The usual surgical distinction between open and closed or blunt injuries is also relevant. But it must be kept in mind that penetrating injuries may cause damage to more than one anatomical structure (Fig. 14.1). To a lesser degree this is also true of blunt impacts.

Incidence

Eye injuries may be seen as isolated lesions, usually due to impacts by small objects, or in conjunction with damage to neighbouring parts of the CMF skeleton, usually as the result of a blunt impact in the orbital region (Gossman et al 1992). Table 14.1 sets out the serious ocular injuries recorded in the series of 839 facial fractures described on p. 88; there were 41 (4.9%) eye injuries of all types, and it is noteworthy that there were very few penetrating injuries of the globe. This series was collected over a period of 3 years: during 1 year of this period, a prospective study of admissions to our chief adult ophthalmological service identified 21 cases of penetrating eye injury (Table 14.2). Thus, penetrating eye injury is much more frequently seen in isolation than in conjunction with other CMF injuries.

CONJUNCTIVAL INJURIES

Surgical pathology

Injuries of the conjunctiva in isolation are uncommon. They are usually associated with more extensive injury and indeed the presence of such a trivial sign as a subconjunctival haemorrhage should always alert the examiner to the possibility of some more serious injury ranging from perforation of the globe (Fig. 6.3) with a retained intraocular foreign body, to skull fracture and intracranial injury. Extensive loss of conjunctival goblet cells is detrimental, since a reduction in mucus production will produce an uncomfortable dry eye. Usually this will recover

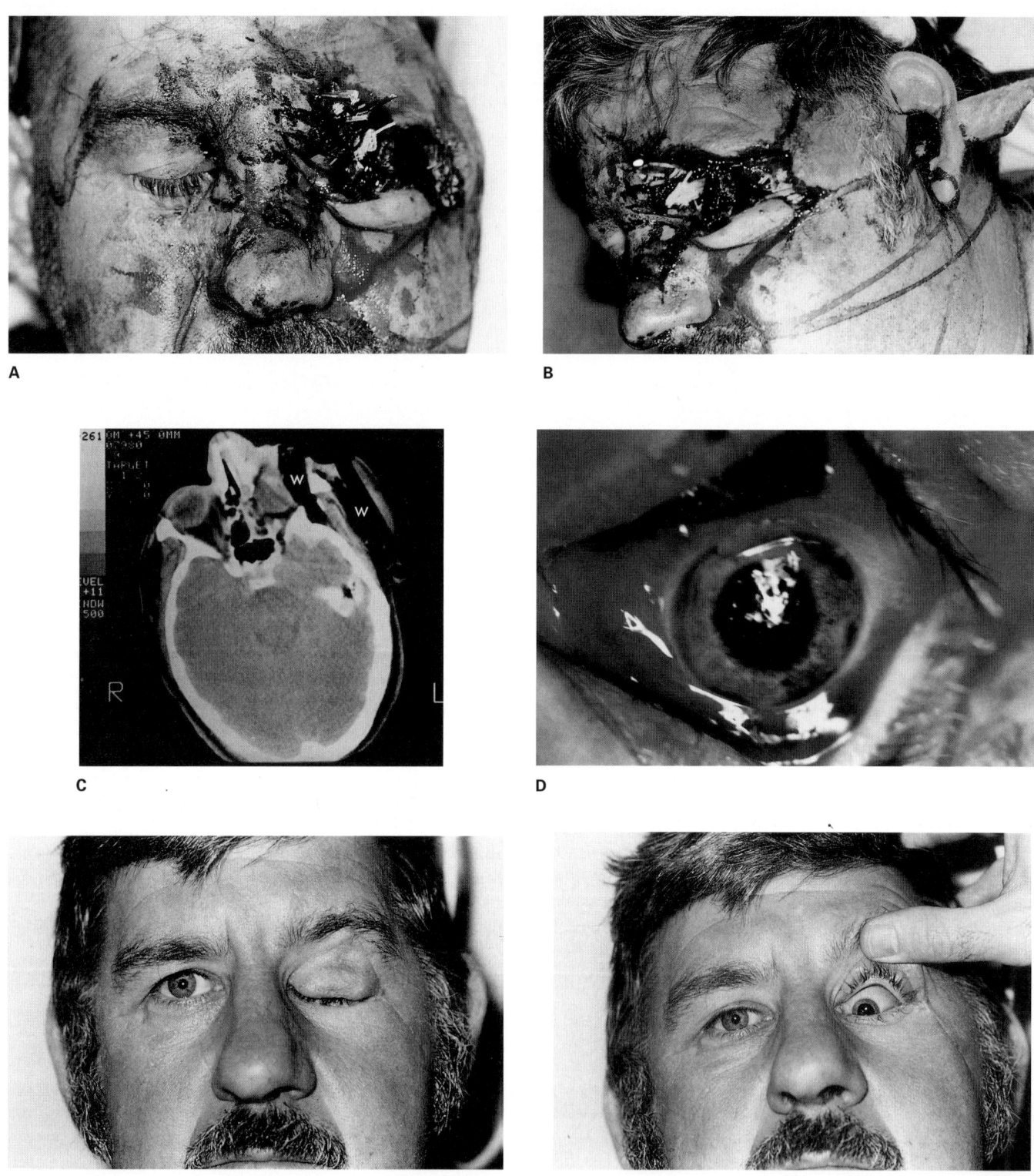

Fig. 14.1 Complex orbital injury. A 39-year-old man was struck in the left orbit by a piece of wood thrown from a circular saw in a timber mill.
A On admission, the orbit was filled with wood fragments. The eye could not be seen. **B** One fragment had transfixed the face and emerged behind the ear. **C** CT showed pieces of wood (W) as black areas in the orbit and under the skin in the temporal region. The globe of the eye was displaced medially. There was no penetration of the cranial cavity. **D** At operation, tracheostomy was performed under local anaesthesia. The zygomatic bone and its arch were temporarily removed; numerous fragments of wood were extracted and the orbital tissues were reconstructed. At the end of the operation, the globe was in correct position; the pupil was dilated and fixed, and there was hyphaema. **E, F** At follow-up, there was ptosis and a blind left eye.

Table 14.1 Ocular injuries in a series of 839 adults with facial fractures

Type of injury	No. of patients
Anterior segment	
Corneoscleral abrasions/lacerations	4
Hyphaema	10
Severe chemosis with infection	1
Increased intraocular pressure	1
Posterior segment	
Vitreous haemorrhage	3
Retinal oedema/tear/haemorrhage	10
Commotio retinae	3
Choroidal haemorrhage/rupture	1
Optic nerve damage	5
Penetrating globe injury (followed by enucleation)	3
Total	41

Table 14.2 Injuries in 21 cases of penetrating eye wound admitted to Royal Adelaide Hospital, Feb. 1990–Feb. 1991

Injured structures	No.
Cornea alone	10
Sclera alone	6
Corneo-scleral wound	5
Uvea	14
Lens	6
Vitreous	4
Retina	4
Residual foreign body	7

with the passage of time but there may be permanent effects.

Clinical assessment

Examination of the conjunctiva requires adequate magnification, which can best be done with the slit lamp microscope. If the patient cannot sit up for this, a portable slit lamp is used. If a slit lamp is not available, a magnifying loupe, together with adequate lighting, is the best substitute. At the same time, the state of the cornea, which may show associated changes, is assessed. Fluorescein, as 1% eye drops or as saturated impregnated paper strips, makes conjunctival ulcerations much more obvious; the examination is helped by a light source, such as a pencil torch or transilluminator, with a cobalt-blue filter. The examiner looks especially for a foreign body, and for damage to the underlying sclera, by using a speculum to hold the lids apart. The adequacy of the tear film is assessed with Rose Bengal eye drops: the dye is taken up preferentially by areas of dry conjunctival and corneal epithelium. Again, adequate light and magnification are needed to identify dry areas.

Management

Simple lacerations of the bulbar or lid conjunctiva often require no repair. Large lacerations involving the bulbar conjunctiva may require suture with absorbable material, when more serious injury has been excluded. Conjunctival injury can result in scarring, contracture and loss of tissue. These complications arise especially in chemical burns of the conjunctiva, particularly those caused by alkali. While the most severe chemical conjunctival burns are produced by alkali, certain organic solvents (e.g. methyl ethyl ketone peroxide) produce ongoing conjunctival dysfunction through their capacity to damage goblet cells (Srivastava & Gupta 1989, Fraunfelder et al 1990). Every effort should be made to prevent contracture and adhesion (symblepharon) by appropriate manipulation and movement of the lids, and possibly by passing a glass rod around the conjunctival fornices under local anaesthesia, to break down adhesions between the bulbar and tarsal conjunctiva. Scleral shells may also be used to maintain the superior and inferior fornices and prevent adhesion. When there is more significant conjunctival tissue loss, and especially when there is ischaemia in the limbal region, grafting of healthy conjunctiva into the limbal region is needed to re-establish the limbal stem cell population which provides the basis of healing of associated corneal epithelial loss (p. 149).

Some surgeons (Reim & Teping 1989) have used hard contact lenses to protect the cornea, providing an artificial epithelium when there is loss of corneal epithelium associated with conjunctival chemical burns. The hard contact lens is glued on to the cornea using tissue adhesive while the conjunctival epithelium recovers at the limbus. When the contact lens is removed the epithelium then regrows over the corneal stroma.

CORNEAL FOREIGN BODIES

Surgical pathology

A foreign body lodged on the cornea is a common and usually trivial injury, but one which causes much discomfort. In a recent Australian study (Kruger et al 1990) a foreign body was involved in 57% of all eye injuries presenting to a Brisbane hospital casualty service.

The pathological consequences of a foreign body depend on its size and shape, position on the cornea, depth of penetration, and chemical nature. The immediate responses are tearing and mucoid secretion by the conjunctival glands, followed by hyperaemia, oedema and a mobilization of white cells from the limbal blood vessels and the tears. Secondary inflammation in the anterior chamber may develop in response to a chronically implanted foreign body, and also suppurative keratitis which may go on to cause scarring of the cornea and even perforation of the globe. Untreated foreign bodies, such as rice husks, are thought to be the leading cause of post-traumatic blindness in some developing countries (B. Thylefors, personal communication). Corneal foreign bodies overlying the visual axis are especially likely to impair vision and must be removed promptly.

Clinical assessment

This requires magnification and a good light, with application of fluorescein; a slit lamp microscope is preferred. If a foreign body is discovered it is essential to exclude any more serious or extensive ocular injury.

Management

Adequate removal of the foreign body, with proper follow-up care, will ensure a quick, complication-free recovery. The corneal foreign body should be removed under magnification and the eye should be observed over the next few days to ensure that the resulting corneal ulcer and abrasion heal satisfactorily without excessive scarring or infection. As a rule it is best to avoid the use of continued topical medications in view of their toxic inhibitory effects on corneal epithelial healing. Kruger et al (1990) assessed the value of using an antibiotic versus a placebo in terms of outcome: no difference was noted. Initially a drop of homatropine (5%) may be used to dilate the pupil and a single dose of antibiotic ointment (e.g. tobramycin) is applied. It is our practice to pad the eye firmly to splint the lids together, and to review the eye daily until the cornea has healed. The firm pad is a well-established method of treatment, but its necessity has not been proven. Indeed some authors have claimed that eyes with pads are more uncomfortable and do not heal more quickly than those without. This probably reflects the way the pad is applied.

If the corneal foreign body is vegetable matter then one must suspect the possibility of secondary infection and especially the possibility of a fungal infection; abrasions produced by vegetable matter often cause a much higher degree of anterior chamber inflammatory reaction.

Some deeply embedded foreign bodies may be difficult to remove and the possibility of producing more corneal scarring and inflammation and introducing infection by excessive manipulation must be borne in mind. When the embedded foreign body is a relatively inert substance such as glass, it may be reasonable to leave it in the cornea and to observe progress. Larger, deeply embedded corneal foreign bodies which do require surgical removal should be cultured in view of the possibility of infective keratitis.

A particularly difficult type of injury to manage is the blast injury in which the cornea and conjunctiva are peppered with multiple (sometimes hundreds) of explosive particles. It is extremely difficult to remove these completely and most are best left alone. The larger, more superficial particles can be removed with patience under the operating microscope but the deeper foreign bodies are extremely difficult to dislodge and again observation may be the best approach rather than risking more damage through attempted removal.

CORNEAL ABRASIONS, ULCERS AND OEDEMA

Surgical pathology

Blunt trauma to the cornea may result in abrasion of the epithelium; this may heal or may go on to form a chronic ulcer. Corneal infection may involve the anterior chamber. Blunt injury which does not cause rupture of the globe may produce transient effects on the cornea, such as oedema resulting from failure of the endothelial pump/barrier function and splits in Descemet's membrane caused by deformation injury. Generally these recover within 3 months.

Clinical assessment

Again, slit lamp microscopy and fluorescein staining constitute the best means of assessing the nature of the corneal damage.

Management

Simple traumatic abrasions and even deeper corneal ulcers are best treated by firm padding to splint the eyelids closed, with daily observation until healing takes place. Again we believe it is essential to limit the use of toxic topical agents applied to the eye. In children a pad is often not needed and is in fact impractical. The natural response of a young child is to keep the eye closed and when more serious injury is excluded, especially a foreign body, the child's eye may be left to heal itself without a pad to the eyelids, which are usually forcibly closed by the child. However, daily review is important.

Superficial abrasions induced by fingernails, vegetable matter such as twigs and leaves or brush hairs are prone to recurrent breakdown and ulceration. It is important in such injuries to promote normal epithelial healing in the first instance. We believe these lesions require firm padding until the ulcer is fully healed. If there is excessive sloughing of loosely adherent epithelium, this should be debrided with a cotton bud; the resultant epithelial defect is treated by firm padding and daily review. Once the epithelium has healed, lubricant eye drops are used regularly by day, with lubricating ointment by night, for the next 6–12 weeks, to ensure that there is no breakdown of the newly epithelialized area. Patients are instructed in management of eye irritation by using lid massage and lubricant drops, particularly in the morning. They are also instructed to use the lubricants more frequently in dry atmospheric conditions, particularly when exposed to air-conditioning or near heaters and when flying.

If on review the abrasion or ulcer seems to be developing corneal infiltrate with associated sloughing of corneal stroma, increasing anterior chamber reaction and increasing pain, then infection should be suspected: corneal scrapings, biopsy and cultures are performed, and on the results of these tests appropriate antibiotic therapy is introduced. This generally means admission to hospital and the use of topical antibiotics on an hourly basis until improvement is seen.

When more extensive craniofacial injury is present corneal ulceration may develop from exposure of the cornea, due to proptosis or loss of lid function. Prevention is the best management and lubricants should be used frequently and copiously. Nurses are instructed to cover the cornea with lubricant ointment frequently and regularly and are instructed to massage the lids over the cornea, thus providing an artificial blink whenever they pass the patient or attend to other needs, such as neurological observations. We have found Glad® wrap (clear plastic food wrap) to be useful in covering the exposed cornea, providing a humid chamber to prevent drying and ulceration (Fig. 9.8).

For recurrent erosions, hypertonic saline drops are sometimes used to promote dehydration of the epithelium if microcysts are present; soft contact lenses may also be useful. When these conventional measures fail, a technique of stromal micropuncture has been described by McLean et al (1986). In this technique the anterior stroma is perforated by a number of micropunctures, done with a 20 gauge hypodermic needle. This is intended to enhance adhesion of the epithelium by producing appropriate areas of scarring.

Photokeratoplasty with the Excimer laser is now a valuable aid in the treatment of recurrent erosion, by providing a fresh anterior stromal surface for support of new epithelium. The laser is used to sculpt the corneal surface. After removal of the corneal epithelium, four to eight laser impulses are used to ablate Bowman's membrane to a depth of a few micrometres, creating a new and more adherent membrane surface, which encourages better healing by the new growth of epithelium. Two cases reported by Vrabec et al (1993) show that normal healing of corneal epithelium may be seen after photorefractive and phototherapeutic laser keratectomy. There are other situations besides recurrent erosion and infected corneal ulceration in which the epithelium fails to heal. Persistent epithelial defects are seen in patients who have poor healing capabilities as in diabetes (p. 538) or where the corneal nerve supply has been disturbed causing neurotrophic keratitis. It is most important to ensure normal lid and tear function in such patients. Any associated lid, lash or periocular skin condition may need treatment.

Agents which promote epithelial wound healing and adhesion, such as fibronectin and epidermal growth factor, are currently under investigation (p. 120). Topical sodium ascorbate drops (10%) and oral ascorbic acid may be beneficial, particularly in cases of corneal damage induced by alkali burns. Topical vitamin analogues have also been used to promote epithelial healing (Tseng et al 1985). If the corneal limbal stem cell region is damaged, grafting of undamaged limbal conjunctiva into the region may be of value in promoting corneal epithelial healing (Thoft 1977, Kenyon & Tseng 1989). If healthy conjunctival or limbal epithelium is not available then an advancement of posterior Tenon's tissue may provide vascular support for the ischaemic limbal region. Thoft (1984) has advocated the use of biogenic kerato-epithelioplasties, done by suturing lenticules of epithelium and superficial stroma from a donor cornea into place.

HYPHAEMA

Surgical pathology

Bleeding into the anterior chamber, whether from penetrating or blunt trauma, may result in the formation of a hyphaema. This is most often caused by blunt trauma to the globe, as from a fist or a ball. Forces transmitted to the aqueous humor push the iris–lens diaphragm posteriorly and tear the iris root or the face of the ciliary body. The bleeding that results is usually self-limiting, being in a closed space, but may form a clot. The intraocular pressure may rise acutely, from mechanical blockade of the trabecular meshwork by red cells. About 48–72 h after the impact, the clot begins to retract, and rebleeding may result; the risk of this continues for another 48 h.

Complications of hyphaema include corneal blood staining and erythrocytic ghost cell glaucoma. Chronic glaucoma may result from angle recession or from peripheral anterior synechiae — adhesion by scar tissue of the iris to the peripheral cornea across the drainage angle. Persistent elevation in intraocular pressure may result in iris ischaemia and atrophy, cataract and optic atrophy, causing visual loss and even blindness. Rebleeding occurs in as many as 25% of patients and is especially likely to lead to complications (Read & Goldberg 1974).

Clinical assessment

A hyphaema may present with clotted or unclotted blood in the anterior chamber (Fig. 14.1D); there may be layering from the effect of gravity. At times the whole anterior chamber is filled with black clot, and the vitreous may also contain blood. As the haemorrhage resolves, whitish fibrin membranes may be seen.

Slit lamp microscopy will detect microscopic hyphaema

in the form of red cells circulating in the anterior chamber. When gravitation acts on more significant haemorrhages, a fluid level of macroscopic hyphaema is seen in the anterior chamber, varying in colour from bright red to black according to the age of the blood clot. The finding of a hyphaema calls for a search for other injuries.

Corneal status and visual acuities are checked daily. Intraocular pressures are measured repeatedly, by applanation (Goldman) tonometry.

Management

The medical management of hyphaema is controversial. No benefit has been proven for hospitalization, enforced bed rest, bilateral eye pads, corticosteroids, miotics or mydriatics (Rakusin 1972, Read & Goldberg 1974). We usually advise rest at home for patients who have a microscopic or mild hyphaema, provided that there is no other intraocular damage. Patients with macroscopic hyphaema are admitted to hospital for bed rest until the period of maximum risk of rebleeding (2–5 days) is over, with gradual mobilization once the clot has resolved. The traumatized eye is covered with a pad: probably this has no effect on the outcome, but does convince the patient that the injury is serious. If there is rebleeding, this regime is contiued for a further period of 5 days, with careful watch for complications such as glaucoma or corneal blood staining. An elevation of the intraocular pressure above 25 mmHg is treated medically, by ½% timolol eye drops and/or acetazolamide tablets (250 mg 6 hourly; 30 mg/kg/day in children, in divided doses). The possibility of optic nerve damage is increased if the pressure remains > 50 mmHg for > 5 days, or > 35 mmHg for > 7 days; if these medications do not keep the pressure below these limits, osmolar therapy with intravenous mannitol (0.5–2 g/kg as a 20% solution) or oral 50% glycerine (2–3 ml/kg) may be required (Romano & Shuster 1990). These osmolar drugs should be used with restraint, to avoid haemoconcentration; if either is employed, the serum osmolality should be monitored.

The use of oral ε-aminocaproic acid in reducing secondary haemorrhage has been demonstrated recently (Kutner et al 1987). This drug prevents fibrinolysis by inhibiting the conversion of plasminogen to plasmin. A regimen of 50 mg/kg every 4 h for 5 days is advised to reduce side-effects, such as nausea, vomiting, tinnitus and hypotension.

Surgical evacuation of the hyphaema is indicated if intraocular pressure cannot be controlled medically, or if corneal blood staining begins to develop. Several surgical techniques have been used; including paracentesis of the anterior chamber, wash-outs with one needle, irrigation or irrigation–aspiration technique, wash-outs with a two-needle technique, clot evacuation with forceps or cryo-probe and clot evacuation associated with trabeculectomy. We usually employ simple paracentesis initially: under topical anaesthesia and with microscopic vision, a 25–30 gauge needle is inserted into the anterior chamber through the limbus. Intermittent pressure on the posterior lip of the needle incision, or reintroduction of the needle, enables drainage of aqueous fluid at regular intervals while the pressure remains elevated. If this technique fails, a two-instrument bimanual wash-out evacuation is performed, with vitrectomy instruments. Surgical clot extraction is dangerous, because the hyphaema limits visibility and uveal tissue may be mistaken for blood clot. Care must also be taken to avoid damaging the iris, the lens or the corneal endothelium. Removal of blood from the anterior chamber usually halts corneal blood staining and alleviates glaucoma.

Patients with sickle cell haemoglobinopathy and traumatic hyphaema have a decreased ability to tolerate modest rises in pressure and may react adversely to acetazolamide. It is recommended that these patients should be closely observed for 24 h, particularly if the intraocular pressure is ⩾ 25 mmHg. If the pressure remains high for > 24 h, surgical intervention is indicated (p. 417).

IRIS INJURIES

Surgical pathology

The iris can be injured by blunt or penetrating trauma. In blunt trauma the most common injuries are sphincter tears and dialyses of the iris root. There is often an associated hyphaema, and anterior chamber inflammation may develop. Iris atrophy and loss of pigmentation, and later iridoschisis, can occur. Penetrating wounds may result in prolapse of iris tissue into the wound (Fig. 5.22). Prolonged prolapse of iris tissue through a penetrating wound leads to ischaemia and devitalization of the iris tissue, increasing the risk of infection.

Clinical assessment

The pupil is often enlarged and poorly reactive, with degradation of the optical image and increase of sensitivity to glare. Slit lamp microscopy may show sphincter rupture, areas of segmental sphincter paralysis, or subtle irregularities in the pupil shape. Intrastromal haemorrhages and microscopic hyphaema may be seen. Pigment loss from the posterior leaf of the iris may be seen by retro-illumination with the slit lamp beam.

Management

Anterior chamber inflammation or iritis should be treated by topical steroid therapy; in the absence of hyphaema, cycloplegics such as homatropine are given.

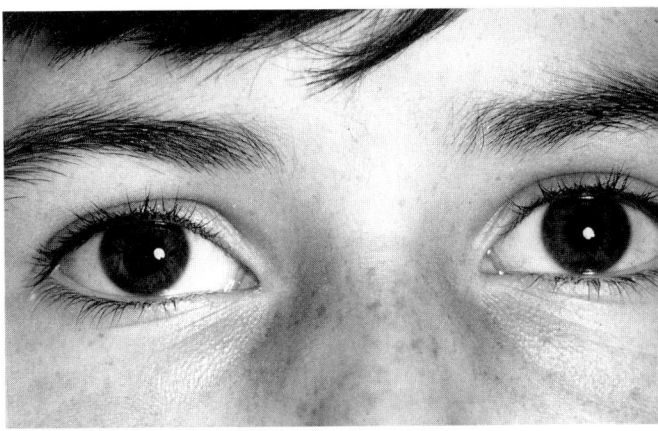

Fig. 14.2 Iris sphincterotomy by a cat's claw. An infant was struck in the right eye by the family cat; a claw perforated the cornea and tore the iris without causing any other intraocular damage; there was no cataract and vision was unaffected. But there was a permanent cosmetic blemish.

A distorted pupil is an aesthetic blemish (Fig. 14.2); wherever possible, normal pupil shape should be preserved. Misshapen pupils often complicate penetrating trauma when iris tissue is prolapsed, or when synechiae form. Wicks of vitreous extending into the anterior chamber towards penetrating wounds may also distort the pupil. If the iris cannot be repaired to provide a normal-looking pupil, cosmetic contact lenses may be used to hide the defect. These may also be of use functionally by limiting pupil size and so reducing optical aberration.

As a general rule, as much iris tissue should be preserved as possible. However, repositioning an exposed iris increases the risk of endophthalmitis, and if iris tissue has been prolapsed longer than 24 h it may wise to excise it. The health of the iris can be gauged by its tone and the appearance of its anatomy under the operating microscope. Irrigation with specially formulated balanced salt solution (Alcon Laboratories) before reposition helps to decontaminate the exposed iris.

Repair of a distorted iris may be left until the primary repair of the penetrating injury has healed. The neodymium: YAG or argon laser permits effective non-surgical repair of distorted pupils, by photodisruption of strands of vitreous, capsule and scar tissue. The laser may be used to enlarge pupils or to create sphincterotomies, thus improving both optical function and cosmesis. Ideally, laser treatment of adhesions and bands should be performed early to prevent prolonged distortion of the pupil.

Surgical repair of lacerations of the iris may be performed by a closed technique (McCannell 1976) or by open operation. 10/0 polypropylene sutures are used. Indications for repair of iris lacerations are functional (multiplopia or glare), or cosmetic. Care must be taken not to induce damage by zealous attempts to achieve a cosmetically perfect result.

LENS INJURIES

Surgical pathology

Trauma to the lens may result in cataract, subluxation, or dislocation. Management depends on many factors including visual acuity, the presence of secondary glaucoma, secondary intraocular inflammation, the presence of other injury to the eye and the necessity to have a clear optical pathway for management of posterior segment injury or disease.

Cataract may be induced in the clear lens either by direct damage to the lens capsule and/or lens fibres or indirectly, by equatorial expansion of the globe during blunt trauma, or by the passage of shock waves through the lens from an impact remote from the lens itself. Cataracts may complicate electrical burns (Fig. 17.2; Johnson et al 1987). Rupture or damage to the lens capsule will permit hydration of the lens structure. Lens opacities can arise in a lens without rupture of the lens capsule from alterations in the physiology and metabolism of the lens. Cataract may occur early or many years after the initial traumatic insult.

Dislocation or subluxation of the lens with rupture of the zonules may be induced by direct trauma to these structures or indirectly by a blunt impact causing distension of the globe in an equatorial direction.

Rupture of the lens capsule and release of lens proteins may induce intraocular inflammation (phako-anaphylactic uveitis: see p. 152). Glaucoma may be induced by high density lens proteins occluding the trabecular meshwork or by macrophages scavenging the lens proteins and blocking trabecular outflow.

Glaucoma may also be secondarily induced by changes in the size and position of the lens leading to relative pupillary block, subsequent peripheral anterior synechiae and shallowing of the anterior chamber angle.

Clinical assessment

The degree of traumatic cataract varies. It may be total, in which case it is clearly obvious to the examiner or it may be relatively minor and non-progressive. Cataract is best detected by examining the eye with an ophthalmoscope and looking for the red reflex. Lens dislocation may also be variable in its degree. At its most subtle, there may be blurred vision induced by astigmatism or alterations in accommodation; dislocation may only be apparent on dilated slit lamp examination and refraction. If the degree of dislocation or subluxation is more marked then a deep anterior chamber with iridodonesis or phakodonesis may be combined with double vision: in these conditions, the iris or lens is mobile, and may wobble. Obvious changes in the position of the lens are seen easily with retro-illumination.

Slit lamp examination may reveal the presence of vitreous in the anterior chamber, indicating that the zonule is ruptured. The presence of secondary glaucoma or inflammation produced by the lens injury is important in helping to decide the appropriate management course. Pressures persistently greater than 25 mmHg demand active treatment but the tolerable pressure may be lower or higher than this, according to the age and health of the patient, or the presence of pre-existing glaucoma.

Management of traumatic cataract

The finding of a cataract may not be an indication for surgery. If there are no visual or medical reasons for removal of the cataract then the conservative approach of observation is better. Some cataracts are non-progressive while others are slowly progressive and may not need surgical treatment for months or years. On the other hand some opacities are rapidly progressive and cause early visual impairment. If secondary glaucoma or inflammation is present and not controlled medically then cataract extraction will be necessary. The approach to removal of the cataract depends on many factors but the most important is the integrity of the lens capsule, particularly the posterior lens capsule. It may be necessary to use ultrasonography to examine the posterior segment of the eye in the presence of lens opacities which prevent an adequate optical view. If the posterior capsule is intact we favour a routine extracapsular cataract extraction approach either using an expression technique for the nucleus in the older patient or phako-emulsification if this is available and appropriate. In children and young adults the lens may be aspirated through a small incision. If at all possible we prefer to replace the lens with an intraocular lens implant; preoperative evaluation includes keratometry and ultrasonography, to determine the parameters of the lens implant.

In children there is the risk of amblyopia (p. 517). In several children under 8 years old, we have used multifocal intraocular lenses in an attempt to give a range of focuses; a careful assessment of amblyopia and management with appropriate patching and spectacles may be necessary. In children the posterior lens capsule may opacify quite rapidly after cataract extraction; a primary capsulotomy performed after the insertion of the intraocular lens may be necessary or neodymium:YAG laser posterior capsulotomy may be done later. If the posterior capsule is not intact then we prefer a lensectomy done through the limbus combined with an anterior vitrectomy. Later a contact lens is used for optical correction.

Management of dislocated or subluxed lens

Once again if symptoms are not severe and if there is no indication such as secondary glaucoma for surgical intervention, then conservative management and observation may be appropriate with correction by either spectacles or contact lenses. Dilating or constricting drops to minimize optic aberration may be appropriate. A dislocated lens need not be surgically removed if it is not affecting the visual axis and is not producing secondary glaucoma or inflammation. When the lens has been removed, either for cataract or subluxation, there is an increased risk of retinal detachment at a later date: both patient and surgeon should be aware of this.

Surgical removal of subluxed or dislocated lenses may be difficult. If there is minimal subluxation of the lens and a predominantly intact zonule and posterior capsule, an extracapsular lens extraction can be attempted. More often, lensectomy with a vitrectomy instrument will be necessary, combined with the removal of anterior vitreous. We prefer an anterior approach through the limbus, although at times a pars plana approach may be necessary. The presence of a hard nucleus in an older patient may require modification of the standard procedure for extracapsular cataract extraction. Numerous techniques have been described in which the lens is impaled with a sharp needle or knife to stabilize it during the lensectomy procedure. We have found that it can be difficult to pierce a mobile dislocated lens, especially in the young child, even with the sharpest of instruments. The use of viscoelastic substances is invaluable in manipulating the lens into manageable positions and to move the vitreous face if this is necessary.

In cases of subluxed or dislocated lenses, it is wise to use hyperosmotic agents such as mannitol before surgery in order to lower the intraocular pressure. Compression of the eye is not recommended as this may further dislocate the lens into the vitreous cavity. The intraocular pressure may be quite variable in children and under general anaesthesia: hyperosmolar agents should therefore be used liberally, though with care.

As mentioned earlier the use of an intraocular lens implant is generally preferable and posterior chamber lens implants are most appropriate. Anterior chamber lenses are probably best avoided and in the presence of significant angle changes they are certainly contraindicated. In patients without posterior capsular support we have sutured posterior chamber implants in place using the modified McCannel technique (Stern et al 1983). Epikeratophakia is an alternative to lens implantation and contact lens use to correct aphakia in children; several authors have reported good success with this procedure, in which a custom-lathed corneal graft is sutured on the child's cornea to correct the aphakia (Morgan et al 1987, Avni et al 1989).

VITREOUS HAEMORRHAGE AND RETINAL DETACHMENT

Surgical pathology

These conditions may follow penetrating ocular injuries;

they are also seen after blunt violence. Intraocular bleeding is often seen in abused infants; sometimes this may be a massive vitreous haemorrhage, going on to retinal detachment and/or glaucoma. Intraocular bleeding has indeed been regarded as typical of the shaken or battered baby, but similar findings may be seen in other types of severe closed head injury in infancy (p. 513). The mechanism in cases of child abuse is uncertain, but a sudden rise in intracranial pressure seems the likeliest explanation (Lambert et al 1986). Harcourt & Hopkins (1971) have described the ophthalmological manifestations of violent child abuse in infancy.

Assessment

Since vitreous haemorrhage may be localized soon after the injury but may later spread diffusely through the whole of the vitreous, it is important to try to examine the retina and posterior segment fully as soon as possible after injury. Ultrasound should be used if a view of the posterior segment is not possible; it is often possible to diagnose retinal detachment, posterior vitreous detachment, scleral rupture, haemorrhagic or serous choroidal detachment and giant retinal tears with ultrasound (Fig. 7.00). If the vitreous haemorrhage results from non-penetrating injury it should be followed for several months before any surgical intervention is considered. Regular ultrasound examinations may be necessary if the retina cannot be viewed clinically. If retinal detachment is detected then pars plana vitrectomy should be performed; otherwise vitrectomy should be deferred for at least 6 months. The presence of vitreous strands emanating from the equator on ultrasound suggests an occult scleral rupture requiring surgical exploration. The prognosis for eyes with vitreous haemorrhage associated with non-penetrating trauma depends on the presence or absence of retinal damage.

Management: vitrectomy

Indications

Vitrectomy plays an important role in the management of severely traumatized eyes with vitreous haemorrhage, with or without retinal detachment. Studies of the histology of penetrating injury show that intraocular cellular proliferation is established within 1 week of injury and membrane formation by 2 weeks. The goals of vitrectomy in these cases are:

- To clear the ocular media
- To remove the vitreous scaffold from the scleral laceration site
- To remove the posterior hyaloid which could provide a future scaffold for epiretinal membrane formation and vitreo-retinal traction
- To identify and treat retinal breaks and detachment.

Timing

This still remains controversial. Some surgeons prefer to operate within the first 48–72 h, others delay the vitrectomy for periods of 4–10 days, or even up to 14 days after injury. Early vitrectomists rationalize that early operation will prevent the development of severe inflammatory changes and at the same time reduce the risk of fibro-blastic proliferation. On the other hand, delaying the vitrectomy beyond 72 h allows further diagnostic evaluation including ultrasound and electrophysiology. Operation is done under better conditions with less risk of severe intraocular haemorrhage during the procedure, since the uveal tissues are likely to be congested and inflamed immediately after the injury or primary repair. Furthermore a posterior cortical vitreous detachment may occur in the delay period, making the vitrectomy easier and more effective. Delaying the vitrectomy beyond 14 days is probably unwise, however, since there is a higher risk of developing sympathetic ophthalmitis.

Techniques of vitrectomy

Vitrectomy varies in complexity from simple ablation of extruded vitreous with scissors and sponges or aspiration through a wide-bore needle, to the use of specialized cutting instruments introduced through ports cut in the wall of the eye. These require the skills of an ophthalmologist dedicated to this field of surgery (p. 245).

For extensive or complicated procedures, it is usually necessary to make three entrance ports for access to the posterior segment (Fig. 14.3). One provides for infusion of fluid into the eye to maintain its shape and pressure throughout the operation. This is usually done by suturing a plug into the eye wall through the pars plana. The flow of fluid is regulated according to the surgeon's requirements, maintaining a balance between the inflow and the aspiration of fluid through the vitrectomy instrument. The two other ports provide access for instruments for each hand of the surgeon. One port admits the vitrectomy instrument, a suction cutting device which removes the vitreous piecemeal, taking also scar tissue and haemorrhage. Through the other port, the surgeon may insert a fibre-optic illumination device, an intraocular cautery or laser, or an intraocular magnet. These instruments are used in various combinations as required in the procedure. The posterior segment is visualized through an operating microscope combined with a corneal contact lens, or by indirect ophthalmoscopy; illumination is either via the fibre-optic endophthalmic light source or by the coaxial light of the microscope. Fine gauge intraocular scissors, forceps, picks and knives have been designed for posterior segment surgery.

Many surgeons routinely use an encircling band for scleral support prophylactically (Fig. 14.3C–E), to decrease the risk of retinal detachment even if no retinal problems

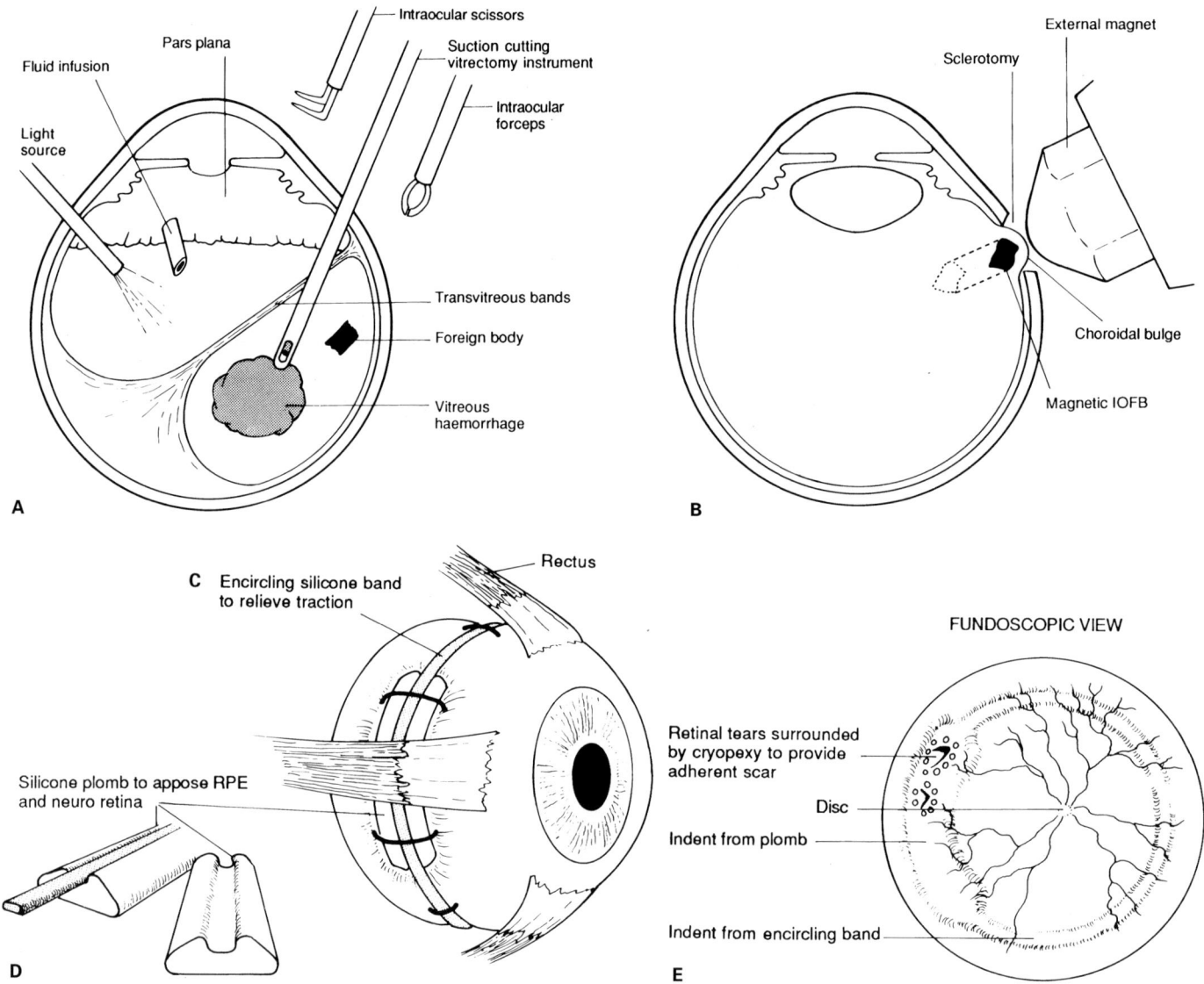

Fig. 14.3 Vitrectomy and other operations on the globe. A Three ports have been made in pars plana of the globe. One is for the introduction of a variety of instruments (scissors, forceps, vitrectomy suction cutting device, cautery and laser). One is for a light source and one for fluid infusion; the last is usually sutured in place, allowing bimanual manipulation of instruments in the posterior segment. **B** Removal of a foreign body with an external magnet. **C** Scleral buckle: a 360° encircling silicone band with a localized silicone plomb overlies retinal tears for which cryopexy is to be performed (**E**). The plomb relieves traction and helps to appose the retinal pigment epithelium (RPE) to the neuroretina. **D** Scleral buckle, showing the plomb held by the encircling band while the cryopen is used to stimulate scarring and fibrosis. **E** Fundoscopic view, showing the 360° indentation produced by the band and the wider indentation produced by the plomb. Two horsehoe tears surrounded by cryopexy lesions are seen sitting on the plomb. Scleral buckling is used in various forms and combinations; this diagram shows only one application — retinal detachment. The technique can be used prophylactically after removal of a foreign body, vitrectomy or posterior segment perforation.

are initially seen at the time of the vitrectomy. Hutton & Fuller (1984) found a detachment rate of 27% of eyes treated by vitrectomy with no scleral buckle; the detachment rate in eyes which were prophylactically buckled was 8%. If retinal detachment is present then tangential and anteroposterior vitreoretinal traction on the break must be relieved by highly specialized techniques which are beyond the scope of this book. If traction cannot be fully relieved, it is necessary to place a scleral buckle to support the break. Subretinal fluid must be drained and fluid–gas exchange undertaken either through a posterior

retinal break or through a posterior retinotomy. Long-acting gases such as sulphahexachloride or perfluropropane will provide prolonged internal tamponade to the detached retina. Silicone oil is generally not recommended in primary vitrectomies for trauma.

Retinal incarceration and scleral laceration may be managed by vitrectomy and scleral buckling, but on occasion posterior incarcerations require retinotomy. Intraocular bleeding during vitrectomies is a significant hazard and this may be managed either by increasing the intraocular pressure by intraocular infusion or by endodiathermy. The fluid–gas exchange may sometimes help tamponade active bleeding. Adrenalin solution may be infused at a concentration of 100 units per ml to attempt to control bleeding also. Occasionally removal of the corneal epithelium and the use of sodium hyaluronate may be of value in improving the view for the operation.

OTHER RETINAL INJURIES

Surgical pathology

Blunt and penetrating impacts on the globe can injure the retina directly or cause a delayed retinal detachment. Retinal oedema (Berlin's oedema), also known as commotio retinae, is usually a reversible impairment of retinal function, but contusive retinal injury may result in jagged holes in the retina and actual fragmentation; similar lesions have been produced experimentally in pigs (Delori et al 1969). Retinal detachment is well recorded as a hazard of boxing.

Transmission of force to the vitreous during injury may lead to acute and often severe vitreoretinal traction. This may produce retinal dialysis with or without avulsion of the vitreous base. Horseshoe retinal tears at the margin of the vitreous base at the edge of a meridional fold or at the equator may occur and operculated retinal tears and macular holes may develop. The most common retinal break from trauma is a retinal dialysis. Most commonly these are superonasal and inferotemporal.

Retinal detachment following a retinal tear due to blunt trauma is uncommon. However, if retinal or vitreous pathology likely to predispose to later retinal detachment is discovered, prophylactic treatment may be advisable.

Clinical assessment

After blunt trauma to the globe, retinal oedema may be seen as retinal whitening around the fovea, giving the appearance of a cherry red spot at the macula. Vision can be markedly decreased but this usually improves when the swelling resolves over 3 or 4 weeks. However, the macula may develop permanent changes in pigmentation and function, associated with reduced vision. Cystoid macular oedema may occur leading to macular hole formation.

Management

The temptation to intervene surgically should be resisted since it is extremely rare that the retina detaches around these holes, presumably because inflammatory changes have caused choroidoretinal adhesion. However, prophylactic cryopexy or photocoagulation may be recommended for any retinal tears that are identified as threatening. In cryopexy, the retina is frozen around the hole by a trans-scleral technique, to produce inflammation and choroido-retinal adhesions. Photocoagulation provokes a similar reaction by direct focal heating with a light source of one wavelength.

PENETRATING INJURIES OF THE GLOBE

Surgical pathology

The primary and secondary effects of penetrating eye injury are often devastating. Depending on the depth of penetration, all the injuries described above may be seen and any component of the globe may be disrupted, with immediate or delayed loss of sight. If the wound is large, the ocular contents may be extruded and the globe may collapse. Secondary complications include infection (endophthalmitis), toxic reactions to implanted metals (p. 153), and autoimmune inflammation in the intact eye — sympathetic ophthalmitis (p. 152). Other complications include corneal or conjunctival scarring, astigmatism, glaucoma, vitreous incarceration associated with inflammation, cystoid macular oedema, pupillary and/or cyclitic membranes and adhesions. Penetrating wounds with a posterior exit may cause inoperable retinal detachment: severe intravitreal fibrovascular and fibroglial proliferation may develop at the exit wound, leading to retinal and ciliary body traction.

Incidence

These are common injuries: Table 14.2 sets our our experience in a 12 month prospective study of adults with penetrating eye wounds. In this small but representative series of 21 documented cases, all were males; only one was wearing appropriate ocular protection when hurt.

Clinical assessment

The history often gives important clues to the nature of the ocular damage, particularly the history of hammering metal on metal (Fig. 14.4). Visual acuity is the most important determinant of final visual outcome. When initial vision was 5/200 or better, a final visual acuity of 5/100 or better was salvaged in 97% of 453 cases reported by de Juan et al (1983). When there is no light perception at presentation, only very rare cases will have useful vision or even light perception, and enucleation may then be the appropriate operation in a severely disrupted eye. But many injured patients are intoxicated or have cerebral injuries affecting their mental status, and it is often not possible to be absolutely sure that there is no light perception. Visual evoked potentials may be recorded in comatose cases or where the eye is closed by orbital swelling (p. 248) but although a strong response is encouraging, the absence of a cortical potential may not always be due to irreversible damage to the globe. So primary enucleation is rarely performed.

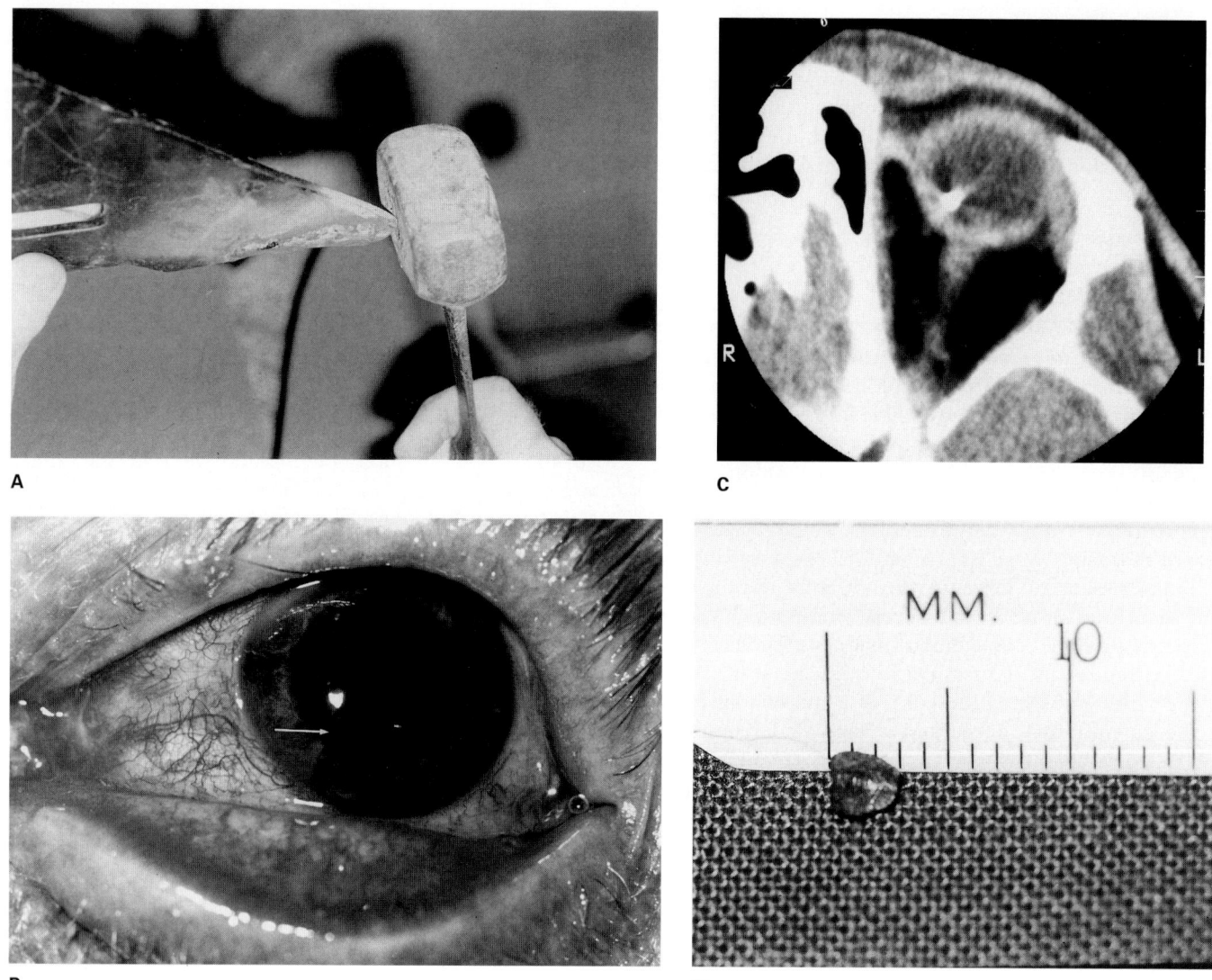

Fig. 14.4 Foreign body removed by giant magnet. A 72-year-old farmer was hammering on a ploughshare. He was not wearing safety glasses. **A** Reconstruction of event: a fragment of metal flew off the point of the plough share. **B** Perforating corneal laceration at 7 o'clock in left eye. **C** CT scan showing metallic foreign body inside the globe of the eye. **D** The foreign body was removed through the pars plana with a giant magnet. A secondary cataract formed and was successfully extracted. 2 years later, a tractional retinal detachment occurred, but the patient declined operation and the eye became blind.

In the preoperative examination it is important not to cause further damage by pressure on the globe itself, and if it is not possible to examine the eye without this risk then examination under anaesthesia may be needed. Immediate repair of any penetrating injury can be undertaken at the time.

Chemosis or subconjunctival swelling often suggests the presence of an occult rupture of the globe; surprisingly the intraocular pressure may be normal or even elevated in such cases, although it is usually low. Signs of a posterior rupture — as in a double perforation of the globe — include poor visual acuity, a shallow or unusually deep anterior chamber, low intraocular pressure, hyphaema, pupillary distortion, bullous subconjunctival haemorrhage and chemosis and brownish subconjunctival discoloration

caused by prolapsed uvea. If an intraocular foreign body is suspected the preoperative assessment becomes more complicated. Sometimes the foreign body may be seen by slit lamp examination or ophthalmoscopy, but if the posterior segment is not clearly seen then other techniques are needed for the detection and localization of the foreign body.

Radiological assessment

Plain X-ray imaging was used in the past. Exact localization was difficult, though Sweet's external localizer and Comberg's contact lens gave significant assistance (Reid 1957). But these procedures were often inaccurate and were of course useless with radiolucent foreign bodies;

they are now of importance only when modern methods of localization are unavailable.

Ultrasonography may be useful, but currently computerized tomography (CT) is the technique of choice for evaluation of intraocular foreign bodies (Fig. 14.4C). Radiologically, wood is the least dense of the non-metallic foreign bodies, followed by plastic and then glass; most metallic foreign bodies have the same densities and are impossible to differentiate by CT. Magnetic resonance imaging (MRI) is dangerous in the investigation of ferromagnetic foreign bodies since the foreign body will change its position when exposed to the strong magnetic impulses of the technique. However, MRI may be very useful in locating wood and other non-metallic foreign bodies.

Management of corneoscleral lacerations

These injuries confront most ophthalmologists, and de-serve detailed discussion. The aim of surgical repair of corneoscleral wounds is complete watertight closure of the globe with restoration of structural and functional integrity (Fig. 14.5). Foreign bodies should be removed if possible, but above all, no further ocular damage should be induced. Secondary procedures may be necessary, such as surgery for cataract and for posterior segment lesions.

Intravenous antibiotics are usually given intraoperatively and continued intravenously for the first 24–48 h after surgery, with oral administration thereafter to complete the course; at present we favour a third-generation cephalosporin and gentamicin. There is evidence to suggest that intraocular gentamicin may be toxic if given in excessive dosage, and we do not instil any possibly toxic bactericidal agent into the eye before operation. Anxiety is alleviated as far as possible by appropriate explanation.

Partial-thickness corneal lacerations may be treated on an outpatient basis with padding and bandage, contact lenses and rarely suturing. Some perforating wounds,

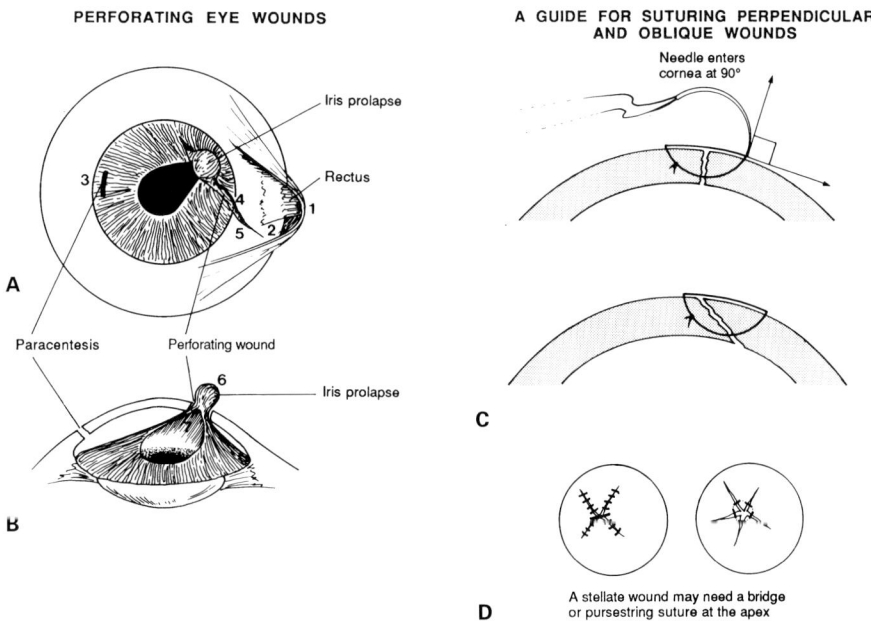

Fig. 14.5 Suture of a penetrating wound of the eye. A, B Frontal and profile views of a perforating corneoscleral wound: the iris is prolapsed as a knuckle or bleb of feathery pigmented tissue (6) protruding through the wound and distorting the pupil into the shape of a teardrop pointing to the prolapse — a classic sign. In repairing a wound like this, the conjunctiva (1) is dissected to show the posterior extent (5) of the scleral wound. If the wound extends under one of the rectus muscles (2), the muscle is detached from the globe, to be reattached with 6/0 Vicryl or 5/0 catgut sutures when the wound has been repaired. The limbal part of the wound (4) is closed first as the limbus is the best landmark for accurate anatomical repair. The corneal wound is sutured with interrupted 10/0 nylon sutures on a bicurved side-cutting needle; the knots are buried. Prolapsed vitreous is abscised and uvea is reposited. A paracentesis (3) may be placed in a position giving access to the anterior chamber for infusion of fluids, including viscoelastics, and to help in freeing the iris from the wound. **C** Technique of suturing a corneal perforating wound. The needle enters the cornea at a 90° angle and should take in at least two-thirds of the thickness of the cornea. If the wound edges are perpendicular, the entry and exit of the needle should be equidistant from the wound; if the wound is oblique the entry site is further from the wound edge than the exit site. The knot is buried in the corneal stroma.
D Suture of a stellate laceration. The wound is sutured in the same way along the limbs of the star, but a purse string or bridging suture may be needed at the apex. If leakage persists, a contact lens, tissue glue, or even a corneal patch graft may be tried.

if they are small and regular, may seal themselves with appropriate bed rest, padding and/or bandage contact lenses. If the anterior chamber does not reform within 24 h, or if there is persistent shallowing of the anterior chamber and leakage, then surgical repair will be necessary. Cyanoacrylate tissue adhesive may be useful, either alone or in combination with surgical repair, for small wounds with tiny degrees of central tissue loss, such as stellate wounds with poor central apposition and selected small lacerations that do not self-seal and are < 2 mm in length. Prompt suture is required for larger corneal perforating lacerations, more complicated lacerations associated with uveal or lens incarceration and particularly for corneal wounds in children.

Operative repair is done under general anaesthesia. The globe is appropriately draped and care is taken not to apply excessive pressure to the eye. In some cases lid sutures will be necessary to give adequate exposure of the globe without placing excessive pressure on the globe, but as a rule a wire speculum suffices. The region is irrigated with sterile normal saline or balanced salt solution, and the lids and surrounding facial area are treated with povidone–iodine half-strength aqueous solution. It is essential to determine the extent of the injury; the laceration should be exposed posteriorly as far as it extends by dissecting off the conjunctiva. It is useful to place initial sutures at landmark points, particularly the limbus, to restore the globe to its anatomical integrity. A step of great importance is the appropriate placement of paracentesis wounds, to allow access to the anterior chamber to instil air or a viscoelastic substance, such as sodium hyaluronate, and to admit instruments to enable iris tissue and/or vitreous to be extricated from the wound. We find that a diamond knife is the best instrument for this, as it causes least pressure on the globe.

Monofilament 10/0 nylon sutures are used on a bicurved side-cutting needle to oppose the corneal wound edges (Fig. 14.5C). If possible, suture bites through the visual axis should be avoided. As the wound is closed it may be necessary to replace some of the earlier sutures which may loosen as the procedure progresses. The use of large cardinal sutures may be useful, particularly in the repair of jagged lacerations. The knots are buried. Purse-string closure may be helpful in stellate or Y-shaped lacerations (Fig. 14.5D). If the centre of such a laceration cannot be apposed and leaks persistently, it may be necessary to use bandage contact lenses, tissue glues or corneal patch grafting.

Scleral lacerations should be repaired with 8/0 non-absorbable sutures or 8/0 Vicryl® sutures. It is essential that the sclera is watertight, in case vitrectomy should be needed within the first 2 weeks after the repair. If the laceration extends under one of the rectus muscles, it may be necessary to detach the muscle temporarily from the globe, re-suturing it at the original insertion at the end of the procedure. Exploration of the sclera behind the muscle insertions should be performed since here the sclera is thinner than elsewhere. If a scleral laceration extends posterior to the ora serrata there may be associated retinal damage; cryopexy is not recommended prophylactically unless the area of retinal damage can be visualized.

Perforations which extend far past the equator are probably best left, since attempts to repair them are more likely to cause more damage. Prolapsed vitreous will require gentle abscision (cutting off) using dry cellulose sponges and scissors, taking care not to place excessive traction on the vitreous. If the laceration extends posterior to the pars plana, the vitreous should not be removed by inserting an instrument into the eye as this risks further retinal damage.

As a rule prolapsing and bulging uveal tissue may be reposited and abscision should be avoided if possible since severe bleeding may often occur. Any excised material should be examined histopathologically to determine its nature; if the retina is found prolapsed then the prognosis is poor.

Blunt injury to the eye may produce scleral rupture in the posterior half of the eye and posterior scleral lacerations may occur as a direct result of double perforating trauma. The more anterior of such lacerations may be repaired but those further posteriorly are best left alone.

Normal uveal tissue should be preserved. The decision to reposit prolapsed uveal tissue is generally made on the appearance and the likelihood of viability. If the prolapsed tissue is macerated, feathery or depigmented it is unlikely to be viable. If on the other hand it appears to have some tone and relatively normal structure it can be reposited with expectation of normal or near-normal function. The advent of viscoelastic agents (see above) has allowed better reconstruction of the anterior chamber and easier repositioning of prolapsed tissue: the viscoelastic material is used to push the tissue into its required position and to hold it in place.

Management of associated lens injury

Buschmann (1993) has reported that small ruptures or perforations of the anterior lens capsule can be sealed permanently by topical application of fibrinogen glue (Tissucol®, Immuno AG Vienna), in the hope of preventing further lens opacification.

If the lens has become cataractous as a result of a penetrating injury a decision has to be made about its management, along the lines already discussed. Rarely does a cataractous lens need to be removed as an emergency. If lens removal is considered in a primary procedure then the surgeon needs to be sure that in fact the opacity he sees is lens material and not fibrin or pupillary membrane. If, however, the lens is grossly disrupted and flocculent cortical material is present in the anterior chamber, this is best removed in the primary procedure through the lensectomy instrument. At the same time any prolapsed vitreous can be removed. If the posterior capsule is intact a standard extracapsular lens extraction may be performed to remove the lens as a secondary procedure, as described above. If, however, the capsule is disrupted, a lensectomy would be appropriate.

An intraocular lens may be inserted if the posterior capsule is intact. Small rents in the posterior capsule need not preclude the use of an intraocular lens in the posterior chamber. As stated earlier, we have inserted intraocular lenses in children down to the age of 4 years, but under this age we prefer contact lens correction of the aphakia. The use of a posterior chamber intraocular lens obviously depends on the ability to ascertain the appropriate power which will require assessment of the opposite eye and knowledge of previous refractive errors. Delaying the surgical removal of a cataract after the primary injury allows better evaluation of the eye in terms of its corneal curvature and axial length, and thus more accurate determination of the power of the intraocular lens.

Management of associated vitreous injury

If the vitreous is involved in the primary injury and has filled the anterior chamber, the primary goal is to remove the vitreous from the anterior chamber and to prevent vitreous incarceration in the original traumatic wound or in any surgical wounds used during repair. This reduces the risk of complications such as inflammation, cystoid macular oedema, vitreous fibrosis and retinal detachment. It also minimizes damage to the corneal endothelium. Viscoelastic agents coloured so as to distinguish them from vitreous may be used to manipulate the vitreous out of the wound or to hold it back into the posterior segment. Air bubbles may also be used to provide a barrier across the pupil, and manipulation of pupil size by constricting with acetylcholine may be of value in holding the vitreous in the posterior segment.

Management of corneoscleral tissue loss

Tissue loss in corneoscleral lacerations will need to be repaired either by tissue adhesives or by some form or keratoplasty, either a penetrating (full-thickness) corneal graft or by lamellar patch grafting. Lamellar grafts may be more appropriate where irregular wound margins, stromal necrosis or both make full-thickness dissections and suturing more difficult; lamellar grafts also find applications when the cornea is severely thinned and leaking, or when there is an anterior stromal scar.

Full-thickness keratoplasty is rarely used in primary repair of perforating injuries. In a period of approximately 6 years, 3608 full-thickness keratoplasties were recorded by the Australian Corneal Graft Registry (Williams et al 1993): only 102 were for the results of trauma, due in 77 cases to mechanical injury and in 25 to burns. Trauma was a primary indication for grafting in only 13 cases. The outcome of such grafts is often poor, though in this series the number of primary grafts was too small to allow any significant comment on prognosis.

Keratoplasty is usually delayed until the eye is uninflamed and free of infection, to optimize the likelihood of graft survival. Moreover, even badly injured corneas may heal well and keratoplasty may not be required; conversely, despite the best possible primary repair, complications may develop after penetrating injuries and these give a poor prognosis for keratoplasty. We reiterate the importance of accurate repair of damaged eyelids since this is vital to the restoration of a healthy ocular surface; if a keratoplasty is to be done, healthy tear and lid function should be present.

Ideally the eye should be free of inflammation and should have a normal intraocular pressure before keratoplasty is undertaken. On occasions, earlier surgery is indicated, as for instance in the case of retained lens material producing uveitis or glaucoma. Keratoplasty may be required for anterior segment reconstruction as a secondary procedure.

Cadaver donor corneal buttons are generally trephined 0.5 mm larger than the host bed. In children who have a high risk of graft rejection and in other patients with high risks, rotating autografts may be used to move a focal scar from the visual axis. On occasions vitreoretinal surgery may be necessary in combination with corneal grafting and vitrectomy may be performed through an 'open-sky' technique. Alternatively, temporary keratoprostheses may be used to allow closed vitrectomy (Gelender et al 1988); we have no experience of this approach.

All vitreous should be cleared from the anterior chamber using a microvitrectomy suction cutting instrument if full-thickness keratoplasty is to be performed. Procedures such as division and separation of peripheral anterior synechiae should be undertaken before proceeding to keratoplasty. Organized fibrovascular membranes and Descemet's hyalinized membranes lying on the anterior surface of the iris in the angle or on the posterior surface of the cornea, should be identified and peeled away, to avoid future fibrosis, synechiae and angle compromise, and ciliary body detachment. Ideally if an intraocular lens is used, as mentioned earlier, a posterior chamber lens should be sutured into the ciliary sulcus. But the long-term outcome of suturing in posterior chamber lenses in this fashion has not been determined.

Iridoplasty may be performed with the aims of restoring a tight iris diaphragm: this improves the likelihood of corneal graft survival by preventing iridocorneal adhesion, as well as preventing glare, improving the appearance and forming a stable iris diaphragm to support an anterior or posterior chamber lens. Polypropylene sutures are preferred for this.

Management of gross ocular disruption

In gross perforating injuries and in injuries involving loss of retinal tissue, the eye cannot be repaired. In such cases enucleation or evisceration should be performed as soon as appropriate counselling has been given and consent obtained. Often this will be delayed to obtain a second opinion: this reassures the patient and allows adjustment to the necessity of losing the eye. Careful observation is necessary to detect the onset of endophthalmitis or sympathetic ophthalmitis.

When the need to remove the eye is accepted, either enucleation or evisceration is carried out. Enucleation (excision of the whole eye) is done when the eye is severely damaged, with no hope of useful vision; it is also done for a blind painful eye. Evisceration (removal of ocular contents) is indicated when there is very severe intraocular infection, e.g. panophthalmitis and an eye full of pus: evisceration avoids the risk of opening the meningeal sheath of the optic nerve and giving rise to bacterial meningitis.

Enucleation

This is done under general anaesthesia. The conjunctiva is incised around the limbus (peritomy), and the rectus muscles are transected at their scleral insertions; the oblique muscles are also transected. We then transect the optic nerve by introducing the wire loop of the Foster snare over the eye as far back as possible; this is facilitated by placing curved artery forceps on the tip of the loop, releasing as the snare is tightened. The transection is usually bloodless. Tenon's capsule and the conjunctiva are closed as separate layers.

Coralline implant

If the orbital and adnexal tissues are not seriously damaged, we recommend the insertion of an integrated hydroxyapatite (coral) implant at the time of enucleation, to give a better aesthetic appearance when an ocular prosthesis is fitted.

This implant represents the most recent advance in the primary treatment of the anophthalmic patient. The technique was first introduced by Perry in 1987 and has now been approved for use as in ocular implantation by the US Food and Drug Administration (Perry 1990, 1991a,b, Dutton 1991). The material is a specially treated coral that is usually placed within the scleral shell of the damaged eye, or if this is not available, in a shell from a donor cadaver. The implant material comes from a specific genus of reef-building coral and is made of calcium carbonate, changed through a hydrothermal chemical reaction to calcium phosphate, the structure of which closely resembles the microarchitecture of normal cancellous bone. When placed in the orbit, it becomes completely ingrown with fibrovascular tissue from the orbit. Once this has happened, a hole can be drilled through the front surface of the implant and a peg placed in the hole which is connected to the ocular prosthesis. The advantages are that the implant will not migrate and, once vascularized, will not extrude even if exposed to the outside environment. The other major advantage is that the prosthesis moves like a normal eye as it still has the rectus muscles attached. However, anecdotal reports suggest that prosthetic support by a peg may not be essential, good movement being imparted to the prosthesis by the coralline implant alone. The chief complication of the procedure is implant exposure, which may take many months to heal.

Evisceration

The cornea is incised at the limbus and removed with scissors; the contents of the eye are then scooped out and the inner surface of the sclera is carefully scrubbed to remove all uveal tissue. This can be done with a gauze swab held in an artery forceps. The pigment layer is usually adherent around the exit sites of the vortex veins. It is often a bloody operation.

If a coralline ball is then to be inserted, the scleral shell is cut so that it can be sutured to hug the ball closely, with no residual dead space. Four windows are cut in the sclera at the sites of the four rectus muscles. These are then sutured into the windows to promote vascularization of the ball. The conjunctiva and Tenon's capsule are then closed over the implant. Some 6 months later, a point corresponding to the desired centre of the new ocular prosthesis is marked on the healed conjunctiva and a hole is drilled at that point in the coralline ball. Into this is fitted an acrylic plug. The epithelium grows under the plug to line the hole in the ball; later, this hole is used to seat a longer plug attached to the prosthetic eye.

Severe intraocular infection contraindicates insertion of a prosthetic sphere into the scleral shell, which is therefore closed with absorbable sutures. These should allow drainage, and the conjunctiva is therefore not closed completely.

When the eye is severely shredded, it is important to search the orbit around the muscles and in the orbital fat for remnants of uveal tissue. It is often easier to enucleate a severely lacerated eye if the scleral tears are held together with sutures.

After enucleation or evisceration, a vaseline gauze pack is inserted into the conjunctival sac, and a pressure dressing is applied for 48 h. An ocular prosthesis is fitted 6–8 weeks later; an acrylic or glass shell is temporarily inserted in the intervening period to prevent adhesions and to maintain a deep inferior fornix to hold the prosthesis.

Management of intraocular foreign bodies

The removal of an intraocular foreign body is best done as early as possible. Inflammation around an intraocular foreign body may rapidly produce a fibrous capsule which can make delayed removal difficult. Foreign bodies containing copper cause immediate severe inflammatory changes, while iron can cause chronic siderotic damage (p. 154). Traumatic endophthalmitis is more often seen as a complication of an intraocular foreign body than after a penetrating injury without an intraocular foreign body.

Preoperatively an attempt should be made to determine the type, size, location and accessibility of the intraocular foreign body. The history may help to determine whether the intraocular foreign body is metallic, and if metallic, whether magnetic or not. Shell and mine fragments are usually ferromagnetic, as are most modern shotgun pellets. Splinters from a ricocheting bullet are unlikely to be magnetic, though steel military bullets intended to fragment may have this property — a small and doubtless unintended benefit of their lethal design.

Intravitreal magnetic foreign bodies may be removed using a magnet through a pars plana sclerotomy (Fig. 14.3B) after repair of the entry site. If there is a vitreous haemorrhage and/or cataract, a pars plana vitrectomy and/or lensectomy may be needed before the intraocular foreign body is removed. The external magnet may be used, but in some cases better control may be obtained by inserting foreign body forceps or a rare-earth intraocular magnet through the pars plana sclerotomy.

Intraretinal foreign bodies are more difficult and more hazardous to remove. If clearly seen, the foreign body may be removed transsclerally through a trapdoor after the choroidal bed has been diathermied and incised. The foreign body may be removed by forceps or by the external magnet. A localized scleral buckle may be needed after the removal (Fig. 14.3C–E). It is sometimes necessary to use cryopexy to reinforce the effects of the previously applied diathermy. If visualization is not good then the foreign body should be removed transvitreally after a pars plana vitrectomy. The foreign body should be gently loosened with forceps before being removed either with the forceps or magnet. A surrounding fibrous capsule may need incision before removal. It is important to remove the posterior hyaloid overlying the area of retinal incarceration, though if a posterior vitreous detachment is already present this is not required. This procedure helps to prevent vitreoretinal traction and/or epiretinal membrane formation leading to retinal detachment.

There is controversy about the need to produce choroidoretinal adhesions at the site of damage caused by an intraocular foreign body (Ambler & Meyers 1991).

The inflammation caused by the foreign body may be in itself enough to produce this adhesion without further cryotherapy or photocoagulation. Some authorities advocate the use of photocoagulation around the intraretinal foreign body preoperatively to decrease the risk of localized detachment of the retina when the foreign body is removed, but this retinopexy may stimulate scar formation in the vitreous, leading to later problems from traction. If retinal detachment does occur at the time of removal then the posterior cortical vitreous should be removed from the retina before fluid–gas exchange is done; the fluid–gas exchange tamponades the retina back in place. If the adherent vitreous cannot be removed completely then a supporting buckle will be necessary. Non-magnetic foreign bodies must be removed with forceps; a pars plana vitrectomy will be needed, with or without lensectomy, depending on the clarity of the lens.

Other foreign bodies, such as glass or plastic, may be observed without immediate removal; however, immediate removal is generally preferable because of the risk of infection. If an intraocular foreign body is too large to be removed through a pars plana sclerotomy then an open technique may be required. Intralenticular foreign bodies may be removed, perhaps by the extracapsular cataract extraction technique with posterior chamber lens implantation. Non-metallic foreign bodies producing little visual deficiency may be treated expectantly especially if the lens is clear. Plasma glue has been used to seal the ruptured lens capsule after extraction of metallic foreign bodies from a clear lens (p. 410).

Management of double perforating injuries

Injuries with both an entry and an exit wound in the globe are often due to small missiles from firearms. In the past, double perforating injuries had a uniformly poor prognosis. This was largely due to an ingrowth of fibrovascular tissue through the posterior exit site; pars plana vitrectomy may limit this process if undertaken early in the second week after the injury. The anterior entry site should be repaired as a primary procedure. It is important to try to create a posterior vitreous detachment during the vitrectomy procedure. Retinal breaks should be managed with gas–fluid exchange and endophotocoagulation or scleral buckling with cryopexy. The eye should be routinely encircled with a scleral buckle (Fig. 14.3C–E).

Complications and results of penetrating ocular injuries

Factors associated with poor final visual outcome are:

- No perception of light on admission
- An afferent pupillary defect
- A wound involving the sclera and/or extending posterior to the insertion of the rectus muscles

- A wound > 10 mm in length
- Severe intraocular haemorrhage
- Severe prolapse of intraocular contents
- Endophthalmitis.

The initial visual acuity is the single most important factor in predicting final visual acuity in patients with penetrating eye injuries. The presence of an afferent pupil defect is also a bad prognostic factor indicating primary optic nerve or severe retinal damage. However, ciliary body and/or retinal function may also be lost later by traction from delayed intravitreal fibrovascular and fibroglial proliferation, or from infection.

Over the last 50 years the prognosis for patients suffering penetrating eye injuries has gradually improved (Fig. 14.6). De Juan et al (1983) reported that some 71% of 453 patients with penetrating injuries had a final visual acuity of 20/50 or better. Eagling (1975, 1976) found that 85% of eyes with anterior segment injuries and 40% of eyes with posterior segment injuries retained 20/40 or better vision.

The prognosis for anterior segment injuries has not improved greatly over the last 20 years but the outcome of posterior segment injury has improved with advances in vitreoretinal surgery. Endophthalmitis is today less frequently seen and fewer eyes are lost to this complication, but it still carries a grave prognosis since it is often difficult to make an early diagnosis and to treat effectively.

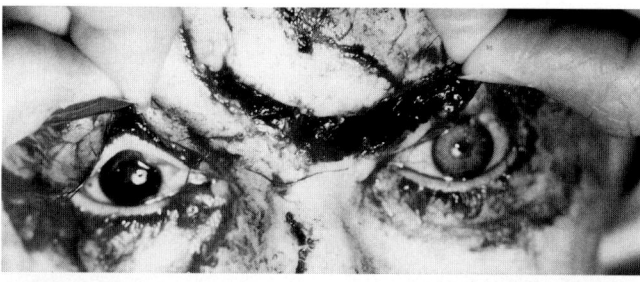

A

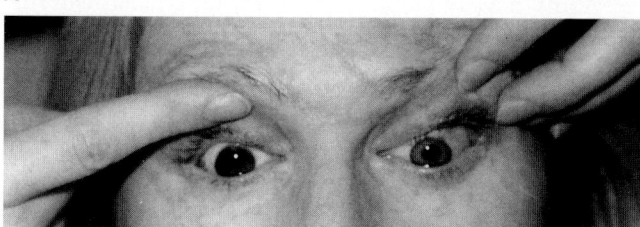

B

Fig. 14.6 Bilateral penetrating ocular wounds. A 19-year-old man suffered penetrating wounds of both eyes from windscreen glass. **A** On admission, there was escape of vitreous from corneo-scleral lacerations of both eyes. On the right, the lens and most of the iris were also injured. **B** With microsurgical techniques, the corneoscleral lacerations were repaired with 10/0 monofilament nylon, and the prolapsing uveal tissue and vitreous gel were abscised, together with aspiration of the damaged right lens. 2 months later, the wounds were well healed. On the right, vision with an aphakic contact lens was 6/9; on the left, vision was 6/5 without correction.

The prognosis for patients with intraocular foreign bodies has improved with improved techniques. Hadden & Wilson (1990) reported that 36 (64%) of 56 cases regained 6/60 vision or better; indeed more than half got 6/6–6/12 visual acuity. Shotgun pellets have a poor prognosis. This is due to the relatively large foreign body travelling at low velocities, producing significant shearing forces on the retina by distension of vitreous base.

ENDOPHTHALMITIS

Surgical pathology

Bacterial endophthalmitis is an inflammation of intraocular tissues resulting from bacterial infection. It can follow any kind of penetrating injury no matter how seemingly innocuous; it may complicate a self-sealing corneal traumatic perforation, or even the cutting of deeply placed sutures weeks after ocular surgery. It may be seen in perhaps 2–7% of such injuries, most often complicating missile or sharp, penetrating injuries.

Under appropriate conditions, almost any organism can cause endophthalmitis, but the organisms most commonly isolated include *Staphylococcus epidermidis*, *Staphy. aureus*, *Proteus* spp., and *Pseudomonas aeruginosa*. *Bacillus cereus* and *Propionbacterium acnes*, as well as *Staph. epidermidis*, have been reported to cause delayed endophthalmitis. Rural accidents may include perforation by objects contaminated with organic matter, causing endophthalmitis from which multiple organisms are grown (Boldt et al 1989).

Sterile endophthalmitis may result from retained lens debris, incarceration of iris or vitreous in a wound, foreign bodies and postoperative iridocyclitis. Blood itself may induce an intraocular inflammation.

Clinical assessment

Endophthalmitis should be suspected whenever the inflammatory signs of a wound are out of proportion to what is expected in the clinical setting. The condition usually presents 1–4 days after injury, though this time base is not invariable.

Signs include chemosis, hyperaemia, corneal oedema and especially anterior chamber reaction with hypopyon (pus level in the anterior chamber) and vitritis. Aqueous or vitreous fluff balls are characteristic of fungal infections. *B. cereus* has been associated with severe traumatic endophthalmitis, rapid in onset and characterized by severe orbital swelling and possibly a corneal ring ulcer.

Bacteriological diagnosis

Whenever there is suspicion of endophthalmitis, aqueous and vitreous tap should be performed to obtain specimens for culture, including fungal culture. The patient is sedated, and if necessary retrobulbar anaesthesia is given. A scratch incision is made under microscopy, partially through peripheral clear cornea (Forster 1991). A 25 gauge needle attached to a tuberculin syringe is inserted through the partial incision into the anterior chamber, and 0.1–0.2 ml aqueous is aspirated. This is immediately sent for microbiological examination. If the patient is aphakic, a 22 gauge needle can be inserted into the vitreous through the same keratotomy, and about ~0.3 ml vitreous can be aspirated, the needle tip being observed under the microscope. Vitreous specimens may require concentration either by centrifugation or passage through membrane filter systems.

If the patient is phakic, vitreous tap is done through a separate sclerotomy 4 mm posterior to the limbus; if an adequate sample of vitreous is not obtained by simple aspiration, the entrance site is enlarged and a localized vitrectomy is done with a vitrectomy instrument. The keratotomy or sclerotomy incision is closed with a suture if necessary.

Management

Intravitreal injections of antibiotics are prepared in tuberculin syringes and injected at the time of the diagnostic vitreous tap. For initial therapy, we use cephalothin (2.25 mg in 0.1 ml) and gentamicin sulphate (0.1 mg in 0.1 ml) or amikacin (0.4 mg in 0.1 ml) In addition to intravitreal antibiotics, systemic topical and periocular antibiotics should be given. Intravenous chemotherapy is given in high dosage, e.g. gentamicin 120 mg 12 hourly (up to 5 mg/kg/day), and cephalothin 1 g 6 hourly, with appropriate corrections for small body weight or poor renal function; this therapy may be continued for 10–14 days, with monitoring of gentamicin levels. Fortified gentamicin eye drops (1%) and cephalothin eye drops are given hourly, with topical cycloplegics such as 1% atropine. Adjustments in the antibiotic regimen are made in the light of the sensitivities of the isolated organism and the clinical response; when the organism is especially virulent, intravitreous injection should be repeated after 48 h. When the organism has been exposed to an appropriate antibiotic regimen for some 24 h, corticosteroids are given topically, subconjunctivally and systemically; we give prednisolone (40–80 mg daily) by mouth, tapering off the course rapidly after 1–2 weeks.

B. cereus is often resistant to cephalosporins and penicillins, and in such cases, clindamycin is probably the drug of choice (O'Day et al 1981), given by intravitreal injection (1 mg in 0.1 ml) with gentamicin, as well as systemic clindamycin and gentamicin.

The role of vitrectomy in the management of bacterial endophthalmitis remains controversial. Vitrectomy is technically difficult in an infected eye, but may be useful in removing inflammatory debris and organisms, and in draining loculated pockets, thereby improving circulation and antibiotic penetration in the vitreous cavity. Vitrectomy samples are more likely to give a positive culture than needle biopsies (Donahue et al 1993). We reserve vitrectomy for those cases of infection which are already advanced on presentation, those not responding to chemotherapy over 36–48 h, and those due to especially dangerous organisms such as *Pseudomonas*.

The outcome depends chiefly on two factors: the virulence of the infecting organism and the rapid institution of appropriate therapy. Failure to worsen or to develop progressive inflammation indicates stabilization and improvement. However, there may be a temporary increase in the inflammatory reaction after intravitreous injection or therapeutic vitrectomy, making clinical decision on further treatment most difficult. Retraction of a fibrin clot or hypopyon after 3–4 days is a sign of a favourable response.

FUNGAL ENDOPHTHALMITIS

Surgical pathology

Fungal infection may follow penetrating trauma to an eye, and in contrast to bacterial infections the endophthalmitis is usually slowly progressive rather than fulminant.

Clinical assessment

Early symptoms may include redness of the eye, pain and visual loss. Slit lamp microscopy may show cells or even hypopyon and fibrin membrane in the anterior chamber; vitreous snowballs and vitreous cells may also be seen. These findings contrast with the effects of endogenous infection in persons with immunological failure, where there is likely to be fluffy white retinal infiltrate, with or without retinal haemorrhages and extension of the infection into the vitreous. Such infections have been seen in cases of AIDS, and also after marrow transplants for leukaemia.

Microbiological diagnosis

Therapy depends on the accurate identification of the organism; a vitrectomy biopsy is preferred to needle aspiration.

Management

Amphotericin B is effective against a wide variety of fungi; if clinical suspicion of fungal infection is high, it may be prudent to give an initial intravitreal injection of amphotericin B (5 μg), and then to withhold further antifungal therapy until the culture or the clinical course gives guidance. If systemic amphotericin B therapy is to be given, an intravenous test dose (1 mg) is first given, followed by a gradual increase in the dosage to 0.5 mg/kg/day. Blood picture, electrolyte screen and renal function should be monitored at 2–3 day intervals. The aim is a total intravenous dosage of 1 g; sometimes toxicity prevents this. Amphotericin B can be given intravitreally, using a dose of 5 µg; this can be repeated after 24 h, but only in an eye that is aphakic and has undergone vitrectomy; if no vitrectomy has been done, the dose should not be repeated for 5–9 days, as the drug has a long half-life.

Flucytosine (5-fluorocytosine) has been successfully used in candida and cryptococcal infections; it penetrates both the aqueous and the vitreous, and can be given orally (100–150 mg/kg/day in four doses); serum levels should be monitored, especially if the drug is given concurrently with amphotericin. Ketoconazole can also be given orally; this drug can cause liver damage. Fluconazole, a similar antifungal drug, may be preferable; it is also effective orally (200–400 mg/day as a single dose), and is reported to penetrate into the ocular tissues and fluids readily, both in the presence of experimental *Candida endophthalmitis* and in normal control animals (O'Day et al 1990). Caution is necessary in the choice of antifungal drugs, and a clinical mycologist should be consulted, especially if there is any possibility of renal impairment.

Corticosteroids should be given after a period of appropriate antifungal therapy. An associated fungal keratitis is treated with hourly topical 0.15% amphotericin, 1% miconazole or 5% natamycin, together with subconjunctival amphotericin B (0.5 mg–1 mg) or miconazole (5–10 mg).

Vitrectomy may help by removing infecting organisms and promoting circulation of the large molecules of the antibiotic; removal of the vitreous scaffolding may reduce the incidence of tractional retinal detachment. If the iris or posterior lens capsule is thought to be infiltrated with fungus, then these tissues can be removed at the same time.

In resistant cases of deep keratitis with retrocorneal/anterior chamber fungal infection, a corneal graft may be needed (Pflugfelder et al 1988).

Results and complications of bacterial and fungal endophthalmitis

The results of treatment of post-traumatic endophthalmitis are poor: in one series of 27 eyes with positive cultures, 20/400 (6/120) or better vision was preserved in only 2/22 (9%) of bacterial infections and 4/5 (80%) of fungal infections (Forster 1991). Our experience is limited, but is in accord with this report: early and appropriate treatment of a penetrating eye injury has not prevented the onset of acute *B. cereus* endophthalmitis 27 h after injury, with eventual loss of sight.

When acute endophthalmitis in a painful blinded eye does not respond to the regime outlined above, the eye should be eviscerated.

SYMPATHETIC OPHTHALMITIS

Surgical pathology

This is a chronic inflammation of the uveal tract characterized by nodular or diffuse infiltration of lymphocytes and epithelioid cells (p. 152). Onset is insidious; a new inflammatory process usually appears in the injured or exciting eye within 2–3 months after ocular injury (Lubin et al 1980), the sympathizing eye becoming involved simultaneously or soon afterwards. Sympathetic ophthalmitis has been recorded as early as 5 days after trauma (Verhoeff 1927) and as late as 42 years (Green 1986); however, in 88% of cases, the onset is within 6 months of the inciting injury (Lubin et al 1980). Accidental ocular injury has been the cause of 54–65% of histologically verified cases reported in the USA (Green 1986, Joy 1935), most of the remainder being secondary to intraocular surgery. Suppuration of the injured eye has long been known to protect against the development of sympathetic ophthalmitis.

Incidence

This is uncertain. Few observers have seen many cases; pathological proof is often lacking, and the diagnosis is frequently only presumptive. Albert & Diaz-Rohena (1989) recently reviewed and tabulated various reported series; it appears that since 1967, the average incidence after non-surgical injury has been 1.5%, while the incidence after intraocular surgery has been 0.04%. Not one case was reported among 3459 victims of ocular trauma in the Korean, Vietnamese and Six Day (Israeli) wars (Hull 1951, Hoefle 1968, Treister 1969). However, these figures are flawed, because many badly damaged eyes were enucleated early as a preventive measure. The true risk rate is unknown.

Males are affected twice as often as females, presumably because they are more often injured; after intraocular surgery, the sex incidences are equal. The condition is said to be rare in the South-West Pacific and among Australian aborigines (Mann 1961) and in Central Africa (Phillips 1961), but is well recognized in Asia as well as in the Western Hemisphere (Kuo et al 1982).

Clinical assessment

Clinically, sympathetic ophthalmitis can be confused with bilateral iritis, or with phakoanaphylaxis — also an immune response, but to lens protein from the injured eye. The diagnosis can only be established by histopathology after enucleation.

The earlier symptoms in the uninjured eye are photophobia and blurred vision. Iritis and cystoid macular oedema are seen on slit lamp examination. A severe granulomatous anterior uveitis usually develops, with formation of 'mutton fat' keratitic precipitates on the endothelial surface of the cornea. A posterior uveitis is also usually seen, characterized by grey/white subretinal nodules, often peripherally sited; these are the Dalen–Fuchs nodules seen on histopathological examination. Similar changes are seen in the injured eye, though it may be impossible to visualize them.

Prevention and management

The only effective prophylaxis is enucleation of the injured eye before the autoimmune response has developed. Reports suggest that the risk of sympathetic ophthalmitis is extremely small if the injured eye is enucleated within 2 weeks of the injury, and early enucleation of a traumatized blind eye should be urged.

There is unresolved debate as to whether enucleation of the injured (exciting) eye has any effect on the course of the disease process after the onset of sympathetic ophthalmitis. Therefore, once the diagnosis has been made, enucleation of the exciting eye should seldom be done since this eye may turn out to have the better vision. Corticosteroids given prophylactically after trauma are reported to be ineffective in preventing the onset of sympathetic ophthalmitis, but do mitigate the severity of the inflammatory process (Lubin et al 1980), and give a better visual outcome. Corticosteroids are therefore the treatment of choice, in the form of high doses of prednisolone, up to 200 mg per day over the first 7–10 days, with frequent topical corticosteroids. It seems logical to give a selective agent that suppresses T-lymphocyte function, and Cyclosporin A has been suggested when corticosteroids are not tolerated or prove ineffective (Jakobiec et al 1983). Azathioprine has also been used effectively (Moore 1968).

Medicolegal implications

When a traumatized eye is blind, we explain the risks to the patient, and obtain a second opinion from another ophthalmologist within a week of the injury. This enables enucleation to be done well before the fourteenth day after injury. The second opinion is both reassuring for the patient and expedient for the surgeon.

SECONDARY GLAUCOMA

Surgical pathology

Blunt impact on the eye compresses the globe from front to back (Fig. 4.11), causing lateral shearing between the uvea and its attachments to the scleral wall. This shearing may cause damage to the structures in the drainage angle — the ciliary muscle, the trabecular meshwork and the iris (Fig. 2.36). Tears through the ciliary musculature often rupture small arterioles, giving rise to a hyphaema. There may be an early rise in intraocular pressure, due either to the hyphaema itself, or to traumatic iritis with inflammation of the trabecular network, or to dislocation of the lens and pupillary block.

Ghost cell glaucoma characteristically follows traumatic vitreous haemorrhage and disruption of the anterior hyaloid face. Degenerated red blood cells (ghost cells) then pass forward into the anterior chamber and obstruct the intertrabecular spaces of the trabecular meshwork, being less pliable than fresh red cells, which can pass through the meshwork.

Delayed glaucoma may occur if there is a gradual closure of a traumatic cleft in the drainage angle, or by endothelial growth over the chamber angle with deposition of tissue resembling Descemet's membrane. In >90% of ocular contusions causing hyphaema, gonioscopy will show angle recession, or other damage in the anterior chamber angle (Morrison 1990). When the angle recession is >180°, glaucoma develops in up to 10% of cases; this usually occurs in the first year after injury.

Management

Traumatic iritis is best treated by topical 1% prednisolone eye drops, together with a cycloplegic agent. Causes of glaucoma other than iritis can be treated with β-blocking agents such as $\frac{1}{2}$% timolol or $\frac{1}{2}$% betaxolol eye drops; 0.1% dipivefrin or 4% pilocarpine may be given to give additional reduction in intraocular pressure. We aim to keep the pressure to <25 mmHg, though other factors may modify this policy: these include pre-existing glaucoma, compromise of the retinal vascular circulation, and decompensation of the corneal endothelium.

If topical medications fail to lower the intraocular pressure, systemic carbonic anhydrase inhibitors may be needed, such as oral or intravenous acetazolamide (250 mg 6 hourly). If maximal medical therapy fails, or if progressive field loss or optic disc cupping appears, surgery may be necessary. Argon laser trabeculoplasty may occasionally induce an acute rise in intraocular pressure, and many ophthalmologists advocate trabeculectomy to improve filtration. Glaucoma complicating the sickle cell trait carries extra risks, and the use of acetazolamide is contraindicated, because the acidosis that may result from this drug can trigger sickling. In these patients Methazolamide or Neptazane should be used instead to reduce intraocular pressure. In sickle-cell anaemia, intraocular pressure remaining >25 mmHg for 24 h is an indication for aggressive intervention.

Long-term follow-up is essential. In particular, patients with >180° of angle recession should undergo annual tonometry and examination of the optic disk for the rest of their lives.

OCULAR MOTOR INJURIES

Surgical pathology

CMF trauma may impair ocular motility by damaging the extraocular muscles, the ocular motor nerves, or the centres in the brainstem or cerebral hemispheres which control ocular movement. Accommodation, convergence and fusion may also be impaired by peripheral injury.

The extraocular muscles may be severed or avulsed by penetrating injuries, and in our experience motor vehicle window glass (p. 89) has been the commonest cause. Knife stabs and more bizarre injuries such as avulsion by a dog's lower incisors or a shop display hook have been reported (Helveston 1990); we have seen avulsion of the inferior rectus by the fingernail of a psychotic man attempting self-enucleation (Fig. 14.7). The tendon of the superior oblique muscle, or its trochlea, is most often injured by stab wounds, and troublesome diplopia is the likely outcome (Fig. 14.8). Blow-out fractures of the orbital floor or medial wall (p. 328) often entrap orbital fat and fibrous septae; less commonly the belly of the inferior or medial rectus muscle is entrapped, resulting in diplopia which may persist despite repair of the fracture, from scarring of the muscle.

Post-traumatic sixth nerve palsies are more common than third nerve palsies, fourth nerve palsies being least common (Rush & Younge 1981). The sixth nerve is vulnerable in its course over the petrous apex, where it may be involved in a skull base fracture; one or both sixth nerves may be paralysed as a non-localizing effect of raised intracranial pressure. The fourth nerve is vulnerable at its origin from the dorsal surface of the midbrain and in its course around the brainstem; paralysis may

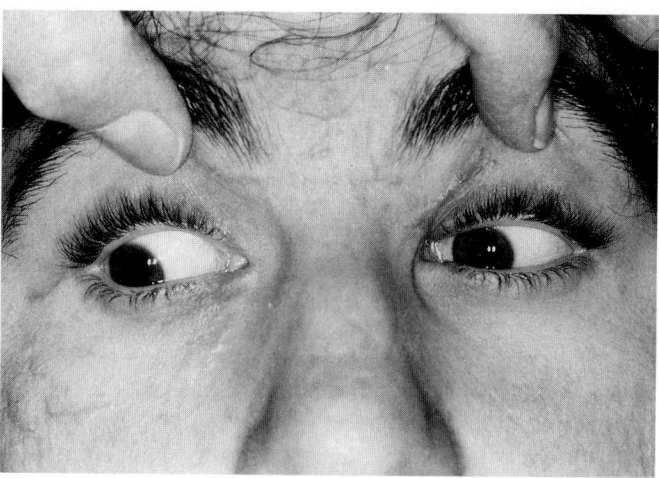

Fig. 14.8 Trochlear detachment: weakness of the superior oblique muscle. The trochlear attachment was injured by a penetrating wound above the left medial canthus. The victim has limitation of eye movement in the line of action of the superior oblique muscle — in gaze down and medially. This is usually associated with troublesome diplopia and a characteristic tilt of the head to the side opposite to the paralysed muscle.

follow seemingly trivial head impacts. Bilateral fourth nerve weakness may be seen as part of a severe closed head injury; the paresis may be asymmetrical and the weakness of the less severely affected superior oblique muscle may only become evident after corrective surgery on the other muscle. The third nerve is most often injured in severe closed head injuries, either as a primary effect, presumably by avulsion (Heinze 1969) in its intradural course, or secondarily by pressure from transtentorial herniation (Fig. 2.28).

Neuroanatomy

Conjugate horizontal gaze palsies are usually due to damage in the pontine paramedian reticular formation, in the vicinity of the nucleus of the sixth cranial nerve; the gaze palsy is usually asymptomatic and recovers spontaneously. Post-traumatic paralysis of upward gaze is usually due to midbrain damage, with other signs of injury in this region (Parinaud syndrome); paralysis of gaze both up and down is associated with lesions in the rostral interstitial nucleus of the medial longitudinal bundle. Skew deviation (vertical malalignment of visual axes on lateral gaze) is due to impaired prenuclear input from the vestibular system, and is a non-specific sign of brainstem or cerebellar dysfunction (Baker & Epstein 1991), though the pons is most often the site of injury (Keane 1975). Skew deviation may be comitant or variable. The nuclei responsible for the near reflex (accommodation, convergence and pupillary constriction) are thought to be in the pretectal midbrain, rostral to the third nerve nuclei. Head impacts may impair accommodation, and this is often mistakenly diagnosed as inattention, lack of effort

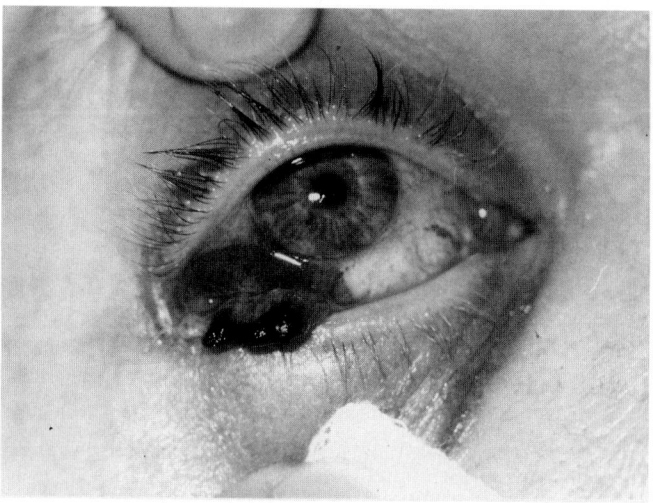

Fig. 14.7 Self-inflicted avulsion of the inferior rectus muscle. A psychotic man attempted to enucleate his own eye, and succeeded in avulsing the inferior rectus muscle before he was restrained. The torn muscle ends were debrided and sutured together, with a good result.

or dyslexia; it is important to make the correct diagnosis, since convex reading lenses may compensate for the impaired accommodation. Convergence insufficiency with intermittent diplopia and blurred near vision have often been noted after head injury, and may be helped by convergence exercises or base-out prisms in reading glasses. The opposite problem, convergence spasm, is rare in our experience. Divergence insufficiency or actual paralysis is also rare (Rutkowski & Burian 1972); divergence is thought to be an active process, not merely a relaxation of convergence (Tamler & Jampolski 1967).

Fusion of the images from the two retinas is mediated in the cerebral cortex, and requires the images to fall on corresponding points in each retina. Fusion defects may be either sensory or motor, the latter being far more common. In motor fusion defects, patients are able to perceive stereoscopic detail when the images are aligned. Inadequacies in vergence reduce the range over which fusion can be maintained. When post-traumatic diplopia is due to an nuclear or infranuclear lesion, vergence is usually unimpaired and correction of the motor defect gives satisfactory fusion. When fusion is not preserved, and a deviation is reduced so that the two images are close together, the patient may be unable to fuse these images and will suffer from persisting diplopia. Such patients, unless able to suppress one image, will have to use an eye patch or wear a contact lens with an opaque pupillary aperture. We have seen six patients with central loss of fusion of this type.

Nerve regeneration

Under favourable circumstances, the ocular motor nerves have the capacity to regenerate completely (p. 136). However, regeneration may be aberrant, resulting in inappropriate movements. This is a well-known complication of third nerve paralysis, and may result in involuntary eye movements and inappropriate pupillary constriction when the gaze of the affected eye is changed. Miller (1985) gives a good overview of this problem. Aberrant cross regeneration between adjacent cranial nerves is also sometimes seen. We have reported an unusual case of trigemino-abducens synkinesis some 2 years after a basal skull fracture in a woman aged 25, who had suffered paralysis of the third, fifth, sixth and seventh cranial nerves on the right side. She showed right facial hemianaesthesia and masseteric paralysis, but found that when she ate or chewed, she developed involuntary abduction of the ipsilateral eye. Electromyography of the lateral rectus muscle supported the diagnosis of aberrant reinnervation. Operation (recession of the right medial and lateral rectus muscles) improved her compensatory head posture and minimized the chewing-induced abduction (McGovern et al 1986). An almost identical case was reported by Nelson & Kline (1990). J. Harrison (personal communi-

cation) has described a case of facial fracture followed by involuntary abduction of one eye on eating, from a different cause: attachment of the transected body of the lateral rectus muscle to the temporalis muscle through a defect in the orbital wall.

Incidence

Although the motility syndromes associated with CMF trauma have been well described, there are few accurate estimates of their incidence (Baker & Epstein 1991, Kowal 1992). Steidler et al (1980) found diplopia in 32.1% of patients with fractures of the middle third of the face. In many cases of CMF injury, residual cognitive or behavioural impairment may impede evaluation of ocular motility, or may impair the ability to tolerate diplopia.

Clinical assessment

A semiconscious individual will not be bothered by diplopia but, when more alert, will tend to close one eye and eventually will complain of the second image. Later, compensatory head postures will be adopted in order to assist fusion of the two images. A patient complaining of double vision should be carefully observed for an abnormal head posture. This happens particularly in cases of incomitant squint where head posture is employed to obtain and maintain binocularity. Thus, a patient with a left lateral rectus paresis will have a left convergent squint (esotropia) due to the action of the relatively unopposed left medial rectus muscle. The patient will turn the face to the left and hold the eyes looking to the right to assist fusion. If fusion is not possible, the patient may turn the head to maximize the image separation, either to facilitate suppression or to use the nose to block one image. A patient with a head tilt to the right shoulder will almost certainly be compensating for a left fourth nerve palsy or trochlear injury.

Trauma can very rarely cause monocular diplopia by damaging the cornea, lens or macula. Much more often, the diplopia is binocular and due to misalignment of the two visual axes. This can be proved subjectively with the red glass test, wherein a red glass is held by the patient in front of the right eye, thereby producing a red image. The patient then fixates on a distant light and is asked if two lights (one red and one white), are seen separated in space. The various cardinal positions of gaze are also tested in the near position. The recognition of two separate images indicates ocular misalignment. Glasses or goggles with one red and one green lens or eye cover are a convenient variant of this test; even poorly cooperative patients can distinguish the red and green images. The best objective test, however, is the cover/uncover test. The patient is asked to fixate on a distant target; one eye is quickly covered and the other eye is observed to see if it moves to pick up fixation. Such movement indicates a manifest squint or tropia. Lack of movement suggests that the eye is fixing on the target appropriately. The occluder is then removed and the uncovered eye observed for movement (uncover test). Such movement indicates a lateral deviation or phoria. This sequence is then repeated by covering the other eye and the process is repeated in the cardinal positions of gaze for both distant and near fixation. One must suspect an intermittent problem if there is a clear history of diplopic similar images and yet there is no ocular misalignment found on the cover test.

When the patient is fixing with the non-paretic eye, the deviation noted is known as the primary deviation, whilst secondary deviation is noted when the paretic eye is fixing. The larger deviation is always when the paretic eye fixates. A subjective difference whilst fixating with each eye in turn indicates nuclear or infranuclear pathology. Secondary muscular contractures occurring over time may lead to lessening of the image separation in the direction of action of the paretic muscle with greater concomitance in the various cardinal positions of gaze. Many patients with weakness of the oblique muscles experience tilting of the image from the affected eye. This may be accompanied by symptoms of nausea and dizziness. Torsional double vision can occur without any vertical separation and is easily measured with the Maddox Rod. Any torsional deviation > 10–12° strongly suggests the presence of bilateral superior oblique palsies.

Post-traumatic strabismus is usually incomitant, in that the angles between the two eyes are different in the different positions of gaze. One must always consider restrictive muscle problems such as entrapment (e.g. blow-out fracture) in the differential diagnosis. It is very important to use a forced duction test to look for mechanical restriction. Topical anaesthetic drops are applied to the eyes and a cotton bud, or better a large plastic contact lens attached to a suction cup on a handle, is applied over the suspect eye. The examiner then tries to rotate the eye in the opposite direction. Thus in down-gaze paresis, duction is applied to the insertion of the superior rectus muscle and the eye is rotated downwards. The two eyes are compared for comparative ease and range of passive movement. One must beware of pushing the globe backwards as this will falsely facilitate movement. Alternatively, toothed forceps can be applied to the muscle insertion, but this is much more likely to induce pain: the patient may flinch and the cornea may be injured by the forceps.

Radiological assessment

A patient complaining of diplopia or any other disorder of ocular motor function usually needs a careful and well-planned neuroradiological assessment. A CT scan with fine cuts through the orbit should confirm the diagnosis if muscle tethering is suspected. It is important to request slices in the coronal plane as these give better pictures than reconstructions from axial images, and show more clearly the relationships between ocular muscles, orbital walls and other structures. When the disorder is thought to be intracranial, MRI is usually the most productive investigation.

Management

General principles

Some disorders of ocular motility require urgent correction. Muscles lacerated by penetrating orbital injuries should be repaired as soon as possible. Orbital fractures complicated by muscle entrapment require early exploration. But in most cases, a period of observation is necessary to allow time for spontaneous recovery.

At least 6 months are usually allowed for recovery of an injured ocular motor nerve; when there has been a severe head injury, 12–18 months will often be allowed. Patients who require secondary bony realignment and grafting to the orbit will often have ocular motility problems; treatment of these should be delayed until at least 3 months have elapsed after all other surgery has been completed. The condition must remain stable and clinical observations unchanged for at least two successive visits before treatment is contemplated. At each visit, the ocular movements and deviations are remeasured, and the field of binocularity and muscle balance charts (Hess or Lee screen) are completed. In a busy clinic, an orthoptist is a cost-efficient delegate for serial screening.

Initial patching or occlusion of one eye will be necessary if the angle is too large to compensate. A compensatory head posture and/or temporary stick-on Fresnel prism may be useful; the prisms may need to be changed for weaker ones as recovery occurs. The patient should be encouraged to return to work when fit enough, provided there is no danger to either self or others; working at heights, with moving machinery or with vehicles should be avoided.

Surgery is used to overcome symptoms and restore concomitance as far as possible, thereby enlarging the field of binocular single vision which preferably should be placed centrally and extending into the lower field, the most used part of the visual field. The decisions as to which muscles to operate on and how much to do are influenced by various factors such as the nature and duration of the palsy, the presence of secondary muscle sequelae and of torsion, and the findings at operation (Crompton 1992).

Sixth nerve injury

Treatment of paresis will differ from that for paralysis. In paralysis there is no activity of the lateral rectus muscle; a simple recession (weakening) of the ipsilateral medial rectus and tightening (resection) of the paralysed muscle (as is done in paretic muscles) will fail, because the unopposed medial rectus muscle will continue to tighten. Traditionally muscles have been split and yoked together or transplanted; the superior and inferior rectus muscles are moved laterally and the medial rectus muscles are recessed. This results in some abduction of the eye and restoration of binocularity in the primary position. The best results can be obtained by using adjustable sutures with temporary knots placed when the muscles are moved under anaesthesia; the position of the muscles can be changed by readjusting the knots once the patient is sufficiently alert to be tested postoperatively.

Botulinum A toxin is a powerful neurotoxin and, when injected into a muscle, blocks neuro-muscular transmission by destruction of muscle endplates (which later regrow). It is now used to prevent secondary contractions of the ipsilateral medial rectus muscle and can hasten the binocular rehabilitation of the patient. The toxin is also used for other ocular motility problems (Lipton et al 1990).

Third nerve injury

Here also, the choice of surgery depends on the degree of weakness. Frequently there is moderate recovery of the medial rectus muscle but not of the other muscles with little ability in elevation and depression. Such cases respond well to simple horizontal recession/resection surgery using adjustable sutures.

The management of complete paralysis is problematic. Accommodation is usually lost and the enlarged pupil may then cause sensitivity to glare; however, miotics can be used regularly to obviate this. Surgery involves adjustable weakening of the intact lateral rectus muscle and disinsertion of the superior oblique muscle tendon, which is shortened and attached just above the insertion of the medial rectus. The ptotic upper lid can be lifted by a sling procedure, though if this is done, the loss of the protective Bell's reflex may lead to corneal ulceration from exposure. Aberrant reinnervation by the regenerating third nerve axons can lead to bizarre eye movement. Third nerve palsies due to severe head trauma may be complicated by central loss of fusion; this will result in intolerable diplopia if surgery for ptosis is successful in opening the eye.

Even if successful, surgery can only give a small central area of binocularity with constant diplopia everywhere else. Many surgeons would therefore hesitate to suggest surgery as the patient can be rehabilitated far earlier and more cheaply with monocular vision, since the complete ptosis prevents diplopia. A frosted spectacle lens can mask unsightly ptosis or strabismus, and will prevent diplopia. One treatment option for those unable to suppress the aberrant images is a contact lens with an opaque pupil.

Fourth nerve injury

In our view, combined torsional diplopia with vertical separation of images maximal in adduction on gaze both upwards and downwards is best treated by shortening the involved superior oblique tendon. Isolated torsional diplopia can be corrected by tightening the anterior half of the superior oblique tendon. Surgery on secondarily contracted muscles such as the ipsilateral inferior oblique or contralateral inferior rectus may also be required. Frequently, further surgery is required after severe head injuries with trochlear nerve injury: a previously unsuspected palsy of the opposite superior oblique becomes unmasked following treatment of the first.

The details of muscle surgery are beyond the scope of this book; Mein & Harcourt (1986) give a good account. In our practice, operation is usually done under general anaesthetic, on a 'day-case' basis. Postoperative infection is rare, but antibiotic ointments are often used for a week, to minimize the scratchiness of the absorbable conjunctival sutures. Eye pads are not usually necessary but corrective spectacles are worn unless they include prisms. Children can return to school within a few days but should avoid swimming and other sports for 2 weeks. Adults can return to office work within a few days but manual workers in dirty environments will require a longer absence.

Diplopia and orbital deformity

The treatment of enophthalmos is discussed in Chapter 21 (p. 559). After correction of enophthalmos, there may be a need for corrective squint surgery for postoperative diplopia. If there is persistent paresis of down gaze of one eye, there will be associated over-action of down gaze of the other eye. This imbalance can be corrected by 'crippling' the overactive inferior rectus to match the paresis in the other eye. This is done by placing Faden sutures to the sclera through the belly of the inferior rectus muscle some 13–14 mm behind its insertion. Vertical separation in the primary position can be corrected by recessing the inferior rectus at the same time. We favour this method, but others prefer strengthening procedures wherein the right medial and lateral rectus muscles are moved to abut on the insertion of the inferior rectus muscle (Lipton et al 1990).

RETROBULBAR HAEMORRHAGE

Surgical pathology

Severe retrobulbar bleeding may complicate blunt or penetrating orbital trauma, or may result from operative exploration or even retrobulbar injection. A rise in pressure within the orbit may compromise the retinal circulation, and vision may be imperilled (p. 74).

Management

Immediate measures are aimed at reducing intraocular pressure within the tense orbit. Lateral canthotomy and inferior cantholysis are usually sufficient, but should these fail, then prompt orbital decompression is needed. There may be no time for a CT scan or for a full haematological examination but the possibility of a bleeding diathesis should be excluded as soon as possible.

Liu (1993) has described a simple and effective emergency decompression. A small opening is made with scissors in the inferior medial fornix, and a small curved mosquito clamp is inserted into the orbit and advanced along the medial orbital wall a distance of ~20 mm. The tip of the clamp is then pushed through the orbital periosteum, the orbital floor and the mucosa of the maxillary sinus; the hole in the orbital floor is then enlarged by opening and rotating the clamp. The author describes successful use of this emergency decompression in five orbits, without any loss of motility or injury to the inferior orbital nerve; there was immediate decrease in proptosis and intraocular pressure, with improvement of vision.

TRAUMATIC OPTIC NEUROPATHY

Surgical pathology

The optic nerve may be injured directly by a missile or other penetrating object, or indirectly by force transmitted through the intact skull (p. 109), when there is usually but not invariably a fracture of the skull base. Such injuries are often seen after impacts in the frontal area.

Many factors have been implicated in the pathogenesis of so-called traumatic optic neuropathy. Walsh & Lindenberg (1963) examined the optic nerves of 70 patients dead after head trauma. Lesions were found in the intraorbital, intracanalicular or intracranial parts of the nerve. They believed that they could distinguish microscopically between primary and secondary lesions. Primary lesions, which were thought to have occurred at the instant of the blow, included:

1. Haemorrhages in the nerve, the dura or the vaginal sheath of the nerve
2. Tears in the nerve, usually in the intracranial segment, but occasionally affecting the whole nerve, and not necessarily associated with a fracture
3. Contusion necrosis from mechanical trauma to the nerve.

Secondary lesions could develop seconds, minutes or even hours after the initial impact, and were thought to be basically circulatory in origin. These secondary lesions included oedema and necrosis of the nerve, presumably due to circulatory insufficiency from vasospasm, primary vaso-occlusion, or external compression.

Crompton (1970) performed similar studies on 84 cases of acute closed head injury. He stressed the importance of ischaemic and shearing axonal lesions at both ends of the optic canal, and also in the intracranial section of the optic nerve; the effects of ischaemia and mechanical shearing could not be distinguished post mortem. He believed that the lesions were inflicted at the time of impact, and therefore his study does not encourage surgical intervention. The few reports of operative biopsies of optic nerve injury (p. 136) have also failed to show lesions likely to benefit from operative treatment. But it can be argued that more favourable lesions are unlikely to be examined by pathologists.

Incidence

In our series of 237 anterior fossa fractures (p. 3.00), there were 32 (13.5%) cases with injuries of one or both optic nerves, or of the optic chiasm. Most were of the indirect type, and in the majority there was blindness of one or both eyes; six patients lost all useful vision. The incidence of blindness due to optic nerve injury in association with CMF fractures has been reported to be in the range 2–33.9% (May 1977, Steidler et al 1980, Holt & Holt 1983); this wide range presumably reflects diversity in case selection.

Clinical assessment

Optic nerve injury may be seen as part of a severe CMF injury, with extensive damage in the anterior cranial fossa and prolonged loss of consciousness. Sometimes however, especially in children, the nerve may be permanently damaged by a comparatively minor impact, typically in the lateral frontal region on the same side; there may be little or no loss of consciousness, and the loss of sight is noticed only when the patient closes one eye, or when the pupillary light reflex is tested. The variable presentation of optic nerve injury justifies the routine of careful tests of visual acuities and fields in all CMF injuries (p. 167). Initial ophthalmoscopy usually shows normal appearances even when sight is permanently lost: Hughes (1962) found that disc pallor does not appear for a

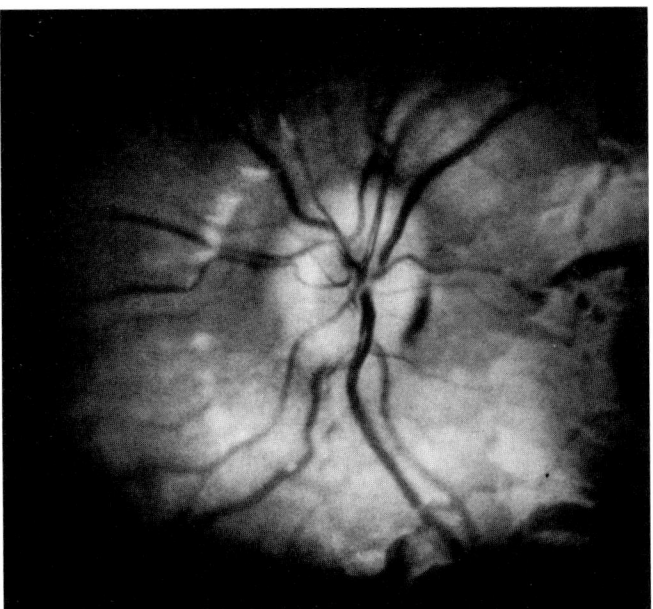

A

Fig. 14.9 Traumatic optic neuropathy with spontaneous recovery. A 10-year-old boy fell 12 feet from a tree and sustained a closed head injury. He was unconscious for some 20 min. Some days later, he complained of poor vision in his left eye, with which he could only 'count fingers'. To confrontation, there was a large central scotoma extending to the periphery in the inferonasal field.
A Fundoscopy showed gross disc swelling with scattered intraretinal haemorrhages. **B** Perimetry showed a central scotoma, with breakthrough to the periphery in the inferonasal field. Hypocycloidal tomography showed a fracture through the floor of the middle fossa involving the left optic canal. He was given dexamethazone (8 mg daily). Sight returned rapidly over the next week and he made an uneventful recovery, with final vision recorded as 6/6.

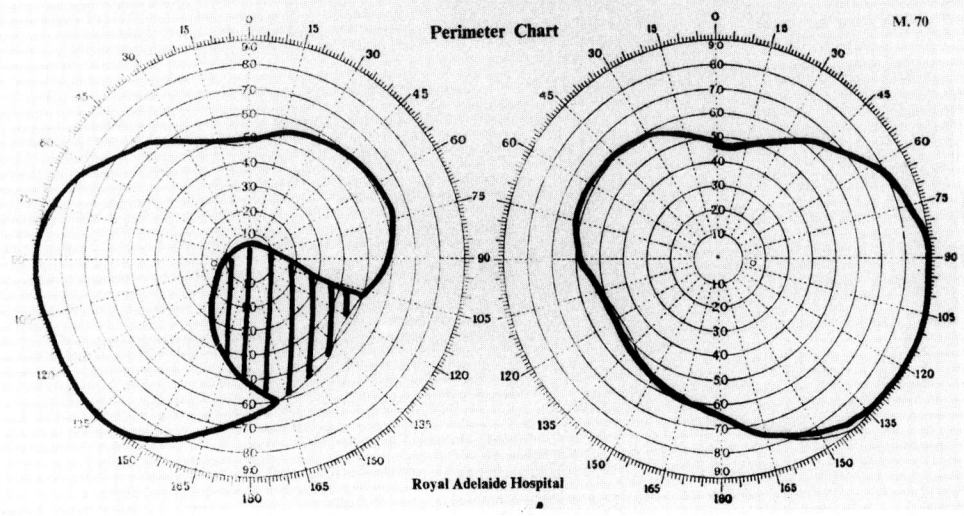

B

period ranging from several days to 3 weeks or more, depending on the proximity of the nerve lesion to the disc. However, ophthalmoscopy may show papilloedema (Fig. 14. 9A), or signs of retinal venous or arterial obstruction especially when the nerve has been injured at or close to its attachment to the globe (Hughes 1962, Kline et al 1984). In a few cases, visual impairment may appear after an interval, and this highlights the need for repeated checks of vision after frontal impacts, done very simply by covering each eye and testing subjective visual function.

Visual field charting is done as soon as cooperation permits; in partial lesions, the findings may give accurate localization of the site of injury (Fig. 2.27). Thus, unilateral altitudinal field loss (horizontal hemianopia) suggests a canalicular injury, while a bilateral defect may indicate an anterior chiasmal or central chiasmal lesion. The initial visual field chart gives a baseline for evaluation of recovery.

Radiological assessment

Fine-cut (1.5 mm) CT scanning of the skull base is the routine means of visualizing the optic foramina. Where there is a fracture with a bone spicule in the canal, coned plain X-ray pictures are sometimes helpful in determining the degree of encroachment on the lumen of the canal. In our series of 32 cases, only five had no CMF fractures; however, cases with no demonstrable fracture of the canal are by no means rare. To visualize the optic nerve itself,

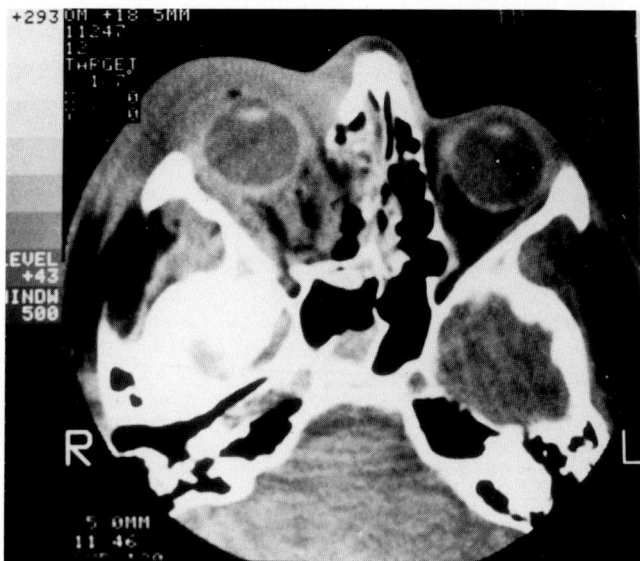

Fig. 14.10 Optic nerve transection. A 19-year-old man suffered facial fractures in a car crash, Axial CT scan showed fractures of the ethmoid complex and soft-tissue damage to the right eyelids and anterior orbit: the right optic nerve appeared swollen and seemed to be transected. This may have been a false impression caused by acute angulation of the nerve; however, axial reconstruction in the line of the optic nerve supported the impression of discontinuity in the nerve, which appeared to have been severed in the posterior orbit.

CT is sometimes satisfactory (Fig. 14.10), but MRI is more effective, and should be done as soon as possible. The finding of an enlarged optic nerve, with signals suggesting blood in the subretinal space, may justify an emergency surgical procedure.

Visual evoked responses (VER)

Mahapatra & Bhatia (1989) reported on the VER in 45 cases of indirect optic nerve injury using checkerboard visual signals; they found that preservation of P-100 waves indicated a likelihood of recovery, while repeated absence of this wave had an unfavourable significance. We have found simpler VER studies helpful in unconscious patients and in children whose cooperation was questionable. The investigation is also useful when orbital swelling prevents testing the pupillary light reflex; for this purpose, we use a hand-held flash stimulator which easily penetrates the closed eyelid (p. 248).

Management

Obviously, nothing can be done when the optic nerve is avulsed or transected. On the other hand, there are rare cases where surgery can be very beneficial. Decompression may be done for intraorbital or intracanalicular compression. A decompressive procedure is certainly indicated when a traumatic optic neuropathy results from damage to the anterior intraorbital portion of the nerve, and is associated with optic disc swelling and signs of

obstruction of the central retinal vein. A tense orbital haematoma causing compression of the optic nerve requires an emergency lateral canthotomy, with drainage of subperiosteal or intraorbital blood, or a decompression into the maxillary air sinus as described above (Liu 1993). In some cases of traumatic visual loss, recovery has followed orbital decompression alone; Radius & Anderson (1981) showed that at least some optic nerve axons can survive total ischaemia for 2 h, and lesser degrees of circulatory compromise might be tolerated longer. Hupp et al (1984) reported dramatic improvement of vision after fenestration of the swollen optic nerve sheath and release of blood. Rarely, compression of the optic nerve by a bone fragment may be rectified by removal of the compressing agent. But the treatment of cases of traumatic optic neuropathy with a normal appearance in the optic fundus is still controversial (Miller 1990).

Some patients with profound visual loss from traumatic optic neuropathy recover spontaneously. Wolin & Lavin (1990) described a patient who had lost all light perception after a blunt impact, and regained 20/50 vision without any treatment. We have seen similar cases, and have learned not to be dogmatic about the outcome for visual recovery until at least 6 weeks have elapsed; thereafter, a definitive prognosis can usually be given.

Despite these occasional gratifying recoveries, the majority of patients do not improve spontaneously. In our series of 32 patients with post-traumatic optic nerve damage, 25 were blinded in one eye or two eyes and seven suffered less severe visual impairments. Only seven (22%) regained normal central vision, and six of these were left with inferior visual field defects; of the 23 who presented with one blind eye, six had a temporal hemianopia in the other eye, probably indicating unilateral optic nerve damage combined with chiasmal cleavage. These deficits were permanent. We could find no differences either in the severity of the CMF disruptions or in the actual facial fracture patterns, and concluded that the force of impact and mechanism of injury were the chief determinants of visual recovery.

Two lines of treatment have been advocated: decompression of the optic nerve within the optic canal, and systemic corticosteroid therapy. The rationale for canal decompression is the hope that this will reduce the effects of haemorrhagic compression of the optic nerve, and improve its blood supply, especially when there is a fracture of the canal wall and a displaced bone fragment. It might be thought that surgical decompression should be reserved for those patients who develop delayed visual loss, with signs of optic neuropathy such as relative afferent pupillary defects, and this has indeed been our policy; however, such cases are rarely diagnosed, and could be missed because of swelling of the eyelids. The rationale for corticosteroid therapy is the hope that traumatic oedema will be reduced, contusion necrosis limited, and vasospasm minimized.

Some impressive recoveries of vision have been reported from both forms of treatment. Thus, Joseph et al (1990) reported improved visual acuity in 11 of 14 patients treated by bony decompression through an external ethmoid approach; whereas only five of 25 eyes showed improvement without any treatment, and one of four cases improved with low dose corticosteroid administration. Lessell (1989) reported improvement in three of four cases treated by external decompression, but the cases treated by bony decompression also received corticosteroids. Anderson et al (1982) found that high dose steroid therapy appeared to be more effective than surgical decompression in a series of seven cases, but this small number does not allow deductions. Mahapatra & Bhatia (1989) treated 45 cases of traumatic optic neuropathy with intravenous dexamethasone (4 mg 6 hourly), followed after 48 h by oral prednisolone; visual improvement was recorded in 23, the recovery being complete in six. These authors found no indication for decompression, even in a case with well-documented progressive failure of vision over 2 weeks. Spoor et al (1990) gave much higher doses of dexamethasone (20 mg 6 hourly), followed by high doses of methylprednisolone (30–15 mg/kg body weight), and reported impressive recovery in 7/9 eyes. Lam & Weingeist (1990) found that repeated intravenous administration of corticosteroids followed by oral dosage may be needed to prevent a relapse.

Our own experience has made us reluctant to advocate optic nerve decompression by the transfrontal route: we have seen partial recovery after this operation, but there are difficulties in unroofing the canal, even with modern high-speed drills, and it would be easy to damage an already compromised nerve. The transethmoid decompression avoids risk of cerebral damage; it too has potential dangers but seems to be the operation of choice. At present, we favour in principle the protocol suggested by Miller (1990) and Joseph et al (1990). Unless there is some contraindication, dexamethasone is given in high dosage (8–10 mg intravenously) as soon as the diagnosis is made. A full neurophthalmological examination is carried out, followed by CT and if possible MRI scan. If there is radiological evidence of an intraorbital or intra-canalicular haematoma, or if the optic nerve looks swollen in the MRI scan, then optic nerve decompression is the logical procedure, and should be done at once. In the absence of such findings, high dose steroid therapy is continued over 3–4 weeks, tapering the course off towards the end. The visual acuity is closely watched, and if it deteriorates, reversion to high dosages may be justified.

Operative techniques

Decompression may be done through an incision below the eyebrow, curving down around the inner canthus of the eye. The ethmoid cells are exenterated. The middle turbinate bone is removed and the sphenoid sinus ostium is identified. With the aid of the microscope, the lamina papyracea is removed back to the region of the optic canal (Fig. 14.11), which often forms a bulge in the lateral

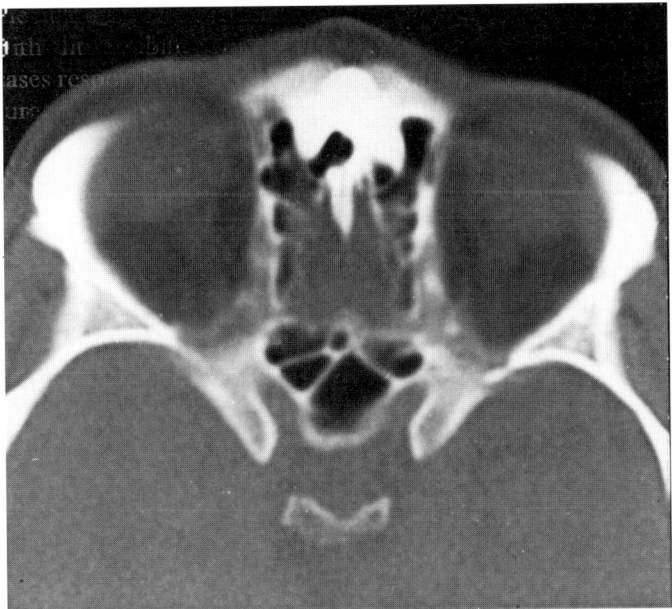

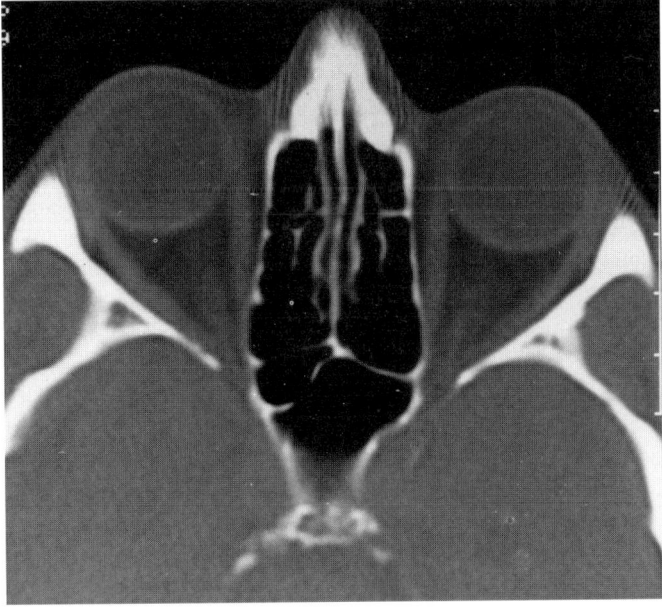

A   B

Fig. 14.11 Transethmoid optic nerve decompression. Axial CT scan shows the anatomy of transethmoid exposure of the optic canal. **A** CT at level of optic canals, showing the close relation of the upper ethmoid air cells to the optic nerves. The nerve can be decompressed by removing the medial wall of the canal, either by open ethmoidectomy or with endoscopic techniques. **B** In a cut 8 mm lower, the sphenoid sinus and the posterior ethmoid air cells are seen; on the right there is a large Onodi ethmoid cell. The orbit can be decompressed through an ethmoidectomy by removing the medial wall of the orbit (lamina papyracea).

wall of the posterior ethmoid and/or anterior sphenoid air sinuses, though in cases with poor pneumatization this may not be evident (Fig. 2.26D). The medial wall of the canal is thinned with a small burr, using copious irrigation; the thin shell remaining is then removed with a small spatula. The nerve is thus decompressed at the orbital end of the canal (Fig. 2.26C). When the decompression has been taken to the intracranial end of the canal, the periorbita may be incised and the nerve sheath slit with microscissors. Dexamethasone (8–10 mg) is given intravenously during operation and continued in progressively reduced dosage for a few days thereafter.

Stammberger of Graz has recently described a transnasal technique of endoscopic decompression of the optic nerve. An endoscopic ethmoidectomy is performed, and the lateral wall of the posterior ethmoid and sphenoid air sinuses is visualized through a 30° angled telescope. The optic canal is located by the bulge in the wall of the sinuses (Stammberger 1991), and the bone over the nerve is removed by a specially modified hooded diamond burr.* The optic nerve decompression can be combined with removal of the lamina papyracea in its entirety when it is desired to decompress the orbit.

Kline et al (1984) concluded that there was an obvious need for a prospective comparison of surgical decompression, steroid therapy and expectant care. This has not yet been done.

EYELID WOUNDS

Surgical pathology

Injuries of the lids represent an important and complex section of CMF trauma. In many eyelid injuries, other parts of the ocular adnexae or indeed of the eye itself are injured; moreover injury to the lids and/or conjunctiva may have secondary effects on the corneal surface.

Eyelid lacerations may be superficial or deep, and may run in any direction; from the aesthetic viewpoint, transverse cuts are favourable, vertical or oblique are unfavourable. Deeper lacerations may involve the orbicularis muscle, the aponeurosis of the levator palpebrae, the tarsoconjunctival layer, the medial and lateral canthal ligaments and the globe itself. Injuries of the lacrimal puncta, canaliculi and sac, and the nasolacrimal duct are common and important; in our experience, the most common cause is dog bites (p. 495). Avulsive injuries, also often resulting from bites, may result in devascularizing segments of a lid, or in full-thickness loss of an eyelid.

Assessment

The wound is obvious, but other injuries must be ex-

cluded, especially an occult injury of the globe (Fig. 6.3). The status of the lacrimal drainage system must be determined: avulsion injuries, especially of the lower lid, are often associated with rupture of the lower limb of the medial canthal ligament and rupture of the lacrimal canaliculus. When there is doubt, fluorescein mixed with normal saline can be injected through the intact canaliculus, to see if the dye comes out through a torn end of the other canaliculus in the wound; alternatively a dacryocystogram may be done.

Management

This depends on the type of laceration, on its site, and on the presence of other ocular or adnexal injuries. The healing processes involved in lid lacerations are the same as those of soft tissues elsewhere, but the prevention of contracture is essential to maintain normal lid contour, function and cosmetic appearance. Lid contour needs to be maintained along the lid margins to ensure that the posterior lid margin is perfectly apposed to the surface of the globe. The lashes should be directed forwards from the lower lid anterior margin, and forwards and slightly downwards from the upper lid margin as in the normal situation.

It is important in maintaining lid apposition to the globe to ensure that damaged lateral and medial canthal ligaments are accurately repaired (pp. 66, 310, 575). The medial canthal ligament especially needs to be reattached to the periosteum of the medial wall of the orbit sufficiently far back. It is also important to ensure that the height of the medial and lateral canthal ligaments is level. If a lateral canthotomy has been necessary, accurate apposition of the tissues is important; inaccurate apposition leads to unsightly ectropion of the lateral part of the lower lid, and often escape of tears (epiphora).

Primary repair

It is important to preserve as much normal healthy tissue as possible and to refrain from unnecessary debridement; secondary procedures can be employed later to improve the cosmetic result. If possible, surgical scars should be placed in the lines of normal skin creases. Repair of lid damage may be performed under local anaesthesia or general anaesthesia as the surgeon and patient prefer.

Lid wounds must be carefully explored, with the possibility of retained foreign bodies in mind, especially in patients who have suffered facial lacerations from windscreen or window impacts. Puncture lacerations involving the upper lid may be associated with more extensive and serious injury including penetration of the roof of the orbit into the anterior cranial fossa (Fig. 13.7). Damage to the trochlea or to the superior oblique tendon is more common, and causes intractable diplopia if not repaired (Fig. 14.8).

---

* The instrumentation for endoscopic surgery described by Messerklinger & Stammberger is manufactured by Messrs Karl Storz.

Lid lacerations which do not involve the lid margin are generally repaired primarily using absorbing sutures for deeper tissue such as orbicularis muscle and tarsal plate and 6/0 silk or nylon sutures to the skin; skin sutures are tied loosely.

If the laceration involves the levator palpebrae superioris every attempt should be made to identify this muscle and to re-suture it into as near normal position as possible on the anterior surface of the tarsal plate. Even with the best possible repair, postoperative ptosis is likely to persist due to damage to the delicate fibres of the levator inserting into the skin. Secondary procedures may then be necessary to repair residual ptosis, often including the creation of a new upper lid crease.

When the lid laceration involves the lid margin the grey line should be apposed accurately with 6/0 black silk mattress sutures to evert the lips of the wound. Further lid margin sutures may be placed in the line of the lashes and behind the grey line. The orbicularis muscle and tarsal plate should then be repaired. Often, the conjunctiva does not need specific repair. If the tarsoconjunctival layer does require suture, 5/0 or 6/0 absorbable stitches are used, the knots being buried away from the conjunctival surface; alternatively a continuous 6/0 nylon pull-through stitch can be used.

Direct primary suture of lid lacerations involving the lid margin can be undertaken even if there is considerable tissue loss or if the tissues at the edge of the laceration are not viable. A defect of a quarter or even a third of the length of the lid can be closed in layers without significant difficulty.

Loss of lid tissue

Severe, avulsive or degloving lid lacerations are most difficult to treat and can produce serious functional and cosmetic deficiencies. The paramount aim of treatment is to provide adequate cover to protect the globe; the eyelids are essential in maintaining a healthy, normal, comfortable seeing eye. If the normal blink reflex is impaired the cornea can be severely compromised.

At the time of primary injury as much tissue as possible should be restored and maintained. Small detached or devascularized segments of eyelid should be replaced as composite grafts after washing with dilute (5%) povidone–iodine and minimal debridement; when the injury was inflicted by a bite, it may be possible to retrieve the morsel and replace it (Fig. 14.12).

Very extensive full-thickness loss of eyelids will require reconstruction by some kind of flap. For reconstructions of this type, Mustardé (1980) has enunciated two principles:

1. The lower lid can be used to reconstruct an upper lid defect, but not vice versa: other sources should be used to reconstruct the lower lid.

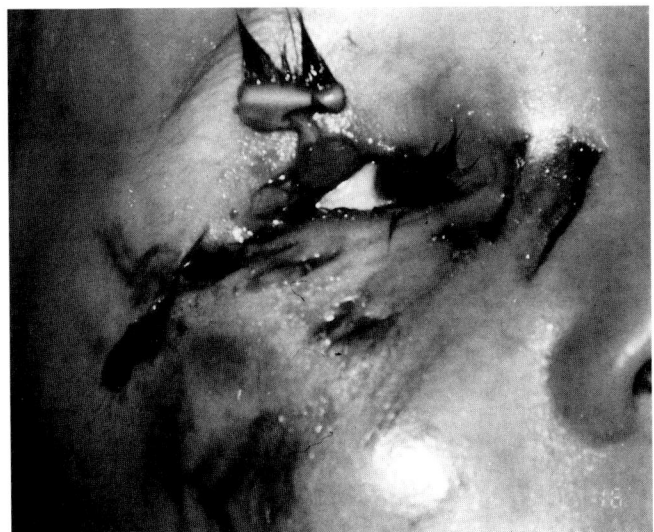

A

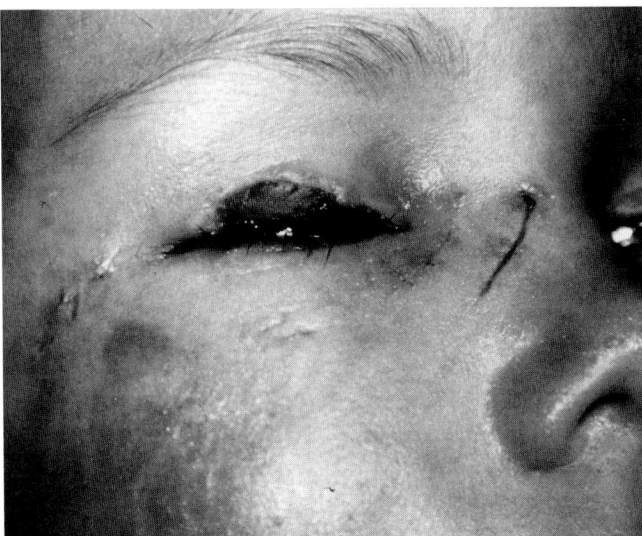

B

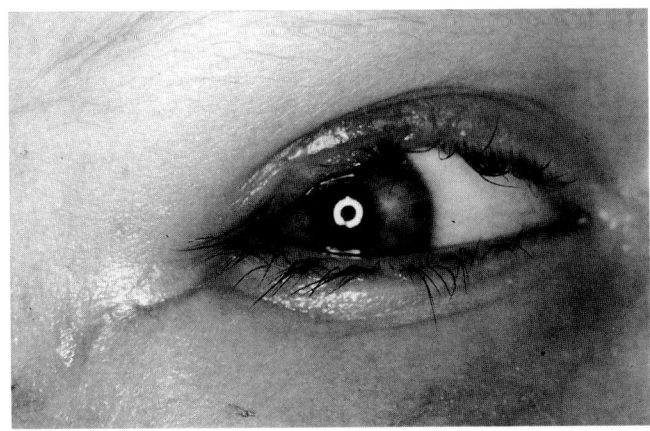

C

Fig. 14.12 Avulsive bite of upper eyelid. A 2-year-old girl was bitten by a dog. **A** A segment of the upper eyelid was avulsed and appeared avascular. **B** The wound was excised carefully and the segment was sutured in place as a composite graft. **C** The graft survived and the final aesthetic result was good.

2. For either lid, it is sufficient to replace three-quarters of the lid length: the lid tissues will stretch.

A little-used technique which can be successful is to insert a free composite graft of a section of healthy lid into a damaged lid, to provide simultaneous replacement of skin, tarsal plate, conjunctiva, lid margin, and lashes. But this may be impossible if the blood supply in the region of the damaged lid is severely impaired, and should not be considered for a large (>1 cm) defect. Plastic surgical opinion argues for pedicled lid repair. Defects of the upper eyelid too large for direct suture can be reconstructed by using the lower eyelid as a skin–muscle–conjunctival flap, rotated through 180° like an Abbé flap for a lip repair. The lower lid is then reconstructed with a rotation cheek flap and a chondromucosal free graft taken from the nasal septum. For larger lid defects, cheek flaps have been used (Fig. 14.13). McGregor (1973) advocated a flap using skin from beyond the lateral orbital area, moved medially to replace a defect of up to two-thirds of either lid. The incision runs laterally from the outer canthus; mobilized skin is moved to cover the lid defect, closure of the secondary defect being facilitated by a Z-plasty. Mustardé (1971) used a rotation cheek flap, designed for use in various lid defects, up to entire loss of the lower eyelid. The incision for this flap also runs laterally from the outer canthus to curve down in the sideburn area as low as the earlobe.

If there is insufficient tarsal plate and conjunctiva to

support and line the reconstructed eyelid, a free chondro-mucosal graft from the nasal septum may be added. Alternatively, sclera from a cadaver bank may be used to replace tarsal plate and provide more rigid skeletal support of the lid; sclera may also be inserted to reduce lid retraction produced by injury. We believe that cadaver sclera can be used if stringent precautions are taken to exclude donors with AIDS, Creutzfeld–Jakob disease or other communicable disease.

Lost or deficient conjunctiva may be repaired by the use of buccal mucosal grafts. A good guiding principle is to use more grafted tissue than you expect to need, perhaps by 50%, as contracture of the graft will occur with time. Because of this tendency to contract, plastic surgical opinion favours nasal mucosa. Subcutaneous fat grafts may be used to provide bulk in a deficient lid.

Rarely, loss of both eyelids may require emergency cover of the cornea by suture of the conjunctiva over it and multistaged repair with a forehead flap; although the result is aesthetically less than perfect, the cornea may be saved (Mustardé 1977, 1980).

Secondary procedures

These are often required to improve the appearance and function of the damaged lids. Attempts should be made to restore tissue loss in a vertical and horizontal sense. Skin may be replaced by using flap pedicle grafts or free skin grafts either from uninjured lids or from the retro-auricular region; however, retro-auricular skin is often too thick, so that a thick split skin graft may be preferred. Loss of eyelashes is often extensive but gaps in the line of lashes along the lid margin can be hidden cosmetically with artificial eyelashes, or may be abolished by wedge excision of the lid and re-suture of the lid margins.

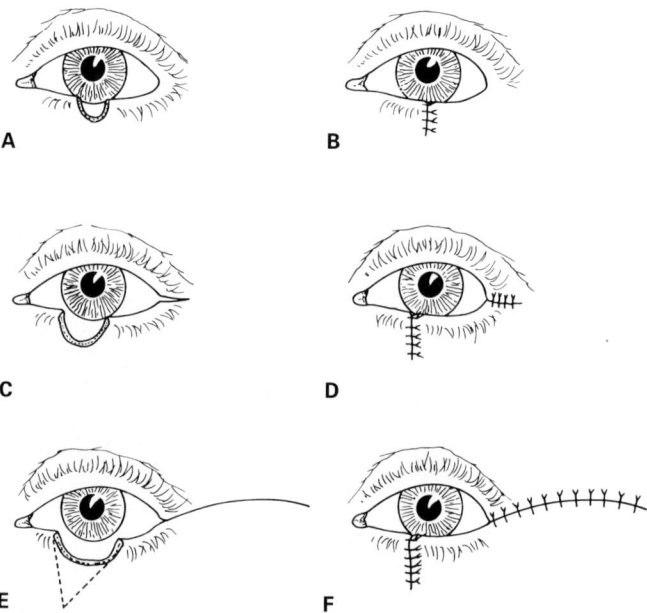

Fig. 14.13 A series of diagrams indicating the principles of repair of the lower eyelid (after Mustardé 1971). A, B Small defect, up to a quarter of lid length, closed directly. **C, D** Defect over a quarter closed by mobilizing the lid on the lateral side. **E, F** Defect between a quarter and a half. Additional tissue is brought from the lateral side by rotating a cheek flap.

Management of lacrimal canalicular injuries

Injury to the superior punctum and canaliculus does not require repair. Some authorities (Crawford 1989) maintain that if the lower canaliculus is involved in a laceration the lid should be repaired as described above, with no specific attempt to repair the canaliculus. Good results are claimed, with few problems from epiphora. Recent studies (Daubert et al 1990, Meyer et al 1990) have shown that effective tear drainage may pass through a single canaliculus. It is also claimed that excessive manipulation of the canaliculi, including intubation of the upper canaliculus, may in fact produce damage, causing epiphora rather than curing it; certainly the use of pigtail probes is not warranted. This is also our experience, and, especially after avulsion injuries involving the medial canthal ligament, we may prefer to marsupialize the medial end of the torn canaliculus into the conjunctival sac. However, there are occasions when repair of the lacerated canaliculus can be undertaken: in clean lacerations, or when both upper and lower canaliculi are wounded.

Repair usually requires microsurgical anastomosis of the two ends of the canaliculus. If it is relatively easy to identify the ends of the canaliculus, we intubate them with 0.64 mm silastic tubing on a malleable 23 gauge probe, or with Crawford's tubes, and reconstruct the lacerated canaliculus with 10/0 nylon around the tube. Care is taken to keep the sutures outside the mucosa of the duct and not to intrude on its lumen; four or five sutures usually suffice.

Wounds in the vicinity of the ampulla and lacrimal sac should be explored; it is usually possible to repair these structures with 9/0 or 10/0 nylon. Injury to the naso-lacrimal duct itself is usually intraosseous, and not amenable to primary repair; when blockage of this duct causes obstructive dacryocystitis, a secondary dacryo-cystorhinostomy is indicated (see below).

Injuries of the lacrimal system may be associated with division or detachment of the medial canthal ligament. This should be reattached or repaired, provided that the lacrimal bone is stable, with sutures passed into the periosteum; when the bone is unstable, it may be necessary to anchor the ligament by transnasal wiring (p. 312).

LACRIMAL OUTFLOW OBSTRUCTION

Surgical pathology

Canalicular lacerations tend to heal well cosmetically and produce surprisingly few long-term problems, but canalicular stenosis is sometimes seen. Maxillary and nasal fractures are often complicated by stenosis of the nasolacrimal duct; at times, this may be iatrogenic, from a maxillary osteotomy in which screws may be placed too high, or from an endoscopic sinus operation. Chronic obstruction of lacrimal drainage is evident as epiphora; mucocele formation may result from obstruction of the nasolacrimal duct, and infection is another likely complication, resulting in dacryocystitis and abscess formation (Fig. 14.14).

Assessment

Epiphora persisting after a period of 3 months or so is investigated by syringing, lacrimal isotope dacryocysto-graphy and macrodacryocystography, which will confirm the diagnosis.

Management

Secondary attempts to repair the canalicular system may be appropriate, but dacryocystorhinostomy with a patent

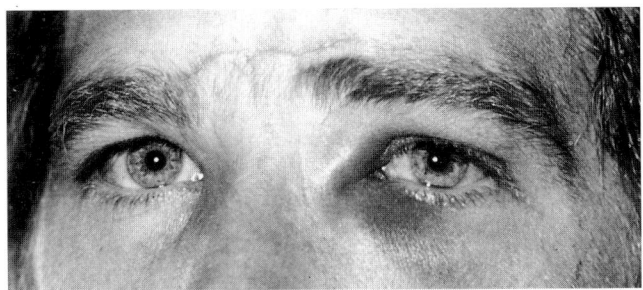

Fig. 14.14 Dacryocystitis. A 25-year-old man suffered fractures in the fronto-ethmoidal complex in a car crash. These were repaired, and both medial canthal ligaments were wired in place. 6 weeks later, he developed mucopurulent discharge from the left eye and an abscess appeared below the left medial canthal ligament. Acute dacryocystitis with abscess formation was diagnosed and treated with broad spectrum antibiotics and local drainage. 3 weeks later, dacryocystostomy was performed and lacrimal drainage was restored.

upper canalicular system may be adequate to produce a dry eye. There are various techniques for this operation. We favour a simple procedure, usually taking less than 30 min. An appropriate area of nasal skin is marked for incision and infiltrated with lignocaine and adrenaline, and the intranasal mucosa is packed with cocaine paste dipped on cotton-tipped applicators; this gives a bloodless field. We then incise the anterior wall of the nasolacrimal sac, which is usually distended, and create an ostium into the nose with a no. 1 Hegar's dilator. The ostium is progressively enlarged with dilators up to no. 9 or no. 10; a Gelfoam pack is left in the ostium and sac, and the anterior walls of the sac are sutured over it. Only rarely have we found it necessary to use bone drills in exposing the sac. Nasendoscopy may be used to carry out dacryo-cystostomy after a previous failure (Orcutt et al 1990).

If the canaliculi have been avulsed from the sac, the resulting epiphora will require conjunctivo-dacryo-cystorhinostomy with insertion of Lester Jones or similar tubes (G. Weiss, Portland, Oregon, USA); in our experience, the results are often disappointing. Laser endoscopic dacryocystorhinostomy and conjunctivo-dacryocystorhi-nostomy have been recently used with good results by Gonnering et al (1991).

Adequate nasal air flow is essential for good tear drainage, and occasionally the nasal septum will have to be straightened, or turbinectomies performed to improve the airflow (Roen 1991).

INJURIES OF THE LACRIMAL GLAND

The lacrimal gland is very rarely injured due to its protected situation under the heavy supraorbital bony ridge. However it may be denervated if secretomotor fibres travelling with zygomatic nerves are destroyed. A micro-vascular submandibular transfer has been described by McLeod & Robbins (1992) for treatment of xerophthalmia.

However, we have seen marked corneal and conjunctival irritation, presumably from the action of salivary enzymes, after this operation, necessitating removal of the transplanted gland.

PTOSIS

Surgical pathology

Ptosis of the upper lid may complicate both penetrating upper lid laceration and contusive injuries of the lids. A penetrating injury may sever the fine aponeurotic slips of the levator palpebrae superioris into the tarsal plate and the skin of the upper lid; deeper lacerations may sever the muscle itself.

Neuroparalytic ptosis may result from a paralysis of the third cranial nerve or the cervical sympathetic innervation of the eyelid. The upper eyelid has a vital role in protecting the eye, and repair of ptosis must be done with great caution in cases with a feeble Bell phenomenon (reflex turning up of the eye on lid closure), and in cases where gaze up is restricted by mechanical tethering or paralysis. Ptosis correction may also be unwise when there is impaired corneal sensation.

Management

Ptosis associated with a penetrating injury requires immediate exploration and repair of the aponeurosis or tendon. The procedure can be done under local anaesthesia so that voluntary action can be used to identify the muscle (Anderson & Dixon 1979).

Minor degrees of ptosis may be repaired after an appropriate delay of perhaps 6 months by a conjunctivotarsal resection (Fasanella-Servat procedure: Collin 1989). More significant degrees of ptosis may require formal levator resection or frontalis suspension, depending on the degree of remaining levator function.

We perform the levator resection through the skin placing the skin incision in the position of the normal lid crease and reforming this at the end of the procedure. Levator aponeurosis dehiscence may be repaired by dissecting the levator muscle and reattaching the aponeurosis appropriately.

Brow suspension procedures may involve the use of fascia lata, though synthetic materials such as Mersilene mesh also work well. Sometimes, to produce the best cosmetic result, the brow suspension procedure should be bilateral.

ECTROPION

Surgical pathology

In cases of CMF trauma, ectropion (drooping of the lower eyelid away from the globe) may result from scarring or paralysis of the facial nerve; scarring may be a sequel of burns or lacerations.

Management

If the cause of the ectropion is a localized area of scarring, a Z-plasty may be used to correct the deformity. In more severe cases the area of scarring may be excised completely by wedge excision.

If ectropion is the result of generalized contracture of the tissue of the lower lid, skin replacement may be necessary, in the form of a pedicle graft, e.g. from the upper eyelid, or as a free graft from the retro-auricular area, placed in the area of deficient skin.

Paralytic ectropion may require temporary or permanent tarsorrhaphy, depending on whether the facial palsy is likely to recover, and if so at what rate and time. The techniques of tarsorrhaphy are discussed in Chapter 9, as it is a procedure of very wide application. Minor degrees of medial ectropion may be associated with ectropion of the lower lacrimal punctum; this may require excision of a diamond-shaped piece of conjunctiva and tarsal plate behind the punctum, with or without a full-thickness wedge excision of the lid. More extensive paralytic ectropion will require a medial canthoplasty, with or without plication or resection of the medial canthal tendon, and a lateral canthal sling. This sling requires a lateral wedge resection of full-thickness lid with preservation of a small strip of the superior tarsal plate which becomes the new lower limb of the lateral canthal ligament. For a fuller description of the management of ectropion, Collin (1989) may be consulted.

REFERENCES

Albert D M, Diaz-Rohena R 1989 A historical review of sympathetic ophthalmia and its epidemiology. Surv Ophthalmol 34: 1–14
Ambler J S, Meyers S M 1991 Management of intraretinal metallic foreign bodies without retinopexy in the absence of retinal detachment. Ophthalmology 89: 391–394
Anderson R L, Dixon R S 1979 Aponeurotic ptosis surgery. Arch Ophthalmol 97: 1123–1128
Anderson R L, Panje W R, Gross C E 1982 Optic nerve blindness following blunt forehead trauma. Ophthalmology 89: 445–455
Avni I, Moverman D, Cahane M, Blumenthal M 1989

Epikeratophakia after ocular trauma. Am J Ophthalmol 107: 268–272
Baker R S, Epstein A D 1991 Ocular motor abnormalities from head trauma. Surv Ophthalmol 35: 245–267
Boldt H C, Pulido J S, Blodi C F, Folk J S, Weingeist T A 1989 Rural endophthalmitis. Ophthalmology 96: 1722–1726
Buschmann W 1993 Fibrinogen glue helps to preserve wounded lens. Ocular Surg News 4: 25–26
Collin J R O 1989 A manual of systemic eyelid surgery, 2nd edn. Churchill Livingstone, Edinburgh

Crawford J 1989 Intubation of the lacrimal system. Ophthal Plast Reconstr Surg 5: 261–265

Crompton M R 1970 Visual lesions in closed head injury. Brain 93: 785–792

Crompton J L 1991 Diagnosis and management of diplopia. Modern Med Aust 35: 84–101

Daubert J, Nik N, Chandeyssoun P, el-Choufi L 1990 Tear flow analysis through the upper and lower systems. Ophthal Plast Reconstr Surg 6: 193–196

de Juan E, Sternberg P, Michels R G 1983 Penetrating ocular injuries: types of injuries and visual results. Ophthalmology 90: 1318–1322

Delori F, Pomerantzeff O, Cox M S 1969 Deformation of the globe under high-speed impacts: its relation to contusion injuries. Invest Ophthalmol 8: 290–301

Donahue S P, Kowalski R P, Jewart B H, Friberg T R 1993 Vitreous cultures in suspected endophthalmitis. Biopsy or vitrectomy? Ophthalmology 100: 452–455

Dutton J J 1991 Coraline hydroxyapatite as an ocular implant. Ophthalmology 98: 370–377

Eagling E M 1975 Perforating injuries involving the posterior segment. Trans Ophthalmol Soc UK 95: 335–339

Eagling E M 1976 Perforating injuries of the eye. Br J Ophthalmol 60: 732–736

Forster R K 1991 Endophthalmitis. In: Duane T D (ed) Clinical Ophthalmology. Harper & Row, Philadelphia, Vol 4, Ch 24, pp 1–21

Fraunfelder F T, Coster D J, Drew R, Fraunfelder F W 1990 Ocular injury induced by methyl ethyl ketone peroxide. Am J Ophthalmol 110: 635–640

Gelender H, Vaiser A, Snyder W B, Fuller D G, Hutton W L 1988 Temporary keratoprosthesis for combined keratoplasty, pars plana vitrectomy, and repair of retinal detachment. Ophthalmology 95: 897–901

Gonnering R, Lyon D, Fisher J 1991 Endoscopic laser assisted lacrimal surgery. Am J Ophthalmol 111: 152–157

Gossman M D, Roberts D M, Barr C C 1992 Ophthalmic aspects of orbital injury. Clin Plast Surg 19: 71–85

Green W R 1986 Uveal tract. In: Spencer W H (ed) Ophthalmic pathology — an atlas and textbook, 3rd edn. Saunders, Philadelphia, Vol 3

Hadden O B, Wilson J L 1990 The management of intraocular foreign bodies. Aust NZ J Ophthalmol 18: 343–351

Harcourt R B, Hopkins D 1971 Ophthalmic manifestations of the battered baby syndrome. Br Med J 3: 398–403

Heinze J 1969 Cranial nerve avulsion and other neural injuries in road accidents. Med J Aust 2: 1246–1249

Helveston E M 1990 Extraocular muscle lacerations. In: Fraunfelder F T, Roy F W (eds) Current ocular therapy, 3rd edn. Saunders, Philadelphia, p 344

Hoefle F B 1968 Initial treatment of eye injuries. First Corps area of Viet Nam. Arch Ophthalmol 70: 33–35

Holt G R, Holt J E 1983 Incidence of eye injuries in facial fractures: an analysis of 727 cases. Otolaryngol Head Neck Surg 91: 276–279

Hull F E 1951 Management of eye casualties in the Far East commands during the Korean conflict. Trans Am Acad Ophthalmol Otolaryngol 55: 885–891

Hughes B 1962 Indirect injuries of the optic nerves and chiasma. Bull Johns Hopkins Hosp 111: 98–126

Hupp S L, Buckley E G, Byrne S F, Tenzel R R, Glaser J S, Schatz N S 1984 Post-traumatic venous obstructive retinopathy associated with enlarged optic nerve sheath. Arch Ophthalmol 102: 254–256

Hutton W L, Fuller D G 1984 Factors influencing final visual result in severely injured eyes. Am J Opthalmol 97: 715–722

Jakobiec F A, Marboe C C, Knowles D M et al 1983 Human sympathetic ophthalmia. An analysis of the inflammatory infiltrate by hybridoma–monoclonal antibodies, immunochemistry and correlative electron microscopy. Ophthalmology 90: 76–95

Johnson E V, Kline L B, Skalka H W 1987 Electrical cataracts: a case report and review of the literature. Ophthalmic Surg 18: 183–185

Joseph M P, Lessell S, Rizzo J, Momose K J 1990 Extracranial optic nerve decompression for traumatic optic neuropathy. Arch Ophthalmol 108: 1092–1093

Joy H H 1935 A survey of cases of sympathetic ophthalmia occurring in New York State. Arch Ophthalmol 14: 773–741

Keane J R 1975 Ocular skew deviation. Analysis of 100 cases. Arch Neurol 32: 185–190

Kenyon K R, Tseng S C G 1989 Limbal autograft transplantation for ocular surface disorders. Ophthalmology 96: 709–723

Kline L B, Morawetz R B, Swaid S N 1984 Indirect injury of the optic nerve. Neurosurgery 14: 756–764

Kowal L 1992 Ophthalmic manifestations of head injury. Aust NZ J Ophthalmol 20: 35–40

Kruger R A, Higgins J, Rashford S, Fitzgerald B, Land R 1990 Emergency eye injuries. Aust Fam Physician 19: 934–938

Kuo P K, Lubin J R, Ni C, Wang K M, Albert D M 1982 Sympathetic ophthalmia; a comparison of the histopathological features from a Chinese and American series. Int Ophthalmol Clin 22: 125–139

Kutner B, Fourman S, Brein K, Hobson S, Mrvos D, Sheppard J, Weisman S 1987 Aminocaproic acid reduces the risk of secondary haemorrhage in patients with traumatic hyphaema. Arch Ophthalmol 105: 206–208

Lam B L, Weingeist T A 1990 Corticosteroid-responsive traumatic neuropathy. Am J Ophthalmol 108: 99–101

Lambert S R, Johnson T E, Hoyt C S 1986 Optic nerve sheath and retinal haemorrhages associated with the shaken baby syndrome. Arch Ophthalmol 104: 1509–1512

Lessell S 1989 Indirect optic nerve trauma. Arch Ophthalmol 107: 382–386

Lipton J R, Page A B, Lee J P 1990 Management of diplopia on down gaze following eye trauma. Eye 4: 535–537

Liu D 1993 A simplified technique of orbital decompression for severe retrobulbar haemorrhage. Am J Ophthalmol 116: 34–37

Lubin J F, Albert D M, Weinstein M 1980 Sixty-five years of sympathetic ophthalmia. A clinico-pathologic review of 105 cases (1913–1978). Ophthalmology 89: 109–121

McCannel M A 1976 A retrievable suture idea for anterior uveal problems. Ophthalmic Surg 7: 98–103

McGovern S T, Crompton J L, Ingham P N 1986 Trigemino-abducens synkinesis: an unusual case of aberrant regeneration. Aust NZ J Surg 14: 275–279

McGregor I A 1973 Eyelid reconstruction following subtotal resection of upper or lower eyelid. Br J Plast Surg 26: 346–354

McLean E N, McRae S M, Rich L F 1986 Recurrent erosion: treatment by anterior stromal puncture. Ophthalmology 93: 784–788

McLeod A M, Robbins S P 1992 Submandibular gland transfer in the correction of dry eye. Aust NZ J Surg 20: 99–103

Mahapatra A K, Bhatia R 1989 Predictive value of visual evoked potentials in unilateral optic nerve injury. Surg Neurol 31: 339–342

Mann I 1961 Bowman Lecture: climate, culture and disease. Trans Ophthalmol Soc UK 81: 261–282

May M 1977 Naso-frontal/ethmoidal injuries. Laryngoscope 87: 948–953

Mein J, Harcourt B 1986 Diagnosis and management of ocular motility disorders. Blackwell, Oxford

Meyer D, Antonello A, Linberg J 1990 Assessment of tear drainage after canalicular obstruction using fluorescein dye disappearance. Ophthalmology 97: 1370–1374

Miller N R 1985 Topical diagnosis of neuropathic ocular motility disorders. In: Walsh & Hoyt's clinical ophthalmology, 4th edn. Williams & Wilkins, Baltimore, Vol 2, pp 676–680

Miller N R 1990 The management of traumatic neuropathy. Arch Ophthalmol 108: 1086–1087

Moore C E 1968 Sympathetic ophthalmitis treated with azathioprine. Br J Ophthalmol 52: 688–690

Morgan K S, McDonald M B, Hiles D A et al 1987 A nationwide study of epikeratophakia or aphakia in children. Am J Ophthalmol 103: 366–374

Morrison J C 1990 Glaucoma after ocular contusion. In: Fraunfelder F T, Roy F W (eds) Current ocular therapy, 3rd edn. Saunders, Philadelphia, p 547

Mustardé J C 1971 The orbital region. In Mustardé J C (ed) Plastic surgery in infancy and childhood. Livingstone, Edinburgh, Ch 10

Mustardé J C 1977 Eyelid reconstruction. In: Converse J M (ed) Plastic reconstructive surgery. Saunders, Philadelphia, Ch 28

Mustardé J C 1980 Repair and reconstruction of the orbital region, 2nd edn. Churchill Livingstone, Edinburgh, Chs 7, 9 and 11

Nelson S K, Kline L B 1990 Acquired trigemino-abducens synkinesis. J Clin Neuro Ophthalmol 10: 111–114

O'Day D M, Smith R S, Gregg C R et al 1981 The problem of *Bacillus* species infection with special emphasis on the virulence of *Bacillus cereus*. Ophthalmology 88: 833

O'Day D M, Foulds G, Williams T E, Robinson R D, Allen R H, Head W S 1990 Ocular uptake of fluconazole following oral administration. Arch Ophthalmol 108: 1006–1008

Orcutt J, Hillel A, Weymuller E 1990 Endoscopic repair of failed dacryocystorhinostomy. Ophthal Plast Reconstr Surg 6: 197–202

Perry A C 1990 Integrated orbital implants. Adv Ophthal Plast Reconstr Surg 8: 75–81

Perry A C 1991a Understanding and treatment of the congenital and acquired anophthalmic socket. Curr Opin Ophthalmol 2: 607–611

Perry A C 1991b Advances in enucleation. Ophthalmol Clin North Am 4: 173–182

Pflugfelder S C, Flynn H W, Zwickey T A et al 1988 Exogenous fungal endophthalmitis. Ophthalmology 95: 19–30

Phillips C M 1961 Blindness in Africans in Northern Rhodesia. Cent Afr J Med 7: 153–158

Radius R, Anderson D 1981 Reversibility of optic nerve damage in primate eyes subjected to intraocular pressure above systolic blood pressure. Br J Ophthalmol 65: 661–672

Rakusin W 1972 Traumatic hyphaema. Am J Ophthalmol 74: 284–292

Read J E, Goldberg M F 1974 Traumatic hyphaema: comparison of medical treatment. Trans Am Acad Ophthalmol Otolaryngol 78: 799–803

Reid R G 1957 The eye. In: Shanks S C, Kerley P (eds) A textbook of X-ray diagnosis by British authors, 3rd edn. Lewis, London, Vol 1, Ch 3

Reim M, Teping C 1989 Surgical procedures in the treatment of most severe eye burns. Revival of artificial epithelium. Acta Ophthalmol Suppl (Copenh) 192: 47–55

Roen J L 1991 Problems and solutions in lacrimal outflow obstruction. Curr Opin Opthalmol 2: 596–600

Romano P E, Shuster J N 1990 Traumatic hyphaema. In: Fraunfelder F T, Roy F W (eds) Current ocular therapy, 3rd edn. Saunders, Philadelphia, p 384

Rush J A, Younge B R 1981 Paralysis of cranial nerves III, IV and VI: cause and prognosis in 1000 cases. Arch Opththalmol 99: 76–79

Rutkowski P C, Burian H M 1972 Divergence paralysis following head trauma. Am J Ophthalmol 73: 660–662

Shingleton B J, Hersh P S, Kenyon K R (eds) 1991 Eye trauma. Mosby, St Louis

Spoor T C, Nesi F A (eds) 1988 Management of ocular, orbital and adnexal trauma. Raven Press, New York

Spoor T C, Hartel W C, Lensink D B, Wilkinson M J 1990 Treatment of traumatic optic neuropathy with corticosteroids. Am J Ophthalmol 110: 665–669

Srivastava A K, Gupta B N 1989 Oculotoxins: effects, implications, and importance in occupational health. Am J Ind Med 16: 723–726

Stammberger H 1991 Functional endoscopic sinus surgery. The Messerklinger technique. Decker, Philadelphia

Steidler N E, Cook R M, Reade P C 1980 Residual complications in patients with major middle third facial fractures. Int J Oral Surg 9: 259–266

Stern W H, Diddie K R, Smith R E 1983 Techniques for the anterior segment surgeon: a practical approach. Grune & Stratton, New York

Tamler E, Jampolski A 1967 Is divergence active? An electromyographic study. Am J Ophthalmol 63: 452–459

Thoft R A 1977 Conjunctival transplantation. Arch Ophthalmol 95: 1425–1427

Thoft R A 1984 Keratoepithelioplasties. Am J Ophthalmol 92: 1–6

Treister G 1969 Ocular casualties in the Six Day War. Am J Ophthalmol 68: 669–675

Tseng S C, Maumenee A E, Stark W J et al 1985 Topical treatment for various dry-eye disorders. Ophthalmology 92: 717–727

Verhoeff F H 1927 An effective treatment for sympathetic uveitis. Arch Ophthalmol 56: 28–41

Vrabec M P, McDonald M B, Chase D S, Aitken P A, Varnell R J 1993 Traumatic corneal abrasions after excimer laser keratectomy. Am J Ophthalmol 116: 101–102

Walsh F B, Lindenberg R L 1963 Die Veränderungen des Sehnerven bei indirektem Trauma. In: Entwicklung und Fortschritt in der Augenheilkunde. Forbildungskurs für Augenärzte, Hamburg. Enke. Stuttgart. Quoted by Walsh F B, Hoyt W F (1969) Clinical Neurophthalmology, 3rd edn. Williams & Wilkins, Baltimore, Vol 3, pp 2378–2379

Williams K A, Muehlberg S M, Wing S J, Coster D J (eds) 1993 The Australian Corneal Graft Registry 1990–1992 report. Aust NZ J Ophthalmol 21: Suppl

Wolin M J, Lavin P J M 1990 Spontaneous visual recovery from traumatic optic neuropathy after blunt head injury. Am J Ophthalmol 109: 430–435

Injuries of soft tissues, ducts and nerves

E. Tan
Contributing author: J. Tomich

INTRODUCTION

Facial soft-tissue injuries vary in severity from very minor superficial wounds to massive avulsions. In a patient with multiple injuries, priority should be given to treating life-threatening conditions, as the treatment of the facial injury can be delayed. However, skin and mucosal wounds should be closed as soon as possible, and to get a good functional and aesthetic end result, meticulous attention to detail and technique is essential. This is equally true of the repair of nerves and ducts.

MANAGEMENT

First aid and life support

This has been discussed in Chapter 8. Massive exsanguinating bleeding from soft-tissue trauma of the face is not a common event. Occasionally a large artery, or vein incompletely divided or with a side hole, may be the cause of uncontrollable haemorrhage. Firm pressure is usually adequate to control bleeding, and the use of clamps and ligature should only be considered if the vessel can be clearly identified. Putting the patient in a sitting position can dramatically reduce venous bleeding.

Assessment

A history of the mechanism of injury, together with the clinical examination, will often provide the diagnosis of the nature and extent of the soft-tissue injury. Documentation of the findings should describe the anatomical site and measurements of surface wounds, and should include diagrams and/or photography. Plain radiography may be needed if there is any concern over skeletal structures; computerized tomography and magnetic resonance imaging can provide visualization of soft tissue and foreign bodies as well as bony abnormalities.

General management of skin wounds

Conditions for treatment

Proper treatment of facial wounds requires the best possible conditions in a well-equipped theatre with good lighting, fine instrumentation, appropriate suture material, and assistance if required from other medical or nursing personnel. The surgeon should also be able to ask for microsurgical instruments, as the use of magnifying loupes or an operating microscope is standard practice in repairing many types of soft-tissue injury.

Timing of closure

The primary closure of open wounds of the face is preferably carried out as soon as practicable, after more serious or life-threatening conditions have been stabilized. Ideally, the timing of closure is decided when priorities have been fully evaluated (see Ch. 9). Far too often this does not happen and one is summoned to an operating room to attend to a patient after the end of a more urgent procedure, without previous discussion or investigation.

If necessary, facial wounds can await repair for up to 48 h without detriment to the end result. When such delay is unavoidable it is best to clean the wound surface and cover it with a sterile dressing. In an obviously contaminated wound, as much foreign matter as possible should be removed by irrigation with sterile normal saline before being dressed. We do not use a topical antibiotic or bactericidal solution as is often done, unless there is very gross contamination. A broad spectrum intravenous antibiotic may be given if delay is likely, or if there is severe contamination. On occasion, a few tacking sutures may be placed to approximate the soft tissue prior to delayed definitive treatment.

Anaesthesia

Most wounds of the face can be treated under local anaesthesia, supplemented with sedation (e.g. diazepam) or narcotic analgesia. Local anaesthesia may be used either as regional nerve blocks or field blocks. Although it is possible to perform adequate blocks of appropriate branches of the trigeminal or cervical nerves, the advantage of field blocks is the reduction in bleeding which is achieved when a vasoconstrictor is incorporated in the local anaesthetic solution. Our preference is for 2% Xylocaine (lignocaine) with adrenaline 1:80 000 (p. 255). General anaesthesia with muscle relaxant and endotracheal intubation is used in more extensive or multiple injuries, in cases where the airway has been secured by intubation, and in children or in uncooperative adults.

Contusions, bruises and haematoma

These injuries are caused by blunt trauma, usually without significant break in the skin, although they may be associated with superficial lacerations or abrasions. Contusions and bruises are due to extravasation of blood and tissue fluids into soft tissues and these resolve spontaneously without sequelae. A haematoma is a sequestrated collection of blood in a tissue space. If large, tense or expanding it can cause skin necrosis, and evacuation of the blood with haemostasis becomes an urgent need. Small haematomas resolve spontaneously but, if the clot has liquefied, aspiration with a large-bore needle hastens the healing process. In all aspirations, very careful asepsis is essential — failure in this may lead to abscess formation and perhaps ulceration.

Abrasions

Abrasions, caused by tangential moving contact against a rough surface can be superficial or deep, and are often contaminated with gravel or other foreign matter. A superficial abrasion can be converted into a deep ulcer by infection. Treatment is by thorough irrigation and cleaning with normal saline or an appropriate aqueous antiseptic solution, scrubbing with a brush to remove foreign matter and applying a sterile occlusive or absorbent dressing. Small superficial abrasions may be painted with 2% aqueous Mercurochrome or povidone iodine

(Betadine); the abrasion can then be left open to form a crust. Deep linear abrasions may be treated as lacerations and sutured, while deep abrasions of some width are best debrided or excised, and then sutured or covered with a skin graft.

Tattooed foreign matter

Foreign matter may be embedded at varying depths in a wound, typically in deep abrasions. On occasion tattooing may occur from an explosion driving in some kind of particulate material (Fig. 22.4). Removal of the tattooed material must be carried out as soon as possible. Oily particles may need to be washed out with solvents such as ether. Thorough scrubbing with a soft nylon brush is needed, and deeply embedded particles require excision with fine tipped scissors or scalpel.

Puncture wounds

These wounds are deceptive (Fig. 6.3). Their external appearances often belie their depth and direction, which exploration with a blunt instrument or a finger will reveal. Deep structures may be damaged or transected some distance away from the vicinity of the surface wound. The object which caused the penetrating injury is usually not sterile and the distal part may break off to be implanted in the depths of the wound. Radiographs are helpful in detecting radio-opaque material but magnetic resonance imaging may be needed to locate wood or glass. Implanted foreign material should be removed wherever possible to prevent later problems of infection, tissue reaction, excessive induration and scarring or pigmentation, as from pencil graphite.

Lacerations

Lacerations can be divided into simple incised wounds, untidy ragged wounds, bevelled or flap lacerations, bursting or stellate lacerations and skin avulsions with or without loss of tissue. In principle, treatment consists of:

1. Cleaning with antiseptic solutions or sterile saline
2. Removal of foreign matter
3. Debridement of devitalized tissue
4. Cutting back irregular or bevelled skin edges to give perpendicular dermo-epidermal edges for suture
5. Accurate layered repair of the wound.

Divided muscles should be identified, and cut muscle surfaces should be matched and sutured with an absorbable suture material like Vicryl® (polyglactin 910), Maxon® (polyglyconate), or polydioxanone sulphate (PDS). Reconstitution of the fat layer is very important in certain sites, such as the malar area and the mental prominence. Separate dermal sutures using 4/0 or 5/0 Maxon/PDS/

Vicryl may be indicated if the wound tends to gape. Skin closure is then effected with interrupted 5/0 or 6/0 nylon sutures: a single subcuticular pull-out nylon or Prolene® (polypropylene) may be preferred. There has been a recent vogue for subcuticular closure using Maxon or PDS with the starting and ending knots buried under the dermis, and the skin surface taped with Steristrips®, Micropore® tape or Hypafix®. This technique may give a finer linear scar without stitch marks but the suture material is extruded in a proportion of cases.

We use Steristrips or Micropore directly over the interrupted skin sutures, as the wounds heal with less redness and inflammatory reaction at the suture line. Sutures on the eyelids can be removed at 3–4 days; on the rest of the face, 4–7 days may be needed.

Bevelled, flapped or avulsed wounds

Small bevelled flaps can be excised, allowing perpendicular skin edge apposition. Larger flaps require debridement of all bevelled edges, which are made perpendicular for edge-to-edge closure. In the head and neck large flaps or partly avulsed tissues sometimes retain blood supply and viability. Even when the length-to-width ratios are large, one should always try to preserve such flaps (Fig. 15.1). Pressure dressings can be applied with care, to reduce oedema and induration without compromising the vitality of the flap; if after 5–7 days the flap looks viable, the pressure dressing is maintained. Pressure may be applied continuously for 2–3 months to achieve a

smoother contour, especially if the flaps are superiorly based.

When there is loss of skin preventing closure without tension, then one is left with the following options: wide undermining and advancement of skin edges, local flap repair by various techniques, and skin grafting. Undermining is sometimes successful for smaller defects but the wound may need to be lengthened at each end as an extended ellipse.

Local tissue is best for colour and texture match, and a local rotation–advancement flap may be possible, taking into account the cosmetic aspects of the region. Transposition flaps may also be worth consideration, especially if the secondary defect can be closed directly; Limberg's multiple transposition flaps have been used in closure of a circular defect (Converse et al 1977). Bilobed flaps for noses, V–Y advancement flaps and pedicled flaps directly brought into place or as an island pedicle have been used; even tubed pedicles (Fig. 17.7) may be appropriate in some situations.

A medium to thick split-skin graft can be used as temporary or definitive skin cover in the larger defects: sometimes a full-thickness skin graft from postauricular or supraclavicular skin may be preferred in a smaller wound with a clean vascular bed. In cases of very large skin loss there may be a case for free tissue transfer, especially if there is a fracture site or bare bone exposed, or where nerve repair with interpositional grafts is needed. The colour and texture match may not be good but this can be acceptable in the circumstances. Split-skin grafting for

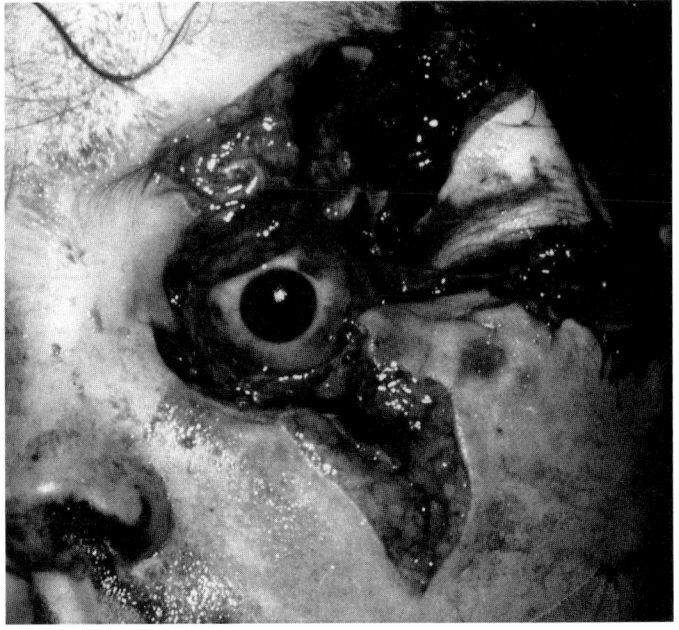
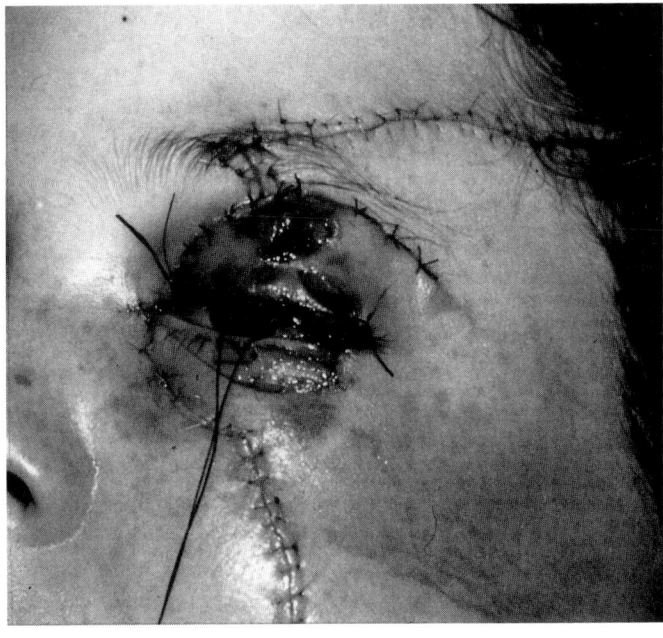

A   **B**

Fig. 15.1 Facial lacerations. A A triradiate laceration exposed the eye and the upper eyelid was almost avulsed. **B** Meticulous repair of the torn skin gave tension-free closure and good eye cover. Despite the questionable viability of the upper eyelid, the final result was satisfactory.

large defects as a temporizing measure has further advantages: the resultant scar may contract and can then be replaced later by adjacent skin advanced after the use of a tissue expander (p. 583).

Nasal injuries

Injuries to the nose may involve the bony skeleton, cartilaginous skeleton, septum and mucosa as well as the overlying skin. Septal haematoma requires drainage, otherwise septal cartilage necrosis and septal perforation or saddle nose deformity may result. Reduction of displaced bony or cartilaginous elements, with some form of fixation if necessary, should precede soft-tissue repair. Mucosal lacerations should be accurately closed with interrupted 4/0 or 5/0 chromicized catgut (CCG) suture and skin closure with 5/0 or 6/0 nylon stitches, taking care to align the nostril margins.

Full-thickness skin loss on the nose will require local flap repair or full-thickness skin grafts. Loss of nostril or ala nasi is best restored with a composite graft from a wedge of helical rim, provided the tissue is no more than 1 cm in width or length; this can be done primarily or at a later stage. Traumatic amputation of the nose or part thereof is most often due to bites whether human or animal (p. 498) but can occur in accidents, as by broken plate glass or motor vehicular crash. Spiteful amputation of a nose still occurs sporadically, but may be self-inflicted during a psychotic state. In avulsion injuries part of the lip or cheek may accompany the nose (James 1976); larger blood vessels may then be available for replantation, if the severed part is recovered. The size of the severed nose and more importantly the size of identifiable arteries and veins will determine whether reimplantation is likely to succeed (Tajima et al 1989, Niazi et al 1990). The vessels are usually very small, being 0.5–0.7 mm in diameter, but an attempt at replanting is worthwhile for any significant sized amputated portion of the nose. At least one artery and one vein has to be anastomosed, and small interposition vein grafts are frequently necessary. When venous reconstruction has been impossible, the application of leeches may control venous engorgement and save the replantation.

Late reconstruction of an amputated nose may be done by a variation of the forehead rhinoplasty (p. 585) or by the microvascular option of a radial, ulnar or lateral arm free flap (p. 626). Skeletal support can be established with an L-strut bone or cartilage graft, or a cantilevered costochondral rib graft.

Injuries of the external ear

Lacerations and amputations

Secondary ear reconstruction is difficult and the results often fall short of expectations. In any individual case, one has to consider a variety of options and decide on the most suitable line of management in the light of the anatomy of the injury and the personal wishes of the injured person.

The ear has abundant blood supply from branches of the superficial temporal artery, the deep auricular artery, and the posterior auricular artery (Fig. 2.16). Often severe lacerations or partial avulsions leave the ear with small or narrow intact skin or soft-tissue pedicles but surprisingly good circulation. Careful debridement of skin and cartilage, and accurate suturing of the skin will frequently give a gratifying survival. Completely avulsed or amputated ears may survive as composite grafts if reimplanted within a few hours of injury (Lewis & Fowler 1979), especially if a bigger area of contact of soft-tissue surfaces is achieved by removal of conchal cartilage or fenestration of the auricular cartilage. Bernstein & Nelson (1982) advocated this line of treatment, using low-dose anticoagulants and measures to reduce venous congestion — surface cooling and multiple stab wounds in the skin of the replanted auricle. Another option is to denude the cartilage framework and bank it in a retro-auricular skin pocket (Mladick 1978). If the retro-auricular skin is missing one may wrap the cartilage with a temporalis fascial flap and apply split-skin graft over the fascia. Successful replantation of amputated ears has been reported (Nahai et al 1978); the success rate is not high due to technical difficulties with short arteries and veins of small diameters, which require vein grafts, but under favourable conditions salvage should be attempted (p. 456). Yet another option is an osseo-integrated prosthesis (p. 481).

Blunt injuries

Otohaematomas commonly occur in contact sport or after blunt trauma to the external ear, and require surgical drainage followed with bolus dressings of acriflavine wool or gauze secured with 5/0 Prolene or nylon sutures. Failure to drain an otohaematoma results in the cauliflower ear so characteristic of professional boxers in the past.

Eyebrow wounds

Lacerations that run through or across the eyebrows should be explored for underlying fractures especially of the frontal sinus, and for damage to the supratrochlear and supraorbital nerves. The underlying muscle should be closed with 4/0 CCG or PDS sutures, and the skin stitched with 5/0 or 5/0 nylon. The hair should not be shaved as it provides a guide for accurate alignment of eyebrow borders. Preservation of hair follicles by careful debridement in an oblique direction parallel with the long axes of the hair shafts, and using fine close stitching, will minimize the bald scar that is usually seen in the eyebrow.

Eyelid wounds

These important injuries are discussed in Chapter 14. Injury to the globe or to the lacrimal apparatus must always be suspected where there has been injury to the eyelids; an ophthalmological consultation is usually needed. Eyelid lacerations are very minimally debrided, if at all, and skin edges should be sutured loosely with 5/0 or 6/0 nylon. Full-thickness skin loss requires local transposition flaps or full-thickness skin grafts, using the contralateral upper eyelid as a donor site. Injuries to the puncta, canaliculi, lacrimal sac and nasolacrimal duct are important, and should be recognized primarily; their repair is discussed on p. 429. Loss of up to one-quarter of the eyelid can be closed directly in layers. Larger full-thickness loss will require reconstructive procedures involving local flaps.

Injuries of the lips, oral cavity and tongue

Soft-tissue injuries of the lips require repair of the mucosa, the musculature and the skin. The areas that require special attention are the vermilion margin or 'white line', the cupids bow and the commissures. The mucosa is repaired with 4/0 CCG or 4/0 silk, orbicular muscle with 4/0 CCG or PDS and the vermilion and skin closed with 5/0 or 6/0 nylon. Vermilion and skin sutures should be removed at the 5th day as the nylon tends to become buried if left longer. Mouth washes three or four times daily with 0.2% chlorhexidine solution, or any other antiseptic mouthwash, are recommended especially after meals.

Intraoral lacerations should be closed primarily, after thorough cleaning, irrigation and debridement. Secondary healing may result in functional problems due to scar contracture. This is especially likely if some soft tissue or mucosal loss has occurred. With significant loss of oral mucosa, a microvascular free flap must be considered as an option for early closure of the defect. The radial forearm free flap is much favoured for intraoral mucosal replacement (p. 628), although the ulnar forearm free flap is equally good. The volar aspect of the distal forearm provides thin fasciocutaneous flaps which are well vascularized by perforating vessels from either the radial or ulnar artery.

For lacerations of the tongue which need stitches, 3/0 or 4/0 silk is the material of choice as it is soft and non-absorbable, and will withstand the constant movement of the tongue. Chromicized catgut tends to undo rapidly, while slowly absorbing sutures like Vicryl or PDS take so long to fall out that they frequently need to be removed.

Scalp wounds

Simple scalp lacerations can be cleaned and sutured with 3/0 or 4/0 nylon sutures under local anaesthesia. Stellate, ragged, avulsed or complicated lacerations with underlying fractures or exposed cranium need assessment as to the vascularity of the injured tissues, followed by debridement of non-viable tissue and appropriate techniques of wound closure. Extensive scalp wounds are closed in two layers, absorbable sutures being used for the galea and nylon or Prolene to approximate the skin edges.

Replantation of large avulsed portions of scalp has been possible since microvascular techniques were used in the early 1970s, with reported successes by Miller et al (1976), Buncke et al (1978), Van Beck & Zook (1978) and Tantri et al (1980). The advantages of scalp replantation are obvious with regard to hair growth and full protective thickness (Fig. 15.2). Massive avulsions may also include the forehead, the eyebrows and the upper eyelids, and all or parts of the ears. The rich cross-anastomoses of vessels in the scalp allow the survival of large portions even on one arterial reanastomosis. However, multiple interposition vein grafts are usually needed to restore the arterial input and as many venous outflows as possible should be constructed. The superficial temporal arteries and veins are the most commonly available and most accessible vessels, but the occipital vessels are also of good size, the arteries being 2 mm in diameter and the veins 3–4 mm in diameter. The superficial temporal artery is apt to go into spasm, when anastomosis may be difficult, especially if the intima becomes folded. If replantation is impossible, the exposed skull must be covered with split-skin grafts; the avulsed scalp may be used as a donor (Micheau et al 1986). In most cases, these grafts can be placed directly on the pericranium, which is usually intact, since the avulsion is in the scalping plane of loose areolar tissue deep to the galea.

If there is a scalp defect with absence of the underlying pericranium, or still more when there is a craniocerebral wound, it is likely that some form of flap closure will be required (p. 373). Loss of pericranium is seen in some missile injuries and in burns of the head (p. 484). When the pericranium is lacking in a small area, it may be possible to bridge the defect by placing a graft directly on the denuded bone. However, large areas of totally denuded bone cannot be closed in this way, and may require a large free flap, or even two free flaps, with microsurgical revascularization; this is especially useful when there is an underlying penetrating brain injury. Where no other means of closure is available, the outer calvarial table is removed with chisel cuts to expose the diplöe; this encourages granulation, on which split grafts can be placed.

SCARS

The aim of good wound management in the face is a fine linear scar, running in the direction of a skin crease and able to blend and 'fade' with the passage of time.

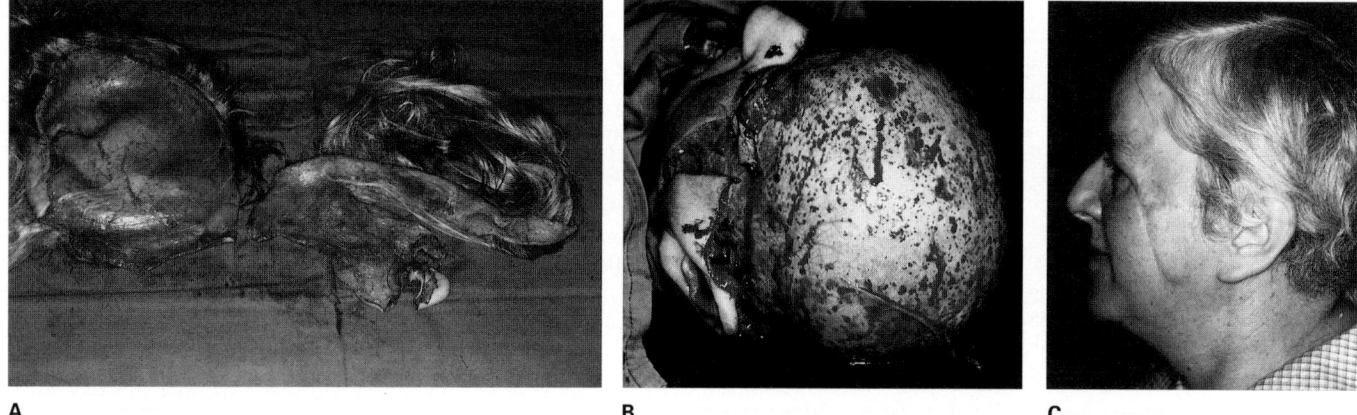

A B C

Fig. 15.2 Scalp avulsion. A 50-year-old woman suffered avulsion of the scalp in an industrial accident. Microsurgical anastomosis was performed within 8 h of injury. **A** Avulsed scalp in two fragments. **B** Denuded calvaria with intact pericranium. **C** Final result.

Scars which are prominent, thickened, raised or contracted frequently result from wounds running across skin creases or folds. Lumpy, raised or irregular scars occur with flap lacerations or when the edges have healed at different levels. Scars under tension contract and hypertrophy, becoming raised, red and widened, and become more prominent by gathering or tethering surrounding skin.

Scars should be left for 6 months or more to mature before revision surgery is considered. The ugly, red hypertrophic scar is still in an immature stage and too early revision will usually result in a similar or larger scar. When mature, the scar can be better assessed as to which portion if any requires revision; the best procedure can then be chosen, whether by excision and resuture, Z-plasty, or W-plasty. Tethered or contracted scars may require release and V–Y advancements, Z-plasty, local flaps or full-thickness skin grafts for correction.

Hypertrophic and keloid scars

Hypertrophic and keloid scars are disorders of scar formation: they are histologically dissimilar in that sections of a keloid show abundant ground substance with large eosinophilic collagen bundles (Fig. 5.2C), whereas hypertrophic scars show scanty ground substance and seemingly normal, mature fibroblasts and collagen bundles. Keloids occur more frequently in pigmented races and in the first two decades of life; they are uncommon in white races and older persons. There are sites of predilection, which were divided into three groups by Crockett (1964):

1. Presternum and back
2. Deltoid, anterior chest, ear, scalp, forehead and beard area
3. Abdomen, lower limbs, face, lower back, genitalia.

Hypertrophic scars are usually limited to the original incision or wound, increasing in thickness or height for 3–6 months and then beginning to regress. A keloid in contrast enlarges beyond the original wound and invades normal skin laterally as well as proliferating vertically. It does not show regression or maturation for many years.

Both types of scar should not be excised without ancillary measures which include Kenacort (triamcinalone acetonide) injections and pressure postoperatively, by elastic garments, Silastic® gel sheets or clip earrings in the case of earlobes. Intralesional injections of Kenacort A40 at 4 weekly intervals for five to six times can usually cause regression and flattening. However, the outcome can then be an ugly depressed scar with dermal atrophy and prominent surface capillary telangectasia. Sometimes excision followed by injections of Kenacort into the edges of the new wound before resuturing can result in a much less prominent scar.

INJURIES OF THE SALIVARY GLANDS AND THEIR DUCTS

The parotid gland

Laceration of the parotid gland may divide minor or major intraparotid ducts, resulting in a sialocele or parotid fistula. Sialography is used to demonstrate whether minor or major ducts have been divided and has some prognostic value. The use of prophylactic antibiotics can be justified in parotid and parotid duct injuries as bacterial infection of the gland is a potential risk; we give flucloxacillin 1 g 6 hourly intravenously for 24 h in an adult followed by oral flucloxacillin 500 mg 6 hourly for a complete 5 day course.

Conservative management was recommended by Landau & Stewart (1985), on the basis of an experience of 14 consecutive cases of stab wounds by knives or bottles, seen in a 4 month period in the Baragwanath Hospital, Johannesburg. Primary duct repair was possible in only three cases. Eleven presented with established sialoceles or fistulas, often infected. They were treated with pro-banthine 6 hourly to inhibit salivation, pressure dressings, and aspiration: in all cases, the leaks subsided.

The parotid duct

The surface marking of the parotid duct is the middle third of a line between the tragus and the midpoint of the interval between the alar base and the facial modiolus. A deep laceration in that area should arouse suspicion of injury to the parotid duct, which should be explored with a view to repair if necessary. The duct ostium is marked by a little ridge in the buccal mucosa opposite the upper second molar and can be probed or cannulated with a fine polythene tube to locate the site of ductal injury. The tube can then be passed into the more proximal duct. Clear fluid can sometimes be seen at the proximal cut end. Magnification with loupes or the operating microscope will facilitate cannulation and repair of the duct with interrupted 9/0 or 10/9 nylon sutures. The polythene cannula should be secured with a 3/0 silk suture in the buccal mucosa, and left for 7–10 days.

If an injured or divided duct is missed, a sialocele or fistula will become apparent. Exploration should then be undertaken to repair the duct, translocate the ostium or ligate the duct proximal to the leakage site.

Submandibular gland

Laceration or injury to the submandibular salivary gland is not common and repair of the duct is not necessary; if a fistula forms it will probably drain into the oral cavity. If duct obstruction causes trouble, the gland can be resected. Sublingual salivary gland injuries are also rare and apart from repair of the associated surrounding soft tissue, no active surgical treatment is required. Mucous cysts may arise from scarring around the ducts of minor salivary glands; an excision or deroofing of the cyst is usually curative.

NERVE INJURIES

The facial and trigeminal nerves are frequently involved in craniofacial trauma. The facial nerve and its branches should be repaired primarily when found to be transected. Peripheral branches of the trigeminal nerve should also be repaired if possible. Injuries to the lower cranial nerves are not often recognized at the time of first assessment or primary treatment.

Facial nerve injury

Surgical pathology

This important nerve may be injured within the posterior fossa, or within the petrous bone, or after it has left the stylomastoid fossa. Division or contusion proximal to the geniculate ganglion results in loss of all motor, sensory and secretomotor function (p. 166). This is sometimes seen in association with fractures of the skull base. Injury of the nerve in its intrapetrous part affects the nerve to stapedius muscle and the chorda tympani, as well as facial motor function. Facial paralysis in this site is not uncommon, and may be associated with longitudinal or transverse fractures of the petrous bone (p. 202); hearing may be affected. Injury beyond the stylomastoid foramen results in motor paralysis of the facial muscles without sensory or parasympathetic involvement.

Injuries distal to the stylomastoid foramen are most often seen in association with lacerations or stab wounds in the vicinity of the parotid gland. The extracranial anatomy of the facial nerve is well described in anatomical and clinical texts. The facial nerve trunk divides into upper and lower divisions, the upper giving temporal and zygomatic branches while the lower division gives the buccal, mandibular and cervical branches (Fig. 2.30). There are plexiform interconnections between the main branches, and variations in the branching pattern. Thus, depending on the site of the injury, the nerve may be divided in its entirety, or there may be localized division of one or more branches.

Assessment

Peripheral (extracranial) facial paralysis is usually obvious at once, and if there is an associated facial wound, the injury is a nerve transection or neurotmesis (p. 137) until proved otherwise. Facial paralysis due to injuries within the petrous bone may also be immediately obvious, or may appear a day or more after injury; presumably these late-onset palsies result from swelling of a contused nerve within the facial canal.

The time of onset of the paralysis is of crucial importance in planning management; the completeness of paralysis also has great significance, and indeed Adegbite et al (1991) see it as even more relevant. When the paralysis appears after an interval, or is incomplete, there is a strong likelihood of spontaneous recovery; this highlights the importance of testing facial movements, even in the unconscious patient (p. 167). A post-traumatic facial nerve paralysis, whether immediate or of delayed onset (and the distinction may be difficult when there is a cerebral injury), demands a clinical evaluation to determine the probable lesion site. If this is likely to be within the petrous bone, or proximal thereto, the evaluation requires:

1. Full audiometry, including impedance studies to test the function of the stapedius muscle.
2. Electrogustrometry to evaluate chorda tympani function.

3. High resolution CT scanning to evaluate the whole length of the nerve, and especially the region of the geniculate ganglion.

4. Electrophysiological tests: facial electroneuronography should be done daily from the fourth day after injury to determine the electrical status of the peripheral axons. If there is progressive degeneration, with the likelihood of complete degeneration, then surgical exploration of the nerve is usually indicated if other circumstances support the decision to do so.

Management

The management of facial nerve injury proximal to the stylomastoid foramen has been well discussed by Fisch (1979) and May (1983, 1986). The details are beyond the scope of this book, but since facial nerve paralysis is often seen in conjunction with CMF injuries, some general comments are appropriate. In late-onset paralysis, exploration of the nerve should only be considered if paralysis remains complete for 6–8 months (McKennan & Chole 1992). Paralysis complete from the time of injury is more likely to be permanent, and — especially if there is a fracture likely to involve the nerve — early exploration is usually warranted, to decompress the nerve or to repair it by grafting. The exploration may be done by the subtemporal route or through the mastoid; for lesions proximal to the geniculate ganglion, posterior fossa craniotomy may be needed. Samii (1983) reported a case in which recovery followed nerve grafting from the proximal stump of the nerve, exposed in the posterior fossa, to the distal portion of the nerve exposed in its mastoid segment.

Nerve repair

Injury to the facial nerve beyond the stylomastoid foramen must be suspected in any deep laceration in the vicinity of the parotid gland and posterior cheek. Clinical confirmation of the injury to the nerve or its branches can be easily observed in signs of complete or partial paralysis of the facial musculature; electrodiagnostic tests may be helpful. Primary end-to-end repair of the nerve or its branches will give the best results: in delayed or secondary repair, the operator may find the cut ends too far separated for direct coaptation or difficult to locate in scar tissue. Exploration of the wound is aided with a Weck 'Pulsatron' disposable nerve locator/stimulator. It has been claimed that the distal motor nerve segment after injury can be stimulated to cause a muscle contraction for up to 72 h after injury, after which it will no longer respond. If the proximal and distal cut ends of the nerve can be approximated, microsurgical repair should be undertaken using 9/0 nylon epineural sutures for the trunk or divisions

and 10/0 or 11/0 nylon perineural stitches for the main branches or smaller branches. Fascicular alignment of the nerve with full contact of the two cut surfaces will encourage maximum axonal regrowth through the repair site (Millesi 1979).

If there has been loss of nerve tissue or a gap due to retraction, as is often seen in delayed repairs, interposition nerve grafts will be preferable to attempting repair under tension (Fig. 15.3). Donor nerve material may be obtained from the branches of the cervical plexus, notably the great auricular or supraclavicular nerves. Alternatively the sural nerve is taken: it can be split into mono- or oligofascicular segments if required.

Interfascicular repair under the microscope using 10/0 or 11/0 nylon should be the aim, and with some knowledge of intraneural topography matching of fascicles

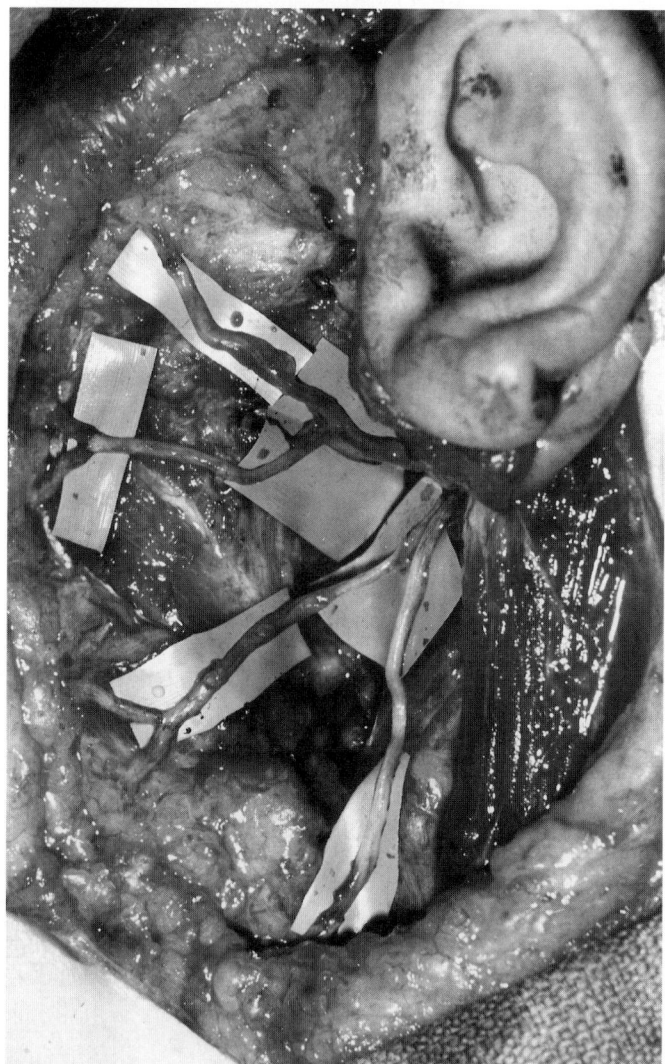

Fig. 15.3 Facial nerve repair with sural grafts. The nerve was repaired after resection of a parotid tumour; the technique is applicable in traumatic injuries.

proximally and distally may be attempted. Results of facial nerve repairs are quite good but synkinesis, mass action and residual weakness are commonly seen.

Faciohypoglossal anastomosis

This nerve transfer may be used as a measure of last resort, when repair is not possible. It is a technically easy operation, and gives good resting tone in the facial muscles (Fig. 15.4). Eye closure is sometimes unsatisfactory, but a lateral angular canthorrhaphy usually gives an acceptable appearance and sufficient corneal protection. Adults rarely achieve a smile, though practice with the tongue before a mirror sometimes gives the capacity

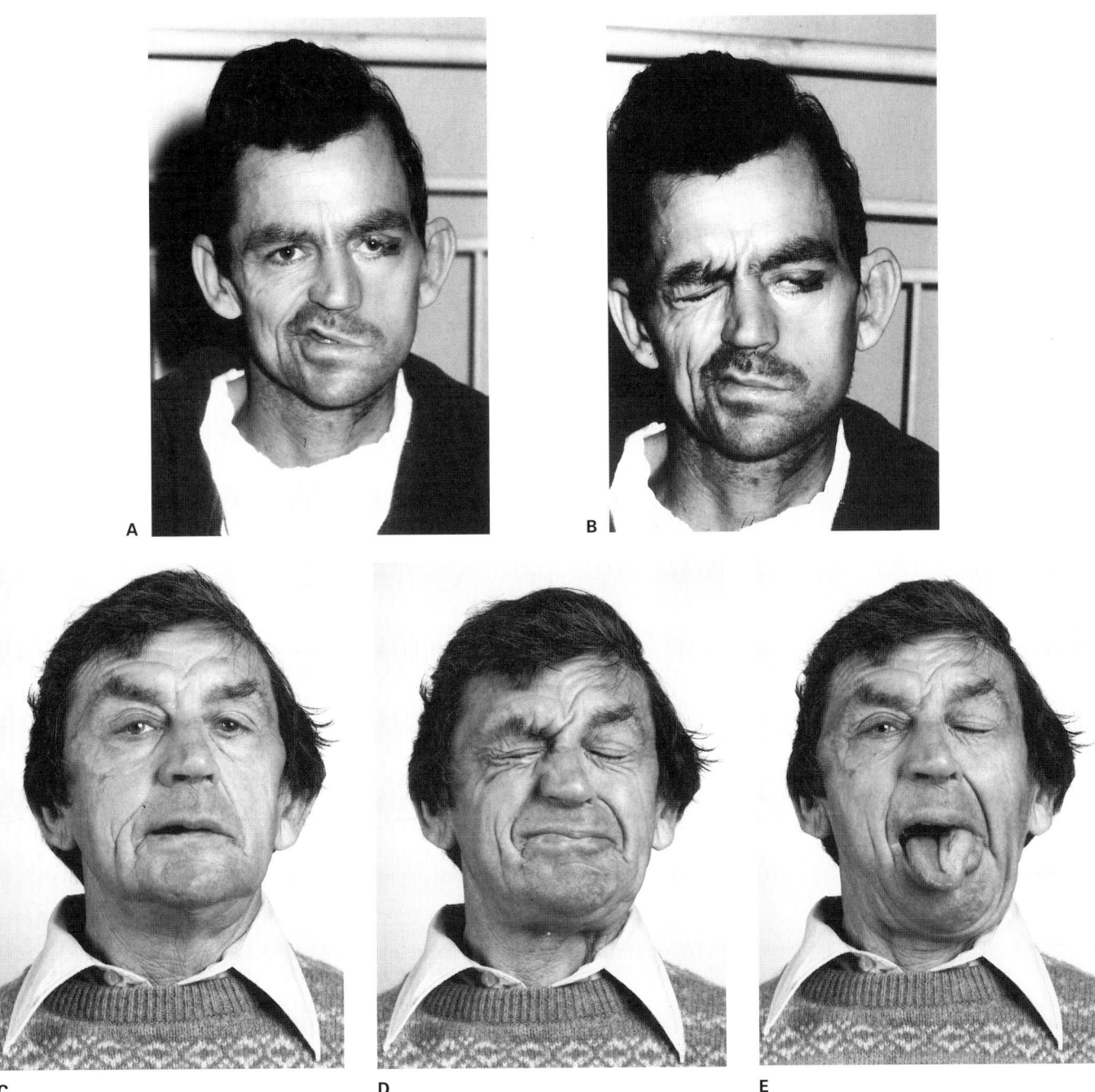

Fig. 15.4 Faciohypoglossal anastomosis. A 35-year-old man underwent removal of an acoustic neurinoma. **A** Postoperatively there was a complete facial paralysis. A lateral tarsorrhaphy was performed. **B** Attempted smiling and eye closure demonstrated the completeness of the paralysis. Faciohypoglossal paralysis was carried out 3 weeks after the initial operation. **C** 30 years later, the resting appearance was acceptable. **D** The patient had learned to carry out mass movements of the whole face by tongue movement, including eye closure. **E** The hypoglossal paralysis was entirely asymptomatic.

to do so. Moderate to severe hemiatrophy of the tongue is seen when the hypoglossal nerve has been used in hypoglossal–facial nerve transfer, though there is usually no subjective disability (Fig. 15.4E). Conley & Baker (1979) reviewed the results of 137 operations of this type, noting that mass facial movements do happen during eating, but in general emphasizing the benefits of the anastomosis, and our experience is similar.

Cross-facial nerve graft, free muscle transfers (Harrison 1985) and other procedures such as static slings, temporalis transfer, and digastric transfer, all have their advocates. However, there are few indications for these procedures in CMF trauma.

Trigeminal nerve injuries

The infraorbital nerve is frequently injured in fractures of the zygoma and maxilla. Bony fragments may transect or compress the nerve in its canal. Most injuries appear to be neurapraxias as recovery of sensation usually occurs within 6 weeks after reduction and stabilization of the fracture, but sensation may return as late as up to one year. Decompression of the nerve may be indicated where there is persistent anaesthesia or dysaesthesia. An elegant method has been described by Converse et al (1967). Direct repair or nerve grafting is usually not feasible.

The supratrochlear and supraorbital nerves may be damaged by lacerations in the eyebrow or lower forehead. Rarely, the fascicles are cleanly cut when they may be sutured with a few 10/0 or 11/0 nylon stitches. They are more likely to be avulsed, stretched or macerated, and repair is then impossible.

The inferior dental nerve is not accessible for repair either proximal to the lingula or in its intraosseous course within the mandible. When injured in a fracture, spontaneous recovery may be anticipated if the fracture has been reduced anatomically and stabilized. At the mental foramen the mental nerve quickly divides into several fascicles which, if cleanly cut across, are amenable to fascicular repair.

The lingual nerve

Lingual nerve injury due to dental drills or the scalpel during submandibular gland excision results in ipsilateral loss of sensation in the anterior two-thirds of the tongue and partial loss and differentiation of taste. A segment is always missing and interposition nerve graft is extremely difficult due to poor access. Results of those few cases that have been repaired have been disappointing.

Combined facial and trigeminal nerve injury

Facial nerve palsy together with anaesthesia of the cornea due to damage to the ophthalmic division of the trigeminal nerve makes a very dangerous combination, which can lead to neurotrophic keratitis, corneal ulceration and secondary vascularization of the cornea, with loss of sight. The eye must be protected by copious regular use of lubricants, such as 2% methylcellulose eye drops and white paraffin ointment, and by a humid eye chamber, in the hope of spontaneous recovery. If this does not take place, a lateral tarsorrhaphy, and perhaps a medial canthoplasty, will be needed to reduce the area of corneal exposure; at times, a central tarsorrhaphy is needed to preserve the integrity of the cornea (p. 246). In the event of a combined facial and trigeminal paralysis, every effort to repair the injured facial nerve is justified

Hypoglossal nerve injury

This nerve is rarely injured except iatrogenically or by a missile wound. If recognized, primary repair may be feasible using 9/0 or 10/0 nylon epineural stitches under magnification.

REFERENCES

Adegbite A B, Khan M I, Tan L 1991 Predicting recovery of facial nerve function following injury from a basilar skull fracture. J Neurosurg 75: 759–762
Bernstein L, Nelson R H 1982 Replanting the severed auricle: an update. Arch Otolaryngol 108: 587–590
Buncke H, Rose E, Brownstein M, Chater N 1978 Successful replantation of two avulsed scalp flaps by microvascular anastomosis. Plast Reconstr Surg 61: 666–672
Conley J, Baker D C 1979 Hypoglossal-facial nerve anastomosis for the reinnervation of the paralysed face. Plast Reconstr Surg 63: 63–72
Converse J M, Smith B, Obear M F, Wood-Smith D 1967 Orbital blow-out fracture: a ten-year study. Plast Reconstr Surg 39: 20–36
Converse J M, McCarthy J G, Brauer R O, Ballantyne D L 1977 Transplantation of skin grafts and flaps. In: Converse J M (ed) Plastic reconstructive surgery. Saunders, Philadelphia, Vol 1, Ch 6
Crockett D J 1964 Regional keloid susceptibility. Br J Plast Surg 17: 245–253

Fisch U 1979 Current surgical treatment of intratemporal facial palsy. Clin Plast Surg 6: 377–388
Harrison D H 1985 The pectoralis minor vascularized muscle graft for the treatment of unilateral facial palsy. Plast Reconstr Surg 75: 206–216
James N J 1976 Survival of large replanted segment of upper lip and nose. Plast Reconstr Surg 58: 623–625
Landau R, Stewart M 1985 Conservative management of post-traumatic parotid fistulae and sialoceles: a prospective study. Br J Surg 72: 42–44
Lewis E C, Fowler J R 1979 Two replantations of severed ear parts. Plast Reconstr Surg 64: 703–705
McKennan K X, Chole R A 1992 Facial paralysis in temporal bone fracture. Am J Otol 13: 167–172
May M 1983 Trauma to the facial nerve. Otolaryngol Clin North Am 16: 661–670
May M 1986 The facial nerve. Thieme, New York, Ch 20

Micheau P, Costagliola M, Chavoin J P, Rouge D, Py N 1986 Le scalp: la greffe mince de première intention, en urgence. A propos de quatre observations. Ann Chir Plast Esthét 31: 351–357

Miller G D H, Anstee E J, Small J A 1976 Successful replantation of an avulsed scalp by microvascular anastomosis. Plast Reconstr Surg 58: 133–136

Millesi H 1979 Nerve suture and grafting to restore the extratemporal facial nerve. Clin Plast Surg 6: 333–341

Mladick R A 1978 Salvage of the ear in acute trauma. Clin Plast Surg 5: 427–435

Nahai F, Hayhurst J W, Salibian A H 1978 Microvascular surgery in avulsive trauma to the external ear. Clin Plast Surg 5: 423–426

Niazi Z, Lee T T, Eadie P, Lawlor D 1990 Successful replantation of nose by microsurgical technique and review of the literature. Br J Plast Surg 43: 617–620

Samii M 1983 Intracranial reconstruction of facial nerve after lateral basal fracture. In: Samii M, Brihaye J (eds) Traumatology of the skull base. Springer, Berlin

Tajima S, Ueda K, Tanaka Y 1989 Successful replantation of a bitten-off nose by microvascular anastomosis. Microsurgery 10: 5–7

Tantri D, Cervino L, Tabbal N 1980 Replantation of the totally avulsed scalp. J Trauma 20: 350–352

Van Beck A, Zook E G 1978 Scalp replantation by microvascular revascularization. Plast Reconstr Surg 61: 774–777

CHAPTER 16

Massive tissue loss

D. J. David   E. Tan

INTRODUCTION

In Chapters 11–15 we presented a plan of multi-disciplinary management of the craniomaxillofacial (CMF) injuries commonly seen in peacetime practice, in which tissue loss is not usually a major factor; this chapter considers the early management of injuries in which there is substantial tissue destruction or ablation. In Chapter 21, we consider the correction of the long-term deformities that may result from such injuries.

Even in peacetime, accidents inflicting massive avulsive tissue loss do occur. Such wounds are seen as the result of gunshots fired at close range, or from industrial explosions. Freak road accidents also sometimes result in avulsive injury and, in some parts of the world, bites by large animals may ablate portions of the face (p. 495). In war, avulsive facial injuries are very common and this has been so since firearms first began to dominate the world's battlefields (p. 2). Military missiles frequently avulse large segments of the face or extensive portions of the frontal scalp and calvarial bone. These wounds, if not immediately lethal, cause frightful aesthetic deformities and often severe impairments of speech, vision and other functions; Fig. 1.15 records some typical cases from World War I. In war, the management of such wounds is likely to be complicated by problems in evacuation, assessment and resuscitation, and definitive management is often delayed.

Our experience of major avulsive CMF trauma (Table 16.1) is based chiefly on peacetime practice, supplemented by study of wounded soldiers referred to us from other centres for secondary repair; in preparing an account of the management of these wounds, we have drawn heavily

Table 16.1 Massive avulsive injuries in the CMF area

Cause of avulsive injury	No. of cases
Gunshot wounds	16 (7 wartime)
Vehicular accidents	11
Other	4
Total	31

The figures give the experience of the Australian Craniofacial Unit during the period 1973–1993. Excluded are cases requiring only neurosurgical management and gunshot wounds not causing significant loss of tissue.

on the published and unpublished experience of other surgeons working in recent wars and civil conflicts.

SURGICAL PATHOLOGY

The pathology of missile injury expresses the nature and velocity of the missile; the anatomy of the impact is also relevant, impacts on bone being especially injurious. Wounds resulting from gunshot are classed as penetrating, perforating and avulsive or ablative. A penetrating wound is typically inflicted by a low velocity missile which remains embedded in the tissues: little damage is done unless a vital structure is hit. Perforating wounds may be caused by higher velocity missiles; in these, there is often a small entry wound, a larger exit wound, and a core of tissue damage between the wounds. Massive avulsive wounds show loss of anatomical structures, with great variety of tissue damage; the damage may be more widespread than the apparent tissue defect, because seemingly intact structures may have been devitalized by the missile impact or may have suffered traction injury from the avulsion.

Avulsive wounds result from very high velocity impacts by missiles of any size, or from large missiles or groups of missiles at lower velocities, or from tearing forces such as the bite of a large carnivorous animal. In war, fragments from mines, bombs and shells and high velocity rifle bullets are likely to cause avulsive injury; in peacetime, such injuries may result from short range (< 6 m) blasts from shotguns or large calibre pistols, or from a variety of rifles used in hunting, civil homicide, or attempted suicide. The ballistics of missile injuries are considered in Chapter 4. Avulsive injuries can also occur from industrial explosions, such as the explosion of a tractor tyre, and from a variety of accidents with machinery. On occasion massive craniofacial injury results from a vehicle accident. Ablative injury may result from tissue destruction by post-traumatic infection; the outcome is often a tissue defect that requires correction by procedures similar to those used in repairing acute avulsive trauma. A severe burn may also constitute an ablative injury.

The permutations of bone and soft-tissue avulsion are infinite, and any part of the CMF area may be damaged as a primary effect of the impact, or as a secondary complication. Soft-tissue injuries caused by missiles are often complicated by the presence of indriven bone and tooth fragments which must be carefully removed; if this is not done, they may be the source of chronic infection and sinus formation.

The eyes and the brain may be injured, either directly or by vascular interference. Extensive damage in the facial region can inflict severe tissue disruption without immediate effect on the central nervous system, yet with delayed cerebral or visual complications of ischaemic type resulting in increased disability (Fig. 16.1).

Wounds of the lower face and mandible

Injuries range from gross destruction of the lower jaw (Fig . 1.15d) to a simple mandibular fracture with soft tissue ablation. In the rifle bullet wound shown in Fig. 16.1, there was gross separation and destruction of the mandibular symphysis, loss of the floor of the mouth and tongue and part of the lower lip; one condylar process was missing, as was the central part of the maxilla. Such injuries are very dangerous: tongue control is lost, and with fading consciousness there may be a lethal airway obstruction. Injuries of the base of the tongue may go on to gross swelling and bleeding and are then an even greater threat to the airway. Loss of the lower lip is a challenging problem because effective reconstruction of the orbicularis oris muscle is a very difficult procedure and repair with distant flaps always gives a second rate functional result.

Missile injuries in the lower face can result in virtually no damage at all, with only a very small entry wound and minimal destruction of the missile tract, with fragments of metal and/or bone dispersed in the tissues or lodged in the palate or adjacent to the base of skull. More frequently, however, we are confronted with some damage to the mandible and lower teeth (Figs 16.1 and 21.73). Banks et al (1985) note that bullets striking the mandible may cause fractures of teeth below the gingival margin at a distance from the impact site, presumably by a shock wave transmitted through the dense bone of the mandible.

Wounds of the midface: maxillae, zygomas and nose

In our practice, the acute midface injuries most commonly seen have been the results of attempted suicide or homicide; we have also had to treat the late problems resulting from war injuries. An avulsive impact from the front, such as a shotgun blast, will frequently produce cone-shaped destruction of the middle third of the face, leaving lateral elements intact. A missile impact from the side may ablate the whole of the upper jaw and nose (Fig. 1.15C), or may tear off half of the upper jaw leaving the other half relatively intact. It is unusual to find a complete loss of the middle third of the face; more often, a segment of palate is missing and the residual fragments are blown aside into abnormal positions. Often the nasal pyramid is completely disrupted. The zygomas are often splayed apart and there may be associated fractures of the coronoid processes of the mandible, or disruption of the temporomandibular (TMJ) joints. If not treated effectively, ankylosis may develop. There are likely to be wide oro-antral and oronasal fistulae, with exposure of the antrum to the outside. According to the direction of the missile(s) there are injuries of adjacent vital structures such as the eyes or the brain; missiles traversing the middle third region may disrupt the middle cranial fossa as well as the anterior fossa, and both temporal and frontal lobe damage have been seen.

In surviving cases of midface regional injury, the structures likely to give long-term surgical problems are the lacrimal apparatus, the facial nerve and the parotid gland. Residual oro-antral and oronasal fistulae, almost inevitable when the hard palate has been widely destroyed, are also important surgical problems. Comprehensive destruction of the nasal structures is extremely difficult to repair in the first instance, and this leads to the necessity for complex secondary surgery. Where there is extensive loss of tissue over the anterior midface with exposure of the maxillary antrum then it is necessary to provide soft tissue and skin cover to this area.

Wounds of the upper face and frontal convexity

A missile wound in the frontal area may show more or less extensive loss of skin and frontal bone. The paranasal air sinuses are often injured; there may be dural penetration and cerebral damage. Such dural injuries may result

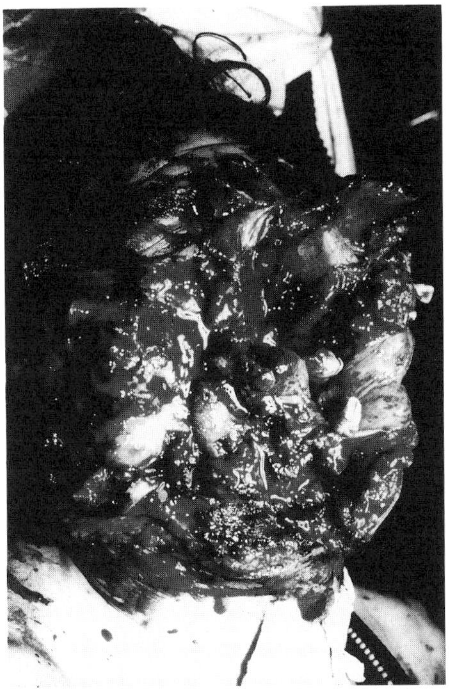

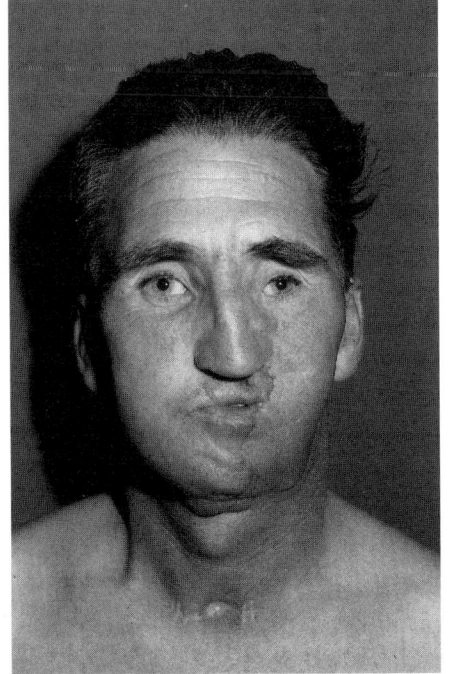

Fig. 16.1 Avulsive facial gunshot wound. A massive soft-tissue and bony injury was inflicted in the face by a Lee Enfield .303 in rifle at close range. The patient drove his car to seek help. Some 8 h later he became blind, presumably from retinal arterial spasm. He was never unconscious. He underwent intubation, tracheostomy, debridement and primary closure of the wound. Subsequently the bone fragments were stabilized with a metal spacer; later, microvascular reconstruction of the mandible was done with other corrective procedures. **A** Initial presentation, with massive tissue loss and bony destruction. Despite the forbidding appearance, he was easily intubated because the tissues could be peeled apart and the laryngeal inlet observed. **B** Semi-elective tracheostomy and repair of the soft tissues were performed. More debridement was necessary to remove damaged muscle and pieces of bone and tooth which had been driven into the wound. **C** The lower jaw fragments were separated by a Bowerman-type prosthesis. At the time of the stabilization of his jaw, the zygomas were reduced and wired into position, establishing the width of the upper part of the middle third of his face. **D** 2 months later, the definitive repair was performed. A composite osteocutaneous free groin flap was raised on the deep circumflex iliac vessels with a skin paddle which was placed in the floor of the mouth coming through the lip and onto the chin. The defect is shown recreated with the bone ends separated and the metal prosthesis removed in readiness for insertion of the graft. **E** The osteocutaneous composite graft on its vascular pedicle. **F** The patient remained blind and had a continuing problem related to the soft-tissue deficit in the orbicularis oris. Since that time he has had a number of operations to sculpture the bone and redrape the soft tissue.

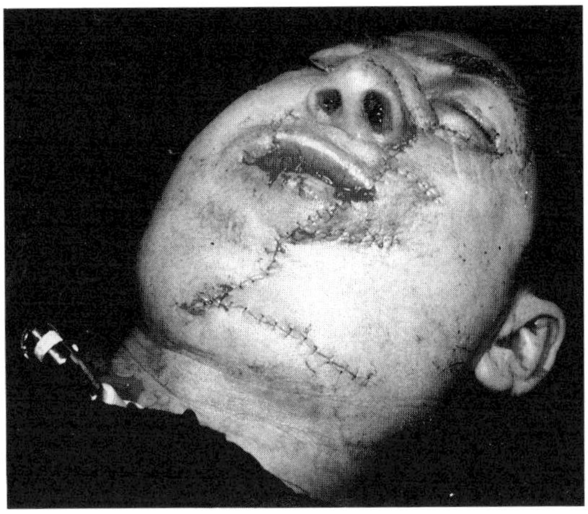

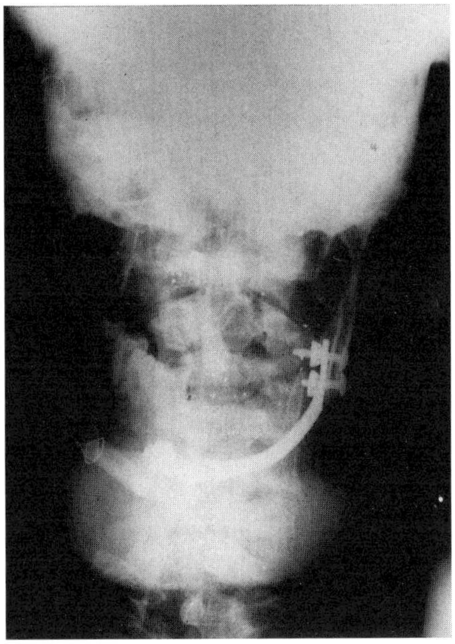

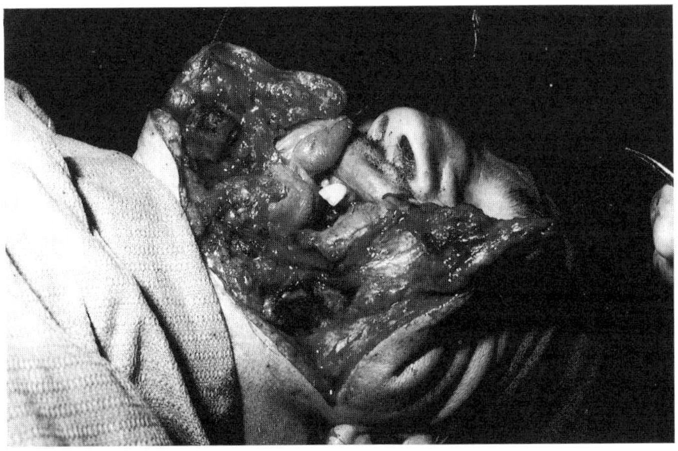

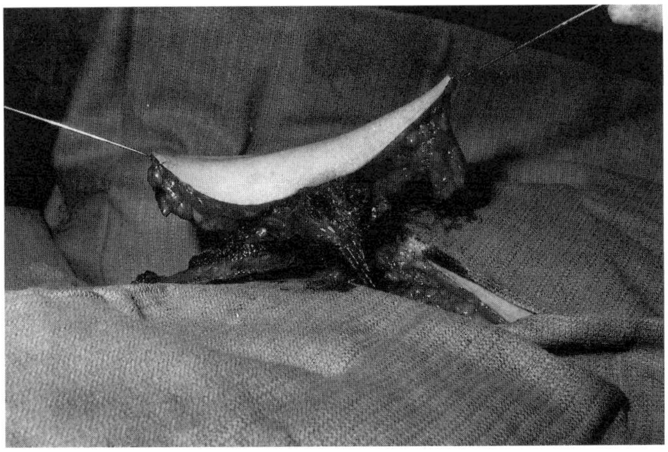

in a permanent cranionasal communication, with risk of early or late meningitis and/or brain abscess. In our view, frontal wounds with proven or probable dural penetration require transcranial exploration and full dural repair; the arguments for and against this policy are discussed on p. 376. This is less necessary when the middle fossa dura is torn, though here too the possibility of a cranionasal or cranioaural fistula must be kept in mind. We have seen delayed meningitis from a missile wound of the middle fossa.

Missile wounds of the upper face are likely to involve the orbit and especially the eye; the inherent anatomical resistance of the mobile globe of the eye to blunt trauma of the facial skeleton, so often seen after in road crashes, does not give protection from a missile (Fig. 1.15B). Injuries of the naso-ethmoidal region are frequently associated with damage to the globe. Reconstruction of the root of the nose and cranial base is often needed, with repair of the nasal pyramid (Fig. 21.48).

Missiles striking the frontal convexity above the orbital level often cause lethal brain damage. However, when the missile path is tangential to the frontal convexity (p. 141), the patient may survive with a variable loss of skin, frontal bone and dura mater; such injuries often entail severe and disabling frontal lobe damage (p. 53).

Frontal ablative defects secondary to bone infection are less serious. Post-traumatic infection may destroy much of the frontal bone, leaving gross deformity; as a rule, there is no associated scalp loss, though sometimes sinus formation may have caused extensive scarring (Figs 21.1 and 21.7).

Scalp avulsion

Frontal scalp avulsion as an isolated injury has been discussed on p. 437). In scalping injuries due to traction on the hair, the plane of separation leaves the pericranium intact, and viable unless it becomes desiccated. In missile injuries, substantial areas of scalp may be avulsed or destroyed, sometimes in conjunction with loss of bone and exposure of dura or brain.

MANAGEMENT

General principles

Vital functions and vital structures must be protected. The vital functions chiefly under threat are the airway and the circulation. Airway obstruction and haemorrhage from large cervical and facial vessels have been the causes of many battlefield deaths, and despite advances in emergency trauma care, preventable deaths still result from peacetime injuries of this type.

After the essential preliminaries of evacuation, together with efforts to save life and to protect function, the pri-

mary management of the wound must be undertaken. The vital structures that need to be covered urgently are the brain and the dura, the eyes and the large vessels in the neck and face. This should be done with the aim of minimizing long-term deformity and disability. The maxillofacial region is different in many ways from other parts of the body in that blood supply of the area is excellent. With the advent of antibiotics, the risk of secondary haemorrhage has been minimized, and one can contemplate a programme of minimum debridement and early closure with a considerable amount of reconstruction being performed in the early phase, if not at the first operation then certainly within the first 10 days to 10 weeks.

Gruss et al (1991) recently reviewed their experience in 37 cases of massive facial injury from gunshots, chiefly suicidal attempts with shotguns or sporting rifles. They argued against traditional programmes entailing early soft-tissue closure and delayed multistaged bone replacement, and advocated early reconstruction with modern craniofacial techniques, notably rigid internal fixation with plates and bone grafts. For severe avulsive injury with loss of bone and soft tissue, Gruss and his colleagues proposed:

1. Immediate conservative debridement, with cover of exposed bone.
2. Delayed (7–10 days) primary definitive repair. Missing midfacial bone should be replaced with split calvarial and rib grafts, with stabilization by miniplates and screws; the correct facial width is restored. The mandible should be reconstructed, fragments being reduced and fixed with miniplates and lag screws. Gaps are bridged with long reconstruction plates. Soft tissue may be replaced with a free vascularized omental graft.
3. Late repair procedures may be necessary: in their practice, these included scar revision, reconstruction of the oral commissure, rhinoplasty and mandibular reconstruction by vascularized or conventional bone grafts.

Two strategies can be considered when one is confronted with the eventual need to reconstruct the mutilations due to ablative midfacial injuries, and they are not mutually exclusive. The first is prosthetic: the defect is replaced as far as possible by an external prosthesis or by an implant of some biocompatible material. The second is truly restorative: the defect is repaired by transplanted autogenous tissue. The advent of microvascular anastomosis (see Ch. 21) has greatly enlarged the utility of restorative transplantation. Indeed, modern reconstructive techniques involving flaps of skin, muscle and bone and free tissue transfer, together with the development of osseo-integrated implantology, have brought the two strategies into a close partnership. By aiming at the best possible early definitive repair, we hope to minimize the need for late correction or prosthetic replacement — and to maximize the success of these forms of management.

Wartime conditions may make compromises unavoidable, and late reconstructions may then be done under more adverse conditions, with established soft-tissue contraction. When one is fortunate in treating the patient in a well-equipped unit from the beginning, the two strategies can be harmonized to facilitate a planned combination of the reconstructive and prosthetic options (Fig. 21.48).

Assessment

In the early assessment of a severe ablative facial injury, an examiner confronted with a mass of unidentifiable bleeding tissues will direct attention to the control of the airway, the circulation and the cerebral status, and other important effects of the injury may easily be missed. Nevertheless, as soon as possible, the systematic clinical, laboratory and radiological work-up described in Chapters 6–9 should be carried out. If there is any reason to suspect vascular damage, such as the trajectory of missile fragments in the lower face and neck, cerebral angiography should be done; if there is any suspicion of blunt or penetrating injury of the brain, computerized tomography (CT) scan is essential. Magnetic resonance imaging (MRI) may also be of great value, but should not be used if there is evidence of a ferromagnetic missile in a dangerous situation. Lead and cupronickel missiles can be disregarded, but the fragments of bombs and shells should be regarded with suspicion and it should be remembered that modern military bullets may have steel components.

In planning the definitive management of a severe ablative injury, the multidisciplinary evaluation and team discussion described in Chapter 9 is of great value. Throughout the course of management, the injury should be repeatedly reassessed. Marx & Stevens (1991) give special attention to:

1. The physiological state, as related to anaesthetic risk
2. The size of the residual soft tissue defects, and the extent of scarring
3. The size and nature of the bone defect(s)
4. The presence of residual pathological conditions, such as foreign bodies or bone chips, perhaps associated with foci of chronic inflammation or fistula formation.

First aid and life support

This has been discussed in Chapter 8; securing the airway and controlling haemorrhage are immediate priorities in most avulsive injuries of the lower and middle face. Clarkson & Walker (1955) vividly described World War II management on the battlefield, emphasizing the occa-

sional need for cricothyroidotomy (p. 226). They noted that injured soldiers often felt little initial pain from jaw wounds, and might survive transection of a major cervical artery: vascular spasm and retraction often provided very effective primary haemostasis. Banks et al (1985) have reviewed more recent wartime practice in Israel, Vietnam, Nigeria, Ireland and the Falkland Islands; they emphasize that early endotracheal intubation is today the mainstay of airway control. Intubation is especially necessary when the conscious level is impaired; cricothyroidotomy may be appropriate when intubation is made difficult or impossible by massive orofacial damage.

Haemorrhage is controlled along the lines set out on p. 227. Banks et al (1985) reported that exsanguinating haemorrhage was not very common in uncomplicated battlefield wounds in the CMF area; however, blood transfusion was often necessary. Delayed bleeding may follow resuscitation and it is likely that emergency carotid angiography and embolization of bleeding arteries will be used increasingly in the management of primary and secondary haemorrhage.

Timing of repair

This is somewhat controversial. There is no doubt that open wounds can and should be closed as soon as possible in civil practice, and also in war surgery; CMF injuries provide one of the few exceptions to the general military rule that soft-tissue wounds should not be closed at the time of the initial wound care (Australian Army Manual of Land Warfare 1985, Whitlock 1985). If properly debrided, the vast majority of CMF wounds will heal well.

There is also little argument when the avulsive wound exposes or penetrates the dura mater. Early closure of the dura and skin is essential, though repair of a subfrontal dural defect may be deferred if there is brain swelling (p. 377). Calvarial bone defects can wait for a much longer period.

It is over the timing of definitive facial reconstruction that discordant opinions are expressed. Many authors see the definitive repair of massive defects as best done late, and only after careful preparation; Marx & Stevens (1991) see reconstruction as 'tertiary care', carried out in stages: in their practice, avulsive missile injuries required 'an average of 7.3 surgeries..., and avulsive motor vehicle injuries... an average of 5.7 surgeries.' Our philosophy is somewhat different, and closely parallels the views of Gruss et al (1991) summarized above.

It is hard to set out a rule of thumb for ablative injuries of the CMF region because each case is unique, and because avulsive trauma has no respect for anatomical boundaries. We talk of the avulsive injuries of the upper middle, and lower thirds of the face, but many such injuries involve all three regions; the treating team is faced with the need to set priorities and to design and implement plans for any permutation of defects. Nevertheless, there is an increased tendency to do more and more, earlier and earlier. It is often necessary to operate on patients in the first few hours after trauma to cover vital structures and to stem haemorrhage and to perform other life-saving manoeuvres; at such operations, as much as possible should be done to facilitate secondary surgery, for example by stabilizing bony fragments of the mandible (Figs 16.1 and 21.86). In less extensive injuries, if all of the surgery can be done in this first stage with little or no extra stress on the patient, then this should be done. There remains a group of patients who will require extensive, and perhaps complex reconstruction of the bony and soft tissues of the face and skull. We see these, not as late reconstructive procedures, but as the continuation of the initial treatment inaugurated by the definitive multidisciplinary team. Where possible, reconstruction should be conducted in the first 7–21 days after injury but there are no hard-and-fast rules, especially when local facilities are inadequate and transfer to a specialized unit is necessary. For example, the microvascular reconstruction of the symphysis and body of the mandible, together with skin and oral lining repair, might well be started very early whereas a cranioplasty for ablated frontal bone in the same patient, if covered with a suitable scalp flap, might be left for some months (Figs 21.1 and 21.73).

The often quoted dictum: 'first the bone and then the soft tissue' attributed to Pichler & Trauner (1948) is a good principle; however, with modern techniques of microvascular flap repair, microvascular tissue transfer and osseomusculocutaneous flaps, much of the reconstruction of bone as well as soft tissue can be performed simultaneously at a single procedure. Where this is done, early problems of scar contracture and difficulty in recreating the defect are not encountered. In all reconstructive procedures, what is done at the first operation often sets the limits on what can be achieved. The first chance is often the best chance. If the patient is fit and free of infection, every effort is made to produce a definitive result at this early phase. However, early operation need not mean immediate operation — it is often prudent to delay surgery for a few hours to stabilize the patient and to prepare a clear, well-planned operative strategy based on good radiological investigations.

Management of soft-tissue avulsions

Because of the favourable blood supply, most CMF wounds can be closed early and will heal uneventfully. This has been the experience in recent war zone surgery (Chapman 1985) as well as in civil practice. However, close-range gunshot wounds with widely disrupted soft tissue may need more extensive treatment by packing, cleaning and drainage, and implanted bone chips or tooth fragments may need to be located and removed.

Cleaning is done chiefly by copious washing with normal saline and a good deal of time should be spent in this, using large syringes with compressive bulbs. The initial debridement may be followed by partial skin closure and packing, with delayed complete closure within a week, at which as much of the definitive reconstruction as possible is carried out. If exposed areas of muscle and bone are left after debridement and suture of skin to mucosa, they should be packed with saline-soaked ribbon gauze. The other indication for packing is bleeding not controllable by diathermy or ligation of vessels. In such cases, the airway is secured by intubation or tracheostomy, and the nasal oral and pharyngeal spaces are firmly packed with 2.5 cm ribbon gauze dampened with saline. The taped ends of the packing are brought out through the mouth and the nose. This packing can be changed at 24–48 h or at the next available opportunity depending on the treatment schedule, e.g. the need for a general anaesthetic for other injuries. Removal of packing should be done under general anaesthesia in the operating theatre with the capacity to control further bleeding and repack if necessary. The insertion of Foley catheters through the nostrils and inflated in the postnasal cavity is a popular way of controlling bleeding in the area. Traction may need to be applied to the catheter to produce the desired effect and this should not be done by tying the catheters together across the columella, which may undergo necrosis — a very unpleasant complication!

In the head and neck, minimal debridement is appropriate because of the good blood supply. The wound edges are excised with a blade and trimmed square with sharp tungsten carbide inset scissors. An experienced surgeon can usually mobilize soft tissues in debrided wounds to produce an effective closure. Equal attention should be paid to suturing the oral mucosa as well as the skin. Mucosal lining must often be sutured to skin in the region of the nose and mouth. The branches of lacerated nerves should be identified and sutured if possible (p. 440); if microsurgical facilities are not available the nerve ends are tagged with black silk sutures in the epineurium, care being taken to avoid damage to the funicles of the nerve.

When there is a raw surface wound uncovered by skin or mucosa which cannot be closed primarily, the exposed tissue may be dressed with gauze soaked in saline, changed every 2–4 h, and later covered with skin grafts when the surface is clean and well vascularized. However, vital structures must be covered as soon as possible. Exposed dura mater is usually covered with a scalp flap (Fig. 21.1); this is even more necessary when brain is exposed, but to minimize adhesions to the damaged cerebral cortex a fascial or pericranial graft is first interposed. Bare vital structures in the neck, such as carotid vessels, are covered by a local flap or by a distant pedicled flap; bare bone may also need to be covered by a local or distant flap (Fig. 16.2). Soft-tissue defects resulting from the transferring of local flaps or from residual soft-tissue injuries in the face can be closed by split skin grafting.

The advantage of having primary closure performed by members of an experienced multidisciplinary team is that at this stage with the team assembled, as much as possible of the reconstruction can be done at once, and an appropriate plan can be made for the intermediate and later treatment.

Replacement of skin in avulsive injury

Restoration of the integument is crucially important to protect vital structures and to cover or form a bed for bone grafting; it is also important in restoring the aesthetic appearance of the face. To this end, the face should be treated as a series of aesthetic units (Fig. 17.10). If possible, muscle and nerve should be replaced, skin giving good colour match should be sought, and a sound skeletal basis should be provided either before or at the same time. An example is seen in total nasal reconstruction: the bony structure is essential to support any soft-tissue reconstruction and planning should be so as to minimize the number of stages. The tissues available for reconstruction of the face are any and all that can be chosen from the entire armamentarium of plastic and reconstructive surgery.

Free grafts

Split-thickness grafts and full-thickness grafts are applicable in the reconstruction of certain cosmetic units such as the upper eyelid, lower eyelid, and the nose where there is a good soft-tissue base; such grafts may be suitable when there is need for replacement of superficial loss of the cheeks and lips.

Wound contracture after early grafting may result in an unsatisfactory result; it may be possible at a later date to excise the grafted area and replace it with skin obtained by tissue expansion (p. 583).

Flaps

The workhorses of traditional plastic surgery have been used in almost every conceivable way to reconstruct various parts of the face. While these find their chief applications in the elective correction of deformities (p. 621), closure by a pedicled or free microvascularized flap is sometimes necessary in the acute phase of management of an avulsive injury.

Scalp flaps

The prodigious blood supply of the region allows the whole scalp to be moved on even one of its major vessels

and there are many variant techniques, e.g. the crane principle of Millard (1969).

Forehead flaps

The central forehead flap is made to include the supratrochlear vessels in its base; it may be used to provide a lining for the nose or a cover for the nose. Recently this flap has gained much advantage with the advent of tissue expansion to provide a large amount of skin for nasal reconstruction. In some cases adjacent tissue can be gained by using tissue expanders to advance forehead tissue after the hairy flap has been returned. Tissue expansion is a valuable method of gaining additional skin of good quality and appropriate colour, with or without hair. However, tissue expansion requires some weeks' delay, and this makes it useless in the early closure of avulsive injury; tissue expansion finds its chief roles in postacute reconstructive surgery. Techniques of tissue expansion, and the occasional complications, are discussed on p. 583.

The 'lateral' forehead flap is based on the anterior branch of the superficial temporal artery; Banks et al (1985) note that this branch alone is inadequate in some 20% of cases, being partially supplanted by the zygomatic branch of the superficial temporal artery (In Fig. 2.16 this vessel is designated as the zygomatico-orbital artery.) They stress the need to assess these vessels before operation by palpation; Doppler ultrasound examination may be more reliable. The value of the lateral flap can be extended by tissue expansion.

The Converse (1942, 1977) scalping flap can be used to provide thin skin for nasal reconstruction. This elegant procedure entails raising the forehead as a full-thickness bicoronal scalp flap; one-half of the forehead is first raised as a thin flap by dissecting it off the frontalis muscle. The thin flap is based superiorly on the main flap, and can be doubled under it to reconstruct the nose. The postauricular flap of Washio (1972) can be used to transfer postauricular skin and some cartilage for reconstruction of the nose. Once again, tissue expansion has enabled small portions of skin to be expanded and transferred on flaps.

Replacement of muscle and skin

There is a wide range of muscle and musculocutaneous flaps; Mathes & Nahai (1979) describe the classical procedures, some of which can be used in avulsive injuries in the CMF region.

Temporalis muscle flaps

The temporalis muscle can be used to cover bone or restore contour to the face; it can be also used to transfer calvarial bone on a vascularized pedicle (Fig. 21.78).

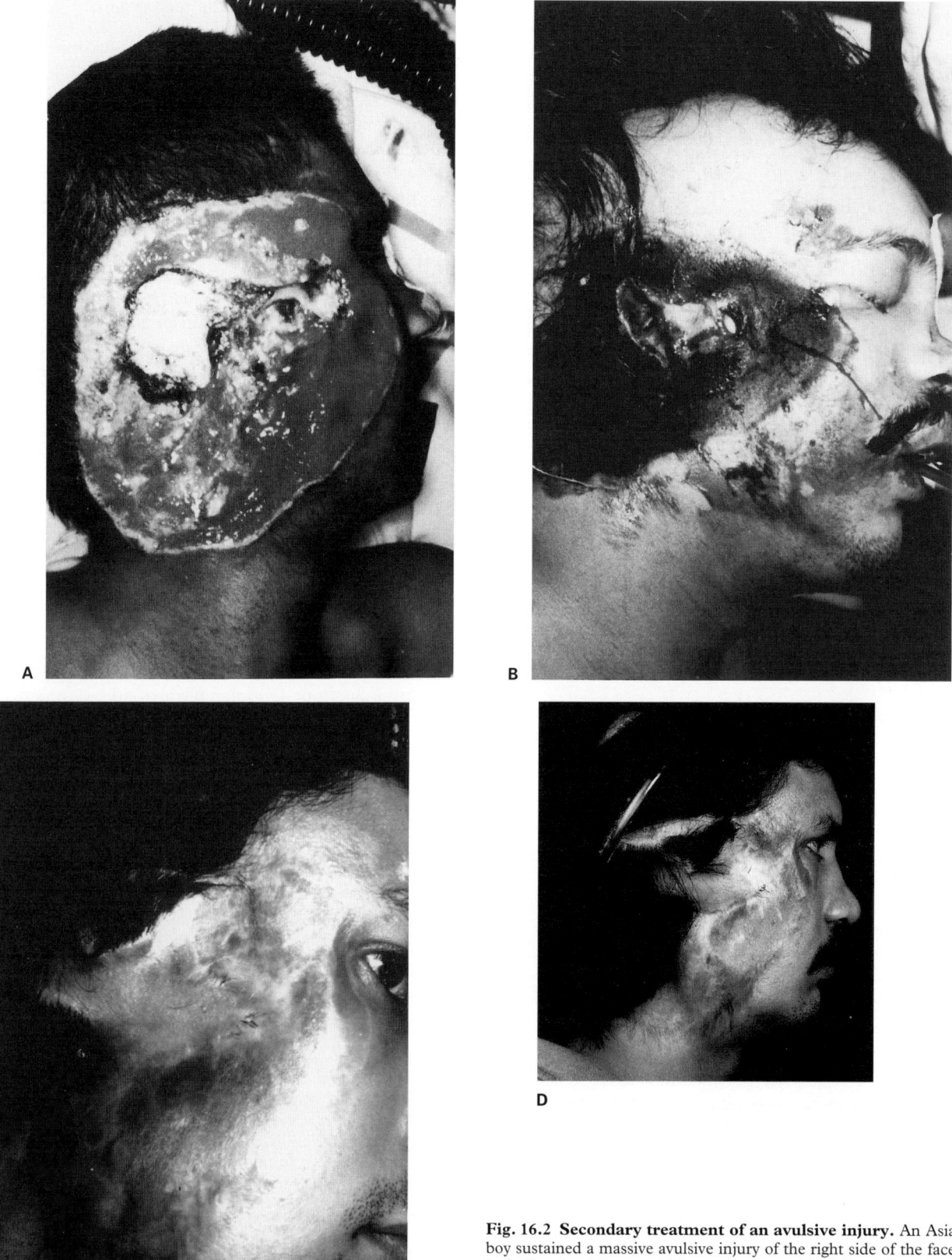

Fig. 16.2 Secondary treatment of an avulsive injury. An Asian boy sustained a massive avulsive injury of the right side of the face including the right ear which was not treated initially. **A** Exposure of the zygoma and temporal bone with extensive soft-tissue loss. **B** An initial attempt was made to cover vital structures with a local flap. **C** The result of inadequate debridement and inadequate soft-tissue cover: multiple sinuses and underlying dead bone. **D** The patient presented for surgery after healing by secondary intention, with some flap cover.

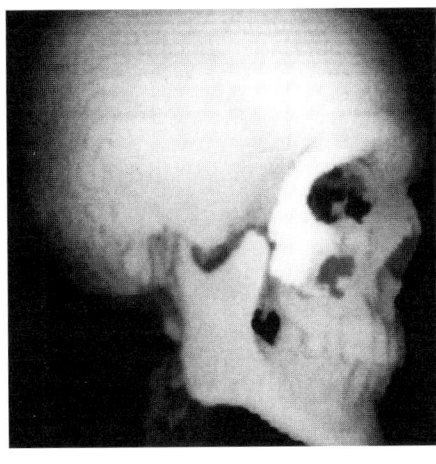

E

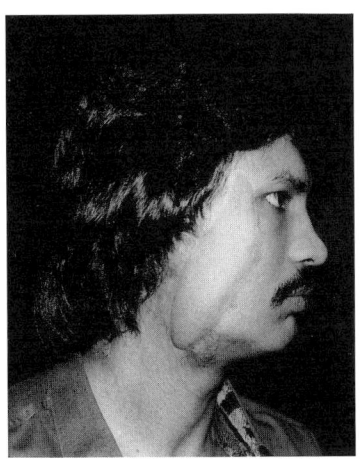

F

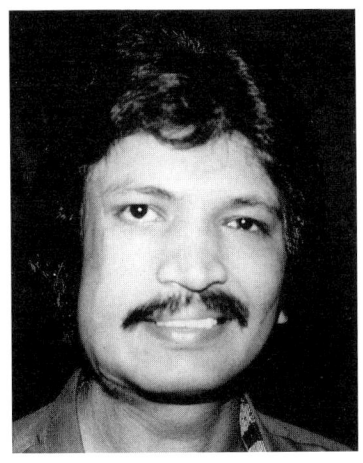

G

Fig. 16.2 Secondary treatment of an avulsive injury. An Asian boy sustained a massive avulsive injury of the right side of the face including the right ear which was not treated initially. **E** Three-dimensional CT showed loss of most of the body of the zygoma and its arch. **F, G** The face in lateral view and anteroposterior views after tissue expansion to advance the scalp hair, free flap (lateral arm) reconstruction of the soft tissues, and underlying bone graft of zygomatic arch.

Galeal flaps

These can be used to cover exposed ear cartilage and to support skin grafts and temporal fascial flaps. The galea must be dissected away from the scalp skin, and its viability depends on the adequacy of supply from the major arteries of the scalp: as they approach the midline, the branches of the superficial temporal artery may fail to meet this need (p. 47).

Deltopectoral flap

First described by Bakamajian (1965) for pharyngo-oesophageal reconstruction, it was for many years the workhorse in the reconstruction of the face and mouth. The flap is transferred on a pedicle raised deep to the deep fascia and supplied by the perforating branch of the internal mammary vessels; it can be moved high enough to replace the cosmetic unit of the cheek. At the height of its usage this flap was manipulated in many ways: it could be tubed, de-epithelialized, turned upon itself and reinnervated by the incorporated supraclavicular nerves.

It is still worthwhile to have this classical flap in the armamentarium although it has been largely replaced by free tissue transfer.

Pectoralis major flap

This is a myocutaneous flap. It is often used in reconstructions after head and neck cancer excision, but not so often for traumatic ablations. The flap is based on the thoraco-acromial branches of the axillary vessels which reach the deep surface of the muscle just below the clavicle and medial to the tendon of the pectoralis minor. The flap may be raised as an island of skin and muscle, with a neurovascular pedicle; the flap may also incorporate bone from the rib or lateral sternal edge (p. 622).

Latissimus dorsi flap

This myocutaneous flap was popularized for breast reconstruction but has versatile applications. The predominant source of supply to the muscle is from the thoracodorsal branch of the subscapular artery; this artery forms a vascular pedicle which is separated from the muscle. The muscle is divided proximal to the insertion of the pedicle, which can support an overlying skin paddle to reach quite high up to the cheek, the pedicle being passed in a tunnel under the skin of the neck.

Trapezius flap

This myocutaneous flap is based on the deep transverse cervical artery and vein; it can be used for defects in the neck and lower part of the face. The lateral third of the clavicle may be incorporated into such a flap as well as the spine of the scapula (p. 622).

Free flaps: replacement of skin, muscle, bone and nerve

A free vascularized flap may be used in postacute reconstruction of an avulsive injury, or may even be performed as an acute procedure; there must of course be a suitable artery and vein in the area to be reconstructed.

Groin flap

This is based on the superficial circumflex iliac artery (SCIA), and is suitable to cover bare bone, dura mater or brain (p. 456). Unless the flap is very large (> 10 cm in diameter), the donor site can be closed directly and a good cosmetic scar can be expected; when this is impossible, a split-skin graft may be necessary. Flaps as large as 20×30 cm have been used, and two flaps will cover the entire calvarial vault. The vascular pedicle has a variable anatomy, which is described by Taylor & Daniel (1981). In 48% of cases, the SCIA rises conjointly with the superficial inferior epigastric artery (SIEA), in 35% the arteries arise separately, and in 17% the SCIA does not arise from the femoral artery. Nevertheless, the SCIA, whatever its origin, is usually 1–1.5 mm in diameter and adequate for an anastomosis. The pedicle tends to be short unless the surgeon puts the skin component of the flap more laterally, when the pedicle can be developed into a longer leash of blood vessels; however, this carries a higher risk of flap morbidity.

An important variant of this groin flap is based on the deep circumflex iliac artery (DCIA). This vessel provides a more dependable blood supply for grafts taken from the ilium; larger bone grafts can be harvested when supplied by the DCIA, and in our practice this free flap is the chief means of reconstruction after massive avulsive injuries of the mandible (David et al 1988). Our operative technique is detailed in Chapter 21 (p. 628).

Latissimus dorsi

This muscle flap, with or without a skin paddle, may be used as an alternative to the groin flap. The transferred muscle must be covered with split skin unless the skin paddle is sufficient to cover the defect. The latissimus dorsi muscle fans out into a wide triangle and may be used to cover a large area of exposed cranium; it is useful in other avulsive CMF injuries when bulk replacement is required.

Omental flap

Gruss et al (1991) have used free vascularized omental grafts to cover bone grafts and to provide bulk in reconstructing gunshot wounds of the lower jaw. We have little experience of the procedure, and have preferred to use the vascularized groin flaps described above.

Intestinal graft

It has been suggested that oral mucosal defects can be replaced with free vascularized intestinal flaps. Again, we have little experience of this technique. One case was treated with a jejunal free flap in this way; the graft survived, but was rugose, friable and productive of excessive mucus, and had to be removed.

The use of free flaps is further described in Chapter 21 and includes many applications of microvascular tissue transfer. The possibility of transfer of muscle, nerve and bone for the reconstruction of all layers and restoration of some function, together with tissue expansion, titanium osseo-integrated implantation and the closely related art and science of computer-aided design/computer-aided manufacture (CAD/CAM) prosthetic reconstruction has advanced reconstruction after ablative craniofacial injury both in quality, result and time saved.

Avulsive injuries of the lower jaw

Avulsive wounds of this region involve bone, teeth and soft tissue. Almost invariably, the bone is extensively comminuted. There is always doubt about the viability of the bone and tooth fragments. Initial debridement involves copious irrigation with normal saline and the meticulous removal of all foreign material; antiseptic solutions may also be used for this essential washing procedure. Loose bone is removed, attached bone is preserved. The dental team decides the fate of involved teeth, the emphasis being on retention, further dissection to remove tooth roots or questionably viable teeth being avoided.

The surgical aim is to prevent or control infection and to produce bone fragment alignment within a sleeve of relatively healthy periosteum. Antibiotics are given as early as possible (p. 236). Where there is extensive comminution, the fragments are united with titanium plates and screws. Where there is loss of bone, particularly in the symphysis, the two sides of the mandible are main-

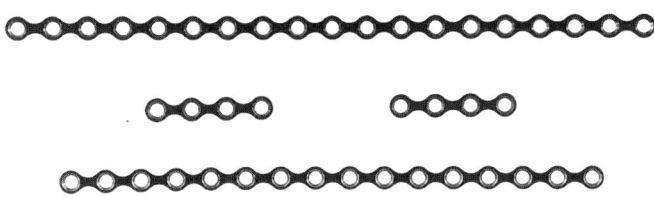

Fig. 16.3 Long titanium plates (AusSystems®). These can be cut into smaller segments when necessary. The full length is useful to bridge gaps in bone for temporary reconstruction.

tained in their normal anatomical relationship using a bridging metal implant. Long titanium plates (Fig. 16.3). are well suited for this purpose; they can be shaped to adapt to the contour of the missing mandible, and fragments of residual bone can be attached to the plate through the screw holes. Alternatively extraoral fixation devices can be used, but in our practice, these have been supplanted by the availability of a wide range of titanium plates. Maximum immobilization is necessary, and where there is an intact maxilla and enough remaining mandibular teeth, intermaxillary fixation can be added to give additional stability.

In ablative injuries of this region, there is often massive skin loss or disruption. Once the bone has been fixed either by reconstituting the mandibular arch or by interposing an appropriate spacer, a water-tight closure of mucosa and a covering of skin is necessary. For this, it may be necessary to undermine the mucosa of the cheek or the structures of the floor of mouth or to mobilize skin from the adjacent cheek and neck. The reconstructed bone must be protected in this way for bone healing to be possible. If skin closure cannot be achieved, then some form of flap repair, whether pedicled or microvascular, must be undertaken. This is probably best done at an intermediate or postacute stage. When hairy skin is needed for the beard or moustache area, tissue expansion (Ohana 1986) may make a scalp flap available.

Avulsive injuries of the midface

When debridement has been completed, the remnants of the maxillary arch should be aligned by manipulation, followed by application of appropriate arch bars and fixation to the mandible by some form of intermaxillary fixation if there is a good mandibular template intact. Titanium miniplates are helpful in stabilizing the zygomas and in attempting to re-establish an attachment of the palatal fragments to the zygomatic buttresses; even at an early stage, the reconstructive principles of Gruss et al (1991) are applicable.

Oro-antral and oronasal fistulae often result from the frequent inability to close the palate. Loss of the specialized nasal tissue — the septum, nasal lining, and nasal cartilages — will necessitate long-term and often difficult

reconstruction in this area. So one should be conservative and should reposition the remnants of these structures with as much care as possible in the primary repair. Where skin cover cannot be completely effected, mucosa to skin suture may be necessary and also grafting with split-thickness skin. The principle that applies in this area is to carry out all the reconstruction that can be done as early as possible, according to the state of the patient and the ability of the treating team; this will facilitate the later reconstructive procedures described on p. 633.

Avulsive frontal and fronto-orbital injuries

In war, many cases of massive injuries in this site survive in good state, and it is often possible to perform much of the definitive treatment as a primary procedure. In a classic review of World War II injuries, Stewart & Botterel (1947) reported on 25 cases of 'cranio-facial-orbital' wounds, and advocated:

1. Radical debridement of the cranial and cerebral wounds
2. Debridement of paranasal sinuses and establishment of drainage through the nose
3. Sealing the subdural and subarachnoid spaces
4. Closure of the scalp without tension and without drainage.

Modern experience has shown that these principles are still valid. However, it is now possible to be less radical in debriding the cerebral wound (p. 373), and to preserve even detached fragments of bone, especially in the fronto-orbital region; these can be replaced and fixed with miniplates, unless there is gross contamination or delay in operation.

If the frontal scalp defect cannot be closed by direct suture, a large frontolateral flap, based on the superficial temporal artery, is rotated forward to cover the sutured dural wound (Fig. 21.1). There must be no tension in the final skin suture line; if there is risk of tension, the posterior margin of the wound is not sutured and the exposed pericranium is covered with a split-skin graft. We have done this even for relatively small (2 × 4 cm) residual skin defects (Fig. 13.1); more experienced war surgeons are sometimes able to cover fronto-orbital defects without flaps, by mobilizing the scalp, but the novice is advised to use flap closure if there is any risk of tension. Emergency skin closure is disfiguring when hairy scalp is advanced onto the forehead or to cover an eye socket; however, the hairy scalp can be later returned using the crane principle described by Millard (1969). This uses the scalp to carry the galea forward. Scalp superficial to the galea can then be returned and split-skin grafts placed over the galeal layer. In some cases adjacent tissue can be expanded using tissue expanders to advance forehead tissue after the hairy flap has been returned.

Scalp avulsion

When a large piece of scalp has been avulsed and that tissue is available then it may be replaced by microvascular techniques (p. 437). Where this is impossible but the pericranium is preserved, split-skin grafts may be applied to the pericranium; care must be taken to ensure that the pericranium does not dry out — this can happen very quickly. When the pericranium is lost but the skull intact, the outer calvarial table can be removed and split-skin grafts placed on the diplöe after granulations have appeared; this temporizing procedure is discussed on p. 437. It is, however, better to cover the exposed bone with a scalp transposition or rotation flap, and this is essential when dura or brain are exposed. On the rare occasions when there is no local tissue with which to cover exposed dura and brain in an emergency, a pedicled flap or microvascular free tissue transfer may be indicated (Fig. 15.2).

Avulsive injuries of the frontal sinus and orbital rim

The general management of fracture of the frontal sinus has been discussed on p. 372. If there is loss of the anterior wall of the sinus or of the orbital rim the defect may sometimes be repaired by a calvarial bone graft at the time of the initial wound closure. However, it is our preference to replace any remaining segments by miniplate or microplate fixation, using bone grafting for an elective repair (Fig. 21.3).

Frontal bone defects

Cranioplasty is a standard neurosurgical procedure and the techniques and problems are well known (p. 548). But in the frontal region cranioplasty presents some special difficulties. The area is not covered by hair and unless contouring is perfect there will be a visible deformity of the forehead. The proximity of the air sinuses makes delayed infection a real threat, especially when a foreign implant is used. In our view, there is no place for cranioplasty in the early management of ablative injuries of the fronto-orbital region. The indications and techniques of frontal cranioplasty are considered in Chapter 21.

Injury to the eye and eye socket

Ablative injury in this site demands consultation with an ophthalmologist; management of the injured eye is considered in Chapter 14. The principles of reconstruction of the eye socket are that the rim should be reconstructed from what fragments are present and that the walls should be primarily bone-grafted, providing there is reasonable soft-tissue cover (Fig. 16.4). The use of foreign material such as Silastic® under these circumstances is not encouraged. When there is insufficient local soft tissue to cover a shattered orbit, it is sometimes necessary to employ a forehead flap or rotation scalp flap.

Ablative injury of the ear

Lacerations, avulsion and destruction of the external ear should be repaired after careful debridement; exposed cartilage should be covered by excising its margins and suturing skin to skin. When an avulsed ear is brought with the patient, it may be possible to suture the ear in place using microsurgical techniques; our colleagues Katsaros et al (1988) reported success in two of three cases of avulsion sustained in road accidents. An artery must first be found in the avulsed ear; when this is perfused from a suitable artery (usually the posterior auricular artery), it is easier to find a bleeding vein. Intraoperative heparin and also haemodilution are advised (Fig. 16.5).

Follow-up care after avulsive injury

The next phase of treatment involves all those measures which are expected to promote mobility and rapid healing: these include wound care, both superficial and intraoral, nutrition, and control of infection. Management aims to prevent or to treat all the systemic problems that may complicate severe trauma and its surgical treatment, notably septicaemia, pneumonia, peripheral vein thrombosis and pulmonary embolism. Also to be treated are the local problems that may complicate these injuries — especially secondary haemorrhage, infection and meningitis

Fig. 16.4 (*Opposite*) **Avulsive facial injury in a car crash.** A 39-year-old man was involved in a freak car accident: a tree fell upon his car and a branch penetrated the front windscreen, piercing the patient's face like a spear, avulsing the right zygoma and leaving it pedicled on soft tissue laterally. Although he was pinned to the vehicle, he was promptly rescued thanks to his mobile telephone. Examination showed that the branch had encountered the anterior border of the mandible, dislocating it laterally. The branch was split by the mandible, with shafts of wood passing medially and laterally into the neck. The medial fragment lay on the carotid vessels. The right orbital floor was destroyed, the right eye was lost, and the anterior wall of the right maxillary antrum was destroyed. There was an extensive soft-tissue deficit of the right cheek. The emergency management involved freeing the patient from the tree and transporting him to a central unit. MRI scan showed the exact relationship of the penetrating shafts of wood to vital structures, and angiographic enhancement indicated the relationships with the vessels. The patient was anaesthetized with care to avoid further damage. The cavities were cleaned and debrided, the zygoma was temporarily fixed and the skin was sutured in place. At a second operation the zygoma was further secured, and at the same time the remnants of the globe were removed and a conformer placed into the eye socket. **A** Manipulation of the foreign body. **B** The zygoma was turned back on a lateral myocutaneous flap, exposing massive destruction of the orbital floor and anterior maxilla. **C** Three-dimensional CT showing the bony deformity. **D** CT scan showing relationship of the shafts of wood to the mandibular ramus. **E** MRI scan showing the relationship of the wood to the mandible and soft tissues (white arrows indicate the wood). **F** The patient demonstrates the residual deformity. **G** Appearance prior to secondary reconstruction of the zygoma, orbit and maxilla.

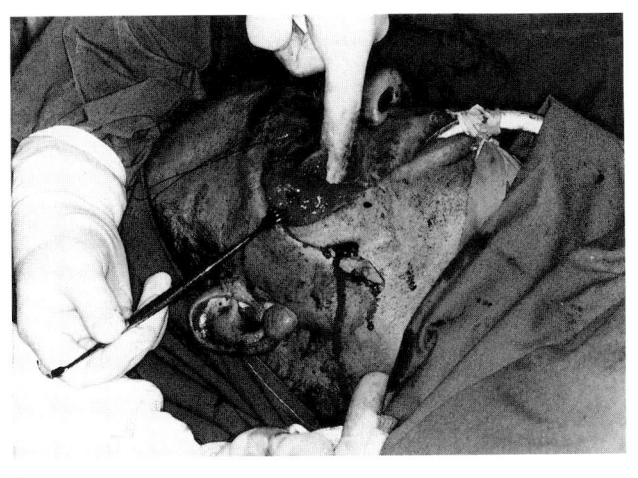

A

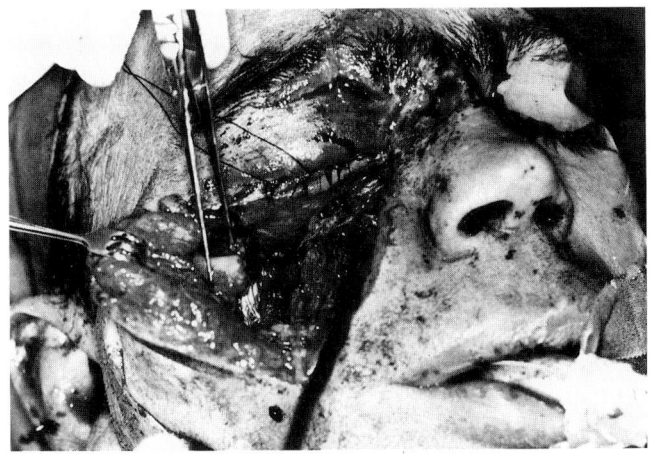

B

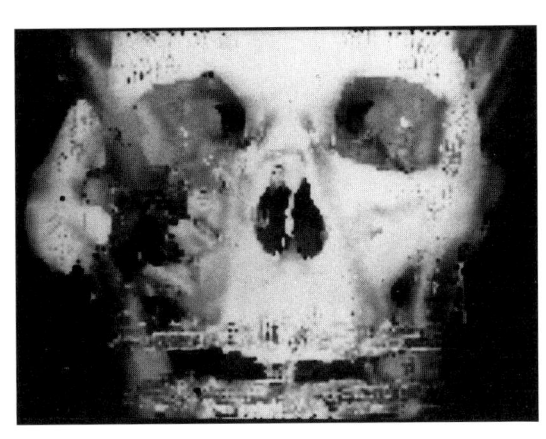

C

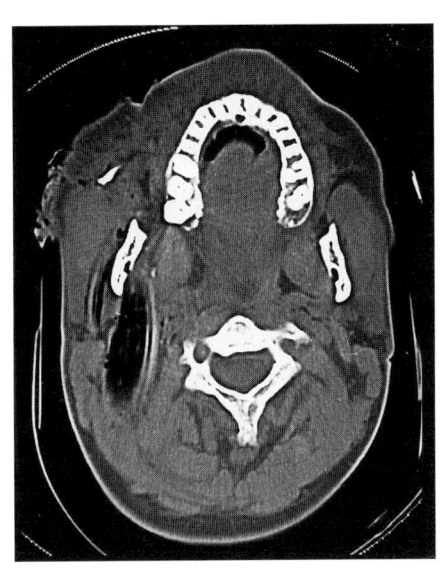

D

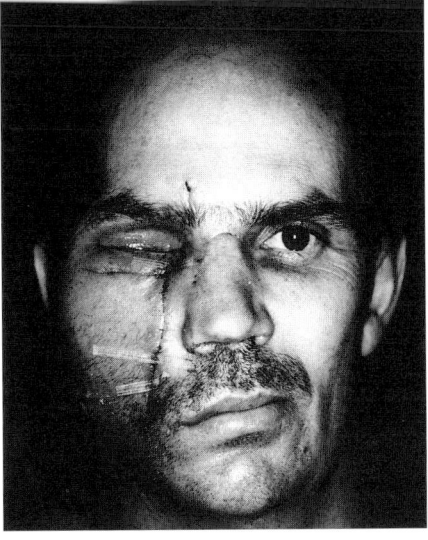

E

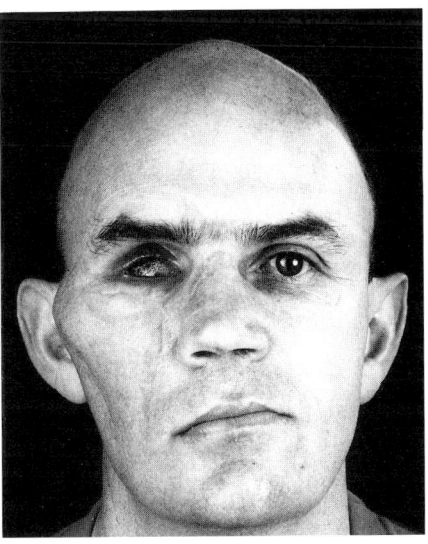

F

G

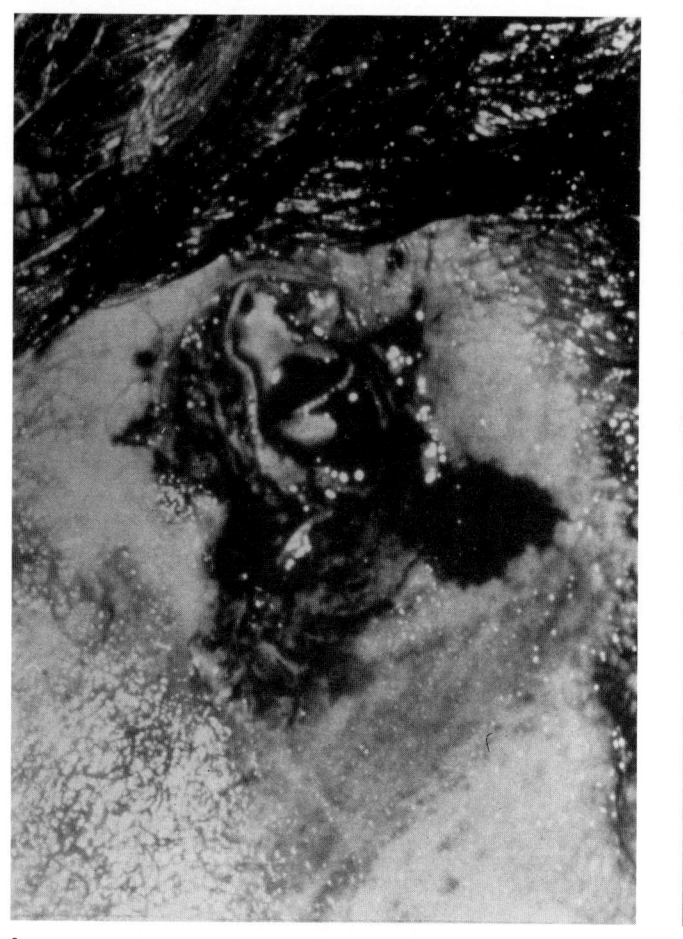
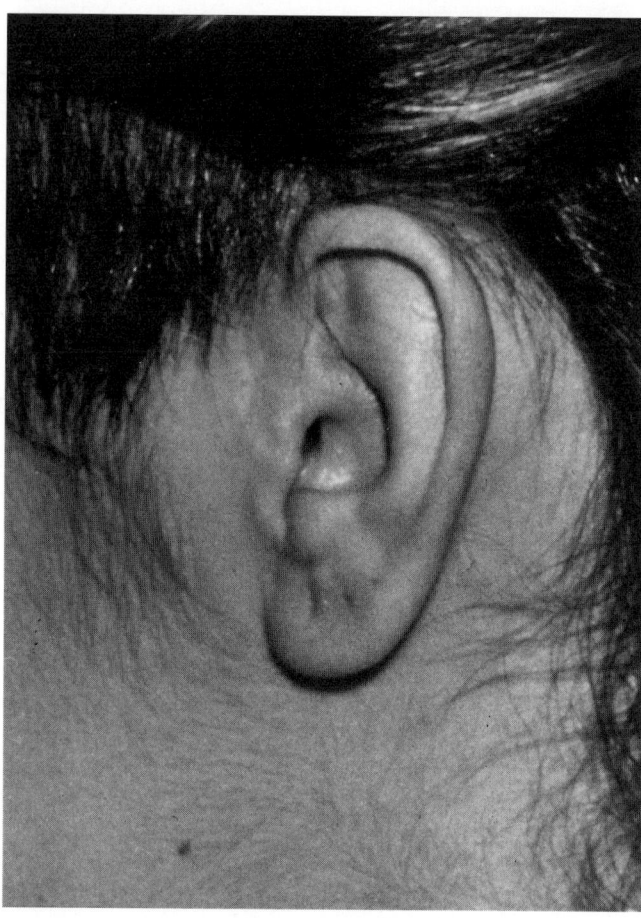

A   B

Fig. 16.5 Traumatic loss of an ear and microvascular replacement. A Initial appearance of the wound with road abrasion and avulsion of the ear. **B** Appearance following reimplantation and successful revascularization.

where there has been a cranionasal fistula in the anterior fossa (p. 387).

When these dangers have been circumvented, and the wounds are well healed, the stage is set for correction of residual deformities. This stage is discussed in Chapter 21.

Complications and results

Wartime experience has shown that if the victim of a massive gunshot wound in the CMF area does not die on the battlefield, the prospects of survival are surprisingly good. Banks (1985) reviewed mortality rates from series of military maxillofacial injuries, and these varied from about 1% in World War II to 26.3% in cases admitted to an intensive care unit in Northern Ireland. These statistics clearly express different chances of early survival and different criteria in selection.

The complications of massive avulsive injury are numerous and diverse. Many are beyond surgical control, but some relate to the quality of management. In the early management of injuries entailing massive tissue loss, it is necessary to use strategies to save life, conserve tissue and commence reconstruction, with a full awareness of what future treatment may be available to complete the job. In a fully equipped craniofacial unit, the processes of management move smoothly from early management to definitive repair, and depending on the nature of the injury it may be possible to carry out the definitive reconstruction at an early date, as urged by Gruss et al (1991). Under other circumstances, the victim of an avulsive injury may have early treatment in a less specialized centre and be transferred elsewhere for the completion of the reconstruction. In this case, a great service is done for the patient if the team giving initial care can adhere to the principles of treatment which will enhance the future reconstruction.

The procedures described in Chapter 21 are aimed to restore function and to correct deformity with as little delay as possible. But with severe avulsive injuries, the phase of reconstruction may be prolonged for months or years, and be subject to the changes of growth, age, degeneration and the emergence of new techniques of treatment.

REFERENCES

Australian Army Manual of Land Warfare 1985 Part II, Medical and dental training, Vol III, Pamphlet No. 2, Field Surgery Handbook

Bakamajian V Y 1965 A two-staged method for pharyngo-esophageal reconstruction with a primary pectoral skin flap. Plast Reconstr Surg 36: 173–184

Banks P 1985 The mortality of maxillofacial missile injuries. In: Rowe N L, Williams J L (eds) Maxillofacial injuries. Churchill Livingstone, Edinburgh, Ch 14, p 690

Banks P, Whitlock R I H, Terry B C et al 1985 Gunshot wounds. In: Rowe N L, Williams J L (eds) Maxillofacial injuries. Churchill Livingstone, Edinburgh, Ch 14, pp 560–694

Chapman C W 1985 Treatment of maxillofacial injuries in various theatres of war. South Atlantic. In: Rowe N L, Williams J L (eds) Maxillofacial injuries. Churchill Livingstone, Edinburgh, Ch 14, pp 683–690

Clarkson P W, Walker F A 1955 Gun-shot wounds of the face and jaws. In: Rowe N L, Killey H C (eds) Fractures of the facial skeleton. Livingstone, Edinburgh, Ch 25

Converse J M 1942 New forehead flap for nasal reconstruction. Proc R Soc Med 35: 811–812

Converse J M 1977 Full-thickness loss of nasal tissue. In: Converse J M (ed) Reconstructive plastic surgery, 2nd edn. Saunders, Philadelphia, Ch 29

David D J, Tan E, Katsaros J, Sheen R 1988 Mandibular reconstruction with vascularised iliac crest: a ten year experience. Plast Reconstr Surg 82: 792–803

Gruss J S, Antonyshyn O, Phillips J H 1991 Early definitive bone and soft-tissue reconstruction of major gunshot wounds of the face. Plast Reconstr Surg 87: 436–450

Katsaros J, Tan E, Sheen R 1988 Microvascular ear replantation. Br J Plast Surg 41: 496–799

Mathes S J, Nahai F 1979 Clinical atlas of muscle and musculocutaneous flaps. Mosby, St Louis

Marx R E, Stevens M R 1991 Reconstruction of avulsive maxillofacial injuries. In: Fonseca R J, Walker R V (eds) Oral and maxillofacial trauma. Saunders, Philadelphia, Vol 2, Ch 30

Millard D R 1969 The crane principle for transport of subcutaneous tissue. Plast Reconstr Surg 43: 451–462

Ohana J 1986 Utilisation du dispositif d'expansion tissulaire de Radovan en chirurgie reconstructive. Ann Chir Plast Esthét 31: 86–93

Pichler H, Trauner R 1948 Mund- und Kieferchirurgie. Urban & Schwarzeburg, Vienna, Vol 2

Stewart O W, Botterell E H 1947 Cranio-facial-orbital wounds involving paranasal sinuses: primary definitive treatment. Br J Surg. War Surgery Suppl 1: 112–118

Taylor G I, Daniel R K 1975 The anatomy of several free flap donor sites. Plast Reconstr Surg 56: 243–253

Washio H 1972 Further experiences with the retroauricular temporal flap. Plast Reconstr Surg 50: 160–162

Whitlock R 1985 Treatment of maxillofacial injuries in various theatres of war. Urban guerilla warfare. In: Rowe N L, Williams J L (eds) Maxillofacial injuries. Churchill Livingstone, Edinburgh, Ch 14, pp 652–682

CHAPTER 17 | Burns

I. O. W. Leitch
Contributing author: E. Tan

INTRODUCTION

Burns of the face occupy a unique place in the field of burn management. Most facial burns heal more quickly than similar burns elsewhere, because of the rich facial blood supply, and because in most areas there are abundant adnexal structures–hair follicles and skin glands– available to provide epithelial cells to regenerate the epidermis (p. 126). But there are parts of the face that do not have these advantages. In the nose and external ears, there is only a thin areolar subdermal layer and the perichondrial blood supply of the underlying cartilage is intimately related to the subcutaneous blood supply.

Burning in these sites can result in necrosis not only of the skin but also of the auricular or nasal cartilages.

Burns of the eyes may also present difficult problems (Fig. 17.1). Destruction of the eyelid may expose the globe; the cornea may then be damaged by desiccation or exposure. The eye may be damaged more directly; this is likely in chemical burns, especially those due to caustic substances.

Healing may be delayed in severe burns of the scalp, especially in the elderly patient, when the scalp is thin and atrophic, and there is a paucity of hair follicles and other adnexal structures to provide a reservoir of epidermal cells for epithelialization. In severe scalp burns,

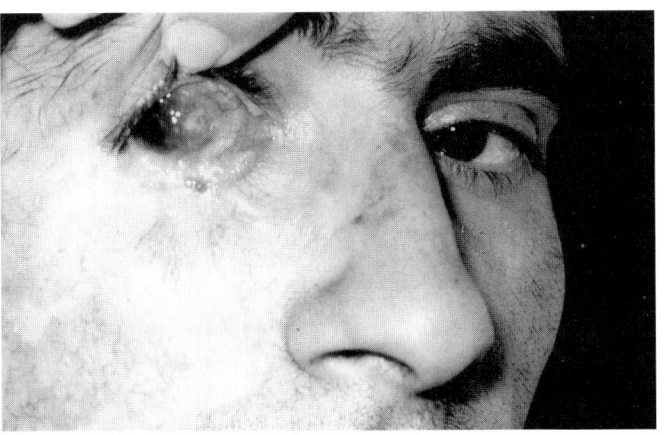

A

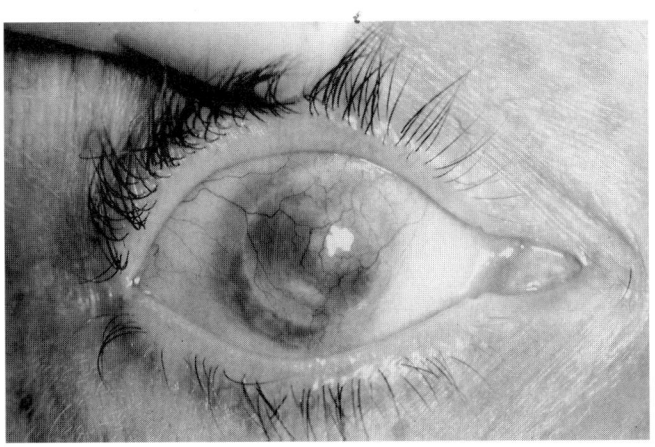

B

Fig. 17.1 Chemical burns. A A 23-year-old man from the Middle East used crushed green walnuts to get rid of an abscess in the cheek. This traditional remedy caused a full-thickness burn of the cheek, destroyed the lower eyelid and damaged the cornea. **B** A 23-year-old man suffered caustic soda burns of both eyes. After 13 operations, including four corneal grafts, there was terrible scarring of both corneas and vision was reduced to hand movements on the right and light perception on the left.

the underlying skull may be exposed, and may even be necrotized. The underlying brain may be damaged. Definitive reconstruction may be difficult because no normally vascularized scalp remains available to cover the injured brain and meninges.

Hypertrophic post-burn scarring is likely to occur in facial burns that do not heal within a 3 week period after burning; this provides the rationale for early excision and grafting in selected cases.

Deep burns of the head and neck may heal with horrific cosmetic deformity, especially when healing is delayed, and hypertrophic, contracting scars are produced. Gross distortion of soft tissue may result, with loss of normal anatomical boundaries. The victim's appearance is often appalling, and the secondary psychological damage may be very great. In addition to the deformities due to con-traction of scars and skin grafts, significant deformity may result from loss of growth potential in children and from loss of function in facial musculature. Pressure from elastic and static face masks can also promote deformity. Secondary growth deformities due to untreated deep burns of the face and neck may cause long-term skeletal deformities in the whole craniofacial region; we have seen young adults who were burned in childhood and have suffered gross cosmetic and functional impairments, requiring complex soft-tissue and skeletal reconstructions.

EPIDEMIOLOGY

Facial burns can result from a wide variety of causes. These include scalding from hot liquids, especially in chil-dren, explosions, and flame burns; particularly common are fires occurring in closed spaces, such as house fires, and motor vehicle accidents.

Facial burns occurred in association with generalized burning in 43.5% of our cases of thermal and chemical burns (p. 96). However, burns to the head and face occurred as isolated injuries in only 2% of our cases. Examples of this included the effects of contact with a hot exhaust muffler box (Fig. 17.2A,B), assault from a domestic iron (Fig. 17.2C), molten metal splash (Fig. 17.2D), a localized explosion, and high tension electrical injury where contact between a metal object, the face and over-head high tension power lines may produce localized deep facial and scalp burns. Causes of electrical burns included contact with power lines by electricity service workers, live power lines draped over road traffic accident victims, and agricultural workers fouling overhead power lines with irrigation pipes or cranes. In some of these injuries, deep burning to the scalp, skull and brain has occurred, requiring elaborate secondary reconstruction. We have seen a frequent pattern of injury resulting from the high voltage ionization of the atmosphere in association with

leakage from high tension cables and installations, causing flash burns involving an electricity worker's exposed face, neck and hands. These burns are often initially diagnosed as superficial but in fact some are deep dermal burns which require surgery to produce healing.

ASSOCIATED INJURIES AND COMPLICATIONS

In the 1940s, it was first realized that burn shock could be treated by intravenous fluid resuscitation. At that time burn shock accounted for up to 20% of burn deaths (Cope & Rhinelander 1943); subsequent development of appropriate aggressive fluid replacement has greatly reduced shock as a cause of death. Burn wound sepsis later received improved treatment with the use of topical antimicrobials, such as Sulfamylon and silver sulphadi-azine (Heggers 1991), and this has led to lower mortality and earlier wound healing, in association with the now widely practised regime of early wound debridement and skin grafting (Heimbach & Engrav 1984).

Moritz et al (1945) studied the experimental pathology of respiratory thermal injury, and this and other work showed clearly the injurious pulmonary effects of inhaled products of incomplete combustion. Phillips & Cope (1962) and Silverstein & Dressler (1970) reported changes in mortality from severe burns from hypovolaemic shock, burn wound sepsis and pulmonary complications: their figures showed a trend of increase in the percentages of death occurring as a result of pulmonary complications. It is now accepted that inhalation injury and subsequent secondary pulmonary pathology account for 20–84% of burn mortality (Sochor & Mallory 1963, Foley et al 1968, Shook et al 1968, Silverstein & Dressler 1970, DiVincenti et al 1971, Davies et al 1983).

Various authors (Phillips & Cope 1962, Stone et al 1967, Trunkey 1978) have shown a significant increase in the likelihood of death in the presence of third degree burns of the face, and an increased morbidity which may be due to the coexistence of inhalation injury. Recent advances in diagnostic techniques have increased aware-ness of inhalation injury and the incidence may be as high as 33% of all major burns (Moylan & Alexander 1978).

It has therefore become increasingly important to diagnose the presence of an inhalation injury during the examination of the patient with facial burns (Fig. 17.3). The history of injury may be significant. Burning in a closed space, or burns from an explosion, should arouse suspicion of inhalation injury. A history of depressed consciousness at the scene of the fire, or subsequently, points to circumstances of burning which may produce an inhalation injury (Wroblewski & Bower 1979). Physical findings of burns to the face, singed nasal vibrissae, soot

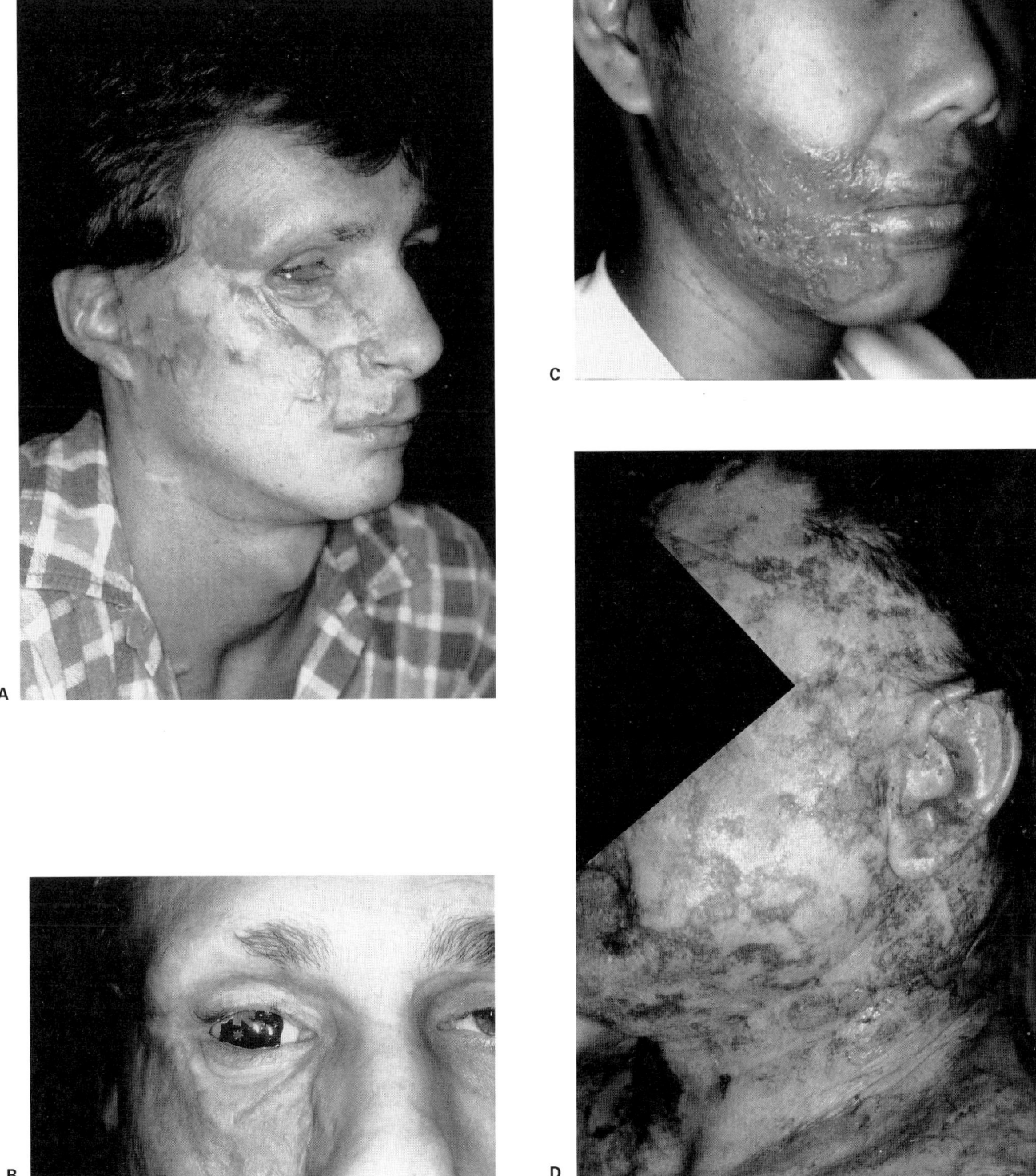

Fig. 17.2 Localized facial burns. These characteristic examples of severe facial contact burns presented difficult problems in reconstruction. **A** A young motor cyclist: a severe localized burn resulted from contact with a hot engine muffler. The burn crossed the boundaries of cosmetic areas, and caused loss of the eye and ectropion of the lower lid. To release the ectropion, extra skin was inset in the upper lip area, but this gave insufficient correction. **B** A full-thickness postauricular skin graft was inserted. An artificial eye was requested; it displays the patient's national flag. **C** A house worker: a contact burn was inflicted with a hot iron in a dispute. The burn was grafted with split skin, and developed the hypertrophic burns scar often seen in Asian patients. The use of both rigid and elastic face masks made little difference in this case. **D** A foundry worker: molten metal was splashed in a foundry accident causing a patchy dermal burn of the face. Many areas had no sensation or evidence of capillary refill; however, with high quality wound care they had largely healed by 14 days, a few punctate residual areas remaining unhealed until 21 days.

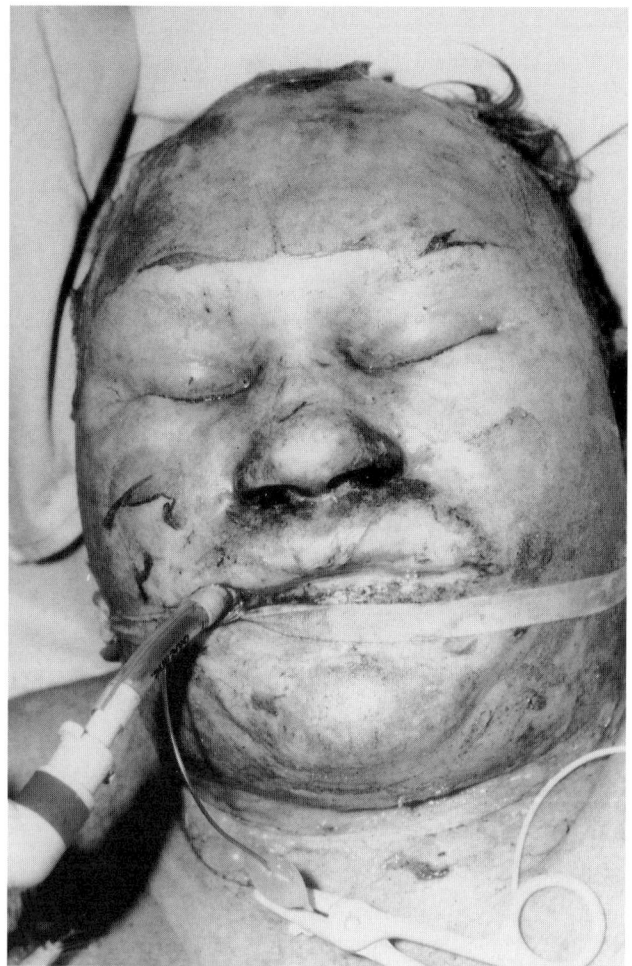

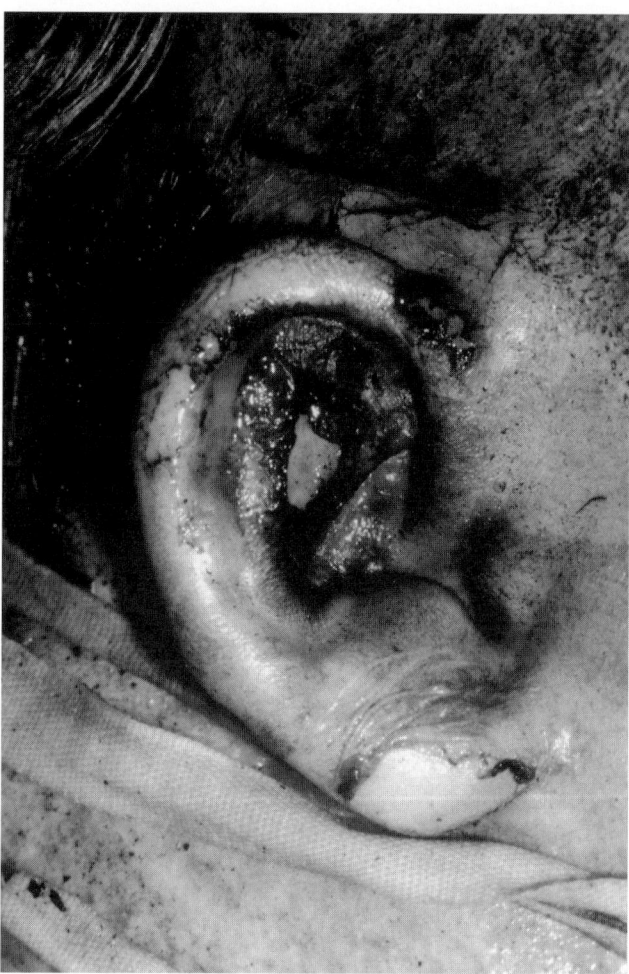

Fig. 17.3 Inhalation burn from petroleum fire. A 54-year-old man sustained deep flame burns of the face. He sustained a severe inhalation burn, and on bronchoscopy there was soot in the air passages to the limits of the bronchoscope. **A** He developed adult respiratory distress syndrome and pneumonia and required mechanical ventilation for 3 weeks. **B** His ear was severely burned; despite dressing with silver sulphadiazine, he developed suppurative chondritis and this required drainage and excision of necrotic cartilage.

particles in the sputum, carbon staining of the tongue and pharynx, and signs of burning (erythema, oedema and blistering) of the pharynx or larynx should suggest sufficient airway exposure to produce an inhalation injury. Inhalation injury from heat alone may cause thermal burns to the pharynx, larynx and trachea resulting in oedema and the onset of supraglottic airway obstruction within 24 h of burning. Parenchymal lung damage on the other hand is produced by the inhalation of irritant chemical by-products of combustion, particularly from burning plastic compounds, and inhaled particulate matter producing infraglottic injury. The onset of symptoms is typically from 72 h onwards. Lung injury may cause pulmonary oedema clinically evident as decreasing gaseous exchange, and may predispose to bronchopneumonia.

In addition to airway and lung damage, there may be a cerebral insult, with symptoms of loss of consciousness due either to hypoxia at the scene of the fire or more likely to carbon monoxide and/or cyanide intoxication

following inhalation (Fig. 17.4). Hypoxia on presentation is rare, as are clinical signs of pulmonary damage, except in patients with severe injury who have a grave prognosis (Stone et al 1967). The presence of pre-existing cardio-pulmonary disease (p. 540) with decreased pulmonary function makes the potential for injury to the respiratory tract much greater (Phillips & Cope 1962, Alpert & Levinson 1970, Carruthers 1978).

A change in the voice, hoarseness, stridor and the coughing up of carbonaceous sputum make the diagnosis of inhalation injury much more likely. The upper pharynx, trachea and main bronchi should be inspected with a fibroptic bronchoscope, which is the investigation of choice to diagnose the severity of injuries to the upper airway, and gives warning of the likely requirement of endotracheal intubation (Wanner & Cutchavaree 1973). Chest radiographs may not show parenchymal damage for 72 h after inhalation injury (Zawacki et al 1977) and the early evaluation of parenchymal injury has been in the

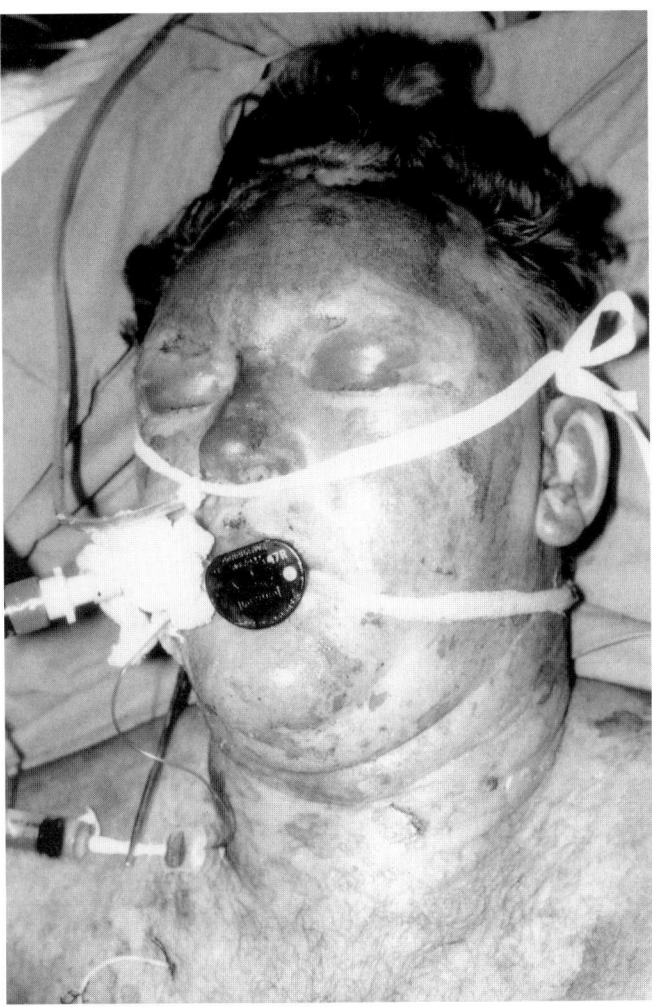

Fig. 17.4 Carbon monoxide poisoning as a complication of severe burns. A 45-year-old man was trapped in a burning house, and suffered 35% TBSA burns. He was dragged unconscious from the fire. He had been overcome by carbon monoxide, and on admission to our unit 2 h later, his carboxyhaemoglobin level was 35%. He required mechanical ventilation for 72 h. He underwent tangential excision of forehead burns and replacement with split skin. The burns of the upper eyelids were treated by early release and split-thickness skin grafting. He made a good recovery.

Table 17.1 Carbon monoxide intoxication

Carboxyhaemoglobin level (%)	Symptoms
0–10	None
15–20	Headache, confusion
20–40	Nausea, fatigue, disorientation, irritability
40–60	Hallucination, ataxia, syncope, convulsions, coma
> 60	Death

past more reliably undertaken by the ^{133}Xe wash-out scan (Moylan et al 1972). We have been unable to undertake this investigation, due to a lack of ready availability of the isotope in Australia, and we have relied instead on repeated clinical assessment of the patient's pulmonary function and arterial blood oxygen concentration. A gradual deterioration in gas exchange capability indicates more intensive respiratory management, including endotracheal intubation and intermittent positive pressure ventilation.

The most likely sign of carbon monoxide intoxication is depressed consciousness or frank coma, but headache and nausea may also be reported (Table 17.1). According to our burn unit protocol, any burned patient with symptoms resembling alcohol or drug intoxication is deemed to be suffering from carbon monoxide intoxication until proven otherwise. Carboxyhaemoglobin levels should be estimated as soon as possible after removal from the fire, as the natural wash-out of carbon monoxide by breathing air halves carboxyhaemoglobin levels after 4 h and breathing 100% oxygen halves carboxyhaemoglobin levels in 1 h. Early emergency treatment may therefore produce blood carboxyhaemoglobin levels on hospital admission that bear no relation to the peak level of carboxyhaemoglobin and the exposure to carbon monoxide at the time of injury. We have developed a series of regression curves to enable more accurate estimation of the carboxyhaemogobin level at the time of injury to assist in the selection of the appropriate treatment regime (R. Webb 1993, personal communication). We consider carboxyhaemoglobin levels up to 10% as acceptable; those above that level require treatment with 100% oxygen by mask or endotracheal ventilation until hyperbaric oxygen therapy (HBO) can be instituted. We have reported on the use of HBO therapy in burns (Gorman & Leitch 1991) and have recently begun a double-blind trial of HBO in burns with particular attention to the role of carbon monoxide intoxication. A trial of normobaric and hyperbaric oxygen in acute carbon monoxide intoxication by Raphael et al (1989) purported to show that HBO was not useful in their group of patients who did not lose consciousness; however, a longitudinal study of 100 consecutive admissions for carbon monoxide intoxication at our institution showed that the long-term sequelae following carbon monoxide intoxication could be significantly reduced by two or more treatments, and the frequency of sequelae was significantly greater if the first HBO treatment was delayed (Gorman et al 1992). For this reason we now treat our patients with suspected carbon monoxide intoxication in association with burns by HBO treatment (Runciman & Gorman 1993) within the first 24 h after burning. Those patients in whom the linear regression tables show carboxyhaemoglobin levels > 10–15% at the time of burning are now routinely treated with HBO therapy at 2 atmospheres for 90 min.

EMERGENCY MANAGEMENT OF FACIAL BURNS

As with all cases of severe trauma, a rapid initial assessment (the *primary survey*) of the injured burned patient is undertaken on admission to ensure that the airway, breathing and circulation are satisfactory. Emergency life-saving attention should be directed to these vital functions; in the patient with burns of the head and neck it is particularly important to assess the adequacy of the airway, as early endotracheal intubation may be required to save life. If endotracheal intubation is needed, or likely to be needed, then the procedure should be done early, before the onset of swelling of the laryngeal and orofacial tissues.

Burn injuries may occur in unusual circumstances, and in association with other trauma which may be difficult to diagnose in the presence of severe cutaneous burns, shock, and absent cutaneous sensation. The examination of the cervical spine should be undertaken at this stage to exclude cervical spine injury; a stiff cervical collar is applied until cervical spine radiographs have been obtained. If it is possible, cervical spine injury should be excluded before endotracheal intubation is undertaken, to avoid the rare tragedy of iatrogenic quadriplegia (p. 225).

Following the completion of the primary survey and appropriate emergency treatment, attention is then directed to a more thorough *secondary survey* in which the patient is examined in the standard head-to-toe manner to determine the extent of injuries. This examination should estimate the percentage surface area of burns, both full and partial thickness, using the 'Rule of Nines'. The Rule of Nines was devised by E. J. Pulaski and C. W. Tennison, and divides the body surface into areas of 9% or multiples of 9% (Moylan 1979); it is a very convenient method of rapid assessment of the burn area (Fig. 17.5).

Lund & Browder (1944) described a more accurate method of assessment of burn area, and we use their tables to reassess the burn area following the initiation of emergency therapy, to make sure that fluid replacement therapy is calculated correctly (Fig. 17.6). The standard vital parameters of height, weight, temperature, blood pressure, pulse and respiratory rate are measured and recorded.

It is important to exclude other non-burn injuries at this stage. In addition, a general medical examination is undertaken to assess the patient's general state of health. An accurate account of any pre-existing medical conditions and medications is obtained, as these may have an important influence on the outcome of the injury.

Following the secondary survey management priorities are established. In patients with burns > 10% total body surface area (TBSA: a total burn of head and neck circumferentially equals 9% TBSA), intravenous resuscitation is started after insertion of a large-bore intravenous needle into a peripheral vein, if possible in an arm. The fluid replacement regime is calculated using the Parkland formula developed by C. R. Baxter of Dallas, Texas (Baxter & Shires 1968); the fluid volume for the first 24 h is estimated at 4 ml per kg body weight per %

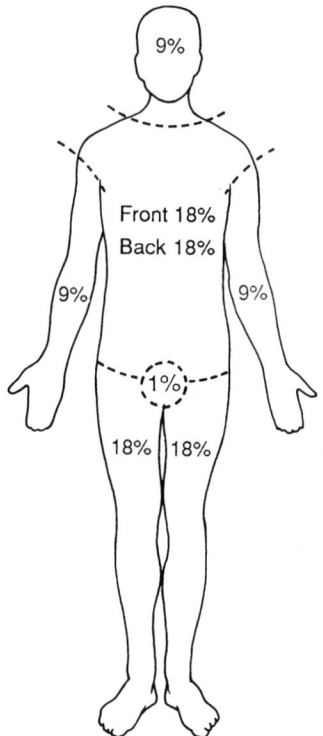

Fig. 17.5 The Rule of Nines. By dividing the surface area of the body into areas of 9% or multiples of 9%, it is possible to rapidly estimate the surface area of the body that has been burnt.

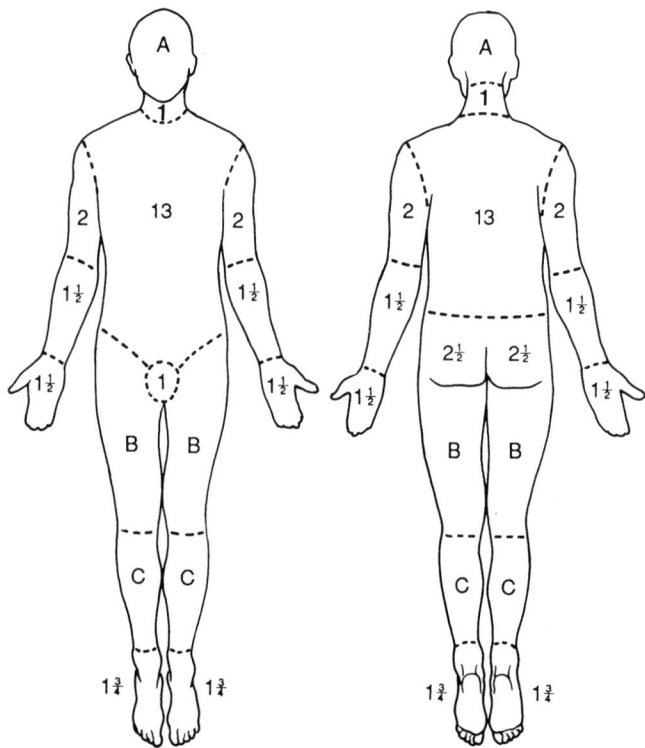

Fig. 17.6 Lund & Browder Chart. This allows a more accurate estimation of surface area burned than the Rule of Nines. The figures indicate percentages of body area. In adults, A (= half head) is 3½; B (= half one thigh) is 4¾; C (= half one leg) is 3½. Correction charts are available for infants and children. After Lund & Browder (1944).

burn of TBSA. The fluid used is Hartmann's solution (compound lactated Ringer's solution); one-half of the calculated volume is infused in the first 8 h, and the other half of the fluid calculated is given in the second 16 h after the burn. This regimen of fluid replacement closely keeps pace with the egress of plasma due to increasing vascular permeability, and cardiac output usually returns to normal by 36–48 h. We previously used the colloid-based fluid replacement formula known as the Odstock formula (Griffiths & Laing 1981) and described more recently by Muir et al (1987) but, as Goodwin et al (1983) showed that colloid conferred no added benefit during the initial stages of resuscitation, and because there has been a need to standardize intravenous resuscitation throughout Australia, we have now adopted the Parkland formula. Its ease of administration and clinical effectiveness have made this formula ideal for our needs. The use of Hartmann's solution has logistic advantages, from the considerations of cost, availability, and portability of plastic 1 litre packs; it is an ideal resuscitation fluid for use in both urban and rural areas, military operations, and road and aeromedical evacuation.

After insertion of the intravenous cannula, blood is drawn for routine laboratory studies. Haematological examinations include haemoglobin, packed cell volume (haematocrit), baseline haematological indices, white cell count, including differential count, platelet count and carboxyhaemoglobin level. Serum, sodium, potassium, bicarbonate, chloride, creatinine, blood urea nitrogen, and osmolarity are also estimated.

Following the start of intravenous resuscitation, an indwelling urethral catheter is inserted to allow accurate hourly estimation of the urine output. The fluid resuscitation rate should be adjusted to produce between 0.5 and 1.0 ml of urine per kg body weight per hour in adults and in children > 20 kg in weight, and 1.0 ml per hour in children < 20 kg body weight.

For those patients who require endotracheal intubation and intensive care, an indwelling Swan–Ganz catheter is inserted to measure pulmonary artery wedge pressures. Estimations of central venous pressure, mean arterial pressure and continuous electrocardiographic (ECG) monitoring, are also undertaken.

Following intravenous resuscitation and stabilization of the patient's condition, attention is turned to primary wound care: cleaning of the head and neck of soot, dirt, and debris from the fire, with shaving of the hair adjacent to the burns to allow clean wound toilet to be undertaken. Blisters and serum are gently removed.

Particular care is taken to examine the eyes, and to perform an adequate eye toilet. Any suggestion of burns to the eyes or eyelids makes a thorough ophthalmological examination necessary, with fluoroscein staining of the cornea to demonstrate corneal ulceration. Desmarres' eyelid retractors may be required in the presence of extremely swollen and oedematous eyelids to allow inspection of the globe, and to enable foreign material to be removed from the upper or lower fornix as part of an eye toilet. The adequacy of the upper lids in protection of the globe should be assessed at this stage. Those patients who have received severe full-thickness facial burns with loss of the eyelids, with or without damage to the globe, need urgent care to ensure that the globe does not desiccate on exposure to the air. An acrylic eye shield, or in emergency a piece of plastic kitchen film (e.g. Glad® wrap: Fig. 9.8A), can be used to great effect to keep the globe moist if appropriate eyelid closure is not possible. Instillation of antibiotic eye ointment under the eye shield provides a good greasy film that protects the cornea from desiccation until definitive lid reconstruction can be undertaken. In the seriously ill patient, exposed corneas can be preserved for several weeks if care is adequate. Frequent irrigation of the eyes may be necessary.

In patients who have suffered chemical burns to the face, emergency treatment to the burned eye consists of copious early irrigation, to remove all traces of residual chemical, followed by full ophthalmological assessment.

ASSESSMENT OF BURN DEPTH

A more accurate clinical assessment of the depth of burning is then undertaken, with particular reference to:

1. The colour of the burn wound.
2. The presence or absence of capillary refill: capillary refill following blanching from pressure demonstrates intact dermal microvasculature and thus a partial thickness burn.
3. In the cooperative patient the presence or absence of pin prick sensation using a hypodermic needle. The presence of pin prick sensation demonstrates the intact nature of the dermal nerve supply, and suggests that the burn is likely to be of partial thickness.

Partial-thickness burns of the face heal spontaneously within 10–14 days. However, difficulties may arise in diagnosing burn depth in the eyelids, scalp, and nose. Reassessment of the burn is undertaken at each daily dressing. It is often initially difficult to judge the depth of so-called indeterminate burns. An obviously superficial or deep burn is easy to diagnose on admission; burns involving the middle and deep areas of the dermis are often initially indeterminate in depth and several days may be needed to establish the diagnosis.

Full-thickness areas on the face generally have a somewhat waxy appearance and often feel rigid. There is no capillary return, and no presence of sensation to pin prick. The facial skin should be examined repeatedly and in detail. Particular attention should be taken to the external ears: there is considerable risk of devitalization of the underlying auricular cartilage with secondary infection producing suppurative chondritis.

GENERAL MANAGEMENT

Patients with facial burns should be nursed in the supine position with the head of the bed elevated to encourage resolution of facial oedema. Patients with burns around the mouth and/or facial swelling may have difficulty in eating; careful assisted feeding by nursing staff may be successful, or it may be necessary to insert a fine-bore flexible naso-enteric tube to provide adequate caloric intake. In those patients with burns > 10% TBSA, it is our practice to institute early enteral feeding via naso-enteric feeding tubes assisted by an enteric feeding pump, the amount of dietary supplementation depending upon the extent of body surface area burned. This is also done in patients who have lost > 10% of body weight.

In the past caloric and nitrogen replacement was assessed by calculation from the Currieri Formula, and the Modified Harris Benedict Equation (p. 384), but recently, with the provision of a Datex Metabolic Monitor, caloric replacement has been managed by weekly measurement of metabolic rate. In our hands, this method of measurement of metabolic rate provides a more accurate basis of energy replacement in the burned patient than older formulas. Measurements are begun 7 days after admission, and repeated weekly thereafter, with a gap of 10 days after each episode of surgery to allow for the effect on metabolic rate of the latent heat of vaporization caused by evaporation of water from unhealed skin graft donor sites.

In the patient with nasal burns, insertion of nasal airways may be required so that transnasal breathing may continue, and also to provide a stent around which healing can occur. Constriction of the nares may occur in the patient with full-thickness burns of the nose which have a prolonged healing time, and also in the patient with loss of nasal lining mucosa and secondary scar deposition. Prolonged wearing of a tube stent may be necessary to retain nasal airways of satisfactory size, even following definitive nasal reconstruction. Similarly, patients with burns to the mouth may require a microstomia splint to provide continuous elastic dilatation as a prevention against scar shrinkage during healing (Fowler & Pegg 1986).

Superficial burns of the face heal spontaneously within 10–14 days and paraffin ointment is a most appropriate covering for these. Where burns involve the full skin thickness, silver sulphadiazine cream is used and the burns are either left exposed or in selected cases closed by application of dressings held in place with elastic net.

In Australia, silver-sulphadiazine with chlorhexidine digluconate cream is used routinely as a topical wound antimicrobial, as this is presently the only topical wound antimicrobial available. Sulfamylon (mafenide acetate), however, may be a more appropriate topical wound antimicrobial, as Moncrief et al (1966) showed that it will penetrate the burn eschar to underlying cartilage, preventing infection in the deep burn and secondary suppurative chondritis. It is especially effective against *Pseudomonas* species (Heggers 1991). The rest of the face is covered initially with paraffin ointment to keep the skin moist while further assessment is undertaken.

It is not our routine practice to use prophylactic intravenous antibiotics in burn management. Apart from the problems noted above with burns to the external ears, infection in the facial burn is uncommon, and with high quality wound care the isolated facial burn rarely requires intravenous chemotherapy. Heggers (1991, 1993) has marshalled very convincing arguments against the indiscriminate use of systemic antibiotics in burn treatment. However, prophylactic chemotherapy is given before burn debridement if there is reason to suspect invasive sepsis on clinical grounds or on the basis of burn culture or biopsy, or of course if there is suspicion of septicaemia. Septicaemia is infrequent in uncomplicated facial burns, but may occur when there is extensive burning and shock, or in pulmonary burns complicated by secondary pneumonia; the possible role of bacterial translocation is discussed on p. 120. Reassessment of the burn at each dressing enables a more accurate diagnosis to be made with time, and an appropriate management strategy can be evolved and revised as the clinical condition changes.

NURSING CARE OF THE FACIAL BURN

Routine nursing care of the facial burn wound is usually undertaken at the bedside. The nurse wears a sterile operating theatre gown, two pairs of sterile gloves, a mask, and protective eye wear.

Wound care is preceded by oral toilet, assisted cleaning of teeth, and shaving of male patients. Shaving is undertaken twice a day; hair is washed daily. Saline gauze is used to clean away paraffin ointment previously applied, beginning with the eyelids, and moving to the remainder of the face, finishing with ears and neck. Using forceps and iris scissors, any blistered skin, debris, foreign material, loose eschar, or dead tissue is debrided. Toilets of the eyes, external auditory canals, nose, and mouth are performed. Fresh sterile soft paraffin is applied to all areas of the burn wound, and is re-applied twice daily, after cleaning as described above.

Because the nose is used as a portal for endotracheal intubation and nasogastric or naso-enteric feeding tubes, which need to be secured with tape, there is a danger that incorrect placement of these tubes may cause nasal damage. Tight cotton tapes used to secure tubes can produce pressure, particularly at the junction of the alar wings and the face, with enlargement of the nasal stoma and destruction of the alar wings. The columella can also be destroyed in the same way (Wachtel et al 1981). It is important for nursing staff to be made aware of this danger; the placement of transnasal tubes should be frequently reassessed to ensure that pressure damage does not occur.

RECONSTRUCTIVE PRIORITIES

In acute and secondary burn reconstruction, as with all other forms of reconstruction, it is most important that a reconstructive plan be formulated to coordinate surgical and non-surgical treatment. This requires a standard method of patient assessment and coordination of members of the burn treatment multidisciplinary team to ensure that the appropriate assessment is undertaken before surgery. Most importantly it requires an accurate evaluation of the extent of the defect to be reconstructed, and the amount of tissue required to undertake that reconstruction. Brou et al (1989) have reported on a reconstructive inventory, used to examine patients periodically, to catalogue their reconstructive needs, and to match these with the quality and quantity of different tissues available. We have used a copy of their proforma, and have found this a most useful way of systematizing the assessment and planning of both acute and secondary burn reconstruction. Because the principles of acute and secondary reconstruction are the same, we recommend this approach for both stages of reconstruction. Bjarnason et al (1992) noted the difference that often exists between the reconstructive goals of the surgeon and those of the child with burns and the relatives, pointing out that it is vitally important that the patient be taken into the surgeon's confidence when reconstruction of the burn is being planned. They noted particularly that children indicated fewer and different desired reconstruction sites than the physicians or parents. Even in adult life, the goals that the patient wishes to achieve are often very different from those that the treating surgeon sees as appropriate. A reconstructive regime based on surgical decisions alone may not necessarily be appropriate to the patient's needs or wishes.

Post-burn reconstruction is divided into *acute or primary reconstruction* (basically measures required to provide primary healing of the acute burn) and *secondary reconstruction*, defined as reconstruction occurring after the acute burn has healed. Whether acute or secondary, the reconstructive priorities should include a consideration of the order in which they should be dealt with, as well as the shortage of tissue, the types of tissue missing (skin, subcutaneous tissue, cartilage, mucosa, bone) and the quantity of tissue missing.

The face relies for its function and appearance on muscular movement, and the earliest reconstructive priority is therefore to restore essential function (Robson & Smith 1987, Robson et al 1992). This will not only contribute to improved appearance, but will also assist the patient to maintain independent daily living activities.

Definitive secondary reconstruction of the facial burn is often made difficult by the lack of appropriate normal facial tissue as a result of tissue destruction during the burn and as a consequence of subsequent treatment. Conservation of tissue is therefore the most important acute primary reconstructive goal (Gillies & Millard 1957, Robson et al 1992). A wound-healing protocol of early tangential excision and skin grafting (see below) should provide the maximum quantity of correctly reconstructed skin based on a good dermal blood supply, for future reconstruction of the whole burned area.

A protocol giving priority to early closure of the acute facial burn can be followed easily when the facial burn occurs in isolation. In the case of the severely burnt patient with life-threatening large area burns elsewhere on the body, management priorities may dictate leaving the facial burn until last, and assigning priority to surgery that will save life, namely closure of the maximum amount of the burn wound in the shortest possible time. After this has been accomplished, attention can be turned to the healing of the facial burn wound, but the unavoidable delay may compromise the cosmetic and functional result that might otherwise be obtained.

Our standard Acute Burn Reconstruction protocol (see below) includes early aggressive wound management, aimed to produce definitive wound healing by post-burn day 14, followed by an active scar management programme, utilizing elastic fabric compression garments (Alvarez et al 1983). This has contributed to the small number of patients requiring secondary reconstruction.

However, the severely burned patient may have a virtually destroyed face with none of the usual sources of normal tissue for nasal or other reconstruction and, if the burn is associated with a severe and deep body burn, donor sites for distant tissue transfer (for example free tissue flaps) may be unavailable. Occasionally 'old-fashioned' tube pedicle tissue transfer may be required (Fig. 17.7D). It is now possible to save patients, particularly children, with very severe burns; the salvage of a child with 99% burns has been reported from the Shriners' Burns Institute, Galveston, Texas (D. N. Herndon 1991, personal communication). In such cases, there are almost insurmountable problems: these include the amount of severe tissue destruction and the lack of available tissue for reconstruction, the splintage of muscle by scar, the secondary impairment of skeletal growth (p. 77) and the significant psychological and social problems that will undoubtedly come from the saving of patients with such

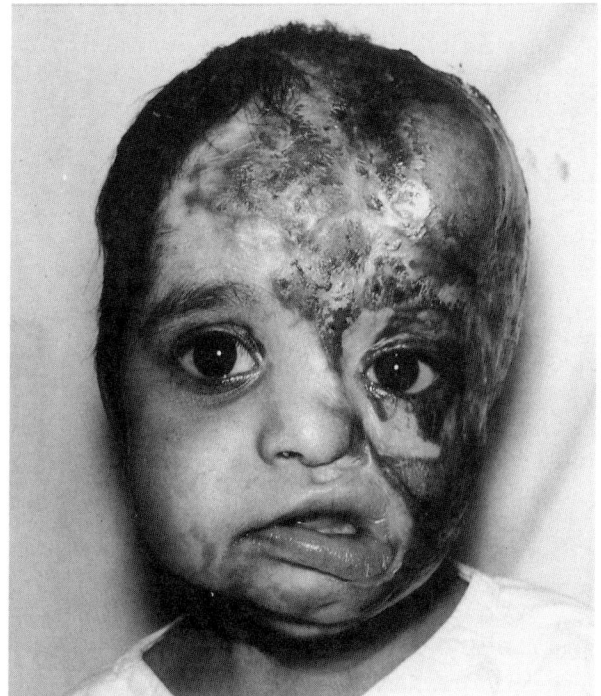

A

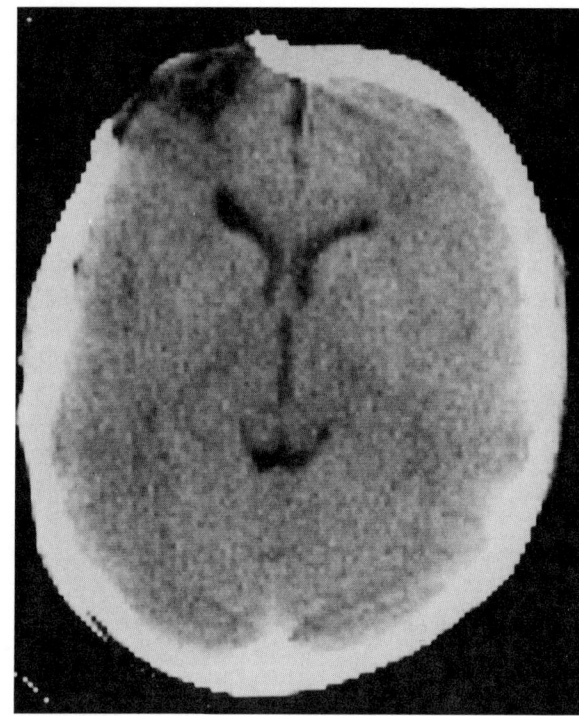

C

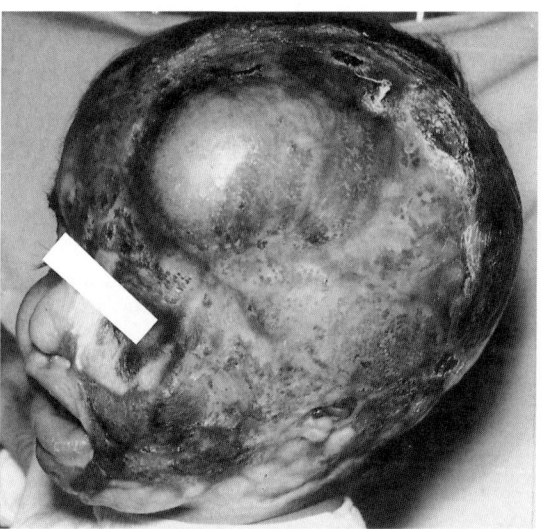

B

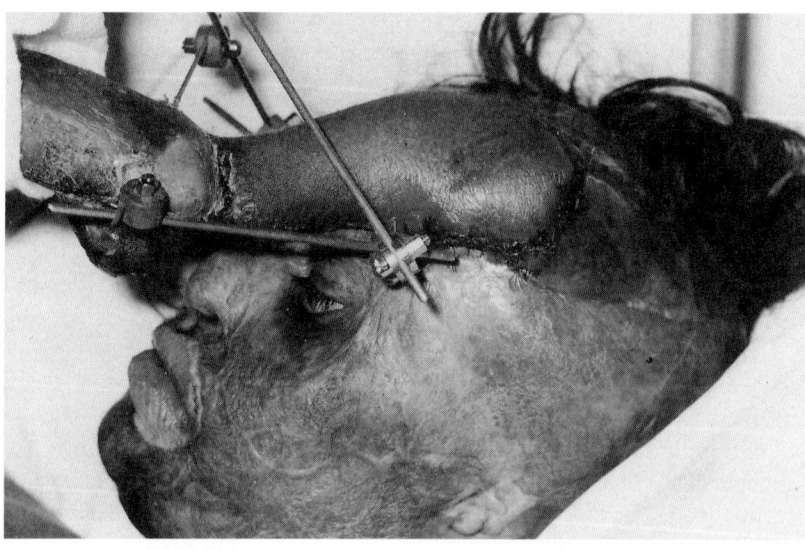

D

Fig. 17.7 Full-thickness craniocerebral burn complicated by epilepsy. A 13-month-old male infant suffered severe full-thickness burns of the head and arms (estimated body area 15%). The hands were mutilated. An area of frontal bone 9 cm in diameter was exposed. The left ear was destroyed. The infant was referred, after some delay, for neurosurgical assessment. The exposed bone appeared necrotic, and there were defects in it through which pus and granulation tissue exuded. On day 55, the necrotic frontal bone was removed, exposing a large extradural abscess. In some areas, the inner table of the frontal bone was preserved because it appeared viable. The exposed dura was later covered with full-thickness skin. **A,B** 4 months after injury, the extensive area of burned face and scalp had been effectively covered with skin grafts; the full-thickness graft on the dural hernia had healed well. There was a bulging pseudomeningocele at the site of bone destruction. Because of the poor quality of the remainder of the scalp, it was considered impossible, in the then state of knowledge, to cover the area with a scalp rotation flap, and the child wore a protective helmet. **C** CT scan (early model) showed an area of low density change, presumably gliosis in the region of the bone defect; a collar of bone had formed around the neck. At the age of 15 years, cranioplasty was performed. **D** An abdominal tubular skin graft was raised and attached to the stump of the mutilated right hand. When vascularization was established, the cerebral hernia was mobilized and the epidermis removed with an abrasive burr. Two ribs were excised, split and fitted into the cranial defect; they were secured with steel wire and silk. The tubular pedicle graft was opened and sutured over the frontal defect. To prevent avulsion, the forearm was secured to the skull by a transfixion pin attached to pegs screwed to the frontal bone. The cranioplasty was successful, but the boy suffered much psychological stress and also epilepsy related to the frontal cerebral scar. This tragic case exemplifies the crippling effects of a domestic fire. It also shows that neurosurgical debridement of a cranial burn should not be delayed unduly, as an extradural abscess is likely to form in the dead space under the necrotic bone.

severe injuries (Fig. 17.8). In some cases of severe burns in the craniofacial region, rehabilitation is further complicated by ocular or cerebral disabilities. In such cases, the support of parents and other family members, vital as it is, may be hard to obtain. In our experience, the majority of severely burned patients come from lower socio-economic groups, and are financially and emotionally least able to rehabilitate from these injuries. More time must pass before correct answers can be given to the moral and ethical dilemmas raised by a treatment regime that promotes survival at all costs.

PRINCIPLES OF BURN MANAGEMENT

The overriding principle of management is to conserve as much tissue as possible and to preserve normal anatomical landmarks. Loss of soft tissue may destroy or distort the anatomy of the face, and may expose vital structures.

Superficial burns of the face epithelialize from the surviving epidermal cells present in the adnexal structures (p. 5.00). If dermal collagen is exposed, it must be protected from desiccation leading to necrosis and increase in burn depth as was shown by Zawacki (1974). Epithelialization must be allowed to proceed in an optimum wound environment.

Deeper dermal burns in which the depth of thermal injury is indeterminate are treated expectantly in some centres and 'allowed to granulate': however, this policy may result in delayed epithelialization, excess collagen deposition, and ugly hypertrophic scar formation (Fig. 17.9).

Sir Harold Gillies noted that when the reliability of skin grafting became established, there was a clear call to carry out primary excision of the burn and immediately to dress it with skin (Gillies & Millard 1957). Gillies performed this in his first case in 1926; it was a debridement and skin graft on the thigh. He subsequently reported other cases of early excision and grafting from his World War II experience. Subsequently Converse et al (1977) reported that early excision was not advisable in facial burns due to the difficulties in diagnosing burn depth. However, earlier work described by Janzekovic (1970) showed that with attention to detail it is possible to diagnose the depth of the dermal burn, the most difficult burn to diagnose correctly. She described the method of tangential excision, in which non-viable tissue is excised until healthy bleeding dermis is seen. Haemostasis is then secured and split-skin grafts are applied. Jackson & Stone (1972) showed that this procedure allows application of a skin graft even on tissue which bleeds sluggishly and is in the zone of vascular stasis: operation may resuscitate the underlying potentially compromised dermis and prevent the development of delayed dermal necrosis. An appropriate dermal framework for split-skin grafting is provided, the reconstructed skin being of better quality than if dermis is not saved.

Later writers (Converse et al 1977, Feller & Richards 1979, Miller 1979) advocated an expectant policy. It was usual to wait until the necrotic dermis had formed an eschar; when this eschar had separated and been replaced by granulation tissue, skin grafts were applied. The earliest advocates of tangential excision were Janzekovic (1970), Jackson & Stone (1972) and Warpeha (1981). Later, Jonsson (1987) from the Karolinska Institute in Stockholm favoured excision of facial burns within 3 days of injury. Encouraging results were reported from the Parkland Hospital in Dallas by Hunt et al (1987). But the strongest proponents of early tangential excision of facial burns have been Heimbach and Engrav of Seattle (Heimbach & Engrav 1984; Engrav et al 1986). We have adopted their policies and method.

The principle that reconstruction of the face should be based on cosmetic or aesthetic units was first enunciated by Gonzales-Ulloa in 1956. He subdivided the face into naturally separate and well-delineated regional aesthetic units (Fig. 17.10). All facial reconstruction should respect these aesthetic units, and skin graft junctions should follow the junction lines of these units to produce an appearance that is normal and natural (Heimbach & Engrav 1984). With these overriding principles in mind, initial reconstructive efforts should be directed towards restoring function to the most active and functionally most important areas of the face, namely the eyelids, the mouth, the nose and the neck. Although a detailed description of the surgery of burns of the neck is outside the scope of this book, burns to the neck occur frequently in association with burns of the face, and subsequent scarring to the neck commonly produces a wide variety of flexion deformities as well as secondary shortage of facial skin. These deformities may act against any facial reconstructive programme by deforming the chin, the mouth, the alar bases and the eyes, by producing secondary skin shortage and contracture, and by posturing the head in an abnormal position, making normal function difficult. For these reasons, attention may need to be directed to early release of neck contractures, with the insetting of good quality skin (either thick partial thickness or dissected full-thickness skin grafts) to minimize subsequent contracture; flap reconstruction may also be used, either by a pedicled graft or by a microvascularized free flap. In addition, elasticized pressure garments will be required to promote early maturation of post-burn hypertrophic scarring. The frequent wearing of a neck brace will hold the head in an appropriate neutral position while the neck skin grafts heal and mature. Following appropriate reconstruction of the functional cervical structures, facial resurfacing can be undertaken to improve the cosmetic appearance of the burned forehead, cheeks, nose, lips and chin.

Resurfacing of the acute burn should be undertaken with reference to facial cosmetic units. A regimen of

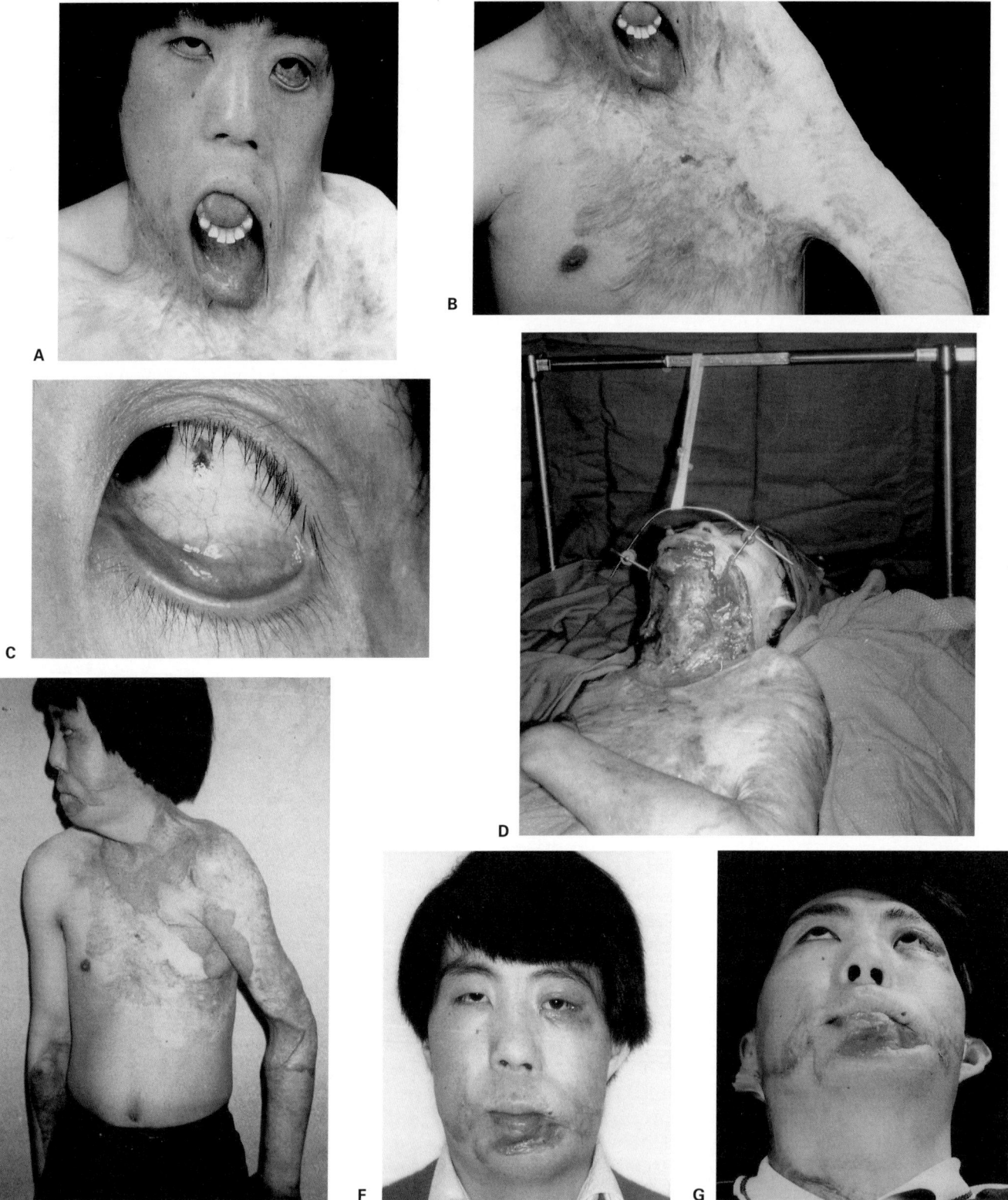

Fig. 17.8 Severe scarring and tissue shortage from burns in childhood. Burns may produce profound growth disturbance and secondary deformity. A young man from another country had suffered burns as a child from a kerosene heater fire. There was severe tissue shortage, partly as a result of the primary burn injury, partly the secondary effect of scar contracture, and partly the tertiary effect of growth. **A,B** Gross tissue shortage in the anterior neck and chest deformed the lower lip and caused secondary growth disturbance in the mandible; there was a gross open bite and mandibular prognathism. **C** A left lower ectropion resulted from the distant tissue shortage. **D** The key to the facial reconstruction was to recreate the original deformity, by excising the scarred area. **E** The submental area was resurfaced with a free radial forearm flap from the right forearm. The anterior neck was resurfaced with a full-thickness skin graft, creating a cervico-mental angle. The secondary shortage of axillary skin was also corrected with a pedicled flap from the scapular region and additional skin grafts. **F, G** The mandibular deformity was corrected by bilateral osteotomies of the mandibular body, and the reconstruction was completed by junctional scar revision and Z-plasty. From Katsaros et al (1990) by courtesy of the *British Journal of Plastic Surgery.*

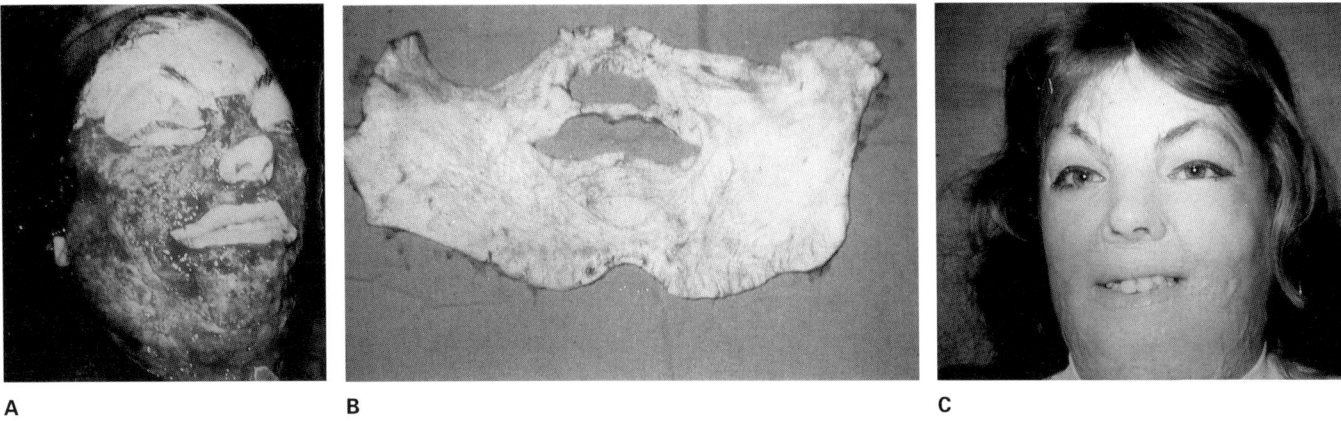

A   B   C

Fig. 17.9 Facial excision for scar formation after split skin grafting. Split-skin grafts were placed on granulating deep facial burns. Ugly scarring resulted, and it was decided to excise the facial scar to restore normal anatomy. (Case by courtesy of Professor Martin C. Robson, MD, Tampa, Florida, USA.) **A** Excision of the facial mask was carried out, down to the surface of the facial musculature, freeing individual muscle units from the splinting effect of the scar tissue. **B** The excised skin mask. A full-thickness skin graft was dissected in the same size and shape, following the pattern of the mask. This was carefully sutured into the defect and held with a contoured pressure mould. **C** In the final result, there was notable restoration of normal facial expression when the facial muscles were liberated from their incarceration in scar. This can be compared with the result achieved with groin flaps (Fig. 17.12C), which are too bulky to allow expression, and with the thinner dorsalis pedis flaps, which conform well to the facial contours but again give less facial expression. The key to success in such operations is absolute haemostasis. Professor Robson has suggested that the procedure might be staged by dressing the excised facial defect with Biobrane® for 24 h before harvesting and applying the skin graft.

tangential excision to debride the acute burn and reconstruction with split-thickness grafting can be used to reconstruct the mid-dermal facial burn, utilizing the remaining dermis as a scaffold for addition of further dermis and epidermis, reconstructing the full thickness of the skin as far as possible.

When there has been destruction of dermis, a split-thickness graft is appropriate for acute resurfacing, to heal the wound as quickly as possible and to minimize secondary scar deposition. Subsequent scar maturation, assisted by elasticized or solid polypropylene appliances, may produce a satisfactory appearance (Shons et al 1981, Powell et al 1985). However, full-thickness skin grafts are often required when the original depth of burning has left no appropriate dermal foundation to minimize contraction of the unsupported partial-thickness skin graft. A lack of availability of large amounts of full-thickness

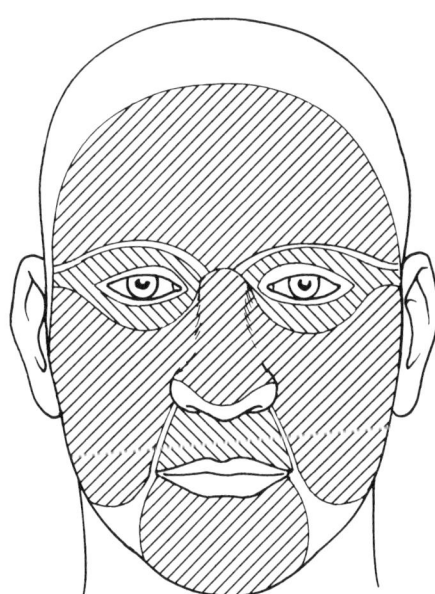

Fig. 17.10 Cosmetic units of the face. The face is subdivided into naturally occurring aesthetic areas, separated by identifiable anatomical boundaries, e.g. the nasolabial fold.

skin may make an aggressive reconstruction programme difficult, but a large full-thickness dissected skin graft can be easily taken from the medial aspect of the thigh, using a pattern prepared from the defect left after excising the scarred areas. This exemplifies the important secondary reconstructive principle of Gillies' 'recreating the original defect' (Gillies & Millard 1957). Robson (personal communication 1992) has used this strategy in totally resurfacing a deformed face grafted with full-thickness skin (Fig. 17.9). Resurfacing the face with homogeneous skin removes the great colour and texture differences that often exist in the burned face which has healed partly by primary healing, and partly after surgery. This method also illustrates Gillies' fundamental reconstructive principle of keeping normal tissue in its normal position, or where necessary moving it back into its original normal position and retaining it there. The true character of the defect can then be estimated, and the retention of the tissues in their correct position calls for the filling of the residual gap with tissues as similar to the lost tissue as possible.

SURGICAL BURN WOUND CARE

Surgical treatment of facial burn wounds should be approached from the point of view of the anatomical aesthetic areas discussed above (Fig. 17.10). If burns which cross the boundaries between anatomical areas are treated without reference to those areas, very ugly deformities will result from breaking up the natural anatomical land marks of the face, and an abnormal appearance is immediately apparent to the beholder's eye. In the acute burn, courage may be required to persuade the patient to have areas of unburned skin within an aesthetic unit excised. This may be especially difficult in the case of a child. Nevertheless some of the most disfiguring cosmetic deformities are seen in those children who have had dermal burns of the face which have been allowed to heal spontaneously. Despite aggressive scar management, ugly hypertrophic post-burn scars may persist for life. Later reconstruction will inevitably involve excision of large areas of normally appearing intervening skin, and this will require counselling that may be much more difficult than the simpler acute decision to extend the initial burn wound excision.

Superficial burns (burns that heal spontaneously by epithelialization from the epidermal adnexal structures within a 10–14 day period) will heal producing skin of normal appearance, apart from early erythema. This erythema fades during the subsequent phase of devascularization, stratification and subsequent cornification of the epidermis. As soon as epithelialization is complete, moisturizing creams are applied: these assist in softening the residual eschar which splints the skin and impairs function and full epithelialization. Skin massage by the patient helps to soften the recently healed skin and to disperse oedema. Destruction of melanocytes in the basal layer of the epidermis may result in areas of reduced skin pigmentation, which can produce unsightly vitiligo. On the other hand, in patients with olive or brown skin, the migration of functionally efficient melanocytes, may result in areas of excessive pigmentation.

Tangential excision

The mid to deep dermal burn on the face will take longer than 10–14 days to heal. While deeper burns may eventually heal, they do so partly by wound contraction, thus producing abnormal masses of hypertrophic scar which produce an ugly deformity that is difficult to treat. Although Hurt & Eriksson (1986) believe that it is preferable to preserve residual facial epithelium for primary healing rather than to excise eschar and use skin grafts, we have chosen to use the method of tangential excision as described by Janzekovic and advocated eloquently for use in the tangential excision of facial aesthetic units by Heimbach & Engrav (1984); we have had considerable success following their technique.

Under general anaesthesia, the patient is positioned in a neurosurgical head rest; depending on the operative plan, it may be useful to begin in the prone position and later in the supine position. The head is shaved if scalp skin is to be used for skin graft.

The facial burns are excised tangentially as cosmetic units, even though some of each excised cosmetic unit may consist of normal unburned skin. Following tangential shaving of necrotic skin, haemostasis is effected by application of cotton laparotomy packs soaked in saline containing adrenaline (1:33 000); careful punctate diathermy is also used. Grafts are then taken for grafting the face; the best colour match is skin from the area of the body above the nipple line in the so-called 'blush area'. No grafted skin can perfectly match the colour and texture of facial skin (Hurt & Eriksson 1986); however, we have found scalp skin quite satisfactory if it is unburned. Even if burned superficially, scalp may be a better colour match for the rest of a superficially burned face than skin from elsewhere. Scalp skin is best harvested after ballooning of the scalp skin by subgaleal injection of saline, using a Pitkin-type syringe. This removes irregularities and allows the harvesting of large strips with the mechanical dermatome (Brou et al 1990). Where skin from the blush area is not available, any available skin must be used, and then the colour match may be less satisfactory.

The skin grafts are applied as complete sheets, care being taken to harvest a sufficiently large piece of skin so that each cosmetic unit can be covered by one graft. The skin grafts are carefully aligned so that their junction lines within each aesthetic unit are parallel to the predominant skin crease lines within that aesthetic unit. The skin grafts are carefully sutured along the lines of junction of cosmetic units, and if more than one adjacent cosmetic unit is involved, the grafts are trimmed so that the junctional scar falls along the line of the junction of the cosmetic units.

Heimbach & Engrav (1984) have described the use of a pre-made moulded plastic mask to provide appropriate pressure on the skin grafts and to immobilize them. These masks promote early adherence to maximize skin graft take. We have treated our facial grafts by exposure, using a regime of hourly graft care, with frequent aspiration of seromas and haematomas. This has proved satisfactory in the hands of our competent staff. However, it is important that pressure be applied to the facial skin grafts, and custom-made elastic face masks or clear acrylic moulded face masks are applied as soon as the skin grafts have become sufficiently adherent to withstand the manipulation of fitting. Engrav et al (1983) have shown that early application of these pressure devices does not interfere with skin graft survival.

Full-thickness burns of the face are treated in exactly the same manner as deep partial-thickness burns, by undertaking a tangential, or rather a sequential, excision until healthy bleeding subcutaneous tissue is exposed, upon which split-thickness skin grafts are placed in the same way. Muir et al (1987) note that early grafting on clean granulating areas is usually very satisfactory and often to be preferred to immediate graft application. Hurt & Eriksson (1986) advocated a protocol of awaiting separation of the eschar from the facial burn before undertaking grafting, their exception to this rule being in full-thickness burns of the eyelids, which are usually excised and grafted as soon as the oedema subsides. We do not wait until granulation tissue has begun to form as delay will promote wound contraction, and the production of excess collagen, which will produce scar tissue and considerable facial disfigurement, is very difficult to treat. Muir et al (1987) admit that any delay in providing skin cover on a fresh granulating wound will be heavily penalized by gross fibrosis and disfiguring contracted scars, especially around the lips and eyelids and on the front of the neck (Fig. 17.9). There is experimental evidence to support this observation.

Prevention of wound contraction

Rudolph (1979) showed that contractile fibroblasts, designated as myofibroblasts (p. 123), are found in an open wound within 4 days, reaching maximum numbers at 3 weeks post-injury. Madden et al (1974) also showed that strips of granulation tissue excised from recent wounds could be made to contract by stimulation with 5-hydroxytryptamine, bradykinin, angiotensin, vasopressin and adrenaline. Abercrombie et al (1954) had shown in small rat wounds that contraction had been completed by 10–15 days. We (Leitch et al 1993) have shown similar results, also in rats. However, wound contraction was inhibited by the commonly used topical antimicrobial applications Sulfamylon (mafenide acetate), silver sulphadiazine and silver sulphadiazine with chlorhexidine. This inhibition of wound contraction was significant ($P < 0.05$) in comparison with a control group of rats.

Apparently paradoxically, we (Leitch & Robson, unpublished) have also shown in further experiments that this in vivo inhibition of wound contraction by antimicrobial drugs is associated with deposition of excess collagen as shown by wound tensile strength measurements. Sulfamylon produced a highly significant ($P < 0.004$) increase in tensile strength; with silver sulphadiazine, the increase was also considered to be significant ($P < 0.049$). These findings support the long-held clinical belief that the wound that is dressed for inappropriately long periods has a higher likelihood of forming unacceptable postburn hypertrophic scar, or even cicatricial contracture and deformity. Stone & Madden (1974) investigated the effects of skin grafting on wound contraction in rabbits, and confirmed that split-thickness skin grafting decreased the amount of wound contraction in recently excised wounds. In their model, grafts were applied on wounds from which full-thickness skin had been excised; in analogous human burn wounds, it is generally accepted that if the skin graft is placed on a dermal framework so as to reconstruct the anatomical layers of the skin, then healing will take place with far less deformity than after grafting on subcutaneous fat or granulation tissue. Because of these findings, and following the work of Heimbach & Engrav (1984), we prefer to treat facial burns more actively, by early excision and grafting, to obtain healing as early as possible. With the application of appropriate pressure garments, this policy gives the best chance of providing minimal deformity. The granulating wound that transgresses the anatomical boundaries of facial cosmetic units produces an ugly deformity which is difficult to correct.

EYELID BURNS

Surgical pathology

Burns of the lids may be caused by thermal (Fig. 17.2A) or chemical coagulation (Figs 17.1 and 17.11). Like other eyelid injuries, burns in this site can have disastrous effects on visual function, even when the globe is not initially damaged.

Some 20–30% of facial burns involve the eyelids. The cornea and conjunctiva are usually spared, testimony to the protective mechanisms of the lids. Loss of an eye from an initial burn injury occurred in fewer than 4% of cases reported by Boswick (1973). Ectropion was the

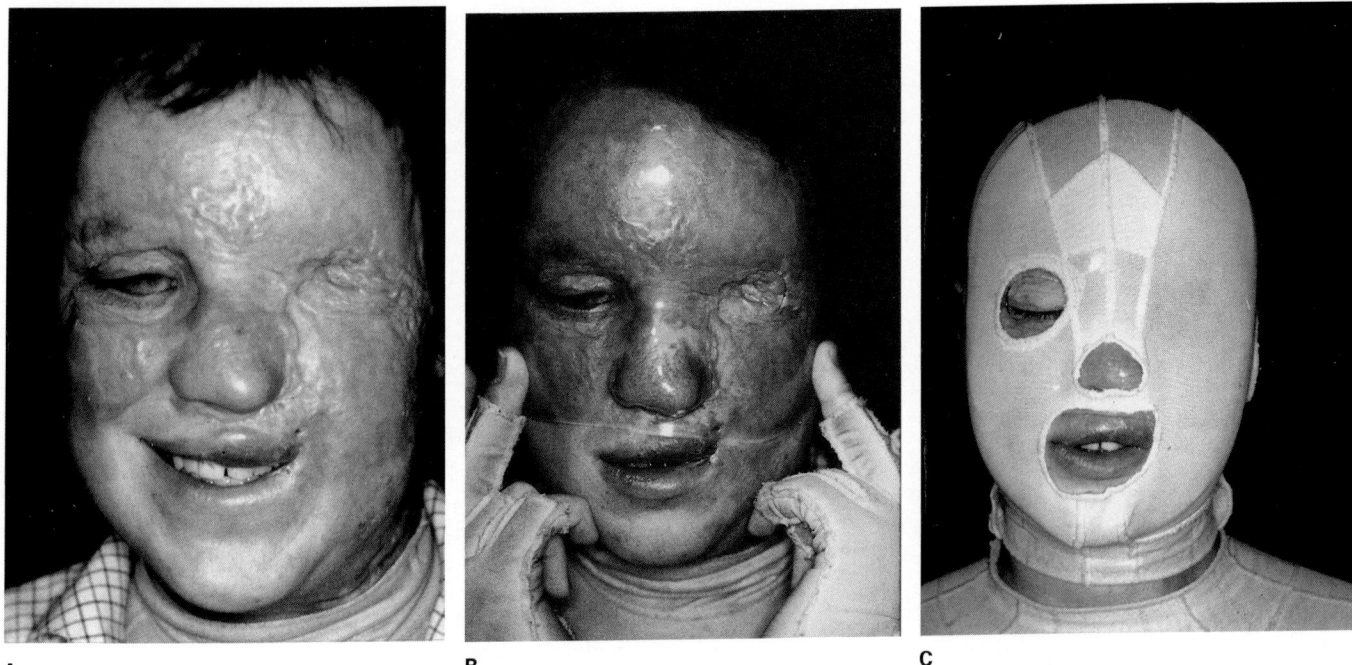

A   **B**   **C**

Fig. 17.11 Facial burns from phosphorus explosion. A young man suffered severe penetrating burns to the face following explosion of phosphorus. He subsequently lost both eyes due to direct ocular damage on the left, and phosphorous toxicity on the right. Severe on-going hypertrophic scarring has produced significant deformity, marked by the loss of the normal anatomical boundaries of aesthetic units. **A** Showing the extent of scarring, the forehead and the right cheek were primarily reconstructed by tangential excision and thick scalp skin grafts. **B** A rigid face mask was worn alternating with **C** An elastic mask, to modify the hypertrophic scar response.

most common late complication of lid burns in this series; primary corneal coagulation occurred in only 1% of patients. Electrical burns may involve every part of the eye; the most common effect seems to be cataract formation (Johnson et al 1987). Full-thickness burns, which are often not very painful, heal with considerable scarring and disfigurement. Granulation tissue forms and develops myofibroblasts which cause severe contracture and eyelid deformity. Burns to the eyelid may also produce a significant management problem because of the delicate nature of the eyelid skin which may suffer severe damage in association with much less severe burns to the rest of the face. The burn itself may destroy the eyelids, exposing the globe which may become damaged from desiccation if not already injured at the time of burning. In addition, loss of eyelid tissue with secondary cicatricial ectropion may produce exposure keratitis which may require emergency management in the early stages of severe burns.

Management

The management of superficial burns of the lids follows the plan of management of burns in general. First aid treatment includes thorough irrigation of the area: if chemicals have been responsible for the injury, copious amounts of water or normal saline are used as soon as possible. In the initial stages, burns to the lids are likely to produce severe oedema which may involve other adnexal tissues. Pressure induced by the oedema on the globe may be deleterious to the optic nerve circulation and canthotomies may be required to relieve this. Lid burns may result in loss of tissue and contractures. Every attempt should be made to preserve tissue, but secondary procedures, including grafting, may be necessary to restore the lids (Fig. 17.2B). The lashes are often singed in thermal burns, and curl in, producing a risk of corneal abrasion; lashes are best removed to prevent discomfort and possibly scarring, ulceration and infection.

The early management of lid burns involves protection of the cornea. Lid hygiene should be used to remove the hard crusts that form on the lid margin. Tarsorrhaphy may on occasions be necessary to prevent exposure keratopathy; this procedure is best performed at the end of the second week following the burn injury but should not be performed on serious burn injuries that extend to the lid margin. Some surgeons have abandoned the use of tarsorrhaphy because severe permanent eyelid margin deformity may result, and instead prefer early excision and grafting of the eyelids.

A tarsoconjunctival advancement flap may be necessary when the lid margins are partially or completely destroyed. Skin is dissected free from the underlying orbicularis muscle, and tarsoconjunctival flaps are advanced over the cornea, the edges being stitched together with a continuous suture which can be removed later. A split-thickness skin graft can then be sutured over the entire defect and a tie-over dressing applied. The newly formed upper and lower lids may be separated 6–8 weeks after the repair. If there is full-thickness loss of tarsus, coverage of the globe may be accomplished by approximating conjunctival flaps advanced from the superior and inferior fornices (Hartwood 1987, Peterson & Boswick 1987). Skin grafting can then be used to reconstruct the anterior lamellar layer. Marrone (1987) has described the use of advancement of the levator muscle and covering it with full-thickness skin to reconstruct full-thickness loss of an upper lid. Definitive reconstruction of the eyelids should be delayed until there is complete resolution of inflammation and after-scar maturation. Efforts are directed at repair of anterior medial canthal displacement, palpebral fissure stenosis, punctal and canalicular obstruction and eyebrow deformities. Skin for grafting may be best obtained from the postauricular and supraclavicular areas. Uninjured eyelid skin is an even better donor site. If none of these areas are available, the inner surface of the arm or thigh can be used.

Because of the thin nature of the eyelid skin a dermal burn may progress rapidly to contracture and acute ectropion with conjunctival and corneal exposure. While it is often necessary to undertake early release and skin grafting of eyelid burns, it may be possible with frequent eye toilets and particularly with the use of antibiotic eye ointment to keep the cornea moist until the patient is in a satisfactory state for semi-elective surgery.

As with surgery elsewhere in the face, the burned eyelids should be treated as a cosmetic unit by releasing the ectropion and insetting an appropriately sized and shaped piece of skin to correct the deformity.

The lower eyelid is best treated by use of a postauricular full-thickness skin graft if this skin is available; if not, a supraclavicular skin graft is the second best choice, followed by skin from the groin (Fig. 17.12). A crescentic defect should be created in the burned eyelid; if the piece of inserted skin is well matched in size and shape, a most satisfactory cosmetic and functional result can be obtained.

Full-thickness skin is not appropriate for reconstruction of a skin defect in the upper lid, as it is too thick to allow the normal visor-like movement of the tarsal plate in eye opening. Partial-thickness skin is used: a graft from the inner aspect of the upper arm is satisfactory. A large defect is created and more skin than is actually required is fed into the defect. A suture of the upper lid is attached to the cheek skin at its junction with the lower eyelid in the method suggested by Gillies & Millard (1957). The tie-over dressings on both upper and lower eyelids are left in place for five days before removal, allowing the patient to begin to use the eyelids.

BURNS OF THE EYEBROWS

Following facial resurfacing, any anatomical landmarks that have been destroyed, such as the eyebrows, can be reconstructed. There are several methods of eyebrow

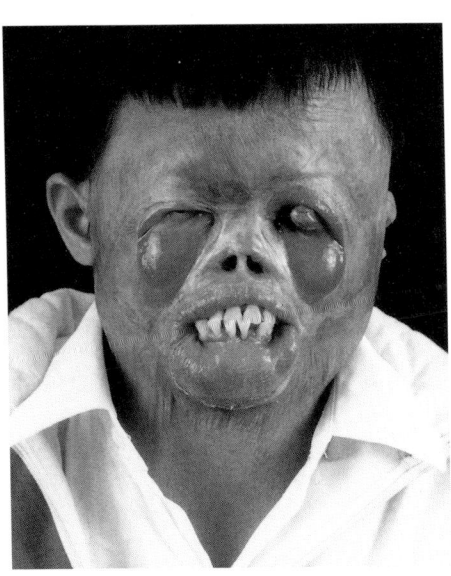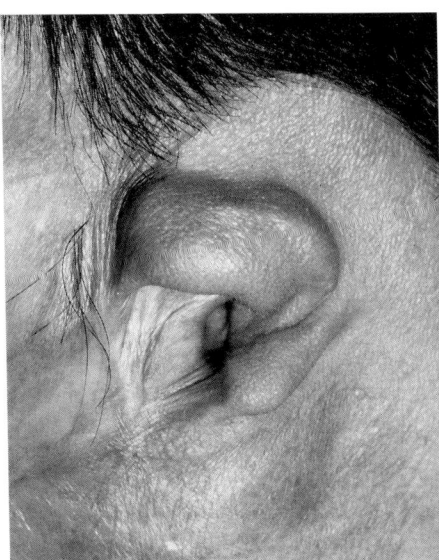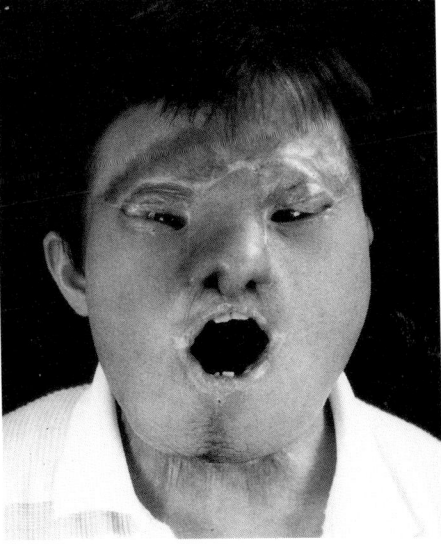

A   **B**   **C**

Fig. 17.12 Gross ectropion, loss of cheek skin, nostril stenosis and mouth deformity from flame burn. The burns were suffered in a house fire some years prior to referral from another country. **A** The deformities were associated with ectropion of the lower lip and loss of the chin point. **B** There was a 'cauliflower' deformity of the external ear as a result of suppurative chondritis. **C** The scar was released, the anatomical landmarks were restored, and free groin flaps were brought to meet in the midline. The nose was reconstructed with a lateral arm flap and bone graft. The reconstruction restored the functions of the eyelids and the mouth, but there was residual excessive bulk which masked the facial movements.

reconstruction. One may transpose a vascularized temporalis flap using a small strip of scalp attached to or vascularized by the posterior branch of the superficial temporal artery. More simply, however, small strip grafts of scalp skin may be inserted into the area of eyebrow loss. These need to be trimmed periodically as scalp hair continues to grow, but provide a much-improved appearance.

BURNS OF THE LIPS AND MOUTH

Surgical pathology

Burns of the mouth may be caused by local scalds, or by chemical or electrical agents, or as part of more extensive facial burns. Small burns of the lips, mouth and oropharynx are often seen in children who swallow caustics accidentally; these usually heal spontaneously, though the possibility of oesophageal injury from a corrosive substance should be kept in mind. Burns of the oral commissure have been reported, but we have not seen local burns affecting this structure except as part of a more extensive burn injury. Burns of the vermilion may produce loss of tissue (Fig. 17.13), but spontaneous healing usually gives a lip of satisfactory appearance. A denuded lip can be reconstructed with advancement flaps of the oral lining, or by use of the mucosa of the under surface of the tongue. Severe facial burns with delayed healing and wound contracture may cause microstomia despite the use of microstomia splints (Figs 17.14 and 17.15). Secondary skin shortage around the mouth may produce ectropion of the lips; burns of the chin may

cause this deformity in the lower lip (Fig. 17.12), and burns causing tissue loss in the neck may produce quite gross deformity of this type, especially when augmented by growth disturbances (Fig. 17.8).

Management

The small mouth may be adequately corrected by reconstruction of the oral commissure (Fig. 17.15). The commissure should lie on a vertical line dropped from the centre of the eye, and skin should be excised to ensure that the size of the oral opening conforms with this ideal. Mucosal flaps (Achauer 1990) can be used to cover the defects created in enlarging the mouth, and these give a satisfactory appearance.

Ectropion of the lips can be corrected by removal of scarred tissue, and replacement with full-thickness skin grafts. It is our policy to wait until the post-burn hypertrophic scar response has undergone resolution before correction is undertaken; if this is not done, there may be further contraction, even of a full-thickness graft. However, the disability suffered by the victim of microstomia may force earlier operation, and then there may be a tertiary deformity requiring later reconstruction.

BURNS OF THE EXTERNAL EAR

Surgical pathology

In the external ear, there is only a thin layer of subdermal tissue and the subcutaneous blood supply is closely related to the perichondrial blood supply of the underlying

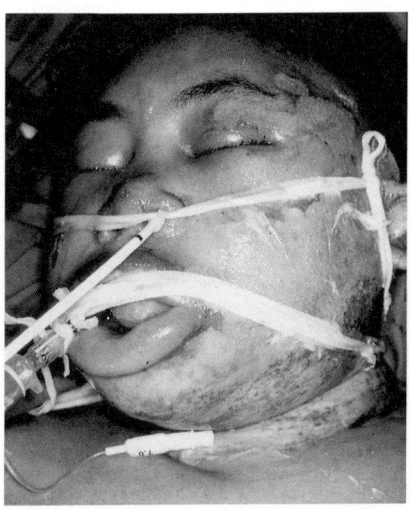
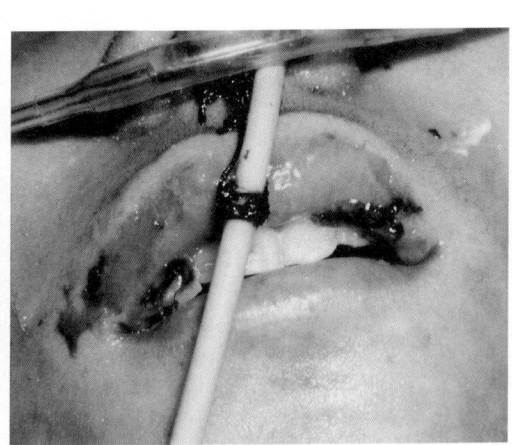
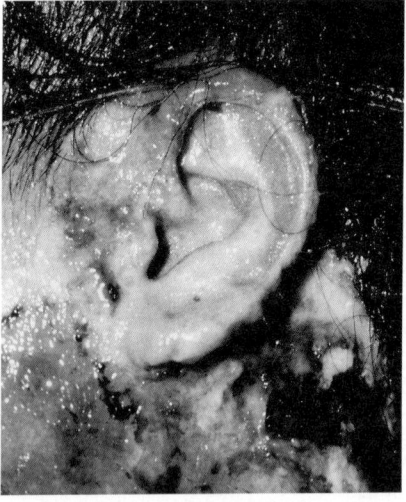

A   B   C

Fig. 17.13 Petroleum burns of the face. A 15-year-old boy suffered severe burns in an accidental petroleum fire. **A** There was an inhalational burn of the upper airway and inflammatory oedema developed, necessitating endotracheal intubation. There was also severe oedema complicating the superficial burns of the cheek, and a dermal burn of the neck. The neck burn was treated with early tangential excision and grafting to provide sound skin healing in case a tracheostomy should be needed. **B** Persistent non-healing of the upper lip vermilion was seen 10 days post-burn, although superficial burns of the cheek had healed spontaneously. The vermilion is thin and lacks adnexal structures; it is surprising that it is not destroyed more often. **C** There was a burn of the ear, largely superficial, which healed spontaneously.

cartilage. Burning can result not only in necrosis of skin, but also of the underlying auricular cartilaginous framework by destroying its cartilaginous blood supply. This causes significant secondary deformity (Fig. 17.16). Necrotic cartilage may become infected, following the establishment of bacterial colonization of the overlying burn whether deep or superficial. This produces painful chondritis, deformity and impaired wound healing (Fig. 17.3). Further compromise of circulation in the damaged ear is produced by oedema, and by pressure from inappropriately placed dressings, or from lying on a pillow. A sponge foam mould can be used to distribute pressure around the skin to avoid this complication.

Management

The key principles of management are to avoid external pressure, and to undertake meticulous gentle cleansing 4–6 hourly with application of topical antibacterial therapy (Kucan & Robson 1984). Surgical debridement is the appropriate way to treat necrotic cartilage, with either suture or application of small split-thickness skin grafts on healthy subcutaneous tissue are the appropriate way of treating these wounds.

The burned ear requires meticulous care. As soon as practicable after admission the ear is cleaned with a saline wash, and a topical antimicrobial is then applied. The optimal topical antimicrobial is mafenide acetate (Sulfamylon: see above) used in a 10% aqueous cream (Kucan & Robson 1984). This substance has the ability to penetrate the burn to the necrotic cartilage, and is recommended as it may prevent subsequent sepsis. Mafenide acetate is not readily available in Australia and we have been forced to use our standard topical antimicrobial, silver sulphadiazine with chlorhexidine digluconate. Dermal or full-thickness burns to the ears will require surgical treatment unless very small. Because of the underlying proximity of the auricular cartilage, burns to the exposed part of the external ear, particularly the helix and antihelix, often destroy the blood supply to the cartilage which becomes necrotic and must be removed before skin grafting can be successful.

Small burns of the external ear, particularly those over the helical rim and occasionally small linear burns over the antihelix, can be treated by excision and suture. If the underlying cartilage is necrotic it is sometimes possible to remove a sliver of underlying cartilage to allow skin closure to occur without tension. Although this decreases the overall size of the ear, it usually produces an ear with satisfactory cosmetic appearance.

When topical antimicrobials are not sufficient to prevent suppurative chondritis, the painful and necrotic cartilage must be widely removed back to healthy cartilage, and any dead space obliterated: split-thickness skin grafts can be used to close the defect. If some cartilaginous framework is preserved, it can be used at a later stage as a framework for auricular reconstruction. The warning symptom of developing chondritis is pain: the uncomplicated burn of the ear is usually not overly painful, but when chondritis supervenes the pain becomes extreme, and can only be improved by surgical drainage.

When a clinical diagnosis of chondritis is made, surgery is undertaken as soon as possible. The suspect area is incised and any pus is drained, with culture to obtain a bacteriological diagnosis. Often the underlying cartilage is soft and frankly necrotic and is not difficult to remove. Careful undermining at the level of the subperichondrium with small scissors should be undertaken to debride back to healthy cartilage. On occasion, considerable undermining of soft tissue is needed to ensure that the remaining cartilage is viable. The wounds are initially left open for drainage. Secondary scarring will often produce a contracted ear of less than optimal cosmetic appearance. Contractions and scarring can partly be overcome by the use of a shaped tie-over mould of wool or foam to decrease the dead space following removal of cartilage, by opposing the anterior and posterior skin edges. It may be thus possible to obtain early healing and to decrease the amount of secondary scarring and deformity.

When the burn is severe, the external ear is completely destroyed (Fig. 17.7); it is then necessary to ensure that the patency of the external auditory meatus is maintained, and to offer an aural prosthesis at a later date.

Results and complications

With proper care, superficial dermal burns of the ear should heal spontaneously leaving a satisfactory result (Fig. 17.13). Small losses of tissue can be reconstructed with single or staged local flap reconstruction. Total loss of the external ear is difficult to reconstruct convincingly by surgery; it is possible, but the end result is

Fig. 17.14 (*Overleaf*) **Deformities produced by contraction of skin grafts.** Facial burns in association with 35% TBSA full-thickness body burns, complicated by respiratory burns requiring tracheostomy, following explosion of a cylinder of natural gas. Life-saving surgery required the treatment of the facial burn to be delayed. Despite grafting wound contraction produced skin shortage, causing ectropion and oral deformity.
A Necrosis of nasal skin and cartilage produced a typical deformity. **B** A release of bilateral upper eyelid ectropion was performed, with reconstruction using split-thickness skin from the upper arm. **C** The extent of correction. **D** A reconstruction of the nose was performed, using free lateral arm flap; this demonstrated the difficulties in matching the colour of the burned face with non-burned tissue.

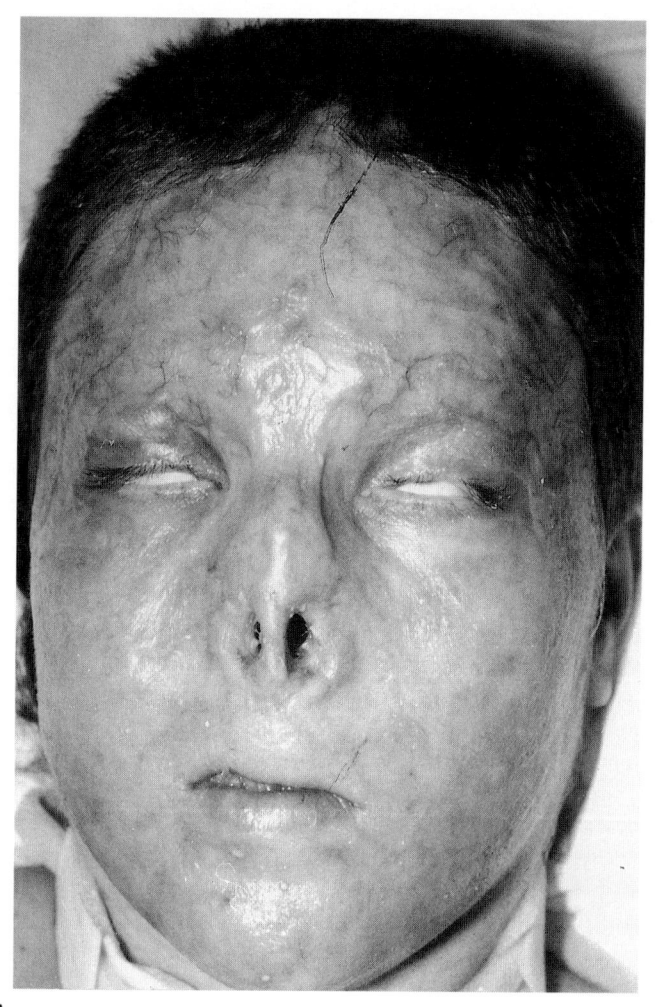

A

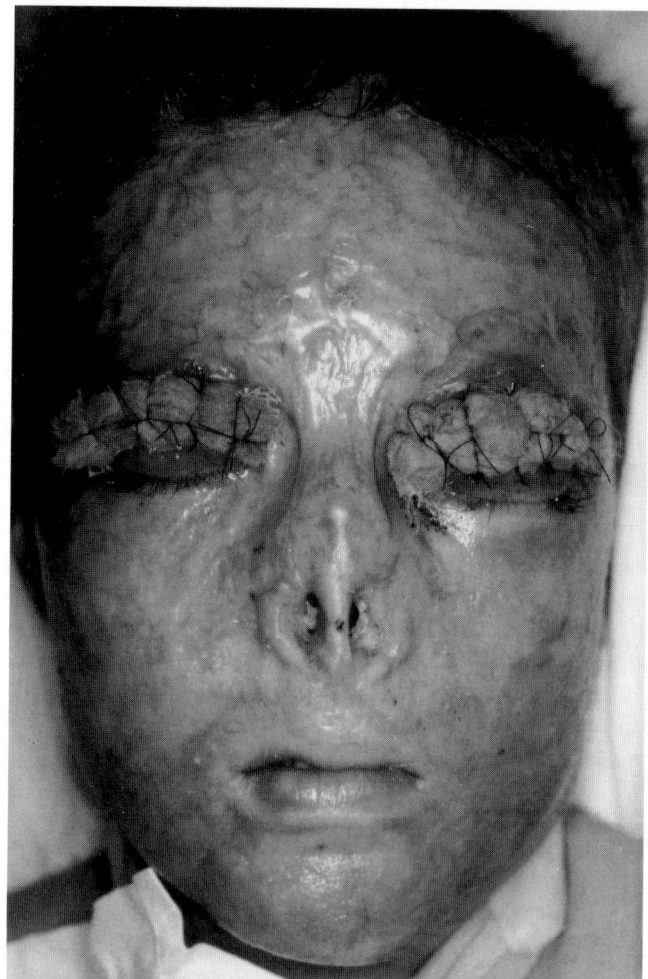

B

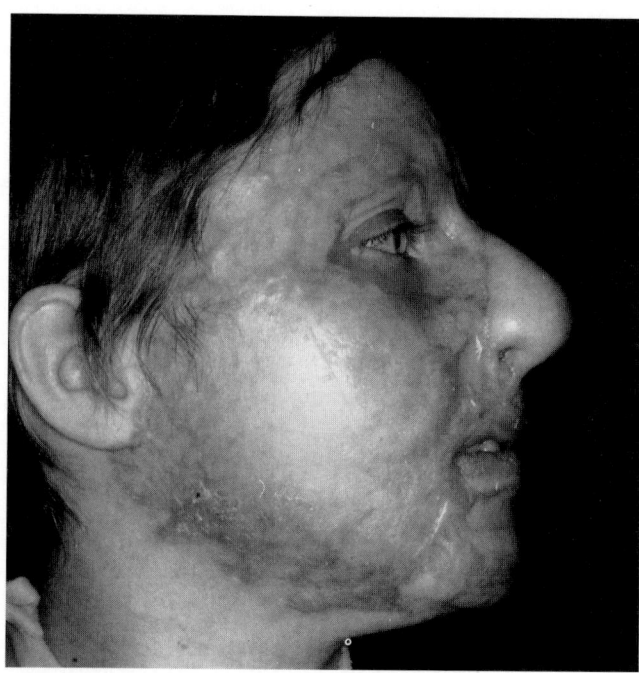

C

D

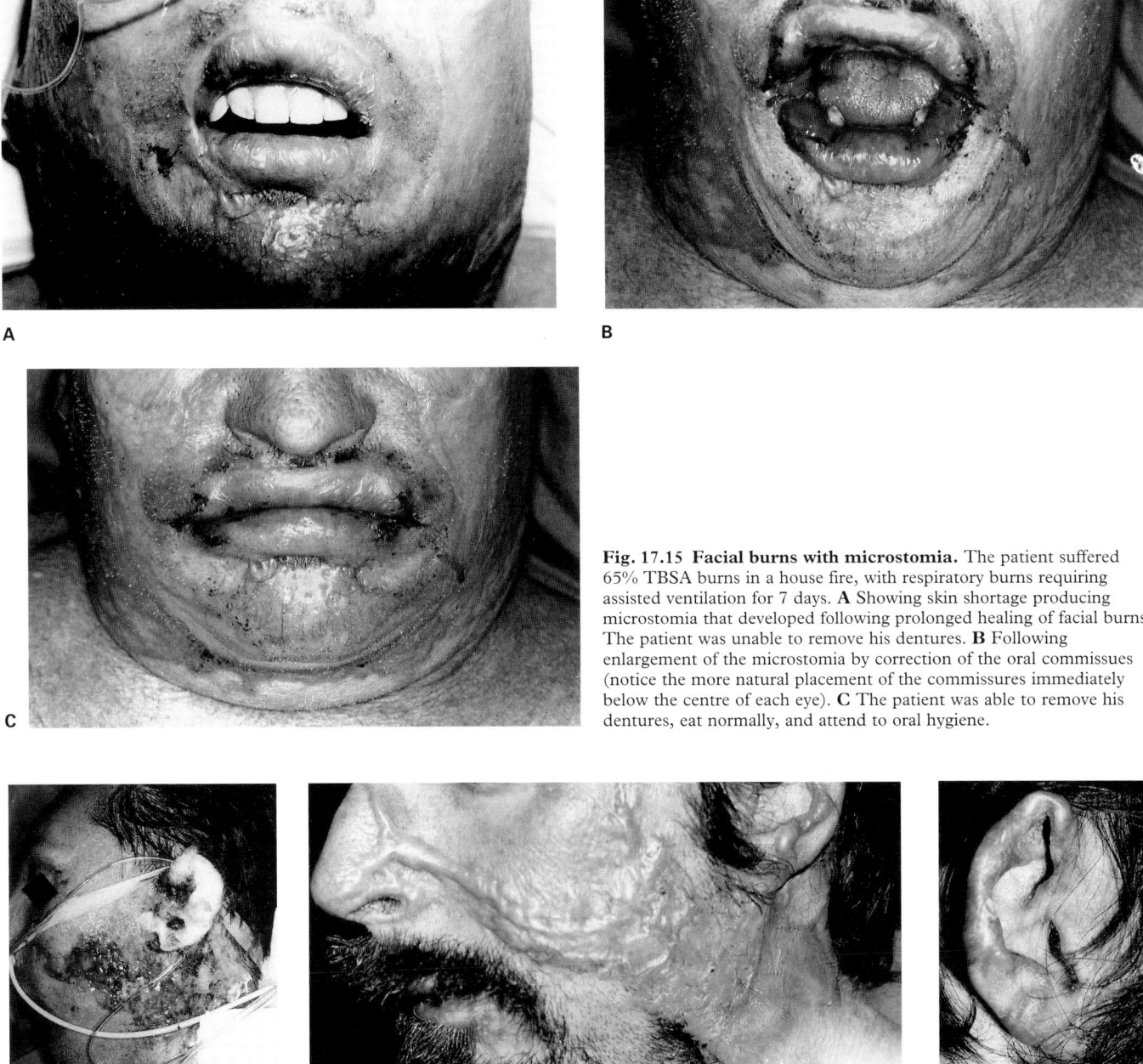

Fig. 17.15 Facial burns with microstomia. The patient suffered 65% TBSA burns in a house fire, with respiratory burns requiring assisted ventilation for 7 days. **A** Showing skin shortage producing microstomia that developed following prolonged healing of facial burns. The patient was unable to remove his dentures. **B** Following enlargement of the microstomia by correction of the oral commissures (notice the more natural placement of the commissures immediately below the centre of each eye). **C** The patient was able to remove his dentures, eat normally, and attend to oral hygiene.

Fig. 17.16 Hypertrophic scars following delayed surgery to facial burns. The patient suffered 55% TBSA petroleum burns to the head, neck, trunk and arms. He required mechanical ventilation, and the facial burns were treated by split-thickness skin grafting of the granulating burns of the nose and cheeks. Skin grafts were applied to the ears following debridement of necrotic skin and cartilage. **A** Showing the extent of the remaining unhealed granulating wound transgressing the boundaries of facial cosmetic units. **B** Showing hypertrophic scar extending across a number of cosmetic units, producing deformity and an unsightly appearance. A beard was grown to minimize the cosmetic deformity of burns elsewhere on the face, making the fitting of a compression mask impossible. **C** Showing the collapsed pinna following healing of skin graft to burns and early post-burn hypertrophic scar.

often poor and requires multiple surgical procedures. With the advent of osseo-integrated prostheses, a more appropriate reconstructive method is the use of a fixed external prosthesis (Eriksson & Vogt 1992). With the help of a skilled prosthetic technician these can be made most convincingly lifelike and are much more satisfactory in appearance than the total plastic surgical reconstruction.

BURNS OF THE NOSE

Surgical pathology

Isolated burns to the nose are uncommon. As a rule, a burn to the nose is less serious than a burn to the ear, because the skin of the nose is thicker and better supplied with sebaceous glands. A superficial or dermal nasal burn will often heal rapidly by epithelialization, usually producing an almost perfect cosmetic result. Burns of the nose are often associated with burns of the cheek and upper lip, and there may in addition be some loss of nasal lining and secondary loss of cartilaginous support of the nose, producing nasal and airway collapse.

Management

In our experience it has only been in severe burns of the whole face, often in association with full-thickness and serious burns of life-threatening proportion elsewhere, that the nose has been burned to the point where significant tissue destruction has occurred (Fig. 17.14). Treatment of the nasal burn then necessarily takes low priority. Under such circumstances we have treated the nasal burn along lines similar to those used for the external ear, using silver sulphadiazine with chlorhexidine digluconate while waiting for secondary wound healing to occur. We accept secondary healing with inevitable scarring and deformity, and undertake nasal reconstruction as an elective interval procedure.

As with burns to the ear, burns to the nose require careful and diligent attention to the burn wound. Skin grafting of a dermal burn of the nose is best undertaken as a cosmetic unit. Exposure of the alar cartilages may occur during tangential excision, and this part of the nose may be best excised carefully using direct excision at the level of the perichondrium, using a small scalpel blade. A thick split-thickness skin graft may provide less contraction if the whole nose is skin-grafted, and can provide an acceptable cosmetic result. Loss of nasal lining and cartilaginous support in a deep full-thickness burn will require secondary reconstruction. Nasal reconstruction in association with other facial burns is difficult, since the usual areas for obtaining tissue for nasal reconstruction in the severe burn are often lost (Fig. 17.14). Again, the reconstruction needs to pay particular attention to the cosmetic unit; the temptation to use a nasal flap reconstruction that does not sit directly at the junction of the nasal and facial cosmetic units will often lead to a less than optimal aesthetic result. The requirement to provide a thin flap of vascularized skin that can be sculptured to form the nose is difficult when most of the usual areas of available thin tissue have been lost in a widespread burn associated with severe and deep facial burns. The best expedient may then be a free flap, such as a lateral arm flap or a radial forearm flap in a relatively hairless person (Figs 17.12, 17.14 and 17.17). However, when facial burning has spared the forehead, a traditional Indian rhinoplasty with a central forehead flap may be used (Fig. 17.18); tissue expansion should permit direct closure of the donor skin defect.

BURNS OF THE FOREHEAD

Management

The forehead can be skin-grafted as a cosmetic unit after tangential excision; we have used scalp skin very successfully for this. Occasionally the forehead is burned very deeply, as when an unconscious patient falls into a fire or on to a hot object. If the periosteum of the skull has been damaged, a split-thickness skin graft cannot be applied. Rotation scalp flaps can be used on the crane principle (Millard 1969). In this, the flap is rotated to cover the defect, left for a week, and then split tangentially; the deep layer is left attached, and the superficial hairy layer is secondarily returned, with skin grafting on the remaining fat and soft tissue, which has by then acquired an adequate blood supply. In the past, tube pedicle grafts have been used (Fig. 17.7D); today, vascularized free flaps are sometimes used to reconstruct a forehead defect in a similar manner to their use in resurfacing large exposed areas of skull in full-thickness burns of the scalp. Tissue expansion (p. 583) provides another source of full-thickness skin, provided the neighbourhood skin is not itself burned.

BURNS OF THE SCALP, SKULL AND BRAIN

Surgical pathology

Burns to the scalp represented 13% of the burns to the head and neck in the series reported by Wachtel et al (1981). The scalp is often protected from thermal injury by the hair, and is rarely involved by thermal injuries associated with blast and explosion, which normally affect the face and anterior neck, since the victim is usually looking forwards when injured.

In patients with hair, the thick hair follicles of the scalp provide an excellent reservoir of epidermal cells. In partial-thickness scalp burns, epithelialization is often rapid and of good quality. This is enhanced by the excellent blood supply due to the extensive vascular plexus with copious anastomoses from front to back and across the midline, fed with large symmetrical named vessels from each side. The scalp can therefore be used with great benefit as a split-skin donor site, and when there are extensive burned areas elsewhere, with few surviving donor sites, the scalp can be harvested repeatedly at 10–14 day intervals. Admittedly, repeated harvesting can

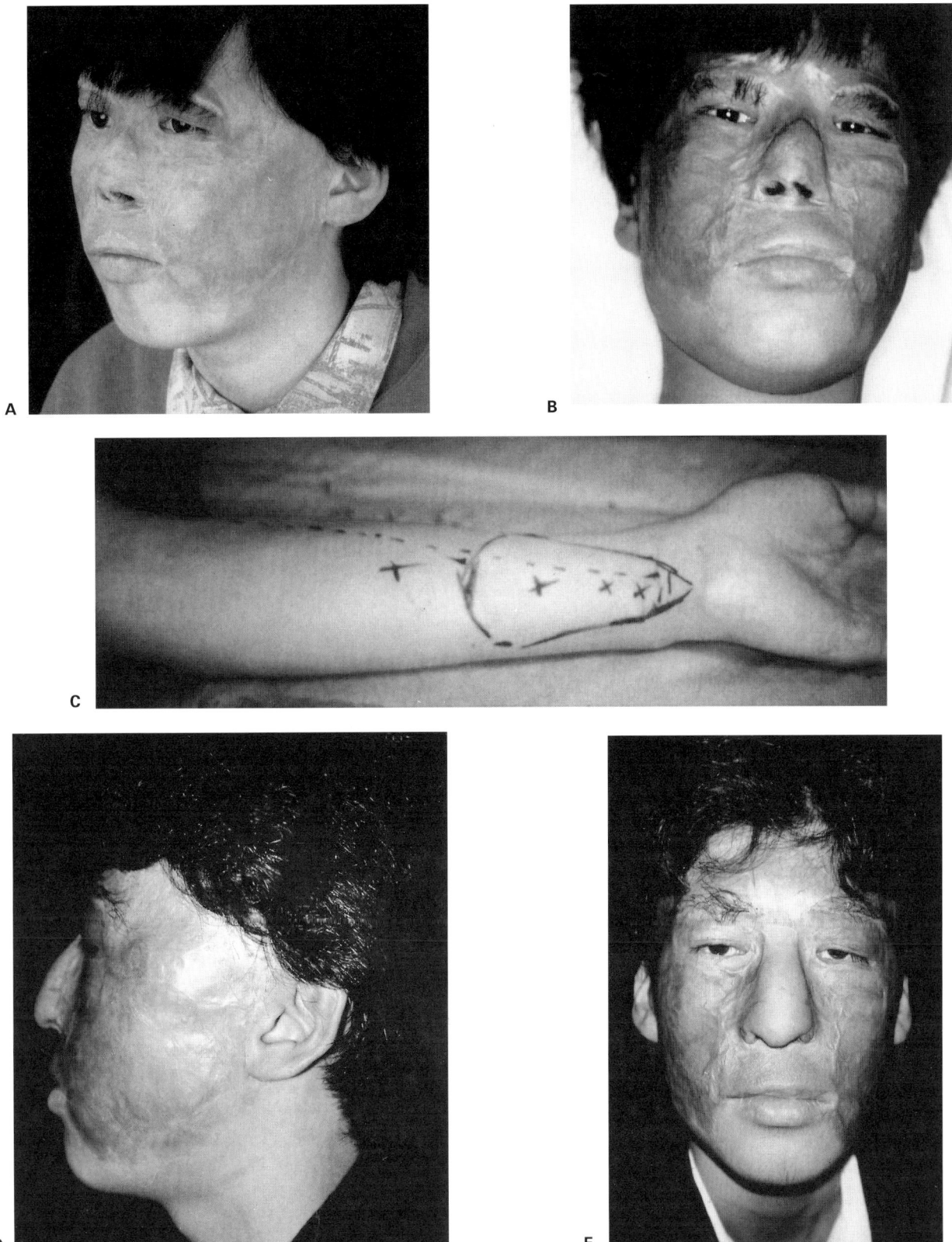

Fig. 17.17 Flame burns requiring rhinoplasty. A 14-year-old boy from another country suffered flame burns as a child. A nasal reconstruction was carried out, using an ulnar forearm free flap. **A,B** Preoperative view of the nose. **C** The free flap design based on the ulnar artery. **D** Postoperative view of the nose: profile view. **E** Postoperative view of the nose: anterior–posterior view. The eyebrows were originally grafted in another country but the result was considered aesthetically unacceptable. The grafts were removed and new composite scalp (hair-bearing) grafts were inserted.

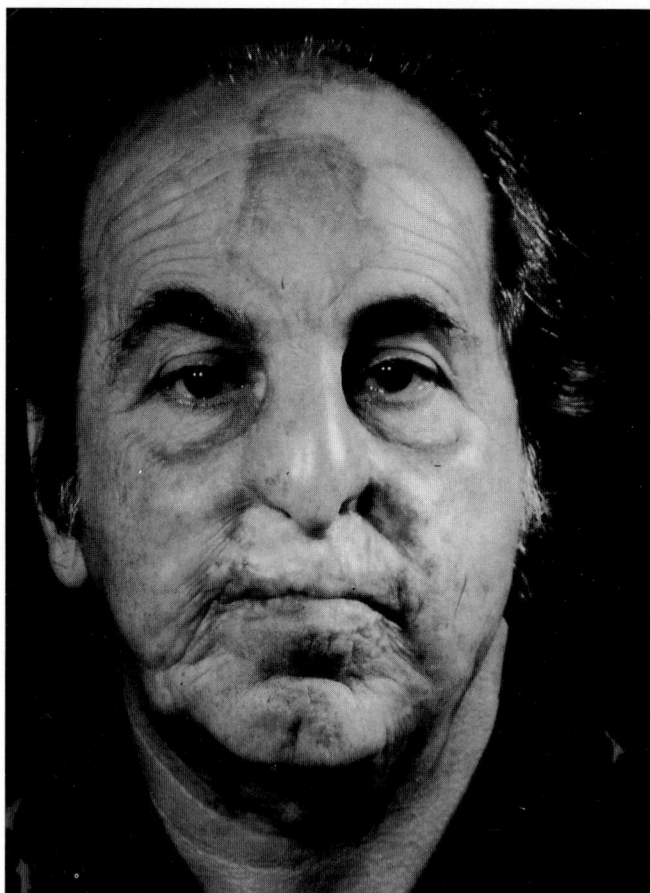

Fig. 17.18 Indian rhinoplasty for radiation burn. This traditional method of nasal reconstruction can be used when the forehead has not been burned. A central forehead or Indian rhinoplasty was performed on one of our patients by Sir Harold Gillies, for fulminating radiation burns caused by overzealous radiation of a benign skin condition. Because like skin was used to cover the burned area, a satisfactory colour match was obtained, the result confirms that a pleasing appearance can be obtained with traditional methods.

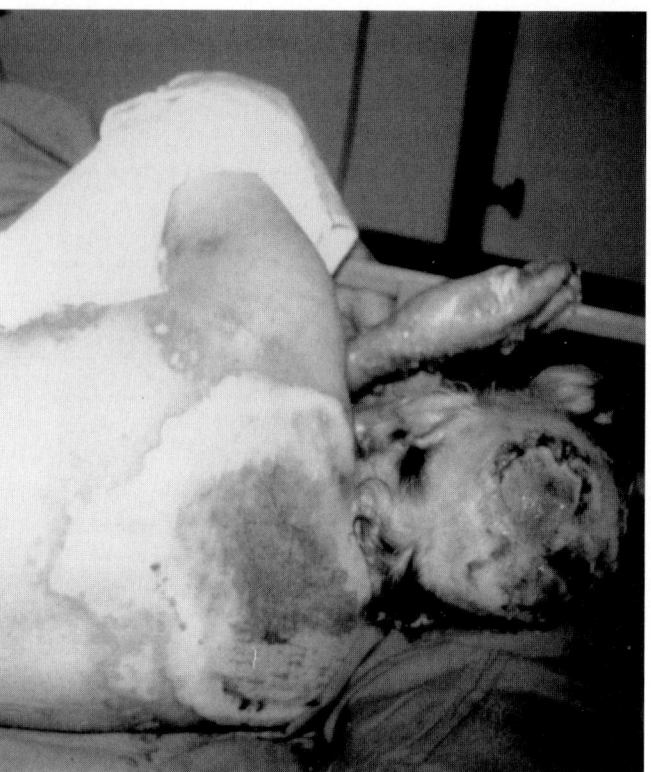

Fig. 17.19 Full-thickness scalp burns. An intoxicated person, resident in a nursing home, sustained flame burns down to the calvaria. After debridement, the defect was repaired with a transposed anterior scalp flap.

cause damage to hair follicles, leading to alopecia (Brou et al 1990), and this is more likely to occur when the scalp itself has healed after superficial burns.

Healing may be delayed in severe burns to the scalp at the extremes of age, due partly to the often thin scalp in the young and the elderly, and also to the sparse hair follicles in young children and elderly patients of both sexes. Adnexal structures may be fewer in these two age groups, so that epithelialization does not occur readily. In addition, burns may be sufficiently deep to cause necrosis of skin and pericranium, exposing the outer table of the skull (Fig. 17.19). Very severe or prolonged thermal injury may devitalize the full thickness of the skull and damage the underlying meninges and brain.

Management

In the presence of a severe burn of the scalp, definitive reconstruction may be difficult from lack of normal vascu-larized tissue as a result of the surrounding burns. When the pericranium is not involved, it may be possible to perform tangential excision of the burned scalp, and to cover the excised area with split-thickness skin. This will result in a bald patch, which can later be excised, closure with full-thickness scalp being facilitated by a subcutane-ous expander. Paletta (1982) advised grafting when the burned area of scalp is >4.5 cm in diameter, even when there is potential for spontaneous re-epithelialization, because of the messy inconvenience of a slowly healing wound in a hair-bearing area.

In very severe burns of the scalp, and in particular high tension electrical burns, in which skull and intra-cranial contents are burned, the same principles of debri-dement and closure apply. Devitalized areas of frontal skull should be carefully removed, and skin grafts can be placed on the dura, as a temporary measure (Fig. 17.7). Alternatively free microvascular cutaneous or myocutaneous flaps may be used to undertake immediate reconstruction (Fig. 17.20). Secondary calvarial reconstructive cranio-plasty is usually undertaken at a second stage as part of long-term reconstruction (p. 548). In these difficult cases, combined neurosurgical and plastic surgical management provides the necessary multidisciplinary expertise.

When the calvarial bone appears to be necrotic, we believe that neurosurgical debridement should not be delayed unduly. In the past, a more conservative approach was often accepted: the exposed calvaria was allowed to exfoliate, or was explored only after many weeks, in the hope that the inner table would remain viable. It was then usual to chisel away the necrotic outer table and to apply split-thickness skin grafts to the granulating diplöe. This method was attempted by us in an infant with severe multiple burns (Fig. 17.7); during the period of delay, a large extradural abscess formed under the frontal bone and although this did not lead to intradural infection, it was potentially a dangerous lesion. It is now our preferred policy to explore the burned calvaria early, no later than 2 weeks, when viability should be evident but before deeper infection is likely. Computed tomography (CT) or preferably magnetic resonance imaging (MRI) should first be done to assess the state of the underlying meninges and brain, and especially the venous sinuses. Debridement begins with trial burrholes in the centre of the suspect bone; if there is no diploic bleeding, the burrhole is enlarged with rongeurs until viable bone is found. If there is reason to believe that the inner table is viable but the outer table necrotic, then the outer table can be removed with a chisel or osteotome; this technique is more time-consuming than the use of a high-speed burr, but is less likely to imperil viability of bone. The dura is not opened, even if it appears to be necrotic, unless there is already clinical or radiological evidence of an intradural abscess. When the bone debridement is complete, the defect is closed with full-thickness skin. Where possible, this is done by advancing or rotating a scalp flap. But this may be impossible and, if this is so, a free myocutaneous graft should be employed. Cranioplasty is deferred until wound healing is complete and the risk of infection is minimal; in practice, a delay of at least 3 months is wise. We have chosen to use rib or calvarial bone grafts for the cranioplasty, rather than a titanium plate, despite the lower protective value of split ribs and their occasional tendency to resorb over time.

Alopecia

Scalp burns may result in alopecia, which may also result from the use of scalp for skin grafts and from closure of scalp defects with flaps from other parts of the body. McCauley et al (1990) have classified the various types of post-burn alopecia and related the anatomy of the alopecia to treatment. When the alopecia is localized and associated with areas of scalp that are unburned, or have healed well, tissue expansion may provide enough hairy scalp to allow excision and closure of the bald area. Patchy global alopecia is not amenable to reconstruction, and in using the scalp as a donor site, the likely aesthetic disfigurement should be balanced against the utility of the grafts in cases needing split skin where other donor sites are lacking.

ELECTRICAL BURNS

Incidence

Electrical burns are a relatively frequent cause of burning in the scalp, largely because of the exposed nature of the head and neck. Monafo & Creekmore (1984) stated that electrical injuries generally account for 3–5% of all admissions to burns centres. Burning may be due to high tension flashes; the scalp may be the site of entrance or exit of electric current. In some countries, lightning strike is the most common source of electrical burns, followed by contact with high tension wires and lastly problems with electrocution from faulty household appliances; however, the incidence of lightning strike is to some extent dependent on climatic conditions, and the incidence of electrocution reflects local safety standards.

Surgical pathology

The effects of electric trauma are firstly flash injury, secondly thermal injury, and lastly more complex physico-chemical changes. The voltages producing burns vary. Electrical injuries are arbitrarily divided into high voltage (> 1000 V) and low voltage. Lightning is direct current with potentials of 1 000 000 000 V or more, and currents up to 200 000 amps. High tension lines have potentials in the range 6600–350 000 V, or even higher (Monafo & Creekmore 1984). Household currents vary between 110 and 415 V in different parts of the world (p. 116). Industrial current is commonly 3-phase a.c. at 415 V.

Electrical injury may be produced by a flash burn, such as a spark from an ionized atmosphere, often found near high tension junctions or fuse boxes, or may result from conduction of current. The effects of current conduction depend on whether the burn is inflicted by alternating or direct current; the skin conductivity is also important and this is determined by skin thickness, moisture and the presence or absence of hair. Initial skin resistance is high, but with continued application of current the resistance decreases, resulting in a surging flow of current. All tissues are conductive but their resistances vary: nerve tissue shows least resistance and bone greatest. The body acts as a volume conductor and current passage causes heating; the heated tissue transmits heat to neighbouring structures. Superficial tissues cool more quickly and this accounts for the finding of more severe burning deeply in proximity to bone; the extent of skin damage therefore does not correlate with the damage found in deep tissues.

In general, the same pathological processes occur as in ordinary thermal burns. However, it must be remembered that at the point of entry, intensely high temperatures are developed, up to 3000°C, but affecting only a very small area. A zone of charring and mummification can often be seen (Fig. 17.20A); in an ordinary thermal burn this would be associated with a lethal injury. Similarly, the zone of demarcation is much better defined, and the characteristic oedema of the thermal burn is much decreased. Unlike a true thermal burn, however, the heat is generated around the point of entry, resulting in much deeper burns that often track along deep tissue planes. Thus, the full extent of the damage may not be fully evident for some time. There is also a degree of cellular physicochemical disruption of the body as a whole which is not yet understood. The most obvious example of these is the disruption to the normal ordered electrical activity of the myocardium and of the brainstem, but more subtle effects have been noted.

Electrical burns may involve only the soft tissues of the scalp or face, but burning may penetrate to the calvaria which may suffer necrosis of the outer table, or even full-thickness bony loss. Further electric current damage may involve the meninges and produce necrosis of part of the underlying brain (see case report).

Neurological effects

The neurological sequelae of electric injury vary in severity from transient loss of consciousness and post-injury confusion, to varying degrees of permanent motor damage including spasticity, paralysis, hemiplegia, obtundation and acute seizures. Late epilepsy may result from scarring subsequent to healed burns. Uncomfortable radiculopathies or neuropathies may occur. The neurological effects of lightning are especially devastating, and may include multifocal intracerebral haemorrhages (Stanley & Suss 1985).

Ocular effects

Situated as it is, the eye is rarely a source of direct contact in an electrical burn. The usual entry and exit points are on the extremities but entry and exit points on the head are not uncommon and sometimes involve the eye in the thermal fringe of the electrical field. The hair and eyelashes are singed and coagulated and there is swelling with oedema and chemosis of the lids and conjunctiva. Conjunctival haemorrhages are often seen. The tarsal plates are relatively resistant to the current but perforation is known, with subsequent lagophthalmos of the upper lid. The cornea may develop interstitial opacities which can be punctate, striate or diffuse. The cornea develops generalized cloudiness and oedema with superficial exfoliation, ulceration and necrosis, leading to secondary ocular perforation. Iridocyclitis is common and

may be mild or severe, transient or recurrent. Synechiae to either the cornea or the lens may occur. The ciliary muscle is often disrupted and may go into spasm. The zonule supporting the lens can also be disrupted, resulting in wobbliness of the lens (phakodonesis). Characteristic electrical cataracts can develop from high tension shock: these are mainly subcapsular, both anterior and posterior and consist of fluid-filled vacuoles. Later, scale-like grey opacities may appear in the capsule itself. The subcapsular lens cortex shows changes varying from indefinite haze to densely crowded punctate opacities appearing as greyish-white linear streaks that bear little resemblance to lens fibre architecture. The retina and choroid are not often affected but can show retinal oedema, papilloedema and haemorrhages. Peripheral lesions resembling traumatic chorioretinitis may lead to secondary patchy chorioretinal atrophy. Tears in the retina and choroid can occur leading to retinal detachment and blindness.

Management

Initial care should include cardiac monitoring. Most patients who survive high voltage electrical injury show cardiac dysrhythmia or ECG changes and in our unit these patients are routinely monitored by ECG for at least 24 h. ECG changes may only consist of mild ST segment abnormalities but conduction of current through the heart muscle may produced appearances associated with muscle damage or even myocardial infarction.

Electrical burns of the scalp can be treated by tangential excision along the general lines of burn management set out above. When the electrical burn includes necrosis of bone, we have considered it necessary to excise non-viable bone and to cover the area with a free microvascularized myocutaneous flap. In one case it was even thought necessary to resect necrotic dura and a thrombosed sagittal sinus (Fig. 17.20B–E); the reasons for this radical procedure are set out in the case report, and the operation was well tolerated. Worthen (1982) has advocated a more conservative approach: impressed by the capacity of calvarial bone to regenerate, he has been prepared to cover necrotic bone with a vascularized scalp flap and to await events. Fear of intracranial infection has made us favour the more radical plan of cranial and even dural debridement; perhaps the availability of MRI will make this unnecessary.

Ocular injuries are treated along the lines set out in Chapter 14; the late development of cataracts often makes lens extraction necessary.

Electrical burn in the frontal region, causing thrombosis of sagittal sinus and bilateral cataracts: a case report.

A 38-year-old tip-truck driver struck a high-tension power cable, and received electric current at an estimated potential of 11 000 V. The entry burn was in the forehead, the exit burn in the left lower leg. He was initially drowsy but responded to commands; he had amnesia of some hours' duration before and after the event. There was a full-thickness burn of the entire forehead, exposing the outer table of the skull in an area 4 × 6 cm in the midline. The left shin was also deeply burned. There were superficial burns of the dorsal surfaces of both hands. The total burned area was estimated to be 15%, and appropriate resuscitation was given, also intravenous penicillin.

The eyes were at first closed by swelling; when they could be examined, there appeared to be complete clouding of corneal epithelium on the right and patchy clouding on the left. However, by day 8, the corneas had cleared, and vision was 6/12 on the right, 6/5 on the left. The fundi appeared normal. On day 6, the leg burn was excised to expose healthy muscle; the tibia and patellar tendon appeared partially necrotic. On day 13, dead frontal bone was removed, exposing the anterior third of the sagittal sinus, which appeared thrombosed; parts of the adjacent dura appeared necrotic. The frontal air sinus was necessarily opened in the debridement. The skin margins were excised and the area was covered with a free groin flap based on the superficial circumflex iliac artery. A cephalic vein graft was placed to drain the flap into the left external jugular vein; arterial supply was established from the left superficial temporal artery by direct anastomosis. Good perfusion was achieved. Postoperatively, CT scan showed low density changes in the brain in the vicinity of the sagittal sinus and loss of the frontal cortical sulcal pattern.

On day 27, the cranial burn was re-explored. Further dead bone was removed until diploic bleeding was seen; eventually a craniectomy 10 cm in diameter was made. There was extradural pus under the foul-smelling bone, from which *E. Coli* and a Klebsiella organism were cultured. It was considered that the CT scan findings indicated a significant risk of subdural infection under the necrotic avascular dura and it was felt that the thrombosed and potentially infected sinus could be removed without risk to the frontal lobes.

Therefore, a 7 cm length of thrombosed sagittal sinus was excised together with the adjacent dura mater. The exposed cerebral cortex was inflamed and swollen; it was irrigated with antibiotic solution. The dural defect was closed with a piece of fascia lata.

This operation was well tolerated. Serial CT scans showed no evidence of abscess formation. On day 39, the burn of the left tibia, which extended through most of the cortex, was excised and covered with a gastrocnemius myocutaneous flap.

On day 49, a complaint of impaired vision in the right eye (6/36) was recorded; ophthalmoscopy showed iritis with a nuclear cataract formation. Extracapsular lens extraction was performed 3 months after injury. Eventually, with a contact lens, 6/6 vision was achieved. A cataract later appeared on the left side. Pterygia developed in both eyes, requiring excision and radiotherapy on the right side.

A cranioplasty was performed 11 months after injury. Three rib segments, each 10–11 cm, were used to cover completely the dural defect under the muscle graft. The rib grafts were wired together and to the margins of the skull defect using the chain link technique. This gave a satisfactory aesthetic result. The scalp flap was later revised and a composite graft was inserted into the right eyebrow. Three years after injury, an intraocular lens was inserted on the left side, and five years after injury this was also done on the right side. Eventually good vision was achieved in both aphakic eyes.

There was clinical and radiological suspicion of resorption of bone in the centre of the cranioplasty. There were problems relating to depression, poor concentration, poor memory and a perceived change in personality. Psychometric evaluation did not indicate any serious cognitive impairment. (Case report by courtesy of Mr P. E. Oatey)

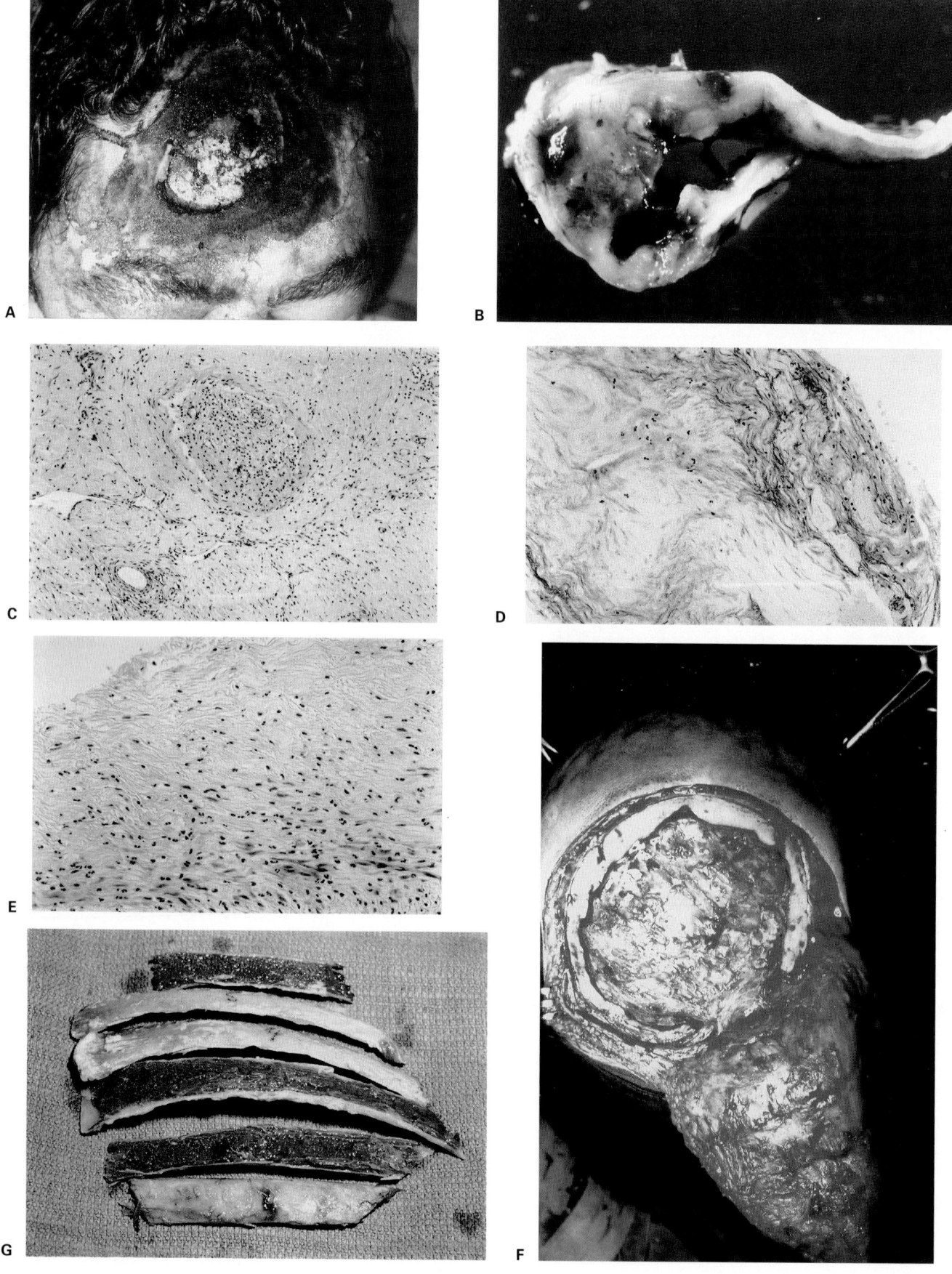

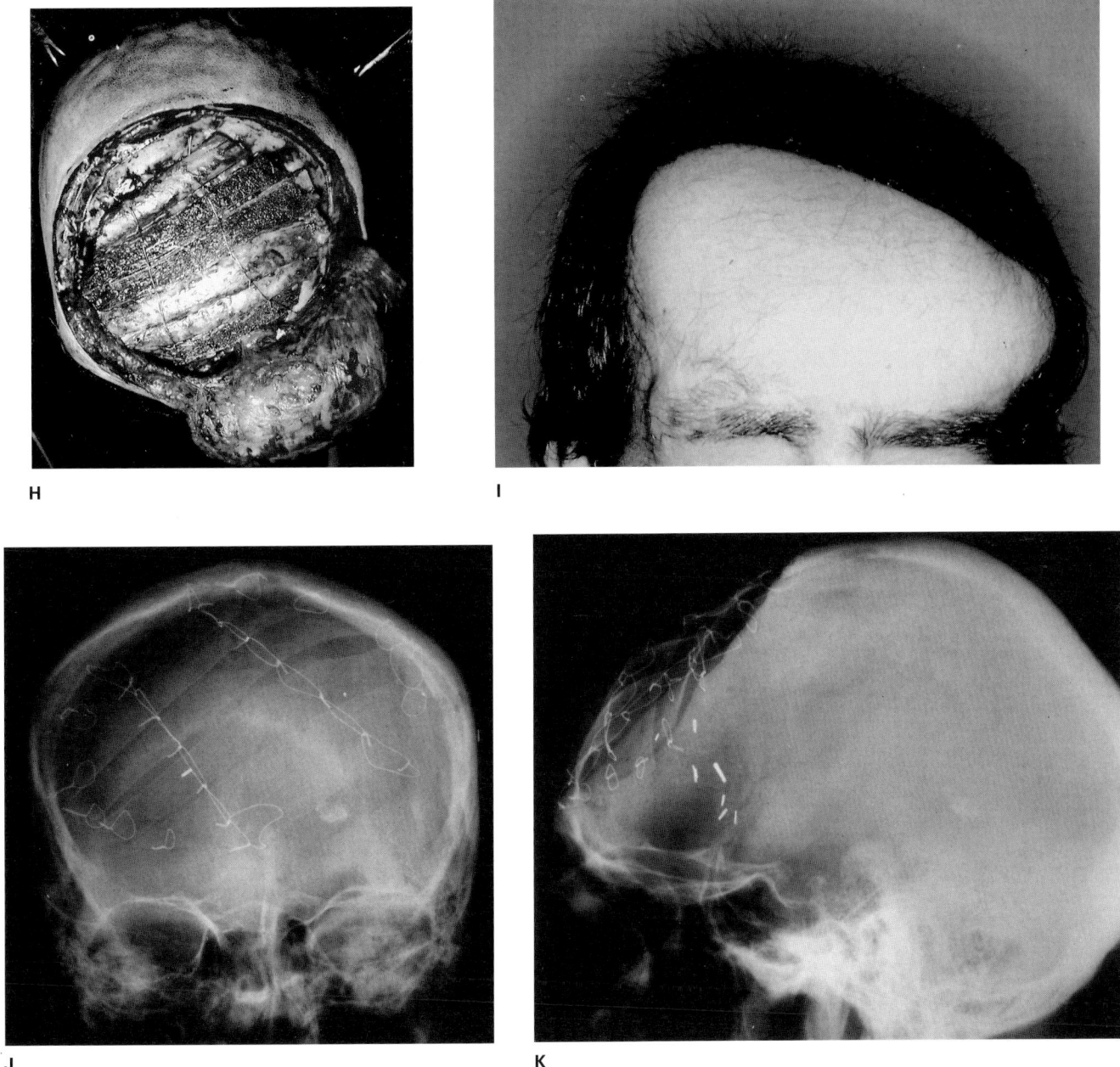

Fig. 17.20 A The frontal burn, with exposed skull. **B** Day 27: the excised sagittal sinus in cross section, flanked by thickened dura. **C** Histological examination of the sinus showed that the thrombosis was partially revascularized; smaller vessels also showed organized thrombosis. H&E × 95. **D** Histological examination of necrotic dura showed masses of denatured collagen with no obvious inflammatory reaction. H&E × 190. **E** In other areas, the dura looked viable, with an inflammatory reaction on the external surface. H&E × 190. **F** 11 months post-burn: the myocutaneous flap was well established. **G & H** Rib cranioplasty. **I** Final appearance of forehead. **J, K** Final appearance of cranioplasty.

POST-BURN DEFORMITIES

Surgical pathology

Burns to the face have always provided some of the most horrific cosmetic deformities particularly when healing is prolonged and hypertrophic burn scar is produced. Scarring is extremely likely to occur in facial burns that do not heal within a 3 week period following burning (Figs 17.16 and 17.21). This underlies the rationale for early excision and grafting of facial burns in selected patients, as discussed above (p. 472).

In addition to the deformity produced by loss of tissue in burning, the secondary scarring that may occur in association with prolonged wound healing of untreated deep facial burns, or the contraction of skin grafts used to heal such burns, may produce distortion of soft tissue and loss of normal anatomical boundaries. It is these two factors which produce the most significant disfigurement associated with facial burns. Early and effective treatment of these burns with particular reference to the anatomical units must be undertaken to minimize the secondary disfigurement that will otherwise occur.

Late growth deformity

Burns in children produce deformity because of acute loss of tissue and contraction of hypertrophic post-burn scars, but considerable additional deformity may be produced by distorted growth. It is well known that normal tissue growth outstrips the capacity for growth of skin grafts and scar, and so disparity between these two growth rates will produce progressive secondary deformity. In the face this is seen most particularly in the neck, around the mouth and nasolabial regions, and around the eyes (Fig. 17.8).

Thus, in addition to the deformity due to contraction of scar and skin grafts, the secondary disturbances produced by restricted growth and by the loss of functioning facial musculature, and sometimes by the pressure of masks used to modify hypertrophic post-burn scar (Fricke et al 1992), will combine to cause impaired craniofacial growth in children, often resulting in gross deformity. Inadequately treated deep facial and neck burns in childhood may produce long-term secondary growth disturbance causing severe anomalies in craniofacial morphology; conversely, anatomical distortions caused by secondary bone deformity further compound the soft-tissue disturbance (Katsaros et al 1990). We have treated several young adults burned during childhood, who had suffered gross secondary bony and other facial deformities in sequel to soft-tissue loss and scarring, who later required sophisticated soft-tissue and bony reconstructions to maximize cosmetic and functional recovery.

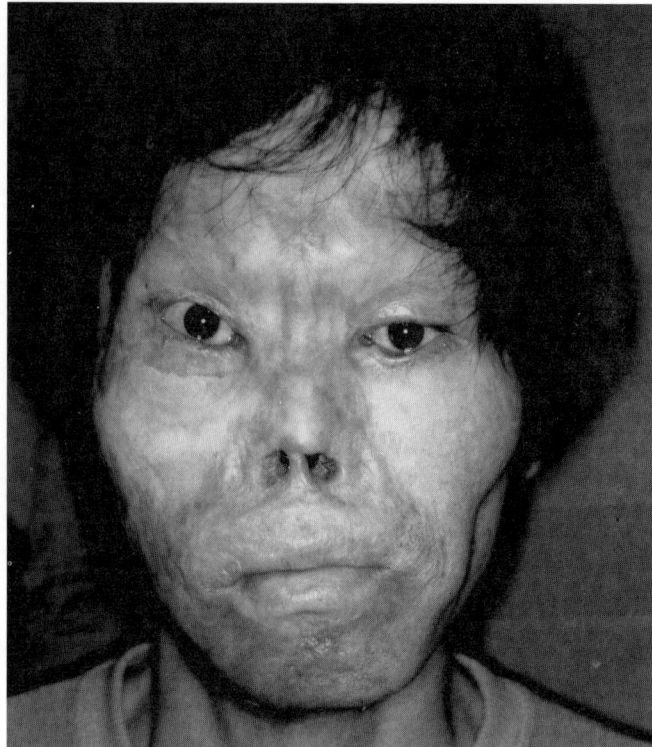

Fig. 17.21 Outcome of conservative treatment with small skin grafts. This man underwent spontaneous healing, supplemented by application of small, non-cosmetic skin grafts. The aesthetic result was poor and he subsequently underwent free flap nasal reconstruction.

Assessment

Accurate assessment of the extent of the deformity is necessary and this can be undertaken satisfactorily by simple measurement in the case of soft-tissue deformity. Secondary disturbance of bone growth and distortion of articulating structures will require integrated planning similar to that undertaken by the multidisciplinary cranio-facial surgery team (p. 234). Three-dimensional CT scan reconstructions provide a visual reproduction of the extent of bone loss or deformity. An integrated planning approach that assesses the deformity, and then step by step sets out to undertake a regime of soft-tissue release and reconstruction, together with appropriate bony reconstruction, gives the best chance of reconstructing the total deformity of the burned child.

Periodic review of growth disturbances may be required; the reconstructive inventory described by Brou et al (1989) is an excellent way of assessing the ongoing nature of the problem, and documenting progress so that an appropriate time for surgery can be selected. As noted above, the reconstructive goals of the surgeon are often in excess of the needs of the patient or the family (Bjarnason et al 1992); these needs must be expressed, discussed and carefully recorded, so that the most appropriate treatment is provided.

Management

The ability to undertake massive one-stage reconstructions, by utilizing modern microvascular and craniofacial techniques of rigid fixation and by importing appropriately large amounts of well-vascularized soft tissue, can be used to great effect but only if planning is done properly (Fig. 17.8). In addition to the aesthetically successful benefits of these reconstructive endeavours, considerable economic advantages have accrued from one-stage reconstructions. For those patients who live remotely from the treating institution, a single one-stage massive reconstruction often provides the only chance for reconstruction, as subsequent transport to the treating institution may be financially impossible. This has been especially evident in those patients referred to us from developing countries.

These massive reconstructive efforts require appropriate anaesthetic and intensive care services to implement the complicated surgical management protocol. Without appropriate anaesthetic support, surgery — however well conceived — is not likely to succeed. Psychosocial support and counselling are also essential (see p. 258).

Conclusions

Underlying all burns reconstruction, whether early or elective, are the timeless reconstructive principles of Sir Harold Gillies of 'recreation of the original deformity' and 'placement of all normal tissues in their correct positions'. In the acute burn, management aims to facilitate spontaneous healing if this is possible. If this is not possible, acute reconstruction by tangential excision and skin grafting is undertaken. As in all reconstructions, like tissue is used if at all possible. The scalp offers good quality skin; skin from other sites, such as the limbs, matches the face poorly in colour and texture, and should not be used except where total facial resurfacing is done. Skin grafting after an acute burn will produce an obvious deformity if the burn is not excised and replaced as a whole cosmetic unit (Fig. 17.9), and, despite distortion of the cosmetic units by severe scarring, it is possible to produce a much more homogeneous appearance in the forehead, cheeks and skin when the boundaries of these units are respected.

The use of like tissue remains important at all stages in the reconstruction. Thus, the Indian forehead flap rhinoplasty pleases because the colour match is excellent. In the past, the forehead donor site was conspicuous (Fig. 17.18) but tissue expansion now answers this aesthetic objection; the match is better than when a free flap from the ulnar forearm is used (Fig. 17.17). As in acute excisions of burns, the principle of covering cosmetic units applies also in secondary reconstructions. In nasal reconstructions, the junctions of the cheek and nasal cosmetic units should be respected. In the free vascularized flap shown in Fig. 17.14, there was insufficient tissue available from the lateral arm — the only relatively hairless skin available — to cover the nasal cosmetic unit completely, and the result was less than satisfactory. Later trimming and advancement of the flap improved this appearance markedly.

After acute reconstruction, post-burn hypertrophic scar may compromise both the appearance and the facial functions; good scar management is needed to optimize the natural improvement that comes with scar maturation. Therefore, secondary surgical reconstruction should if possible wait until the scar has matured. This may always not be possible and it is sometimes necessary to excise immature scar when function is compromised.

From the functional viewpoint, untethering the facial musculature allows the return of expressive facial movement. The illustrations in this chapter show the advantages of resurfacing the facial muscles with full-thickness skin (Fig. 17.9). In contrast, a free vascularized flap reconstruction (Fig. 17.12) may by its bulk mask facial expression. Severe tissue destruction may make a free flap necessary; if so, a thin vascularized flap from the ulnar forearm (Fig. 17.17) or a flap vascularized by the dorsalis pedis artery may provide the best possible result.

All reconstructive strategies entail excision of scar, recreation of the original defects, and quantitation of the skin, subcutaneous tissue, bone, cartilage and muscular defects. The defects must then be replaced, perhaps by application of a soft tissue flap, and/or a mixture of grafts and flaps of lining material and skin, together with the importation of appropriate amounts of skeletal support in the form of microvascularized or non-vascularized bone grafts. In cases where regional shortage of tissue has occurred as a result of severe burning both of the face and elsewhere, the associated regional tissue shortage may be increased by the use of part of the tissue to reconstruct other parts of the face, and this may potentiate the seriousness of the secondary defect. This additional lack of tissue in the secondary defect may of itself require sophisticated reconstruction.

Management of severe facial burns is difficult and often frustrating. The emotional importance of the face makes it essential to strive for an optimal aesthetic result, but by the nature of the injury, some deformity is inevitable. There may be conflicting management priorities, such as the claims of associated burns or other injuries elsewhere in the body, or the requirements of hypertrophic scar maturation. Management requires meticulous attention to detail — and throughout attention to the principles of reconstruction with which Gillies' name will always be associated.

REFERENCES

Abercrombie M, Flint M H, James D W 1954 Collagen formation and wound contraction during repair of small excised wounds in the skin of rats. J Embryology Exp Morphology 2: 264–274

Achauer B M 1990 Burn reconstruction. Thieme, New York, p 69

Alpert S, Levenson S M 1970 Respiratory tract injury associated with burns. NY J Med 70: 1633–1637

Alvarez O M, Mertz P M, Eaglestein W H 1983 The effect of occlusive dressings on collagen synthesis and re-epithelialization in superficial wounds. J Surg Res 35: 142–148

Baxter C R, Shires T 1968 Physiological response to crystalloid resuscitation of severe burns. Ann NY Acad Sci 150: 874–894

Bjarnason D, Phillips L G, McCoy B et al 1992 Reconstructive goals for children with burns: are our goals the same? J Burn Care Rehabil 13: 389–390

Boswick J A 1973 Burns of the head and neck. Surg Clin North Am 53: 97–104

Brou J A, Robson M C, McCauley R L et al 1989 Inventory of potential reconstructive needs in the patient with burns. J Burn Care Rehabil 10: 555–560

Brou J A, Vu T, McCauley R L et al 1990 The scalp as a donor site revisited. J Trauma 30: 579–581

Carruthers R 1978 Airway complications of burns in children. Med J Aust 11: 258

Converse J M, McCarthy J G, Dobrkovsky M, Larson D L 1977 Facial burns. In: Converse J M, McCarthy J G (eds) Reconstructive plastic surgery, 2nd edn. Saunders, Philadelphia, Ch 33

Cope O, Rhinelander F W 1943 The problem of burn shock complicated by pulmonary damage. Ann Surg 117: 915–928

Davies L K, Poulton T J, Modell J H 1983 Continuous positive airway pressure is beneficial in treatment of smoke inhalation. Crit Care Med 11: 726–729

DiVincenti F C, Pruitt B A Jr, Reckler J M 1971 Inhalation injuries. J Trauma 11: 109–117

Engrav L H, Heimbach D M, Walkinshaw M D, Marvin J A 1986 Excision of burns of the face. Plast Reconstr Surg 77: 744–751

Engrav L H, MacDonald L B, Corey M H, Heimbach D M, Marvin J M 1983 Do splinting and pressure devices damage new grafts? J Burn Care Rehabil 4: 107–108

Eriksson E, Vogt P M 1992 Ear reconstruction. Clin Plast Surg 19: 637–644

Feller I, Richards K E 1979 Early management of the face and lips. In: Feller I, Grabb W C (eds) Reconstruction and rehabilitation of the burned patient. National Institute for Burn Medicine, Ann Arbor, p 182

Foley F D, Moncrief J A, Mason A D Jr 1968 Pathology of the lung in fatally burned patients. Ann Surg 167: 251–264

Fowler D, Pegg S P 1986 Modified microstomia prevention splint. Burns 12: 371–373

Fricke N, Dutcher K, Omtel L, Engrav L, Hollender L 1992 Effects of pressure garment wear on facial and dental development. Proc Am Burn Assoc 24: 15

Gillies H, Millard D R 1957 The principles and art of plastic surgery. Little Brown & Co., Boston

Gonzalez-Ulloa M 1956 Restoration of the face covering by means of selected skin in regional aesthetic units. Br J Plast Surg 9: 212–221

Goodwin C W, Dorethy J, Lam V et al 1983 Randomized trial of efficacy of crystalloid and colloid resuscitation on hemodynamic response and lung water following thermal injury, with discussion by C R Baxter, F T Caldwell and W W Monafo. Ann Surg 197: 520–531

Gorman D F, Clayton D, Gilligan J E, Webb R K 1992 A longitudinal study of 100 consecutive admissions for carbon monoxide poisoning to the Royal Adelaide Hospital. Anaesth Intensive Care 20: 311–316

Gorman D, Leitch I 1988 The role of hyperbaric oxygen in the treatment of thermal burn injuries: a brief review of the literature and the results of a pilot study. South Pacific Under Water Med Soc J 18: 121–123

Griffiths R W, Laing J E 1981 A burn formula in clinical practice. Ann R Coll Surg Engl 63: 50–53

Hartwood C E 1987 Methods of reducing burn scar deformity. In: Stark R B (ed) Plastic surgery of the head and neck. Churchill Livingstone, New York, Vol 1, pp 282–285

Heggers J P 1991 Antimicrobial Agents. In: Heggers J P, Robson M C (eds) Quantitative bacteriology: its role in the armamentarium of the surgeon. CRC Press, Boca Raton, p 115

Heggers J P 1993 Antimicrobial therapy for the plastic surgeon. In: Morain W D (ed) Adv Plast Reconstr Surg 9: 156–185

Heimbach D M, Engrav L H 1984 Surgical management of the burn wound. Raven Press, New York, pp 115–131

Hunt J L, Purdue G F, Spicer T, Bennett G, Range S 1987 Face burn reconstruction—does early excision and autografting improve aesthetic appearance? Burns 13: 39–44

Hurt A, Eriksson E 1986 Management of the burn wound. Clin Plast Surg Reconstr Surg 13: 57–67

Jackson D M, Stone P A 1972 Tangential excision and grafting of burns. The method and a report of 50 consecutive cases. Br J Plast Surg 25: 416–426

Janzekovic Z 1970 A new concept in the early excision and immediate grafting of burns. J Trauma 10: 1103–1108

Johnson E V, Kline L B, Skalka H W 1987 Electrical cataracts: a case report and review of the literature. Ophthalmic Surg 18: 283–285

Jonsson C E 1987 The surgical treatment of acute facial burns. Scand J Plast Reconstr Surg 21: 235–236

Katsaros J, David D J, Griffin P A, Moore M H 1990 Case report. Facial dysmorphology in the neglected paediatric head and neck burn. Br J Plast Surg 43: 232–235

Kucan J O, Robson M C 1984 Care of the burned ear. In: Wachtel T L, Frank D H (eds) Burns of the head and neck. Major problems in clinical surgery. Saunders, Philadelphia, Vol 29, Ch 9

Leitch I O W, Kucukcelebi A, Robson M C 1993 Inhibition of wound contraction by topical antimicrobials. Aust NZ J Surg 63: 289–293

Lund C C, Browder N C 1944 Estimation of area of burns. Surg Gynecol Obstet 79: 352–358

McCauley R L, Oliphant J R, Robson M C 1990 Tissue expansion in the correction of burn alopecia. Classification and methods of correction. Ann Plast Surg 25: 103–115

Madden J W, Morton D, Peacock E E 1974 Contraction of experimental wounds. I. Inhibiting wound contraction by using a topical smooth muscle antagonist. Surgery 76: 8–15

Marrone A C 1987 Thermal eyelid burns. In: Hornblast A, Hanio C T (eds) Oculoplastic orbital and reconstructive surgery. Williams & Wilkins, Baltimore, Vol 1, pp 433–447

Millard D R 1969 The crane principle for transport of subcutaneous tissue. Plast Reconstr Surg 43: 451–462

Miller T A 1979 Burns of the face. In: Artz C P, Moncrief J A, Pruitt B A (eds) Burns: a team approach. Saunders, Philadelphia, Ch 20

Monafo W W, Creekmore H 1984 Electrical injuries to the scalp. In: Wachtel T L, Frank D H (eds) Burns of the head and neck, Vol 29, Major problems in clinical surgery. Saunders, Philadelphia, Ch 11

Moncrief J A, Lindberg R B, Switzer W E, Pruitt B A 1966 The use of a topical sulfonamide in the control of burn wound sepsis. J Trauma 6: 407–419

Moritz A R, Henriques F C, McLean R 1945 The effects of inhaled heat on the air passages and lungs — an experimental investigation. Am J Path 21: 311–315

Moylan J A 1979 First aid and transportation of burned patient. In: Artz C P, Moncrief J A, Pruitt B A (eds) Burns: a team approach. Saunders, Philadelphia, Ch 9

Moylan J A, Alexander L G 1978 Diagnosis and treatment of inhalation injury. World J Surg 2: 185–191

Moylan J A Jr, Abib K, Birnbaum M 1975 Fiberoptic bronchoscopy following thermal injury. Surg Gynecol Obstet 140: 541–543

Moylan J A, Wilmore D W, Mouton D E, Pruitt B A 1972 Early diagnosis of inhalation injury using [133]Xenon lung scan. Ann Surg 176: 477–484

Muir I F K, Barclay T L, Settle J A D 1987 Burns and their treatment, 3rd edn. Butterworths, London, Ch 5

Paletta F X 1982 Surgical management of the burned scalp. Clin Plast Surg 9: 167–177

Peterson H D, Boswick J A 1987 Eyelids: the art and science of burn care. Aton Publishers, Rockfield, MD, pp 339–345

Phillips A W, Cope O 1962 Burn therapy. II. The revelation of respiratory tract damage as a principal killer of the burned patient. Ann Surg 155: 1–10

Powell B W E M, Haylock C, Clarke J A 1985 A semi-rigid transparent face mask in the treatment of post-burn hypertrophic scars. Br J Plast Surg 38: 561–566

Raphael J C, Elkarrat D, Jars-Guincestre M C et al 1989 Trial of normobaric and hyperbaric oxygen for acute carbon monoxide intoxication. Lancet 2: 414–419

Robson M C, Barnett R A, Leitch I O W L, Hayward P G 1992 Prevention and treatment of post-burn scars and contracture. World J Surg 16: 87–96

Robson M C, Smith D J 1987 Reconstruction of the burned face, neck and scalp. In: Boswick J (ed) The art and science of burn care. Aspen, Rocksville, MD

Rudolph R 1979 Location of the force of wound contraction. Surg Gynec Obstet 148: 547–551

Runciman W W, Gorman D F 1993 Carbon monoxide poisoning: from old dogma to new uncertainties. Med J Aust 158: 439–450

Shons A R, Rivers E A, Soleni C D 1981 A rigid transparent face mask for controlling scar hypertrophy. Ann Plast Surg 6: 245–248

Shook C D, MacMillan B G, Altemeir W A 1968 Pulmonary complications of the burn patient. Arch Surg 97: 215–224

Silverstein P, Dressler D P 1970 Effect of current therapy on burn mortality. Ann Surg 171: 124–129

Sochor F M, Mallory G K 1963 Lung lesions in patients dying of burns. Arch Pathol 75: 303–308

Stanley L D, Suss R A 1985 Intracerebral haematoma secondary to lightning stroke: case report and review of the literature. Neurosurgery 16: 686–688

Stone P A, Madden J W 1974 Effects of primary and delayed split skin grafting on wound contraction. Surg Forum 25: 41–44

Stone H H, Rhame D W, Corbitt J D, Given K S, Martin J D 1967 Respiratory burns: a correlation of clinical and laboratory results. Ann Surg 165: 157–168

Trunkey D D 1978 Inhalation injury. Surg Clin North Am 58: 1133–1140

Wachtel T H, Frank D H, Frank H A 1981 Management of burns of the head and neck. Head Neck 3: 458–474

Wachtel T H, Frank D H (eds) 1984 Burns of the head and neck, Vol 29, Major problems in clinical surgery. Saunders, Philadelphia, Ch 11

Wanner A, Cutchavaree A 1973 Early recognition of upper airway obstruction following smoke inhalation. Am Rev Respir Dis 108: 1421–1423

Warpeha R L 1981 Resurfacing the burned face. Clin Plast Surg 8: 255–267

Worthen E F 1982 Surgical treatment of electrical burns of the scalp and skull. Past and present. Clin Plast Surg 9: 161–165

Wroblewski D A, Bower G C 1979 The significance of facial burns in acute smoke inhalation. Crit Care Med 7: 335–338

Zawacki B E 1974 Reversal of capillary stasis and prevention of necrosis in burns. Ann Surg 180: 98–102

Zawacki B E, Jung R C, Joyce J, Rincon E 1977 Smoke, burns, and the natural history of inhalation injury in fire victims. Ann Surg 185: 100–110

Bites

E. Tan   J. Crompton
Contributing authors: M. Hammerton   D. Simpson

INTRODUCTION

Human and animal bites have certain peculiarities. Like gunshot wounds, they may present unfamiliar technical problems, especially when brought late for treatment of an avulsive injury. There may be unusual psychosocial problems. Most importantly, bite wounds may be infected by organisms causing virulent infections, including the uniquely terrible disease rabies.

Surgical pathology

Depending on the ferocity and anatomical characteristics of the biter, the bite may be perforating, lacerating, crushing, avulsive or any combination of these. A snap from a provoked pet dog may inflict a deep perforation, even through a child's skull; however, the dog will often withdraw at once, and not tear or worry as a wild carnivore might. A crocodile on the other hand may seize and crush, being eager to drag its whole victim under water rather than to bite off a portion. Other carnivores may avulse substantial parts of the face. Our experience relates chiefly to domestic dog bites, children being often the victims of family pets, and to a lesser extent to human bites.

Human bites are inflicted in close combat or in sexual passion. The prominent parts of the face are usually bitten; the lips, nose and ears are often attacked, and loss of tissue is common. The amount of tissue removed is limited by the size of the human mouth and the anatomy of the dentition: in general, relatively small pieces of the face are bitten off, sometimes in sharply defined morsels. In an African series of 72 facial bites (Venter 1988), there was loss of soft tissue in more than half. The hairy scalp is rarely bitten. Human bites of the eye and its adnexae have been reported, and even penetration into the orbit (Patel & Collin 1991).

Animals often bite some part of the face or scalp and the orbital and periorbital tissues are frequently involved. Dog bites are likely to cause lacerations and puncture wounds; these bites are often very serious, especially when inflicted on a child by a large dog of ferocious breed (p. 96) and powerful jaws (p. 113). Most severe facial dog bites occur in children, especially under the age of 5 years; in a study of severe facial bites in the Bristol area, Palmer & Rees (1983) found that 80% were in children under 15 years old, and Karlson (1984) found a similar proportion in a series from Wisconsin. Dog bites involve a combination of penetrating and avulsive injuries. Dog bites may be very disfiguring, and may also cause serious damage to the eye and its adnexae. Injury in the region of the medial canthus is common, and damage to the lacrimal system was found in 15 of 16 periorbital dog bites studied by Gonnering (1987). The extraocular muscles may be injured, even avulsed. Cats inflict punctures without tearing or avulsing, and like other Felidae they may scratch as well as bite (Fig. 14.2).

In some parts of the world, large carnivores may inflict gross mutilations on their victims, and treatment is often complicated by delay in seeking expert management. Govila et al (1989) reported a case in which a bear bit off 8 cm of jaw from the mandible of an Indian woman, the avulsed jaw was brought to a surgeon, but too late for replantation. Davis (1993) states that North American bears typically bite the face or scalp; one of his illustrations shows very extensive avulsion of the scalp by a grizzly bear. Ilukol (1990) has described her own experience as a small girl in the Karimojong tribe in northern Uganda. She was attacked by a hyena, and her lips, nose and right maxillary region were avulsed, with loss of much of the scalp. After reconstructive plastic surgery in Kampala she made a new life as a trained nurse. Her story gives a vivid picture of the impact of mutilation and cultural disruption.

Clinical assessment

The wound or wounds should be carefully inspected. In view of the possible medicolegal implications of bites by humans and domestic animals, it is wise to obtain photographs, with a standard metric scale in the plane of the bite (Davis 1993); in such cases, consultation with a forensic odontologist may also be desirable.

If the eyelids are involved, the lacrimal drainage should be examined under the microscope; the canaliculi may be probed, under anaesthesia in children. In all cases of facial bite by an animal, careful search should be made for a bite elsewhere in the body.

Radiological assessment

Teeth can penetrate the skull, and the associated scalp wound may not be very alarming. It is therefore necessary to obtain X-ray pictures of the skull or facial skeleton in cases of facial or calvarial bites. Computed tomographic (CT) scans with appropriate window settings visualize small calvarial punctures well, and show the depth of cerebral penetration and the presence of indriven bone fragments.

Microbiological assessment

It is wise to consult a microbiologist as soon as possible. Different species have different oral microbiota and some animal pathogens may be hard to culture by standard laboratory methods. Human bites often become infected. Goldstein et al (1977) found anaerobes (chiefly bacteroides) in more than half of 20 cases and staphylcocci in only five; *Eikenella corrodens*, a normal human oral inhabitant, was seen in three. In human bites, the possibility of human immunodeficiency virus infection may arise, and, if possible, serological tests should be done on the biter (see p. 535). Various microbes have been implicated in infection from dog bites, including *Staphylococcus aureus*, *Pasteurella moltocida* and the anaerobic cocci, *Pseudomonas aeruginosa*, *Staph. epidermidis* and various streptococci. *P. multocida* may cause acute local cellulitis and lymphangitis (Shanson 1989), and also has the capacity to cause meningitis and cerebral abscess (Weber et al 1984). *Capnocytophaga canimorsus* (formerly known as Dysgonic Fermenter-2), a common isolate from the dog's mouth, may produce fulminant septicaemia in patients who are immune-suppressed. Penicillin must be included in the prophylaxis (Stevenson et al 1976, Gonnering 1987). The septic complications of dog bites have a bad reputation, though with modern methods of treatment, serious complications are rare. Cat bites and scratches are also liable to infection, and Goldstein (1992) found *P. multocida* in some 50% of cases.

Immunoprophylaxis

When a bite is the cause of a facial injury it is important to determine the immune status of the patient including the record of tetanus immunization and whether the patient may be immunocompromised, as by acquired immune deficiency syndrome, splenectomy, or alcoholism (see Ch. 20). Tetanus immunization should be given unless the patient is known to have been immunized within the last 5 years. If there is doubt, tetanus immunoglobulin should be given. In countries where rabies is prevalent, it is important to determine whether there is any possibility that the animal responsible for the bite may be rabid. Rabies is endemic in most parts of the world, with the exceptions of the UK, Ireland, Sweden, Taiwan, Japan and Australasia, which are at present supposedly free (Bek et al 1992). The virus is commonly transmitted by dog bites, though other mammals — foxes, bats, cats, wolves, and monkeys — have been incriminated. A rabid animal may be unbelievably ferocious, and can attack the head or face, when the incubation period is likely to be relatively short; in the past, the mortality was high even when antirabic vaccine was given. Baltazard et al (1955) reported 29 cases of wolf bites, all bitten by a single rabid wolf in the course of one night: 18 sustained severe head wounds (Fig. 18.1). This series gave an opportunity to compare the preventive value of antirabic vaccine with and without high titre antibody serum: there were no deaths in five who received two injections of serum, one death among seven who received a single injection of serum, and three deaths among five who received vaccine alone.

In some developed countries, domestic dogs and cats are routinely vaccinated, and in these countries it is important to determine whether the animal responsible for a bite has not received rabies vaccination. If this cannot be determined, then it must be assumed that the animal has not been immunized. If the animal has behaved abnormally before biting, or if there are any other suspicious circumstances, it is recommended that the animal's decapitated head should be sent refrigerated — not frozen — to a laboratory able to make the diagnosis of rabies (Flanigan et al 1985); immunofluorescent staining for rabies antigen is a reliable method. Unvaccinated dogs or cats responsible for a bite are isolated for 10 days: if there are no signs of illness, the animal is assumed to be healthy, and prophylaxis is not advised. This assump-

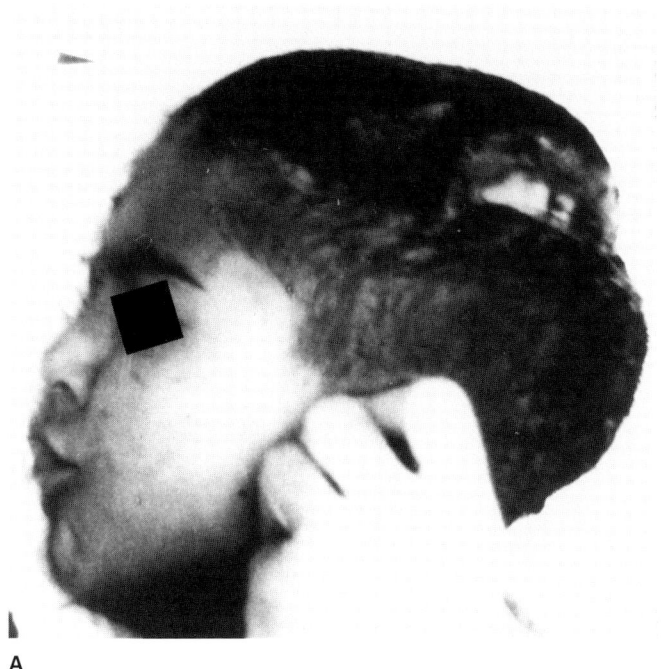

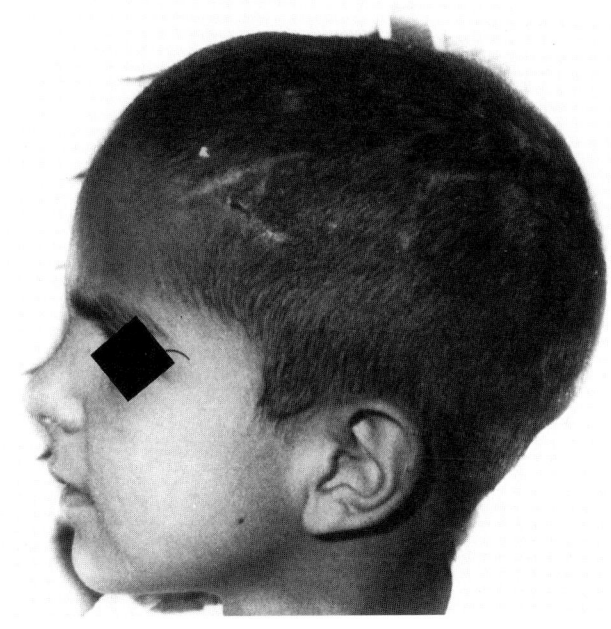

Fig. 18.1 Compound skull fracture from wolf bite. A 6-year-old boy was bitten by a rabid wolf; he was given antirabies vaccine and six injections of antirabies serum. **A** Open craniocerebral wound in the parietal region. **B** He made a good recovery after antirabic treatment and surgical closure of the wound. By kind permission of Dr D. Carleton Gajdusek and the Editor of the Bulletin of the World Health Organization.

tion has been challenged by reports of dogs which have remained well for a month or longer after transmitting rabies to human victims (Dutta & Dutta 1994). Wild animals are assumed to be rabid unless proven to be free by laboratory tests.

If there is proof or suspicion that the bite could have been infected with rabies virus, rabies vaccine is administered at once, and also rabies hyperimmune globulin (RIG) to give protection during the 8 days needed for antibody response to the vaccine. At present, the recommended procedure is to give Mérieux inactivated rabies vaccine by intradeltoid injection on days 0, 3, 7, 14 and 28. RIG (20 IU/kg) is given on day 0, and it is advised that half of the dose should be infiltated around the bite wound, and the rest given into the gluteal muscle (Bek et al 1992, Goldstein 1992). Other less expensive vaccines are available, and their merits are discussed by Hyde et al (1994) in an excellent review of rabies prevention. These authors report a regimen of intradermal vaccination developed in Thailand and now approved by the World Health Organization; they caution that this regimen should not be used by staff inexperienced in the technique.

The incubation period for rabies is typically 2–8 weeks, but much longer periods have been reported. A person bitten by a rabid animal will obviously be under prolonged emotional strain, and should be counselled and as far as possible reassured.

Management

General

All bite injuries should undergo early wound decontamination unless there are obvious signs that infection is already present. The single most important step in prevention of infection is decontamination by forced irrigation using at least 200 ml of normal saline through a 19 gauge needle. This has been shown to reduce wound infections very substantially; in one study, the infection rate fell from 69% to 12% (Callaham 1980). Lavage with dilute povidone–iodine (Betadine®) or chlorhexidine solution may also be used. If rabies is in question, a viricide should be used.

Prophylactic antibiotic therapy is usually given, though the evidence for its use is questionable; one trial with oral oxacillin failed to show any benefit (Elenbaas et al 1981). The choice of antibiotic for initial use is debatable. *P. multocida* is usually sensitive to penicillin, but oral staphylococci are often resistant. Venter (1988) gave ampicillin and flucloxacillin in a series of human bites and reported excellent results, and we have given these antibiotics. Dog bites often have such diverse microbial contamination that a broader spectrum cover may seem appropriate, such as ceftriaxone. However, the regimen at present recommended by our advisers is amoxycillin and clavulanic acid, or if there is penicillin allergy, cotrimoxazole and metronidazole.

Surgical repair should be undertaken using the standard soft-tissue repair techniques described in Chapter 15. In the past, fear of infection often led to a policy of delayed wound closure, with poorer aesthetic results. With antibiotic cover, primary closure is usually successful even when there is significant tissue loss (Venter 1988), and this is recommended unless there is overt infection. If the bite has amputated a piece of tissue, replantation is sometimes possible: the amputated fragment should be washed in warm sterile saline and taken as soon as possible for consideration by the microsurgeon. If there is any delay, the tissue should be kept cool but not frozen.

General management should always include attention to the cause of the bite. A domestic pet which has bitten a child may do so again, and should as a rule be humanely killed. Human bites may also be repeated, and demand a full psychosocial enquiry, especially when the victim was a woman or child.

Periorbital bites

Standard ocular plastic techniques are used to repair eyelid wounds if less than 6–8 h old (Gonnering 1987). If there is marked tissue oedema, haemorrhage or suspicion of infection, operation must be postponed for 2–3 days. If the orbital septum is damaged it may be best left unrepaired, with a small drain placed through it for 24 h. The lacrimal system is often involved, and should be repaired if possible (p. 428). Injury to the upper lid may involve the levator muscle and trochlea as well as the orbicularis muscle; these should be repaired with 6/0 catgut. Amputated eyelids should be preserved, for possible use as a composite graft (Fig. 14.12). Spinelli et al (1986) reported five cases in which large pieces of eyelid had been bitten off in passion or combat; the morsels were replaced and survived though loss of cilia was seen when there was delay in replantation. When operation was done within 14 h, the cilia survived. The authors recommended 'an aggressive search' for missing morsels.

Bites of the lips

The lips were the leading site of dog bites in the series reported by Palmer & Rees (1983), being lacerated or amputated in 63/148 bites. Lip bites should be treated along the lines set out in Chapter 15 (p. 437). It is sometimes possible to replant an amputated lip: Jeng et al (1992) replaced the vermilion area of a lower lip after 8 h by reanastomosing one inferior labial artery and joining the other to a vein.

Bites of the nose

These are very disfiguring (Fig. 18.2), and in some communities carry cruel implications of punishment for a domestic or political crime (p. 8). Primary treatment is discussed on p. 436 and the case for microvascular

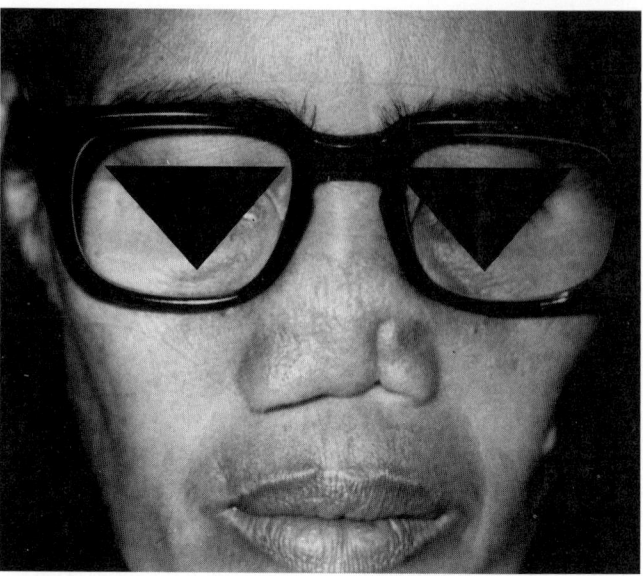

Fig. 18.2 Partial amputation of the nose. This wound resulted from domestic aggression. Initial treatment was inadequate, and permanent deformity resulted.

replantation has been argued. Strategies for rhinoplasty are described in Chapter 21 (p. 582).

Bites of the ear

These are relatively less disfiguring, and indeed may be a source of mild pride when sustained in combat. The bite usually amounts to cropping rather than avulsion. Primary treatment is discussed in Chapter 15. Scott & Klaassen (1992) have emphasized the value of immediate reconstruction of the helical rim with a posterior auricular skin flap; these authors had little success from replanting the fragment of helix as a composite graft. We have had some success in replanting ears avulsed in road accidents (p. 456) and, when a large piece of ear has been bitten off, microvascular repair may be warranted. But for many people, cover by hair may be sufficient aesthetic management.

Massive avulsive bites

We have no experience of bites by an animal large enough to ablate large segments of the face. Reports in the literature suggest that such injuries should be repaired along the lines indicated in Chapter 16. In the case of bear bite reported by Govila et al (1989), the lower jaw was successfully reconstructed with a pectoralis major island flap containing a length of rib.

Craniocerebral bites

The sharp teeth of a dog may perforate the infant's

calvarial bone and pierce the underlying cerebral cortex. Wilberger & Pang (1983) reported four such cases, aged from 7 weeks to 12 months, and we have treated a case. The entry wound may seem insignificant, but exploration is always essential; Klein & Cohen (1978) reported a case where failure to explore the wound led to the later development of a brain abscess, the organism responsible being *Pasteurella multocida*. Alpert & Sutton (1984) reported a similar case of abscess complicating failure to diagnose and treat a craniocerebral dogbite; a *Peptococcus* organism was cultured from the abscess. Treatment of craniocerebral bites should be along the lines set out in Chapter 13 (p. 372). Deep cerebral penetration is unlikely, but in the case treated by us, an indriven bone chip was missed at exploration, and had to be removed at a second operation.

REFERENCES

Alpert G, Sutton L N 1984 Brain abscess following cranial dogbite. Clin Pediatr (Philadelphia) 23: 580

Balthazard M, Bahmanyar M, Ghodssi M, Sabeti A, Gajdusek C, Rouzbehi E 1955 Essai pratique du sérum antirabique chez les mordus par loupes enragés. Bull WHO 13: 747–772

Bek M D, Smith W T, Levy M H, Sullivan E, Rubin G L 1992 Rabies case in New South Wales: public health aspects. Med J Aust 156: 596–600

Callaham M 1980 Dog bite wounds. J Am Med Assoc 244: 2327–2328

Davis J H 1993 Injuries due to animals. In: Mason J K (ed) The pathology of trauma. Arnold, London, Ch 18

Dutta J K, Dutta T K 1994 Rabies in endemic countries. Problems with canine carriers of the virus and the cost of safe post-exposure prophylaxis. Br Med J 308: 488–489

Elenbaas R M, McNabney W K, Robinson W A 1981 Prophylactic antibiotics and dog bite wounds. J Am Med Assoc 246: 833–834

Flanigan T J, Rippert E T, Nieusma G E 1985 Rabies therapy for animal bites in the head and neck region. J Oral Maxillofac Surg 43: 704–706

Goldstein E J C 1992 Bite wounds and infections. Clin Infect Dis 14: 633–640

Goldstein E J C, Caffee H H, Price J E, Citronbaum D M, Miller T A, Finegold S M 1977 Human bite infections (letter) Lancet 2: 1290

Gonnering R S 1987 Ocular adnexal injury and complications in orbital dog bites. Ophthal Plast Reconstr Surg 3: 231–235

Govila A, Rao G S S, James J H 1989 Primary reconstruction of a major loss of lower jaw by an animal bite using a 'rib sandwich' pectoralis major island flap. Br J Plast Surg 42: 101–103

Hyde H, Chutivongse S, Hemachudha T 1994 Rabies and its prevention. Med J Aust 160: 83–87

Ilukol M 1990 Child of the Karimojong. Macmillan, India.

Jeng S-F, Wei F-C, Noordhoff M S 1992 Successful replantation of a bitten-off vermilion of the lower lip by microvascular anastomosis: case report. J Trauma 33: 914–916

Karlson T A 1984 The incidence of facial injuries from dog bites. J Am Med Assoc 251: 3265–3267

Klein D M, Cohen M E 1978 Pasteurella multocida brain abscess following perforating cranial dogbite. J Pediatr 92: 588–589

Palmer J, Rees M 1983 Dog bites of the face: a 15 year review. Br J Plast Surg 36: 315–318

Patel B C, Collin J R O 1991 The management of human and animal bites of ocular adnexa. Curr Opin Ophthalmol 2: 590–595

Scott M J, Klaassen M F 1992 Immediate reconstruction of the helical rim after bite injury using the posterior auricular flap. Injury 23: 333–335

Shanson D C 1989 Microbiology in clinical practice, 2nd edn. Wright, London

Spinelli H M, Sherman J E, Lisman R D, Smith B 1986 Human bites of the eyelid. Plast Reconstr Surg 78: 610–614

Stevenson T, Thacker J, Rodeheaver G 1976 Cleansing the traumatic wound by high pressure irrigation. J Am Coll Emerg Physicians 5: 17–21

Venter T H 1988 Human bites of the face. Early surgical management. S Afr Med J 74: 277–279

Weber D J, Wolfson J S, Swartz M N, Hooper D C 1984 Pasteurella multocida infections: report of 34 cases and review of the literature. Medicine (Baltimore) 63: 133–154

Wilberger J F, Pang D 1983 Craniocerebral injuries from dog bites. J Am Med Assoc 249: 2685–2688

Immaturity and senescence

A. Hanieh   M. Moore
Contributing authors: T. Brown   M. Hammerton   D. Simpson

INTRODUCTION

In Chapters 11–15, we have considered the management of craniomaxillofacial (CMF) injuries in the period of maturity. When injury is sustained at either of the extremes of the age range, there are age-related peculiarities in the injury patterns, and these must be taken into account in clinical management. Consideration must also be given to the psychosocial characteristics of the young and the old. No one questions that 'children are different', and paediatric surgery is accepted as a specialty in its own right, requiring special expertise and often a separate trauma service. No such claims are made for geriatric trauma, nor do we suggest that it is necessary to do so. But with the increasingly large number of elderly persons in most modern communities, it is appropriate to give attention to the peculiar features of trauma in old age as well as in youth.

Children generally tolerate injury well, but interference in normal growth and development can have tragic long-term consequences: this is true not only of brain injuries but also of certain facial skeletal injuries. Old people on the other hand tolerate both the general and the local effects of CMF impacts badly, yet there are some complications of head impacts in the elderly that can be treated with success.

INFANCY AND CHILDHOOD

FRACTURES OF THE FACIAL SKELETON

Effects of immaturity

Whereas adult fractures occur in a relatively stable, unchanging structure, in the child both the skeleton and the dentition are an evolving entity. The paediatric craniofacial skeleton is a dynamic, growing structure which changes qualitatively as well as quantitatively with time (p. 76); the development of skeletal and soft tissues is interrelated and dependent on the functional status of the matrix in which the tissues are growing. Both trauma and surgical intervention can interfere with the growth process in ways that may not be apparent until years later, and management must take the stage of growth into account (p. 489). While the relevance of growth is generally recognized, there is a tendency to lump together into one category all children from birth to 18 or some other upper age limit, on the basis — indisputable but not very discriminating — that they are not adults. This obscures important age-related differences (Bartlett & DeLozier 1992): only by distinguishing subgroups of the paediatric population, based predominantly on structural anatomical changes, can consistent age-related patterns of fracture be identified. Techniques of fracture reduction and fixation can then be standardized, and the effects of both fracture pattern and means of stabilization on subsequent craniofacial growth can be better understood.

At birth, the facial skeleton contains relatively more cancellous bone and cartilage than the adult facial skeleton. It contains all the unerupted teeth, and it has not yet been weakened by the development of the paranasal sinuses (Fig. 2.10). It is covered by a relatively thick layer of adipose tissue. In consequence, the infant's mandible and still more the midfacial complex are resilient on impact: comminution is unusual, and greenstick fractures common. The postnatal acceleration of facial growth is accompanied by the development of the paranasal sinuses and the eruption of teeth (Tables 2.4–2.6), producing regions of relative weakness and relative strength. Before the completion of the eruption of the permanent dentition (5–12 years), the presence of unerupted teeth weakens the bone of the midface and mandible and predisposes to more oblique and sagittal fractures through the developing tooth crypts, which are not of adult type (Moore et al 1990).

Orbitocranial growth is very nearly completed by 7 years. After the age of 12 years, sinus aeration maximizes, adult dentition is established and mineralization of the skeleton becomes complete; the facial skeleton has changed from a solid resilient mass into the complex system of robust but rigid pillars and thin plates described in Chapter 2 (Fig. 2.15). Thereafter, the patterns of fracturing in the CMF skeleton approximate those seen in adults.

Incidence

Several authors have emphasized the low frequency of facial fractures in children, compared to adults. Rowe (1968) recorded that 1% of a series of 1500 facial fractures occurred in children < 6 years old and 5% < 12 years. Conventional reasoning relates the low incidence to the protected environment of childhood; other factors include the child's small facial mass relative to the calvarial vault, the thicker overlying soft tissues and the structural resilience of the facial skeleton. However, the rarity of facial fractures should not be exaggerated. Carroll et al (1987) found 241 (23%) children aged < 16 years in a series of 1044 patients referred to an oral–faciomaxillary unit in Great Britain. In our combined series of 984 facial fractures (Fig. 3.1) collected over a 3 year period, there were 120 (12.2%) cases in the age range 1–14 years; many of these had nasal fractures mostly of minor clinical significance, but the series included cases of mandibular and maxillary fractures potentially capable of causing long-term disabilities. Similarly, in our series of 237 fractures of the anterior cranial fossa (p. 377), there were 37 (15.6%) children; 10 (4.2%) were < 5 years old, and four of these had fractures of the midface as well as frontal fractures.

Some fracture types are uncommon in early life: isolated fractures of the midface, including complex naso-ethmoid and orbital fractures are especially rare, but isolated orbitozygomatic fractures including blow-out fractures are less so. The nose and the mandible are the two most frequently fractured facial bones in childhood; in published series of paediatric fractures, the relative proportions vary greatly, perhaps because of case selection. McCoy et al (1966) reported the mandible to be involved in 41% of paediatric facial fractures, nasal fractures being seen in 23%. Fractures of the mandible comprised 32% and nasal fractures 45% of the cases reported by Kaban et al (1977); Hall (1972) reported a similar proportion

(24.2% mandibular fractures, 46.6% nasal fractures). In our paediatric series, which includes all cases treated by the ENT department and the craniofacial unit, but excludes some fractures of the frontal bone, nasal fractures (59.2%) greatly outnumbered mandibular fractures (22.5%). Taher (1993) subgrouped his series according to involvement of the upper or lower third of the face, and reported a 63.2% incidence of injury to the lower third region. This series included children who were civilian casualties of missile warfare.

Emergency assessment and management

Management in children with major CMF injuries begins, as at any age, with securing the airway and controlling haemorrhage. The smaller airway diameter increases the danger of upper airway obstruction from bleeding, foreign bodies or loss of anterior tongue support. Posturing and appropriate drainage with suction will, however, maintain oxygenation in most circumstances. When these simple measures are not adequate an oral airway may be inserted, or orotracheal intubation may be performed; if the child is comatose from associated cerebral injury, intubation is usually mandatory. But it should be remembered that intubation in children is sometimes difficult and a misplaced tube can be disastrous (Fig. 19.1). Tracheostomy in young children is a last resort, because it may be a difficult procedure and more importantly the morbidity and mortality are considerable.

The child's circulating blood volume is small in comparison with the adult, and also small in relation to the child's surface area. Blood loss from extensive soft-tissue injuries of the head and neck and especially from the scalp may cause hypovolaemia very rapidly. Local pressure will as a rule control haemorrhage before definitive treatment is undertaken. Blood replacement is often needed, especially if there is blood loss from other associated injuries; loss from long bone and pelvic fractures is often underestimated.

Because the blood volume of a small child is disproportionate to the relatively larger surface area, there is an increased risk of hypothermia, and this is dangerous when large volumes of banked blood are transfused; a cold, poorly perfused child may be unable to cope with the potassium load in banked blood, and hyperkalaemia may develop unless the child is warmed and kept well perfused.

Infants and small children are also vulnerable to hyponatraemia; this may result from unrecognized sodium loss, imprudent infusion of hypotonic fluids, or increased secretion of antidiuretic hormone, whether appropriate or inappropriate. If the serum sodium is < 120 mEq/l, and especially if the child is drowsy, irritable or fitting, then urgent medical treatment is required (p. 382).

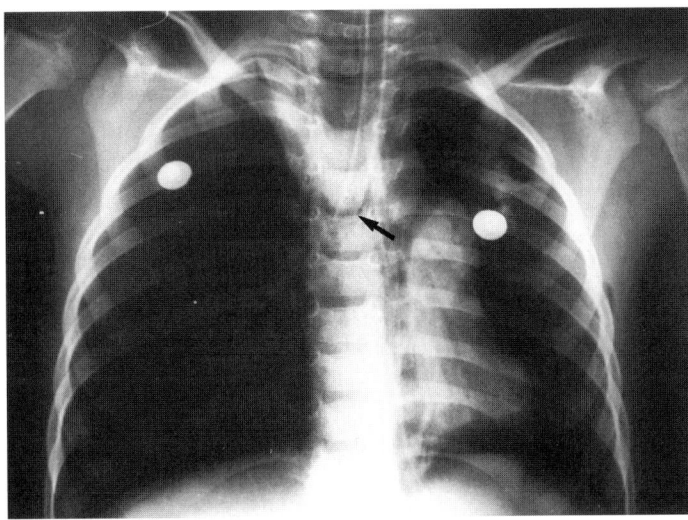

A

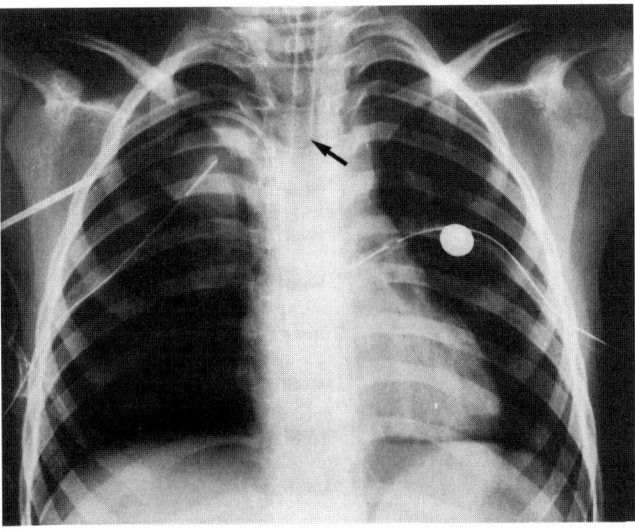

B

Fig. 19.1 Misplaced endotracheal tube. A 4-year-old boy was injured in a country road crash: he sustained a severe fronto-orbital wound and was unconscious. An endotracheal tube was inserted and he was transferred to the metropolitan paediatric trauma centre for neurosurgical treatment. He arrived in respiratory distress. **A** Chest radiography showed collapse of the left lung and hyperinflation of the right lung; the tube (arrow) is in the right main bronchus. **B** Reinsertion of the endotracheal tube (arrow) and insertion of an intercostal pleural tube restored respiratory function.

Clinical assessment

The injured child is generally poorly communicative and uncooperative. An adequate history may only be obtained from a parent or other observer. However, parental truthfulness cannot be assumed, and the possibility of child abuse should always be considered, especially when an injured infant shows an unusual pattern of injury, or when the history is implausible.

The clinical manifestations of craniofacial fractures in children are similar to those in adults, but the relatively thicker overlying soft tissues limit the clinical information available from palpation; so does the low level of cooperation given by a frightened child, in pain and perhaps unable to see because of periorbital swelling. Sedation or even general anaesthesia may be employed to facilitate examination; this should only be done after all other injuries have been assessed.

In deciding whether there is any post-traumatic change in the child's facial appearance, parental observations or photographs taken in the past may help to decide whether the child looks different as a result of the injury.

Radiological assessment

Plain radiological examination in the child yields relatively less diagnostic information than in the adult. The small size and the lack of pneumatization of the paranasal sinuses reduce the contrast in tissue densities, leading often to false negative findings. It is therefore mandatory to maintain a high index of suspicion for facial fracture, and to obtain axial and direct coronal CT scans of the craniofacial region if there is any doubt at all. Only then will the true incidence of facial skeletal injury be recorded. The relationship between an undisplaced or minimally displaced fracture, initially thought not to require acute treatment, and a later growth disturbance may then be better foreseen and understood.

Associated injuries

As in other age groups but perhaps even more in the paediatric population, the presence of an associated injury whether local or distant must be suspected. McCoy et al (1966) recorded associated injuries other than facial in 57% of their series. Kaban et al (1977) reported an incidence of 29% of other non-facial injuries; in their series 70% of associated injuries occurred in patients with mandibular fractures. Taher (1993) reported associated non-facial injuries in 36% of cases in his series, almost half of which occurred in patients with lower third fractures.

MANDIBULAR FRACTURES

Surgical pathology

The infant's very small mandible is rarely fractured. If fractures occur in infancy, they are usually of greenstick type and will heal in 2 or 3 weeks. Older children do suffer fractures with considerable displacement; Converse & Dingman (1977) note that the fracture lines are often long and oblique. The state of the dentition is relevant both to management and to the long-term effects of injury. Internal fixation by plating is undesirable early in

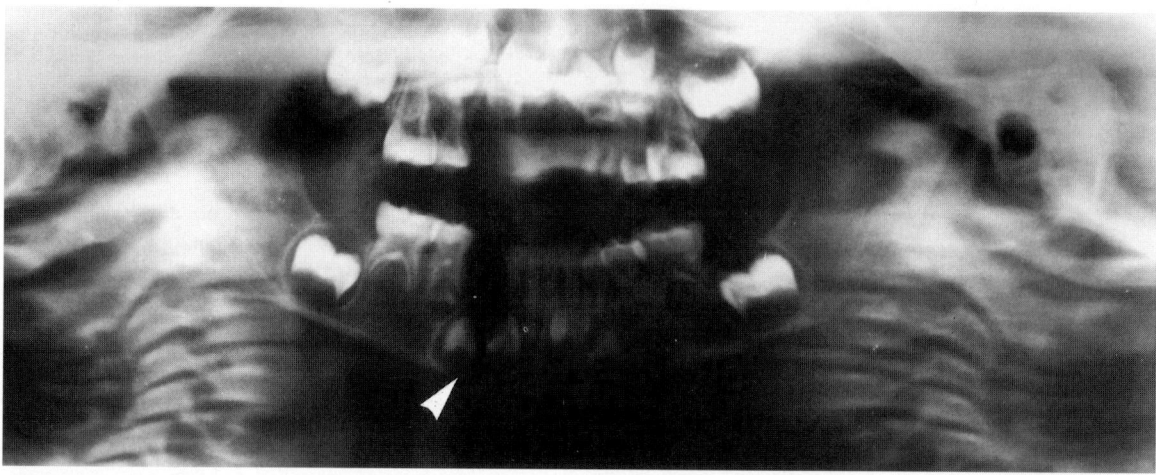

Fig. 19.2 Mandibular fracture. A 3-year-old child was kicked by a horse. There was a significantly displaced compound right parasymphyseal fracture (arrow head) for which intermaxillary fixation might be inadequate. Careful placement of miniplate or microplate and monocortical screws at the lower border will provide stability of fracture reduction with minimal damage to the unerupted secondary tooth buds.

the stage of mixed dentition: the buds of the secondary teeth may be injured by drilling the adjacent cortex. Fortunately, provided that the roots of the deciduous teeth are fully formed, or their resorption not yet advanced, one may use these teeth to support ligation to arch bars. Usually this is the case in the age range 3–8 years, but palpation of the teeth and dental radiographic examination should be undertaken to verify their suitability for this purpose. Late in the stage of mixed dentition, the roots of the deciduous teeth may have absorbed, and ligation is then impossible. In such older children, the cortical bone is likely to be thicker and it may be safe to insert monocortical screws in the lower border of the mandible (Fig. 19.2).

Management

In children, it is possible to accept small discrepancies in the accuracy of fracture reduction in the expectation that the occlusion will adjust spontaneously with further growth. Therefore, in the rare event of an unstable mandibular fracture occurring before the eruption of significant elements of the primary dentition, it is usually best to immobilize the mandible by an acrylic splint secured by circumferential wires. The splint can be removed after 2 or 3 weeks, when the fracture is united.

In the early part of the stage of mixed dentition, it may be best to use closed reduction and to stabilize the fracture by simple intermaxillary fixation, either by arch bars or by wires wound around teeth and twisted into eyelets, which can secure intermaxillary wires. This avoids the risk to the tooth buds entailed by cortical drilling. The intermaxillary fixation can be dismantled after 3 weeks, and a less than perfect reduction can be accepted. But in the late part of the stage of mixed dentition, inter-

maxillary fixation is difficult, because the dental roots are being absorbed, and it is hard to secure arch bars to the teeth; fixation with miniplates secured by monocortical screws is therefore preferable. If the plate and the screws are inserted in the lower border of the mandible, sound healing is usually achieved.

However, it has been argued that miniplates may have an adverse effect on the growth of the mandible. At present the evidence for this is not decisive (Lin et al 1991, Bartlett & DeLozier 1992), but as a rule we remove the plates after 3 months.

FRACTURES AND DISLOCATIONS OF THE CONDYLE

Surgical pathology

Paediatric fractures of the condylar neck are often of greenstick character and heal with no after effects. Even quite severe fractures of the condyle often heal and remodel completely with minimal treatment (Fig. 19.3). Leake et al (1971) followed 13 children with untreated displaced fractures over the period of maximum growth, and found no cases of residual deformity. However, in the first 3 years of life, the condyle may be crushed by a fall on the chin point, and this injury may have long-term consequences: asymmetrical facial growth and ankylosis of the temporomandibular joint. Rowe (1969) has related these occasional disasters to the anatomy of the infant's condyle: short, vascular, and apt to be crushed within the capsule (Fig. 4.6B). He has emphasized the role of growth centre damage as a cause of facial distortion; however, current thinking (p. 77) now gives the condylar cartilage a less commanding role in the dynamics of facial growth, and it is still somewhat uncertain how seriously the crush-

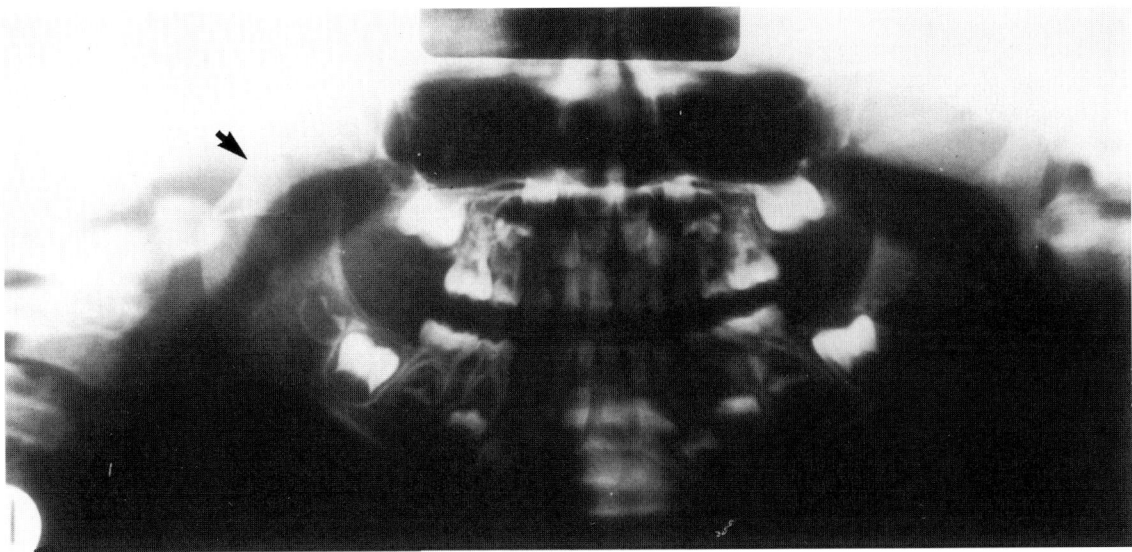

Fig. 19.3 Condylar fracture. An 8-year-old child fell on the chin. Orthopantomogram demonstrated a displaced, dislocated right condylar fracture (arrow) managed conservatively with initial short period of intermaxillary fixation.

ing of a condylar cartilage should be taken. Certainly, efforts to replicate in animals the deformities supposedly due to condylar or subcondylar fracture have been inconclusive (Boyne 1967, Beckler & Walker 1969). But the adverse effects of ankylosis are indisputable, especially if it develops during the first 3 years (p. 598).

Management

This is discussed in Chapter 11 where we have reviewed the work of Lund and Lindahl on the remodelling of the condyle and the glenoid fossa after fracture dislocations of the head of the mandible in childhood, and the compensatory growth of the ipsilateral mandible. These authors advocated conservative treatment and their arguments have been assessed (p. 282). The outcome in children may be affected by the age of the child when injured as well as by the anatomy of the fracture: the pubertal growth spurt may play a part. In some cases treated conservatively, we have seen significant growth disturbances, with hypoplasia of the ipsilateral mandible and the development of a bimaxillary tilt of the occlusal plane. Ankylosis has been noted.

Because of these unfortunate experiences, our management policy in paediatric condylar fractures includes operative reduction under certain circumstances. Miniplates are used; with these, the mandibular condyle presents special grounds for concern, since its growth is endochondral, and to ensure that plating in this part of the mandible does not interfere with growth, we remove the plate(s) after 3 months.

When a disorder of condylar growth has become apparent, surgical intervention should be considered before the deformity is increased by further growth. While osteo-

tomy of the ramus or subcondylar region may correct deformity for the time being, it is unlikely that correction of this nature will prevent recurrent deformity in the long term. There is evidence to suggest that it is better to replace the deformed condylar head with a shaped costochondral graft designed both to reconstruct the temporomandibular joint and to increase the posterior height of the mandible: the costochondral graft is intended to give continued growth- and sometimes does so to excess (Peltomäki & Isotupa 1991). Where possible, an attempt is made to attach the lateral pterygoid muscle to the cartilage of the reconstructed condyle to help the graft to function in unison with the contralateral joint. The operative technique is considered on p. 604.

ORBITOZYGOMATIC FRACTURES

Surgical pathology

The orbitozygomatic skeleton appears to be more resilient in the paediatric age group, no doubt because of the abundant spongy cancellous bone and the limited development of the paranasal air sinuses (Fig. 2.10). The facial pillars are thus broader and more stable, and the points of weakness in this region are more resistant to fracturing than in the adult facial skeleton.

Zygomatic fractures and orbital blow-out fractures are uncommon in infants, less so in older children. Supraorbital rim and orbital roof fractures are considered below, in relation to frontal calvarial fractures; they are usually seen only after high energy impacts.

Although zygomatic fractures are far less frequent in the infant than in adults, they may present more difficult problems. As an isolated fracture the zygoma is often greensticked or impacted, causing difficulties in both diagnosis and management. The most frequent clinical finding is marked periorbital swelling and bruising, frustrating diagnosis by palpation. Plain radiography of an impacted fracture may not be diagnostic in the absence of significant sinus pneumatization; axial and coronal computerized tomography (CT) will best document the degree of displacement in all dimensions. An isolated zygomatic arch fracture in children is rare, but may result from severe localized trauma to the arch; the treatment is as in the adult (p. 320).

Management

The ideal time for treatment is at 4–8 days post injury. This allows the soft-tissue swelling to reduce, permitting assessment of skeletal symmetry, as well as giving ample time for appropriate radiographic evaluation and planning. Treatment follows the same principles as in adults, although open reduction may be more frequently required because the fractures are often impacted. Internal fixation with miniplates at the frontozygomatic region produces adequate fixation where the reduction is unstable. Microplate fixation at two or three points provides stability with less potential for the plates to be palpable or visible. Nevertheless, increased soft-tissue dissection is necessary and this may be undesirable. Wangerin & Kiesbye (1991) showed that in young rats, dissection and plating of the zygoma caused marked asymmetry of facial growth, though this largely disappeared after 4 months. Extensive dissection and exposure of the zygomatic arch is indicated only when the zygomatic fracture is associated with major midfacial or panfacial disruption.

ORBITAL FLOOR FRACTURES

Management

These are rare fractures in childhood, and occur most commonly in association with zygomatic fractures. They are explored and repaired as in adults. Orbital blow-out fractures can occur despite the small size of the maxillary sinus. This is because the size and shape of the orbit reaches adult dimensions relatively early: the orbit in a 10-year-old approximates in size to an adult orbit (p. 76). Management entails primary repair of the orbital floor, with reconstruction by grafting with autogenous bone, as in an adult injury of similar type: failure to reconstitute both orbital floor and medial orbital wall adequately risks the development of post-traumatic enophthalmos (p. 558).

NASAL FRACTURES

Surgical pathology

A broken nose is not only the commonest but also the most frequently undiagnosed and inadequately treated facial fracture in children (Olsen et al 1979). Many adult nasal deformities are traced to untreated childhood injuries.

The child's nose is characterized by small nasal bones and proportionally larger cartilaginous elements. Injury is consequently more likely to be primarily cartilaginous (Moran 1977). Perhaps more extensively documented than for any other facial region, childhood injury of the nose, and in particular the nasal septum, has the potential for later growth retardation. Many animal studies have identified nasal septal injury or removal as a potent cause of growth inhibition in the nose and anterior maxilla (Wexler & Sarnat 1965, Sarnat & Wexler 1966, Kemble 1973). The nasal suture remains open in children, predisposing to 'open-book' types of nasal fracture: these are characterized by lateral displacement and overriding of the nasal bones on the frontal process of the maxilla. The upper lateral cartilages, loosely attached to the deep surface of the distal portion of the nasal bones, may be detached or displaced, often associated with haematoma formation. Posterior dislocation then permits buckling and dislocation of the nasal septum, again with the risk of septal haematoma formation.

Assessment

In children with nasal fractures, external examination and radiographic investigation are often of limited value as the nasal bones are small and the cartilaginous elements proportionally larger. With a history of a fall or local injury to the nose, nasal and/or periorbital swelling and bruising should be assumed to be due to nasal fracture until proved otherwise. Early examination is mandatory as healing is rapid. General anaesthesia with appropriate vasoconstriction of the nasal lining may be required in the child to confirm the presence or absence of nasal fracture.

Intranasal examination will identify septal fracturing or dislocation and the presence of a septal haematoma, which is common in children.

Management

Treatment of nasal fractures in childhood is essentially as for adults. Displaced bony elements are reduced in a closed fashion as accurately as possible. Care is taken to avoid operative trauma. Open reduction is seldom necessary, being used chiefly where there are extensive associated midfacial injuries. Septal haematomas require early aspiration or incision and formal drainage to avoid septal cartilage necrosis, growth disturbance, saddle-nose deformity and columella retraction. Septal dislocations are treated conservatively by closed relocation of the displaced septum; any associated septal haematoma is evacuated at the same time. Late septal deformity is common and convention has it that definitive correction is performed during middle and late teenage years or even later as an elective procedure. This is discussed further in Chapter 21.

NASO-ORBITO-ETHMOID FRACTURES

Surgical pathology

In children, these fractures are extremely rare. They are seen in association with severe panfacial or craniofacial fractures, caused by high energy impacts. When such injuries do occur, and cause severe anteroposterior crushing in a very young child, there may be a disfiguring disturbance of growth including true hypertelorism (p. 571).

Assessment

The clinical features of injuries in this region are no different from those of comparable injuries in adults. But in a frightened child with an injury causing pain and periorbital and nasal swelling, clinical examination is of limited value. Where this pattern of injury is anticipated axial and coronal CT scan assessment is mandatory.

Management

Exposure by a coronal scalp flap, as for an adult, is employed where there is naso-ethmoid depression and telecanthus. Fracture reduction, including all frontal elements is necessary, with rigid internal fixation, preferably with microplates. These plates require removal at a later stage if placed in areas where they could interfere with later facial growth. In infants interosseous wiring may produce sufficient stability; in the older child, miniplates have been used in the past without significant complications. The medial canthal ligaments are repaired in the same fashion as for an adult injury (p. 312).

MIDFACIAL FRACTURES

Surgical pathology

The midface (middle third) is a proportionally small region of the paediatric face. It is protected by the overriding and relatively prominent upper face and forehead, and fractures in this region are not very numerous; Neukam et al (1991) found 16 cases of children (< 15 years) in a series of 589 midfacial fractures treated in Hanover in a 10 year period.

Nevertheless, paediatric midfacial fractures are more common than fractures in the naso-ethmoid region. High energy impacts are necessary to produce major midfacial injuries, the pattern of which seldom mimic the classical Le Fort adult types. A more oblique pattern of fracture with inferior extension into the midface from the fronto-naso-orbital region (Fig. 19.4) has been identified (Moore et al 1990).

Assessment

Despite these differences in fracture patterns, the clinical symptoms, signs, and radiographic investigations are as for the adult.

Management

Where midfacial displacement is noted, as evidenced by facial contour changes or occlusal disturbances, reduction is required early because healing is rapid — usually within 4–8 days.

With minimally displaced impacted greenstick fractures, reduction may be all that is required. Alternatively a wide range of techniques of external and internal fixation is available. In choosing between different techniques, the remodelling potential of the growing facial skeleton should be kept in mind, and here again there has been debate on the pros and cons of miniplate fixation.

During the period of mixed dentition, treatment may be complicated by the instability of arch bars or eyelet wires. Direct osseous fixation of the arch bars has been used to overcome this problem. Internal wire suspension and external cranial traction devices have been similarly used but are now largely superseded by interosseous wiring, miniplate and microplate fixation. External appliances require frequent repositioning and are poorly tolerated by children, while suspension wiring suffers from the problem also seen in adults — the direction of pull is orientated wrongly.

Microplate or miniplate fixation is now preferred because of the greater stability afforded. Care in plate positioning and application is essential in the younger child to avoid damaging unerupted tooth buds.

Subperiosteal dissection is necessary for plate insertion, and while potentially associated with growth disturbances this has not occurred in our experience. Denny et al (1993) in a small series record similar findings even when the internal fixation plates were not subsequently removed. The belief that all plates inserted in the growing craniofacial skeleton should be removed because of the potential for growth impairment has been adopted without much valid research. The whole question of late growth disturbance after paediatric midfacial fracture (Ousterhout & Vargervik 1987), and the relative contributions in this which are made by the initial injury, the adequacy of reduction and the technique of exposure and fixation are issues which are largely unresolved. The risk of very small internal fixation plates on the anterior maxilla contributing to growth changes seems slight, but the further disruption to the soft-tissue matrix needed for plate removal could be more damaging. While interosseous wiring or plate fixation across facial sutures has a theoretical capacity to retard growth, the rapid early bone remodelling around the wires and screws minimizes any significant compressive forces that may have been generated.

We believe that facial growth alteration following midfacial injury is minimized by stable and accurate reduction of all fractures, careful repair of the surrounding soft tissues, and an operative technique which limits subperiosteal dissection to what is necessary for fracture reduction. Neukam et al (1991) also believe that the fear of disturbances in dental and facial growth should not deter surgeons from operative intervention when there is significant skeletal dislocation in the midfacial region.

INJURIES TO THE TEETH IN CHILDHOOD

Effects of immaturity

Young children are prone to injuries involving both the deciduous teeth and the underlying permanent teeth in various stages of development. If the germ of a permanent tooth is damaged, aesthetic and functional impairments may result from disruption of normal developmental processes. These effects may not be predictable at the time of injury.

Surgical pathology

In children, dental injuries commonly result from a fall or other impact on the anterior aspect of the face, and the anterior teeth are therefore most often damaged (Fig. 12.1). The types of injury to the deciduous dentition include fractures, subluxation, extrusion, intrusion and exarticulation of a tooth or teeth. The treatment of injuries of the deciduous teeth is aimed at the need to ensure preservation of the underlying and developing permanent teeth.

Radiological assessment

Dental radiography (p. 347) is used to determine whether or not the root of the deciduous tooth has penetrated the underlying permanent tooth follicle. If invasion of the follicle has occurred then the deciduous tooth is removed. In the event of misdiagnosis of luxation of the tooth follicle, malformation of the developing tooth crown is likely to follow.

Management

Removal of a deciduous tooth must be carried out with care to avoid damage to the permanent tooth which lies in close proximity. For this purpose forceps should be used rather than elevators. The deciduous tooth should be grasped on its proximal surfaces so that the beaks of the forceps do not slip down the labiolingual surfaces to

the region of the developing follicle. The tooth should be removed from its socket in a labial and axial direction, after which the labial and lingual bony plates should be held firmly between the fingers and a suture placed in the gingival tissues.

Most tooth fractures in the young child consist of small incisal edge enamel fractures which can be treated by smoothing with a fine diamond stone in a dental handpiece. Where the crown and the root of the tooth are fractured there will be bleeding from the pulp chamber and in such cases extraction is usually advisable.

Treatment of deciduous tooth avulsion differs from that for avulsion of permanent teeth in that replantation of the deciduous tooth is to be avoided as the pulp will become necrotic. In the case of the permanent dentition, replantation can be successful if the lapse of time between avulsion and replantation is short (p. 353).

Tooth injuries resulting from a fall by a young child usually involve lateral luxation: the crown is pushed back (palatally) and the root apex forward (labially), thus avoiding damage to the underlying tooth follicle. No treatment is indicated in these instances unless there is a resultant occlusal interference.

Occasionally young patients are seen with intrusion of the deciduous maxillary incisors, resulting from a fall during which the teeth are impacted in an axial direction. As the roots of deciduous incisors have a natural labial inclination, they will usually be pushed into the labial bone when forcibly intruded. Normally the tooth will re-erupt within a few months but if this does not appear likely, the buried tooth can be mechanically extruded and cemented to adjacent teeth in its original position. This procedure requires anaesthesia.

CALVARIAL FRACTURES

Effects of immaturity

In early life, the calvarial component of the head is more prominent and relatively more exposed to direct injury. This is reflected in the vault-to-face volume ratio which is 8:1 at birth, and still 4:1 at age 5 years; thereafter the vault shows relatively little growth, while the face continues to grow until age 21 years (Fig. 2.39), when adult proportions are established.

The infant's frontal bone is a thin plate of woven bone, easily indented like a ping-pong ball (Fig. 19.5). As growth progresses, the frontal bone becomes thicker and shows a sandwich structure of inner and outer tables separated by cancellous bone containing haematopoietic marrow. This structure gives greater biomechanical resistance to injury, especially in the absence of the frontal air sinuses, but impacts of sufficiently high energy will cause frontal fractures, often depressed, and often radiating into the orbit (Fig. 19.6).

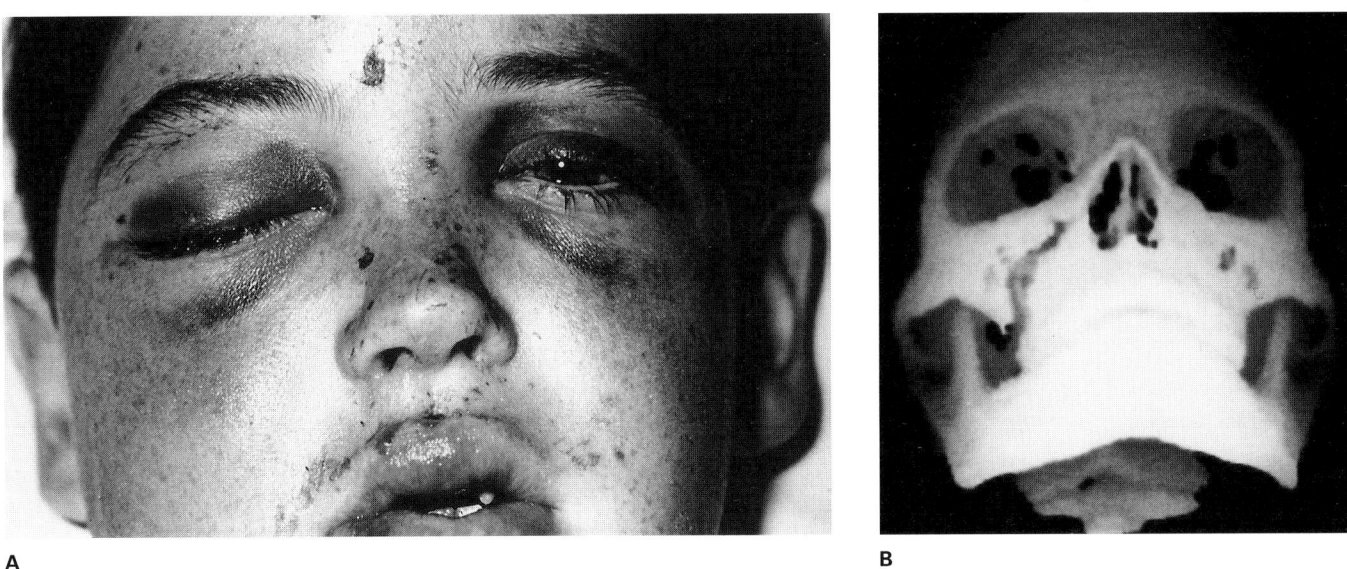

Fig. 19.4 Midface fracture. A 10-year-old cyclist was struck by a motor vehicle. **A** He presented with diffuse facial swelling, periorbital ecchymoses, and malocclusion. **B** 3D CT reconstruction revealed depressed fracture of the right zygoma, and an oblique midfacial fracture.

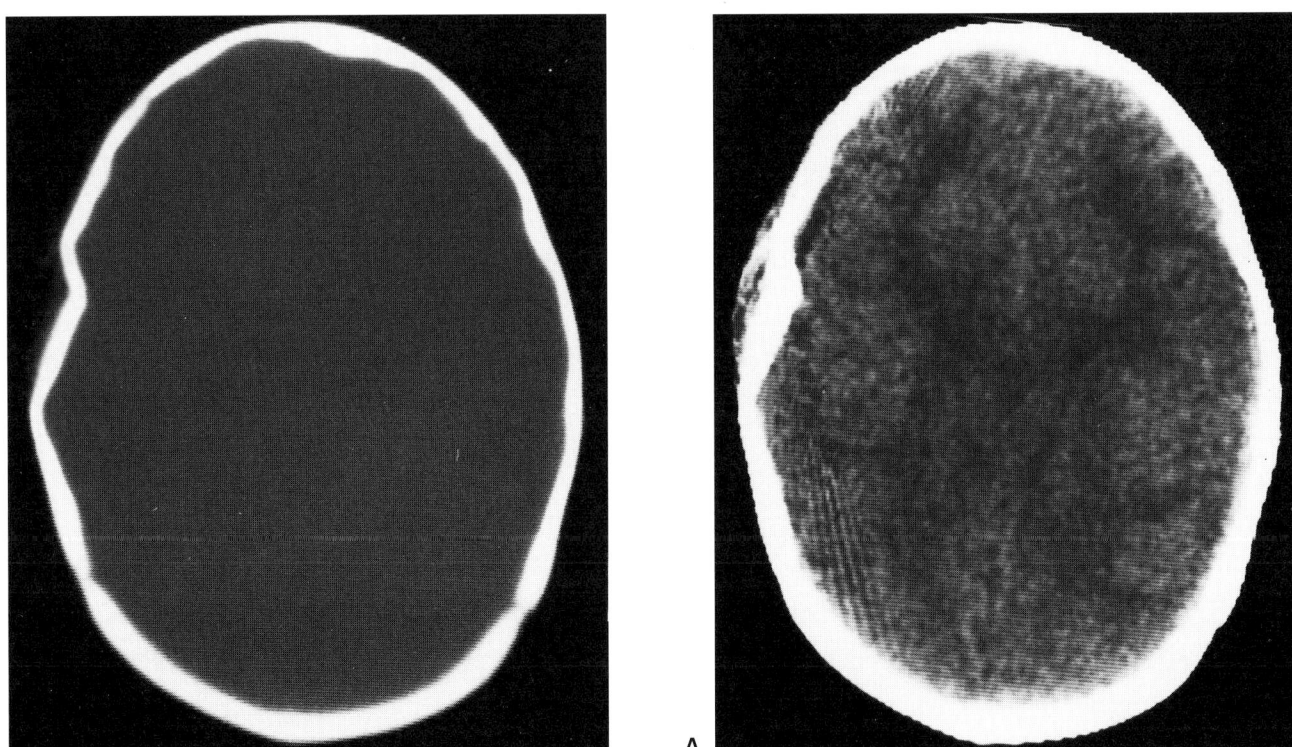

Fig. 19.5 Depressed fracture of pond (ping-pong) type. An 11-month-old infant's head was crushed by a tyre when a car reversed on to him; he appeared unaffected apart from bruises on the head. **A** CT scan (bone setting) showed a depressed fracture in the left anterior parietal bone, with no comminution. **B** CT scan (brain setting) showed a minor degree of indentation of the brain. The fracture was elevated. There were no detectable effects.

Incidence

In a consecutive series of 60 skull fractures in hospitalized children, we found the frontal bone alone to be fractured in 12; in seven others there was extension from the frontal bone into the facial skeleton. All frontal fractures with facial involvement were inflicted in road crashes. The temporoparietal region was most frequently involved by linear fractures. Infants rarely suffer frontal fractures.

Selley & Fränkel (1961) found only two frontal fractures in a series of 50 infants with skull fracture, and our experience is similar. If linear frontal fractures do occur in infancy, they are likely to be the result of severe impacts sustained in car crashes; involvement of the orbit and lower face is then often seen.

Radiological assessment

The paediatric calvarial fracture may be difficult to diagnose in skull radiographs where the bone is thin, while false positive diagnoses arise because of confusion with normal structures, such as cranial sutures, synchondroses, Wormian or sutural bones and accessory sutures. CT is invaluable in showing the degree of calvarial depression, and visualizes many basal fractures not seen in plain radiographs (Fig. 19.6); CT is indispensable in diagnosing the associated cerebral pathology.

Linear calvarial fractures

These course toward the cranial base and may involve

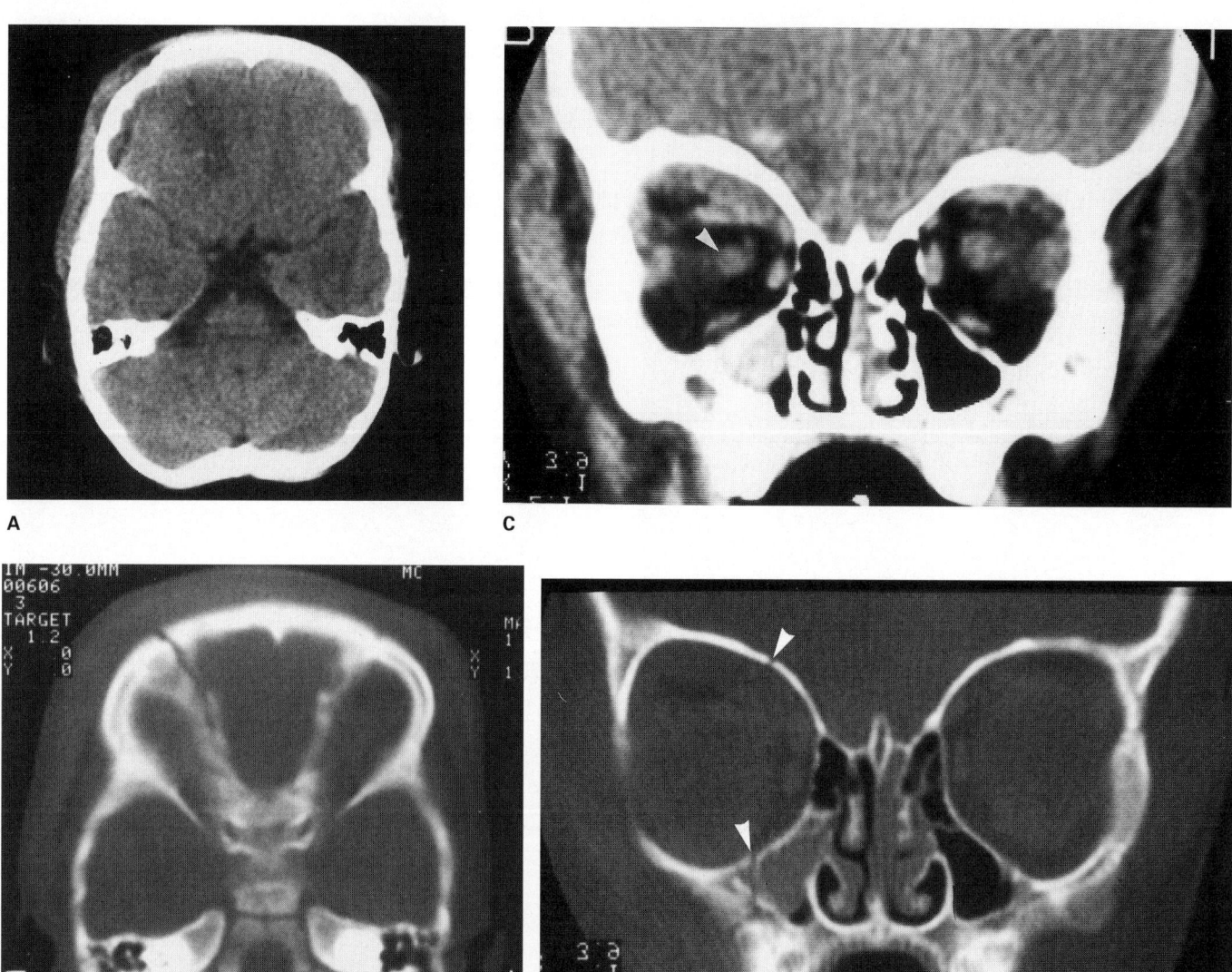

Fig. 19.6 Craniocerebral effects of a frontal impact. A 2-year-old boy fell down a flight of stairs and landed on his head. There was loss of consciousness for about a minute. He had a right periorbital haematoma, and the right eye was pushed downwards. **A** Horizontal CT of brain showing low and high density lesion in the right frontal lobe, presumably a haemorrhagic contusion. **B** Horizontal CT of skull base showing linear fracture extending from the right supraorbital margin into the roof of the orbit. **C** Coronal CT view showing intraorbital haematoma adjacent to the fracture in the orbital roof, with haemorrhagic cerebral contusion on the other side of the fracture line. The intraorbital haematoma caused downward displacement of the right eye and optic nerve (arrowhead). **D** Coronal CT view of the orbits, showing fracture of the roof (arrowhead) and a corresponding fracture (arrowhead) involving the orbital floor, with opacification of the right maxillary sinus.

the roof of the orbit, as a 'blow-in' or 'blow-out' fracture (Messinger et al 1988). Basal skull fractures, which are less common, course toward the calvarium. There is a tendency to follow and indeed extend into sutures which are readily diastased.

Depressed skull fractures

Though less frequent than linear fractures, depressed fractures often occur, as pond or ping-pong fractures in infants (Fig. 19.5), and as more or less comminuted areas of depression, often oval or circular, in older children (Fig. 5.8); unlike the pond fractures, these are usually compound and often associated with dural and cerebral damage. They are most often seen in the parietal and frontal regions.

Basal skull fractures

These occur somewhat less frequently, usually in association with high velocity impacts where there are obliquely orientated patterns of fracturing of the entire craniofacial skeleton (Fig. 19.7). Basal fractures were present in seven of our series of 60 cases of paediatric cranial fractures. Only one was associated with cerebrospinal fluid rhinorrhoea requiring dural repair. In the paediatric age group, basal skull fractures are often associated with cranial nerve lesions (Kitchens et al 1991).

Sutural diastasis

This usually occurs by extension of an adjacent fracture into the suture and is most common in younger patients where the sutures are completely unfused. The coronal or lambdoid sutures are most frequently involved, often with extension to the contralateral side. Multiple sutures are seldom involved.

Growing fractures

These curious lesions constitute a pathological process peculiar to early life. They are rare, occurring in less than 1% of paediatric cranial fractures. Most (90%) occur under 3 years of age, two-thirds being under 1 year old. The parietal region is the commonest site, but cases in the frontal and occipital regions have been reported (Lende & Erickson 1961, Till 1975).

In the presence of underlying brain injury and a dural tear, an expanding bone defect may appear at the fracture site. A leptomeningeal cyst forms; osteoblastic activity is inhibited, the bone does not heal and the fracture margins undergo resorption and reshaping. The fracture enlarges, its edges take on a scalloped appearance and a pulsatile central bulge is found. The underlying brain may suffer progressive atrophy and a porencephalic dilatation of the

lateral ventricle may be seen in the CT scan. Although the mechanism of production of this uniquely paediatric injury is uncertain, it seems likely that it represents the dynamic expansion of the growing brain acting on an area of deficiency in its capsule. Chronic raised intracranial pressure may be a factor in some cases.

Management

Linear skull fractures need no special consideration unless there is wide separation of the bone edges. The possibility of a growing fracture then arises. In infants and younger children, plain radiographs should be repeated a few months later and, if the fracture is not healing, a dural tear should be suspected and operative repair may be needed. Certainly this should be done if there is any sign of expansion or the formation of a pulsatile defect. An appropriate scalp flap is turned, and the dural defect — which is often larger than the bone defect — is exposed and repaired with a pericranial graft. Duhaime & Sutton (1992) recommend lyophilized cadaver dura as an alternative to pericranium, but we have abandoned this very convenient homograft from concern over the risk of slow virus transmission (p. 138). A free bone graft is then cut from another area of the skull and wired into the defect over the graft. In an infant, the donor area will usually close without the need for a cranioplasty: bone regenerates from the intact dura, especially if this is covered with bone dust and chips.

Simple depressed frontal fractures, if more than 5–10 mm below the line of the outer table, should be elevated for aesthetic reasons. This view has been challenged (Steinbok et al 1987), and certainly these fractures are usually benign. But we have seen an untreated frontal pond fracture sustained in infancy which was permanently visible many years later, and such fractures can be easily elevated through a burrhole or small craniectomy.

Compound depressed fractures, penetrating brain wounds and cranionasal fistulae (Fig. 19.7) are treated as in adult neurosurgical practice (Ch. 13).

BRAIN INJURIES

Effects of immaturity

It is frequently said that infants and children recover from cerebral injury better than adults. The overall mortality from severe closed head injury certainly tends to be lower (Bruce et al 1985), and the clinical recovery from impaired neurological function is often dramatic. The immature brain shows some characteristic reactions to injury which are not seen in adults; these are poorly understood, but suggest instability in vascular and neuronal physiology. In children who have suffered a complete aphasic arrest of speech after injury to the dominant hemisphere, one frequently sees sudden, seemingly complete recovery after days or weeks; similar dramatic recovery has been documented after decerebrate rigidity or prolonged mutism associated with a CMF injury (Todorow 1975). These observations suggest that in some so far unexplained way, the child's neural function has been thrown into a state of reversible paralysis or diaschisis. It also seems that the immature brain has greater capacity for functional substitution after structural brain damage than the mature brain; the clinical and experimental evidence for this has been critically reviewed by LeVere et al (1988). But there is a dark side to these pleasing recoveries. Alajouanine & Lhermitte (1965) studied 32 children with acquired aphasia; most of them regained normal or near normal speech, but all of them had significant difficulties in later school work. In infants especially, one is often saddened by the late appearance of learning difficulties long after seemingly good recovery from head injury. Plasticity in the infant's brain has negative aspects: Teuber (1975) has shown that recovery of speech function after damage to the dominant hemisphere may be achieved at the cost of stunted function in the non-dominant hemisphere. Moreover, the favourable aspects of craniocerebral immaturity may be balanced by adverse factors, such as the poorer degree of protection afforded by the skull. Luerssen et al (1988) found that the lower mortality of head injury seen in paediatric practice is least evident in the first 5 years. They found a mortality rate in excess of 40% for comatose (Glasgow Coma Scale ≤ 8) infants and children in that age group, falling to under 20% at the age of 14 years.

Surgical pathology

In children, the primary neuropathological effects of head impact are in general much as in adults. Because the child's skull is thinner, there is a tendency for blunt impacts to cause relatively more local ('coup') cerebral damage (Fig. 19.6) and relatively less diffuse injury. There are, however, some peculiarities in the child's pathophysiological responses to impact and in the incidence of secondary complications.

Benign traumatic encephalopathy

This term describes a group of striking but transient disorders of cerebral function often seen in children who have sustained a relatively minor impact (Guthkelch 1979). A child falls or is struck on the head, does not at first lose consciousness, and then in half an hour or more suffers a grand mal epileptic seizure, or some non-convulsive loss of cerebral function such as dysphasia or cortical blindness, or merely becomes very drowsy. These very alarming effects subside completely in a few hours. Snoek et al (1984) found a mean age of 7.3 years (range 1–17) for convulsive cases and 6 years (range 2–13) for non-convulsive cases; in our experience, children under 5 years old are most often affected. Unstable vascular responses may underlie the clinical syndrome.

Diffuse cerebral swelling

Supposedly due to post-traumatic hyperaemia (Bruce et al 1981), this is a characteristic effect of severe head impact in children, and can sometimes be the cause of dramatic delayed clinical deterioration (Fig. 19.8). In such cases, it is important to exclude a metabolic cause of cerebral oedema, such as hyponatraemia. Aldrich et al (1992) reviewed data from 111 cases of severe head injury in childhood (age ≤ 16 years) and found 19 cases with CT evidence of cerebral swelling in the absence of the multiple small cerebral haemorrhages, which are considered to be marker signs of diffuse axonal injury. Their findings confirmed that this phenomenon is commoner in children than in adults; however, only one child showed delayed clinical worsening. Muizelaar et al (1989) carried out cerebral blood flow (CBF) studies on 32 children (3–18 years, mean age 13.6) and confirmed that cerebral hyperaemia is often found in severe childhood head injury; 24 h after injury, there was a correlation between increased depth of coma and impaired cerebral blood flow.

Intracranial haemorrhage

Acute subdural haemorrhage is less often seen in children, but extradural haemorrhage is by no means rare. In a community-based study of 680 traumatic intracranial haemorrhages (Fig. 19.9), Dan et al (1986) found that about one-third of the extradural haematomas were in the age range 0–14 years, whereas only about 10% of 290 uncomplicated acute subdural haematomas were in this age range (Stening et al 1986b). Chronic subdural haematomas of adult type are very rare in children, though infants — especially the victims of repeated battery by an adult — are often found to have large subdural collections of serous or bloody fluid.

Cranionasal fistulas

Because the paranasal air sinuses do not develop their adult size until adolescence (Fig. 2.10), cerebrospinal fluid (CSF) rhinorrhoea and post-traumatic meningitis are less common in childhood. Nevertheless these serious complications do occur and can be lethal (Caldicott et al 1973).

Obstructive hydrocephalus

Progressive ventricular dilatation is sometimes seen as

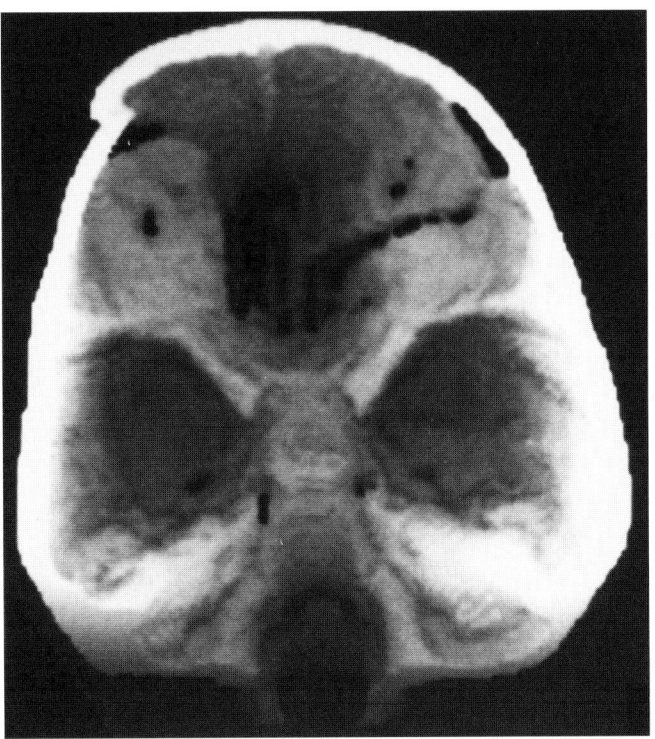 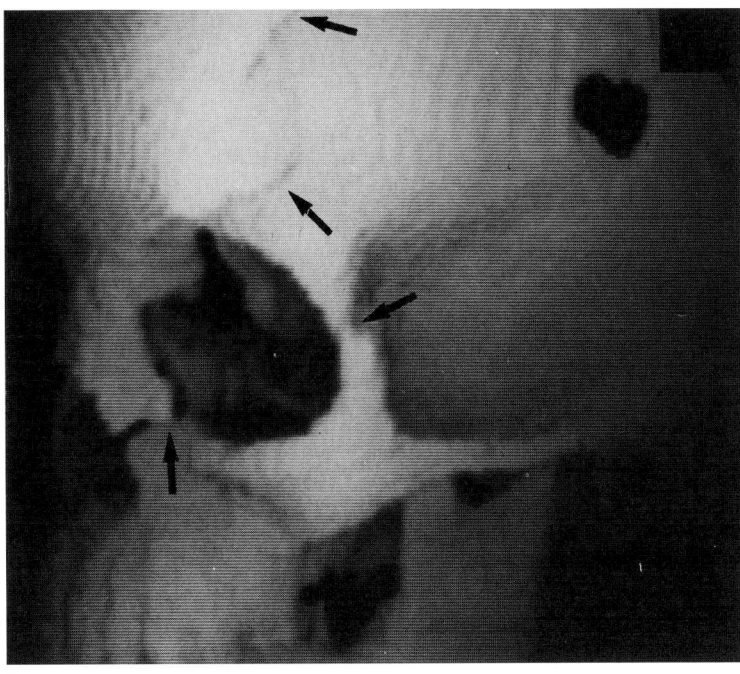

Fig. 19.7 Basal skull fracture with orbital and midface fractures. A 3-year-old boy was injured in a road crash. He suffered a right frontal compound skull fracture, and also extensive disruption of the roof of the left orbit and nasal region; the injury may have been of crushing type. The right eye was blind, from optic nerve damage. 3D CT scan showed: **A** A fracture crossing the anterior cranial fossa, with displacement of a left frontal segment; **B** Multiple fractures of the left frontal bone and orbit (arrows), with an oblique extension across the midface. On day 21, the anterior fossa was repaired: a large defect in the roof of the left orbit was found, with dural tears and frontal lobe damage on both sides. The anterior fossa was covered with a graft of pericranium and fascia. The left orbital fractures were reduced into anatomical position and immobilized by wiring.

a sequel of severe closed head injury in childhood, and presumably represents blockage of CSF circulation in the subarachnoid spaces or arachnoid villi by bleeding (p. 148), though delayed atrophy and brain shrinkage must be considered in the diagnosis, especially when the ventricular dilation is of only moderate severity and associated with other evidence of atrophy (Fig. 19.8). Rarely, there are signs of raised intracranial pressure, (ICP) and the hydrocephalus may require treatment by a ventriculoperitoneal shunt. It is not clear whether the immature CSF pathways are more easily blocked than those of an adult.

Clinical assessment

In the acute period, older children are examined by the general methods set out in Chapter 6. In assessing the conscious level in young children and still more in infants, the adult Glasgow Coma Scale (GCS) is inapplicable. The paediatric version (PGCS: see Fig. 19.10) gives age-related norms for the responses to be expected in the first 5 years of life (Reilly et al 1988); the scale has been used by us for some 15 years, and has received independent support from a comparative study by Yager et al

(1990). However, it is important to ensure that the medical and nursing staff who use it have some instruction in its application, and in developmental neurology generally (Simpson et al 1991). The staff of a paediatric trauma unit are usually proficient in assessing the responses of injured infants and young children, but this cannot be assumed in a general trauma ward. Fundoscopy should never be omitted in a head-injured infant. Papilloedema is a rare finding, but retinal haemorrhages are often seen after severe impacts, especially in the victims of child abuse. Retinal haemorrhage, however, is not diagnostic of abuse, being sometimes seen after falls from a considerable height (> 1 m) or after vehicular accidents (Duhaime et al 1992).

In the older child the systematic methods of examination used in adult neurological practice (p. 163) can be applied. The assessment of intelligence is related to the child's age and school progress, and tests of reading competence standardized by educational authorities (Schonell 1961, Jastak & Wilkinson 1984) are very helpful in detecting previous subliteracy as well as post-traumatic impairments. In the infant or toddler, developmental responses are studied in relation to the age. It is often impossible to elicit the classical developmental reflexes

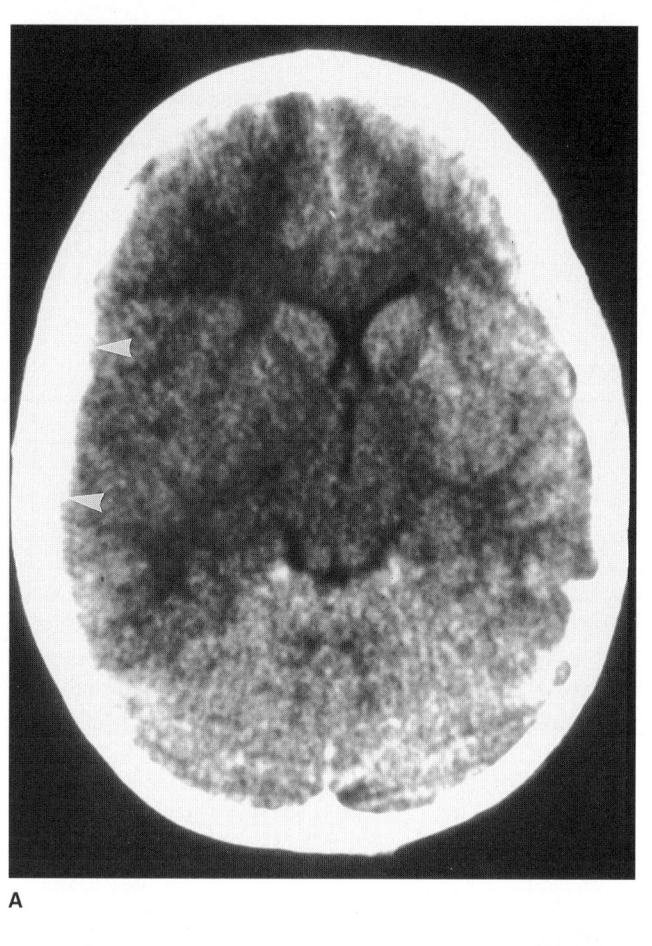

A

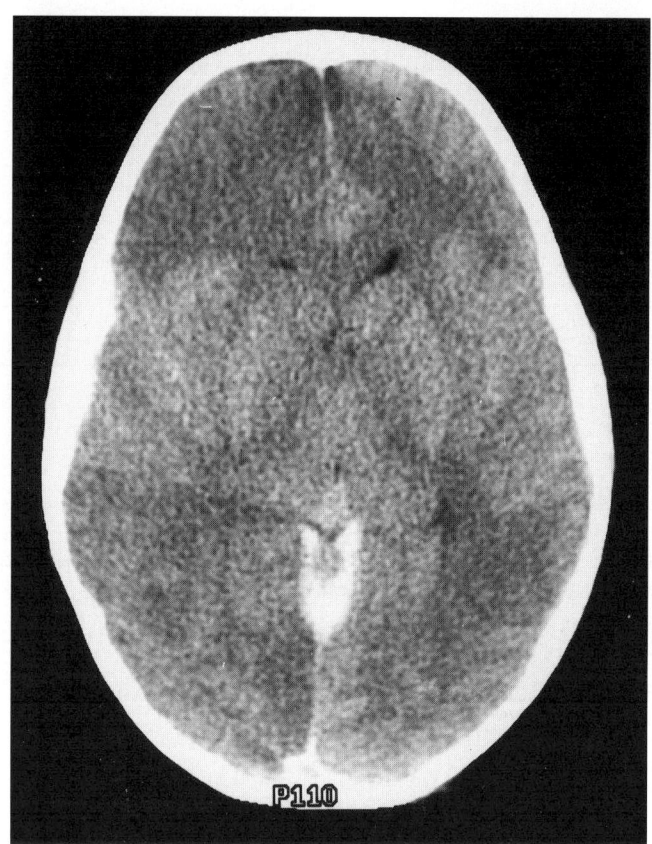

B

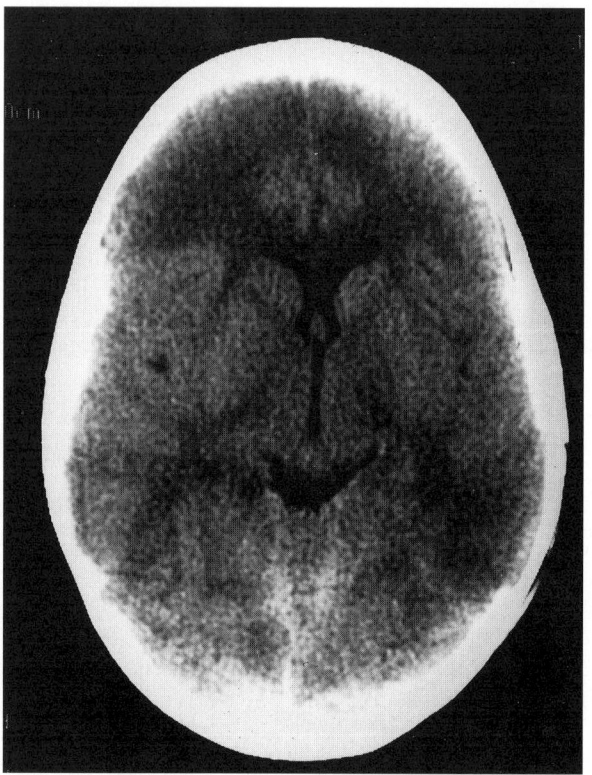

C

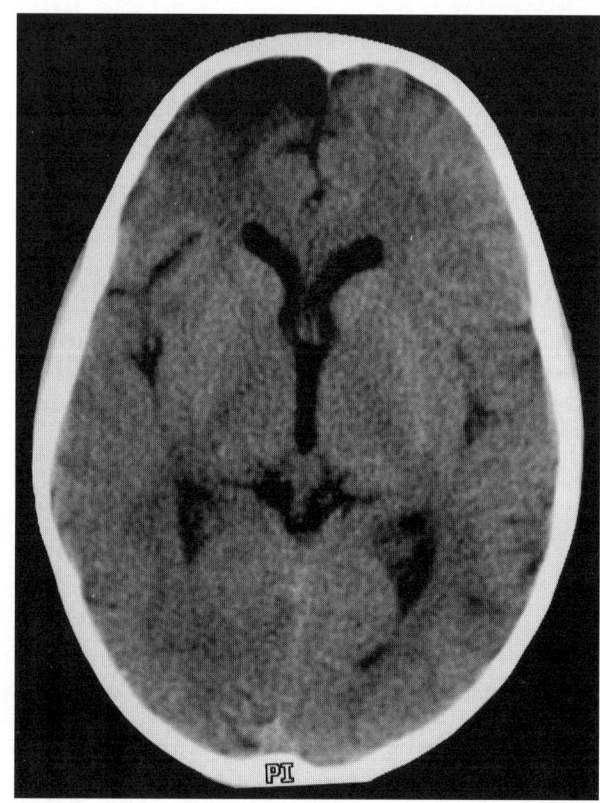

D

Fig. 19.8 Acute subdural haematoma and severe brain swelling. A 5-year-old boy was hit by a truck in a remote part of Australia. He was unconscious, and was intubated in a country hospital. He was paralysed and ventilated, and then transferred a distance of some 250 km to a hospital with a CT scanner but no neurosurgical facilities. **A** CT scan (day 1) showed a small right-sided acute subdural haematoma (arrows) and brain swelling, especially in the right frontal lobe. The quadrigeminal cisterns were well seen. He was immediately transferred by air a distance of > 2000 km to a paediatric neurosurgical unit. On day 3 he was extubated and began to talk. On day 4, the conscious level worsened. **B** CT scan (day 4) revealed more marked brain swelling, obliteration of basal cisterns and some subarachnoid blood. He was again intubated and ventilated. **C** CT scan (day 7) showed a dramatic improvement in brain swelling and good visualization of the ventricles and cisterns. The subarachnoid haemorrhage had resolved. **D** The child made a good recovery, but developed behavioural problems. 5 months later, CT showed atrophic changes in the right frontal area. The rapid onset of brain swelling and dramatic recovery are characteristic of head injuries in the first few years of life. So, unhappily, are the late psychological effects.

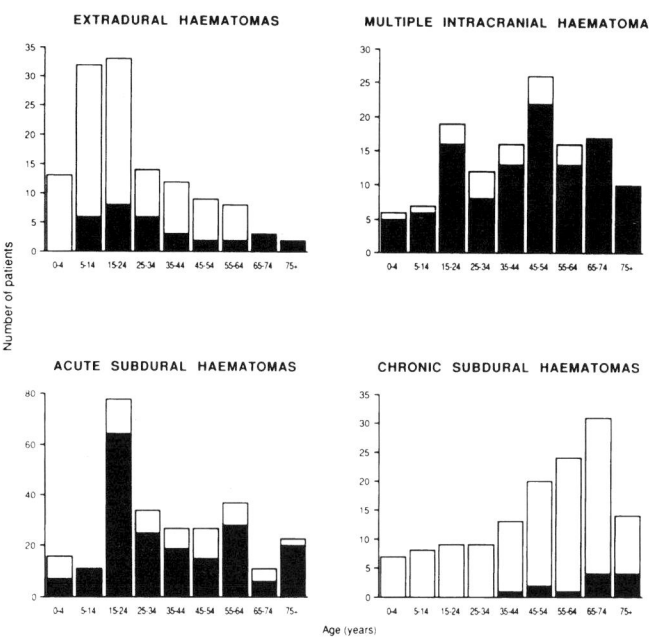

(Moro, Landau and parachute automatisms) in an injured infant, and their value is in any case not great. A full developmental assessment (Griffiths 1970) requires patience and some experience; for routine purposes, the examiner may use a simple check list such as the norms set out in Tables 19.1 and 19.2. However, in the early post-traumatic period, fear and pain usually make a definitive assessment of the developmental age unreliable. Parents can often help by calming the patient, and by comparing the responses to his/her attainments before injury.

Fig. 19.9 Age incidence of intracranial haematomas. The histogram shows the age distributions of the four chief categories of extracerebral haematoma in a population-based series of 680 intracranial haematomas reported by Dan et al (1986), Stening et al (1986a,b) and Vanderfield et al (1986). The category of multiple haematomas represents cases with two or more of the other three haematoma types or with an intracerebral haematoma; in 82% there was an acute subdural haematoma. Solitary intracerebral haematomas are not included. Black bars indicate deaths.

			BIRTH	> 6 MONTHS	> 12 MONTHS	> 2 YEARS	> 5 YEARS	
Eyes Open	4	Spontaneous	■	■	■	■	■	Eyes Closed by Swelling = C
	3	To Speech						
	2	To Pain						
	1	None						
Best Verbal Response	5	Orientated					■	Endo-tracheal Tube or Trach-eostomy = T
	4	Words			■	■		
	3	Vocal Sounds		■				
	2	Cries	■					
	1	None						
Best Motor Response	5	Obeys Orders				■	■	Record Best Arm Response
	4	Localise Pain		■	■			
	3	Flexion to Pain	■					
	2	Extension to Pain						
	1	None						
		TOTALS						

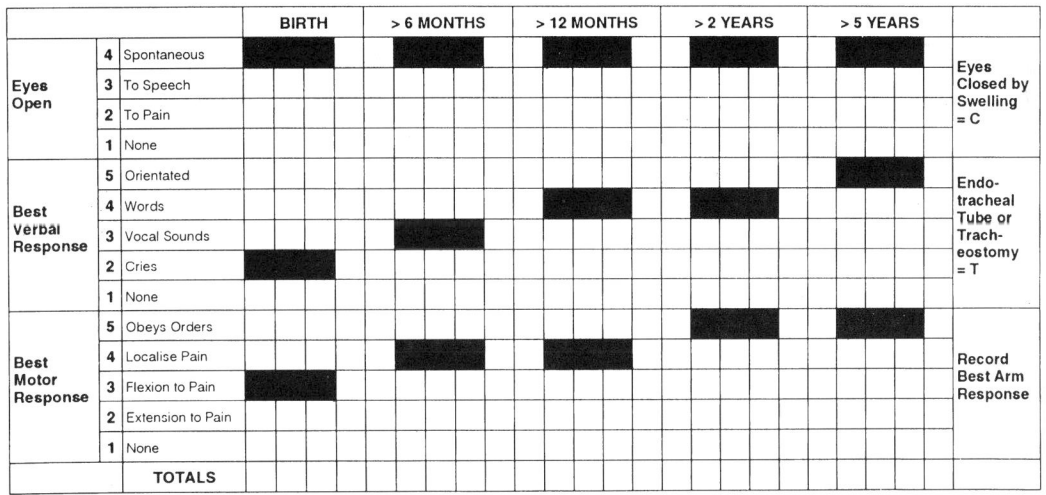

Fig. 19.10 Paediatric version of the Glasgow Coma Scale. In this scale, minor changes are made in the Best Verbal Response, to accord with the range of normal responses in the first years of life: the expected responses at different ages are marked as black bars. After Reilly et al (1988).

Table 19.1 Verbal and social milestones, related to the expected norms in the Paediatric Glasgow Coma Scale (PGCS)★

Age	Normal milestones	PGCS norms
Birth	Cries	Cries (0–26 weeks)
8 weeks	Vocalizes — chiefly vowels Smiles	
16 weeks	Laughs, uses consonants	
28 weeks	Syllables: ba da ka mu	Vocal sounds (26–52 weeks)
48 weeks	Word with meaning	
52 weeks	2–3 words with meaning	Words (1–5 years)
18 months	Jargon, many intelligible words	
24 months	spontaneous 2–3 word sentences	
3 years	Asks questions, uses pronouns	
4 years	Talks fluently, often fabricates or fantasizes	
5 years	Gives age, knows name, draws man, answers questions	Orientated (> 5 years)

★ The norms are taken from various standard textbooks (references given by Simpson et al 1991).

In cases of loss of consciousness, it is exceptional for a child to give the duration of the period of amnesia. The serial records of conscious level give a better measure of the duration of impaired awareness, if made by trained staff. However, PGCS scores should be used with caution as measures of the severity of a head injury in infancy: the infant's range of responses to external stimuli is narrower than an adult's, and a quite severe cerebral injury may underly a seemingly well-preserved conscious level.

Parents are involved in the care of the head-injured infant or child at all stages, and parental observations of altered behaviour are often of much diagnostic value, both initially and later. When the injured child's condition is stable, an assessment by a clinical psychologist is of great value in determining whether there are any neuro-psychological deficits and in planning educational rehabilitation. Psychological tests used in our service are listed in Appendix III.

Radiological assessment

CT scanning is the mainstay of diagnosis of intracranial haematomas and the indications are much as for adults (Teasdale et al 1990), though, in our practice, CT is used even more readily because the clinical signs of cerebral injury, especially cerebral compression, are often missed in frightened uncooperative children. In infants with open anterior fontanelles, ultrasonography is a very useful alternative. Magnetic resonance imaging frightens some children, and anaesthesia is often needed; nevertheless, this method of investigation is much used, especially in elucidating the long-term sequelae of head trauma.

Management

The principles of management outlined in Chapter 13 are relevant in infants and children with CMF injuries involving the brain, but certain aspects of craniocerebral immaturity have to be taken into account.

Intracranial haemorrhages present no very peculiar features, but one must keep in mind that volumes of blood loss which would be insignificant in adults may represent a very large depletion of the infant's blood volume: this is especially important with extradural haemorrhage. An infant with a clot of 50–100 ml volume may present pale and shocked, having lost perhaps 20–40% of its circulating blood; urgent blood transfusion must be given while operation is under way, and we have been prepared to use unmatched O– blood in such circumstances, as an acceptable risk.

In the child comatose after a CMF injury, control of airway and ICP are paramount. The policies of coma treatment set out on p. 381 are relevant, but it should be reiterated that endotracheal intubation in young people can be difficult if the operator lacks paediatric experience.

Table 19.2 Motor and psychomotor milestones, related to the expected norms on the Paediatric Glasgow Coma Scale (PGCS)★

Age	Normal milestones	PGCS norms
Birth	Spontaneous flexion and extension; reflex limb extension on neck extension (Moro startle response)	Flexion (0–26 weeks)
12 weeks	Selective movement of pricked limb; some head control when pulled to sit up	
20 weeks	Voluntary grasp	
26 weeks	Voluntary hand-to-hand transfer. Head extends when body is held in prone posture (Landau response)	Localizes pain (6 months – two years)
32 weeks	Directs gaze at pricked limb	
48 weeks	May give toy to examiner. Usually crawls	
52 weeks	Localizes pain exactly. May walk. Protective arm extension when lowered head forward (parachute response)	
18 months	Walks well. Obeys simple orders	
2 years	Runs. Obeys orders, points to parts of the body	Obeys orders (> 2 years)

★ These are deliberately simplified and set later than the usual milestones (references given by Simpson et al 1991).

In skilled hands, endotracheal ventilation is very satisfactory for periods of days or even weeks; a period of 2 weeks is certainly acceptable. Tracheostomy is rarely needed, except when there is severe orofacial trauma; in small infants, endotracheal intubation is the safer option regardless of the expected duration of coma. Brain swelling is often a serious problem, and it is believed that this is in large degree due to cerebral hyperaemia (p. 512) though other causes can often be identified. ICP manometry (p. 369) is therefore instituted in children who remain in coma after resuscitation. If the initial CT scan is entirely normal, the risk of serious cerebral complications is less; nevertheless, it is still wise to monitor ICP for the first 24–48 h. If ICP is persistently elevated despite ventilation, it will be necessary to give intravenous mannitol and/or frusemide. Bruce et al (1981) suggested that a bolus dose of mannitol may cause a detrimental increase in the hyperaemia so characteristic of paediatric head injuries. We have not been impressed by this contention, though we have sometimes chosen to give frusemide first, especially when ICP measurement had not yet been installed. Muizelaar et al (1989) did not find evidence to suggest that mannitol increases ICP.

General nursing of the comatose child is usually easier than in adult cases. Nasogastric feeding is in most cases satisfactory, and gastrostomy is rarely indicated. Urethral catheterization can cause later stricture formation, and should be done with care and without any force; small catheters must be available. As soon as possible the catheter is removed, incontinence being usually easily managed.

It is in the period of recovery and rehabilitation that paediatric CMF injuries present most challenges. Physical problems, such as joint contractures and myositis ossificans, are rare, but intellectual and behavioural disorders are common and unhappily may lead to permanent disabilities. In the early stages, irritability or mutism may be seen, especially after frontal lobe damage; later, poor school performance and changed personality are common and often tragic sequels. In the rehabilitation process, which begins early, many people are involved: nurses, physiotherapists, speech and occupational therapists, social workers, play therapists, and most importantly the educational psychologist may all be engaged at appropriate phases of recovery (Simpson & Yeo 1982). But in most cases, the parents play the crucial role. If properly counselled — the neurosurgeon is usually best able to do this effectively — the parents can relate best to the injured child, they can provide a continuous familiar presence, and can detect changes in responsiveness. And their inevitable sorrow and anger may be mitigated if they have been responsible team members as well as victims of the accident.

EYE INJURIES IN CHILDHOOD

Effects of immaturity

Humans have two overlapping frontal visual fields. The advantage of this is stereopsis; the disadvantages include the troublesome symptom of diplopia if the mature binocular visual system is disturbed and the serious problem of amblyopia after injuries affecting the immature visual system.

Because the visual system is immature up to approximately 8 years of age, any disturbance of its normal development, including injury, can lead to failure to reach maximum visual potential. The outcome of an ocular injury may be opacification of the cornea or lens, or alterations in the refractive power, or deviation of the visual axis induced by paralytic strabismus or restrictive strabismus. All these conditions may lead to amblyopia (reduced visual acuity) produced by failure of cortical cell maturation.

To grasp the concept of amblyopia, one must realize that for normal binocular vision with a high level of stereopsis, both eyes need to receive equal and symmetrical visual stimulation from the time of birth until the visual system reaches maturity. The visual cortex contains populations of cells which require binocular input to develop to maturity. If anything disturbs normal visual development by producing an asymmetrical input into the binocular system, these cells fail to develop their full potential. If an injury occurs in this amblyogenic age period, the effects are more far-reaching than loss of vision in one eye. The developing visual cortex also suffers and may be irreversibly affected, if the condition is not adequately managed.

The sensitivity of the visual system to these disturbances varies with the age of the children. It is most sensitive between the ages of 6 and 18 months and becomes less sensitive as the child nears the age of 8 years.

Management

In general, the principles and techniques of management described in Chapter 14 are relevant in childhood eye injuries. However, the problem of post-traumatic amblyopia requires special consideration (Elston 1990).

When there is a remediable impairment of the eye's optical system, then correction by appropriate spectacles, contact lens or intraocular lens correction is necessary. When this is not the case, we treat amblyopia with adhesive occlusive patches. This seems most effective when a concentrated effort is made to maintain full-time occlusion. Occlusion therapy of the uninjured eye is not innocuous, and should not be too prolonged; there are reports of occlusion-induced amblyopia in the covered eye. In general total full-time occlusion should not be prescribed in excess of 1 week per year of age: thus, a

4-year-old child should have 4 weeks of occlusion and then a reassessment of fixation patterns and visual acuity, whereas a 6-month-old infant should have only a few days' occlusion before the reassessment.

There are very few occasions when adhesive patches cannot be used. These include severe allergy to the adhesive, proptosis or corneal exposure which could be aggravated by the patch, and the presence of other periocular injuries which prevent the use of the patch. In cases where patches cannot be used we resort to atropine drops or ointment applied to the uninjured eye on a daily basis. If spectacles are worn and an occlusive patch cannot be used, the spectacle lens of the unaffected eye may be blurred or totally occluded using adhesive contact. In some cases, atropine cannot be used because there is an allergic sensitivity.

While the recognition of the risk of amblyopia and the appropriate management of amblyopia, if it is present, are important, we believe that patching should not be pursued so aggressively as to limit the child's development and rehabilitation generally. A child suddenly forced to rely on an amblyopic eye may lose confidence in everyday activities at school, or be ostracized by peers. Success in patching depends very largely on the parents.

SENESCENCE

FACIAL INJURIES

Effects of skeletal ageing

Bone loss is a part of the ageing process. After the age of 45 years, some degree of osteoporosis is usual, though there is much individual variation. Osteoporosis is more severe in postmenopausal women and in persons leading a sedentary life; it is also more severe when nutrition is poor and in persons given long-term corticosteroid therapy (p. 537) or anticonvulsant drugs. Cancellous bone is especially affected: thinning or loss of trabeculae reduce tensile strength and osteoporotic bones break easily.

Loss of teeth has an even more dramatic effect on the facial skeleton. There is a striking and progressive resorption of alveolar bone when a tooth is lost; this is most evident in the mandible but the maxillary alveolar bone is also resorbed (Figs 19.11 and 19.12). The nature of alveolar resorption is still poorly understood. Ageing is associated with narrowing or occlusion of the inferior dental artery (p. 49), and this is of surgical importance in relation to the healing of edentulous mandibular fractures; however, Pogrel et al (1987) did not find an association between absence of this artery and loss of teeth. The wearing of conventional dentures does not prevent alveolar resorption (Tallgren 1967). However, alveolar bone height is preserved if osseo-integrated titanium implants for prosthesis fixation are inserted into the edentulous maxilla or mandible immediately following tooth loss (p. 637).

Incidence of edentulism

In a consecutive series of 1074 cases of facial fractures treated by us, a quarter occurred in persons who were

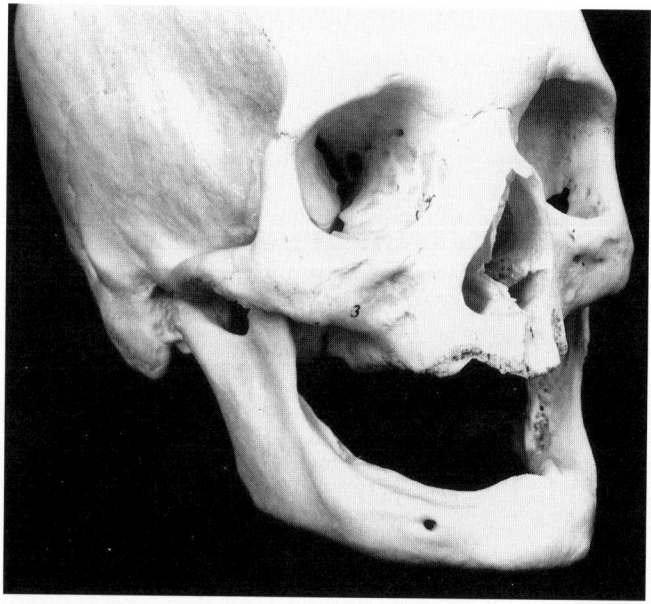

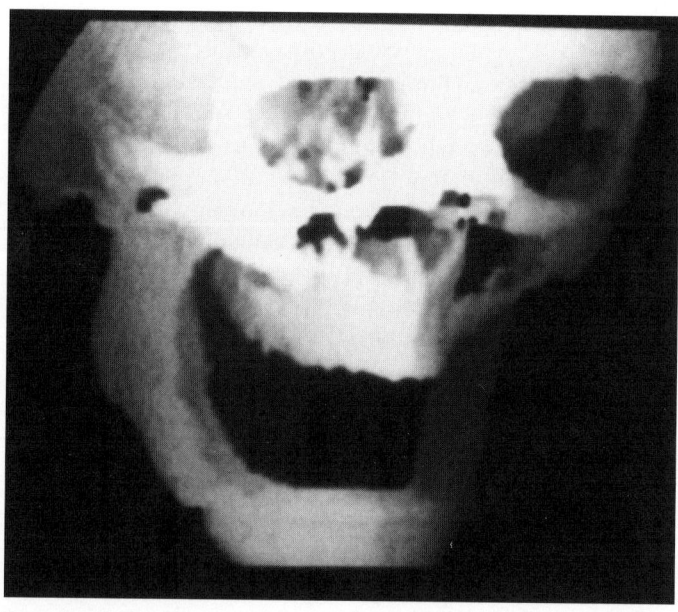

A   B

Fig. 19.11 Edentulous jaws. The atrophy of the edentulous alveolar margins is most evident in the mandible, but is also evident in the maxillae. **A** Dried skull of an octogenarian. **B** 3D CT scan of same skull.

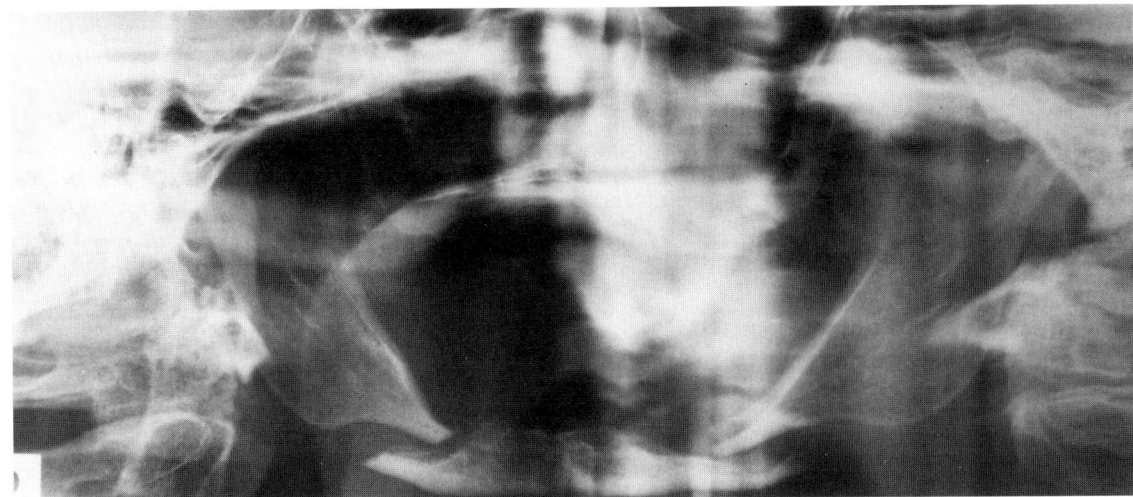

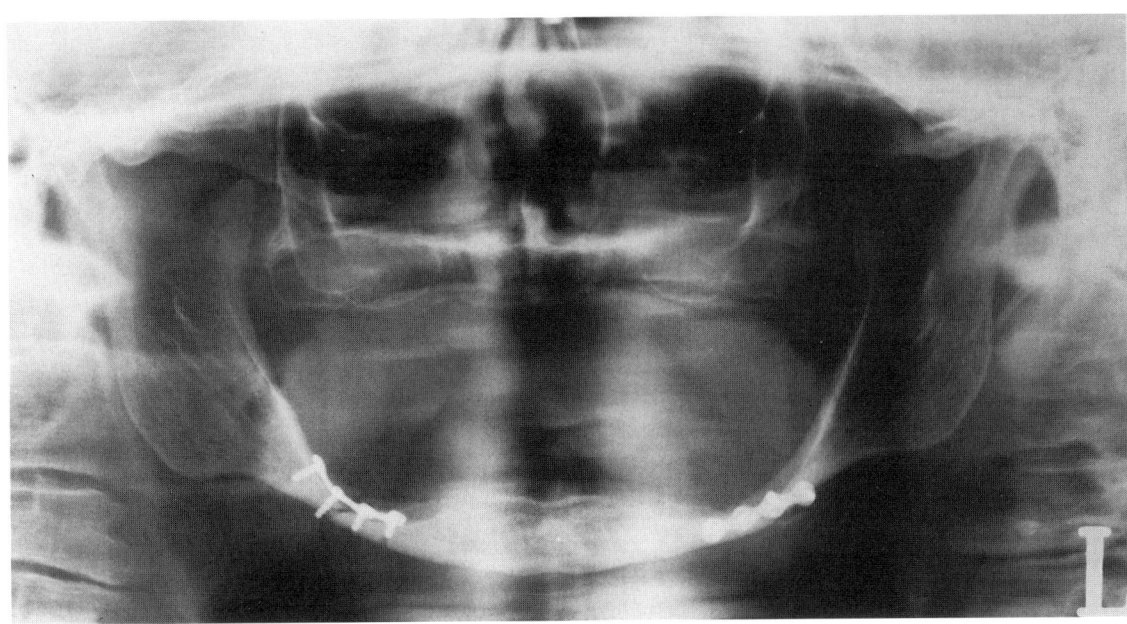

Fig. 19.12 Classical bilateral mandibular body fracture in the edentulous mandible. A An 86-year-old woman was assaulted by an intruder and sustained bilateral mandibular body fractures. **B** These were immobilized with lower border miniplates. Despite fracture of the left miniplate, there was progress to bony union, permitting the wearing of dentures.

partially or totally edentulous. Complete or partial loss of teeth is of course very common in geriatric populations, but can occur at any age. Today great emphasis is placed on oral health and on the benefits of retaining the natural dentition; the percentage of edentulous persons in developed countries has been declining in recent years. A recent report on oral health in Australia showed a substantial reduction in edentulism during the decade 1979–89 (Australian Institute of Health Dental Statistics and Research Unit, 1992). This reduction was noted in all age groups from 15–24 to 75+ (Table 19.3). In the 75+ age group edentulism fell from 78.6% to 63.4% but the reduction was most striking in the younger age cohorts, particularly in the four groups between 25 and

Table 19.3 Prevalence of edentulism expressed as percentages by age in Australia, 1979 and 1989*

Year	Age group (years)						
	15–24	25–34	35–44	45–54	55–64	65–74	75+
1979	1.3	5.4	14.0	26.5	40.2	60.7	78.6
1989	0.6	1.4	5.7	14.9	28.9	43.2	63.4

*Data from Australian Institute of Health Dental Statistics and Research Unit (1992).

64 years. Projections based on these data indicate that only a minority of older adults will be edentulous after the year 2000. A further survey of Australians aged ≥15 years who had partial or complete dentures was carried

Table 19.4 Distribution of persons with partial or complete dentures by age and sex: Australia, 1989–90*

	Age group (years)						
	15–24	25–34	35–44	45–54	55–64	65–74	75+
Males	1.6	9.0	22.9	40.4	57.2	73.6	84.6
Females	1.5	9.5	26.3	50.3	70.8	83.9	92.0
Total	1.6	9.2	24.6	45.2	64.0	79.2	89.3

* Values expressed as percentages of all persons examined. Data from Australian Bureau of Statistics (1992).

out in 1989–90 (Australian Bureau of Statistics, 1992). Over 13 million persons were surveyed to produce the results summarized in Table 19.4. The percentage of persons with either partial or complete dentures ranged from 1.6% in the 15–24 year age group to 89.3% in the 75+ age group. In all but one age group females exceeded males in the percentage of persons wearing dentures of any type. This may reflect a higher priority placed on facial appearance by females than males.

Incidence of facial fractures in the elderly

Zachariades et al (1984) noted that facial fractures in edentulous patients accounted for 5.2% of cases in their large experience; of these, half were aged between 50 and 70 years. Orbitozygomatic fractures accounted for 29%; most of the remainder occurred in the mandible. In the elderly, mandibular fractures are often multiple, apparently with an increased incidence of fractures in the body and the angle (Zachariades et al 1984, Thaller 1993).

Le Fort-type midfacial fractures are relatively rare, and occur (if at all) at the higher levels; Zachariades et al (1984) recorded no examples of classical Le Fort I fractures in their series. A modified Le Fort I pattern of fractures of the maxilla, which is displaced upward following the line of the upper border of the denture, has been seen when injury occurs while an upper denture is being worn (R. Cooter, personal communication: Fig. 19.13).

Assessment

The elderly patient with a facial fracture may have some pretraumatic illness likely to affect management (Ch. 20), or may be taking a drug that could have adverse effects on surgical management. Careful interrogation and medical examination are always needed, and a general or specialist medical consultation may be called for. Compromised cardiovascular or respiratory function may influence the choice and duration of anaesthesia and the tolerance of postoperative intermaxillary fixation. The social circumstances should be discussed, with special attention to the patient's abilities in self-care after discharge and the networks that may provide support.

If dentures were worn at the time of the injury, they should be inspected. Dentures indeed may be the impacting agent, causing more or less characteristic fracture patterns in the edentulous jaws (see above).

Principles of management in old age

In some respects, management is easier than in younger patients. Facial fractures with displacement producing aesthetic changes but not functional disturbances may be tolerated more readily by elderly people, and this allows a more conservative approach. Minor occlusal disturbances in the edentulous patient may be overcome by prosthetic remodelling, rather than by surgical intervention. And finally, the elderly patient is often more observant of postoperative instructions, and less inclined to generate disruptive forces in mastication, as compared with younger people.

Fractures of the edentulous mandible

The treatment of these fractures presents a number of special problems, particularly in old age. Loss of alveolar bone, with reduction in total bone mass and impaired blood supply, results in poor union between bone ends in patients who may also be elderly and/or medically compromised, factors which increase the potential for delayed or impaired healing. Bruce & Strachen (1976) identified a non-union rate of 20% in fractures of the edentulous mandible irrespective of the treatment employed. This high rate of bony non-union is comparatively constant when compared to the varying figures for healing in the dentate mandible.

Various methods of management have been used in the treatment of edentulous mandibular fractures. None is wholly satisfactory. Fracture reduction and fixation by circumferential wiring was much used in the past, with additional splinting effected by wiring the patient's dentures or by a fabricated splint (Gunning splint: p. 16) to the mandible, with or without intermaxillary fixation to provide increased stabilization. Intermaxillary fixation is often poorly tolerated in the elderly, and may significantly compromise respiratory function. Moreover, there may be pre-existing degenerative changes in the temporomandibular joint and in the associated muscles and ligaments; the addition of a period of prolonged immobilization may induce irreversible changes in masticatory function. Extraoral pin fixation and percutaneous Kirschner wire fixation have been advocated; these achieve a variable level of osseous stability.

Many authors have favoured techniques of open reduction and internal fixation, ranging from transosseous and interosseous wires to a variety of meshes, lag screws and miniplates. Early bone grafting has been advocated to increase the area of bony contact and hence better fracture stability and bone healing, while augmenting the

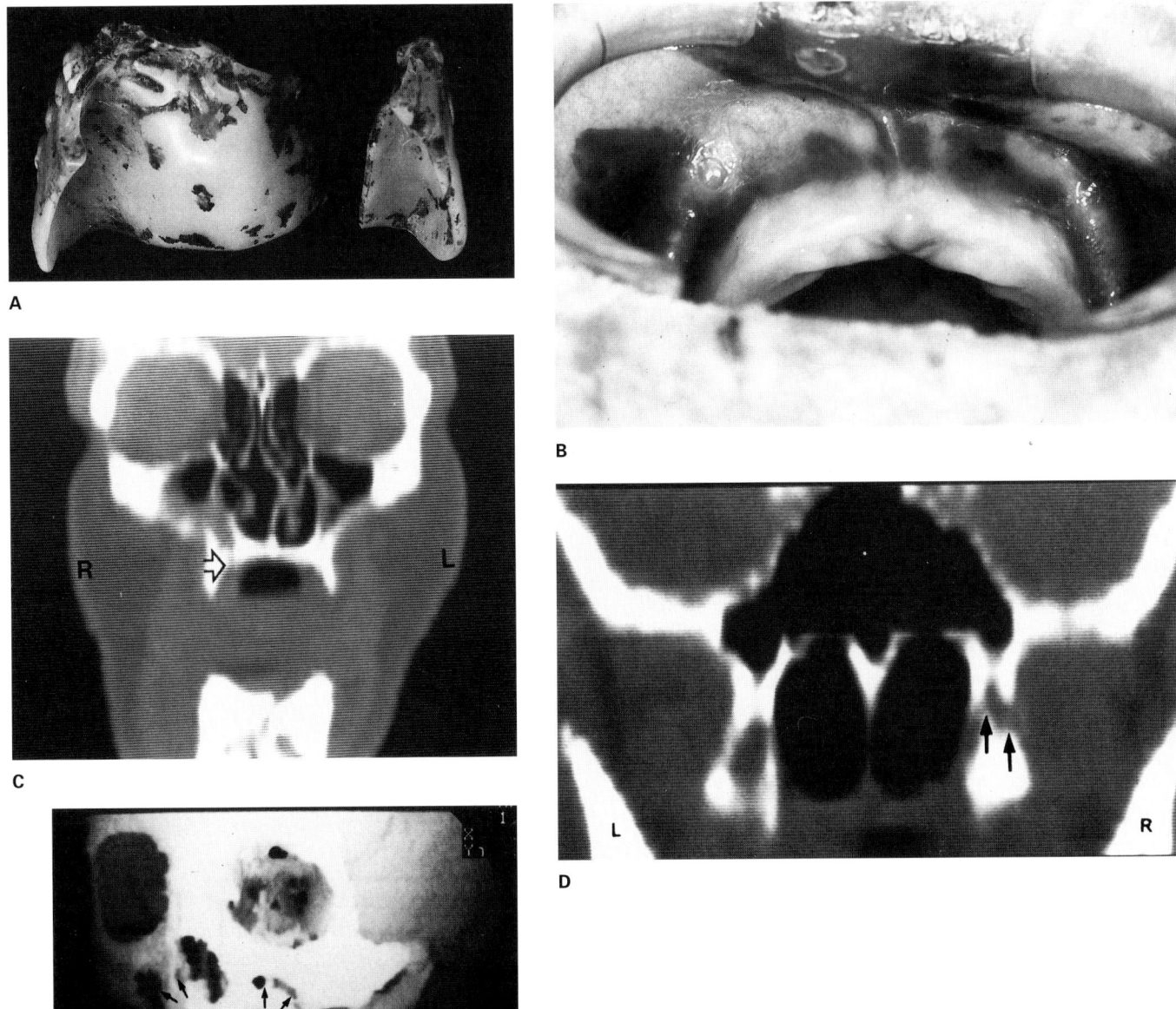

Fig. 19.13 Le Fort I fracture related to use of dentures. A 50-year-old edentulous man suffered a lower facial impact against the steering column while wearing dentures. The treatment consisted of open reduction and internal fixation of the maxillary fractures. **A** Broken denture. **B** Bruised upper alveolus. **C, D** 2D views of the fracture (arrows). **E** 3D view showing Le Fort I type fracture (arrows). By courtesy of Dr R. Cooter, from thesis accepted for Doctorate of Medicine, University of Adelaide.

alveolar ridge and thus improving the potential for post-operative denture rehabilitation (Obwegeser & Sailer 1973).

Rigid miniplate screw internal fixation of facial fractures now finds much support (Thaller 1993). All types of plate, ranging from large mandibular compression-type plates to the smallest microplates and micromesh, have been utilized. The reduced bone volume, relatively poor blood supply and positioning of the inferior alveolar nerve serve as biological limitations on the use of plating techniques. The exit of the inferior alveolar nerve from the crest of the resorbed mandibular body makes intraoral exposure and plate placement more difficult and more hazardous; upper border placement of plates by the

Champy technique (p. 273) in the edentulous mandibular body risks an increased incidence of plate exposure, and plate prominence may interfere with later prosthetic rehabilitation.

We favour exposure and fixation of the edentulous mandibular body fracture via an extraoral submandibular approach. Miniplate and bicortical screw fixation on the labiobuccal cortex and inferior border maintains a stable reduction of the displaced fracture and avoids intermaxillary wiring. Bilateral body fractures in the edentulous mandible are treated in the same way (Fig. 19.12).

Undisplaced fractures can be treated conservatively, with a liquid or non-chew diet and a soft foam collar to support the chin. Close follow-up with radiographs is mandatory to ensure early intervention if there is any evidence of subsequent fracture displacement.

Fractures of the edentulous maxilla

In cases where displacement is minimal, conservative non-operative management may be appropriate. Even if union occurs with some degree of anterior open bite, remodelled dentures may be sufficient to achieve an acceptable occlusion.

Where mobility or displacement is marked, operative reduction and fixation by either closed or open methods are necessary. The mobile maxillary arch can be immobilized with the patient's own dentures or with a Gunning-type splint secured to the palate, or suspended by wires from the zygomatic arch or frontozygomatic region. Intermaxillary fixation aids in maintaining a stable though non-rigid fixation. The relative deficiency of bone support in comminuted fractures risks upward compression and posterior relapse of the midface position.

Open reduction and miniplate fixation is our preferred approach, particularly for the higher-level midfacial fractures (Le Fort II and III) where bone volume is little changed from the situation in dentate persons, and hence the treatment plan need not be different. Loss of alveolar bone produces difficulties with miniplate fixation of the low level (Le Fort I) fractures. To find sufficiently strong bone for miniplate fixation one must often utilize the alveolar ridge bone for plate positioning, or import new bone as a primary bone graft. Both these manoeuvres may prevent denture wearing, or if dentures are worn may result in mucosal erosion and exposure of the plate. Under these circumstances, reoperation to remove the plates and screws may be necessary after fracture healing, before new dentures can be constructed and worn.

Despite the changes in the bony skeleton and the attendant variations in technique of reduction and fixation, the outcome both functionally and aesthetically is comparable to that achieved in the dentate state. Fibrous union or malunion has not been a clinical problem in our unit. The commonest complication, as noted above, has been a demand to remove prominent or exposed miniplates to allow definitive denture fitting.

DENTAL INJURIES

The problems resulting from loss of the teeth are discussed above. In those elderly persons who do retain their teeth, dental injuries are treated along the lines set out in Chapter 12.

CRANIOCEREBRAL INJURIES

Effects of ageing

The vulnerability of the ageing brain to trauma is well known. Jennett & Teasdale (1981) studied outcomes in a large number of severely head-injured persons who remained in coma for at least 6 h. There was a linear relationship between age and bad outcome (death or vegetative survival), and in patients > 70 years there were no good recoveries. Luerssen et al (1988) also found an increase in mortality rates with advancing age; for comatose (GCS $\leq$ 8) patients, the death rate rose dramatically in the 45–49 year age group, and remained between 60% and 80% thereafter. This failure to recover from the initial impact must be attributable to an age-related vulnerability to primary brain injury; it does not appear related to a higher incidence of secondary complications (Vollmer et al 1991).

With advancing age, the brain shrinks (Fig. 19.14). This change is usually seen, even in intellectually normal people, after 60 years, and becomes more marked in the seventh and eighth decades; it is still more marked if there is overt evidence of Alzheimer's disease or other form of dementing disease. The basis of this reduction in cerebral volume is in debate, but it seems to result both from a loss of neurons and a reduction in the number of dendrites and dendritic spines; some parts of the brain are less affected than others (Tomlinson & Corsellis 1984). Reduction in the neuronal population and in the complexity of the dendritic connections may explain why the aged brain tolerates trauma so badly, though other factors, such as vascular fragility and impaired cerebral blood supply, may be concerned. Sullivan et al (1987) reviewed the literature, and concluded that there is a reduction in resting CBF with advancing age; Hoyer (1984) suggested that both CBF and brain glucose metabolism are reduced in the elderly. However, it is still unclear what relevance this age-related change may bear to the outcome of cerebral impact in old age.

Surgical pathology

Haemorrhagic cerebral contusions are often seen in old people who have suffered blunt head impacts, sometimes

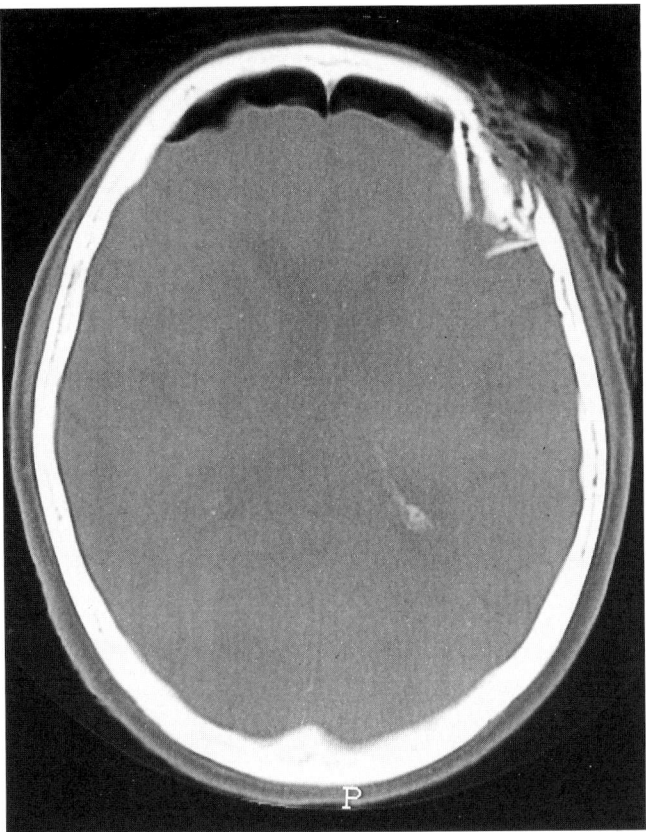

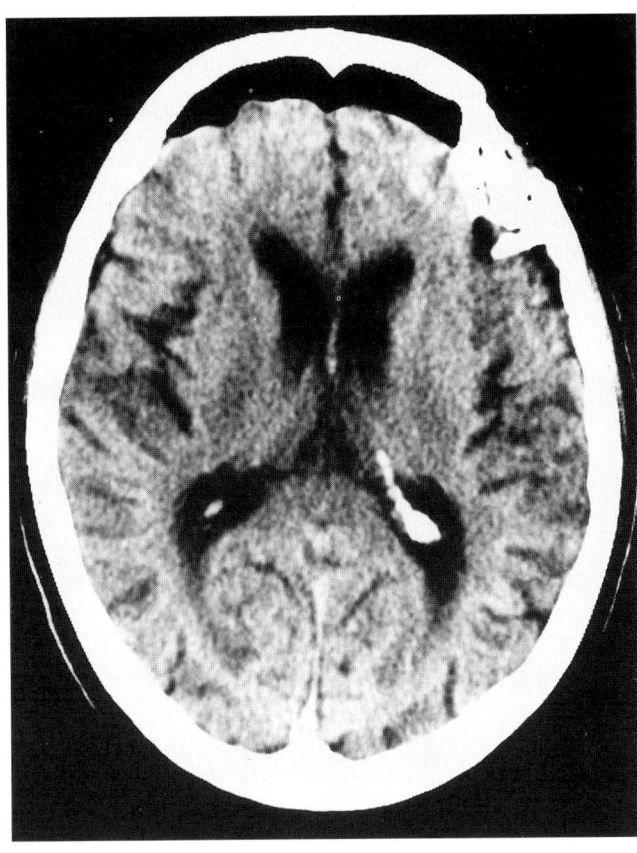

A

B

Fig. 19.14 Compound frontal skull fracture in an old man. A 79-year-old man was struck in the left frontal region by a flying piece of a grinding machine. When admitted, he had a speech impairment and a mild right hemiparesis. **A** CT scan (bone setting) shows a severely comminuted depressed fracture. There is a subdural aerocele. **B** CT scan (brain setting) shows marked dilatation of the ventricles and subarachnoid space, suggesting cerebral atrophy. The fracture was elevated and the wound was closed in standard manner. His hemiparesis improved, but his family think that his mentality has deteriorated. The finding of a subdural aerocele in association with a compound fracture is unusual, and may be related to cerebral shrinkage.

of relatively low energy; it is reasonable to postulate vascular fragility as a factor.

Extradural haemorrhage is relatively uncommon over the age of 60 (Fig. 19.9); this has been correlated with the greater adherence of the dura mater to the calvarial bone in the elderly. Subdural haemorrhage by contrast is often seen in old people. Acute subdural haematomas are often seen in patients over the age of 65 years (Stening et al 1986b), and chronic subdural haematomas show a peak incidence in the decade 65–74 (Vanderfield et al 1986). This can be related to cerebral shrinkage: the shrivelled brain presumably does not tamponade bleeding into the subdural space.

Cranionasal fistulas occur at all ages, and we have seen no special features in nine cases of anterior fossa fracture presenting at ages in the range 60–92 years. One may theorize that a shrunken brain would promote the entry of air into the skull through an anterior fossa fracture; this complication was indeed recorded in four of our nine cases. Fig. 19.14 shows a large subdural aerocele in

association with a shrunken brain, though in this case the unusual portal of entry was a compound skull fracture.

Assessment

Old age does not present any special difficulties in neurological evaluation, unless there is an associated dementia. However, there are several aspects of the ageing process that must be kept in mind.

The high incidence of delayed subdural bleeding demands careful observation and follow-up, even after seemingly minor CMF injuries. Chronic subdural haematoma typically presents weeks or months after a head impact, and the presentation may be insidious.

Second, viability always enters into the assessment of the elderly victim of a CMF injury with cerebral involvement. It is not as a rule a question of the anaesthetic and operative risks, though these are certainly increased in the elderly. Cardiac complications (Lutz & Georgieff 1984) and postoperative thrombo-embolic complications are more numerous over the age of 60 years, but rarely contraindicate a necessary neurosurgical procedure. Rather, the question of the likelihood of the injured brain making an acceptable recovery may deter the neurosurgeon from recommending some major operation. It is always necessary to know the previous level of function, and a psychosocial evaluation is very necessary: if there was pretraumatic Alzheimer's dementia or other cerebral disability, the likelihood of survival, still less a good recovery, is substantially reduced.

Management

Compound frontal fractures and cranionasal fistulae may be treated along the lines described in Chapter 13: in our small series of nine elderly patients with fractures of the anterior cranial fossa, the outcomes were considered good or moderate in six. Nevertheless, the case for conservative management of these injuries is surely stronger in the elderly.

In cases of acute intracranial haemorrhage, the decision to operate may be difficult. In elderly patients who present in coma from an acute subdural haematoma, and even in those with an extradural haematoma, good recovery is rare and prolonged survival in a state of severe disability is not unknown (Howard et al 1989). Similarly, in elderly patients who remain in coma after diffuse cerebral injury, there is little likelihood of a good outcome from prolonged intensive care. Ethical issues of great complexity can arise in counselling the family, especially when the patient has previously recorded strong wishes against treatment that might promote survival in a state of cerebral impairment.

The management of chronic subdural haematoma in association with CMF impacts is important enough to justify separate consideration.

CHRONIC SUBDURAL HAEMATOMA

Surgical pathology

Chronic subdural haematomas are characteristically seen in the elderly. In most cases, it is believed that the source of bleeding is a torn bridging vein, and vascular fragility or inelasticity may be causative factors. In the acute phase, the haematoma is solid but, over a week or more, the clot liquefies, and may eventually be absorbed. However, the haematoma may be augmented by repeated small haemorrhages under low pressure, together with serous exudate, into a cavity lined by granulation tissue formed from the dura mater. If not dealt with in time, subdural haematomas may expand and cause death from brainstem compression.

Alcoholism and anticoagulant medication (p. 532) often promote the bleeding process. Bilateral haematomas are frequently seen, being recorded in 10.4% of the cases studied by Vanderfield et al (1986).

Assessment

These haematomas commonly present weeks or months after a fall or minor blow to the head. The association with impacts in the CMF area is not especially high, but is sometimes seen: in the series of 135 cases reported by Vanderfield et al (1986) there were four cases associated with facial fractures.

The patient usually complains of headache, followed by mental changes and increasing drowsiness. Focal signs such as hemiparesis are sometimes seen; in the later stages, there are often typical signs of posterior transtentorial herniation: ptosis and inability to look up (Fig. 2.28). Diagnosis is usually by CT scan (Fig. 19.15) though, when the haematoma is isodense with brain tissue, MRI may be much more informative (Fig. 19.16). Bilateral chronic

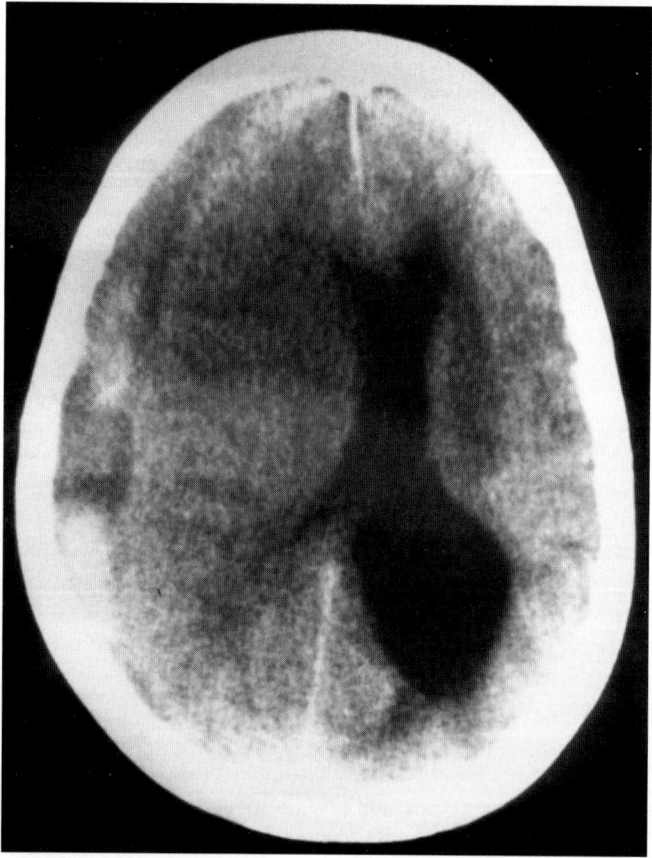

Fig. 19.15 Chronic subdural haematoma in old age. An active 82-year-old woman fell on a number of occasions, and in one of these falls she suffered a frontal impact. She became drowsy and incontinent. CT scan showed a chronic subdural haematoma the haematoma contained solid clot, seen as hyperdense masses. There was gross midline displacement. The haematoma was drained and she made a good recovery.

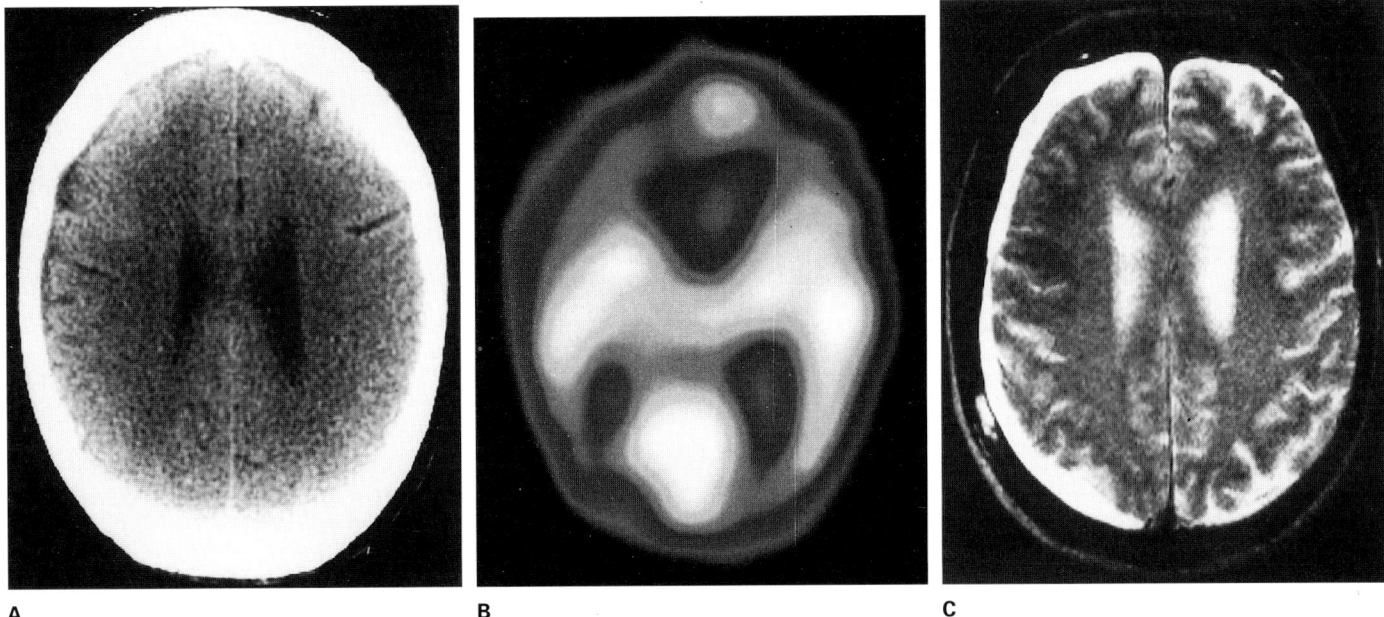

Fig. 19.16 CT, single-photon emission CT (SPECT) and MRI diagnosis of a chronic subdural haematoma. A 65-year-old male pedestrian was struck by a car and thrown into the windscreen. He was unconscious when admitted, and had a skin laceration near the right orbit, with a right subconjunctival haematoma. Initial CT showed multiple focal haemorrhages in both frontal lobes and in the corpus callosum. Progress was slow. On day 14, as part of a research study, he underwent CT, SPECT and MRI scans. **A** CT scan showed a small, seemingly insignificant, isodense collection in the right subdural space. **B** SPECT scan showed a significant asymmetry in metabolic activity in the same area. **C** MRI scan showed a signal-intense lesion in the T2-weighted image, suggesting a larger subdural collection. Operation was performed and a fluid subdural haematoma was drained. He made a good recovery, but remained blind in the right eye, presumably from an unsuspected optic nerve injury.

subdural haematomas may indeed be entirely unsuspected in a CT scan if the fluid is isodense, though obliteration of subarachnoid cisterns should suggest the possibility; MRI scan is then diagnostic. However, in comatose patients with a suggestive history, it may be legitimate to avoid delay by carrying out immediate bilateral burrhole exploration.

Management

Except in cases presenting in deep coma, or previously severely demented, the possibility of a good recovery is strong, and urgent operation can be recommended. The haematoma is usually fluid and can be drained through one or two burrholes; even when there are some solid clots, craniotomy is rarely needed. Usually there is rapid clinical recovery after simple evacuation of the fluid component of the haematoma. The brain may not expand after the escape of fluid; however, we have not seen this as

an indication for prolonged external drainage. Formerly, if the patient was in coma before operation, and especially when there were clinical or radiological signs of transtentorial herniation, it was usual to re-expand the brain in the theatre by slow intrathecal injection of Ringer's solution until the brain almost reached the dura mater; today, most neurosurgeons do not see this as necessary.

Results and complications

Vanderfield et al (1986) reviewed a total of 803 cases reported in eight published series, and added 135 cases of their own. Their survey confirmed that this is the most benign type of intracranial haematoma. Mortality rates ranged from 2% to 13%, and good recoveries (when reported) ranged from 65% to 83%. Delay in diagnosis seems to be an important cause of bad outcome, though pre-existing disease is often significant.

REFERENCES

Alajouanine T, Lhermitte F 1965 Aquired aphasia in children. Brain 88: 653–662

Aldrich E F, Eisenberg H M, Saydjani C et al 1992 Diffuse brain swelling in severely head-injured children. J Neurosurg 76: 450–454

Australian Bureau of Statistics 1992 1989–90 National health survey. Health related actions. Australia. Catalogue No. 4375.0

Australian Institute of Health Dental Statistics and Research Unit 1992 The dental labour force and oral health status in Australia, 1992

Bartlett S P, DeLozier J B 1992 Controversies in the management of pediatric facial fractures. Clin Plast Surg 19: 245–258

Beckler D M, Walker R V 1969 Condyle fractures. J Oral Surg 27: 563–564

Berger M S, Pitts L H, Lovely M, Edwards M S B, Bartowski H M 1985 Outcome from severe head injury in children and adolescents. J Neurosurg 62: 194–199

Boyne P J 1967 Osseous repair and mandibular growth after subcondylar fractures. J Oral Surg 25: 300–309

Bruce R, Strachen D 1976 Fracture of the edentulous mandible. J Oral Surg 34: 973–979

Bruce D A, Alavi A, Bilaniuk L, Dolinskas C, Obrist W, Uzzell B 1981 Diffuse cerebral swelling following head injuries in children: the syndrome of 'malignant cerebral oedema'. J Neurosurg 54: 170–178

Caldicott W J H, North J B, Simpson D A 1973 Traumatic cerebrospinal fluid fistula in children. J Neurosurg 38: 1–9

Carroll M J, Hill C M, Mason D A 1987 Facial fractures in children. Br Dent J 163: 23–26

Converse J M, Dingman R O 1977 Facial injuries in children. In: Converse J M (ed) Reconstructive plastic surgery, 2nd edn. Saunders, Philadelphia

Dan N G, Berry G, Kwok B et al 1986 Experiences with extradural haematomas in New South Wales. Aust NZ J Surg 56: 535–541

Denny A D, Rosenberg M W, Larsen D L 1993 Immediate reconstruction of complex cranioorbital fractures in children. J Craniofac Surg 4: 8–20

Duhaime A-C, Sutton L N 1992 Delayed sequelae of pediatric head injury. In: Barrow D L (ed) Complications and sequelae of head injury. American Association of Neurological Surgeons, Park Ridge, IL, Ch 12

Duhaime A-C, Alario A J, Lewander W J et al 1992 Head injury in very young children: mechanisms, injury types, and ophthalmologic findings in 100 hospitalized patients younger than 2 years of age. Pediatrics 90: 179–185

Elston I 1990 Epidemiology of visual handicaps in childhood. In: Taylor D (ed) Pediatric ophthalmology. Blackwell, Boston

Griffiths R 1970 The abilities of young children: a comprehensive system of mental measurement for the first eight years of life. Child Development Research Centre, London

Guthkelch A N 1979 Benign post-traumatic encephalopathy in young people and its relation to migraine. Neurosurgery 1: 101–106

Hall R K 1972 Injuries of the face and jaws in children. J Oral Surg 1: 65–75

Howard M A, Gross A S, Dacey R G, Winn H R 1989 Acute subdural haematomas: an age-dependent clinical entity. J Neurosurg 71: 858–863

Hoyer S 1984 Plasticity of the brain in old age. In: Piotrowski W, Brock M, Klinger M (eds) Neurosurgery in the aged. Adv Neurosurg 12: 109–116

Jastak S, Wilkinson G S 1984 Wide range achievement test. Level I. Jastak Associates, Wilmington, Delaware

Jennett B, Teasdale G 1981 Management of head injuries. Davis, Philadelphia

Kaban L B, Mulliken J B, Murray J E 1977 Facial fractures in children. An analysis of 122 fractures in 109 patients. Plast Reconstr Surg 59: 15–20

Kemble J V H 1973 The importance of the nasal septum in facial development. J Laryngol Otol 87: 379–386

Kitchens J L, Groff D B, Nagaraj H S, Fallat M E 1991 Basilar skull fractures in childhood with cranial nerve involvement. J Pediatr Surg 26: 992–994

Leake D, Doykos J, Habal M B, Murray J E 1971 Long-term follow-up of fractures of the mandibular condyle in children. Plast Reconstr Surg 47: 127–131

Lende R A, Erickson T C 1961 Growing skull fractures in childhood. J Neurosurg 18: 479–489

LeVere N D, Gray-Silva S, LeVere T E 1988 Infant brain injury: the benefit of relocation and the cost of crowding. In: Finger S, LeVere T E, Almli C R, Stein D G (eds) Brain injury and recovery: theoretical and controversial issues. Plenum, New York

Lin K Y, Bartlett S P, Yaremchuk M J, Grossman R F, Udupa J K, Whitaker L A 1991 The effect of rigid fixation on the developing craniofacial skeleton. Plast Reconstr Surg 87: 229–235

Luerssen T G, Klauber M R, Marshall L F 1988 Outcome from head injury related to patient's age. A longitudinal prospective study of adult and pediatric head injury. J Neurosurg 68: 409–416

Lutz H, Georgieff M 1984 Risk in anaesthesia with particular reference to the elderly patient. In: Piotrowski W, Brock M, Klinger M (eds) Neurosurgery in the aged. Adv Neurosurg 12: 122–127

McCoy F J, Chandler R A, Crow M L 1966 Facial fractures in children. Plast Reconstr Surg 37: 209–215

Messinger A, Radkowski M A, Greenwald M J, Pensler J M 1988 Orbital roof fractures in the pediatric population. Plast Reconstr Surg 84: 213–216

Moore M H, David D J, Cooter R D 1990 Oblique facial fractures in children. J Craniofac Surg 1: 4–7

Moran W B 1977 Nasal trauma in children. Otolaryngol Clin North Am 10: 95–101

Muizelaar J P, Marmarou A, DeSalles A A F et al 1989 Cerebral blood flow and metabolism in severely head-injured children. Part 1: relationship with GCS score, outcome, ICP, and PVI. J Neurosurg 71: 63–71

Neukam F-W, Schliephake H, Berten H L, Hausamen J-E 1991 Verletzungen des Mittelgesichtes im Kindesalter. Fortschr Kiefer Gesichtschir 36: 234–237

Obwegeser H, Sailer H 1973 Another way of treating fractures of the atrophic mandible. J Maxillofac Surg 1: 213–221

Olsen K D, Carpenter R J, Kern E B 1979 Nasal septal trauma in children. Pediatrics 64: 32–35

Ousterhout D K, Vargervik K 1987 Maxillary hypoplasia secondary to midfacial trauma in childhood. Plast Reconstr Surg 80: 491–497

Peltomaki T, Isotupa K 1991 The costochondral graft: a solution or a source of facial asymmetry in growing children. A case report. Proc Finn Dent Soc 87: 167–176

Pogrel M A, Dodson T, Tom W 1987 Arteriographic patency of the inferior alveolar artery and its relevance to alveolar atrophy. J Oral Maxillofac Surg 45: 767–769

Reilly P L, Simpson D A, Sprod R, Thomas L 1988 Assessing the conscious level in infants and young children: a paediatric version of the Glasgow Coma Scale. Child's Nerv Syst 4: 30–33

Rowe N L 1968 Fractures of the facial skeleton in children. J Oral Surg 26: 505–515

Rowe N L 1969 Fractures of the jaws of children. J Oral Surg 27: 496–507

Sarnat B G, Wexler M R 1966 Growth of the face and jaws after resection of the septal cartilage in the rabbit. Am J Anat 118: 755–768

Schonell F J 1961 The psychology and teaching of reading, 4th edn. Oliver & Boyd, Edinburgh

Selley I, Fränkel F B 1961 Skull fracture in infants. A report of 50 cases. Acta Chir Scand 122: 30–48

Simpson D A, Yeo P H 1982 Rehabilitation after head injuries in a paediatric neurosurgical unit. In: Garrett J F (ed) Australian approaches to rehabilitation in neurotrauma and spinal cord injury. International exchange of information in rehabilitation, monograph 19: 8–19. World Rehabilitation Fund, New York

Simpson D A, Cockington R A, Hanieh A, Raftos J, Reilly P L 1991 Head injuries in infants and young children: the value of the Paediatric Coma Scale. Child's Nerv Syst 7: 183–190

Snoek J W, Minderhoud J M, Wilmink J T 1984 Delayed deterioration following mild head injury in children. Brain 107: 15–36

Steinbok P, Flodmark O, Martens D, Germann E T 1987 Management of simple depressed fractures in children. J Neurosurg 66: 506–510

Stening W A, Berry G, Dan N G et al 1986a Experience with multiple intracranial haematomas in New South Wales. Aust NZ J Surg 56: 543–548

Stening W A, Berry G, Dan N G et al 1986b Experience with acute subdural haematomas in New South Wales. Aust NZ J Surg 56: 549–556

Sullivan H G, Kingsbury T B, Morgan M E et al 1987 The rCBF response to Diamox in normal subjects and cerebrovascular disease patients. J Neurosurg 67: 525–534

Taher A A Y 1993 Pediatric facial injuries in Tehran: a review of 87 patients. J Craniofac Surg 4: 21–27

Tallgren A 1967 The effect of denture wearing on facial morphology: a seven year longitudinal study. Acta Odont Scand 25: 563–592

Teasdale G M, Murray G, Anderson E, Mendelow A D, MacMillan R, Jennett B, Brookes M 1990 Risks of acute intracranial haematoma in children and adults: implications for managing head injuries. Br Med J 300: 363–367

Teuber H-L 1975 Recovery of function after brain injury in man.

In: Outcome of severe damage to the nervous system. Ciba Foundation Symposium 34 (NS). Elsevier, Amsterdam

Thaller S R 1993 Fracture of the edentulous mandible: a retrospective review. J Craniofac Surg 4: 91–94

Till K 1975 Paediatric neurosurgery. Blackwell, Oxford, Ch 3

Todorow S 1975 Recovery of children after severe head injury: psychoreactive superimpositions. Scand J Rehab Med 7: 93–96

Tomlinson B E, Corsellis J A N 1984 Ageing and the dementias. In: Adams J H, Corsellis J A N, Duchen L W (eds) Greenfield's neuropathology, 4th edn. Arnold, London, Ch 20

Vanderfield G K, Berry G, Kwok B et al 1986 Experience with chronic subdural haematomas in New South Wales. Aust NZ J Surg 56: 577–583

Vollmer D G, Torner J C, Jane J A et al 1991 Age and outcome following traumatic coma: why do older patients fare worse? J Neurosurg 75: S37–S49

Wangerin K, Kiesbye W 1991 Einfluss operativer Frakturversorgung auf das Wachstum des Mittelgesichts. Fortschr Kiefer Gesichtschir 36: 255–258

Wexler M R, Sarnat B G 1965 Rabbit snout growth after dislocation of nasal septum. Arch Otolaryngol 81: 68–71

Yager J V, Johnston B, Seshia S S 1990 Coma scales in pediatric practice. Am J Dis Child 144: 1088–1091

Zachariades N, Papavassiliou D, Triantafyllou D et al 1984 Fractures of the facial skeleton in the edentulous patient. J Maxillofac Surg 12: 262–266

Systemic disease

R. M. Edwards   D. A. Simpson
Contributing author: J. Trott

INTRODUCTION

The victims of craniomaxillofacial (CMF) trauma are typically young adults in good health; even in old age, accidents are more likely to happen to people who are still fit and active. It is therefore easy to forget that some trauma victims have serious antecedent illnesses which may be very relevant when a plan of management is prepared. The systematic clinical assessment outlined in Chapter 6, and especially the clinical history, should detect most of the medical conditions likely to prejudice the treatment of a CMF injury. In many countries, it is usual for persons with a serious medical condition to wear a Medic Alert wrist bracelet (Fig. 20.1) engraved with the diagnosis and any long-term medication being taken;

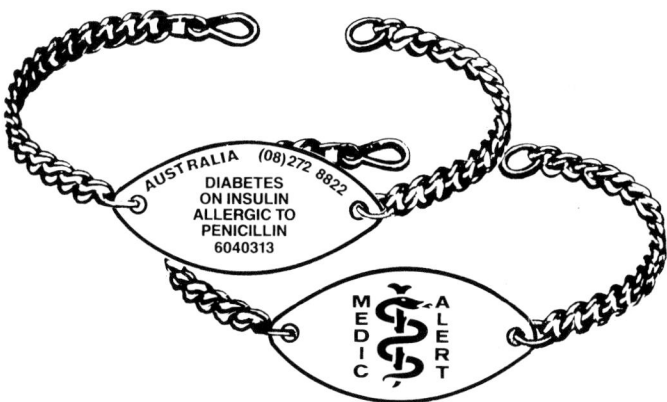

Fig. 20.1 Bracelet identifying medical problems. Medic Alert foundations provide these bracelets in the USA, Japan, Canada, Australia and many other countries. By courtesy of St John Ambulance and Australia Medic Alert Foundation.

this is very helpful when the accident victim is admitted unconscious. But some people resent or deny their illnesses and may not accept the need to wear the bracelet.

A long list could be made of the systemic illnesses which have the potential to affect the outcome of a CMF injury. This chapter considers only those which, in our experience or in the literature, are common and important.

ALCOHOLISM

Significance

Ethyl alcohol plays many roles in relation to CMF trauma. It is the cause of many road crashes, assaults, suicidal attempts and falls. It is an important confounding factor in the evaluation of the conscious level after head injury (p. 170). It is almost certainly a potentiator of acute brain injury. Experimental studies in cats (Flamm et al 1977) and dogs (Albin & Bunegin 1986) have shown that alcohol in intoxicating quantities promotes post-traumatic brain swelling and bleeding; direct cell membrane damage by free radicals has been postulated. Brooks et al (1989) found that cognitive recovery after head injury was poorer in those who had been drunk when injured, and their data suggested that this was due to an acute toxic effect rather than to chronic alcoholism; however, the series was not large and there were many variables. Waller et al (1986) have shown that drunk drivers are more likely to die or suffer serious injury than sober drivers, even when allowance is made for other variables known to influence outcome. Alcohol impairs immune functions, and promotes infection; Gurney et al

(1992) found an increased incidence of pneumonia in head-injured patients who were intoxicated. Excessive alcohol consumption has well-known toxic effects on the liver, the brain and other organs; chronic alcoholic liver damage is an important cause of haemostatic failure. Acute alcohol withdrawal may follow CMF trauma in alcoholics, causing epileptic seizures and/or confusional states, of which delirium tremens is the most characteristic and most dangerous. Chronic alcohol dependence is therefore to be regarded as a systemic illness likely to affect the management of CMF injuries in many ways.

Assessment

There has been debate as to when acute alcoholic intoxication becomes an alcohol problem and when an alcohol problem becomes chronic alcohol dependence. We take the pragmatic view that any alcohol-related injury is an alcohol problem and demands an enquiry into the injured person's drinking habits and nutritional status, especially when the blood alcohol level on admission exceeds 100 mg/dl. AUDIT, a 10 item questionnaire prepared by the World Health Organization, is recommended as a screening procedure to identify problem drinking (Babor et al 1989). Elevation of the serum gamma glutamyl transferase (GGT) suggests chronic hepatocellular damage, and is widely used as a marker of harmful alcohol consumption; as a screening test, it will identify some 35–45% of heavy drinkers (Whitfield 1991). However, an elevated serum GGT is a non-specific finding, and may result from sepsis, poor hepatic perfusion, or drugs such as barbiturates or dilantin (Mihas & Tavassoli 1992). Computed tomography (CT) may show cerebellar atrophy: this is also a non-specific finding, but when the atrophy is most evident in the superior cerebellar vermis, suspicion should be aroused (Fig. 20.2).

Clinically, delirium tremens must be distinguished from other similar confusional states; hallucinosis is strongly suggestive of delirium tremens, but occasionally results from other causes. Airway obstruction and chronic hypoxia may cause confusion, especially in elderly patients; hypercarbia and hyponatraemia are said to have similar effects. A brain injury may also cause restless confusion. In any victim of CMF injury who develops symptoms suggesting delirium tremens or alcoholic withdrawal fits, the possibility of a different metabolic cause should be excluded by appropriate investigations. It is especially important to consider the possibility of uraemia, hypothyroidism and liver failure before administering sedatives to a presumed case of delirium tremens.

Management

If there is reason to suspect chronic alcohol dependence

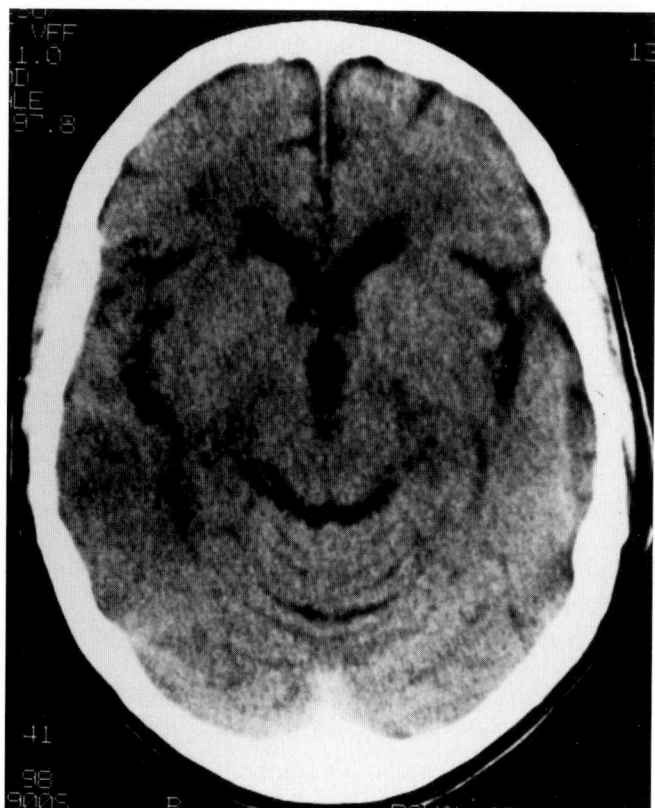

Fig. 20.2 Alcoholic cerebellar atrophy. A middle-aged man was admitted complaining of post-traumatic headache. Subdural haematoma was suspected, but CT scan showed signs of cerebellar atrophy. There was a history of excessive alcohol consumption.

or excessive alcohol consumption in a comatose patient, particular care is taken to monitor the metabolic state and the intracranial pressure (p. 369). Thiamine, alone or in a multivitamin preparation, is given by intravenous injection; in severe alcoholism, it is important to give thiamine before infusing a glucose solution, to prevent Wernicke's encephalopathy. The screening tests for impaired bleeding and clotting are performed.

In conscious patients recovering from CMF trauma, alcohol withdrawal may result in a grand mal fit or a confusional state, usually 12–48 h after cessation of alcohol consumption. These are dangerous complications after surgical fixation of jaw fractures, especially if intermaxillary fixation has been used. When the history suggests alcohol dependence it is usually wise to defer maxillofacial surgery for 10 days, while the possibility of alcohol withdrawal is monitored; oral benzodiazepine medication (e.g. diazepam up to 60 mg) is given (Romach & Sellers 1991).

If a seizure does occur, treatment by intravenous diazepam (2 mg/min to 20 mg) is recommended to control the seizure, together with phenytoin (Dilantin) or phenobarbitone. A CT scan should be done to exclude intracranial bleeding. Fitting after alcohol withdrawal does not require long-term anticonvulsant medication. There is often associated fluid retention, which should be corrected by fluid restriction; frusemide or mannitol should be used sparingly because these agents tend to promote electrolyte loss in the urine and metabolic alkalosis. If there is hyponatraemia (< 120 mmol/l Na), hypertonic (e.g. 5%) saline infusion should be given (Ayus et al 1987).

Delirium tremens may appear in the first few days after injury, and is a very serious complication of CMF trauma. The control of delirium tremens is somewhat controversial. Bakay & Glasauer (1980) advocated treatment by intravenous 25% glucose, thiamine and a small dose of insulin; however, most surgeons rely on oral or intravenous diazepam as a means of sedation, with precautions against the transient apnoea that sometimes follows intravenous injection of this drug. Haloperidol (0.5–5 mg by intramuscular injection) has been advocated for rapid control of hallucinosis, but we do not advise this drug in head injury management as it has unpredictable neurological side-effects.

In all injuries complicated by alcoholism or alcohol dependency, there is a possibility of previous nutritional inadequacy. Thiamine is given in the initial stage of management; thereafter, a dietetic consultation is desirable to get a full dietary history and to ensure that a good diet is maintained.

Alcohol addiction complicates rehabilitation, especially when there are behavioural disorders due to frontal lobe damage, and alcohol may potentiate post-traumatic epilepsy. Langley et al (1990) offer a comprehensive counselling programme adjusted to the apparent severity of the pretraumatic alcohol problem. It is common to find that patients with cerebral injury experience an inability to tolerate previously acceptable quantities of alcohol, and awareness of this has helped some to abstain or to take alcohol only in low doses. It is important to warn all head injured persons of this lowered tolerance, and to advise great restraint in the future. It has in fact been urged that the aftermath of a severe injury offers a window of opportunity for counselling on alcohol consumption. It is our practice to refer persons — especially young persons — who are admitted with a high blood level of alcohol to the counselling service of our hospital Drug and Alcohol Resource Unit. But we have no statistical evidence to show that this practice is effective.

BONE DISEASES

Significance

Any disease process which weakens bone by expansion or destruction renders that bone liable to pathological fracture. This is more likely to happen in a bone subject to high tensile or compressive forces; it follows that in the CMF area, the bone most often affected by pathological fracture is the mandible. The facial skeleton and calvarial bones are often involved by generalized bone diseases, or invaded by metastatic tumours, primary tumours and tumour-like conditions; nevertheless, pathological fractures are uncommon and it is extremely unusual for a pathological fracture to be the first sign of bone disease in the CMF skeleton.

Fractures through dental or dentigerous cysts have been reported (Partridge & Towers 1987) and have been seen in association with primary or secondary infiltrative tumours (MacMillan et al 1991). Rowe & Killey (1955) noted that the mandible is a rare site for metastases, in comparison with the rest of the skeleton; in their experience, the condylar neck was the favoured site when metastasis did take place. In our practice, pathological fractures have been rare; in a study of 324 consecutive mandibular fractures seen over a 3 year period, there were none attributable to malignant disease. We have, however, occasionally seen pathological fracture due to radiation necrosis when the mandible was included in the field of external beam irradiation of an adjacent squamous cell carcinomas of the oral or pharyngeal mucosa. Mandibular radiation necrosis tends to progress slowly and may become septic (Millett et al 1990).

Assessment

In most cases, there is a history of local or generalized bone disease. Pathological fractures may occur relatively silently, or more acutely with pain and swelling. Even when there is no relevant history of neoplasm or bone disease, the radiographs should be diagnostic, or at least suspicious, of the disease process. The clinical assessment will include attention to the general health in cases of malignant bone disease, and to oral hygiene and possible local infection.

Management

This will be dictated by the nature of the disease process. Benign tumours should be excised, with restoration of the facial skeleton by some appropriate technique; malignant tumours may respond to combined therapy.

In cases of septic osteoradionecrosis, intravenous antibiotics (usually flucloxacillin and metronidazole) are given, and the necrotic area is debrided, with removal of sequestra and any involved teeth and dental roots. Satisfactory fibrous union may take place, allowing function without the need for anatomical reconstruction. However, where pain or dysfunction demand restoration of the bone, a vascularized bone graft should be inserted by microvascular methods (p. 626) after resecting all the bone involved by radiation. In those rare cases in which the fracture is associated with primary malignant disease

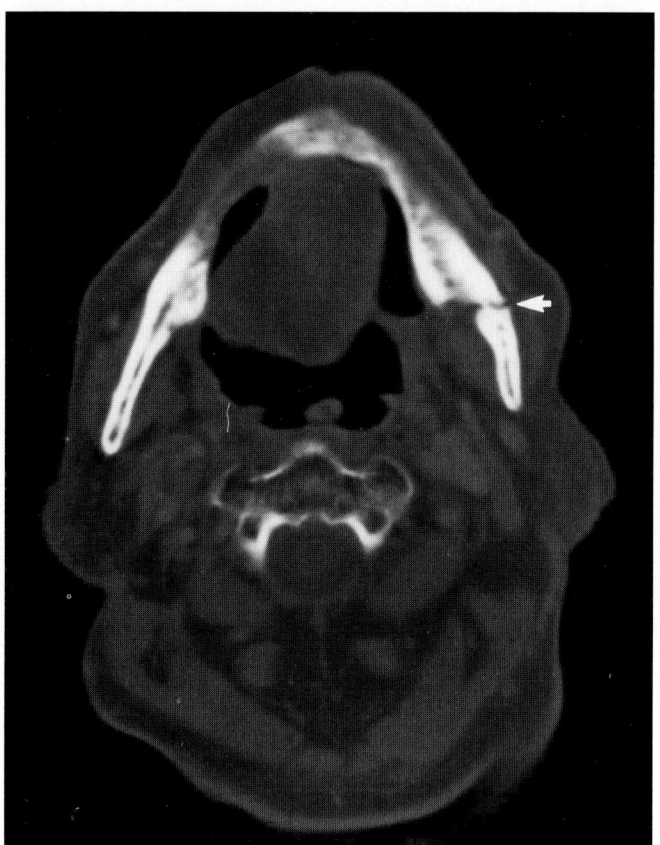 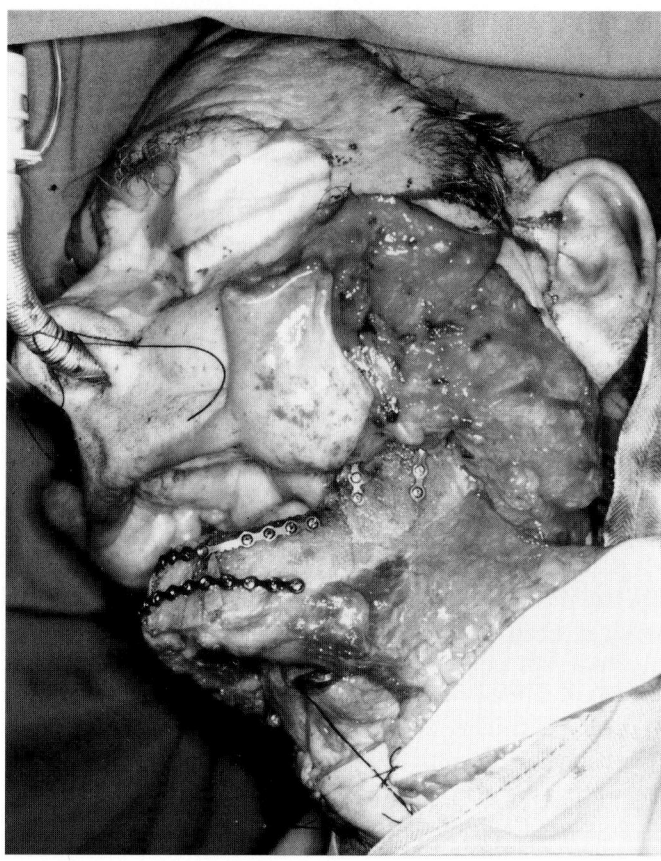

A   **B**

Fig. 20.3 Pathological fracture of the mandible. A 58-year-old man presented with pathological fractures of the left angle and right body of the mandible. He had undergone excision and postoperative radiation of a squamous cell carcinoma of the floor of the mouth 8 years earlier. **A** CT scan showing fracture of angle (arrow). **B** The mandible was excised from mid-ramus to mid-ramus, with immediate microvascular reconstruction using two bone grafts taken from the iliac crests and supplied by the deep circumflex iliac arteries. The man lived six months, with relatively good jaw function.

(Fig. 20.3), then one may carry out block resection of the disease and the surrounding bone and soft tissue, including the fracture, restoring function with an appropriate bone graft (Sadoff & Rubin 1990).

COAGULOPATHIES AND OTHER BLEEDING DISORDERS

Significance

Haemostatic failure can be a disastrous complication of CMF injury, especially when there is intracranial bleeding. When there is a major coagulopathy such as haemophilia, or a severe platelet defect, even a minor head impact can cause progressive intracerebral, subdural or less commonly extradural bleeding. Our experiences before the advent of potent specific therapy were very unhappy (Simpson & Robson 1960); even now, management can be very difficult. Our neurosurgical experience includes 15 cases of head injury in which a pre-existing systemic disorder of haemostatic function led to a life-threatening intracranial haematoma; seven died, five after seemingly minor head impacts. Haematomas in the neck or mediastinum may complicate minor injuries (Fig. 20.4), or appear after some injudicious attempt to cannulate one of the cervical vessels; airway obstruction may be a disastrous consequence. Although some defects of haemostasis are more serious than others, we have seen trouble from almost all the common coagulopathies and purpuric syndromes (Table 20.1).

Haemostasis may also fail in a healthy individual if post-traumatic bleeding depletes the haemostatic capacity: massive transfusion may promote this, since stored blood may be deficient in some essential factors, especially platelets and factor VIII. This form of post-traumatic haemostatic failure is termed washout coagulopathy. Another acquired cause of haemostatic failure is disseminated intravascular coagulopathy (DIC), a common sequel of sepsis and/or major trauma, and sometimes seen as a complication of severe cerebral injury, presumably because brain thromboplastic agents enter the systemic circulation (Kaufman & Mattson 1985, Simpson et al 1991). Iatrogenic haemostatic impairments are common as a result of anticoagulant prophylaxis against thrombo-embolic disease, and liver disease may also result in a coagulopathy.

Assessment

In any CMF injury, one should ask about previous abnormal bleeding after a wound or surgical or dental procedure, especially if blood transfusion has been needed. The patient is asked about medications likely to cause haemostatic failure, such as warfarin or aspirin. If the injured person is unconscious, the relatives should be questioned: in one of our cases, a history of abnormal bleeding was only given after death. The clinical examination should note skin bruising disproportionate to the supposed violence, which suggests a platelet/vascular disorder, and bleeding from small wounds and punctures, which suggests a coagulopathy.

Routine screening tests of haemostatic efficiency (Table 20.2) will detect most but not all clinically significant abnormalities. Normal screening tests and a history of unremarkable recovery after dental extraction or surgical procedure together virtually exclude a long-standing coagulopathy. But haematological tests are no substitute for a careful history and examination, since the relevance of a laboratory finding depends very largely on the clinical context. If abnormal haemostasis is diagnosed or even suspected, a haematological consultation is mandatory; in a peripheral hospital this may mean an urgent telephone call, since the necessary expertise is not widely available.

Management

The surgeon and the haematologist must plan treatment together. The haematologist must not only make the

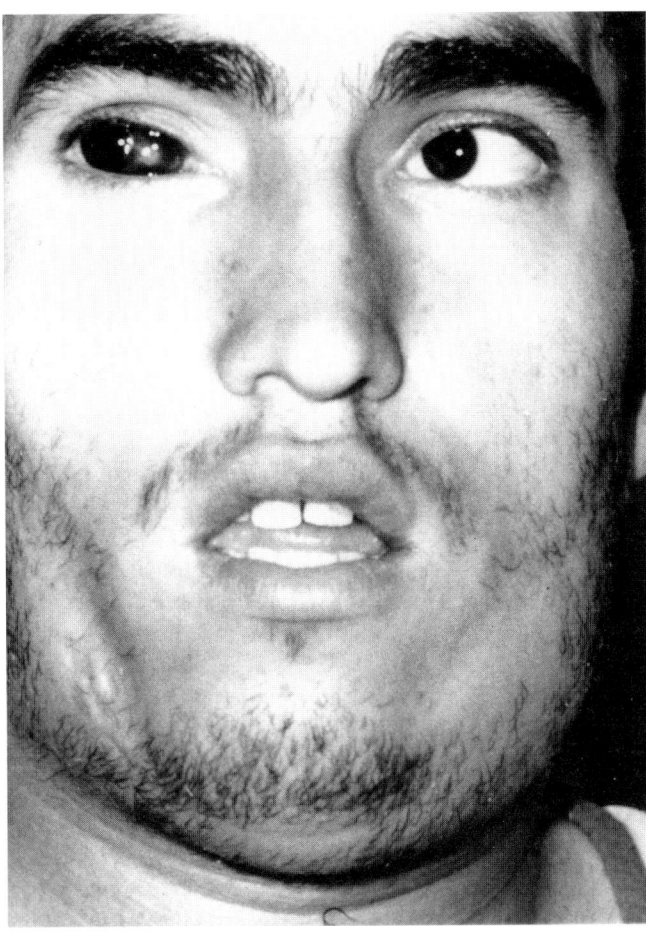

Fig. 20.4 Conjunctival and cervical haematomas in haemophilia. A young man, known to have haemophilia, consulted an ophthalmologist because of a large conjunctival haematoma. During the examination, a cervical swelling was noted. This rapidly increased in size and caused bradycardia and respiratory embarrassment.

Table 20.1 Common causes of haemostatic failure and their correction

Disease	Defect	Significance	Therapy
CONGENITAL			
Haemophilia A	Factor VIII	Always serious	Factor VIII concentrate or cryoprecipitate
Haemophilia B (Christmas disease)	Factor IX	Always serious	Factor IX or Prothrombinex
Von Willebrand's disease	Factor VIII and platelet defect	Less severe	Factor VIII concentrate or cryoprecipitate
Fibrinogen defects	Fibrinogen	Usually mild; may show impaired healing	Cryoprecipitate or fibrinogen concentrate
Glanzmann's disease	Platelet dysfunction	Can be serious	Platelets
ACQUIRED			
Washout coagulopathy	Multiple – especially V and VIII	Serious but preventable	Fresh frozen plasma? Prothrombinex
Liver disease	Multifactorial, especially vitamin K-dependent factors	Usually manageable	Vitamin K_1, fresh frozen plasma? Factor concentrates? Platelets?
Disseminated intravascular coagulopathy	Multifactorial	Varies; can be serious	Fresh frozen plasma, platelets? Factor concentrates.
Coumarin (Warfarin therapy)	Factors VII, IX and X	Easily managed	Cease Warfarin; Vitamin K1
Idiopathic thrombocytopenia	Platelets low	Easily managed	Corticosteroids; platelets
Aspirin therapy	Platelet dysfunction	Easily managed	Cease aspirin; platelets?

The estimates of clinical significance are based on personal and published experience in cases of intracranial bleeding; however, there is considerable variation in the severity of the defects.

Table 20.2 Tests of haemostatic function. The tests marked with an asterisk★ are done routinely if the surgeon requests a coagulation screen; the other tests are done if there is any clinical suspicion of a defect

Test	Normal values
Prothrombin international normalized ratio (INR)★	< 1.2
Activated partial thromboplastin time (APTT)★	22–37 seconds
Fibrinogen	1.5–4.0 g/L
Thrombin clotting time	12.0–16.0 seconds
D-dimer fibrin degeneration products (FDP)	< 0.25 mg/L
Bleeding time	2–8 minutes
Platelet count★	150 000–350 000/microlitre

diagnosis and give appropriate therapy, but must also follow the clinical progress and assay the haematological response; unhappily, severe coagulopathies do not always respond to treatment in the expected way and bleeding may continue long after the surgical wound has been closed. The surgeon must avoid operation if there is an acceptable form of non-operative management. Conservative management may be possible in many facial fractures; while the haemostatic defect is corrected, the patient is given antibiotics, a soft diet and appropriate oral hygiene. Even in non-progressive intracranial bleeding (Fig. 20.5), conservative management may be wise. But if there is progressive intracranial bleeding with deepening conscious level, the clot must be evacuated with every care to secure perfect haemostasis by local and systemic treatment (Yoshida et al 1979). Drainage is usually futile; any procedure likely to cause deep bleeding, like brain puncture,

should be avoided. Factor replacement must be given at once and continued until the wounds are healed.

Table 20.1 lists the specific replacements for the chief congenital and acquired haemostatic defects.

Haemophilia A is best treated with large doses of factor VIII concentrates (up to 50 IU/kg), heat-treated to prevent viral transmission; cryoprecipitate is cheaper but less effective, and with more risk of disease transmission. Fresh frozen plasma is inadequate and should not be given. Von Willebrand's disease, though surgically often less alarming, usually also requires factor VIII concentrates.

Haemophilia B (Christmas disease), which we have found as terrible in its cerebral effects as haemophilia A, is best treated by prothrombinex, which contains factor IX and significant levels of prothrombin and factor X (Beal & Isbister 1985, Beal et al 1988).

The thrombocytopenias are likely to need platelet transfusions. When the thrombocytopenia is thought to be an autoimmune effect, prednisolone (50–70 mg/day) and intravenous immunoglobulin are indicated. We have found no difficulty in managing head trauma in association with platelet defects, except in a case of Glanzmann's disease, where cannulating a dilated ventricle led to disastrous deep bleeding.

Wash-out coagulopathy should be anticipated and prevented (p. 228). If blood replacement exceeds one body blood volume, it has been usual to give fresh frozen plasma (2 units, approximately 550 ml), though Cohen (1993) has expressed doubt on the value of this relatively small volume. Platelets are given if the count falls below 60 000 /μl. If larger volumes of blood have to be replaced, Beal et al (1988) advise the use of fresh blood.

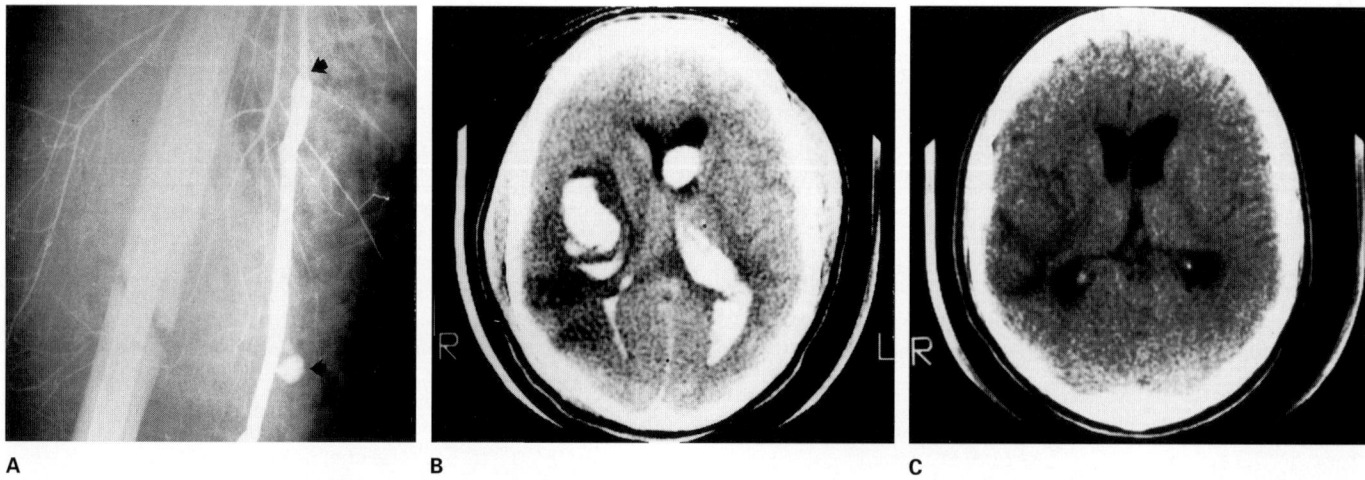

A   B   C

Fig. 20.5 Intracerebral haematoma in consumption coagulopathy. A 17-year-old pedestrian was hit by a car. He suffered a head injury and a fracture of the right femur, with rupture of the superficial femoral artery. An arterial repair by grafting was done at once. The graft leaked; reoperations followed and he received about 65 l blood. Despite administration of coagulation factors and platelets, he developed a severe wash-out coagulopathy. **A** Aortogram showing venous graft (upper arrow) with bleeding from a vein arising from the graft (lower arrow); there was also intrapelvic bleeding, which was arrested by embolization. **B** CT scan on day 5: large deep right-sided temporal haematoma, with intraventricular haemorrhage. Because of the coagulopathy, conservative treatment was adopted. **C** CT scan on day 35: the haematomas absorbed spontaneously and he made a good recovery, with a residual sensory hemiparesis.

The treatment of DIC in cases of CMF trauma is somewhat controversial. Fresh frozen plasma has been used with good effect, but additional support by other concentrates may be necessary. Unhappily the effects of the thrombotic process can include devastating cerebral infarction (Simpson et al 1991).

The haemostatic failure in hepatocellular liver disease is multifactorial and may include deficiencies of the vitamin K-dependent factors prothrombin, VII, IX and X in variable proportions; thrombocytopenia is not unusual. Vitamin K alone is often ineffective; fresh frozen plasma and platelets may be needed. We have found it easy to secure peroperative control of the bleeding tendency in alcoholics, but postoperative bleeding has sometimes been troublesome.

HIV INFECTION AND AIDS

Significance

The acquired immune deficiency syndrome (AIDS) pandemic has challenged surgical thinking and practice in many ways. In the management of CMF trauma, there are two aspects of infection by human immunodeficiency virus (HIV) that demand consideration, even by those surgeons who, like ourselves, work in communities with a low prevalence of this infection. The first is the risk of transmission of the HIV virus to a member of the surgical/dental team — or vice versa. This has received much attention in the recent literature (Sim & Jeffries 1990). The second aspect of HIV infection, which has received far less attention, is the possible adverse effect on wound healing and on resistance to postoperative infection.

Assessment

Persons at high risk may be identified by discreet enquiry into their sexual activities, previous blood transfusions, or use of intravenous drugs. Travel in geographic areas where HIV infection is very prevalent has been mentioned as a risk factor; the World Health Organization provides biannual reports on the prevalence and incidence of AIDS, and these identify many countries in Africa and America where the incidence is alarmingly high. However, there are obvious limitations on the value and applicability of such enquiries. The injured person may resent the enquiry, or may have forgotten some relevant experience in another country. Often in CMF injuries, the injured person may be unconscious, or in no state for delicate interrogation.

Physical examination may arouse suspicion. The oral examination (p. 345) may disclose thrush, hairy leukoplakia of the tongue or severe gingivitis (Greenspan et al 1990). Anal warts or an unusually lax anal sphincter may be pointers. Multiple unexplained needle punctures or superficial venous thromboses may be evidence of intravenous drug abuse. However, serological tests are needed to confirm the diagnosis.

The HIV-1 virus, the chief cause of AIDS, evokes serum antibody responses detectable by enzyme-linked immunosorbent assay (ELISA); the test usually becomes positive from 2 weeks to 3 months after infection. False positive results may occur, and a positive ELISA test must be confirmed by the very sensitive Western blot test. HIV-2, a cause of AIDS in West Africa and elsewhere, can also be diagnosed by serological tests. Persons known to have one or more risk factors should be strongly encouraged to undergo serological examination. However, there are ethical and practical limitations on the use of this diagnostic procedure. In the USA, the UK, Australia and some other parts of the world, it is likely that a doctor who fails to obtain informed consent before carrying out this examination would be liable to a civil law suit, and perhaps even a criminal charge (Gibbs 1990, Palmer 1990). Victims of acute CMF trauma may be unwilling or unable to give informed consent and it may be unwise to imperil a patient's confidence in the surgeon by raising this issue when urgent surgery is being recommended. A negative serological test for HIV antibody does not exclude recent infection; furthermore, some patients with clinical signs suggesting advanced AIDS may show negative tests for antibody, when tests for HIV antigen are advisable (Bayley 1990).

The CD4 lymphocyte count is accepted as a useful monitor of immune depletion; counts below 200/ml are now considered to justify the diagnosis of AIDS.

Prevention of infection

It is agreed that surgeons and other health workers may contract HIV infection by needlestick transmission. Conjunctival transmission is also possible; it has been shown that high-speed motorized instruments, such as drills and saws, can aerosolize HIV-infected blood, which could infect the conjunctiva (Hughes & Bailey 1993). The surgery of facial fractures is fraught with risks of finger injury, from interdental wires and spicules of bone as well as from needles and other sharp instruments. The risk from a single prick is thought to be low; estimates below 1% have been given, well below the risk of contracting hepatitis B. Nevertheless, the fact of AIDS as a surgical hazard has stimulated a review of surgical and dental theatre practice.

Since latent HIV infection may be entirely asymptomatic, and since routine serodiagnosis has limitations, it has been argued that stringent surgical safety measures should be enforced in all cases of acute trauma. In a low-incidence community, the need for this is questionable. But the risk of viral infection in the theatre has stimulated a general change in surgical techniques, towards minimizing the chances of transmission by finger prick or other accident. No-touch techniques have been advocated: for craniomaxillofacial surgeons, there are limits to this precaution since, in many procedures needed in CMF repair, the operator must rely on fine finger touch sense. The mobilization of facial fractures requires finger pressure, and if there are spikes of bone, the risk of skin perforation is high.

In trauma victims known to be HIV positive, or who have a history of risky activities and have not undergone testing, world surgical authorities have formulated standard management protocols. Measures to prevent intraoperative HIV infection are also effective precautions against hepatitis B, though of course members of surgical teams ought to be immunized against this infection.

Our theatre protocol for high-risk cases, based on recommendations by the Royal Australasian College of Surgeons (1987), is as follows:

1. All members of the team should be aware of the hazard of infection and of the precautions to be taken. Team members with open skin lesions will not participate in the operation.
2. Shaving of the operative field is omitted.
3. All theatre personnel will wear protective eye shields and face masks, long-sleeved waterproof gowns with wrist cuffs, and waterproof shoe covers; those who are scrubbed will use double surgical gloves. Where eye splash is likely, a visor may be used (Kinninmouth & Hutchinson 1991).
4. Anaesthesia is induced in the theatre rather than in the anaesthetic bay or room.
5. Operative techniques are designed to minimize the risk of injury to members of the team in handling needles, knives and dental instruments, especially in their transfer between operator, assistant and patient. Interdental wiring is considered to be especially likely to result in finger pricks, and should be avoided if possible.
6. Impervious wound dressings are used, with closed wound drainage if this is indicated.
7. Appropriate sterilization procedures are used for anaesthetic equipment, blood–contaminated waste and instruments. HIV is heat sensitive; chemical sterilization is less reliable, but 2% glutaraldehyde or 0.2% sodium hypochlorite solutions are thought to be effective.
8. In the event of accidental inoculation of blood, saliva or other infectious material from a patient known to react positively for HIV (or hepatitis B), whether in the conjunctiva, mouth, open skin wound or needle puncture, the affected area should be washed with a skin disinfectant; it may be appropriate to encourage local bleeding with a venous tourniquet. The accident should be reported and a specialist physician with an interest in AIDS should be consulted. Some authorities recommend prophylactic chemotherapy, such as zidovudine.

The patient must also be protected against iatrogenic infection. Surgeons and other theatre staff should undergo periodic serological tests for HIV, both for the protection of their patients, and as a baseline in case of later work-related infection. A health worker who has positive HIV serology should seek expert advice before undertaking any procedure, surgical or otherwise, that could put a patient at risk; as a rule, such a health worker should cease operating. The risks of transmitting HIV to a patient also include infection from blood transfusion or from banked bone (Buck et al 1989) or other organs; serological tests on donors are mandatory and should be repeated, since such tests may be misleading in the early weeks after infection.

Wound healing and post-traumatic infection

HIV invades the CD4$^+$ subset of helper/inducer T-lymphocytes, and also affects macrophages and other cells relevant in tissue repair and defence against infections (p. 121). As is well known, the first manifestation of AIDS is often infection by an opportunistic protozoal or fungal organism that would not ordinarily cause significant disease. HIV infection may also cause thrombocytopenia, even in the early stages of the disease (Yarchoan & Broder 1989). It might therefore be supposed that HIV infection would seriously complicate the management of CMF trauma. However, it is hard to find in the literature any clear guidance on the extent to which this is the case, or on the policies to be adopted in injured persons who are seropositive. It is clear that a therapeutic distinction must be made between those injured persons with asymptomatic HIV infection, and those in the later stages of the disease. It is reported that clinical immune failure has developed in 30–50% of persons with HIV infection followed over a 5-year period (Gibbs 1990), but the latent period is measured in years, and injuries may present long before immune failure is clinically evident.

Early reports suggested a high incidence of wound complications in AIDS (Robinson et al 1987). However, Schecter (1990) and Burke et al (1991), working in San Francisco, an area of very high AIDS prevalence, have concluded that asymptomatic patients with HIV infection do not have a significantly increased surgical morbidity or mortality from surgery, at least in the anorectal region. If this is confirmed, it appears reasonable to treat CMF injuries in such patients along routine lines; in particular, there would appear to be no special reason to prefer conservative management of facial fractures over the methods of internal fixation described in Chapter 11. When the infected patient is losing weight and showing signs of organ involvement, the risks of impaired wound healing and postoperative infection do become significant, and it may be appropriate to refrain from advising operations that are not clearly essential to the patient's short-term well-being, especially those entailing surgical implants. Bayley (1990), working in Zambia for a population with a very high prevalence of HIV infection, comments on the high incidence of wound infection, even after clean elective surgery, and records late infection of orthopaedic implants. Possibly the apparently better results reported from the USA reflect a difference in the facilities available for supportive care and correction of associated malnutrition and anaemia.

It is to be hoped that an effective antiretroviral drug will resolve the surgical dilemmas arising from HIV infection. In the meantime, surgeons who work in societies in which this infection is rare must await guidance from those who are less fortunate.

STEROID MEDICATION AND IMMUNOSUPPRESSIVE THERAPY

Significance

Any person who has taken cortisone or one of its synthetic analogues for long periods may show impairment of the normal hypothalamic–pituitary–adrenal (HPA) response to stress. The degree of suppression of adrenal function is roughly measured by the time taken for recovery after cessation of therapy, and this varies with the dose and duration of corticosteroid treatment. But anyone who has taken a glucocorticoid in pharmacological doses for 1 month may have clinically significant adrenal suppression. In such cases, there is a real risk that hypotension, or even a lethal Addisonian crisis, may develop after an injury.

Corticosteroids may also impair wound healing, especially the synthesis of collagen (p. 122). Chronic steroid medication is often associated with osteoporosis and bone fragility; it appears that osteoblastic activity is inhibited and parathormone secretion stimulated, with consequent increase in osteoclastic activity and impaired bone formation.

The success of many forms of organ transplantation depends on potent immunosuppressive drugs, including cyclosporin, azothioprine and corticosteroids in various combinations. These drugs obviously render the patient vulnerable to microbial infections.

There are thus important theoretical risks from trauma in this heterogeneous group of patients, quite apart from those related to the underlying disease. In our experience, the practical consequences of steroid medication and even immunosuppression have not been very difficult to manage: anaesthesia has been well tolerated and wounds have healed. Nevertheless, management must take into account all the possible adverse consequences of adrenal cortical failure, impaired immunity and defective collagen formation.

Assessment

There will usually be a history of both the original illness and the medication given; however, when a patient is admitted unconscious, the history may be unavailable or incomplete. Signs of Cushing syndrome should alert the examiner to the possibility of steroid medication, especially in asthmatics. It is important to remember that the signs of acute adrenal failure may not take the form of a classical Addisonian crisis, with nausea and vomiting accompanied by hyponatremia and hyperkalemia; in the patient with suppressed adrenal function, the clinical manifestations may be limited to confusion, circulatory collapse and hyperthermia (P. Harding, personal communication). It would be easy to attribute these to a head injury.

The serum electrolytes should be measured. The serum cortisol level should also be estimated. Normally, there is a rise after the stress of trauma or recent surgery, and a person who has undergone such a stress would be expected to have a serum cortisol level of at least 500 pmol/l and probably much higher. The finding of a lower level may point therefore to chronic suppression of the HPA axis, or some other form of adrenal failure; however, the administration of replacement corticosteroid therapy need not wait on the results of this test.

Management

The trauma victim who has been taking corticosteroids should receive at least the equivalent of the regular daily dose by the parenteral route; additional medication is needed if a long or especially stressful operation is undertaken. In such situations, we have given hydrocortisone, up to 300 mg daily in four divided doses. Vitamin A is reported to reverse the adverse effects of corticosteroids on wound healing, and can be given both systemically and locally; the recommended daily systemic dose is 25 000 IU (Lawrence 1992). We have no experience of the utility of vitamin A in this role.

DIABETES MELLITUS

Significance

It is generally believed that diabetics heal poorly after wounds, and are prone to bacterial infections, especially by staphylococci. Diabetics are often obese and arteriosclerotic, but it appears that the tendencies to poor wound healing and to microbial infection are directly related to uncontrolled hyperglycaemia and/or insulin deficiency. McMurray (1984) reviewed experimental studies on animals rendered diabetic by various means. In these experiments, epithelial wound healing was satisfactory, but there was a defect in collagen synthesis resulting in poor healing in the deeper wounds and reduced tensile strength. Granulocyte activity was also reduced, and this could relate to the predisposition to infection, especially as Gram-positive cocci flourish in the presence of hyperglycaemia. Fahey et al (1991) have reported a specific impairment in production of the cytokine interleukin-6 in experimental diabetes, which could underly the defective healing seen in human diabetics. There is now a large literature on the relevance of growth factors, hypovitaminosis A and C, and insulin deficiency in wound healing in experimental diabetes mellitus, recently reviewed by Leveson & Demetriou (1992). This experimental work suggests that efforts to maintain normal blood sugar control are justified in injured persons, both to support the immune responses and to promote wound healing. In our experience of CMF trauma, problems in wound healing attributable to diabetes mellitus have in fact been rare, no doubt because the face and scalp have an excellent blood supply. However, occasional cases of impaired healing have occurred (Fig. 20.6).

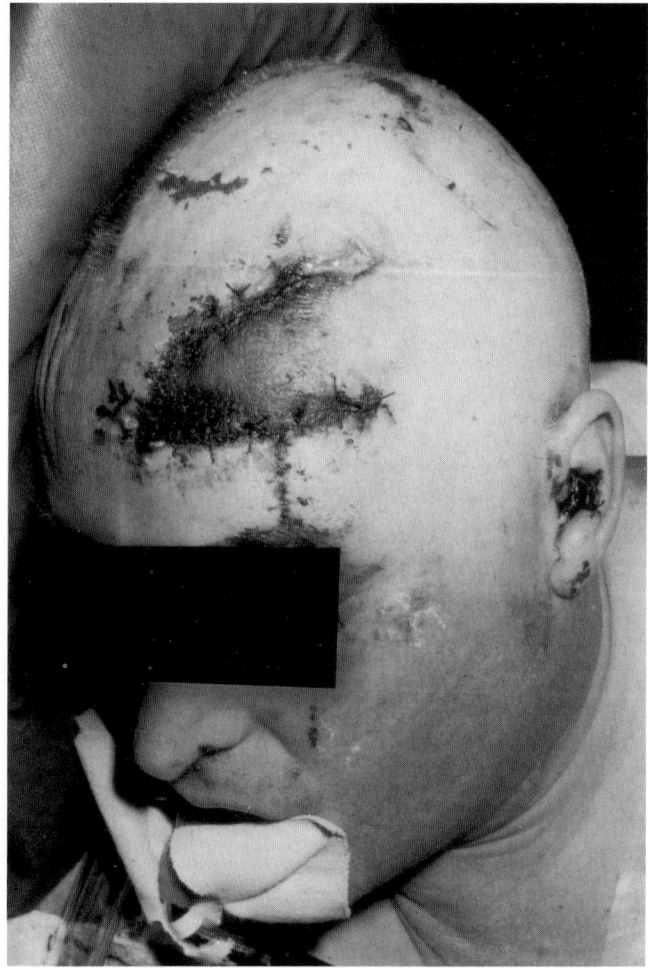

Fig. 20.6 Diabetes mellitus and wound healing. A 50-year-old man suffered a frontal skull fracture, with multiple scalp lacerations, which were sutured. Diabetes mellitus was first diagnosed on day 4. The frontal scalp wound became necrotic on day 8, and a large subgaleal abscess was drained. Secondary skin grafting was done when the diabetes had been controlled. In this case, the diabetes seemed to have contributed to the skin necrosis, though poor primary wound management was probably also a factor.

Diabetes mellitus may complicate the management of CMF trauma more directly, especially when the traumatized patient requires anaesthesia, or is comatose from a cerebral injury. Head injury and other forms of severe trauma are often complicated by hyperglycaemia and lactic acidosis. This stress-induced sympathoadrenal effect usually subsides in 48 h (De Salles et al 1987) but, if there is pre-existing diabetes, the hyperglycaemia and lactic acidosis may reach detrimental levels (Moossy & Nelson 1992). Keto-acidosis impairs consciousness and induces hyperventilation: the hyperventilation is a compensatory response to acidaemia, but under anaesthesia or respiratory paralysis, this response is abolished, and a dangerous degree of dehydration and electrolyte derangement may ensue, with sudden onset of cerebral oedema. Hyperglycaemia is less overtly dangerous, but there is much evidence to show that hyperglycaemia is associated with bad outcomes after head injury (Lam et al 1991); experimental studies have suggested that high serum glucose levels potentiate the effects of cerebral ischaemia. Very high blood sugar levels, even in the absence of ketosis, may cause a severe hyperosmolar state, and the association of hyperglycaemia and hyperosmolality in a comatose patient should always arouse concern. On the other hand severe hypoglycaemia is also dangerous especially when the patient is in coma or anaesthetized: the hypoglycaemia may pass undetected, and cause permanent brain damage.

Assessment

In the injured person with a history of diabetes mellitus, the blood glucose and pH should be monitored closely. In cases of juvenile-onset (Type I) diabetes, fingerprick glucose levels are done every 4 h or oftener, and the level should be kept in the range 4.0–16.0 mmol/l. Hyperglycaemia is a common finding in the early stages of recovery from a severe head injury and, in the absence of a history of pre-existing diabetes, high serum glucose levels may not be significant; however, the possibility of undiagnosed subclinical disease should be kept in mind and glucose levels should be frequently monitored. Serum insulin levels are of little utility, except in the unlikely event of an undiagnosed Type 1 diabetes; in the more common mature-onset (Type 2) diabetes, it is likely that the serum insulin level will be elevated. In all cases of diabetes mellitus, the diagnosis should give attention to possible complications of the disease that may have an adverse effect on management and outcome. These include:

- Atherosclerosis, causing myocardial ischaemia or peripheral gangrene
- Diabetic retinopathy, glaucoma or cataract
- Diabetic autonomic neuropathy, which may denervate the heart (Lloyd-Mostyn & Watkins 1975) or impair the baroceptor reflex response; the denervated heart

may arrest, and the impaired baroceptor system may fail to cope with the adverse effects of positive pressure ventilation on the circulation
● Diabetic nephropathy, especially when associated with bacterial pyelonephritis.

Management

When the injured person is known to have diabetes mellitus, the details of the diabetic regime should be ascertained as soon as possible. The patient with Type 2 diabetes mellitus may not be insulin-dependent, and will often have been treated by diet or by oral hypoglycaemic drugs (Table 20.3). Such diabetic states may nevertheless decompensate under the stress of trauma, and may then require insulin in large doses. The patient with Type 1 diabetes mellitus is likely to be insulin dependent and liable to ketosis.

In all cases of diabetes complicating CMF injury, a suitably experienced physician should be consulted at once. When the injuries are of minor degree and occur in patients who are expected to be able to eat, the previous medication may be continued. However, oral hypoglycaemic drugs should be discontinued one half-life of the dose before operation. Operations on patients who are receiving insulin should ideally be done in the morning after the morning dose of insulin has been omitted. All diabetic patients should be protected from hypoglycaemia during anaesthesia by an intravenous infusion of 5% dextrose.

Diabetic patients with major CMF trauma require close collaboration between physician, anaesthetist, intensivist and surgeon. In such patients, energy intake is erratic and the metabolic requirements may fluctuate markedly according to the metabolic response to trauma. Bacteraemia from compound intraoral fractures may occur; traumatic cerebral swelling may require treatment

Table 20.3 Oral anti-diabetic drugs. The action times are variable and the figures given are not guaranteed. Modified from Holman & Turner (1991)

Name	Dose range	Action time	Comment
Tolbutamide	1–3 g/day	6–8 h	Short-acting
Chlorpropamide	100–500 mg/day	32 h	May cause nocturnal or prolonged hypoglycaemia
Glipizide	2.5–20 mg/day	6–8 h	Short-acting
Glibenclamide	2.5–20 mg/day	24 h	May cause hypoglycaemia especially in the elderly
Gliclazide	80–320 mg/day	12 h	
Metformin (Biguanide)	0.5–3 g/day	5–6 h	May cause lactic acidosis; preferred in obese young diabetics

Table 20.4 Insulin preparations in common use. The figures for the time courses are arbitrary; the time course is affected by the dosage

Generic name	Source	Time course
Rapid onset insulins		
Insulin acid-soluble	bovine	2–6 h
Insulin soluble	bovine, porcine, or biosynthetic human	1–6 h
Mixed insulins soluble/isophane in varying proportions	porcine or biosynthetic human	2–16 h
Intermediate onset insulins		
Insulin isophane (Neutral protamine Hagedorn-NPH)	bovine, porcine or biosynthetic human	4–16 h
Insulin zinc suspension (Lente and Semilente)	bovine, biosynthetic human, or mixed porcine and bovine	6–24 h
Slow onset insulins		
Insulin zinc suspension – crystalline (Ultralente)	bovine or biosynthetic human	6–32 h
Insulin protamine zinc	bovine	6–24 h

with hyperosmolar agents such as mannitol. To maintain the serum glucose in the desired range, insulin (Table 20.4) is given either by intravenous infusion, or intramuscularly, or subcutaneously. A variable flow-rate pump can be used to infuse insulin through the side arm of an intravenous drip route, with careful monitoring of the serum glucose level. It has been suggested that subcutaneous administration may be safer when wild fluctuations in the serum glucose level are recorded; however, in a shocked patient, subcutaneous insulin may not be absorbed, and this can lead to poor control initially, followed by later insulin excess when circulation is restored. Soluble human recombinant insulin has been in routine use for some years; it is thought to be faster in action and less immunogenic (The 1989). Parenteral nutrition may be required (p. 383).

During operation or in cases of prolonged coma, sufficient insulin must be given to enable glucose to pass across the cell membrane and into the cell to be metabolized via the Emden–Meyerhof pathway and the citric acid cycle. This energy cycle does not result in the accumulation of ketones and metabolic acidosis, and protects the hepatic stores of glycogen. Hypokalaemia may result from the action of insulin in transporting potassium across the cell membrane, and a potassium infusion is often needed.

Bowen et al (1984) give a practical routine of intraoperative management of insulin-dependent diabetics. They advise a continuous intravenous infusion of 10% glucose, insulin and potassium given through a separate intravenous line, and monitored by hourly glucose analyses; as stated above, we have been satisfied to use 5% glucose in most cases. Throughout the operation, and during the period of intensive care, the serum glucose is kept within the range 5.0–10.0 mmol/l; infusion of dextrose is maintained to ensure that hypoglycaemia is avoided, and the serum electrolytes are monitored closely. In the later phases of management, long-term diabetic control is planned in conjunction with a consultant physician.

HYPERTENSIVE VASCULAR DISEASE

Significance

Surgery and anaesthesia may be deleterious in the uncontrolled hypertensive patient; stroke, congestive cardiac failure and coronary artery disease may be precipitated or become clinically evident while a CMF injury is being dealt with. Various procedures may evoke reflex hypertension and tachycardia: these include laryngoscopy and dissection of the orbits and root of the nose. The hypertension may persist after the stimulus has ceased.

Essential hypertension commonly develops in middle or old age. However, reactive hypertension may be seen at any age in cases of severe head injury, often as a response to raised intracranial pressure, and pre-existing hypertension may complicate management. Normal cerebral autoregulation (p. 148) is likely to fail, locally or generally, in severe cerebral injuries: when this happens, an increase in arterial pressure may promote cerebral oedema without improving cerebral perfusion. On the other hand, arterial hypotension can be disastrous in the presence of impaired cerebral perfusion.

Management

When an injured patient has been treated for essential hypertension before the accident, therapy should be continued. In undiagnosed or inadequately treated patients, it is wise to defer surgery until control has been established. Prys-Roberts (1981) recommended that, if possible, operation should be postponed when the diastolic arterial pressure is > 110 mmHg, to allow trial of medical treatment.

Except in the elderly (> 75 years), it is wise to bring the diastolic arterial pressure to the normal level, and consultation with a physician is advisable: in the traumatized patient, there are many possible drug interactions. In the operative and postoperative management, and in the intensive care of severe head injuries, anaesthetists will select a short-acting drug or drugs likely to maintain normal blood pressure; Robertson et al (1983) favour intravenous propanolol.

MYOCARDIAL DISEASE

Significance

In patients older than 50 years who have survived a previous myocardial infarct, there is a 10 times greater risk of a second infarct if a surgical procedure has to be performed. This risk diminishes as time passes, from 40% during the first 3 months after the infarct, to 15% after 6 months, falling to the general risk of the coeval population by 1 year (Prys-Roberts 1977). Myocardial ischaemic disease may have caused cardiac failure before injury, or this may supervene subsequently.

Assessment

In most cases, a history should be forthcoming, even if the patient is in coma. However, in older patients the possibility of unsuspected myocardial disease should be kept in mind. The electrocardiogram (ECG) may be diagnostic, but changes in the ST take-off and other ECG abnormalities are often seen in severe head injuries in the absence of myocardial injury or ischaemia (Clifton et al 1983).

Management

A cardiologist should be consulted and should join in the management of the injury. If operation is not urgent, medical preparation is possible: cardiac failure can be controlled, antihypertensive medication can be given, and digitalis may be given. In urgent situations, the surgeon and the anaesthetist must balance the benefits of such preparatory treatment against the risks of delay.

During anaesthesia, the blood volume must be carefully maintained; central venous manometry is particularly important, and if there is evidence of left ventricular failure a Swan–Ganz catheter and pulmonary artery wedge pressure recording may be useful. Autonomic reflexes should be depressed by deep anaesthesia. A nitroglycerine infusion may be given during and after operation to improve the myocardial circulation. Above all, hypoxia must be avoided; the oxygen saturation should be kept to > 95%.

PULMONARY DISEASE

Significance

Patients with chronic lung disease tolerate severe CMF trauma very badly, especially if there is a coexisting chest injury causing atelectasis and impaired ventilation. In trauma victims, lung function may be further impaired by aspiration pneumonia, fat embolism, pulmonary embolism, neurogenic pulmonary oedema and iatrogenic fluid overload; patients with facial burns may suffer lung damage from inhaled smoke (p. 462). In elderly patients with severe chronic lung disease, management is always difficult, and complications such as septicaemia and multiple organ failure are frequent.

Assessment

The history and physical signs of chronic lung disease are usually diagnostic; interrogation is needed to determine the previous exercise tolerance, tobacco use and sputum production.

Chest radiographs, ECG and blood gas estimations are obtained but, in most cases, a pulmonary physician should be consulted on the need for detailed evaluation of lung function before any elective surgical procedure is undertaken (Branthwaite 1977).

Management

Pulmonary function must be optimized at once. If operation can be deferred, sputum production should be reduced and any infection should be controlled by antibiotic therapy and by chest physiotherapy. Unfortunately, many CMF injuries need urgent operative treatment. When this is so, endotracheal intubation and ventilation should be instituted at once, and combined with coma supportive management along the lines set out in Chapter 13. This is especially necessary when there are concurrent chest injuries. Pneumothoraces, even if small, should be treated by intercostal underwater sealed drainage. During operation, and in the intensive care of comatose patients, attention to respiratory function is along standard lines; pulmonary arterial pressure is measured with a Swan–Ganz catheter, and great care is taken to avoid fluid overload or dehydration. Gallagher & Colohan (1992) have reviewed the general management of nosocomial pneumonia after head injury and stress the importance of Gram-negative organisms, especially *Pseudomonas aeruginosa*, *Klebsiella* and *Enterobacter* species and *Escherichia coli*. These authors recommend multiple antibiotic regimens, combining an aminoglycoside with a cephalosporin, semisynthetic penicillin or clindamycin; the β-lactam aztreonam may be used when there is resistance to these antibiotics. They also discuss the role of local instillation of an aminoglycoside into the lungs by endotracheal catheter.

MALNUTRITION

Significance

In developed countries, chronic malnutrition is seen as a consequence of alcoholism, anorexia nervosa and other less common causes; in severely injured persons, it may be the result of inadequate or inappropriate parenteral nutrition, or abdominal injury. In many developing countries, malnutrition is often the dietary effect of poverty or war. In the management of CMF trauma, malnutrition is chiefly important in two contexts: stress tolerance and wound healing.

Stress tolerance

The malnourished person may not tolerate stress, especially anaesthesia. In severe states of malnutrition, cardiac failure may occur; this is characteristic of wet beri-beri (vitamin B_1 deficiency).

Malnutrition and wound healing

An adequate protein intake is needed for normal collagen synthesis and in the inflammatory response to injury. Vitamin C is essential in collagen synthesis; it has long been known that in scurvy, wounds will not heal and fractures will not unite, or may even become ununited. Vitamin A is essential both in epithelialization and in collagen synthesis.

Though not usually a sequel of trauma, cancrum oris (noma) exemplifies the failure of healing and liability to chronic infection seen in cases of malnutrition. It is a necrotizing ulceration of the lips and mouth seen in malnourished children, once prevalent in European slums and in armies, and still well known in Africa (Tarpley & Meier 1991); it may lead to ankylosis of the temporomandibular joint and to orocutaneous fistulas.

Assessment

Malnutrition may be global, as in starvation, or selective, as in the hypovitaminoses. In areas where malnutrition is endemic, clinicians will usually know what forms of malnutrition to expect; where it is rare, a careful dietetic history should indicate the protein intake, and whether there is some special causative factor, such as alcoholism, extreme vegetarianism, or unwise cooking practices. The growing child is especially vulnerable to protein deprivation.

In most forms of malnutrition, hypoproteinaemia and anaemia are common, and should be evaluated by appropriate laboratory tests, including haemoglobin, serum albumen and transferrin levels (p. 384).

Management

Our experience of cases of CMF trauma complicated by malnutrition of any kind is too small to justify personal comment. Jelliffe & Jelliffe (1991) recommend liquid or semisolid diets rich in calories, protein and other nutrients; if there is clinical evidence or suspicion of a specific vitamin deficiency, it should be supplied in large quantities and as soon as possible. When oral food intake is impossible, parenteral nutrition is necessary; Haydock & Gill (1987) confirmed the efficacy of intravenous nutrition on wound healing, and noted that it was best given before operative treatment.

REFERENCES

Albin M S, Bunegin L 1986 An experimental study of craniocerebral trauma during ethanol intoxication. Crit Care Med 14: 841–846

Ayus J C, Krothapulli R K, Arieff A I 1987 Treatment of symptomatic hyponatremia and its relation to brain damage: a prospective study. New Engl J Med 317: 1190–1195

Babor T F, de la Fuente J R, Saunders J, Grant M 1989 AUDIT: the alcohol use disorders indentification kit. Guidelines for use in primary health care. World Health Organization, Geneva

Bakay L, Glasauer F E 1980 Head injury. Little, Brown & Co, Boston, Ch 20

Bayley A C 1990 Surgical pathology of HIV infection: lessons from Africa. Br J Surg 77: 863–868

Beal R, Isbister J P 1985 Blood component therapy in clinical practice. Blackwell, Melbourne

Beal R W, Kimber R J, Ludbrook J, Schiff P 1988 Surgical haematology and transfusion practice. In: Marshall V, Ludbrook J (eds) Clinical science for surgeons, 2nd edn. Butterworth, Sydney, Ch 7

Bowen D J, Daykin A P, Nancekievill, Ml, Norman J 1984 Insulin-dependent diabetic patients during surgery and labour. Use of continuous intravenous insulin-glucose-potassium infusions. Anaesthesia 39: 407–411

Branthwaite M A 1977 Lung disease. In: Vickers M C (ed) Medicine for anaesthetists. Blackwell, Oxford, Ch 3

Brooks N, Symington C, Beattie A, Campsie L, Bryden J, McKinley W 1989 Alcohol and other predictors of cognitive recovery after severe head injury. Brain Inj 3: 235–246

Buck B E, Malinin T I, Brown M D 1989 Bone transplantation and human immunodeficiency virus. An estimate of risk of acquired immunodeficiency syndrome (AIDS). Clin Orthop 240: 129–136

Burke E C, Orloff S L, Freise C E, Macho J R, Schecter W D 1991 Wound healing after anorectal surgery in human immunodeficiency virus infected patients. Arch Surg 126: 1267–1271

Clifton G L, Robertson C S, Kyper K, Taylor A A, Dhekne R D, Grossman R G 1983 Cardiovascular response to severe head injury. J Neurosurg 59: 447–454

Cohen H 1993 Avoiding the misuse of fresh frozen plasma. Br Med J 307: 395–396

De Salles A A F, Muizelaar J P, Young H F 1987 Hyperglycemia, cerebrospinal fluid lactic acidosis, and cerebral blood flow in severely head-injured patients. Neurosurgery 21: 45–50

Fahey T J, Sadaty A, Jones W G, Barber A, Smoller B, Shires G T 1991 Diabetes impairs the late inflammatory response to wound healing. J Surg Res 50: 308–313

Flamm E S, Demopoulos H B, Seligman M L, Tomasuda J J, DeCrescito V, Ransohoff J 1977 Ethanol potentiation of central nervous system trauma. J Neurosurg 46: 328–335

Gallagher M, Colohan A R T 1992 Infectious complications of head injury. In: Barrow D L (ed) Complications and sequelae of head injury. American Association of Neurological Surgeons, Park Ridge, IL, Ch 5

Gibbs C J 1990 Acquired immune deficiency syndrome. The biological, ethical, and moral dilemmas of this twentieth-century plague. In: Walton C C (ed) Enriching business ethics. Plenum Press, New York, Ch 9

Greenspan D, Greenspan J S, Schiødt M, Pindborg J J 1990 AIDS and the mouth. Munksgaard, Copenhagen

Gurney J G, Rivara F P, Mueller B A, Newell D W, Copass M K, Jurkovich G J 1992 The effects of alcohol intoxication on the initial treatment and hospital course of patients with brain injury. J Trauma 33: 709–713

Haydock D A, Gill G L 1987 Impaired wound healing response in surgical patients receiving intravenous nutrition. Br J Surg 74: 320–323

Holman R R, Turner R C 1991 Oral agents and insulin in the treatment of non-insulin-dependent diabetes mellitus. In: Pickup J C, Williams G (eds) Textbook of diabetes. Blackwell, Oxford, Ch 48

Hughes L A, Bailey M H 1993 Human immunodeficiency virus status in facial fracture patients. Plast Reconstr Surg 91: 577–580

Jelliffe D B, Jelliffe E F P 1991 Protein-energy malnutrition.

In: Strickland G T (ed) Hunter's tropical medicine, 7th edn. Saunders, Philadelphia

Kaufman H H, Mattson J C 1985 Coagulopathy in head injury. In: Becker D P, Povlishock J T (eds) Central Nervous System Trauma Status Report. National Institute of Neurological & Communicative Disorders & Stroke, National Institutes of Health, Washington, DC, Ch 11

Kinninmouth A W G, Hutchinson J D 1991 Full face protection in orthopaedics. Injury 22: 117–118

Lam A M, Winn H R, Cullen B F, Sundling N 1991 Hyperglycemia and neurological outcome in patients with head injury. J Neurosurg 75: 545–551

Langley M J, Lindsay W P, Lam C S, Priddy D A 1990 Programme development. A comprehensive alcohol abuse treatment programme for persons with traumatic brain injury. Brain Inj 4: 77–86

Lawrence W T 1992 Clinical management of nonhealing wounds. In: Cohen I K, Diegelmann R F, Lindblad W J (eds) Wound healing. Biochemical and clinical aspects. Saunders, Philadelphia, Ch 33

Leveson S M, Demetriou A A 1992 Metabolic factors. In: Cohen I K, Diegelmann R F, Lindblad W J (eds) Wound healing. Biochemical and clinical aspects. Saunders, Philadelphia, Ch 15

Lloyd-Mostyn R H, Watkins P J 1975 Defective innervation of the heart in diabetic autonomic neuropathy. Br Med J 3: 15–17

MacMillan A R G, Oliver A J, Radden B G, Lacy M F 1991 Langerhans cell disease associated with pathological fracture of the mandible. Aust Dent J 36: 451–455

McMurray J F 1984 Wound healing with diabetes mellitus. Surg Clin North Am 64: 769–778

Mihas A A, Tavassoli M 1992 Laboratory markers of ethanol intake and abuse: a critical appraisal. Am J Med Sci 303: 415–428

Millett D T, Chapple I L, Hirschmann P N, Corrigan A M 1990 Septic osteoradionecrosis of the mandible associated with pathological fracture: report of two cases. Clin Radiol 41: 408–410

Moossy J J, Nelson P B 1992 Metabolic abnormalities in head-injured patients. In: Barrow D L (ed) Complications and sequelae of head injury. American Association of Neurological Surgeons, Park Ridge, IL, Ch 10

Palmer R N 1990 Legal aspects of AIDS: hospitals and doctors. In: Sim A J W, Jeffries D J (eds) AIDS and the surgeon. Blackwell, Oxford, Ch 16

Partridge M, Towers J F 1987 The primordial cyst (odontogenic keratocyst): its tumour-like characteristics and behaviour. Br J Oral Maxillofac Surg 25: 271–279

Prys-Roberts C 1977 Vascular disease. In: Vickers M C (ed) Medicine for anaesthetists. Blackwell, Oxford, Ch 2

Prys-Roberts C 1981 Vascular disease and anaesthesia (editorial). Br J Anaesth 53: 673–674

Robertson C S, Clifton G L, Taylor A A, Grossman R G 1983 Treatment of hypertension associated with head injury. J Neurosurg 59: 455–460

Robinson G, Wilson S F, Williams R A 1987 Surgery in patients with acquired immunodeficiency syndrome. Arch Surg 122: 170–175

Romach M K, Sellers E M 1991 Management of the alcohol withdrawal syndrome. Annu Rev Med 42: 323–340

Rowe N L, Killey H C 1955 Fractures of the facial skeleton. Livingstone, Edinburgh, Ch 31

Royal Australasian College of Surgeons 1987 Management of AIDS (HIV) and hepatitis "B". Melbourne

Sadoff R S, Rubin M M 1990 Fibrosarcoma of the mandible: a case report. J Am Dent Assoc 121: 247–248

Schecter W P 1990 Surgery of AIDS and related conditions. A San Francisco perspective. In: Sim A J W, Jeffries D J (eds) AIDS and the surgeon. Blackwell, Oxford, Ch 4

Sim A J W, Jeffries D J 1990 AIDS and the surgeon. Blackwell, Oxford

Simpson D A, Robson H N 1960 Intracranial haemorrhage in disorders of blood coagulation. Aust NZ J Surg 29: 289–303

Simpson D A, Speed I E, Blumbergs P C 1991 Embolism of cerebral tissue: a cause of coagulopathy and infarction? Surg Neurol 35: 159–162

Tarpley J, Meier D E 1991 Surgery. In: Strickland G T (ed) Hunter's tropical medicine, 7th edn. Saunders, Philadelphia, Ch 12

The M-J 1989 Human insulin: DNA technology's first drug. Am J Hosp Pharm 46 (Suppl 2): S9–11

Waller P F, Stewart J R, Hansen A R, Stutts J C, Popkin C L, Rodgman E A 1986 The potentiating effects of alcohol on driver injury. J Am Med Assoc 256: 1461–1466

Whitfield J B 1991 Biological markers of alcoholism. Drug Alcohol Rev 10: 127–135

Yarchoan R, Broder S 1989 Immunology of HIV infection. In: Paul W E (ed) Fundamental immunology, 2nd edn. Raven Press, New York, Ch 38

Yoshida M, Hayashi T, Kuramota S, Hiyoshi Y, Yokoyama T 1979 Traumatic intracranial hematomas in hemophilic children. Surg Neurol 12: 115–118

CHAPTER 21 | Deformities

D. J. David   J. R. Abbott   M. Jay   M. A. C. Nugent
Contributing author: S. B. Cantrell

INTRODUCTION

Merville et al (1974) wrote that in the treatment of facial fractures, one should strive for 'rearchitecturalisation of the facial skeleton . . . one should try at the outset to reduce everything to perfection, since each osseous element determines the position of its neighbours . . . one should thus try to leave nothing for secondary restoration.' This view has been eloquently reinforced in the most up-to-date way by the work of Gruss, who goes to great lengths to achieve a perfect initial reconstruction. This very desirable strategy is exemplified in the management plans set out in Chapters 11–19; it is made easier by good X-ray assessment, good exposure, very good fixation, and modern grafting techniques including the use of free grafts vascularized by microsurgery. Nevertheless, serious residual deformities do occur either because of the severity of the initial injury, or because of inadequate primary reconstruction.

Sir Harold Gillies (1968) divided post-traumatic facial deformities into those with substantial loss of tissue and those without. When there is no serious loss of tissue, residual deformities are due to:

1. Failure to diagnose correctly, i.e. to assess the nature and extent of the original acute injury
2. Failure to disimpact or wholly replace displacements from such an injury and/or to provide adequate fixation.

Deformities often entail visible contour defects, even when there is no severe tissue loss. Contour defects may be treated by:

1. Osteotomy and repositioning

2. Onlay or inlay of bone grafts or alloplastic material
3. Prostheses which may be intraoral (maxillary or mandibular) or extraoral, such as prosthetic eyes, ears or noses.

This chapter deals with those deformities for which primary treatment might have been better, and with those where even, in retrospect, primary treatment was appropriate, but where there was still unavoidable uncertainty about the final result, such as enophthalmos, temporomandibular joint (TMJ) injury, childhood injury and many soft-tissue injuries with scarring. Also to be considered are those injuries which from the beginning were destined to need secondary surgery, such as the massive avulsive defects considered in Chapter 16, not all of which can be adequately corrected in the primary and postprimary reparative procedures.

The aim of secondary surgery for deformity is to restore the patient to functional and aesthetic wholeness, always taking into account the pretraumatic appearance. This may entail another sequence of operations, often performed over a long period of time. Although the ideal of full correction must be kept constantly in mind, complete restoration of form and function may in fact never be possible.

Classification of major post-traumatic deformities

These can be broadly grouped as:

1. Forehead contour deformities

The frontal sinuses may be involved, and loss of integument (bone and/or scalp) may expose the brain to risk

545

of future injury (Fig. 21.1). Forehead deformities can be considered in two groups: frontal and temporal.

2. Orbital deformities

These include:

- enophthalmos
- exophthalmos
- orbitozygomatic and naso-orbital deformities
- telecanthus
- orbital dystopia (including hypertelorism).

These may be associated with nasolacrimal dysfunction, abnormalities of eye movement or impaired lid closure (Ch. 14). Orbital injuries sustained in early life are likely to result in deformities which become progressively more marked as growth advances. Many orbital deformities involve significant deformity of the anterior and/or middle cranial fossae, and can be described as cranio-orbital.

3. Nasal and naso-orbito-ethmoid deformities

In this category, which is poorly defined from the preceding group, one can identify a common type of post-traumatic deformity localized to the nasal bones and cartilages, and a group of more complex deformities involving the bridge of the nose and the ethmoid bone. There may be associated problems related to the nasal airway and paranasal sinuses.

4. Deformities of the facial skeleton involving the upper and lower jaws

These deformities are intimately related to occlusal problems and may be affected by post-traumatic TMJ pathology, including ankylosis. Distortions of the facial skeleton may be in three dimensions; in children, distortions are affected by time and growth, constituting a fourth dimension.

5. Soft-tissue defects

Deformities resulting from hypertrophic scars and keloids are briefly discussed on p. 438. Other deformities result from avulsive soft-tissue injury (Ch. 16). The loss of an eye constitutes a soft-tissue deformity of much aesthetic and psychological significance (p. 641).

Our computerized records of post-traumatic deformities give details of 385 cases referred to the Australian Craniofacial Unit over a period of 18 years; although this figure underestimates the number of such cases seen in that

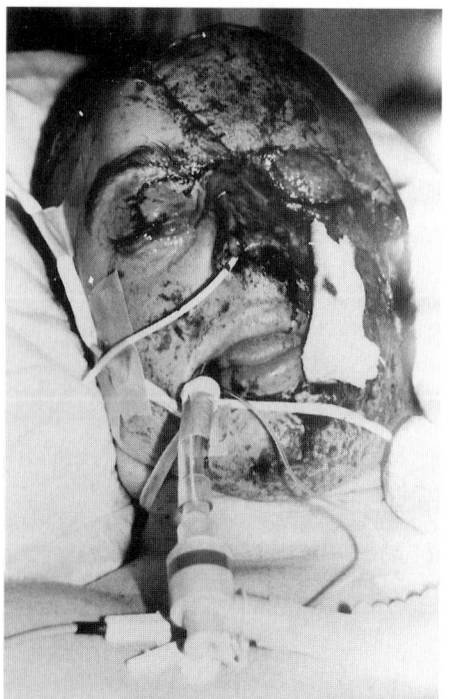 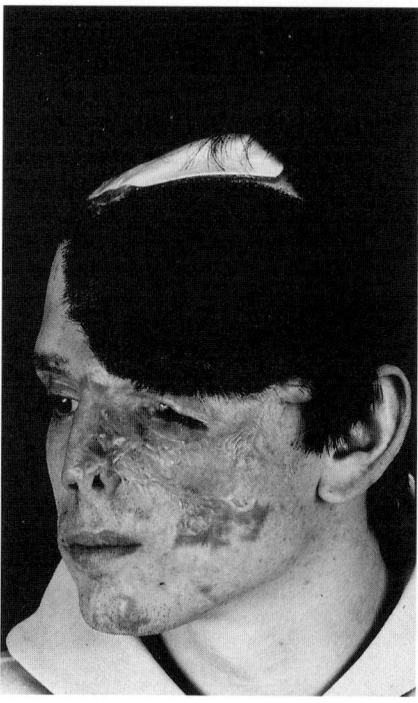 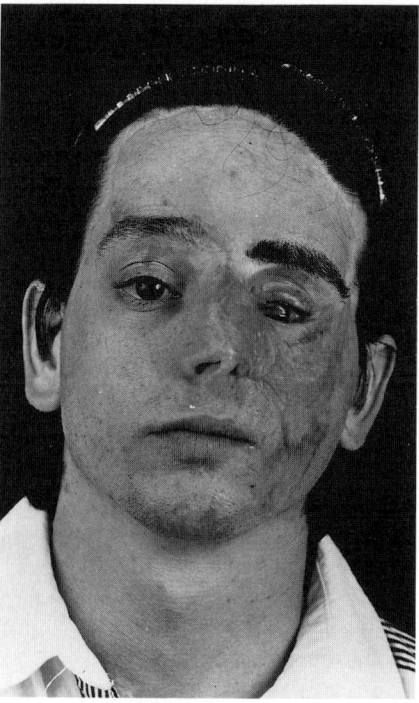

A **B** **C**

Fig. 21.1 Cranial trauma with exposure of the brain. A A teenage male was involved in a vehicular accident, in which the frontal lobe was exposed and damaged on the left side. There was severe orbito-frontal skeletal damage and after debridement the brain required urgent skin covering. This was done by mobilizing a scalp flap which was brought forward to the eyebrow level. The posterior defect was covered with split-skin graft. **B** The flap, seen some months later as hairy scalp extending to the eyebrow. The nose and face are badly scarred. **C** The scalp has been returned superficial to the galea. The galea was left intact and the frontal defects grafted with iliac bone. The forehead was replaced as a cosmetic unit using a groin flap vascularized with microvascular techniques.

period, it seems likely that the series is representative of the experience of a tertiary craniofacial unit such as ours. Of these cases, a detailed review of 205 records shows that approximately half were classed as orbital or cranio-orbital. Mandibular and/or maxillary deformities with malocclusion constituted ~24% and naso-orbito-ethmoid deformities only ~8%; in >10% the deformities were complex and had to be described as panfacial. The series excluded localized post-traumatic nasal deformities, but a separate series of 185 such cases has also been reviewed (see p. 579).

FRONTAL DEFORMITIES

Surgical pathology

The most common post-traumatic frontal deformities

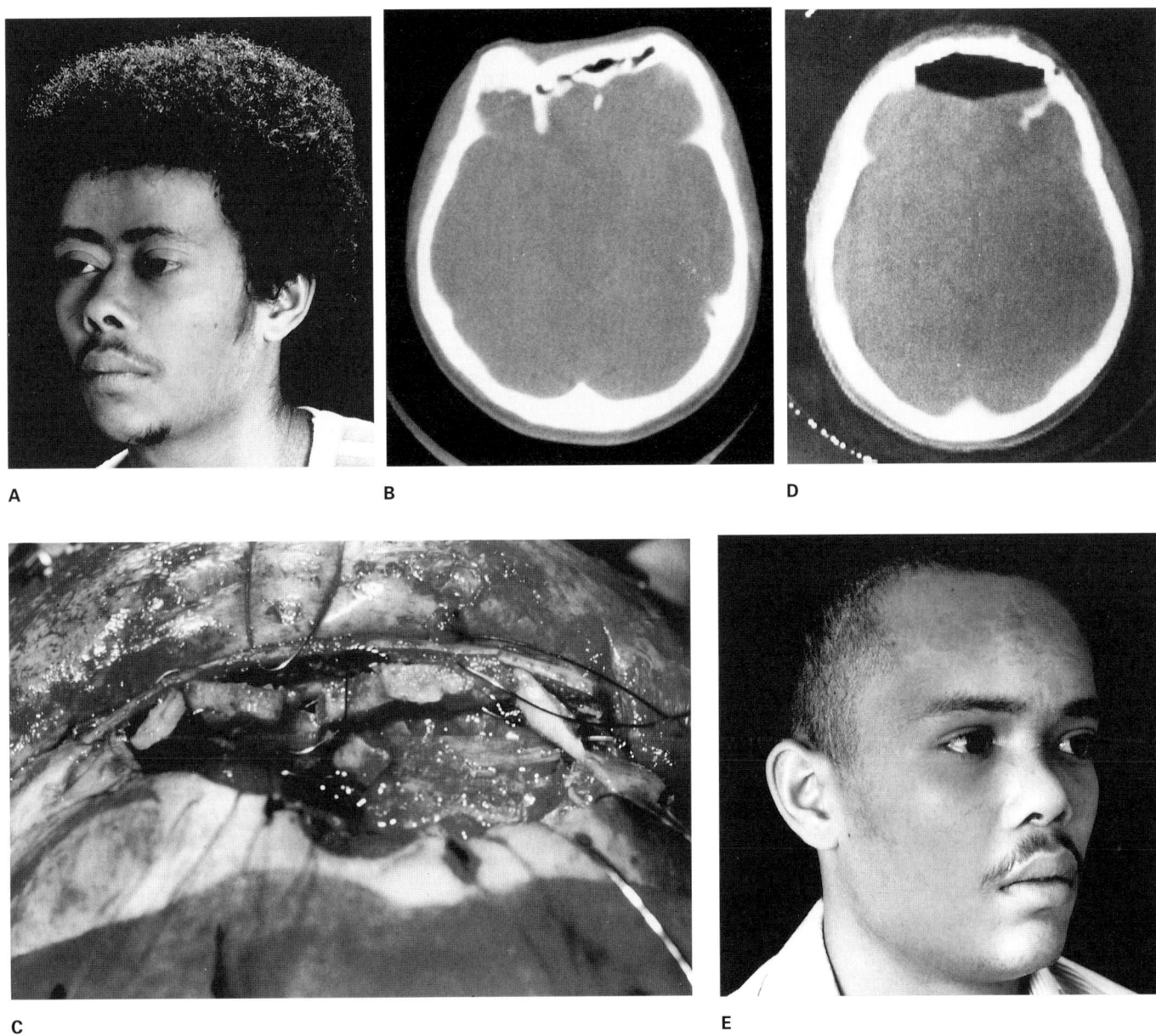

A   **B**   **D**

C   **E**

Fig. 21.2 Delayed correction of cranial deformities. A 20-year-old man was involved in an accident in a cane field in which his motorbike ran into a post. The post struck him in the forehead inflicting severe central frontal and frontonasal fractures. He did not receive any primary treatment, and presented some years later with an uncorrected fracture involving both walls of the frontal sinus and the glabella region. **A** Depression of the frontal bone, producing a contour defect and an obtuse frontonasal angle. **B** CT scan of the deformity as it affects the frontal sinus and its relationship to the frontal lobes. **C** Surgical exposure via bicoronal scalp flap and subperiosteal dissection to expose the fragmented and depressed skull. A craniotomy was performed above the affected region and the scarred dura was separated from the back of the damaged frontal sinus. Following repair of the dura, the frontal sinus fragments were replaced and augmented with split calvarial graft. All fragments were firmly wired into place and the frontal sinus was obliterated by cranialization. Additional bone graft was placed into the nose and the nasofrontal region. **D** Postoperative CT scan with extradural air. **E** The young man at time of discharge with a properly contoured frontal bone and reconstituted frontonasal angle.

are traumatic bone deficits, displaced supraorbital rims, flattening or concavity of a shattered frontal sinus and postoperative deformities such as sunken bone flaps and burrholes. Loss of bone secondary to osteitis is also a cause of disfigurement and often exposes the frontal lobes to the risk of future trauma. Wires or plates used in previous repairs may be prominent or even exposed by ulceration.

Management

Post-traumatic frontal recontouring can be achieved by bony advancement, autogenous bone grafts, bone allografts, metal plates or mesh, or implants of Silastic®, methyl methacrylate or other biocompatible material (p. 154). All methods of frontal cranioplasty have merits and demerits.

Correction by osteotomy

Forehead remodelling by osteotomy is often recommended for congenital deformities of the superior orbital margin and frontal bone resulting from craniosynostosis, and similar osteotomies can be performed for neglected post-traumatic deformities. But in traumatic cases, correction by osteotomy is a long operation that usually involves the adherent dura (Fig. 21.2) and occasionally the brain. The mucosa of the frontal sinuses must be eradicated down to the frontal recess; the osteotomized bone should be fixed rigidly and any defects grafted with calvarial bone graft. The potential for complications is high: these include infection in an inadequately vascularized bone, haematoma in the dead space between advanced bone and dura, and bone resorption from avascular necrosis. Epilepsy presumably caused by disturbing an underlying meningocerebral scar is a particularly serious complication.

It is not uncommon to see a lateral fronto-orbital contour deformity resulting from an uncorrected or poorly corrected fracture in this site. The fracture can be osteotomized and repositioned and fixed with miniplates. Exposure is through the bicoronal scalp flap with limited dissection of the temporalis muscles from the skull and lateral orbital wall to expose the old fracture. A small craniotomy or enlarged burrhole can be made to expose and protect the dura during the osteotomy. After contour restoration and fixation any remaining defect is filled with split calvarial bone.

Contour restorations by osteotomy can produce excellent results. The most frequent complications in our experience result from the dead space created by the advancement of the fronto-orbital margin when the connection with the nose has not been adequately obliterated. Care must be taken to cranialize the frontal sinus and to separate the extradural space from the nose. This can

be effected by cutting a galeofrontalis flap from the undersurface of the bicoronal scalp flap. If the dead space is small, it can be filled with this flap or by a pericranial flap based laterally on the temporalis muscle. More massive extradural dead space cavities may be filled with a free muscle transplant either from rectus abdominis or latissimus dorsi vascularized by microvascular techniques (Fig. 21.3).

Correction by bone grafts

Bone is a logical material to use to fill a traumatic bone defect, and is often initially very successful. When the defect results from the removal of a frontal bone flap as an emergency neurosurgical decompressive procedure, it is usual to preserve the flap in a bone bank and to replace it when the patient's condition permits. Frozen bone flaps sometimes resorb, but success is achieved often enough to justify this very simple and innocuous procedure.

Fresh autogenous bone harvested at the time of a reconstructive procedure gives early vascularization, excellent capacity for immobilization, lack of immune rejection and freedom from disease transmission. However, there is much increase in the operative time and some increase in morbidity (Laurie et al 1984). Small post-traumatic defects are commonly filled with calvarial bone, bone dust, rib or iliac crest (Fig. 21.4). Calvarial grafts can be taken through the exposure of the frontal bone defect; for very large defects, parietal bone can be transferred and the posterior defect filled with another bone graft, or with bone obtained by splitting the calvarial plate. When split calvarial bone is used, the inner plate is left in the parietal region and the outer plate is transferred to the frontal region. Split-rib grafts have been much used to fill large calvarial defects (Fig. 17.20). Medium-sized defects can be filled with a bone plug removed by trephine or a graft of cortical and cancellous bone cut to shape from the ilium (p. 240). Split inner table of ilium can be used as a vascularized graft for very large defects where the vascularization is at risk because the overlying scalp has been compromised (Taylor et al 1979a,b, McCarthy et al 1987) (Fig. 21.5).

Apart from grafts revascularized by microsurgery, bone grafts are unpredictable and may resorb. A single grafting does not always suffice, though Phillips & Gruss (1991) have shown that fixation renders the survival of bone grafts more predictable than was previously thought. The degree of overgrafting necessary to produce an acceptable result varies and is hard to estimate. Rib and iliac crest grafts have been successfully used by many surgeons, and once they are incorporated, long-term infection or skin breakdown is unlikely. But it is not easy to get a perfect aesthetic result with split-rib grafts: Körlof et al (1973) reported uneven, depressed or prominent contours in half their cases. It is common experience to

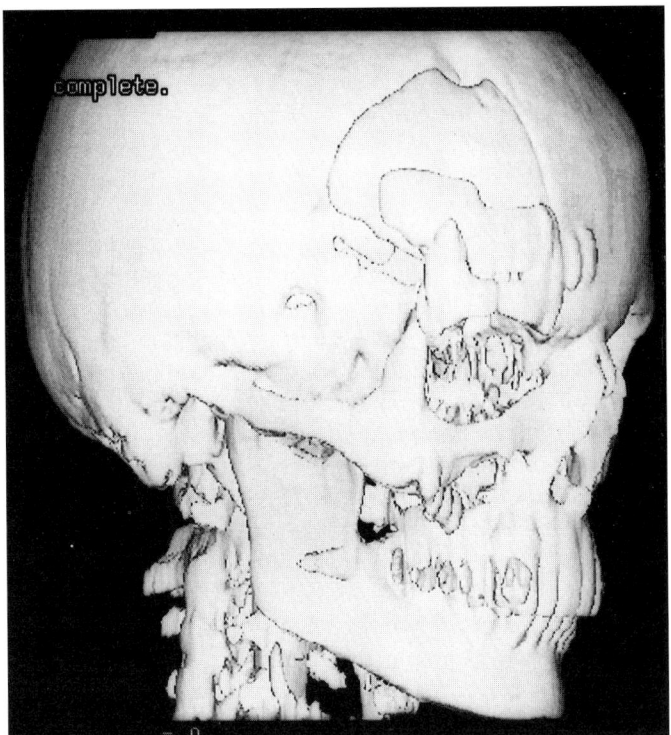

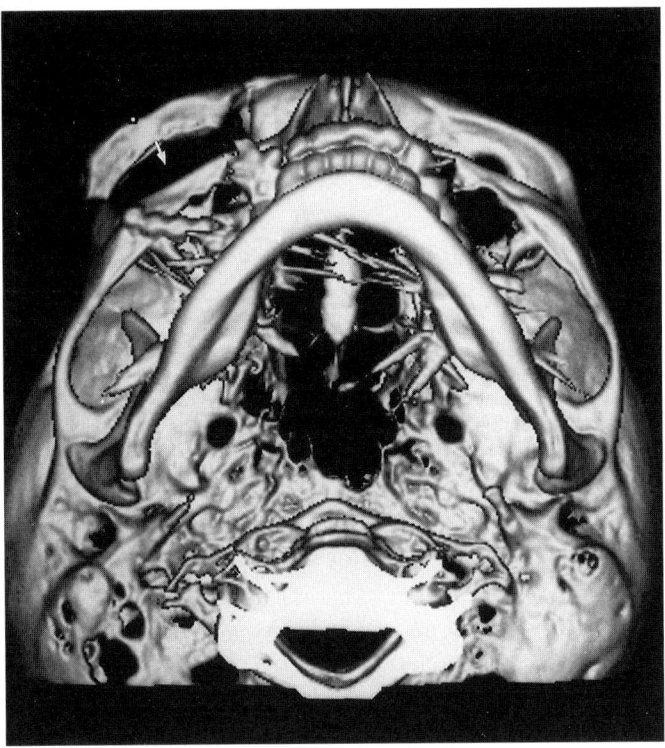

A **B**

Fig. 21.3 'Dead space' from cranial fracture. A middle-aged woman suffered a compound, comminuted fracture of the right fronto-orbital region affecting the shape of the orbit and producing a flattening of the right eyebrow region. **A** CT scan showing the relationship of the distorted fronto-orbital crown and orbit. **B** Fronto-orbital advancement was performed on the right side with an osteotomy, repair of the underlying dural defect, cranialization of the frontal sinus and blocking of the nasofrontal ducts. Postoperatively she blew her nose violently and produced an extradural air pocket which became filled with fluid.

be obliged to reoperate to smooth the surface of a frontal bone graft and to remove wires and screws which have become prominent from partial resorption (Fig. 21.6). It is also questionable whether free bone grafts have the impact resistance of a metal plate: Timmons (1982) noted progressive loss of bone density in later X-ray pictures.

Metal and plastic implants

These are often used for large frontal cranioplasties (Fig. 21.7). Titanium plates offer excellent protection and are easily screwed to the skull. The Belfast technique of shaping titanium plates in a high-pressure hydraulic forming chamber (Gordon & Blair 1974, Blair et al 1980)

makes it possible to give a nearly perfect aesthetic effect; the plates are radiolucent and we have not found the thermal conductivity of the titanium plate to be a cause of complaints. The application of three-dimensional computed tomography (3D CT) has provided an even more elegant method of producing titanium plates: with the aid of 3D CT data, a model of the defect is sculpted and from this a plate of the desired thickness and shape is cast in titanium (computer-aided design/computed-aided manufacture: CAD/CAM technique). Titanium has high biocompatibility (Fig. 5.28), and in the short term we have been well pleased with metallic cranioplasties. Unfortunately the long-term results are not always satis-factory. We have records of some 150 patients with post-traumatic skull defects repaired with tantalum or (since

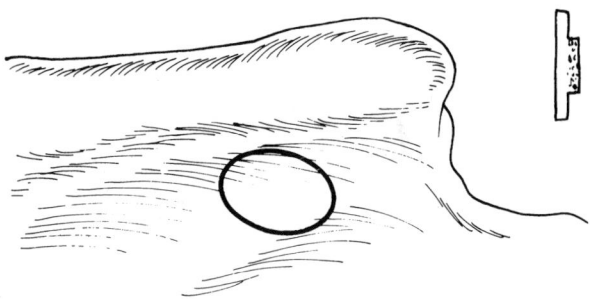

Fig. 21.4 Post-traumatic cranial defects. Medium-sized post-traumatic defects in the frontal region can be effectively closed with a 'bath plug' graft from the inner table of ilium. Cortical and cancellous bone is harvested and shaped as a bath plug so that the cortical bone overlaps the frontal bone adjacent to the defect and the cancellous bone fits as a plug into the defect. Two small screws provide rigid fixation.

1961) titanium plates, and in at least 16 (11%) it has been necessary to remove the plate because of infection or ulceration of the skin. The incidence of such complications may indeed be higher as many patients have left our area and their plates could have been removed by neurosurgeons too kind to tell us the bad news. In some cases the complication can be blamed on preventable errors in technique, but we have seen infection supervene

20 years after a satisfactory cranioplasty, from a superficial scalp wound.

Acrylic (methyl methacrylate: p. 155) is cheap and easy to shape; Ousterhout & Zlotolow (1991) have reported good results. Manson et al (1986) have found a low incidence of infection though, when this does occur, the results can be devastating. The plates are less resistant to impact than titanium and may fracture (Otto 1958, Henry et al 1976). This can be rectified by reinforcing the acrylic with metallic mesh (Galicich & Hovind 1967), though in our hands these reinforced plates have been aesthetically disappointing: when the skull is thin, the wire-reinforced plate margins are hard to inlay and are palpable and visible when fitted as an onlay prosthesis. Long-term complications, such as infection, are not rare, and we have the impression that these complications are not less frequent than with titanium plates, though to our knowledge no comparative clinical trials have been reported.

We have only rarely used silicone rubber (Silastic®) as postoperative reconstructive material in the craniofacial skeleton; however, we have removed many pieces of silicone rubber used by others (Fig. 21.8). Lash et al (1964) and Courtmanche & Thompson (1986) have reported

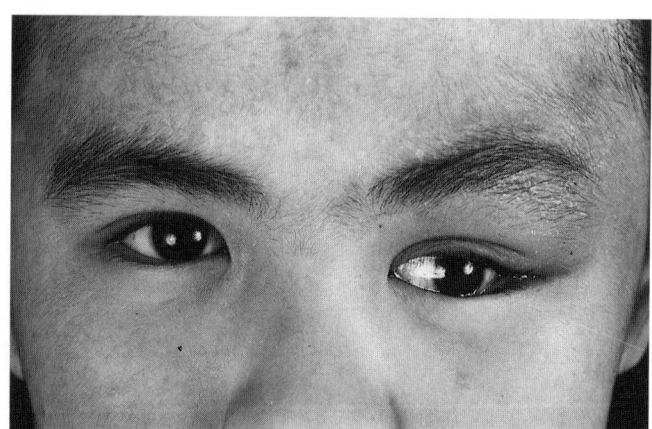

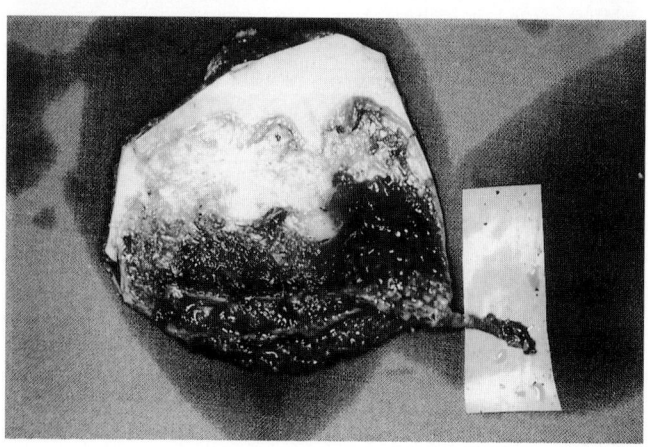

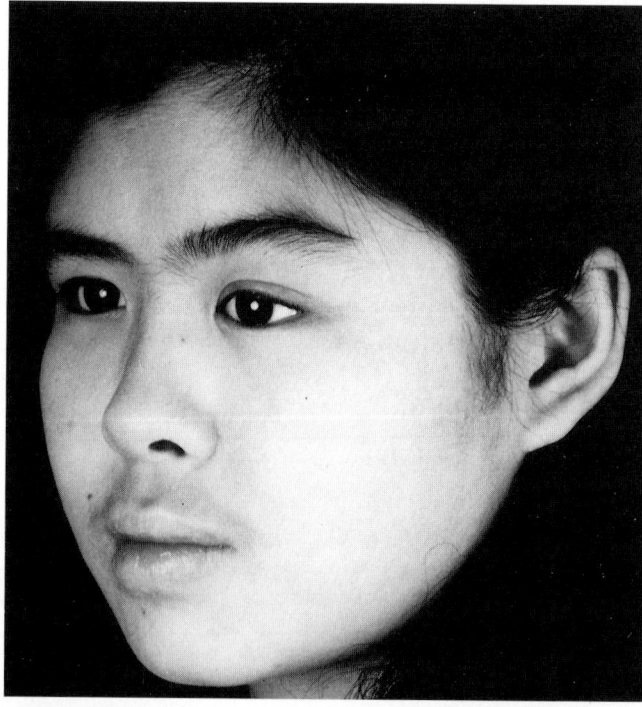

Fig. 21.5 Vascularized graft reconstruction of cranial defects. Split inner table of ilium, in the form of a free flap based on the deep circumflex iliac vessels, has been used to reconstruct the frontal bone defect. **A** Distorted frontal region with some degree of global dystopia. **B** Inner table of ilium with attached periosteum and vascular pedicle. The quite pliable inner table has been cautiously bent and fixed into the defect peripherally with titanium screws, the pedicle placed within reach of the temporal vessels. **C** The patient 1 year after the reconstruction.

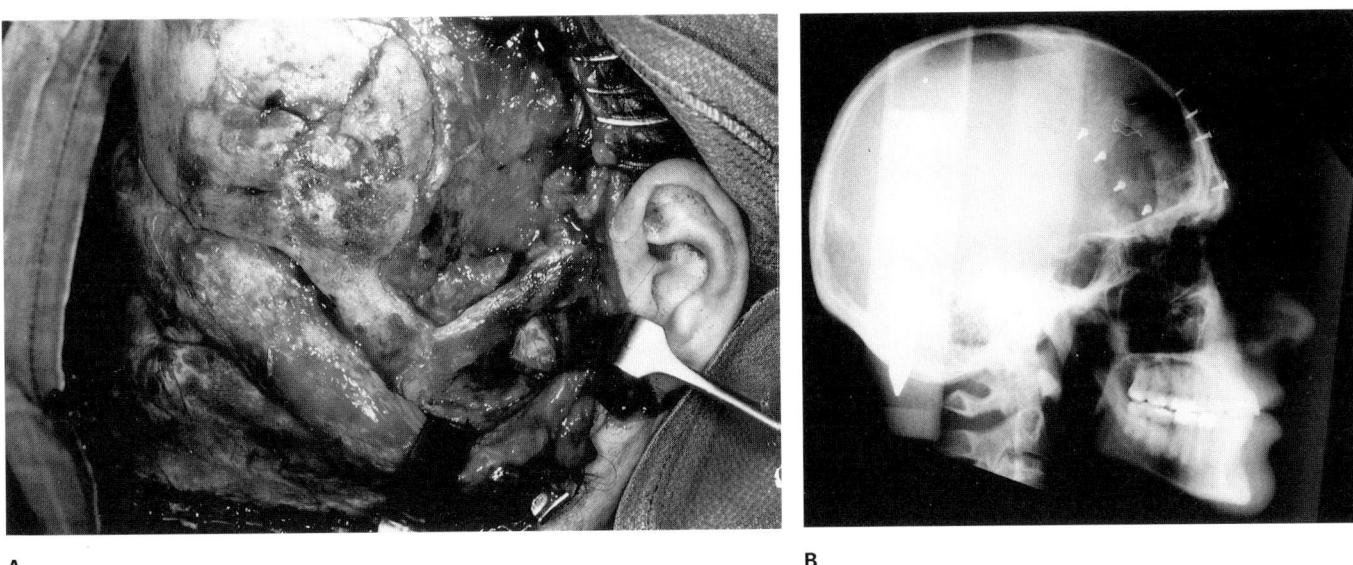

A   **B**

Fig. 21.6 Rib grafting for cranial defects. A woman was involved in a vehicular accident and suffered severe fronto-orbital and left facial fractures. **A** Primary reconstruction performed with split-rib grafting of the frontal region. Later, the grafted area became rough and uneven, with resorption resulting in palpable grooves and wires. **B** Split-ribs used for frontal cranioplasty and fixed with titanium screws.

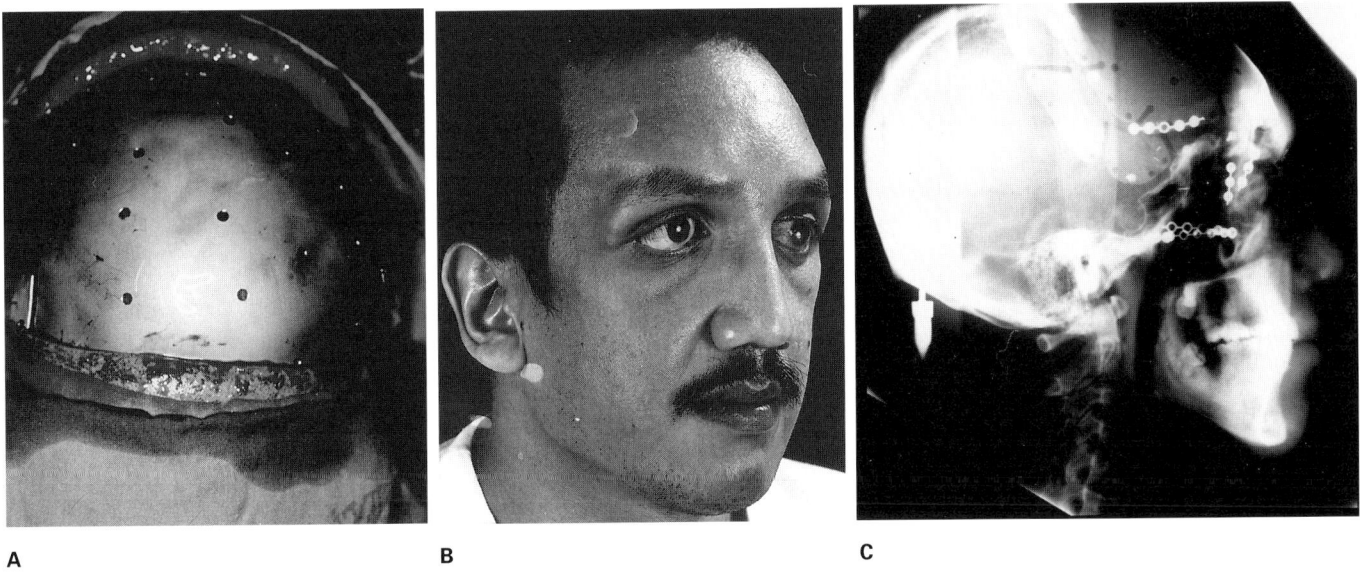

A   **B**   **C**

Fig. 21.7 Frontal cranioplasty using a large titanium plate. A Operative view showing plate in position. **B** Half-face view showing the frontal contour produced by the plate. **C** Lateral X-ray view showing radiolucency of the plate.

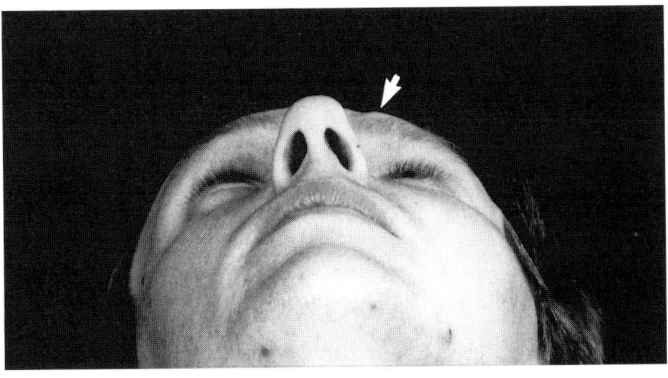

Fig. 21.8 Silastic implants in craniomaxillofacial trauma. A 19-year-old man suffered a severe left fronto-orbital fracture in a motor vehicle accident, leaving him with a depressed left supraorbital margin and frontal bone. This was inadequately treated at the first operation and subsequently managed by inserting a carved block of Silastic into the plane between the galea and the skin. The resulting soft-tissue capsule (arrow) was bulky and mobile on palpation.

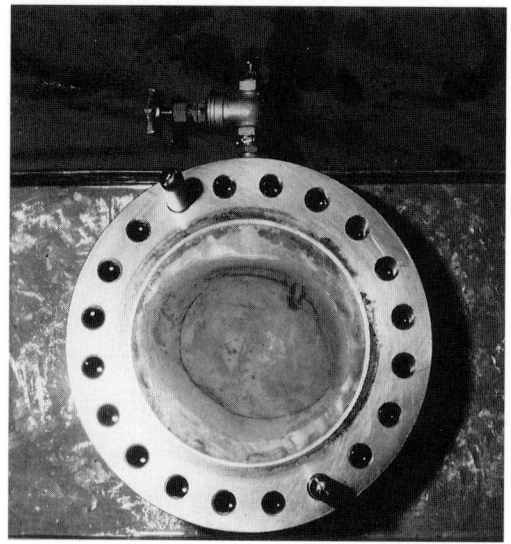

A

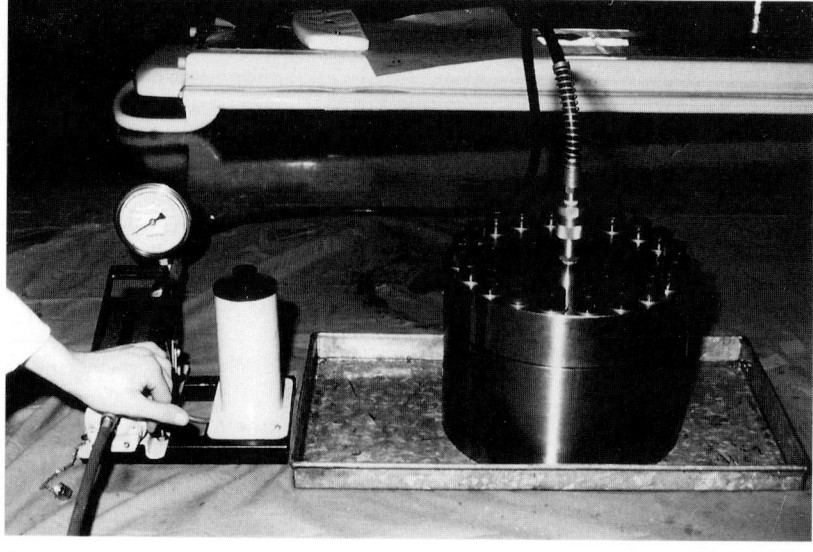

B

Fig. 21.9 Contouring a plate in a pressure chamber: Belfast technique. An impression of the bone defect is taken in wax; from this a plaster model of the calvarial region is made. **A** A Matrix of the plaster model is made in dental stone and fitted into the cylindrical pressure chamber. A titanium blank plate, cut to be larger than the bone defect and of approximately the same shape, is than placed in the chamber on the matrix. **B** The chamber is closed with 20 screws and a hydraulic pump raises the pressure to 6000 psi. **C** Diagram of action. Above, the titanium blank is lying on the matrix under a thick rubber diaphragm; below, it is forced by high pressure to conform with the contours of the matrix. The moulded plate is trimmed and polished, and holes are drilled.

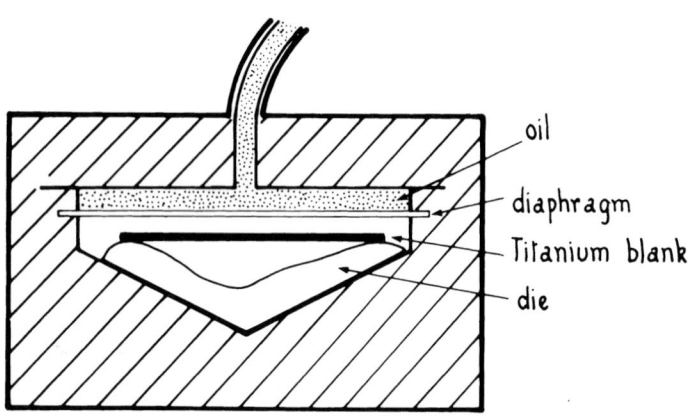

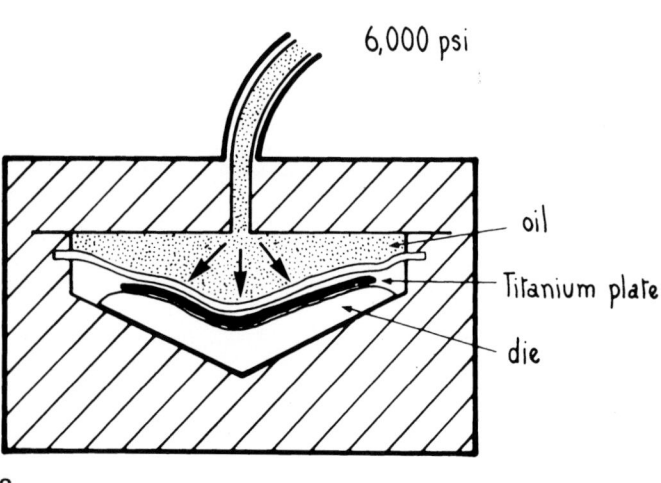

C

good results, but in some of their cases the follow-up periods were short. Silastic® implants are hard to sculpt, do not unite with the underlying skull and often erode through the overlying tissue which may itself be compromised by the original injury. It is our experience that these implants are often placed within the soft tissues by inexperienced surgeons: a capsule forms around the implant, which becomes prominent and may migrate under gravity, producing an unsightly frontal appearance.

Alloplastic cranioplasties will continue to show complications until a material is found which is permanently incorporated in the tissues. Hydroxyapatite may be such a material (p. 155). Waite et al (1989) have reported on a small series of cranioplasties done with blocks of hydroxyapatite; they report some difficulties in contouring the block, which can be overcome by preforming with the help of a model prepared from a 3D CT scan. Hydroxyapatite is brittle, but is said to become acceptably impact-resistant when invaded by fibrous tissue. Demineralized allogenic or xenogenic bone prepared by freezing, lyophilization and irradiation has been advocated. We have no experience of treating frontal contour defects with these substances. We note that Ousterhout (1985) reported that there was considerable implant resorption and that the results of contour restoration were unsatisfactory.

Implants are *contraindicated* within 6 months of any local infection; a previously damaged paranasal sinus increases the risk. No cranioplasty should be attempted unless there is good skin cover over the area to be repaired. The dura mater should be intact, and if the paranasal air sinuses were involved, then the area of involvement should have been covered with soft tissue. These requirements sometimes necessitate a staged sequence of operations over 6 months or more.

Cranioplasty with titanium

The plate is made before operation. Blake et al (1990) use plates shaped and contoured by hand, with the help of a model of the defect prepared from CT scan data; where necessary, plates are welded together. In our experience, plates made by hand are satisfactory for closing defects when simple contours are needed; a wooden mallet and a concave anvil can be used to form a convex plate, final shaping being done with pliers and a metal ball hammer. However, plates made in this way are sometimes unsatisfactory when complex defects have to be closed.

We now prefer the Belfast technique of preforming the plate in a pressure chamber (Blair et al 1980). When this method is used, an impression of the defect is made through the intact skin with dental alginate or wax, and a model of the forehead is then made in dental plaster. From this, a matrix is made in dental stone; the matrix is placed in the forming chamber. A sheet of 0.6 or 0.7 mm titanium is cut to cover the defect with a clearance of at least 15 mm, and laid on the matrix; the sheet of titanium is placed between two sheets of mild steel to avoid crumpling of the plate in the chamber (Fig. 21.9) The chamber is sealed and a hydraulic pressure of ~6000 psi is applied. The plate is moulded by the pressure to conform with the impression in the dental stone matrix. The shaped plate is removed from the chamber; screw holes can then be drilled and slots cut to allow bending of the plate margins, since a perfect fit is rarely obtained when the frontal bone has been modelled through the intact skin. Finally the plate is polished and its edges smoothed. It is sterilized by autoclaving. The bone defect is exposed by a coronal scalp flap, possibly modified to include an earlier scar (Fig. 21.10A). The scalp is elevated by sharp and blunt dissection, care being taken not to open the dura or the frontal air sinuses. The plate is then made to conform with the exposed bone exactly; this usually entails some swaging and bending. Pericranial flaps are elevated to define the margins of the bone defect. The bone is prepared for the plate by raising a thin

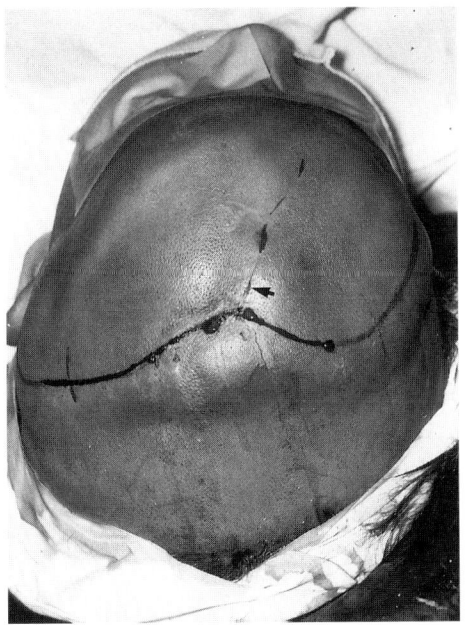
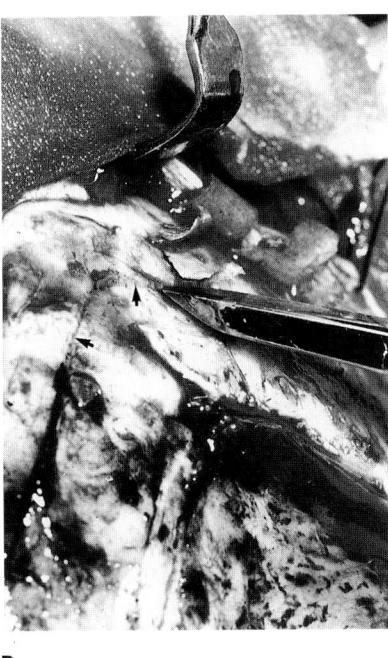
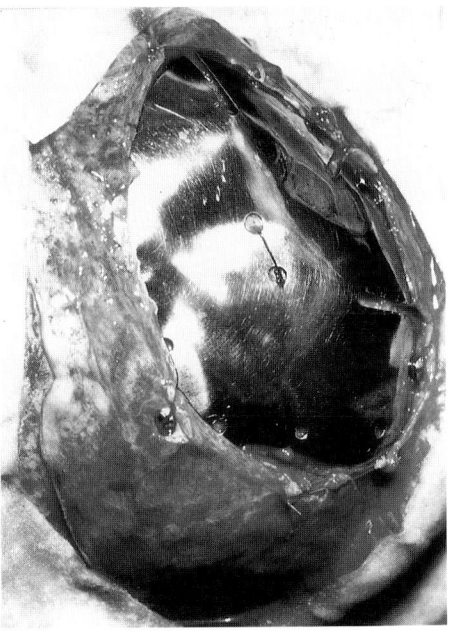

A   B   C

Fig 21.10 Fitting a moulded titanium plate. A 4-year-old boy suffered a compound depressed frontal fracture. Scalp closure was difficult, and the bone fragments were not replaced. The wound healed well. **A** 7 months later, the bone defect was explored through a coronal scalp flap, modified to ensure that the incision would not lie directly over the defect. One limb of the original scar (dotted line: arrow) was not reopened.
B The defect was defined and pericranial flaps were reflected from it. The preformed plate was fitted to lie on the bone. A line (arrows) was marked on the bone, and shavings were elevated with a chisel along this line to overlap the margin of the plate. **C** The preformed plate was secured with four slotted screws and the pericranial flaps were brought to cover the edges of the plate. Recovery was uneventful. This technique has been shown to promote osseo-integration of the plate.

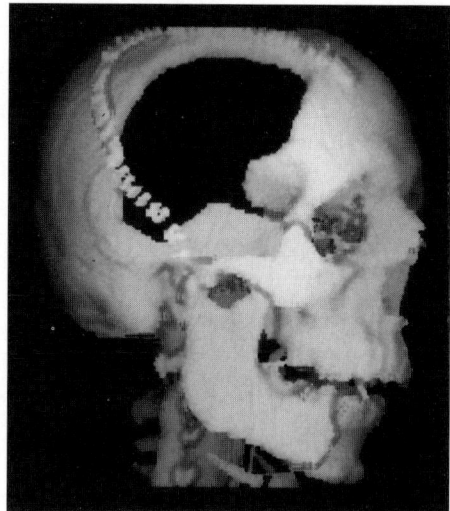

A

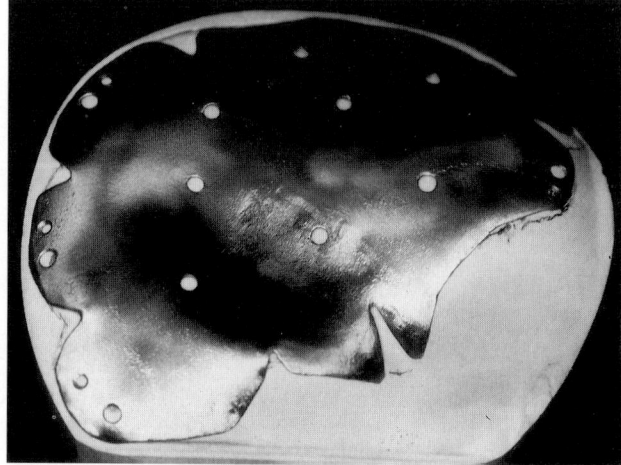

B

C

Fig. 21.11 Casting a plate: CAD/CAM technique. A CT scan shows a post-traumatic frontotemporal craniotomy defect; the scan was obtained soon after operation. Scalp clips outline the wound. **B** Using PERSONA software analysis, a computer-milled model of the defect was obtained and from this a mould for a plate was made. **C** A titanium plate was cast in this mould in an inert atmosphere at 1720°C with Tycast 2000 centrifugal casting equipment. (Jeneric Pentron 53N, Plains Industrial Road, Wallingford, CT 06492, USA.) The cast plate is shown fitted to the model.

shaving of bone all around the outline of the plate (Fig. 21.10B): this covers the edges of the plate and is intended to promote osseo-integration (Fig. 5.28). The plate is secured with at least four titanium screws; in the past, the slotted 5 and 6 mm screws made to our design (Simpson 1965) have been preferred to the smaller screws used to hold miniplates, but the heads of these smaller screws are less conspicuous and recent experience suggests that they may give adequate fixation. In drilling tapping holes for the screws, care is needed not to tear the dura; it may be wise to put oxycel gauze in the extra-dural plane under the site of the screw. The pericranium is pulled over the edge of the plate and the skin flap is replaced with or without suction drainage.

With the advent of 3D CT scanning and the ability to cast titanium implants using the CAD/CAM technique,* the plate can be shaped with much more precision (Fig. 21.11), and a perfect fit can be achieved (Fig. 21.12).

Cranioplasty with autogenous bone

When a frontal defect is closed with autogenous bone, the exposure is similar. The bone edges must be more fully exposed and freshened with a chisel or large dental burr designed for shaping acrylic; bone wax is not used in situations where it might delay bone growth. If rib is to be used, a suitable number of ribs is harvested and the ribs are split as described on p. 241. The ribs are cut to appropriate lengths and secured to cover the defect: the end of the rib can be inlayed into the freshened margin of the bone defect, and secured with steel or titanium wire. However, small titanium screws make rigid fixation possible with greater speed and simplicity. Bone dust obtained from the calvaria near the defect can be used to improve the contour of the repair. A plate of iliac bone may be preferable for a smaller defect or may be used in conjunction with rib grafts for a larger defect.

Split calvarial grafts (p. 241) may be used for smaller defects when X-ray has shown that there is a good calvarial thickness. For larger defects and a superior cosmetic result, a temporoparietal bone flap is removed by a neurosurgeon and the inner table is split off in one or more segments (Fig. 21.13). These segments can be used to repair the secondary bone defect created by the craniotomy while the outer table can be used for the frontal defect. If a vascularized graft is needed, the bone of choice is the inner table of the ilium. This can be split, providing a large area of bone and leaving little contour defect in the hip. The indications are not common but occur in situations where the defect is large, the overlying scalp much damaged or after failure of other methods.

---

*For modelling these plates, we have used Persona software, available from Maptek Pty Ltd, 350 Indiana St (Suite) 530, Golden Colorado USA.

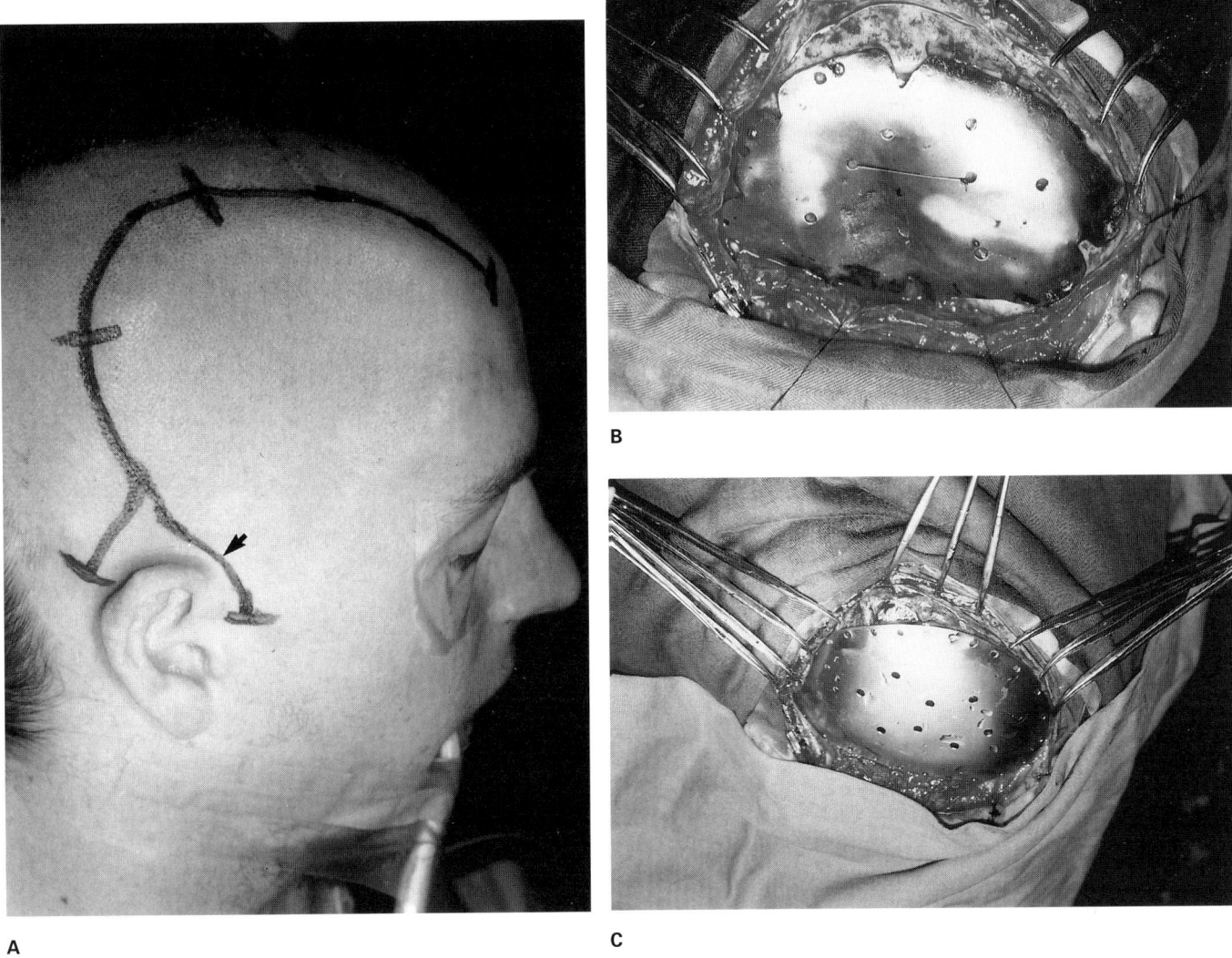

A

C

Fig. 21.12 Fitting a cast plate made by CAD/CAM technique. A 19-year-old man suffered a compound depressed fracture in the right frontotemporal area. Decompressive craniotomy was performed to relieve cerebral oedema. The bone fragments were shattered and it was decided that they were unsuitable for a future cranioplasty. (Fig. 21.11 shows the resulting bone defect and the preparation of the plate.) **A** 7 months later, the bone defect was explored through the original incision with a postauricular extension; the lower limb of the incision (arrow) was not reopened to ensure that the plate was not under the final scar. **B** The bone defect was defined, and flaps of pericranium and temporalis fascia were elevated. A pocket in the temporalis muscle received the lower margin of the plate. The precast plate conformed perfectly to the margins of the bone defect and was secured with screws. The concavity in the temporal fossa is seen as a shadowed area in the plate. **C** By contrast, a plate moulded in the pressure chamber is shown in the same patient: it had not been possible to make a matrix with such an exact replication of the temporal contour, and the temporal concavity was not reproduced. This plate was discarded. Case report by courtesy of Mr M Stoodley.

The technique demands the skills and experience of a microsurgeon. A separate surgical team exposes the ilium (p. 240). A free flap of split ilium vascularized from the deep branch of the circumflex iliac artery is detached from the inner table of the bone and anastomosed to one of the scalp arteries; a cuff of muscle is transferred with the bone to protect the arterial supply. The flap of bone is firmly fixed in the defect. The maximum area of bone that can be taken is about 12 × 8 cm; however, larger defects can be filled by a combination of vascularized iliac bone and conventional rib or calvarial grafts. The procedure has the advantages of vascularized bone and the ilium gives a reasonably appropriate contour, which can be further improved by bending. But the dissection is difficult, and the need to establish an anastomosis with the superficial temporal artery restricts its use somewhat. It seems to be most useful in the frontotemporal area. We have done this in four cases, only one of which was post-traumatic.

Choice in cranioplasty

At present, our preferences are divided between autogenous bone and titanium for cranioplasty when a large frontal defect has to be repaired, but we are not blind to the occasional failures with both materials. Results appear

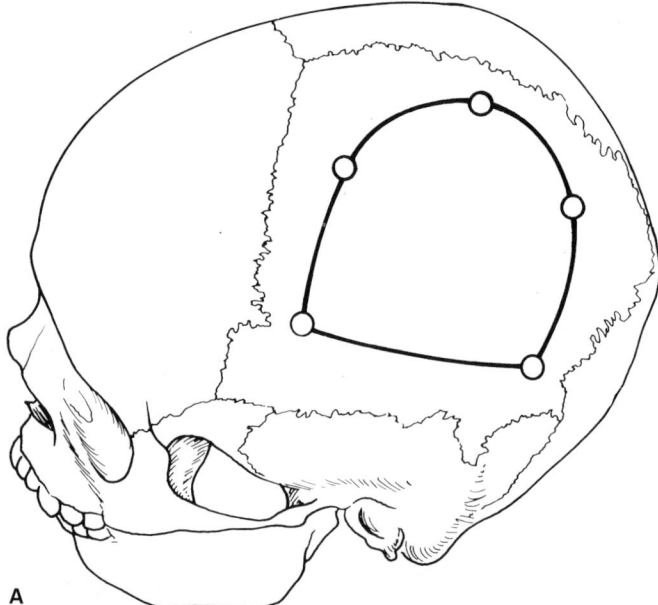

A

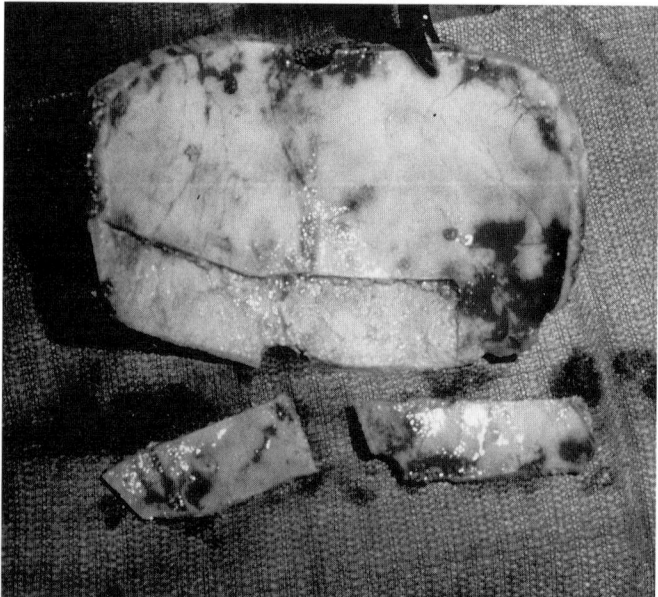

B

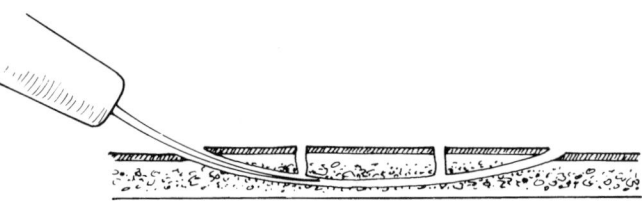

C

Fig. 21.13 Split calvarial bone grafting. A Frontal defects are exposed by turning the bicoronal scalp flap forwards; the parietal region is exposed by turning the flap backwards. A parietal bone flap is raised and split. **B** Strips taken from the inner table are replaced to fill the secondary defect, and the outer table is placed into the primary defect and screwed or plated into position. Thin two-hole plates with low profile screws are used. **C** Smaller defects can be filled with the outer table of calvarium, split through the diplöe.

to be better where fresh autogenous bone is used, and have been further improved with the use of rigid fixation by miniplates and screws. But in almost all cases, plates, screws and wires become prominent when swelling subsides and bone resorption takes place. Except for small defects, the best aesthetic results have been obtained with large fragments of split calvaria and with titanium. Calvarial cranioplasty seems to be more satisfactory in the long run. Split-rib cranioplasty tends to remain uneven and this may show in the frontal region (Fig. 21.6).

Therefore, as a general rule, we favour autogenous bone grafts. Small defects are plugged with inner table of ilium, having some cancellous bone attached — the so-called bath-plug graft. Medium-sized defects are closed with split calvarial grafts. Large defects with compromised soft-tissue cover are repaired with the split ilium free flap. Nevertheless, titanium plates remain very popular, especially when the patient requires maximum protection against recurrent cranial trauma.

TEMPORAL DEFORMITIES

Surgical pathology

Hollowness in the temporal region can be due to a sunken

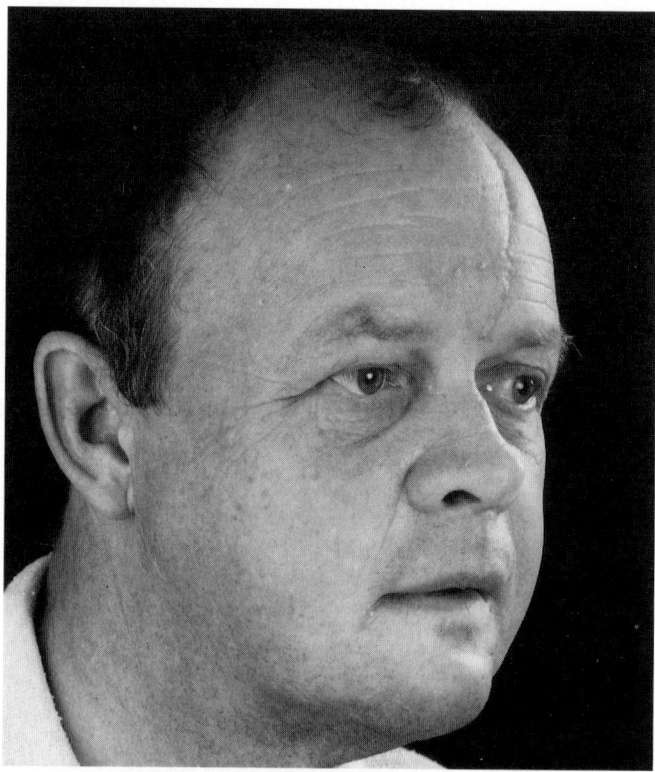

Fig. 21.14 Temporal hollowing. A 50-year-old man involved in a flying accident required a bicoronal scalp flap for exposure of the upper and middle face. Several months after the initial surgery, temporal hollowing resulted from displacement of the temporalis muscle from its normal attachments.

or displaced temporal bone flap. More commonly in post-traumatic cases, the deformity follows a surgical procedure in which the temporal muscles have been elevated from their calvarial attachments above and from their orbital attachments anteriorly, when exposed through a bicoronal scalp flap (p. 238). When this occurs the lateral margin of the lateral orbital rim and the zygomatic arch often appear very prominent and angular.

Management

The temporal concavity resulting from elevation of the temporalis muscle from its attachments can be prevented by careful reattachment of the temporalis fascia to the superior temporal line, the lateral orbital margin and the superior surface of the zygomatic arch. When an established deformity has to be corrected (Fig. 21.14), the area is best exposed by the bicoronal scalp flap. The temporalis muscle is dissected out of the temporal fossa down to the level of the zygomatic arch. The temporalis muscle must be reattached, but it is often also necessary to fill the temporal hollow by placing bone or some other

substance underneath the muscle. Bone is preferred, with rigid fixation. Repair is completed by suturing the superior margin of the temporalis muscle to the pericranium above as well as to the lateral orbital rim using a few holes drilled along that margin.

ORBITAL DEFORMITIES

Surgical pathology

These deformities generally involve some or all of the following:

1. Enophthalmos due to expansion of the orbital walls, floor and/or roof, expanding the orbital volume; there may also be damage to or loss of orbital contents (Fig. 21.15)
2. Rarely exophthalmos, with or without pulsation due to loss of the roof or caroticocavernous sinus fistula (p. 392)
3. Naso-ethmoid deformity, often with loss of function of the nasolacrimal apparatus (Fig. 21.16)
4. Extra ocular muscle dysfunction.

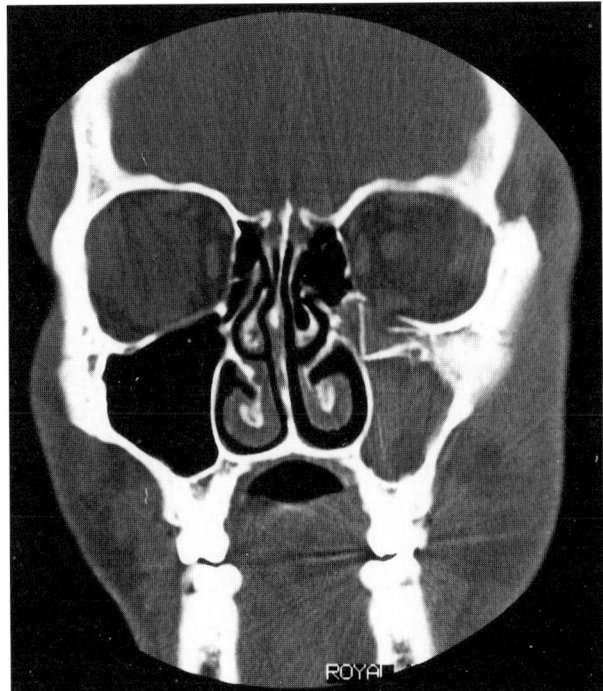

A

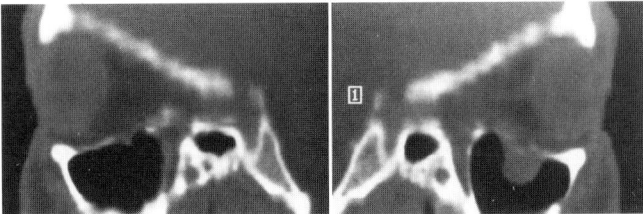

B

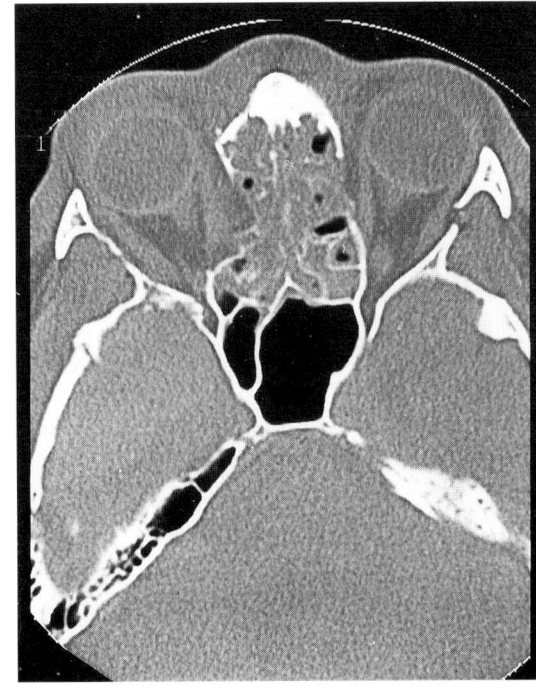

C

Fig. 21.15 Enophthalmos secondary to traumatically increased orbital volume. A Coronal CT scan showing damage to the orbital floor, lateral orbital wall, and medial orbital wall, producing expansion of the orbit. **B** Sagittal reconstruction showing the expanded orbital floor. **C** Axial view showing the medial orbital wall collapsed into the ethmoid, expanding the orbit in this direction. The effect of the malar displacement on orbital volume is also evident.

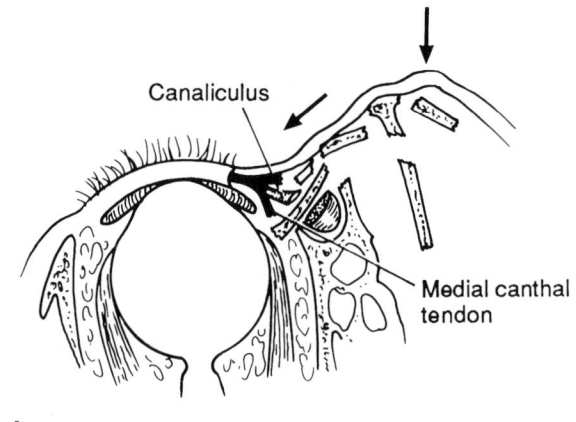

A

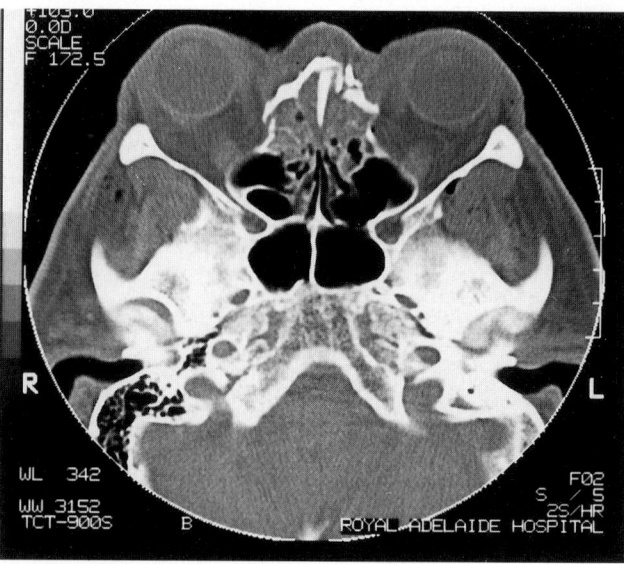

B(i)

Fig. 21.16 Injury to the nasolacrimal apparatus. A Relationship of the nasolacrimal apparatus to the lacrimal fossa and the medial orbital walls in crush injury of this area. Not only is the bone disrupted but the delicate nasolacrimal apparatus is endangered. **B** CT scan of a crush injury to the naso-orbital-ethmoid region: (i) axial view showing the complete disruption at the level of the canthal attachment; lacrimal drainage is impaired; (ii) coronal view showing the buckle in component of the deformity.

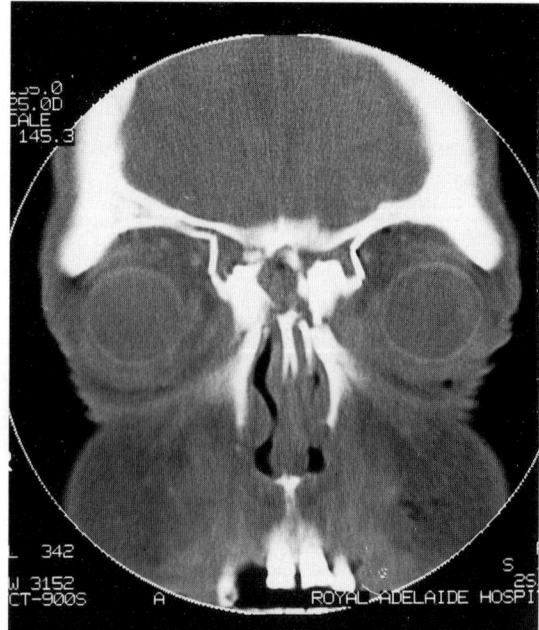

B(ii)

Orbital deformities established in childhood

Naso-orbital and orbito-zygomatic fractures are rare in young children, less so in the older child. Post-traumatic orbital deformities in the younger child have special features resulting from interference with normal growth.

True hypertelorism may result from an anteroposterior crush injury in infancy, causing genuine separation of the orbits (Fig. 21.17). More often, naso-orbital fractures cause traumatic telecanthus which tends to become more prominent as growth proceeds; there is often an associated depression of the nasal bridge and lacrimal drainage dysfunction (Fig. 21.18).

Loss of an eye during the phase of growth of the globe and orbit results in reduced orbital size, presumably because the orbit is deprived of its functional matrix (p. 77).

Management

The results of treatment of established post-traumatic orbital deformities in the paediatric population depend on the age of the patient and the timing of treatment. As a general principle, surgical treatment should be delayed until growth is complete; malunited fractures should not be treated in the period of craniofacial growth by refracturing or bone grafting (Manson et al 1986). Definitive surgical corrections are best performed when orbital growth is complete. If it is necessary to intervene earlier then multiple surgical interventions will probably be required. Most orbital growth is complete by the age of ~6 years and osteotomies in the orbital region can be performed at or after this time. However, onlay bone grafting of the region is likely to need later repetition because of resorption.

ENOPHTHALMOS

Surgical pathology

Residual orbital deformities can result from inadequate primary treatment or from massive loss or damage in the orbital margins and walls. Lesions of the orbital contents such as the globe, muscles, fat and lacrimal apparatus are frequently associated with malunited orbital fractures.

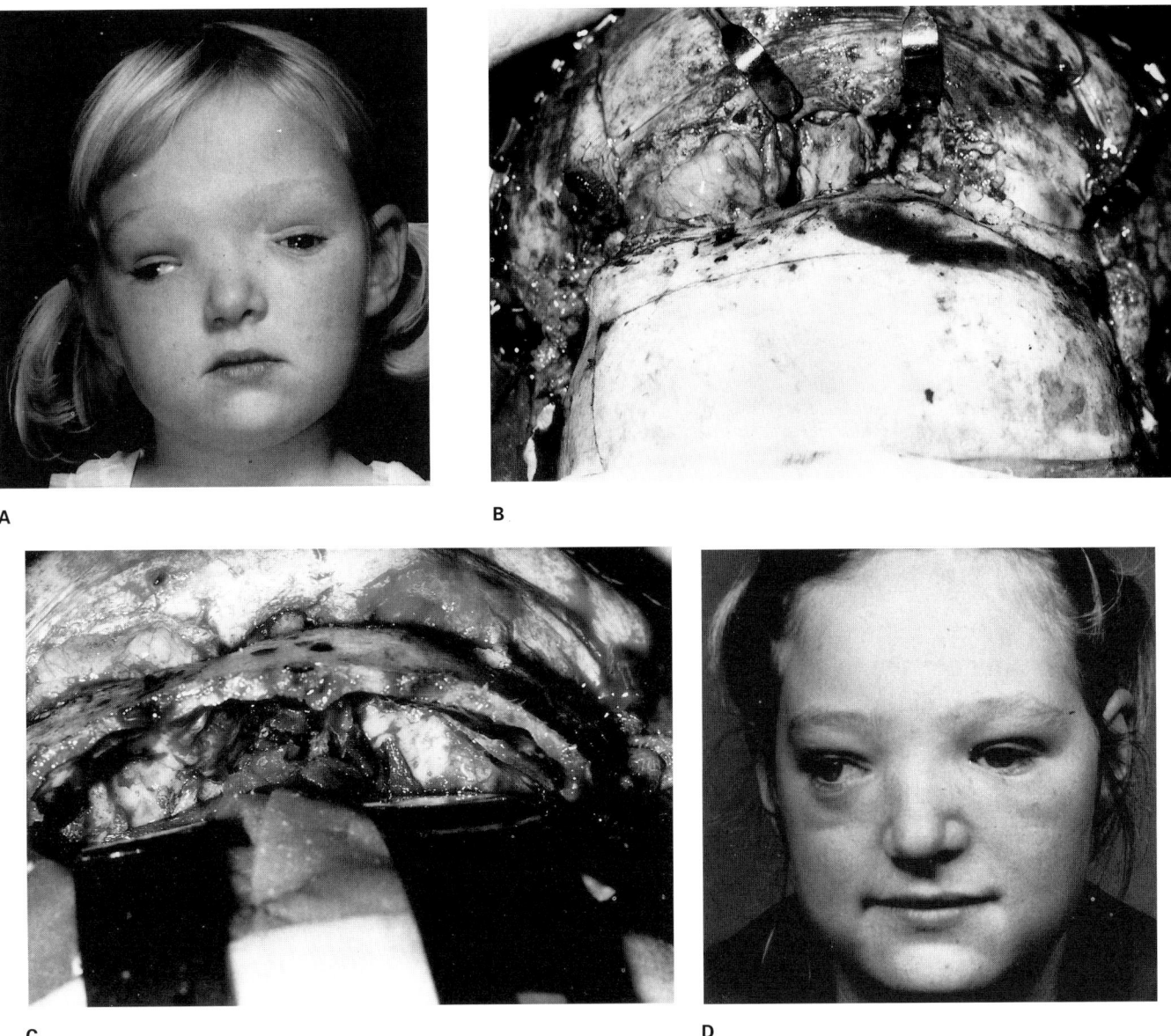

Fig. 21.17 Traumatic hypertelorism. A 3-year-old girl presented with traumatic hypertelorism having been run over by a tractor as a neonate. In spite of the heavy weight, the pliable skull and soft ground saved her life but compression produced a splaying of the orbits, including the lateral wings of the sphenoid bone, reminiscent of congenital defects with hypertelorism. This is a very rare situation and, we believe, only occurs under similar conditions. **A** The child on presentation with obvious traumatic hypertelorism and increased lateral canthal distance, medial canthal distance, and interpupillary distance. **B** The left orbit is displaced laterally. **C** When the anterior fossa is exposed the shape and direction of the roof of the orbit can be seen to be rotated to the left, and the widened interorbital distance is reflected in the midline of the anterior cranial fossa. **D** 10 years later she still has a squint on the right side, widening of the intercanthal region and some tearing due to the disruption of the nasolacrimal apparatus on both sides.

If the orbital deformity expands the orbital volume, or is associated with a bone defect into which orbital contents can herniate, then there will be enophthalmos; the recession of the globe will be exaggerated if there is loss or atrophy of any part of the orbital contents.

Management

The late correction of enophthalmos should be possible if the orbital contents can be replaced and the walls of the orbit reconstructed. This has in the past been considered extremely difficult if not impossible (Converse et al 1977, Dingman 1978). Today, the better understanding given by CT scanning and the capability of 360° circumferential access and full dissection of the orbit have together made the correction of enophthalmos possible — but not always certain. Prevention of orbital deformity by initial operative reduction is always desirable, and with good imaging, wide exposure and primary bone grafting, the need for late correction has receded.

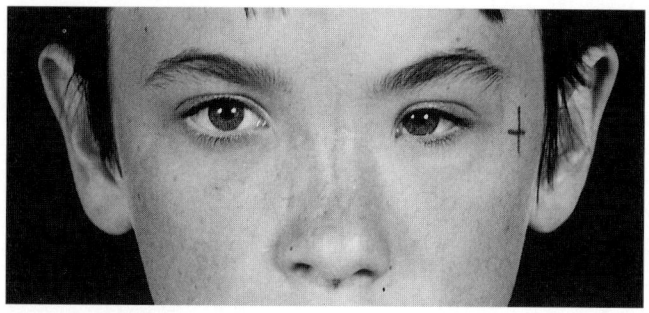

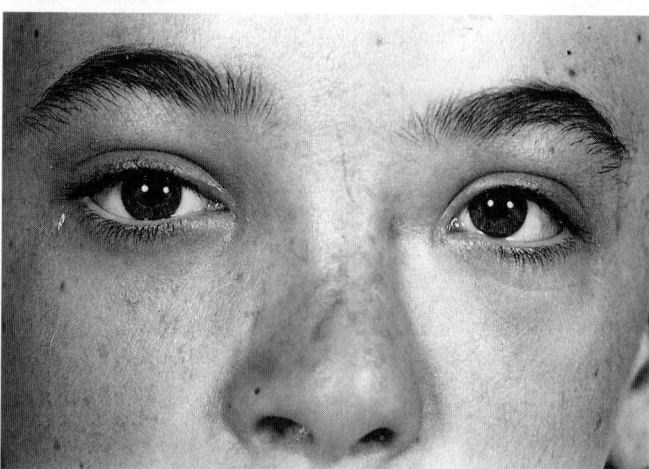

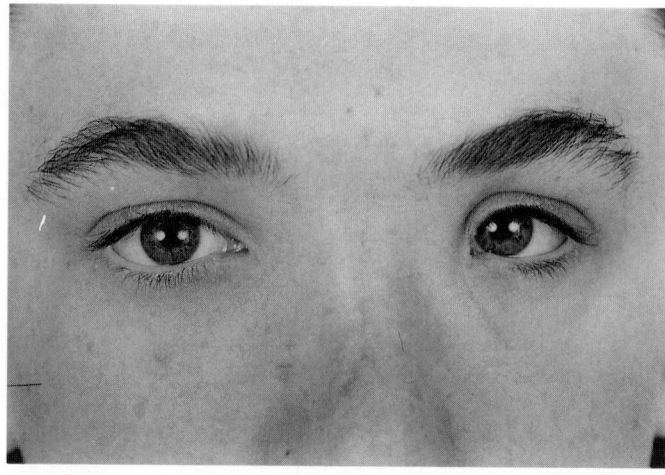

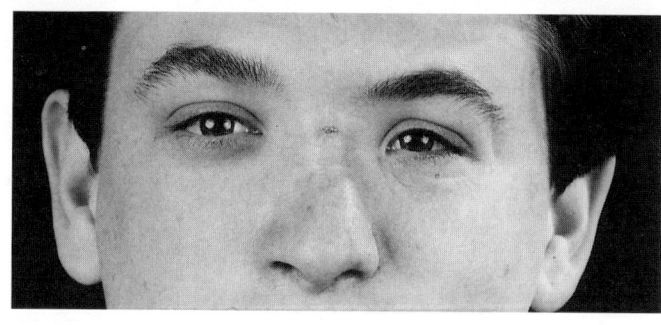

Fig. 21.18 Orbital fracture in childhood. A 6-year-old boy fell from a cliff. He presented with a distorted nasal bone and medial orbital wall area around the nasolacrimal apparatus. In spite of appropriate primary correction the damage and obstruction persisted. When growth was completed he required definitive surgery. **A** Appearance shortly after medial canthopexy and orbital wall and nasal reconstruction. **B** The naso-orbital region a month later, with signs of tearing and canthal drift. **C** Appearance 2 years later with the canthal drift worsening and the shape of the palpebral fissure markedly changed. **D** Appearance 8 years after the original injury. Further corrective surgery has been performed to replace the canthus and build up his nasal bridge, as well as dacrocystorhinostomy.

Orbital floor defects

Floor defects, on which all attention was previously focused, are often associated with medial wall defects or with an enlarged inferior orbital fissure; the orbital contents prolapse into these defects and adhere to them.

The damaged orbital floor can be exposed by the approaches described in Chapter 9 (Fig. 21.19). For the simplest problems, such as a small 'blow-out' fracture, the transconjunctival approach to the orbital floor is adequate; a proximal conjunctival flap is elevated and held out on a stay suture to protect the cornea (Tessier 1973, David 1974) (Fig. 9.5). For more extensive exploration when wiring or plating may be necessary, the incision may be extended by a lateral canthotomy. However, care must be taken in repairing this as inaccurate restoration can produce tethering and sometimes a thickened scar.

The blepharoplasty incision incorporating a musculo-cutaneous flap also gives wide exposure but results in an external scar albeit a usually excellent one. In this approach, a small incision 3–4 mm long is made in the crow's foot crease from the lateral canthus downwards and laterally, through skin and muscle. The points of curved iris scissors are inserted deep to the muscle and the musculocutaneous flap is developed across the whole width of the lid and up to the lid margin. The scissors can then be inserted with one blade deep to the musculo-cutaneous flap and a cut made 1–2 mm below the lid margin. This musculocutaneous blepharoplasty flap provides very wide exposure to the upper anterior maxilla and the orbital floor. We rarely use lower lid incisions because of the resultant scarring and potential lower lid oedema.

Where the orbital floor exploration is part of an orbito-cranial operation, an experienced surgeon can approach the floor via the bicoronal scalp flap. The periosteum is mobilized from the lateral orbital rim and the zygomatic arch. The periorbital dissection is as extensive as possible, though of course avoiding the apex of the orbit. The margin of the defect must be clearly defined; the mis-placed orbital contents are often fibrotic and dissection

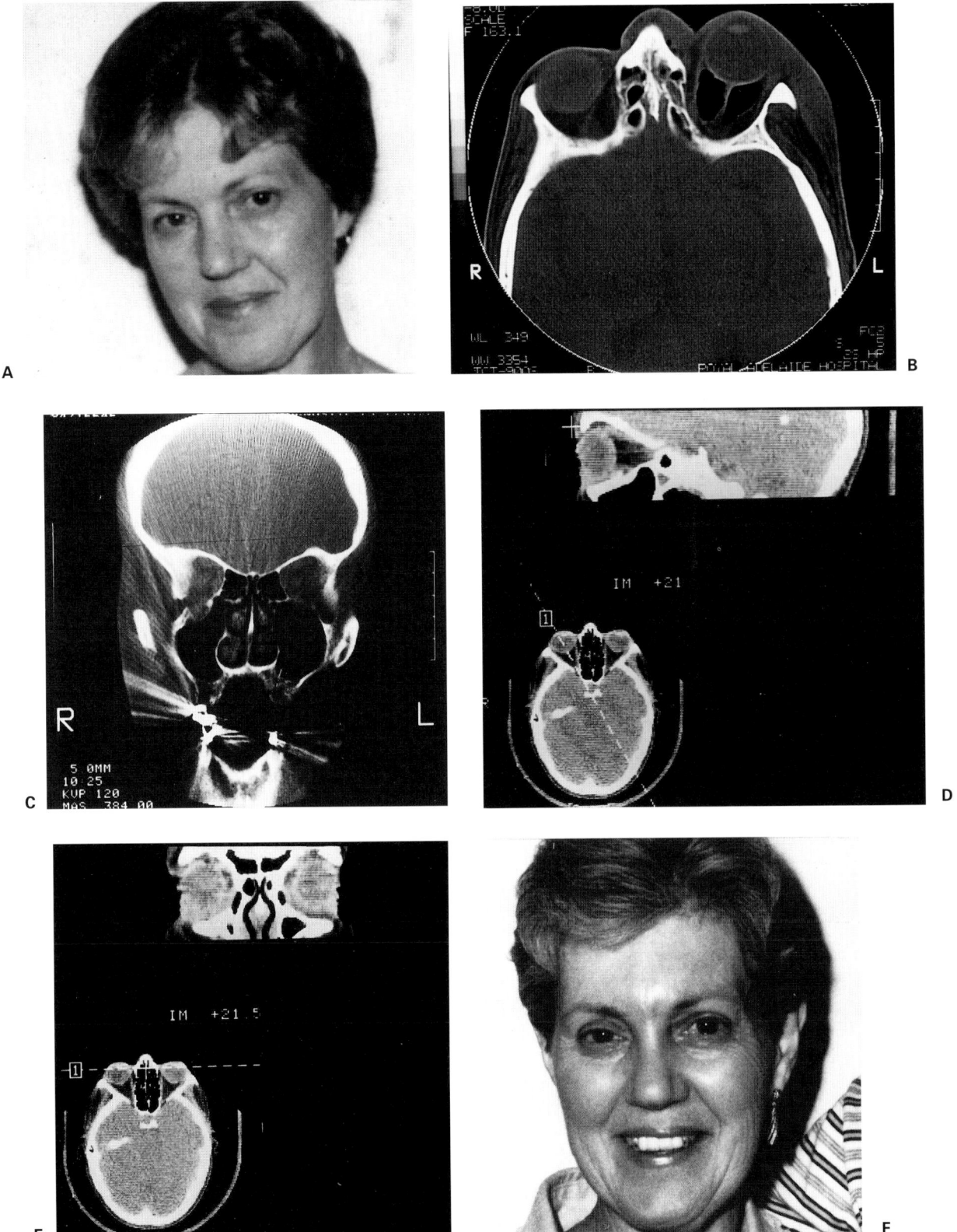

Fig. 21.19 Complications of orbital trauma. Depressed orbital floor, uncorrected for almost 10 years. The patient had enophthalmos and persisting diplopia. **A** Initial presentation with enophthalmos, slight global dystopia on the right side, and the head tilted to compensate for diplopia. **B** Axial CT shows the enophthalmos, with intact medial and lateral walls. **C** Coronal CT shows the downward expansion of the orbital floor with orbital contents prolapsed into the antrum. **D** Sagittal reconstruction demonstrating how iliac crest cortical bone graft to the orbital floor sits over the defect and supports the globe. **E** 2D reconstruction in a coronal plane, showing the globe supported on the newly grafted orbital floor. **F** Postoperative appearance. There is still a slight deepening of the supratarsal groove, but the enophthalmos and diplopia are almost completely resolved.

may be difficult. Care is needed to avoid excessive pressure on the globe, yet the surgeon must be able to extend the exploration to the posterior aspects of the orbit and discover the posterior margin of all defects. Considerable experience is needed for competence in this. Wolfe & Berlowitz (1989) enthuse over Tessier's technique for inferior orbital marginotomy to facilitate this difficult dissection (Tessier 1982) and to allow the defect in the orbital floor to be bone-grafted precisely under direct vision (Fig. 21.20). We rarely find this procedure necessary.

When the defect or defects are fully visualized, the defect is repaired. The architecture of the orbital floor may be restored by means of bone grafts, inorganic implants, or osteotomies. Except when a malunited orbito-zygomatic complex can be corrected by osteotomy alone, we unreservedly support the use of bone grafts alone for reconstructing the orbital floor, having removed all shapes and sizes of Silastic® and other foreign material inserted in earlier days by ourselves and latterly by others. Silastic®, in particular, in time seems to find its way into the paranasal sinuses.

Medial orbital wall defects

These are identified and defined exactly by CT scanning. Often, some of the orbital contents are prolapsed into the ethmoid sinus, and the volume of the orbit is thus enlarged. The intact ethmoidal sinus with its 'Chinese lantern' structure can be seen on the normal side and its delicate contribution to the orbital wall contour and hence the volume can be estimated and compared with the injured side.

The approach is best made via a bicoronal scalp flap, giving wide exposure of the fracture in the lateral plate of the ethmoid; the defect can then be dissected and the contents reduced. To do this effectively the posterior aspect of the fracture must be identified. The anterior ethmoidal artery is encountered en route to the fracture and should be coagulated. Defects can then be repaired, usually with a thin piece of split calvarial bone, harvested through the bicoronal scalp flap, which allows exposure of the parietal region (Fig. 21.21). Not only must the defect be bridged but the volume of the orbit must be reduced; however, the normal anatomy is not easy to reconstruct and bone graft replacement is always a little imprecise.

Lateral orbital wall defects

Isolated fractures of the lateral wall are rare: damage in this area is usually associated either with total orbital disruption with multiple wall defects, or more commonly with an uncorrected or inadequately corrected fracture of the zygomatic complex. Enophthalmos resulting from the displacement of the zygomatic complex is caused by downward and outward displacement of the bone, enhanced by the pull of the masseter muscle, producing an expanded orbit. The zygomatic component of the orbital floor may be disrupted, allowing the orbital contents to prolapse into the maxillary antrum. Similarly the thin bone behind the lateral orbital rim, which articulates with the greater wing of the sphenoid bone, may be disrupted with prolapse of orbital contents into the temporal fossa. Once the malar fracture has been reduced by osteotomy (Gruss et al 1990) then any persisting enophthalmos is due to the depression of the orbital floor (see above) or to outward bowing of the lateral orbital wall. Surgical

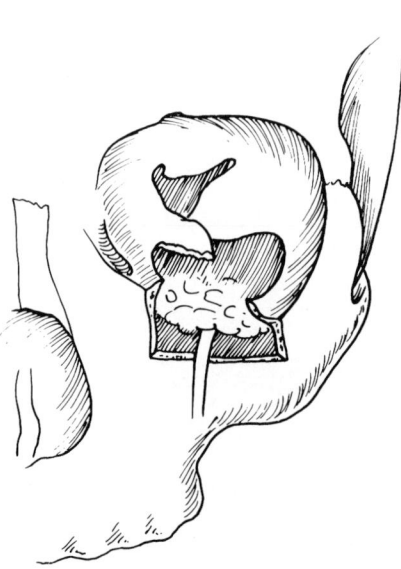

Fig. 21.20 Surgical exposure of the orbital floor. Technique recommended by Tessier (1982) for resection of the inferior orbital margin above the infraorbital nerve, providing increased exposure for retrieving orbital contents from the antrum and subsequently reconstructing the orbital floor.

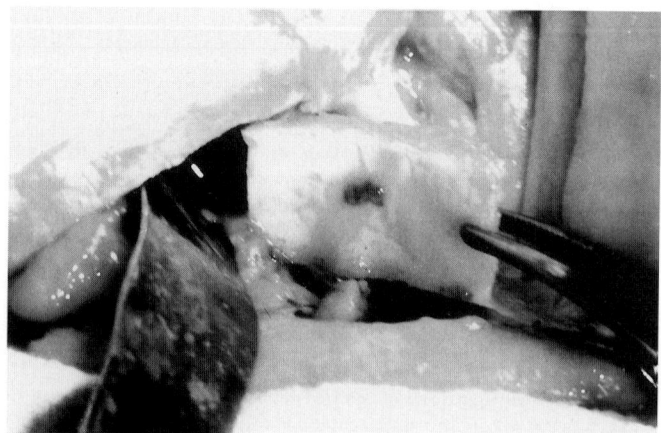

Fig. 21.21 Post-traumatic enophthalmos. Patient presented with enophthalmos following orbital trauma. Split calvarial bone graft is placed into the medial orbital wall via the bicoronal scalp flap.

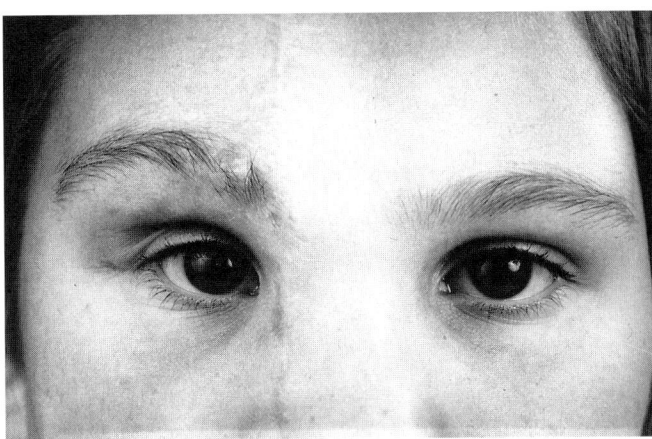

A

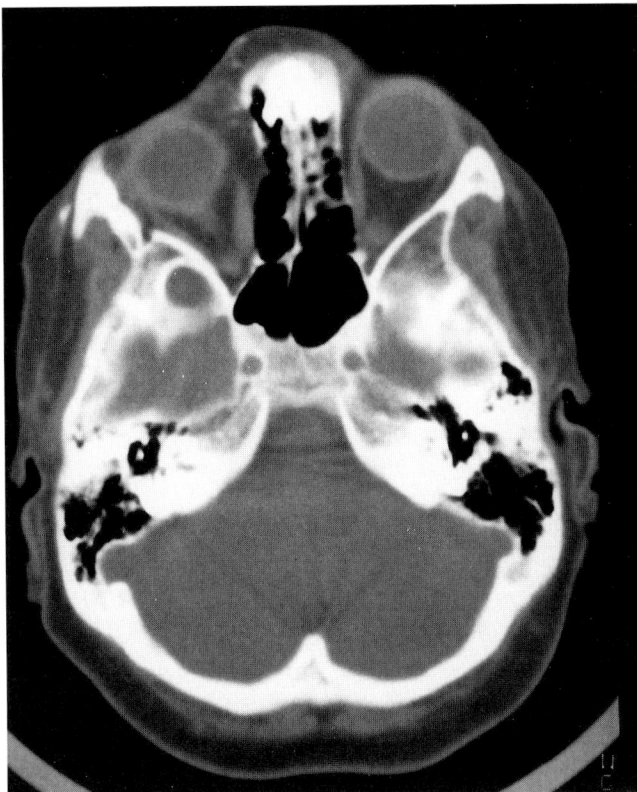

B

Fig. 21.22 Displacement of the orbital complex. There are rare cases in which the globe and orbital box are displaced but the relationship between the globe and box is maintained. It is our experience that this occurs when there is an injury early in childhood with force directed to one side such that a 'unilateral hypertelorism' results. **A** Distorted asymmetrical retrodisplacement of the orbit and globe. **B** CT scan showing some retrodisplacement of the globe within the expanded orbit, with the whole complex positioned posteriorly.

strategy and operative techniques are as for enophthalmos caused by massive destruction of one wall only: wide exposure of the orbital skeleton, restoration of the zygomatic complex, rigid fixation, identification of areas of bone loss in the walls of the orbit, reduction of all herniated orbital contents and restoration of orbital volume, with careful reconstruction of the orbital wall defects by autogenous bone grafting. Usually this is done with split calvaria but rib and iliac bone can be used. If more projection of the globe is necessary smaller grafts can be placed behind the axis of the globe to produce forward projection. In the past diced cartilage and other materials have been used to pack the orbits, and even glass beads, Silastic® blocks, Teflon®, Supramid® etc. They are no substitute for the direct visualization and accurate repair of the defects by bone graft. However, we are beginning to use porous polyethylene (Medpor®) in the hope that this will obviate the problems of harvesting and resorption of bone grafts (Nguyen & Sullivan 1992).

There are some rare cases where the globe and the surrounding orbit are retrodisplaced but the relationships of globe to orbital rim are maintained (Fig. 21.22). Such a deformity is the result of injury in childhood, causing posterior displacement of the whole orbital box: correction is properly done by transcranial advancement of the orbit with the contained globe, using the osteotomy patterns described below for the correction of orbital dystopias. After such an osteotomy it is likely that the orbital contents will need some further augmentation by bone grafting the defect and packing some bone on the walls behind the axis of the globe. This troublesome deformity has received insufficient attention in the literature.

DEFORMITIES OF THE ORBITOZYGOMATIC COMPLEX

Surgical pathology

These deformities commonly result from untreated or inadequately treated depressed fractures of the zygomatic bone and lateral wall of the orbit. The zygomatic bone makes a key contribution to facial morphology, connecting as it does by its radiating processes to the frontal, maxillary and temporal bones, and depressions of the zygomatic bone are often very noticeable. The clinical signs and symptoms of secondary deformation of the orbitozygomatic complex are similar to those following acute injury:

1. Alteration of facial contour
2. Displacement of the orbit and/or globe
3. Diplopia
4. Residual sensory nerve damage
5. Limitation of mandibular movement.
6. Aesthetic problems from a damaged globe, absent globe or empty socket; these are considered on p. 641.

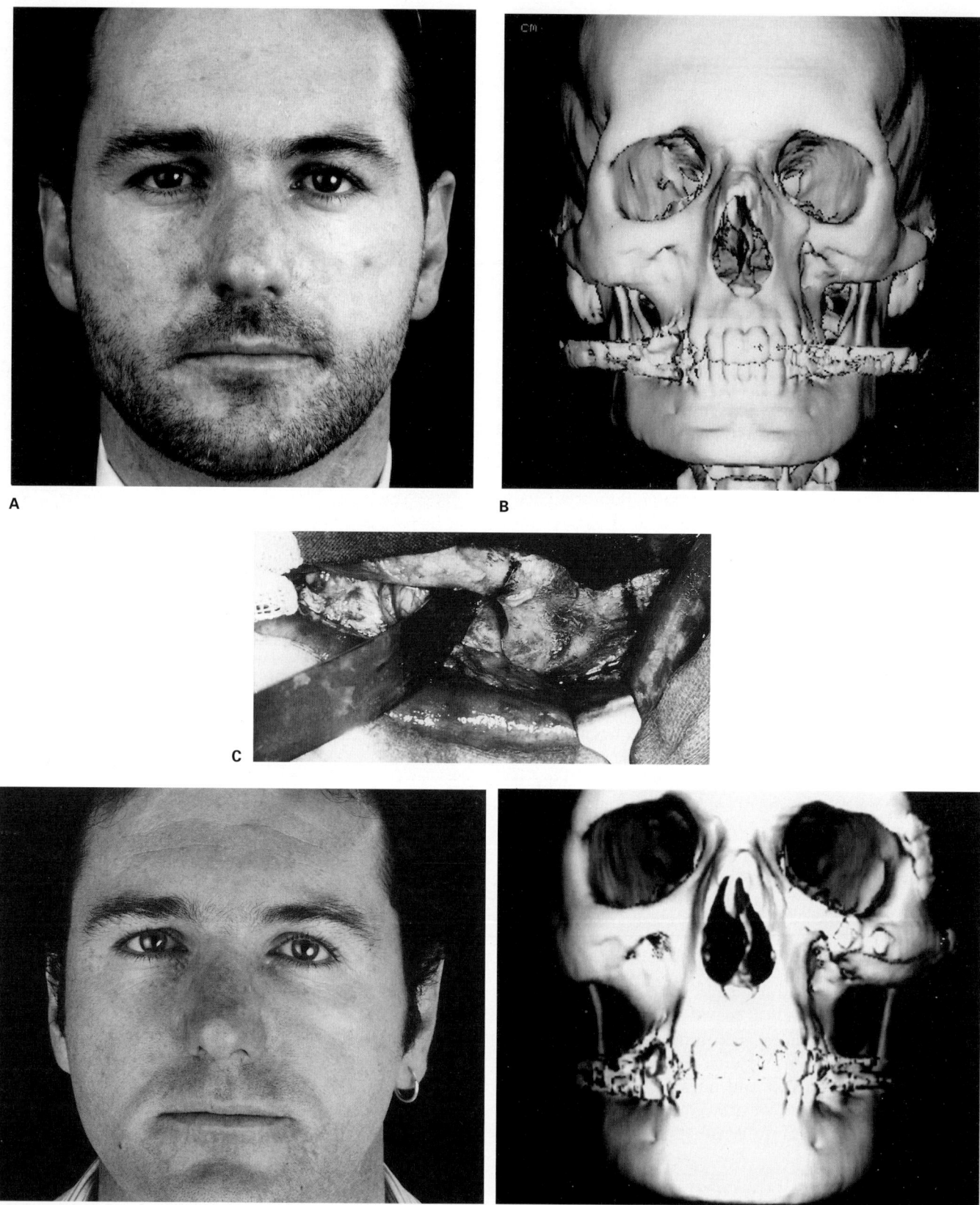

Fig. 21.23 Zygomatic osteotomy. A Patient with a fractured zygoma expanding the orbit and producing flattening of the cheek. **B** CT scan showing the bony deformity in three dimensions. **C** Operative photographs showing deformity of the zygoma. **D** Postoperative CT scan. **E** Postoperative appearance.

Alteration of facial contour

This may be due to bony displacements and/or soft-tissue damage (Fig. 21.23). The range of deformity varies from a hardly noticeable bony displacement which blends with natural facial asymmetry, to gross displacement of the whole bone with or without comminution, overlying scarring and loss of the fibrofatty malar cheek pad.

Bony deformity may result from severe comminution and subsequent resorption of small fragments of bone, or from displacement caused by scar contracture in skin and muscle. Inadequate primary fixation may result in displacement due to the action of the masseter muscle during mandibular movement. Segments of bone may be lost from the orbital rims and zygomatic arch. The zygomaticomaxillary buttress area is often subjected to compression forces, resulting in movement. Segments of bone may be lost from the orbital rims and zygomatic arch. The zygomaticomaxillary buttress area is often subjected to compression forces, resulting in comminution and later fibrosis: these, if uncorrected in a primary repair, add to the orbital deformity.

Orbital and/or ocular dystopia

In these deformities, the orbit and globe may be displaced in any or all of the three dimensions, and displacement of the globe may be independent of orbital rim displacement. Horizontal and vertical dystopias are especially disfiguring, as is orbital hypertelorism, which is a form of horizontal dystopia. Hypertelorism was one of the first challenges for pioneers in the surgery of craniofacial deformities (Fig. 21.24).

The whole orbital complex may be enlarged inferiorly or inferolaterally by a downward and lateral displacement of the zygoma. The floor of the orbit is thereby involved and there is vertical orbital dystopia. The globe itself may be displaced downwards when the floor of the orbit is deficient as in a 'blow-out' fracture. Lateral displacement of the globe may occur in fractures of the naso-orbito-ethmoid complex, but true lateral displacement of the whole orbit is in our experience a rare deformity. Also rare is an inferior displacement of the orbit due to trauma. When the compressive forces occur in infancy, the bones are soft and injury results in a splaying out of the orbits, which is maintained or accentuated with further growth (see below). Superomedial displacement of the malar bone is rare but may produce a decreased orbital volume with superior positioning of the globe and exophthalmos.

Diplopia

Double vision may result from displacement of the globe, damage to the cranial nerves, damage resulting in scarring of the extraocular muscles or prolapse and entrapment of orbital soft tissue. Because there are so many factors involved in diplopia, reconstructing the orbit and repositioning the globe may not in themselves overcome double vision. It is wise to wait a considerable time (at least 1

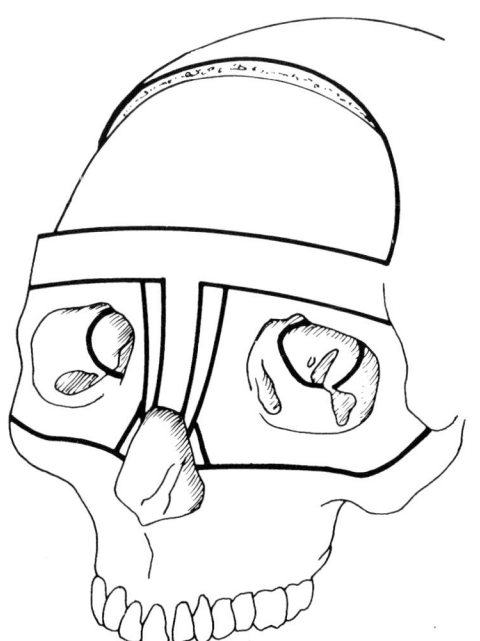 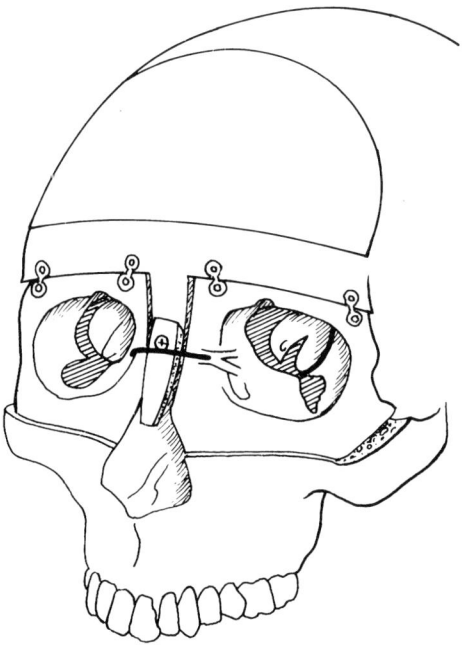

Fig. 21.24 Hypertelorism correction. Hypertelorism correction according to Converse et al (1970). Midline structures are preserved wherever possible. The cuts are made behind the axis of the globe so that the globe is translocated with the orbital box.

year) after reconstructive surgery before surgery on the extraocular muscles is undertaken. Multiple surgical interventions may be necessary and the muscles of the other eye may indeed need adjusting to achieve fusion. The assessment and management of post-traumatic diplopia are considered in Chapter 14 (p. 418).

Sensory nerve damage

Anaesthesia, paraesthesia or hyperaesthesia of the zygomaticofrontal, zygomaticofacial and infraorbital nerves may express nerve injury resulting from the initial trauma or from dissection during the surgical correction.

The nerves passing through the body of the zygoma (p. 61) may take well over a year to recover and the numbness of the cheek and temple must be explained to the patient. The recovery phase is often accompanied by dysaesthesiae — 'funny feelings' — and shooting pains. Recovery is usually complete after 2 years.

Infraorbital nerve lesions affecting the gums and teeth are present in a minority of patients and in a very few give rise to neuralgia which is persistent and hard to treat (p. 659).

Limitation of mandibular movement

This occurs when the zygomatic arch impinges on the excursion of the coronoid process of the mandible.

Assessment

Nothing surpasses thorough clinical assessment and the critical eye of the skilled surgeon. In addition to the plain radiographs listed in Chapter 7, namely the occipitomental view, postero-anterior views of the orbit, submentovertical view and orthopantomogram, the CT scan has given a new dimension to assessments of deformities of this region. The ability to view the orbital walls in detail has been supplemented by attempts to quantify the orbital volume on the basis of CT data (Manson et al 1986). The techniques for this have their limitations but do indicate that changes in the size and shape of the bony orbit constitute the most important factor in the problem of enophthalmos (p. 193). Whitaker (1987) has given an excellent analysis of the midface malar region in three zones, which is very applicable to the assessment of contour restoration after trauma, no matter what technique of repair is used. These three zones extend from the nasolabial fold outwards and onto the zygomatic arch. The medial zone is just lateral to the nasolabial furrow. The middle zone is the prominence of the zygoma and the outer zone is the zygomatic arch (Fig. 21.25).

Management

The indications for surgical correction can be inferred

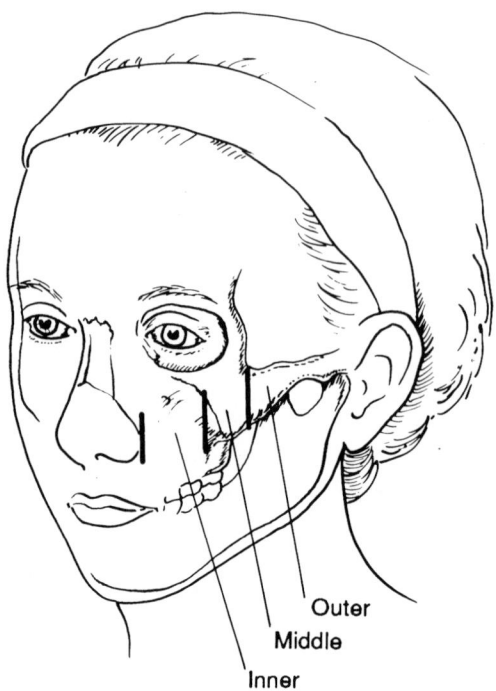

Fig. 21.25 Midface malar region. The three regions of the malar midface region as identified for the purposes of augmentation by Whitaker (1987). By courtesy of *Plastic and Reconstructive Surgery.*

from the pathology. The chief is obvious facial deformity resulting from bony displacements and/or soft-tissue scarring. Diplopia due to orbital or global dystopia is an indication when persistent. Enophthalmos, often combined with deformity and diplopia, may be an indication, as is impingement of the zygomatic arch on the coronoid process.

Long-term paraesthesia or hyperaesthesia of the infraorbital nerve may be an indication when the patient persists with the complaint, though the likelihood of symptomatic relief may not be good.

Operative correction

Success depends largely on determining whether the deformity results from a deficit in the bone, or from a pure malposition, or from a combination of both. Segmental bony deficits are usually corrected by bone grafts, whereas malposition of the orbitozygomatic complex with normal adjacent bones is corrected by osteotomizing the bone, thus recreating the fracture, and then repositioning the bone with or without onlay grafts.

The most appropriate exposure must be used: the choice of exposures includes the bicoronal approach, the periorbital (eyebrow, lid and conjunctival) incisions, and approaches through existing scars. Whichever approach is chosen, access should not be compromised. When contour restoration by onlay or inlay techniques is indicated,

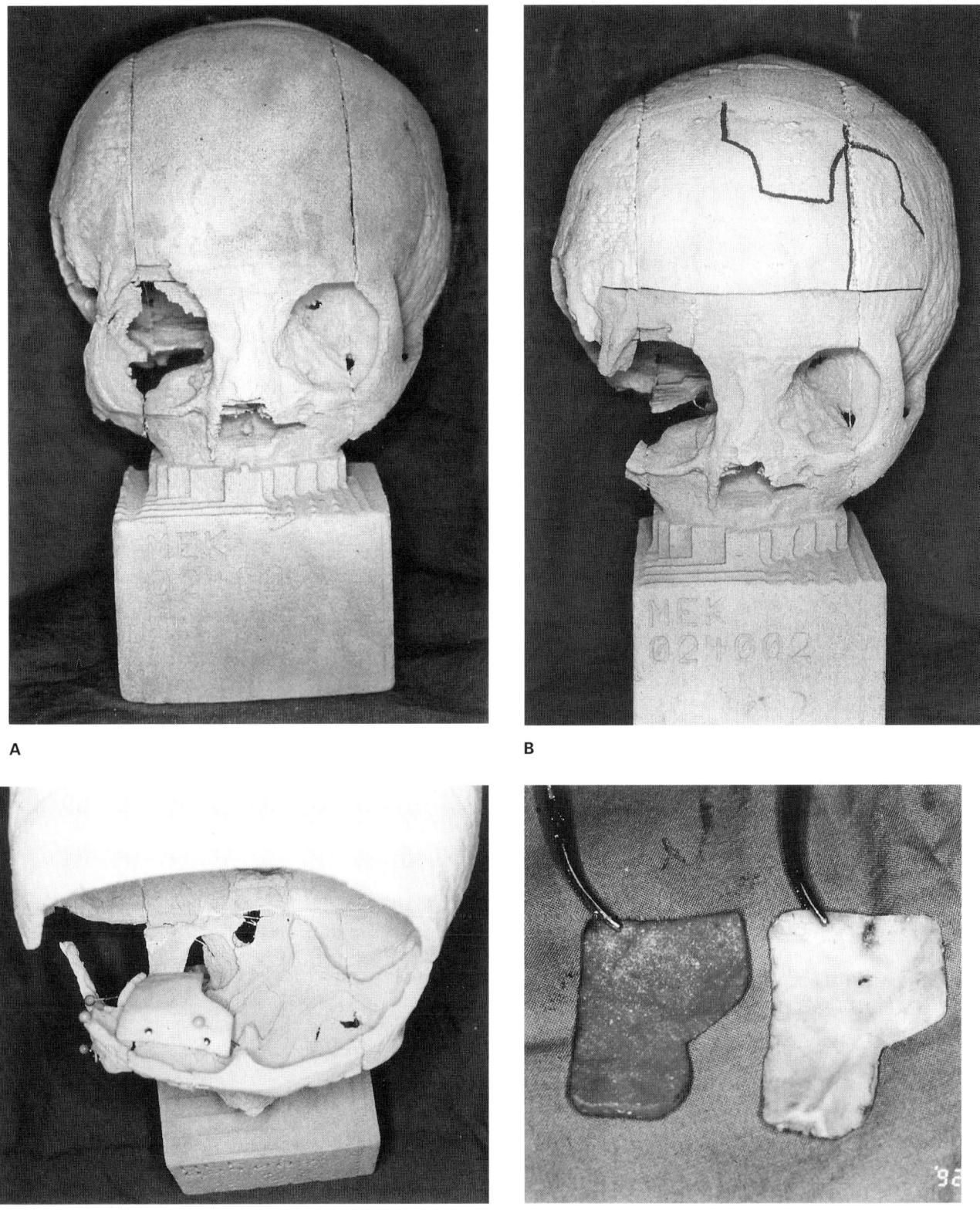

A

B

C

D

Fig. 21.26 Solid models for preoperative planning. A Solid model of a case of sphenoid resection due to neurofibromatosis. (The technique may well be used for trauma.) **B** Exterior view. **C** Anterior fossa view, enabling templates to be prepared so that the bone can be cut absolutely accurately at operation. **D** Templates with the carved bone at the time of surgery. (Photos courtesy of Dr S. Tajima.)

a choice of material needs to be made. Segmental bone losses around the orbital rims, zygomaticomaxillary buttress and zygomatic arch are replaced with autogenous bone onlay and/or inlay, fixed with titanium screws or miniplates (Gruss 1992). The bone graft of choice is split calvarial bone (p. 241), but rib or hip bone can be used. The bone may be screwed into place and recontoured in situ or preshaped. Maejima et al (1993) and Yab et al (1993) have developed 3D solid models which can be used to prepare templates from which bone grafts can be modelled in a precise fashion to repair defects in the cranium and orbit. Figure 21.26 shows such models being used in a case of neurofibromatosis, by a method equally applicable to post-traumatic deformities. Countersinking screw heads adds to rigidity and makes the head less palpable through the skin when the inevitable — though usually slight — bone resorption occurs. The finest possible plates consistent with stability should be used in this region. While we prefer bone even for the most subtle onlay restoration of the malar prominence, other substances are available. Silastic® has been used for this purpose, but it is difficult to carve exactly; the tendency to migrate has been noted. Hydroxyapatite is likewise difficult to contour to the complex curves of the cheekbone. Whitaker (1991) championed the use of Proplast® (polytetrafluoroethylene combined with aluminium oxide or other structural substance) in this area and supported its use in spite of some claims of increased infection. However, recent studies suggest that Proplast® is often associated with adverse local reactions (p. 155). Polyethylene (Medipor®) may be more satisfactory. The frequent necessity of having to remove previously placed plates and screws, the distortion or loss of tissue planes, the presence of fragments of bone and scar often containing sinus mucosa, all combine to make the use of alloplastic material very problematic.

In almost all cases, operation is done under general anaesthesia with oral endotracheal intubation. The surgical field is cleaned with povidone–iodine solution; local anaesthetic with adrenaline (p. 255) is injected at the subperiosteal level. The patient is given intravenous antibiotics before the incision is made.

When the lateral rim of the orbit and zygomatic arch are involved then the bicoronal approach is preferable; this can be combined with buccal and eyelid incisions if necessary. The upper buccal sulcus incision can be used in cases where there is an aesthetic deformity affecting the prominence of the zygoma and the anterior maxilla. Exposure from above allows detachment of the temporal fascia from the lateral orbital rim and the zygomatic arch, and this enables the periosteum to be elevated from the orbitozygomatic complex (Fig. 21.23). Exposure from below is done via an incision in the buccal mucosa 5 mm above the apex of the sulcus, and the cut is made directly to bone beneath the infraorbital nerve: the periosteum

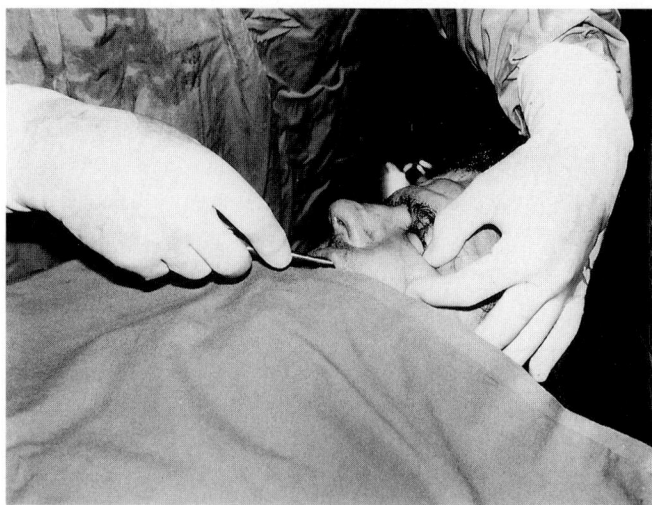

Fig. 21.27 Dissection of the orbitozygomatic complex via the transoral approach. The forefinger and thumb of the non-dominant hand protect the orbit during the dissection.

and attached muscles can then be elevated with a sharp periosteal elevator. The right-handed surgeon can protect the globe of the eye by grasping the orbital margin, zygomatic arch and body junction between the finger and thumb of the left hand, dissecting between the two digits (Fig. 21.27).

When bone is used to re-establish a pre-existing contour by replacing lost bone, there is always a problem as to how to shape the graft and how thick it should be. Even when appropriate bone, e.g. calvaria, is secured with rigid fixation, judgement at operation is often compromised by soft-tissue swelling, and as there is always some resorption of bone there is a necessity for overgrafting. It is this uncertainty that inspires the continuing search for a satisfactory bone substitute.

When the whole orbitozygomatic complex is malpositioned, treatment is by osteotomy. Wide exposure is desirable, and the bicoronal scalp flap is preferred. Osteotomies are made at the frontozygomatic suture, and in the lateral orbital wall, inferior orbital rim, lateral maxillary buttress and zygomatic arch (Figs 21.28 and 21.29). To perform these cuts, the periorbita is stripped from the lateral wall and floor of orbit. Additional exposure may be necessary through the eyelid (p. 238). The exposure extends to the infraorbital fissure and orbital floor. The periosteum is stripped from the arch and body of the zygoma, avoiding and protecting the infraorbital nerve. The masseter muscle may be detached from the body of the zygoma to achieve movement after osteotomy. In old traumatic cases this dissection may not be easy. The tissue planes that are so readily stripped in congenital or purely cosmetic deformities are lost or interrupted and scar from trauma or previous surgery bleeds unduly. Fragments of bone are often displaced into soft tissues; on the orbital

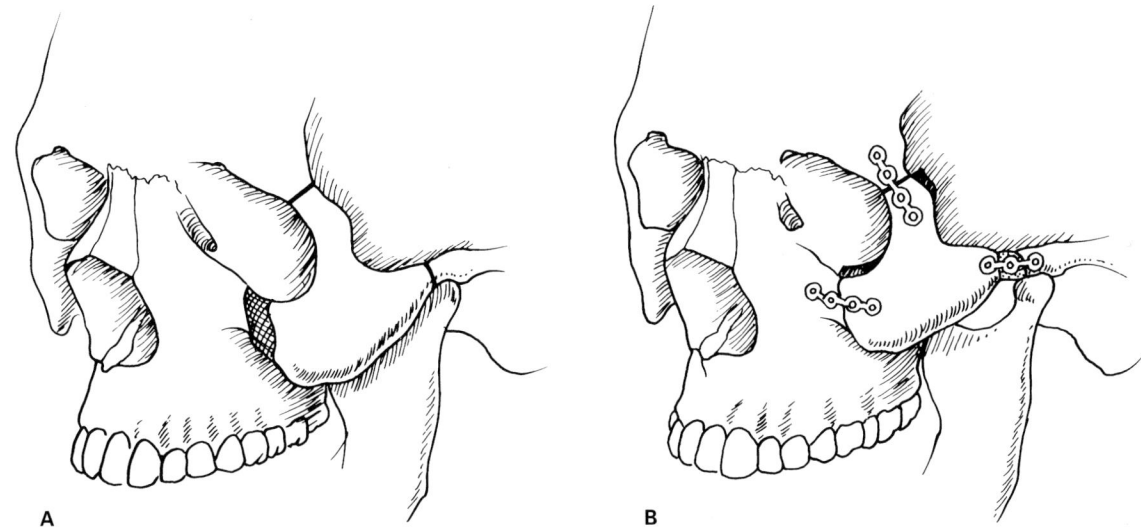

Fig. 21.28 Zygomatic osteotomy. A Depressed and malpositioned zygoma. **B** Three-point osteotomy and repositioning with miniplate fixation and bone grafting.

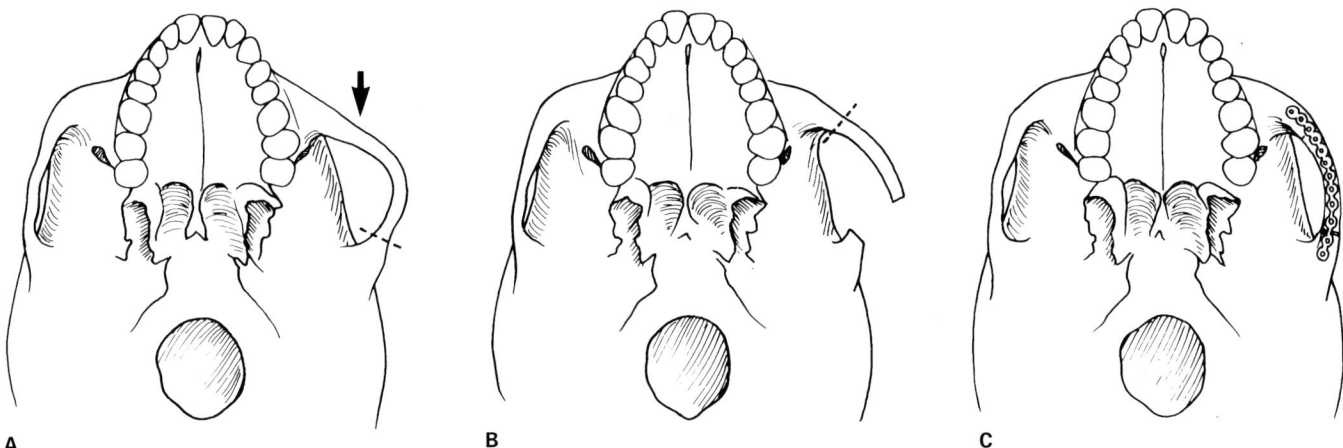

Fig. 21.29 Zygomatic osteotomy. A Depression of the zygomatic body and bowing of the zygomatic arch requiring osteotomy for correction. **B** The orbitozygomatic complex is freed at the frontozygomatic suture, the infraorbital margin, and the lateral maxillary buttress. **C** After repositioning the arch, forward projection is maintained by grafting the gap in the arch and fixation with a long miniplate.

side of the dissection the periorbita has often been previously breached and there may be little but scar between the orbital contents and the maxillary antrum. Careful persistence is needed, with good surgical assistance, taking care to avoid too much pressure on the globe but not failing to get the adequate exposure that the surgery demands.

The osteotomies are made with power saws; a reciprocating saw is preferred, held like a pen. Malleable metal retractors protect the orbital contents. Osteotomies are made through the arch, through the frontozygomatic suture and from the temporal fossa into the orbit; in cutting into the orbit, the saw blade is held flat against the temporal fossa surface, and the surgeon views the point of the blade on the orbital side and the base of

the blade on the temporal fossa side, to avoid entering the middle cranial fossa. The cut extends to the inferior fissure and across the orbital floor to the rim, respecting the infraorbital nerve; it is extended laterally to separate the zygoma from the maxilla. Once these cuts have been successfully made, a slightly curved osteotome is inserted into the section of the cut in the zygomatic buttress; gentle rotation of the osteotome will usually separate the bone quite easily.

As Gruss (1992) has rightly pointed out, the key to the correct positioning of the orbitozygomatic complex is the zygomatic arch. Once the distorted arch's shape and length are restored, an accurate overall positioning is possible with restoration of correct orbital volume. In old malunited fractures the shape of the arch may have to

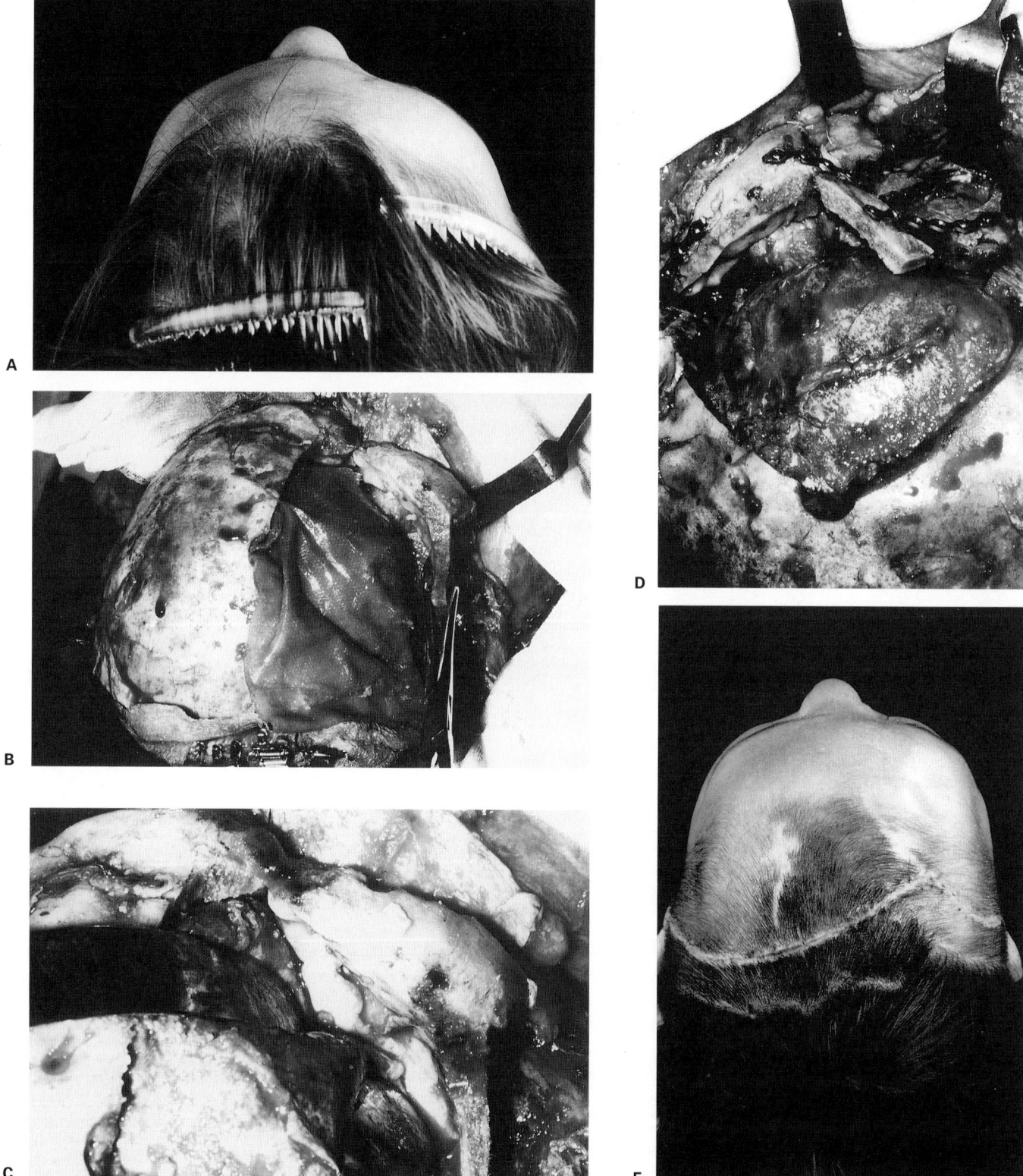

Fig. 21.30 Secondary alterations in facial contour. Patient shown in Fig. 21.22, who had a severe post-traumatic deformity of the right side of the face following a complex fronto-orbital, orbitozygomatic and naso-ethmoid injury sustained in a vehicular accident 6 years earlier. The initial treatment consisted of a frontal craniotomy, reduction and fixation of the zygoma, and soft-tissue repairs. **A** View from above, illustrating deficiency of the forehead and right side of the face. Enophthalmos is mild because the position of the globe within the orbital box has been relatively well maintained while the whole of the orbital complex is displaced posteriorly. **B** Operative appearance of the deformity with the frontal craniotomy removed to reveal the shattered and depressed fronto-orbital complex. **C** Dissected anterior fossa with the old fracture represented at the junction of the anterior and middle cranial fossae. **D** Fronto-orbital complex replated in its new position. **E** The postoperative appearance highlights the repositioning of the zygoma and forehead to restore and slightly overcorrect the contour on that side.

be changed by osteotomy; appropriate basal CT cuts will show the distortion of the arch and guide the surgeon as to how it should be cut and reshaped. Without the wider exposure given by a coronal flap and complete arch dissection, this manoeuvre is very difficult. Long fine miniplates or microplates are used to stabilize the newly shaped zygomatic arch and bridge the zygomaticotemporal gap; similar plates are applied to the frontozygomatic suture, lateral maxillary buttress and inferior orbital margins. Autogenous bone grafts are used to fill the gaps in the arch, buttress and orbital walls.

Correction of deformity in the orbitozygomatic complex is an essential first step in correcting a malunited panfacial fracture, utilizing the same planning principles that are applied in the primary management of a recent panfacial fracture (p. 339). In reconstructing such an extensive deformity, correct positioning of the orbitozygomatic complex on each side is followed by establishment of the occlusion and correcting malunited jaw fractures; this enables the relationship of the correctly occluded jaws to be established with the zygomatic complex. The naso-orbital component can then be attached medially, enabling the anterior maxillary walls to be built out and the nose constructed on the platform of the face (Fig. 21.29).

When there is massive disruption of the orbitozygomatic complex with extensive destruction of bone, then osteotomy is out of the question: the whole orbitozygomatic complex must be rebuilt. This can be achieved with split calvarial bone grafts. If enough bone cannot be harvested from the skull, then the calvarial grafts should be augmented with split-rib grafts. A long piece of bone is shaped and fixed into position with plates and screws to replace the zygomatic arch, being attached medially to the maxilla and laterally to the zygomatic process of the temporal bone. The lateral orbital wall is reconstructed with a series of longitudinally placed struts from the frontal bone, attached to the newly formed zygomatic arch. Further onlay bone graft may be needed to shape the orbital rim laterally. The cheek prominence may be further enhanced with bone screwed to the longitudinal graft used for reconstruction of the zygomatic arch. Such reconstructions are often compromised by damaged skin and other soft tissues; further surgery may be necessary to smooth out the bone, to remove screws which have become prominent from resorption or to add additional bone or other material to enhance the contour.

Post-traumatic orbital dystopia may require correction by moving the 'whole orbit': in reality, this means moving the anterior two-thirds of the orbital pyramid. As has been previously stated, it is rare that post-traumatic hypertelorism or vertical orbital dystopia requires mobilization of the orbital box; in our experience this occurs only with deformities resulting from injuries suffered in infancy and early childhood. When such a mobilization is required, it is to move that part of the orbit which

carries the globe with it, and this is the anterior two-thirds of the orbital pyramid. The mobilization is in part done by a transcranial approach, and the bicoronal exposure is of course necessary; the neurosurgeon is added to the craniofacial team. The distances of the planned orbital movement are determined by examination of the patient and by appropriate radiography.

In vertical dystopia (Fig. 21.31), a frontal craniotomy, in size less than the width of the orbit, is performed on the side to be displaced, and the intracranial extradural dissection is limited to part of the anterior fossa to be protected during the cutting of the roof, and the medial and lateral orbital walls. Additional incisions in the eyelids or upper buccal sulcus can be performed, but usually the whole osteotomy can be done from above. The upper osteotomy is made 1 cm above the supraorbital rim and the lower is made across the anterior maxilla just beneath the infraorbital foramen. The posterior lateral orbital cuts are made vertically through the lateral orbital wall, flush with the temporal fossa base. The lateral orbital wall osteotomy is extended across the orbital roof and inferiorly across the orbital floor into the inferior orbital fissure. The medial orbital wall is cut at about the level of the anterior ethmoidal foramen and we now prefer not to dissect the medial canthal ligament as it is difficult to reattach this ligament again.

If the orbit is being repositioned superiorly, a measured amount of bone is removed from the frontal bone. The orbit is gently mobilized and fixed superiorly. The removed bone can then be used to graft the horizontal defect in the maxilla beneath the infraorbital nerve to maintain the vertical translocation; additional bone grafts are placed in the inferior defects if necessary. The new position can be determined very accurately.

When the orbit is being moved medially, as in hypertelorism, we prefer to maintain the midline structures wherever possible, namely the vertical plate of the ethmoid and the central part of the anterior fossa (Converse et al 1970), and in our experience this has always been possible in post-traumatic hypertelorism. Medial translocation of the orbits is achieved after the removal of the appropriate amount of nasal bone, frontal bone and anterior fossa, parasagittal to the cribriform plate. The medial translocation is stabilized by insertion of bone in the lateral osteotomy. It is prudent to place a thin overlay of bone on the horizontal maxillary cut, to prevent prolapse of soft tissue into the defect, which might result in a sunken appearance in the mid-face. The medial canthus must be aligned as accurately as possible and if necessary canthopexies are performed (Fig. 21.24). It is our experience, and we believe this is generally shared, that vertical dystopias are easier to correct than horizontal dystopia. Hypertelorisms, particularly in the rare post-traumatic cases, are likely to require bone grafting to the nose, canthopexies and often secondary surgery to the

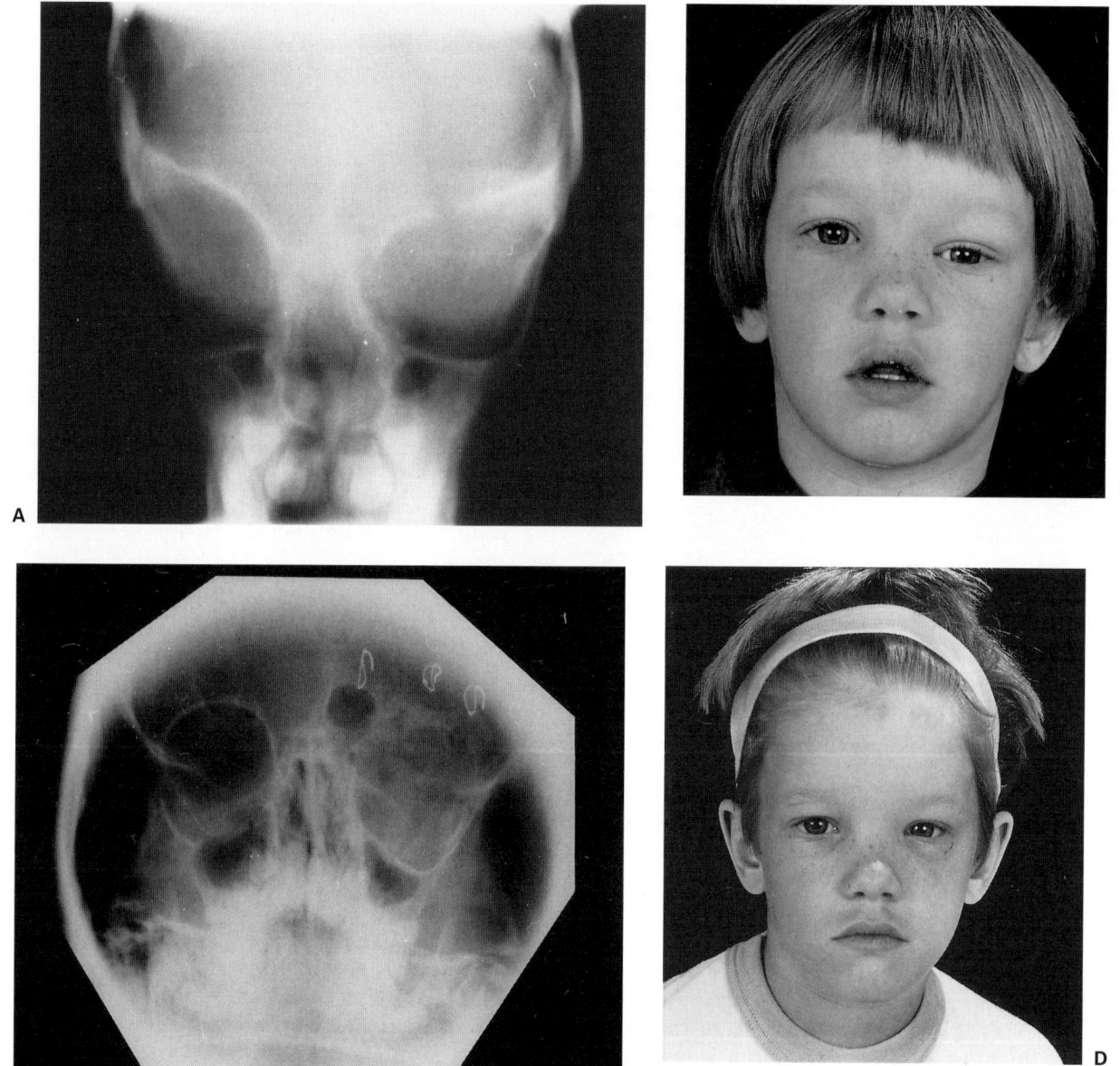

Fig. 21.31 Translocation of the orbit. A 6-year-old boy fell 20 feet from a balcony at his home onto cement, suffering concussion, nasal fracture, and left orbital fracture. He developed a CSF leak into the orbit which was repaired by a neurosurgical team. He presented two years later with left orbital dystopia of 1 cm and mild traumatic hypertelorism with a left divergent squint. **A** Tomogram taken at initial treatment showed a depressed and expanded left orbit. A residual fracture was evident in the orbital roof. **B** Photograph at the time of his presentation for craniofacial surgery showed orbital dystopia. **C** Post-operative X-ray picture showed the orbit after elevation, with three wire ligatures holding the elevated orbit to the frontal bone. **D** Post-operative photograph of the child showed the correction two years later with virtually no residual enophthalmos or orbital dystopia.

nasolacrimal apparatus. In our experience, multiple operations are necessary during the growth period and even later to overcome the persistent telecanthus component of these horizontal dystopias.

Complications and results

Haematomas and infection may occur. Infection is often associated with implanted materials such as plates and screws, and with operative exposure of the maxillary sinus. Pre-existing sinusitis should always be treated before reconstructive surgery; any indications of sinusitis from the history or preoperative X-ray findings may be an indication for endoscopic examination and subsequent drainage of the infected sinus, especially when the maxillary antrum is involved. In our experience screws presenting into the maxillary antrum after primary surgery have sometimes appeared to be a focus of infection.

More serious complications relate to eyesight. Compression of the optic nerves may result from implanted

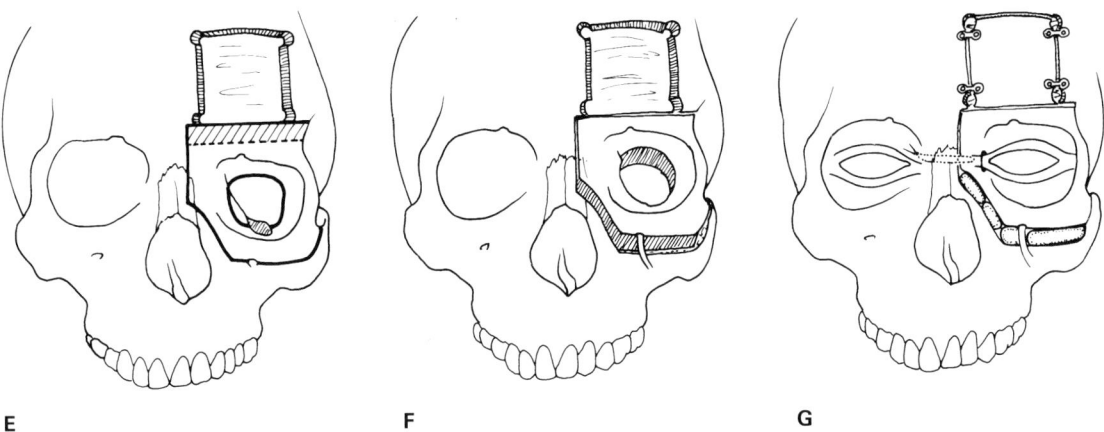

Fig. 21.31 Translocation of the orbit. E Diagrammatic representation of the small frontal craniotomy and removal of bone superior to the orbit used in such cases. Intraorbital and anterior cranial fossa cuts are made behind the axis of the globe to facilitate movement of the globe with the orbital box. **F** After repositioning, the bone removed superiorly can be used to augment the maxilla inferior to the orbit. The bone removed for the frontal craniotomy can be split to provide additional graft if necessary. **G** Canthopexy is necessary to re-establish the lid shape and relationships.

bone, from manipulation of the fracture or from retro-bulbar haematoma. In our experience, the patients susceptible to this complication are those with massive destruction of the orbit, where there has already been some compromise in optic nerve function; such patients are in danger of losing some or all of their residual vision. Fortunately, this is not common but does occur. Wolfe & Berlowitz (1989) refer to one case of blindness in 1600 orbits dissected and one case of loss of visual field. We have had one case in which vision decreased after an orbital dissection, in an experience of more than 100 translocations for post-traumatic orbital dystopia. This misfortune occurred in a patient with pre-existing visual impairment; eventual visual loss was not complete. It appears that, in traumatic cases, it is the damaged optic nerve that is more at risk. Trauma to the sixth cranial nerve is also common in cases where there is much scar and dissection is difficult.

In our experience, the aesthetic results are often indifferent, and often the reasons for this are beyond the control of the surgeon.

The controllable factors are the repositioning of the zygoma by osteotomy and the reconstruction of the orbital walls by bone graft. The variables are the restoration of the orbital volume to produce accurate positioning of the globe in three dimensions and the status of damaged soft tissues; loss of orbital fat, damage to muscles, eyelids and lacrimal drainage apparatus may impair the correction.

Initially good results can deteriorate with time. Resolution of postoperative oedema confounds early assessments. Bone grafts used to increase the projection of the globe may slowly resorb; tissues scarred by trauma and/or surgical intervention go through phases of hypertrophy and maturation. Even when a good early result has been obtained, and with the best possible surgical experience and judgement, the ultimate result with respect to the position of the globe may leave something to be desired. Because of these unpredictable factors, it is necessary to monitor the results of correction for a number of years.

Some patients have prolonged postoperative infraorbital nerve anaesthesia. The area of sensory loss usually extends from the lower lid over the cheek and lateral alar region to the upper lip. If sensation has not recovered after 3 months then it is most likely that the nerve is permanently damaged. We have not found release of the nerve as a secondary procedure to be of any benefit. In those cases where the numbness has progressed to a neuralgia — a very rare but distressing situation — exploration of the nerve and relief of pressure in the canal has not produced satisfactory symptomatic improvement in our hands (Fig. 21.32). The management of intractable facial neuralgia is further discussed in Chapter 22 (p. 557).

NASAL AND NASO-ORBITO-ETHMOID DEFORMITIES

Surgical pathology

Secondary deformities of this type range from malunited fractures involving the nasal bridge (i.e. the nasomaxillary region) together with the nasal cartilages and septum, to complex lesions involving the entire naso-ethmoid and orbital regions (Manson & Sargent 1992). The symptoms may be functional as well as aesthetic: nasal airway patency and sinus drainage may be affected, the sense of smell is often lost and impaired nasolacrimal drainage may cause

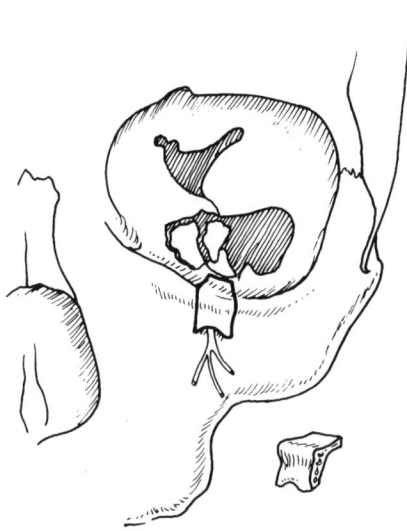

Fig. 21.32 Technique for decompression of the infraorbital nerve. A portion of the bone is removed above the nerve and into the orbital floor. The nerve may be traced back to the fracture area and dissected from the orbital content, and the fragments of bone removed or replaced. A bone graft may also be used to overlay the area (after Converse et al 1977). This approach observes the principle that nerves should be explored from a normal area to the abnormal. It is not a very satisfying procedure as far as results are concerned.

epiphora. There may also be risks of late intracranial infection, arising from proximity to damaged meninges (pp. 147 and 379).

Localized nasal deformities

These deformities may be confined to the nasal bones and cartilages or may be seen in conjunction with a more extensive deformity. When untreated or inadequately treated there may be resorption of bony fragments, fibrous union or malunion with excessive callus formation. Depending on the direction of the deforming force, the nasal pyramid may be deviated or flattened. An anteroposterior defect results from crushing of the supporting walls and collapse of the supporting bony structures. The nasal septum may be buckled by the impact and displaced according to the direction of the force, and buckling may obstruct one or both nasal passages.

An unacceptable appearance due to distortion of the nasal pyramid is the most common presenting symptom. The nature of the injury determines the type of deformity, which may involve only the bony portion of the nose above, or both bony and cartilaginous parts (Fig. 21.33). The bony nasal skeleton may be deviated to one side, or one nasal bone and maxillary process may be depressed more than the other; the cartilaginous lower nose may be displaced in conformity with the displacement of the bone, or may be deviated in the opposite direction. The cartilages may be torn from the bone and displaced.

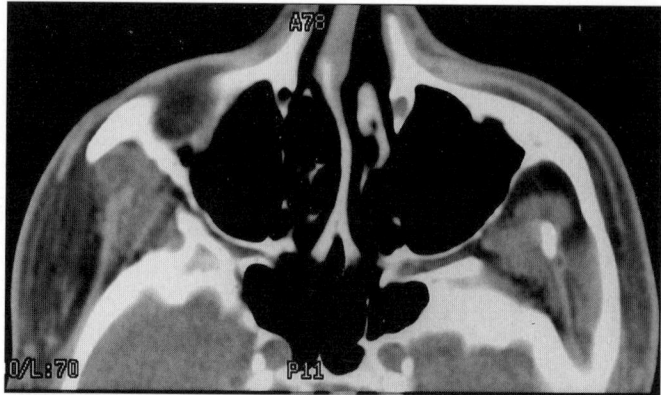

A

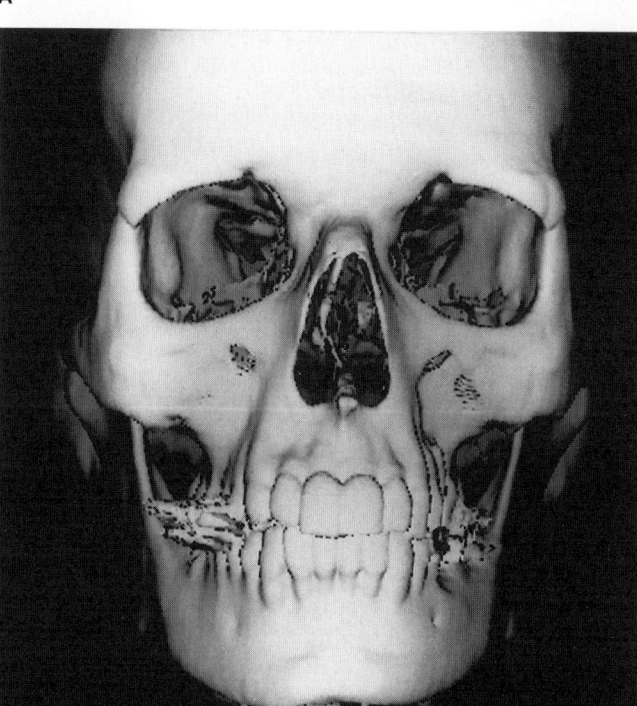

B

Fig. 21.33 Nasal septal deformity. A Septal architecture shown on axial CT. **B** Deformity of the bony septum.

The dorsum may be depressed in either its bony or its cartilaginous portions.

Malposition of the septum is responsible for deformity, not only in the dorsum but also at the columella level. There may be retraction of the columella or displacement of the caudal septum so that it presents in one or other nostril. The septum is often responsible for alteration in the patency of the nasal airway, the other common presenting symptom. It is the underlying deformity of the nasal septum which produces airway obstruction; obstruction may also be due to adhesions between the middle and inferior turbinates and the septum. Underlying developmental variations of the middle and inferior turbinates, particularly bullous enlargement on the contralateral side of a pre-existing deviation, will further complicate the obstructive picture. Septal damage may also be associated with a nasoseptal perforation, giving a whistling noise in breathing, and causing crusting in the nose.

Disruption of the lateral wall of the nose and consequent stenosis and obstruction of the normal ventilation and drainage of maxillary ethmoidal and frontal sinuses can lead to infection. This usually becomes apparent some time following injury and needs active treatment only if symptoms persist that are not controlled by medication, or if further surgery is planned.

The nasal valve area is the narrowest part of the nose and nasal airway and is the most important site of airway obstruction. Trauma can produce deviations of the septum in this area and also stenosis and webbing of the attachment of the upper lateral cartilage to the septum producing very troublesome obstructive symptoms. Trauma to the lower lateral cartilages may cause not only cosmetic deformities but also collapse of the lateral vestibular wall particularly on inspiration which is a most distressing symptom.

Naso-orbito-ethmoid deformities

Where a nasal fracture extends into the orbit, the term naso-orbito-ethmoid fracture is appropriate (p. 308). Malunited fractures of this type are complicated by the presence of the lacrimal system and the medial canthal structures; they also cause problems with orbital volume and contour and may result in an abnormally shaped palpebral fissure by disturbing the attachments of the medial canthal ligaments. There may be posterior displacement of the comminuted fragments of the nasal bones and the frontal process of the maxilla which may protrude into the orbital cavity as well as injure the lacrimal sac.

There is characteristically a flattened bridge of the nose and telecanthus; the eyes appear to be apart, there is often canthal dystopia, and if infection is present the tell-tale swelling of a blocked and infected lacrimal sac is seen. There may be cutaneous scars and prominent epicanthic folds. The deformity may be unilateral or bilateral (Fig. 21.18A). The abnormal 'eye' slope is due to the disconnected medial canthal ligament (and attached bony fragment) being distracted by the continuous pull of the orbicularis oculi muscle (Fig. 21.34).

LOCALIZED NASAL DEFORMITIES

Assessment

These deformities present with a history of nasal injury, often not of great severity. Examination reveals a malunited fracture involving the nasal bridge and the lateral

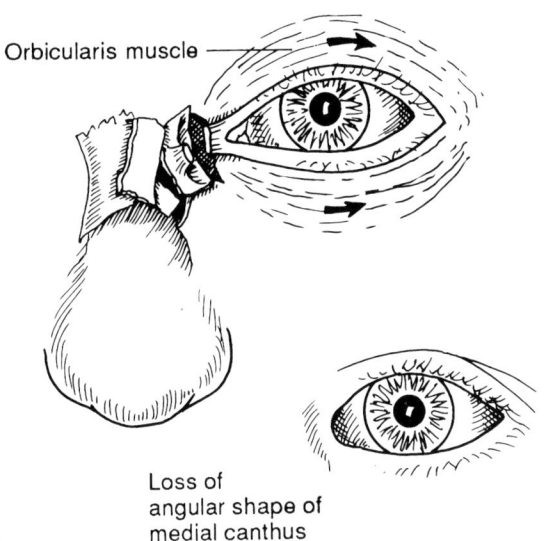

Fig. 21.34 Canthal dystopia. The shattered medial canthal region is distracted laterally by pull of the orbicularis oculi muscle, giving the rounded appearance of the medial canthus which is typical of the deformity (after McCarthy et al 1990a).

walls of the nasal cavity, with no extension into the adjacent frontal or orbital regions. The causative fracture involves the nasal bones, the frontal process of the maxilla and the septal cartilage, and these are deformed in varying degrees (Fig. 21.35).

A complete internal examination by the team ENT surgeon is mandatory. The internal physiology of the nose and paranasal sinuses must be examined, as well as the external form of the nasal pyramid. Photographs are taken to show front profile and basal views of the nose. Plain X-ray pictures demonstrate the anatomy of the septum and the state of the paranasal sinuses (p. 198). CT scan shows the details of septal deformity and nasal architecture in general very well (Fig. 21.33); CT scans will also show the details of the distorted architecture in the medial orbital walls in the canthal region.

The ENT assessment may indicate a need for sinus drainage; chronic suppurative disease of the sinuses needs to be dealt with before major reconstructive surgery, particularly if it is intended to insert free grafts of cartilage or bone.

In the more complex injuries, assessment of the lacrimal drainage apparatus is important and a dacryocystogram may be useful (p. 178).

Management

Emphasis must be placed on the correction of both function and form. Ideally, both dysfunction and deformity are corrected in a single operation. It is our experience, however, that 10–20% of cases will need some later 'touch-up' operation because of the tendency for scar tissue to produce unpredictable results as it forms and

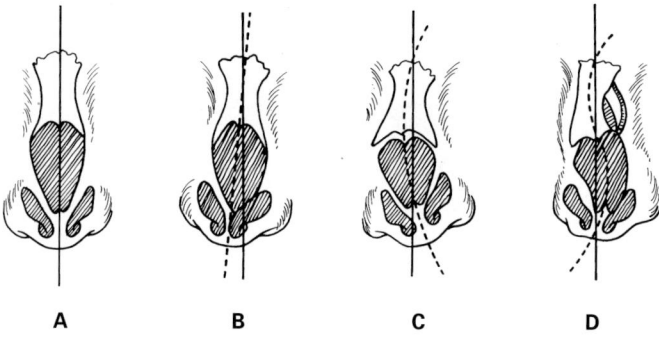

Fig. 21.35 Post-traumatic nasal deformity. A Normal shape of the dorsum of the nose. **B** Lateral deviation after trauma. The whole nose is deviated to one side and the displacement is uniform. **C** Deviation with convexity of the crest on the right side, while the tip of the nose is displaced to the opposite side. **D** A ''double curvature' of the dorsum.

matures: there is much variation in the endpoint of healing in this facial region. In very badly damaged nasal pyramids where the anteroposterior crush element is combined with a nasoseptal deviation, it is often wise to plan a two-stage operation: a first stage to centralize the nasal pyramid and reconstruct the septum and a second stage to graft the nose to obtain the desired definitive shape.

Correction of deviation

The nasal skeleton must be exposed and this can be done intranasally (Fig. 21.36). In severe deformities of the septum and nasal skeleton, the open external approach provides the necessary exposure, not only to appreciate all the underlying deformities but also for their correction. For lesser deformities the intranasal or classical aesthetic

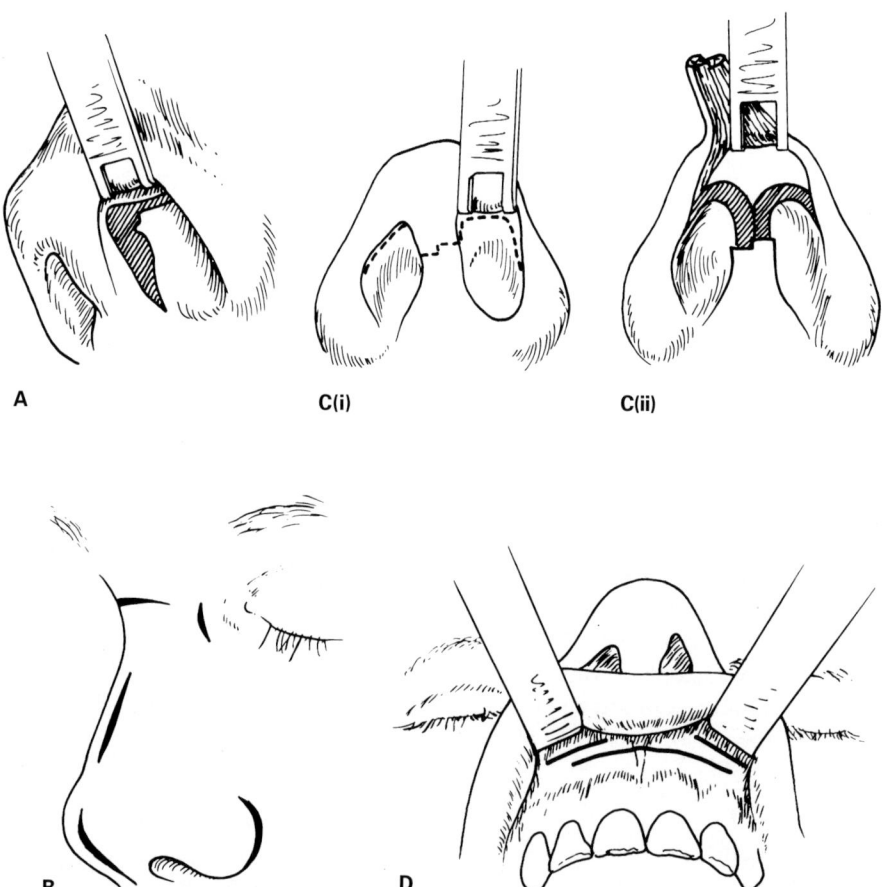

Fig. 21.36 Surgical approaches to the nasal skeleton. A Transseptal incision extended into the intercartilaginous plane. **B** Various skin incisions available for achieving complete dissection of the nasal framework (Tessier 1991). **C** (i, ii) Open rhinoplasty technique with a transcolumella step incision leaving the nasal cartilages intact. **D** Intraoral transbuccal approach for exposure of the nose, either bilateral or unilateral.

rhinoplasty incisions suffice. The greater the deformity the more extensive the exposure necessary.

Dissection is facilitated by careful injection of 2% lignocaine and 1/80 000 adrenaline solution through a fine needle into the appropriate tissue planes, producing hydrodissection as well as vasoconstriction. The skin is widely freed from the bony and cartilaginous skeleton. Wherever possible the upper lateral cartilages are left attached to the septum and the septal mucosal dissection is not carried over onto the lateral cartilages. However, in more severe cases the upper lateral cartilages are freed from the septum, leaving the upper lateral cartilage attached to the nasal lining mucosa.

The mucoperichondrium and periosteum are dissected off both sides of the nasal septum through an incision at the mucocutaneous junction or via a hemitransfixion incision at the caudal border of the cartilaginous septum. This will give complete exposure of the entire septum, and correction of both anterior and posterior deformities can be addressed. Removal of non-supporting parts of the septum can be undertaken. These include part of the posterior cartilaginous septum as well as most of the perpendicular plate of the ethmoid and vomer. As much as possible of the anterior cartilaginous septum is preserved as it has important supportive and physiological functions. It is most important that even minor deviations of the septum in the region of the valve are corrected. Small amounts of cartilage in this area can be removed but enough must be left to provide satisfactory support for the anterior nose. Occasionally the entire cartilaginous septum may need to be removed and then replaced in a number of smaller but straight pieces. At the end of the procedure, replacement of bone and cartilage between the mucosal layers reduces the likelihood of perforations, stabilizes the septum by reducing lateral movement or flapping and enables any subsequent surgery on the septum to be performed without too much difficulty.

Fracture lines in the cartilaginous septum should be excised; there is no place for scoring of cartilage on one or other side of the deviation in the expectation that this will correct the deformity. Adhesions or scarring in the region of the nasal valve can usually be treated by simple division and insertion of Silastic® stents between the septum and outer lateral cartilage. These are left sutured in situ for ~10 days to prevent recurrent adhesions.

There are many variants on the basic operative plan. Occasionally split-skin grafts or composite grafts of ear cartilage and skin may be needed. The septal incision can be extended into an intercartilaginous incision, through which the skin can be separated from the bony and cartilaginous framework. A direct approach can be made through the nasal skin by midline incisions through the columella, dorsum of the nose, glabella, alar base and lateral nose. We frequently use the dorsal nasal incision for fixation of bone grafts and the columella incision

for reconstruction of the cartilaginous nasal framework. The vestibular incisions are very useful to completely free the scarred soft tissues from the piriform aperture; this is necessary when a columella strut is being used to obtain nasal projection. Once the airway is restored and the septum centralized by septal resection or septoplasty, the bony skeleton is osteotomized to reduce any displacement, and the nasal cartilages are repositioned and reshaped to produce a new centralized and symmetrical appearance (Fig. 21.37).

Osteotomies are made laterally at the base of the nasal pyramid and medially parasagittal to the midline. The superior attachment of the nasal bone can be osteotomized percutaneously with a tiny 2 mm osteotome or broken across by in-fracture or out-fracture. The lateral osteotomy is performed via a stab incision in the nasal vestibule laterally; the soft tissues are elevated from the frontal process of the maxilla with a Joseph elevator. The cut from the piriform aperture to the glabella is made with a saw and/or an osteotome; the thickening and distortion of previously fractured bones often make this manoeuvre difficult.

The paramedian osteotomies are performed with the saw and/or osteotome; the superior bridge of bone is cut with a small osteotome percutaneously or fractured by digital pressure. When the cuts have been made the nasal pyramid can be centralized. Any bony or cartilaginous excess is then rasped or trimmed away. The central position of the septum is maintained with two Silastic® sheet splints, fixed with two sutures through the septum to produce a sandwich effect. The internal support of the nasal pyramid is provided by packing and the external moulding by a plaster of Paris splint (Fig. 21.37).

Correction of depression

The treatment will differ according to the degree and the site of the depression. Depression of the bony dorsum demands bone grafting. Depression of the lower cartilaginous part of the nose may also benefit from bone or cartilage grafting but other procedures can be used.

In principle, three strategies are available for repair of the lower cartilaginous part.

1. The bony pseudo-hump may be removed from above the dorsal depression, thus flattening and smoothing the profile. It is often also necessary to perform an osteotomy of the nasal pyramid to narrow it.
2. Small cartilage grafts taken from the septum, ear or costal cartilage can be used to build up the lower depression as well as to augment a recessed columella and deficient alar cartilages.
3. After flattening the bony dorsum with a rasp a very fine split-rib and costochondral-junction graft can be fashioned, the graft being fixed above to the nasal bone with a single screw for rigidity.

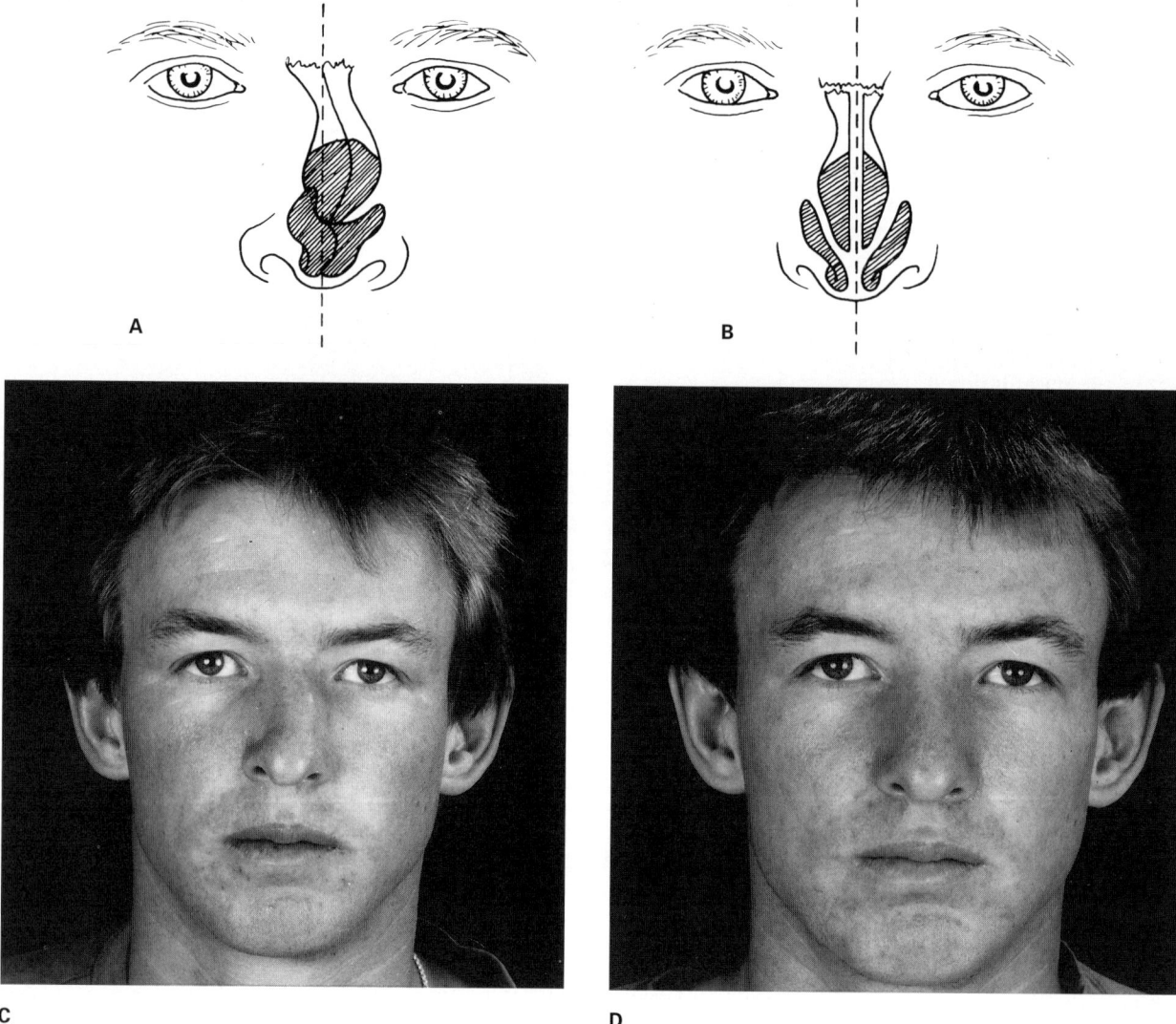

Fig. 21.37 Post-traumatic nasal deformity. A Diagrammatic representation of the nasoseptal deformity. **B** The desired correction.
C Appearance of the post-traumatic deformity. **D** Appearance 6 months after correction.

The principles for correction of total depression of the nasal body are well described by Tessier (1991). He stated that this reconstruction should always be done with bone, and that the bone must be fixed in the right environment, namely bone-to-bone surface. This dictum has been given scientific substance by Phillips & Rahn (1988, 1990). The nasal mucosa must be intact.

Bone grafting in the nasal region may be carried out through a variety of incisions, each with its merits:

1. An intercartilaginous incision is suitable for smaller distal deformities and does not facilitate rigid fixation of the grafts; it may need to be combined with a dorsal puncture or incision, to allow insertion of screws for fixation.
2. A vertical columella incision gives access to the alar domes and one can insert grafts of costal cartilage, septum or ear to augment the recessed columella.
3. An open rhinoplasty incision gives wide access to the lower cartilages as well as the bony dorsum.
4. An oral vestibular approach helps to free the piriform aperture.
5. A midline incision on the nasal dorsum: in our practice, this is the most common route by which bone grafts are inserted and fixed with screws. Pre-existing scars on the nasal dorsum may be used as access incisions. The bicoronal flap when used for other purposes provides good access.

To reconstruct the depressed nasal dorsum we agree with Tessier (1991), Merville et al (1983) and others in preferring to use autogenous onlay bone grafts taken at the time of operation. Iliac crest is preferred by Tessier, calvarial bone graft by Gruss et al (1985). Our preference is for rib and cartilage taken at the costochondral junction. Through the dorsal midline incision, together with a

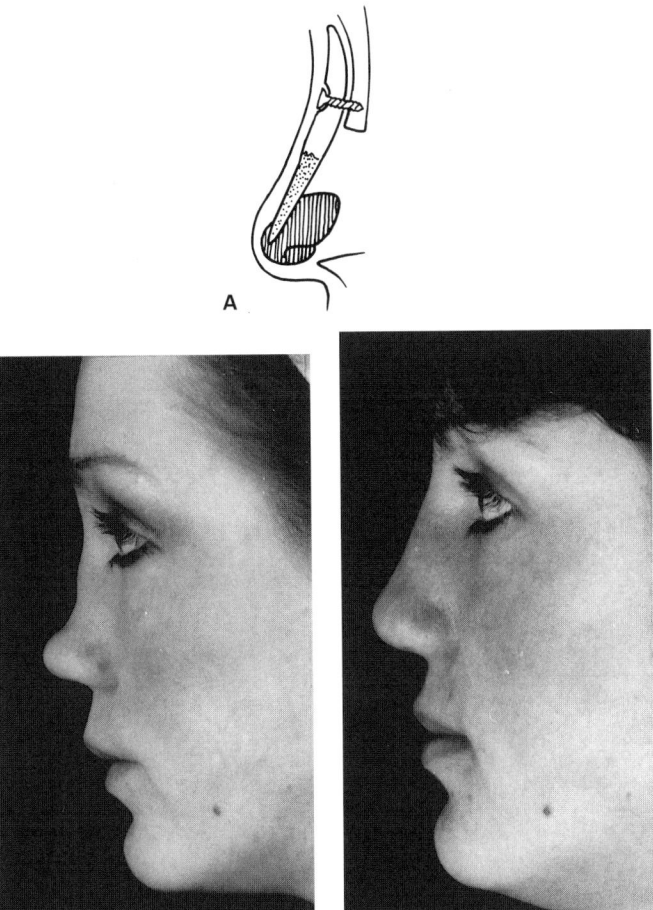

Fig. 21.38 Nasal bone grafts. A Diagrammatic representation of the bone graft overlying the freshly rasped nasal bones as far as possible. This is fixed with a countersunk screw or, if required for stability, two screws. B A typically depressed nasal septum. C Appearance after bone grafting.

columella incision if necessary, the nasal bones are freshened and the graft is fashioned so that the rib bone overlies the nasal bone and the shaped cartilage lies at the nasal tip. The graft is secured with one or two countersunk titanium screws (David & Moore 1989), giving rigid fixation and allowing bone-to-bone union, while the cartilaginous component of the graft overlies the cartilaginous area of the nose (Figs 21.38 and 21.39).

Tessier and Merville both use transnasal wire to fix a shaped iliac bone graft, which is usually slotted into the glabellar region (Fig. 21.40). When the bicoronal scalp flap is used, or if an extended glabella incision has been employed, a titanium plate and screws can fix the graft and give the appropriate projection. An L-shaped graft may be preferred (Fig. 21.41), with a columella strut placed via the buccal sulcus incision or through a columella incision to help with projection of the nasal tip and to give bulk to a recessed columella. Since the advent of miniplate and screw fixation in the glabella region we do not use this technique.

Complications and results

Minor post-traumatic nasal deformities are common, and can be corrected by relatively simple surgical techniques. Rhinoplasty for localized post-traumatic nasal deformities is generally a satisfactory procedure. In a personal series of 185 consecutive rhinoplasties for post-traumatic nasal deformities of all types, early complications were listed in only 4.9%; these were chiefly secondary haemorrhage and persistent blockage of the nasal airway. Of those patients who required a nasal bone graft, it was necessary to remove the screw in some 10%; in 2.8% removal of the bone graft was necessary.

COMPLEX NASO-ORBITO-ETHMOID DEFORMITIES

Management

Correction of an established deformity is often very difficult. Once again, an early operation provides the best opportunity for repair (p. 311). Fundamental to the correction is restoration of the bony contour of the region. As has been pointed out by Gruss (1992), in most cases the canthal ligament is attached to a large fragment of bone. In these cases, restoration of the bony contour involves osteotomy, repositioning of the bone, fixation with miniplates or microplates, possibly bone grafting of the dorsum of the nose and reconstruction of the medial orbital wall where this is either protruding into the orbit or is absent (Fig. 21.42). The dorsum of the nose often needs bone grafting; this can be done with the costochondral graft described below, screwed into the underlying residual nasal bone or attached by an angulated plate to the frontal bone. Where it has been judged that there is too much scarring and the skin over the dorsum of the nose is tight, we have preceded this manoeuvre by inserting a small wedge-shaped tissue expander of 1–2 cc capacity which is blown up slowly over the next month. This has given very satisfactory results (Fig. 21.43).

Where there is an infected mucocele caused by obstruction of the nasolacrimal drainage it is important to clear up any infection beforehand. Having done this, it is probably best to proceed with the correction of any epicanthic folds which can be done by the Converse technique (Converse et al 1977) or the Mustardé 'jumping man' technique (Mustardé 1959). When these techniques are employed in post-traumatic cases, they are invariably associated with a canthopexy; if this cannot be achieved by repositioning the bone, then transnasal insertion of the canthus into the bone will be necessary. At the same time, all residual scar tissue around the medial canthus should be removed. It may be necessary to pass the canthal tendon into or through a bone graft and fix it to the other side of the nose (p. 312). Complete periorbital

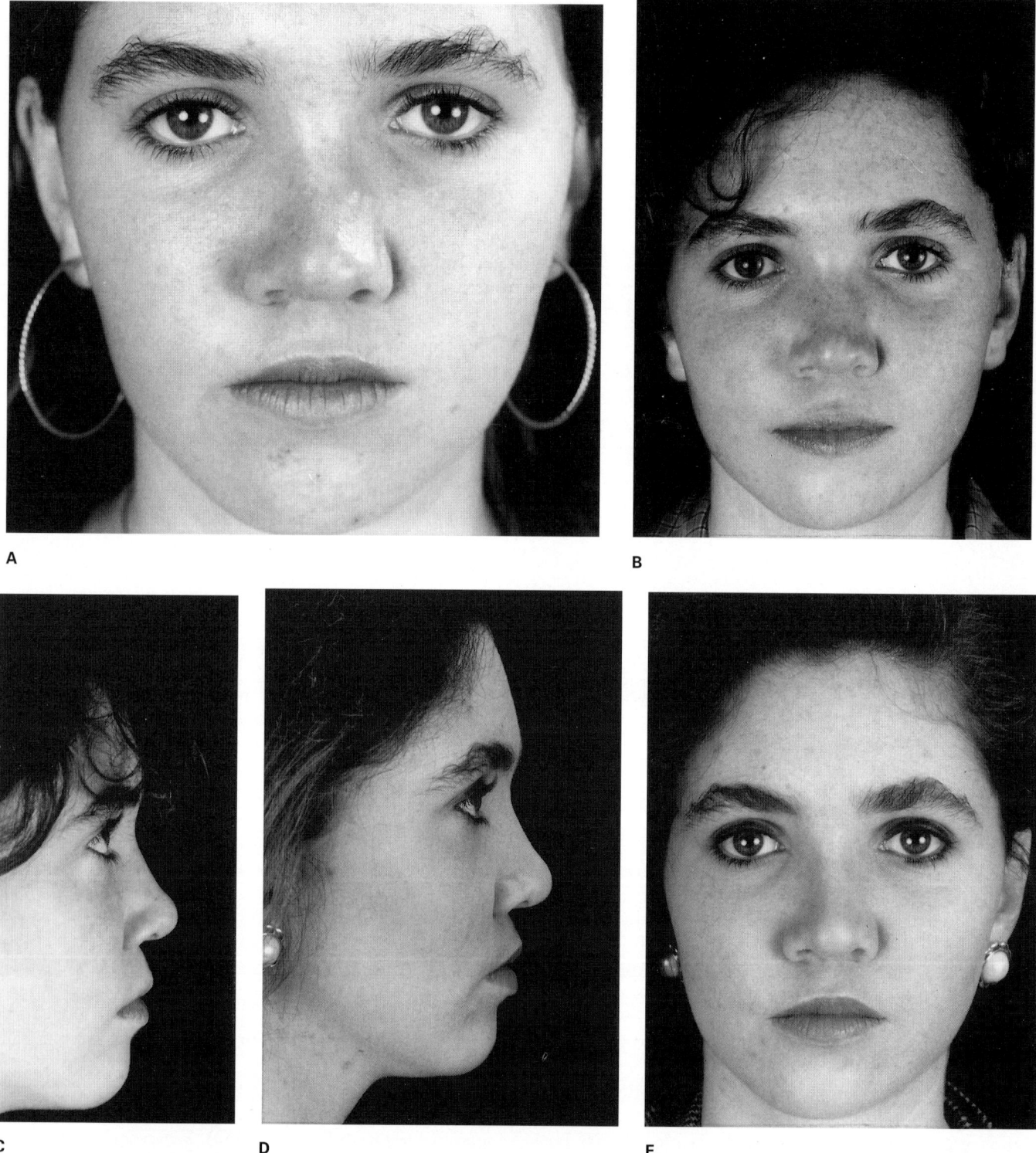

Fig. 21.39 Post-traumatic nasal deformity. A teenage girl sustained a severe nasoseptal crush earlier in life with nasal deviation and blockage. **A** Initial presentation with a flattened, aesthetically unacceptable nose and blocked nasal airway. **B** Appearance following septorhinoplasty which has produced a narrower nasal pyramid, some projection of the pyramid, and a clear airway. **C** Postoperative lateral view. **D** Profile view after the next stage, in which a very fine costochondral graft was placed onto the dorsum of the nose as described. **E** Final appearance, with the small midline incision hardly visible.

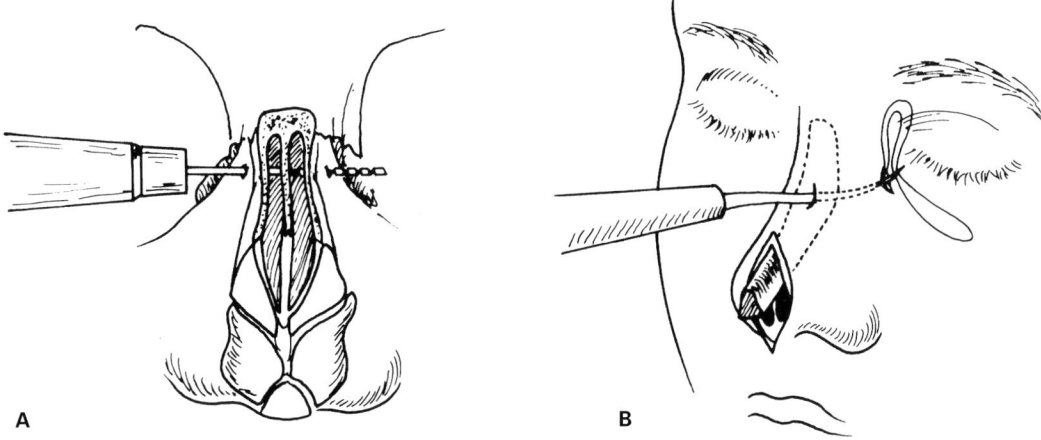

Fig. 21.40 Bone grafting the dorsum of the nose. This technique is described by Tessier (1991). **A** Burrholes are placed in the frontal process of the maxilla. The bone graft, fashioned to produce a natural looking hump, is secured with a wire passed through the burrholes. **B** The graft is seated on freshened dorsal bone of the nose. The alar domes may be sutured over the bone graft.

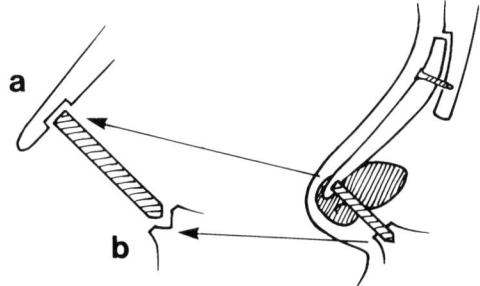

Fig. 21.41 Nasal columella support. If the surgeon contemplates the need for a columella support, it is formed from cortical bone which may be embedded in a small groove (a) at the lower end of the graft. The base of the supporting strut is firmly embedded in a hole (b) prepared at the level of the anterior nasal spine. The screw fixation technique has obviated the need for this more cumbersome and less rigid form of reconstruction.

stripping is necessary to achieve movement of the medial canthus in post-traumatic cases.

Operative correction

The preferred approach for secondary deformity is a one-stage procedure in which osteotomies, bone grafting, rigid fixation, canthopexy and dacrocystorhinostomy are performed in a single operation. Surgical exposure may be via existing scars or through a glabella incision, vertical or horizontal, together with lower eyelid incisions. However, these are now almost invariably supplanted by the bicoronal scalp flap.

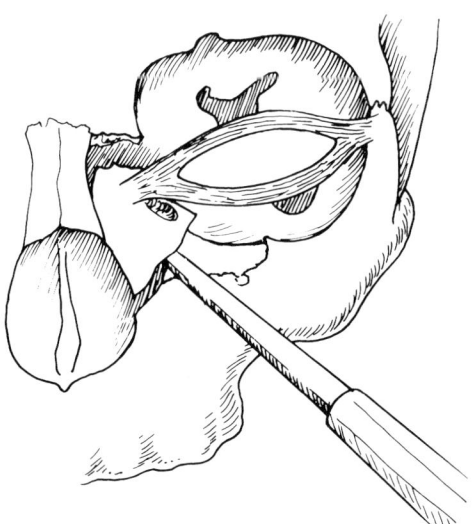

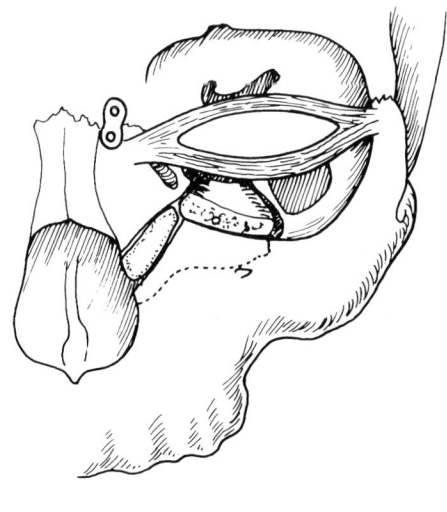

Fig. 21.42 Displacement of the medial canthal ligament. When the medial canthus is distorted and the canthal ligament is attached to a displaced bony fragment, it may be possible secondarily to identify the fragment and perform a repositioning osteotomy. After repositioning, the fragment is best stabilized with a mini- or microplate, and any resulting defects bone grafted.

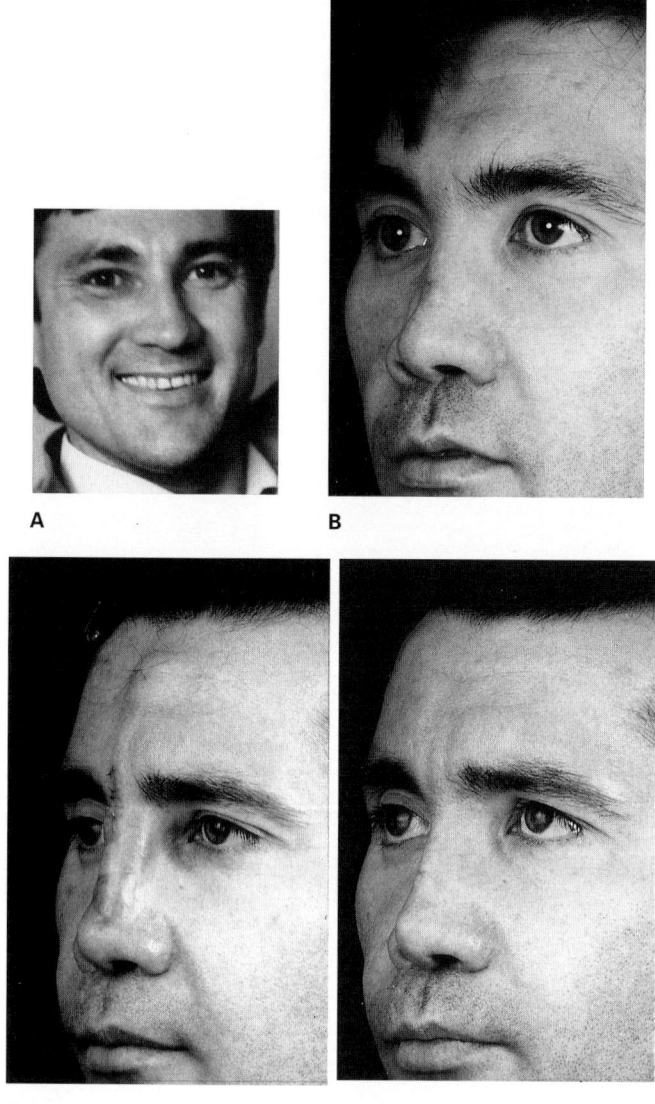

Fig. 21.43 Tissue expansion prior to nasal bone grafting.
A Patient seen before his massive naso-orbital-ethmoid fracture.
B Postoperative appearance. He complained of a change in nasal shape. **C** Due to the tight skin and scarred dorsum, a small tissue expander has been placed under the nasal skin and gently expanded over a month. **D** Replacement with a costochondral graft fixed at the glabella.

It is often wise to inject the nasolacrimal drainage apparatus with methylene blue. The medial orbital walls are dissected, the orbital floor is dissected in its medial part, the canthal ligament is identified where possible, and if attached to an identifiable fragment of bone, it is osteotomized. Those who have experienced this form of surgery know how tedious it is and how unrewarding the dissection of the scar and fragmented bone can be. The reconstruction proceeds from the posterior aspect forwards, the medial orbital wall being repaired with bone grafts first, and the dacrocystorhinostomy is performed

before the medial canthus is attached (Fig. 21.44). If the canthus is not attached to a fragment or fragments of bone which can be plated back into place, then the canthus itself is plicated with wire, which is then passed well posterior to the lacrimal groove or its supposed position, to anchor the canthus. In the past, the wires have been used to assist in the fixation of the dorsal bone graft; however this has been supplanted by screw fixation. It is often necessary to correct a downward displacement of the medial canthus, particularly in long-standing cases, and this may be corrected by repositioning a bony fragment. Often a Z-plasty of the soft tissue is required (Fig. 21.45).

Complications and results

It is our experience that satisfactory results in these complex deformities are rarely achieved in the ideal of a single corrective procedure. Complications include:

- canthal drift, giving a wide flattened appearance between the eyes
- prominent wires and screws
- persistent infections resulting chiefly from blockage of the nasolacrimal drainage system.

MASSIVE ABLATIVE DEFORMITY OF THE NOSE

Management

Massive deformity of the nose involves significant loss of cover, support and lining. Techniques to achieve reconstruction under these circumstances are as old as plastic surgery itself, nasal reconstruction using the forehead flap being first mentioned in the Sanskrit writings of Susruta, thought to be no later than 600 BC and very possibly earlier (p. 8). Ever since, the forehead has been the most common source of skin cover; an excellent historical review of the development of techniques of nasal reconstruction of the forehead has been made by Adamson (1988). Gillies' 'up and down' flap was further developed by Converse (1942) as a scalping flap (p. 453). Since Tagliacozzi's brilliant use of the arm in the sixteenth century (p. 12), other sources of skin have been used. Distant flaps have been advocated by Washio (1972), bringing postauricular skin onto the nose. Free flaps have been used, vascularized by microsurgical techniques, nice results being produced at the 9th People's Hospital in Shanghai with radial forearm flaps (T. S. Chang, personal communication, 1986). Nevertheless, forehead skin remains the best substitute for nasal skin replacement as it is adjacent, of good colour and good texture though often of limited area (Fig. 17.18). The use of tissue expanders in the forehead as part of total nasal reconstruction has been advocated by Adamson (1988) and is now widely accepted.

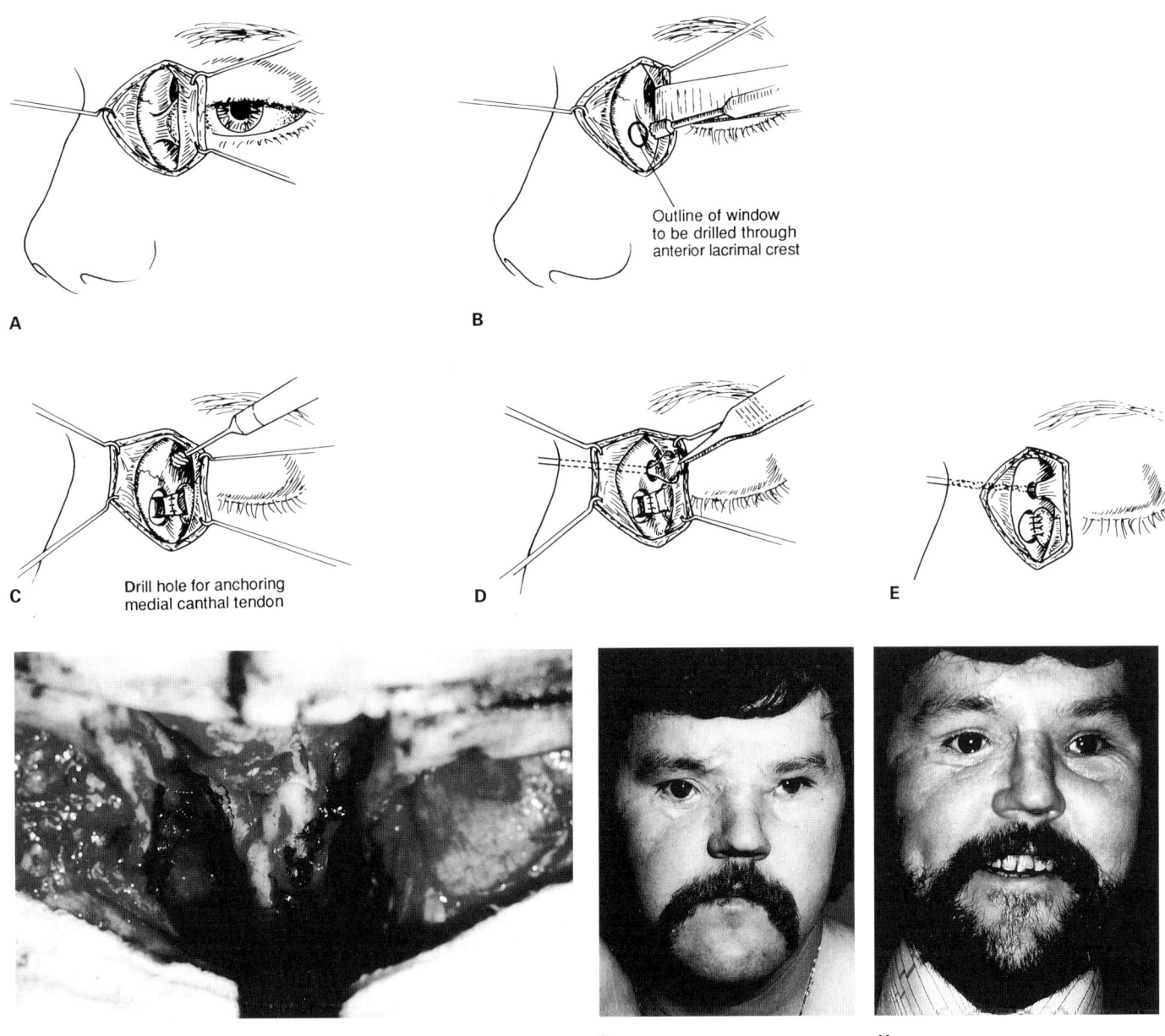

Fig. 21.44 Combined dacrocystorhinostomy and medial canthopexy (after McCarthy et al 1990a). **A** Medial canthal incision. Alternatively, access can be gained from a bicoronal scalp flap. **B** Window to be drilled through the area of the anterior lacrimal crest, which may be significantly distorted. **C** When possible, the sac lining is sutured to nasal lining and a drill hole for anchoring the medial canthal tendon is performed above. This is done usually transnasally. **D** Medial canthal ligament fixed into a burrhole in the bone by wire passed across the other side. **E** Reattached canthus after the completed procedure. **F** Bicoronal view indicating the exposure for bone grafting the medial orbital wall and dorsum of the nose, canthopexy, and dacrocystorhinostomy. It is important that the operative sequence proceeds from the back forwards: reconstruction of the medial orbital walls and orbital floors completed, canthopexy started, repair of the lacrimal passages completed, canthopexy completed, dorsal nasal bone grafting completed, and skin closure with appropriate Z-plasties or W-plasties. **G** Patient with a gross naso-orbital-ethmoid fracture. Approached by the bicoronal scalp flap, the medial orbital walls and dorsum of the nose were grafted and medial canthopexies and dacrocystorhinostomy were performed on the left side. **H** Appearance 1 year after surgery.

Tissue expansion

This has been with us since the beginning of the human species, in the form of the expansion that results from pregnancy. The phenomenon is also seen when skin, nerves and muscles and even bone expand over an under-lying haematoma or a slowly growing tumour. Neumann (1957) first used artificial expansion to facilitate a surgical reconstruction; more recently Radovan (1982, 1984) introduced surgical expansion for a wide range of recon-structive purposes. The technique enables tissue adjacent

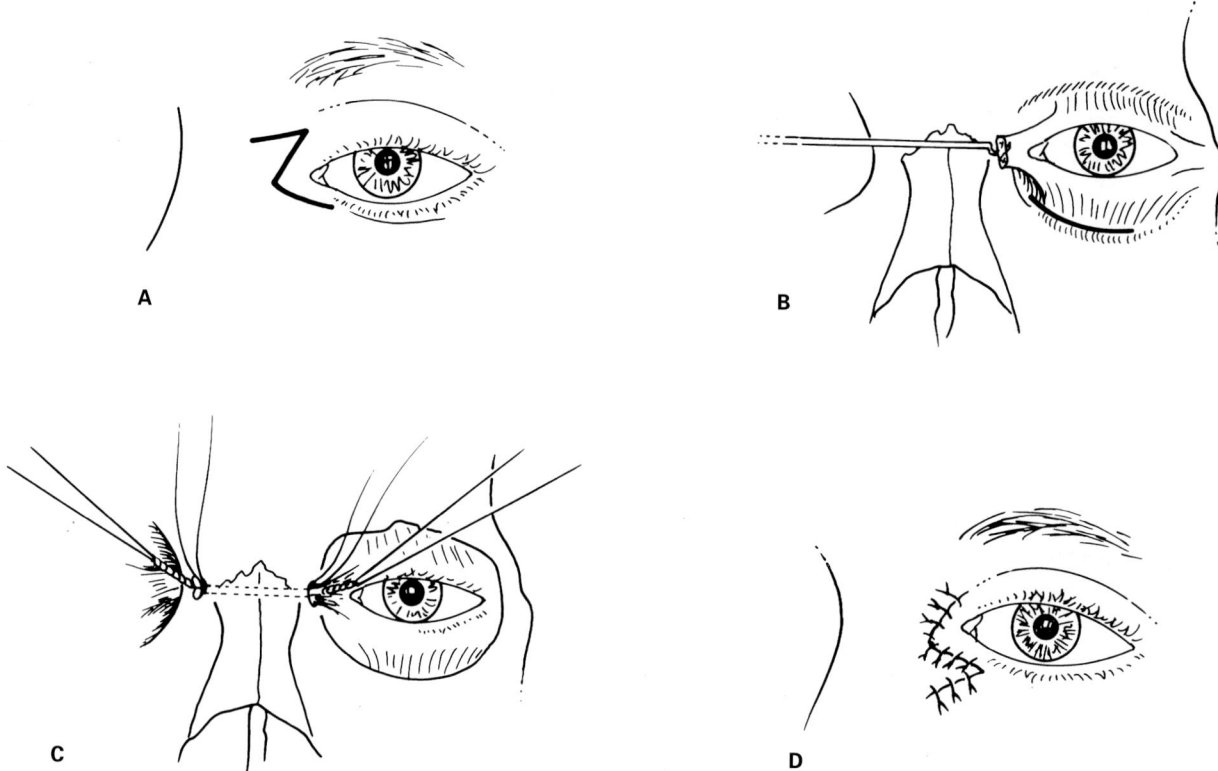

Fig. 21.45 Medial canthus repositioning with Z-plasty. Z-plasty in the medial canthus for correction of canthal dystopia. The medial canthus is reattached into the bone and through to a toggle on the other side, thus creating an inferior defect which is filled from the flap above. **A** Design of the incision. **B** Repositioning of the canthus. **C** Medial canthus attached to the toggle on the opposite side, but well inserted into the bone. **D** Completion of the procedure with closure of the Z incision.

to a defect to be expanded, thus providing donor tissue of similar colour, texture and sensation with minimal scar formation. A temporary expander, capable of being filled with fluid by injection through a valve system, creates a pressure which exerts force on the overlying tissue; this gradually expands, providing the additional tissue for reconstruction. In replacing traumatic defects in the craniomaxillofacial (CMF) area, this technique may be used to expand scalp, face and neck tissue or tissue around the ear for secondary auricular reconstruction. Tissue expansion may also be used for the preforming and pre-expanding of a distant flap prior to its transfer by microvascular techniques to the head and neck region (Homma et al 1993).

Tissue expanders are now produced in a wide variety of sizes and shapes. The first stage is the insertion of the expander. Radovan in his earlier articles indicated that the base of the expander should be of similar diameter to the defect which is to be closed. A smaller pocket is developed for the reservoir dome. Initially, a small amount of normal saline is injected into the expander through the connecting tube — approximately 10–15% of the capacity can be introduced. Further injections are generally commenced after 10 days; each is monitored by watching for blanching of the skin and by the pain tolerance of the patient (Marks et al 1987). When the tissue has

been completely expanded, and after allowing ~14 days between the last expansion and the planned time of operation to consolidate the effects of the expansion, the expander is removed and the tissue is transferred to close the defect.

Haematoma, infection and tissue necrosis are the chief complications (Austad 1987, Steenfos et al 1993). Insertion of a suction drain into the cavity will help to avoid these problems. If infection develops, it normally spells the end of that phase of the expansion, which may have to be abandoned. Necrosis is a rare occurrence; monitoring the expansion and deflating the expander if there appears to be a threat of ischaemia will usually prevent or control this complication.

Nasal lining

There are many techniques for providing nasal lining. They include inversion of the forehead flap to produce the nostrils and columella, lining the inner surface of the forehead flap with medium-thickness split skin, turning down local flaps of residual nasal skin, and the use of local flaps from the face, such as nasolabial tissue in patients where this is abundant. In total nasal reconstruction, it is essential to have good cover and good lining, and the skeleton must be reconstituted to provide good support:

expanded forehead skin and free flaps will contract mightily if not draped over an adequate skeleton. With the use of plates and screws, the cantilever costochondral graft secured to the glabella region has proved in our hands to be an excellent method of securing skeletal support.

In post-traumatic cases, complete nasal reconstruction requires multiple interventions over a long period of time. There are often difficult scars in the region which make tissue expansion more hazardous, and may indeed necessitate a free flap reconstruction, which itself is often made difficult by damaged recipient vessels. Therefore there is need for precise preoperative planning.

Timing of reconstruction

When the patient has been managed by the CMF team since the time of injury, it may be difficult to decide when to do the definitive nasal reconstruction. Initially, the patient's life must be preserved and the principles of acute care of a massive avulsive injury are set out in Chapter 16. Nasal reconstruction is best performed on a face that has been otherwise fully reconstructed: the procedure is therefore done towards the end of a reconstructive programme. In our practice, the decision is usually easier, because the vast majority of patients present late, with well-established problems for secondary correction — unhappily often after many earlier attempts at reconstruction.

Operative correction: rhinoplasty

The preferred technique of rhinoplasty is a staged sequence of procedures, using forehead skin with tissue expansion of this region where necessary and where wound patterns permit.

In the first stage, the forehead skin is expanded by inserting a 200–300 cc rectangular expander in the forehead under the galea via a bicoronal approach where the scar is sited well behind the hairline to ensure that the suture line is not compromised by tension generated by the expander. The valve of the expander is placed over the temporoparietal region. Haematoma formation around the expander is reduced by a suction drain left for 48 h postoperatively, and generally brought out on the side opposite to the valve. After 3 weeks, expansion is begun and continued over the next 2–3 weeks until enough expanded skin is obtained. Necrosis and exposure of the expander are avoided by careful siting of the scar and by great care in expanding the prosthesis, using pain and skin blanching as indications of the limit of saline injection. Superior results are obtained if there is a further delay of 2–4 weeks after full expansion.

Nasal reconstruction can now be planned 'in reverse'. The nasal lining is often fashioned from a residual nasal skin flap based on the margins of the defect and turned over so that the raw surface is exposed. The forehead skin flap is planned to be based on one or other of the supratrochlear vascular pedicles.

In the next stage, the forehead flap is raised. The skin is cut with a knife and the capsule that forms around the expander is incised with cutting diathermy to avoid rupture of the expander. The expander is then removed and the flap is cut so that it can be rotated downwards to cover the nose on one or other of the supratrochlear vascular pedicles. The fibrous capsule that has formed around the tissue expander is carefully dissected away to provide a thinner flap and to mobilize the rest of the scalp for straight-line closure.

The next stage involves fashioning of the nasal lining. Our preference is to use local nasal remnants where possible. The distal flap turnover techniques, in which the distal end of the flap is turned in to form the nasal lining, nostril margins and columella, work quite well. Skeletal support is usually a costochondral graft, two-thirds bone, one-third cartilage, screwed into the glabella with one or two titanium screws sunk into the bone. Where there is not enough residual bone to give the right angle of the cantilever, an angled titanium plate can be used with the plate bent to give the right projection. The flap is then set in over the graft and the nostrils are held patent by shortened Silastic® 'trumpet' nasal airway tubes. After a few weeks these can be replaced by Silastic® nasal splints used for cleft palate nasal reconstruction. The forehead defect is closed by direct suture; if necessary a small split-skin graft can be used to cover any raw area at the glabella where the base of the flap may be exposed.

There is always a third stage, and possibly more stages, necessary for division of the forehead pedicle, thinning of the flap, possible re-augmentation of the skeleton and re-establishing an adequate nasal airway. The third stage is best left at least 3 months after the reconstruction and ideally for much longer if possible.

Complications and results

Complications of rhinoplasty include skin necrosis and recurrent deformity. To minimize the risks of skin necrosis as a complication of tissue expansion we choose the subgaleal plane and thin the flap later, though Adamson (1988) reports superior results by subcutaneous dissection. During the expansion process care must be taken to avoid haematoma formation, which is generally disastrous. If skin breakdown and expander exposure are threatened one may retrieve the situation by slowing the rate of expansion without abandoning the procedure.

The cartilaginous tip of the graft may produce necrosis of the overlying nasal skin. This should not cause alarm as the necrosed skin can be excised and the underlying cartilage pared down to a suitable size.

Recurrent deformity may result from shrinkage or collapse of the reconstructed nose. To prevent this, skeletal

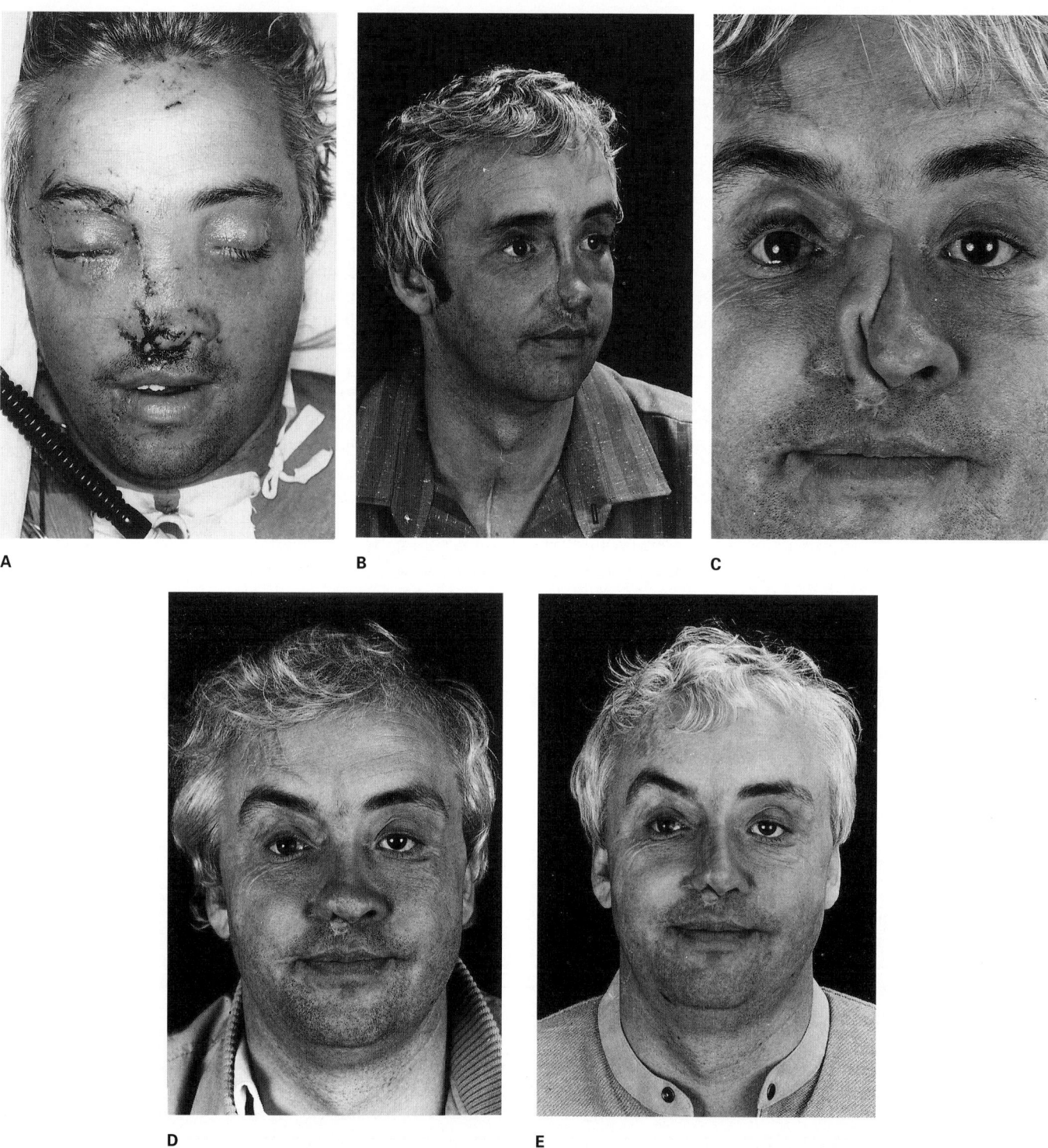

Fig. 21.46 Nasal reconstruction. A 45-year-old male was involved in a motor vehicle accident in which he sustained multiple limb fractures and extensive fractures of the middle third of the face involving loss of nasal tissue and compound comminuted naso-ethmoid fracture. The soft-tissue loss included almost two-thirds of the right ala and part of the cartilage and skin of the right side of the nose with a laceration extending up to the medial canthal region. A series of operations were planned using a forehead flap based on the glabellar region, which was rotated down to provide extra tissue, turned over to provide an alar rim, and divided at a second stage. The local tissue was refashioned and ultimately the dorsum of the nose was expanded with a small tissue expander. A costochondral graft was fixed to the glabellar region with a single 9 mm titanium screw. **A** Initial appearance. Tracheostomy has been placed and the avulsion injury of the right side of the nose has been closed primarily. **B** Appearance following fixation of his facial fractures. The residual nasal deformity is evident. **C** Forehead flap rotated down to add soft tissue to the nose. **D** Penultimate stage in which the right ala has been refashioned and the nasal dorsal skin replaced in part. **E** After tissue expansion of the dorsal skin with a small cylindrical expander, a costochondral graft gives greater nasal projection.

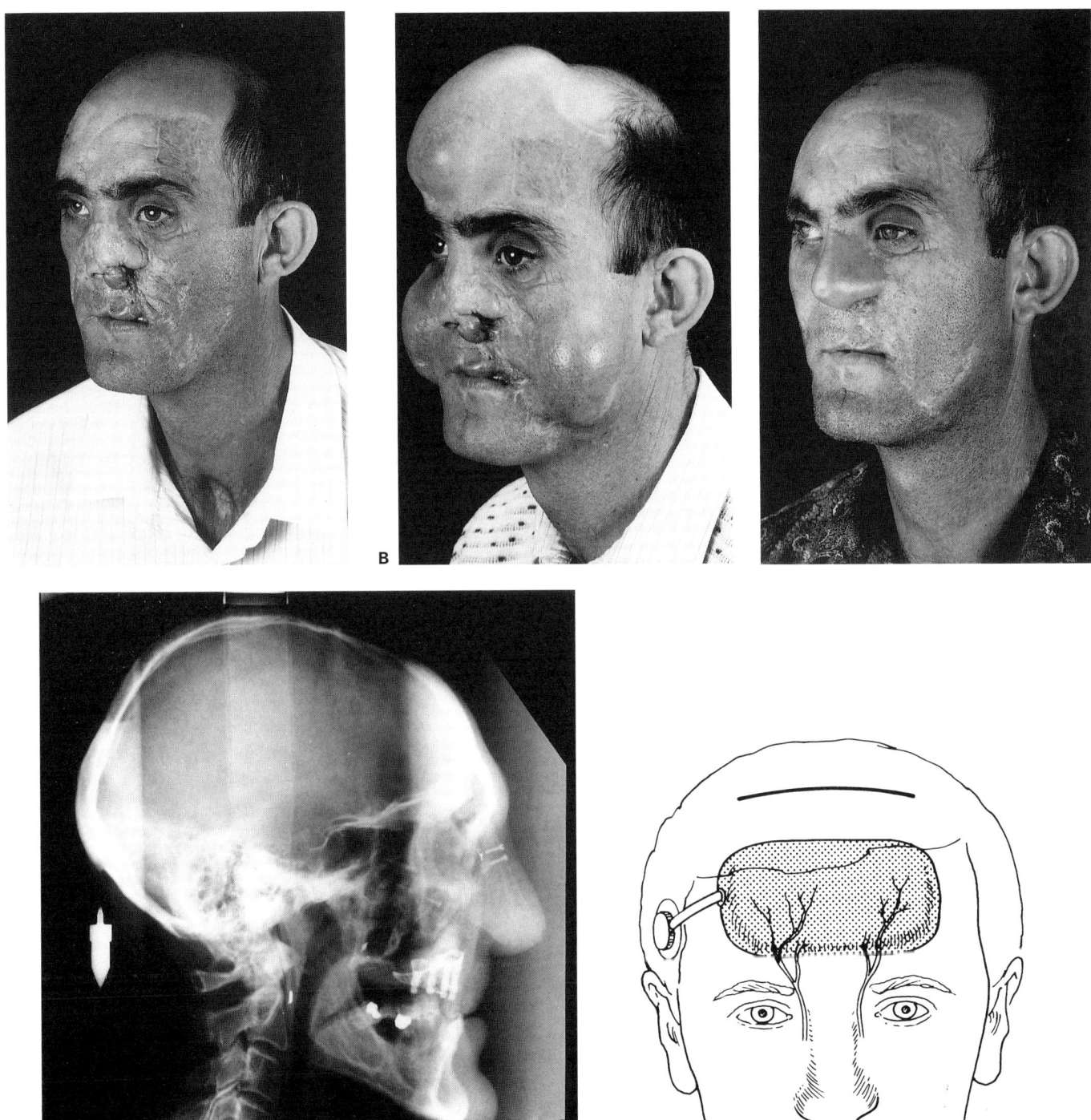

Fig. 21.47 Nasal reconstruction. A young civilian male involved in a rocket attack in Beirut suffered a massive injury to the middle third of the face. While the reconstruction of the nose should not be seen in isolation from the rest of his deformities, it is illustrative of the use of tissue expansion, as there had been at least ten previous attempts to reconstruct his nose. A large tissue expander was placed into the forehead, with the port placed well into the parietal region, and the expansion was continued over 2 months. The whole nose was replaced as a cosmetic unit using the residual nasal skin for lining. The subsequent nostril patency was maintained by a pair of Silastic trumpet splints for 2 weeks postoperatively; then these were replaced by the smaller splints typically used for rhinoplasty associated with cleft lip repair. **A** Initial presentation. **B** Three tissue expanders have been placed to move undamaged skin medially from both cheeks and inferiorly from the forehead for nasal reconstruction. **C** Appearance following nasal reconstruction and simultaneous costochondral cantilever bone grafting. **D** Lateral radiograph demonstrating the nasal reconstruction as well as the subsequent ÇAD/CAM produced osseo-integrated implant in the deficient maxilla. **E** Position of a forehead tissue expander used for nasal reconstruction. The injection port can be placed in the parietal region, and the incision for insertion of the expander is kept sufficiently far away from the edge of the expander and behind the hairline if possible. Care must be taken to preserve the arterial supply to the expanded skin.

reconstruction is mandatory as the flaps, whether expanded or free, will shrivel if there is no underlying skeleton. Rigid fixation is necessary and bone grafting may need to be repeated to get the required nasal projection. Nostril contraction is a considerable problem requiring secondary surgery; this complication is best obviated by the use of nasal splints for up to 6 months (Figs 21.46–21.48).

Despite this intimidating list of possible complications, restorative rhinoplasty is in general a satisfactory procedure. Aesthetic perfection cannot be promised, but the result should be a great improvement on the appearance of a mutilated nose.

MAXILLARY AND MANDIBULAR DEFORMITIES

Principles of management

The established post-traumatic deformity may be due to malposition of bone, loss of bone or soft tissue, loss of specialized structures such as teeth, or these in any combination. The result is a loss of form, function and aesthetic appearance.

The aim of aesthetic reconstruction is of necessity measured against the pretraumatic appearance of the patient and this is often impossible to restore (p. 83). The functions of speech, swallowing, mastication, and respiration may be compromised in a way that makes comfortable living very difficult. The complex anatomy of the region, interwoven with vital functions, and the need for aesthetic acceptability make secondary surgical correction of deformity in this part of the craniofacial skeleton very challenging, and nowhere are the needs for precise planning more evident.

Initial failure to achieve a correct functional and cosmetic restoration of the dentofacial complex can be caused by at least three factors:

1. The severity of the initial injury may necessitate prolonged maintenance of life support systems, and healing can occur before definitive surgical steps can be taken to restore normal form and function to the face. This is seen particularly in the maxilla and in young patients. Untreated displaced fractures of the jaws can be regarded as united at any time after 3 weeks from injury.
2. Accidents often occur in remote areas so that early treatment is not carried out in units that have the necessary expertise in the different specialty areas to provide the optimum result. Often the appropriate diagnostic radiographs are not easily available and so the extent and severity of facial injuries is not correctly assessed.
3. Finally, poor initial management can result from incorrect assessment of the extent of injury, or failure to reduce and fix bone fragments adequately.

Hopefully, we believe that the integrated multi-disciplinary approach to initial CMF injury management is today minimizing the frequency and severity of secondary deformity. Improved fixation methods reduce the number of patients requiring secondary facial correction: the use of miniplates rather than interosseous wires gives very accurate union of fractured facial bones. Again hopefully, the number of secondary deformities resulting from delayed or incorrect management should become less as better retrieval systems are in place to serve remote areas and as the primary treatment of trauma by general surgeons and general medical practitioners is improved. But it is important to understand that with almost all severe injuries, some residual disabilities will result. This must be accepted. Failure to recognize and to accept some reduction in the cosmetic and functional result may lead to repeated wasteful and futile surgical interventions and other treatments.

While one of the most important aspects of reconstruction of the middle and lower face is occlusion of the teeth, the more complex comminuted fracture may produce noticeable aesthetic changes even after malocclusions have been corrected.

MAXILLARY DEFORMITIES

Surgical pathology

The most common deformity caused by a comminuted fracture of the upper jaw is flattening of the profile and shortening of the vertical dimension. There is often associated perialar flattening, widening of the alar base of the nose and flattening of the nasal bridge. The result is a significant change from the premorbid appearance which is most distressing to the patient (Fig. 21.49). Less common is the elongated face where the disconnected maxilla has been distracted downwards and fixed in a low position, seen occasionally when craniomandibular fixation has been misused. Asymmetrical deformities result from twisting of the maxillary segment as a whole or splitting of the palate with malposition of other segmental fractures.

Clinical assessment

The victim of an accident often has difficulty in adjusting to an altered appearance and frequently complains of feeling and looking like a different person. Malocclusion is a common symptom. This may be severe and obvious, expressing a wide fracture displacement. In other cases the changes may be subtle and limited to the dentoalveolar complex; malocclusion may result from loss of teeth and alveolar bone or from changes produced by prolonged application of interdental and intermaxillary fixation. One of the main difficulties is to determine what the occlusion was prior to the injury, and old dental records may be very helpful.

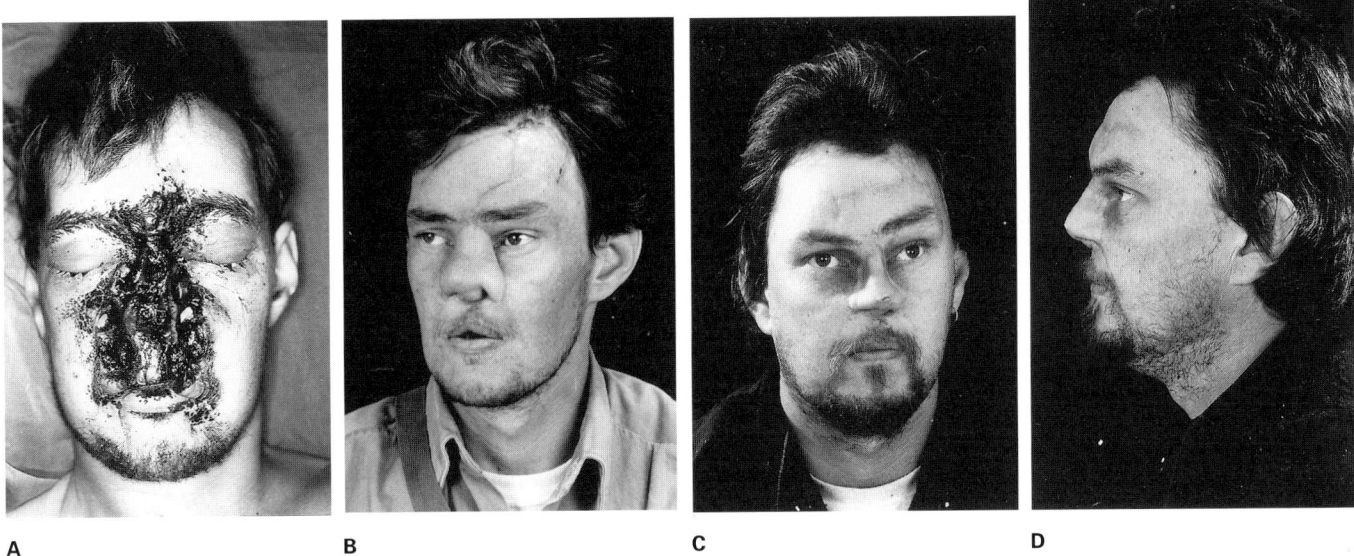

Fig. 21.48 Total loss of the nose and part of upper lip from a gunshot wound. The nasal soft tissue has been replaced by a forehead flap and the distal end has been turned over to make the columella and nostril margin. Subsequently this complex needed to be radically thinned and supported with further bone grafting. This was secured at the glabella region with a four-hole titanium plate, with two screws into both the nasal bone graft and the frontal bone. **A** Initial presentation, with total absence of the nose and centre part of the upper lip. **B** Appearance after initial fashioning of the nasal soft tissue. **C & D** Appearance after subsequent thinning and bone grafting.

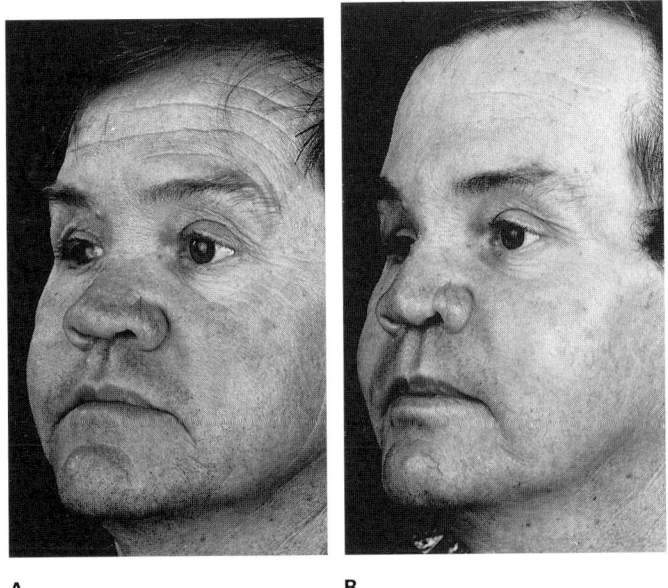

Fig. 21.49 Post-traumatic changes in nasal anatomy. A A patient suffered a panfacial fracture in which most of the impact was taken on the middle third of the face. The midface is retrodisplaced and foreshortened, with widening of the alar base. **B** Appearance following advancement of the maxilla, replacement of the zygoma, and augmentation of his nose. The emphasis has been on elongation of the maxilla and autorotation of the mandible.

Radiological assessment

Complete radiological assessment is necessary before planning correction. This includes the views necessary for planning orthognathic surgery (p. 177), including an orthopantomogram and biplanar cephalometric X-ray analysis. The pattern of the fractures must be identified and CT scanning is indispensable in this. Fracture sites and the extent and nature of any previous surgical interventions must be assessed. 3D data obtained by CT can be used for diagnosis of the deformity and for surgical planning (Abbott et al 1990). These data establish the shape of the maxilla and its spatial position with respect to the adjacent bones, and define any absence of bone. Such data are also used in construction of a maxillary prosthesis when necessary, by the CAD/CAM technique (p. 637).

Dental assessment

Detailed assessment of the dentition is important, and includes testing for viability of the teeth. The condition of the periodontal tissues must be known and any necessary treatment of caries and other inflammatory conditions performed. Dental models are taken and mounted on an articulator to facilitate operative planning (Fig. 21.50).

Photographic assessment

This is an important record and is part of the routine work-up for any surgery on the face. Lateral, frontal, basal and occlusal views are taken. It is important, whenever possible, to have pretraumatic photographs of the patient. An understanding of the state to which the patient wishes

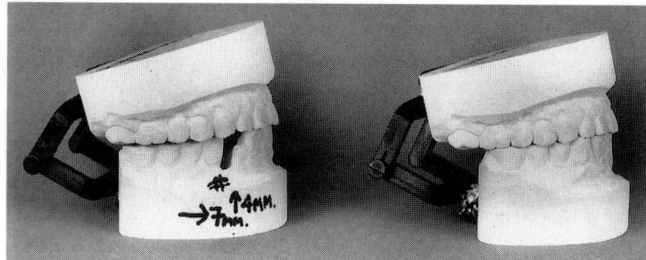

Fig. 21.50 Dental models mounted on disposable articulators.
The model on the left shows the traumatic occlusion, with written notes on the dental stone indicating the degree of displacement. The model on the right is produced by sectioning the lower model and re-establishing the occlusion. The interdental wafer is then produced from these prediction casts.

to be restored is of vital importance to the treating team; examination of old photographs is quite often startling and the change brought about by the trauma and subsequent treatment may be alarming to the surgeon as well as the patient. Photography also provides the basis for a discussion about what is possible in each case.

Speech assessment

Trauma affecting the jaws, teeth, oral and nasal cavities must of necessity affect speech and mastication. The possible effects of nasal obstruction and neurological deficit due to head injury must also be taken into account. Each patient should have a speech assessment to document the situation with respect to hypernasality, hyponasality, lateral escape, and tongue position during speech; any problems with mastication and swallowing must also be recorded before secondary surgical intervention. A full ENT examination documents the state of the maxillary antrum, nasal physiology and middle ear function; if necessary endoscopic examination of the maxillary antrum may be done.

Management

Treatment aims at restoration of function (occlusion, airway and sinus drainage) as well as restoring the displaced or deformed maxilla to its correct position in relation to the other facial bones.

Planning

The information gathered from the clinical examination and special investigations is discussed at a multidisciplinary planning meeting which usually includes the patient. Decisions are made as to whether surgical intervention is needed or not, and whether orthodontic or prosthodontic treatment is needed, or combinations of each of these, in order to re-establish the occlusion and facial form. Priorities are established and a treatment plan formulated.

The first step may be dental restoration and orthodontic alignment of teeth, followed later by further dental model analysis and X-ray analysis in preparation for surgical movement of bony segments.

Surgery performed on the dental model precedes the actual intervention and determines the desired position of the maxilla or its segments; this is recorded with an occlusal wafer. The desired vertical dimensions are established in the model surgery but must be related to possible problems with overlying scarred soft tissue. For example, when lengthening an impacted maxilla, one must be careful when the lips are very scarred as the soft tissue will not follow the bone readily under these circumstances, and an ideal maxillary reconstruction may expose too much tooth and gum. Compromises may be unavoidable.

At this stage the design of the fixation is determined (Fig. 21.51). The planning meeting also considers the possibility of secondary surgery, such as a second 'tidy up' operation after the initial major surgery with additional bone grafting or soft-tissue revision.

Correction of maxillary deformity

The pattern of osteotomy obviously depends on the pattern of the fracture and the nature of the deformity, and the surgical team should be prepared to do any manoeuvre necessary to restore the bony skeleton as nearly as possible to its original condition. To re-establish normal occlusion, surgical repositioning of the upper jaw may involve mobilizing the whole maxilla, or only one or more segments of the dental arch. The whole jaw may be moved at the Le Fort I, II or III levels, with lengthening, rarely shortening, rotation or other segmental movement according to the needs established in the planning.

The most common surgical manoeuvre is the Le Fort I osteotomy. While it has been, and to a certain extent remains, convenient to describe a midface osteotomy by reference to the fracture pattern described by Le Fort (p. 18), post-traumatic deformities rarely correspond exactly to his classical lines.

Before operations of this type, most patients are fitted with orthodontic bands. Just prior to surgery, arch bars are fabricated for the intermaxillary fixation needed at the time of the operation. Sometimes orthodontic treatment is not possible, either because of the nature of the injury or because of the unsuitability of the patient for orthodontic treatment on the grounds of age, state of dentition, or personality; in these cases, the operation has to be done using arch bars designed by the maxillofacial technician. These are then wired to the upper and lower teeth after induction of anaesthesia to provide intermaxillary fixation. An occlusal wafer manufactured according to the model planning and pretreatment surgical assessment determines the position of the maxilla in respect

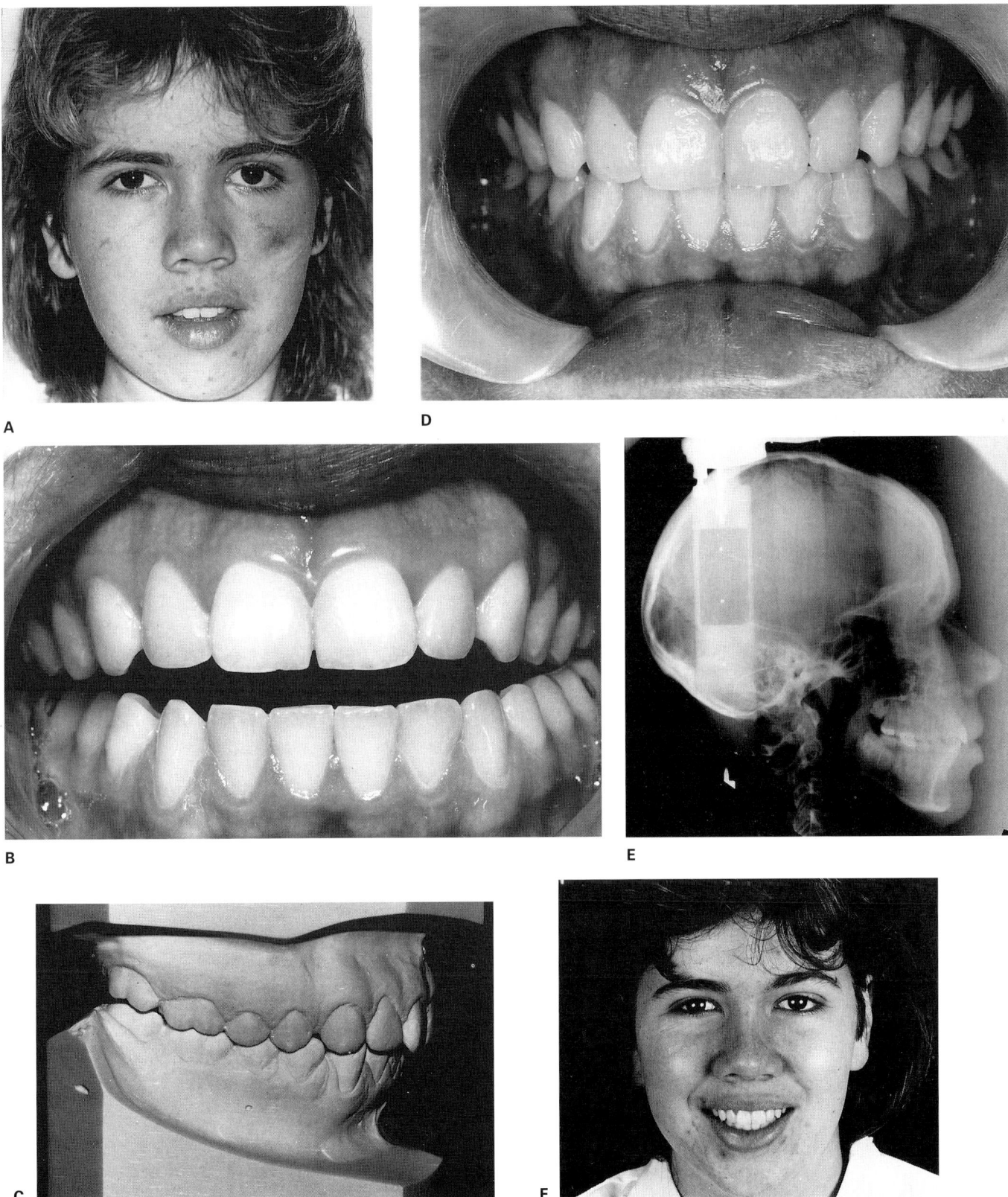

Fig. 21.51 Preoperative planning. A 19-year-old girl was involved in a motor vehicle accident; she sustained a Le Fort I fracture which was initially not detected. 6 months later, she presented with a malocclusion. The models show the deformity and the planned surgical intervention. **A** Initial presentation with anterior open bite. **B** Close-up view of the malocclusion and anterior open bite. **C** 'Plaster model surgery' predicts correction of the occlusion by 4 mm forward advancement and 5 mm downward displacement. **D** The occlusion 6 months postoperatively. **E** Cephalometric X-ray, taken at the same time, shows the restoration of her maxillary form. **F** Postoperative facial appearance. Nasal length and position have been restored.

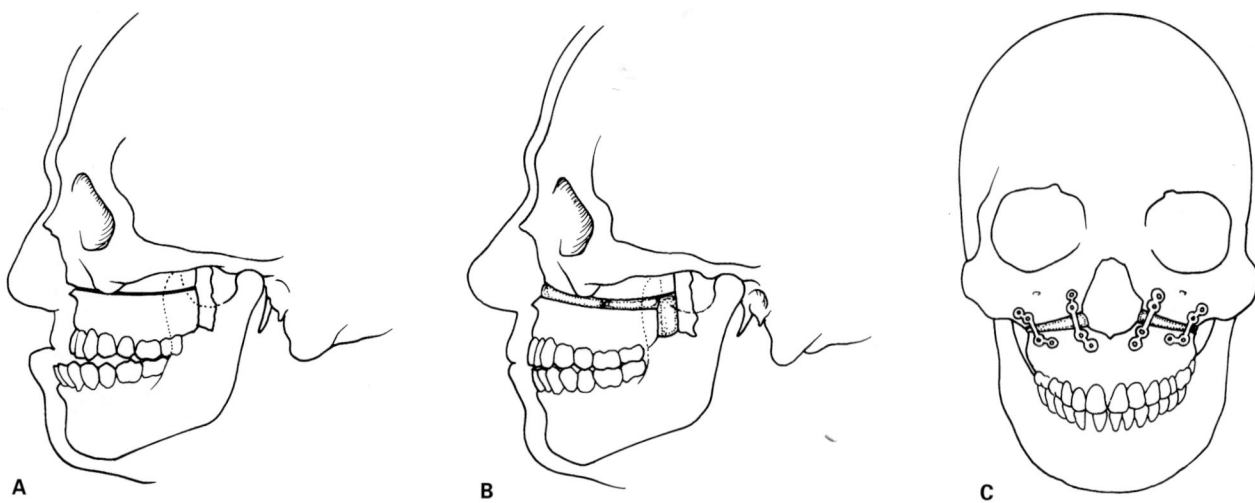

Fig. 21.52 Le Fort I osteotomy. A The horizontal osteotomy is placed above the tooth roots along the anterior wall of the maxillary sinus and carried through the buttresses at the pyriform margin, zygomatic, and pterygoid regions. **B** Bone grafts are placed in the horizontal aspects of the cut if the advancement is more than a few millimetres. We have never placed these grafts between the maxillary tuberosity and the pterygoid plates although many surgeons follow this practice. **C** Four miniplates of the softer variety (without memory) are placed at the zygomatic and pyriform buttresses. These can be easily bent to shape.

to the lower arch. When the face has been shortened the length must be increased, taking into account the relationship of the front teeth and the length of the upper lip, and bearing in mind where possible the premorbid appearance. Soft-tissue scarring of the lips and face may modify the surgical plan, as may loss of teeth.

Correction of deformity is not easy. Measurements taken during the planning of surgery are transferred to the patient at operation by callipers. These measure from a fixed point on the forehead to the teeth; and the measurements are important to obtain a precise position of the jaw segments. But there is always a role for the eye of the surgeon who has been engaged in the work-up and who is closely familiar with the case — the art of surgery.

A horizontal osteotomy is placed above the tooth roots along the anterior wall of the maxillary sinus and carried through the buttresses at the piriform margin, zygomatic and pterygoid regions (Fig. 21.52). This enables 3D repositioning of the tooth-bearing part of the maxilla. Previous

fragmentation of the area must be taken into account and the bony fragments are studied carefully on the CT scan. Scars of the buccal and palatal area must be noted lest a wide soft-tissue exposure compromise the blood supply of the osteotomized segments; a tunnelling technique with minimal soft-tissue elevation may then be necessary. The usual way to effect the Le Fort I osteotomy is to separate the maxillary tuberosity area from the pterygoid plates; this may not be easy as previous trauma often leaves very indistinct planes obscured by a mixture of dense scar and bony fragments. After completing the osteotomy in the anterior maxillary wall, medial wall of the maxillary sinus, nasal septum and pterygoid plates, the mobilizing manoeuvre of down-fracture completes the osteotomy of the posterior sinus wall osteotomy. This manoeuvre must be done with care and patience as the scar tissue is often very extensive and too much force may do unnecessary damage. We have long since ceased to use instruments such as Rowe's disimpaction forceps which grab the segment like tongs; in post-traumatic cases these forceps risk damaging soft tissues and compromising blood supply. Instead the fracture is gently levered open with an elevator or osteotome, or on occasion formally osteotomized to free the fragments.

Bone grafts (iliac crest, ribs, and/or calvarial bone) are used to fill the gaps in the osteotomy lines and fixation is secured with titanium miniplates of such malleability as to be easily bent without later recoil. If possible, the plates are placed at the zygomatic and piriform buttress areas on each side, with two screws on each side of the osteotomy, and are used to fix the interpositional bone graft as well to give rigid fixation. Extensive damage in the region of the osteotomy may make it necessary to compromise this ideal pattern of fixation. When this is so, segments of cortical bone can be fashioned as a 'bone plate' and used to bridge areas of the bone and scar in-adequate for fixation, by securing the 'bone plate' to solid bone at each end. We have never used the pterygoid region for interpositional bone grafting.

To establish the desired occlusion, the occlusal wafer is fixed to the maxillary segment. In most cases it is possi-ble to dispense with intermaxillary fixation at the end of the operation; however, the occlusal status must be closely supervised and intermaxillary fixation re-established if necessary. Often intermaxillary elastic bands are useful to stabilize the occlusion and to give guidance on its long-term stability. This essential measure of control is lost if arch bars or dental appliances are removed too early.

In cases with a comminuted perialar extension of the Le Fort I pattern fracture, en bloc osteotomy is not only difficult to perform but does not produce good results. This type of deformity is therefore treated by a Le Fort I osteotomy plus onlay bone grafting in the region of the medial buttress; grafting extends in the perialar region from the lower part of the piriform aperture superiorly to the frontal process of the maxilla, with a bone graft to the nasal dorsum fixed with a screw in the glabella region. This can be combined with nasal septal surgery when necessary.

Secondary corrections sometimes require osteotomies more or less corresponding to the Le Fort II and III lines. However, as with the Le Fort I fractures, it is very rare for these lines to be well defined in facial fractures of the types seen today. The panfacial fractures for which secondary surgery is performed typically consist of a Le Fort I segment displaced to cause malocclusion, and a naso-ethmoid segment comminuted and retrodisplaced or concertinaed to produce the characteristic flattening and altered features, with one or both zygomas displaced. In fact, a deformity representing an en bloc Le Fort II or III fracture requiring the classical osteotomy is almost never seen.

If an en bloc osteotomy of the Le Fort II variety is to be performed, the area can be exposed through the buccal sulcus. Additional exposure may require vertical or hori-zontal incisions over the dorsum of the nose and lower eyelid or conjunctival incisions. Our preference is to make the approach through a bicoronal scalp flap in combination with the buccal approach. After forward advancement and any rotation or lengthening which may be needed, the gaps are filled with bone grafts and the segments stabilized with miniplates. The points of fixation are usually the zygomas laterally and the frontal bone medially. There have been many variations to these oste-otomies. Where the Le Fort II osteotomy involves the orbital rim the cut must go behind the lacrimal fossa and

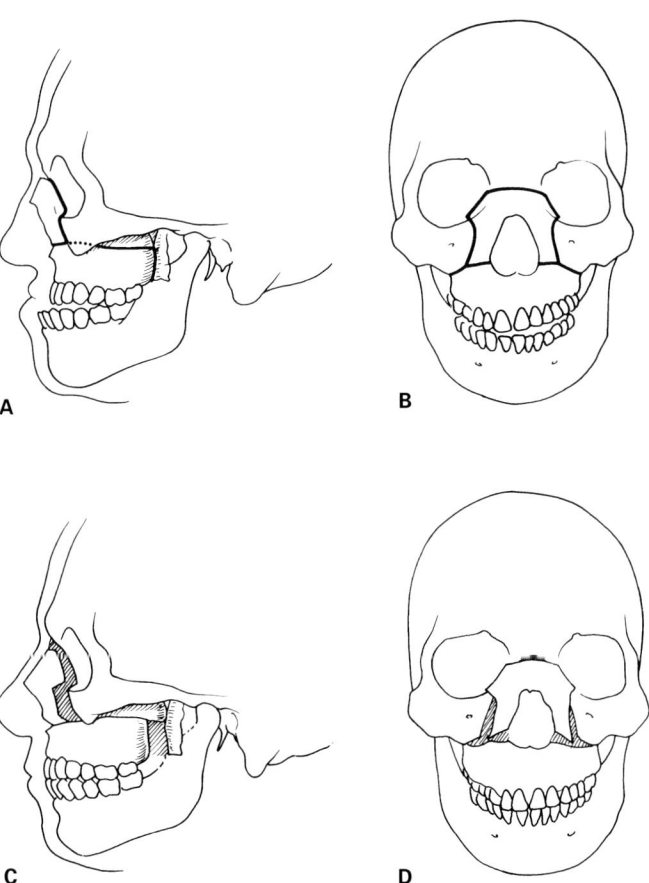

Fig. 21.53 Le Fort II osteotomy. A The Le Fort II osteotomy can be done in combination with other osteotomies, either with the zygoma or a Le Fort I section. **B** We believe it important to have the upper part of the osteotomy behind the nasolacrimal apparatus to protect it, and to swing the osteotomy down medial and inferior to the infraorbital foramen to the line previously recommended for the Le Fort I osteotomy. **C** The gaps are bone-grafted and secured with miniplate fixation. **D** There is often a step in the infraorbital rim which needs to be grafted or smoothed over. The step at the glabella can be burred down and the gap grafted. Canthopexy and the addition of bone graft for nasal support are further options. In our experience it is best not to detach the canthal ligaments if they are reasonably well seated.

this may cause a step in the glabella region which should be burred down (Fig. 21.53).

The old displaced Le Fort III fracture is also a rare deformity (Fig. 21.54). The osteotomy lines have been described in the context of congenital deformities by Gillies & Harrison (1950), Tessier (1971) and Murray & Swanson (1968). The approach is via the bicoronal scalp flap and all the osteotomies are performed from above. In the frontal region care must be taken to cut below the level of the anterior cranial fossa, being mindful of the possibility that fragments of bone and scar tissue in this area may provide only a flimsy barrier between the nose and the cranial contents. Occasionally, the anterior cranial fossa needs to be exposed by the neurosurgeon to close a cranionasal fistula. A full transcranial approach is then necessary via a bifrontal or occasionally unifrontal craniotomy, with dissection of the anterior fossa and intra-dural (rarely extradural) repair of the fistula (pp. 339 and 379). This is done before the osteotomies are performed, and watertight dural closure is secured. After complete orbital dissection, each medial orbital osteotomy is made behind the lacrimal fossa, extended into the orbital floor and connected to the lateral osteotomy, which separates the zygoma from the greater wing of sphenoid and extends into the inferior orbital fissure. The zygomatic arch is disconnected. The osteotomy between the maxillary tuberosity and the pterygoid plates is well done from above; a finger in the mouth placed over the maxillary tuberosity will feel the cut being made in the correct position.

It is more usual for the component bones to be sepa-rated and moved differentially according to the pattern of the deformity produced by the original fractures. Thus, the zygomas may be moved separately from the horizontal maxillary segment. Each zygoma can be repositioned and fixed with miniplates taking into account Gruss's strategy of accurate reduction of the zygomatic arch with attention to both its length and shape (Fig. 21.55). The segment mobilized by Le Fort I osteotomy can be located into the occlusal wafer and fixed to the mandible; the appropriate degree of lengthening is then produced by opening the mandible and so establishing the necessary downward displacement of the attached maxillary seg-ment. The resulting gap can then be grafted. When deal-ing with the orbitonasal components of these complex midface deformities, there is a difficult judgement to be made in deciding whether to perform an osteotomy or to solve the problem with bone grafting alone. Similarly, the naso-ethmoid area can be osteotomized or more usually grafted (Figs 21.38–42).

Isolated dento-alveolar deformities

It is possible to reposition the anterior and lateral seg-ments of a deformed maxilla as a secondary correction by applying the planning and operative manoeuvres described in Chapter 11. With appropriate X-ray exami-nations, the fracture site can be delineated; dental casts are cut and repositioned accurately and the appropriate osteotomy is performed on the model, from which a wafer is made. At operation, the segments are cut and located in the preformed wafer and fixed with miniplates and bone grafts where necessary. It is most common for such segments to derive their blood supply from the palatal segment and, as with other low maxillary osteotomies, great care must be taken to preserve this: there must be full knowledge of any previous scars in the mucosal and palatal attachments that might compromise the blood supply of the mobilized segments.

Maxillary deformity in edentulous patients

When the degree of displacement is minimal, then com-pensation can be built into the manufacture of new prostheses. There are, however, two situations that may call for secondary surgery for deformity.

The first arises in younger patients who have recently become edentulous, perhaps during the accident that has precipitated the call for treatment. Such patients may wish to have titanium implants for fixation of dentures. Dental titanium implants are a sophisticated form of denture fixation, best achieved when the maxillary (or mandibular) base bone is thick enough and so placed that the implants can be positioned vertically. If the maxilla is deformed significantly in any of its three dimensions then it should be repositioned with the aid of miniplate fixation and Gunning splints (Fig. 21.56). A work-up is done as described above; model surgery on an articulator will indicate when the splints are located, what the posi-tion of the maxilla should be and what resulting bone defect needs to be grafted. If there is much loss of alveo-lar bone, autogenous bone graft(s) should be inserted. Planned insertion of titanium implants to fix a dental prosthesis (p. 637) can then be considered (Fig. 21.57).

Secondly, correction may be considered when there is an old and displaced fracture in an atrophic maxilla, so severe as to prevent successful denture retention whether with fixed or removable prostheses. Reduction is more difficult and repositioning of such a maxilla needs exten-sive bone grafting with the aid of miniplate fixation. The subsequent prosthetic management is the key to the success of secondary surgery in such cases, whether it be by simple removable prosthesis, clip-on prosthesis, or with osseo-integration and a fixed prosthesis. In all such cases, patients must be fully informed of both the surgical and technical requirements that will be necessary to ensure a satisfactory result.

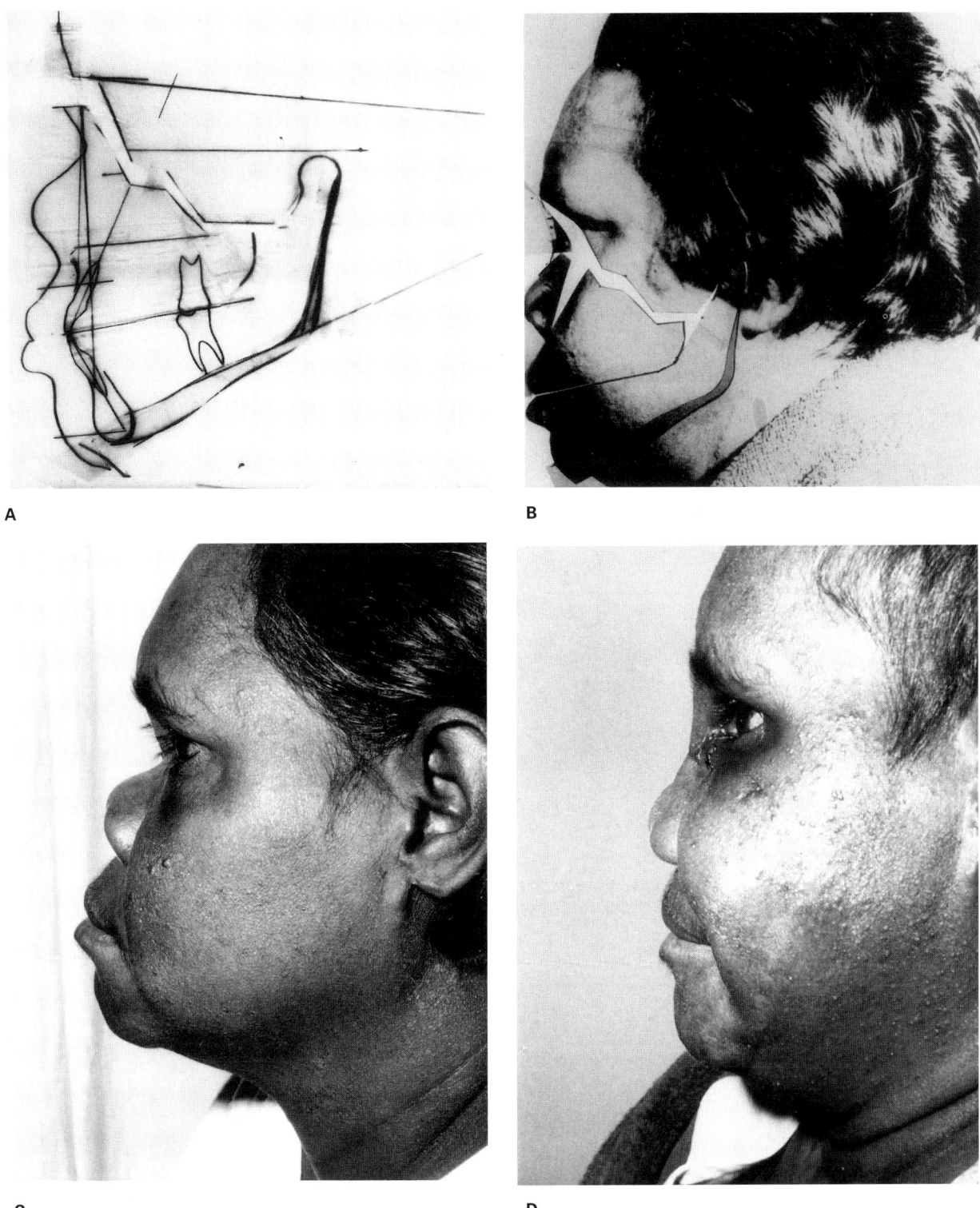

A

B

C

D

Fig. 21.54 Le Fort III osteotomy. The midface can be moved forward en bloc as a Le Fort III osteotomy with the lines of disconnection from the upper skull made through the frontozygomatic suture, lateral orbital wall and anterior part of the zygomatic arch. More commonly the osteotomy is comprised of multiple segments, perhaps as many as a Le Fort I segment plus two zygomas and the naso-ethmoid complex. The latter procedure leaves much to be desired because of the instability of the previously fractured components. **A, B** Photocephalometric analysis has been used in this case (Henderson 1974), in which a life-size transparent photograph is superimposed on the cephalometric tracing and cut to reproduce the planned osteotomy and repositioning. **C** Patient with a previously uncorrected Le Fort III fracture. **D** Postoperative appearance, with the elongated and advanced middle third after subcranial Le Fort III osteotomy.

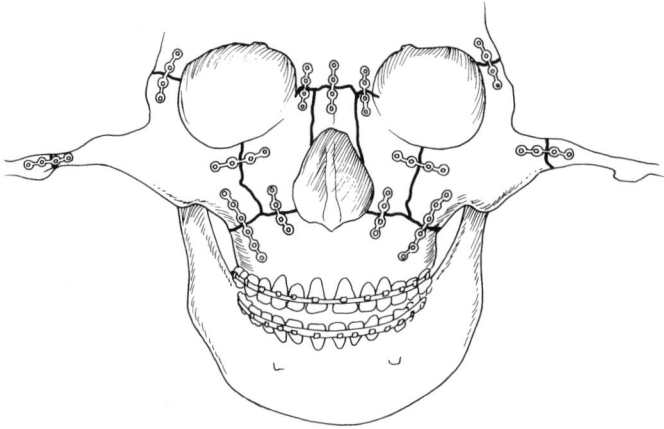

Fig. 21.55 Reconstructive technique. After Gruss et al (1990). At the beginning the zygomatic arch and frontozygomatic suture line are secured giving anteroposterior projection and transverse facial width. The naso-ethmoid region may be reconstructed within this outer frame, and if the occlusion is then established onto a normal or accurately reconstructed mandible, the lower face will fit in harmony with this upper framework. If pieces of bone are missing, immediate bone grafts can be used to replace them with the same sort of rigid fixation.

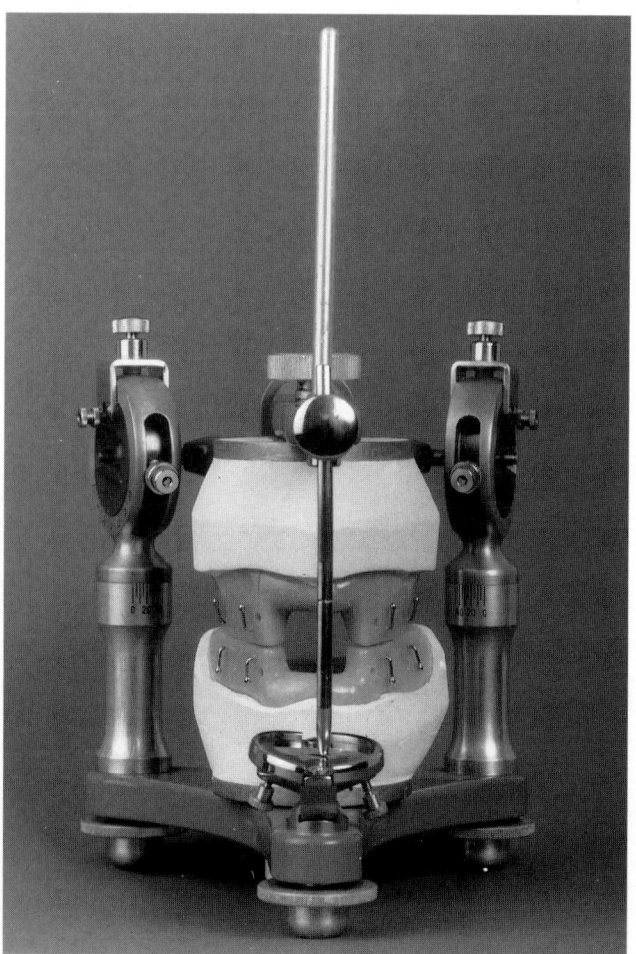

A

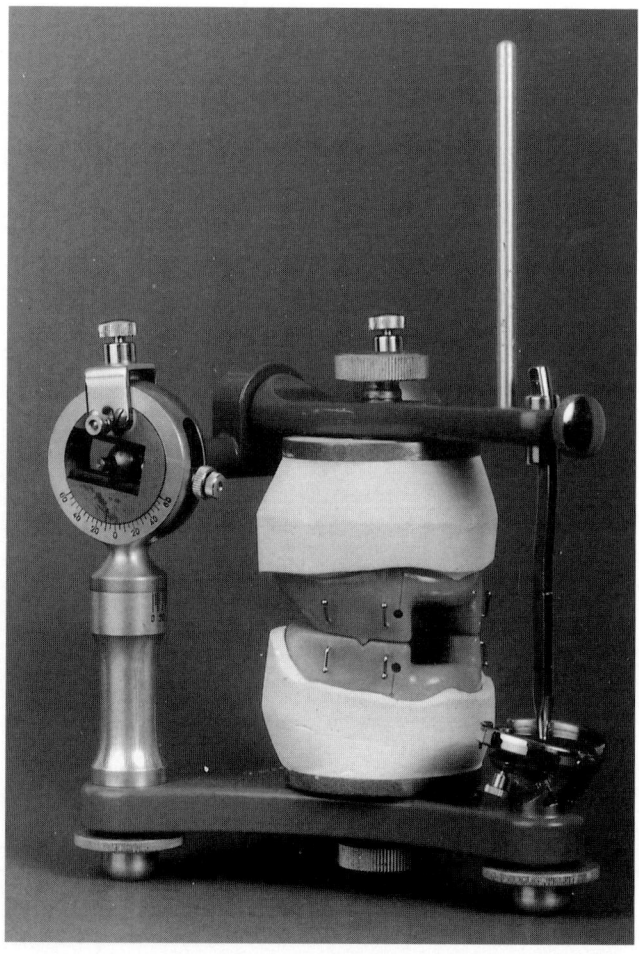

B

Fig. 21.56 The Gunning splint. Example of a Gunning splint mounted on the articulator to indicate the planning necessary by the prosthodontist for the repositioning of the edentulous maxilla, with a goal of creating a denture suitable for cosmetic and functional purposes.

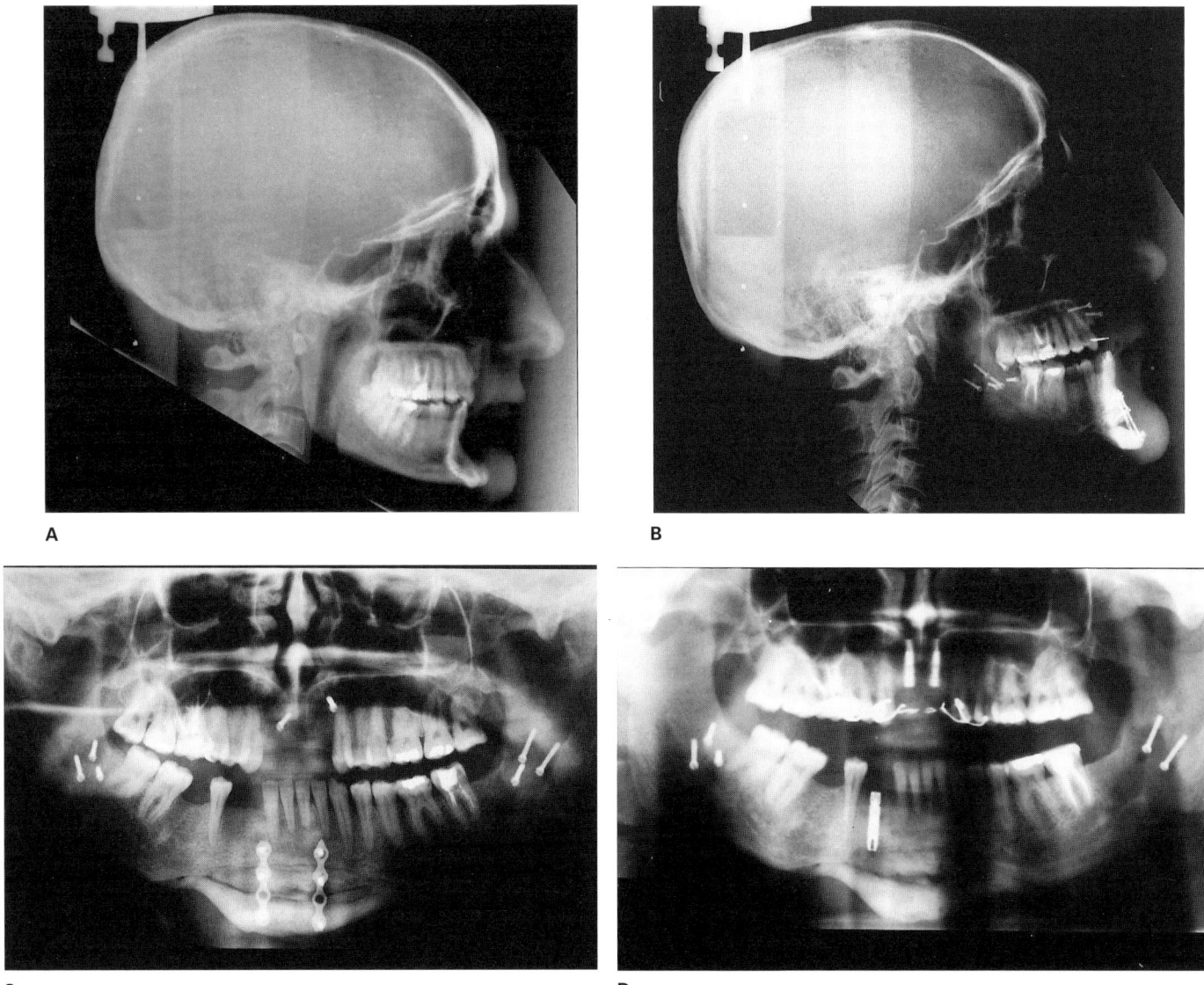

Fig. 21.57 Titanium osseo-integrated implants for dental rehabilitation. A man with a previously fractured mandible, new alveolar fracture of the anterior maxilla, and loss of mandibular teeth. **A** Lateral X-ray before secondary treatment. **B** Appearance after advancement of the mandible and genioplasty. **C** Bone graft into the anterior maxilla held with two titanium screws to increase the bone mass in this area. **D** Osseo-integrated implantation supporting the anterior dental prosthesis as well as a single implant into the mandible.

TEMPOROMANDIBULAR JOINT ANKYLOSIS

Surgical pathology

Classification

Ankylosis of the TMJ may be fibrous or bony, intra-capsular or extracapsular. Kazanjian (1938) was one of the first authors to classify these disorders in a logical way, and his terms remain useful. 'False ankylosis', called pseudo-ankylosis by many later authors, includes any mechanical obstruction to mandibular movement which does not represent pathology within the TMJ capsule. True ankylosis results from intra-articular disease processes which lead to bony or fibrous adhesions of the joint itself. Rowe (1982) also used the term pseudo-ankylosis to describe limited joint movement resulting from the indirect influence on joint mobility caused by depression of the zygomatic arch and subsequent fibrous adhesions; a similar situation arises where there is post-traumatic shortening of the ramus of the mandible, relatively greater length of the coronoid process and shortening of the temporalis muscle.

Pathogenesis and nature of deformity

Post-traumatic ankylosis of the TMJ may develop in childhood or in adult life (p. 286). The long-term consequences of facial skeletal trauma are nowhere more dramatic than the effects produced by fractures of the mandibular condyles in children, which may result in ankylosis and mandibular growth restriction (Fig. 21.58), often causing secondary deformity elsewhere in the face. In cases of traumatic ankylosis of the TMJ, secondary deformities of the upper jaw are admittedly not so common or severe as in hemifacial microsomia, where absence or hypoplasia of the condyle is often associated with severe secondary deformities of the upper jaw. But in the few cases suffering from very early onset bilateral ankylosis, there is some deformity of the upper jaw also.

The pathogenesis is often controversial, and indeed there are many causes of reduced mobility of the mandible. Some cases of true ankylosis certainly result in early childhood from trauma to the developing mandibular condyle, perhaps complicated by secondary infection, and there is often an associated failure of mandibular growth (p. 504).

Intracapsular crushing and haemarthrosis in an area that is highly osteogenic and capable of being a focus of infection may produce a nasty combination of bony ankylosis and deformity. Not only does complete bilateral fusion of the bones lead to difficulty in opening the mouth but there is gross malocclusion and in extreme forms

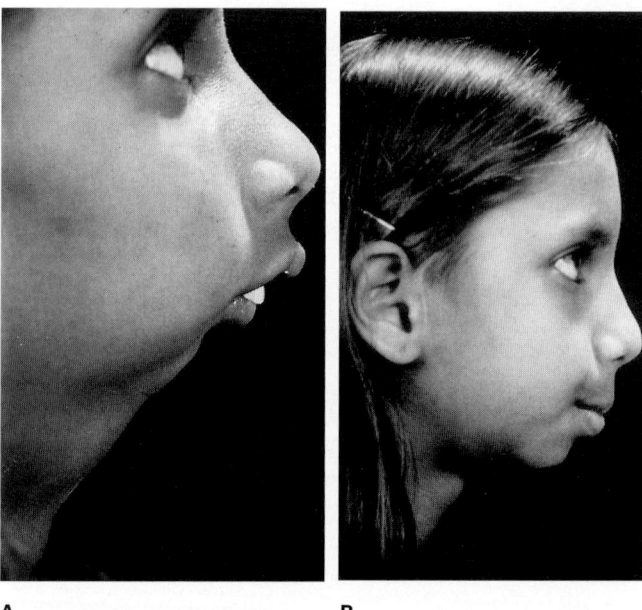

A   **B**

Fig. 21.58 Temporomandibular joint ankylosis. A 10-year-old child sustained mandibular trauma in infancy, with infection of the temporomandibular joints, giving rise to the dramatic 'bird face' deformity with severe retrognathia and trismus. This child was fed by forcing food behind the posterior dentition with a finger — first by the parents and later by the patient. **A** Initial presentation. **B** After reconstruction of the temporomandibular joints with costochondral grafts, inverted 'L' osteotomy, interpositional bone graft and genioplasty as a one-stage operation.

the 'bird face' deformity shown in Fig. 21.58. The effects on airway and nutrition are significant as are the psychosocial problems. Less severe TMJ ankylosis can also occur in children. When seen late there may be some destruction of the mandibular condyles, trismus and a mild malocclusion, with varying degrees of growth disorder.

The relation between condylar damage and mandibular growth is still obscure (p. 80). There are cases in which, despite considerable condylar destruction, mandibular growth is almost normal. Perhaps the reason that such patients suffer minimal growth abnormalities following severe condylar injury is because ankylosis did not occur. It would therefore seem that the critical treatment objective in condylar fractures is early mobilization to prevent condylar ankylosis and therefore subsequent growth deformity.

The majority (69%) of cases reported by Lello (1990) were consequences of trauma, and this finding is consistent with most contemporary studies (Posnick & Goldstein 1993). Rowe (1982) supports the view that trauma has succeeded infection as the principle cause of ankylosis in children. The cases that we have seen of this gross deformity have come from developing countries and we have formed the view that lack of health services resulted in failure to treat these children for an initial traumatic event.

Older authors have given more weight to the causative role of inflammation of one type or another (Topazian 1964). Norman (1978) suggested that the differential diagnosis of mandibular hypomobility may include pseudoankylosis (under this heading he includes fibrosis secondary to burns, radiation treatment, and infection), as well as union of an enlarged coronoid to the maxilla or zygomatic arch and a depressed fracture of the zygomaticomaxillary complex. Other less convincing causes include 'trismus' secondary to an elongated styloid process and an ossified sphenomandibular ligament.

Re-ankylosis after TMJ arthroplasty is held to be a postoperative consequence of the proximity of raw, uncovered bone surfaces as well as insufficiency or absence of immediate postoperative mandibular movement to disrupt the formation of bone bridges and maturing fibrous tissue.

In adults, TMJ ankylosis is usually due to intracapsular comminuted fractures. These may be associated with extra-articular fibrous ankylosis (Kazanjian's false ankylosis). Uncorrected fracture dislocations with subsequent fibrosis may also produce reduced mandibular mobility. Very severe crush injuries to the area can result in a fibro-osseous response of massive proportions with a block of bone extending from the ramus and coronoid process to the zygomatic arch and base of skull. Fortunately cases of such complete ankylosis in adult life are rare.

Finally, an unfortunate cause of post-traumatic iatrogenic ankylosis results from enthusiastic exploration of

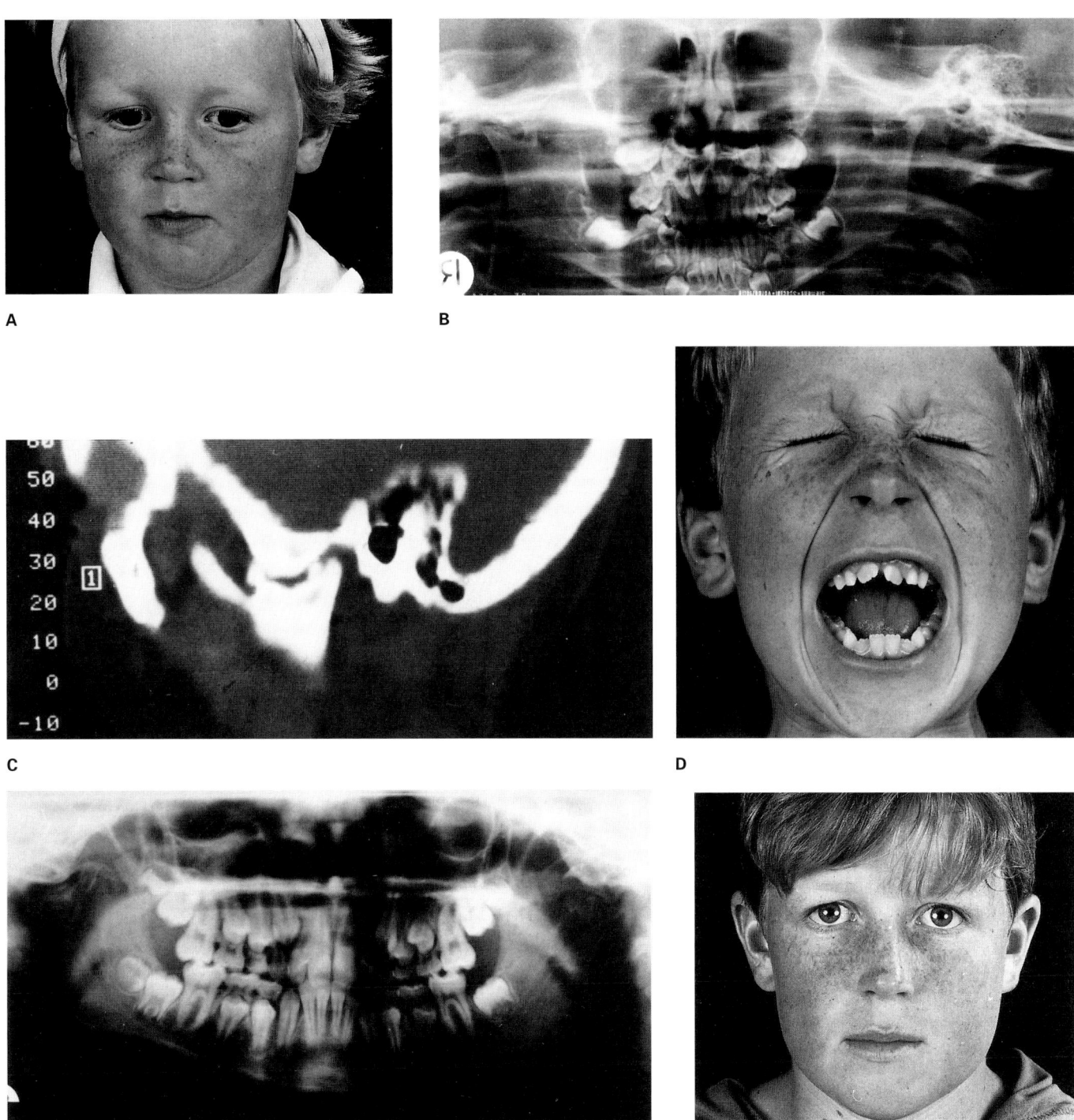

Fig. 21.59 Temporomandibular joint ankylosis. A 3-year-old boy was run over by a tractor, suffering bilateral condylar fractures. These healed with a grossly shortened and flattened morphology. He was treated conservatively for 4 years but by then demonstrated restricted mandibular opening and X-ray evidence of bony ankylosis. He had problems when eating and cleaning his teeth. Removal of the bony ankylosis and interposition of perichondrium over the smoothed condyle restored the ability to open the mouth much wider. His facial growth has developed relatively normally in spite of the distorted temporomandibular joints. **A** Initial presentation. **B** Orthopantomogram (OPG) taken at the time of presentation, several years after the original accident. **C** CT scan showing the bony ankylosis. **D** Opening (with effort) after surgery. **E** OPG taken at 12 years of age with distorted temporomandibular joints. **F** Good facial growth has been maintained.

the joint for TMJ dysfunction, with a resulting increase in fibrosis.

Clinical assessment

The age of the patient at the time of the injury will determine the clinical symptoms and signs. In severe bilateral ankylosis, no movement of the jaws is possible: the victim may be undernourished and may suffer from chronic airway obstruction. In younger patients there may be characteristic secondary deformities. Symmetrical retrognathia may occur with bilateral joint involvement; with unilateral ankylosis, there is a variable degree of retrognathia and deviation of the jaw to the side of the ankylosis. There is compensatory adjustment of the occlusion and compensatory maxillary growth deformity. The birdlike facies with grossly retruded mandible, the small featureless chin and the antigonial notching of the mandible are characteristic. There is a Class II malocclusion. Dentoalveolar growth attempts to compensate for the lack of jaw bone growth and the mandibular teeth are proclined. In unilateral ankylosis in younger patients there is a marked degree of facial asymmetry, the ramus and body of the mandible being chiefly affected. The chin point is distorted in shape due to the asymmetrical muscular pull on it and is deviated to the affected side. However, the dental occlusion may show good interdigitation of teeth due to adjustment at the dento-alveolar level. Nevertheless, dental hygiene may be impaired, with all the consequences that this brings: caries, periodontal disease and dental abscesses have been recorded as the usual concomitants of complete TMJ ankylosis (Georgiade 1977). In cases of fibrous ankylosis, the signs are less obvious. The main symptom is reduced mobility and the growth deformity is not gross. In the adult the symptoms of lack of movement, possibly pain, and malocclusion are usual in both intra-articular and extra-articular ankylosis; the history and examination will help to make this important diagnosis.

Radiological assessment

Radiological investigations include plain X-ray views, orthopantomogram and CT scanning to demonstrate the nature and extent of the ankylosis and the presence of extra-articular components such as coronoid–zygomatic bone fusion. The condylar fusion may extend medially, forming a bone block several centimetres wide, which may obliterate the sigmoid notch; it is therefore important to have 3D views of the region before any surgical venture, and modern applications of CT scanning are most helpful here. Magnetic resonance imaging (MRI) is useful in delineating the intra-articular soft-tissue pathology (p. 189).

Management

Principles of conservative and operative treatment

Treatment is indicated where there is a significant problem with function or form. In bilateral ankylosis in childhood, there are likely to be serious difficulties in feeding, airway obstruction and impaired dental hygiene, in addition to the deformed appearance resulting from cessation of growth. As has been noted above, the nature and degree of the secondary facial deformity are related to the time of onset of the ankylosis, its duration throughout the patient's growth phase and whether the lesion is unilateral or bilateral.

In less severe cases of fibrous ankylosis in an adult or older child, the indication for surgical or non-surgical treatment will depend on the outcome of a preliminary trial of exercise treatment. In some cases, progressive mobilization by conservative treatment may be successful: the gap is gradually widened with increasing numbers of wooden spatulas, or with an acrylic screw in the shape of a carrot (Fig. 21.60). In younger patients with fibrous ankylosis causing restricted movement but with no gross problem with growth, there is also a place for conservative management: this involves monitoring growth, physiotherapy and patience. However, as Munro et al (1986) have pointed out, the response to conservative treatment may be deceptive: even with complete ankylosis there is often sufficient elasticity in the jaw to allow some movement, and attempts to manage complete ankylosis by exercises, passive or active, are in vain.

Surgical intervention should not be undertaken lightly because the intervention itself may contribute to ankylosis. The aim of surgical treatment is to re-establish movement of the joint, to maintain movement, to facilitate growth and to reduce deformity, especially in the child since impaired mandibular growth may produce a cascade of

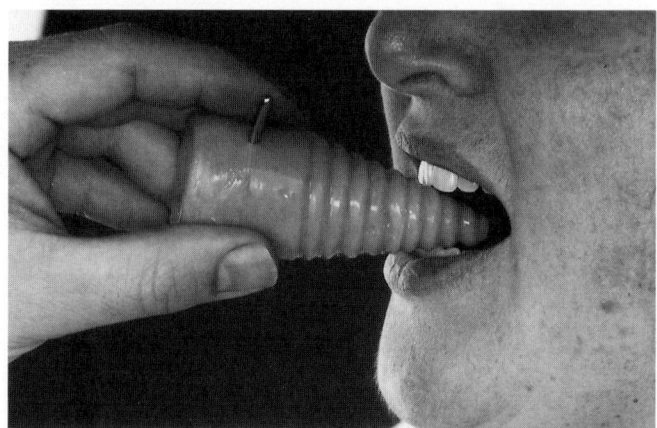

Fig. 21.60 Acrylic 'carrot' used to assist with progressive mouth opening.

secondary deformities in the upper jaw. In the adult a distinction must be made between ankylosis that has developed in childhood when there are secondary deformities of the chin, maxilla and dentition and ankylosis of recent origin when release of the joint will produce an acceptable occlusion.

The surgical challenge is not only to reconstruct the joint, but also to maintain function and preserve the reconstruction from postoperative re-ankylosis. The difficulty in producing satisfactory results from reconstruction of TMJ ankylosis is reflected in the many and varied procedures described to achieve these ends. Autogenous grafts have included metatarsals, calvarial bone, pieces of iliac crest, and costochondral grafts. Alloplastic substances used include metal (Vitallium) or acrylic prostheses, and sculpted Silastic® and Proplast® blocks, inserted to maintain joint mobility and mandibular height. MacAfee & Quinn (1992) used a polyoxomethylene condylar head fixed to a pure titanium mesh. The copious literature relating to alloplastic implants in the TMJ joint is reviewed by Kent & Misiek (1991) and there is a disappointingly high incidence of complications. Gallagher & Wolford (1982) reported on the better long-term stability of Proplast® when compared with Silastic®. However, Smith et al (1993) have confirmed what has become a common experience that Teflon®–Proplast® implants may generate an osteoclastic giant cell reaction that can erode bone even as far as the middle cranial fossa. The propensity for alloplastic materials to develop late problems including displacement, erosion of bone, and failure of the prosthetic joint as well as the suspected local and systemic responses to silicone, make autogenous costochondral joint replacement our procedure of choice (Kent et al 1983, Dolwick & Aufdemorte 1985).

Anaesthesia

In those cases where there is some movement of the jaw it may be possible to intubate orally. If it proves possible to ventilate the patient with a face mask then paralysis may be achieved with suxamethonium prior to intubation. A range of stylets, bougies and laryngoscopes should be at hand. The wide but flat Seward blade has been most useful.

If the teeth are firmly opposed to one another then the nasal route is used. The nose should be cocainized (10% plain cocaine paste) allowing plenty of time for good anaesthesia (20 min). Then 4% lignocaine (3 ml) is injected into the trachea through the cricotracheal membrane. The patient is encouraged to cough after the injection. Sedation with a narcotic (fentanyl) and a benzodiazepine (midazolam) is helpful. Anaesthesia is then induced with oxygen and a volatile agent. A fibrescope with an armoured tube passed over the scope is introduced through the nose and into the larynx and trachea. The tube is then slipped down over the scope and into the trachea.

Anaesthesia may then be formally induced. Blind nasal intubation is an alternative option (Edwards 1993).

While in general we do not advocate hypotensive techniques, it is desirable to suppress the reflex tachycardia and hypertension sometimes induced by dissection in the TMJ area. Occasionally the surgeon will be impeded by oozing from tissues around the joint capsule and modest hypotension may be induced for this portion of the operation.

If the facial nerve is at risk during the dissection then muscle relaxants should be omitted so that the nerve and the muscles it supplies are active and can respond to a nerve stimulator.

Exposure for arthroplasty

Surgical approaches to the TMJ are described on p. 285. It is very important to have wide access, and the approach offered by the bicoronal scalp flap, extended into the pre-auricular region and combined with release of the temporal fascia from the zygomatic arch and division of the masseter muscle, makes this the exposure of choice in difficult cases. In less difficult unilateral cases the flap need not be extended quite so far to the other side, though it must go far enough to make access easy. The insertion of the costochondral graft has been described as best performed via a combination of the pre-auricular and submandibular approaches (Evans et al 1985, Crawley et al 1993); we have used this combined approach when inserting a costochondral graft. However, the extended bicoronal flap may offer sufficient exposure of the condyle and ramus to facilitate the whole operation. Where complex osteotomies are needed together with joint exploration and reconstruction, Crawley et al (1993) use a neck incision below and behind the angle of the mandible as well as the bicoronal approach.

The capsule of the joint is identified and divided. The bony mass enveloping the joint and condylar neck is exposed, together with the base of skull above and the condylar neck and ramus of the mandible and the sigmoid notch below. Subperiosteal dissection is continued down as far as the angle of the mandible and beyond if necessary. Where possible this dissection is extended to secure the posterior aspect of the condylar neck and a curved retractor is placed around the neck to protect the maxillary artery which lies medial to the joint (p. 47). However, this protective manoeuvre may not be possible and one must then proceed with caution in dividing the bone. When the retractor is in place, it is possible to use a large burr to release the bone at the level of the fused joint space which may be partly visible. The bone can be burred away medially leaving a thin shell intact above;

lower down toward the condylar neck, the curved retractor protects the soft tissue and the cut can be made more aggressively. Once the bone is removed the ends are smoothed over and the base of skull is also smoothed. The mandible can then be tried for movement. Fibrous contractures may need to be divided or a coronoidectomy performed. To obtain sufficient mobilization, further dissection may be necessary to detach the medial and lateral pterygoid muscles, the temporalis muscle, the stylomandibular and sphenomandibular ligaments and the pterygomandibular raphe.

Interpositional arthroplasty

The aim of the operation is the creation of a gap, and it is in effect an extended condylectomy. There has been a persistent belief that this gap alone is sufficient treatment of the ankylosis. However, experience has shown that to prevent re-ankylosis, some form of interpositional arthroplasty is necessary. This may be with autogenous tissue, such as fascia lata, muscle, bone, cartilage or dermis (Tajima et al 1978), or alloplastic material, such as Proplast®, Teflon®, silicone rubber or metal.

In less severe cases we have inserted a sheet of perichondrium taken from the costal cartilage and sutured over the reshaped condylar process with small burrholes into the bone to aid fixation. Above this a disc of reinforced Silastic® sheet is similarly sutured into the area of the condylar fossa. Lello (1990) reported the successful use of a minimal gap arthroplasty with insertion of a graft of composite free auricular skin and a cartilage graft to prevent re-ankylosis; however, Yih et al (1992) report that auricular cartilage has proved disappointing in the long term. In the more severe cases the bone ends may need to be widely separated: Topazian (1964) recom-

mended a gap at least 1 cm wide, and Rowe (1982) even more separation. Munro et al (1986) have stated that there should be a bone-free gap of at least 3 cm between the glenoid fossa and the ramus if recurring ankylosis is to be avoided. When a wide gap has been produced some form of support for the vertical height is necessary, or there will be deviation of the mandible and/or open bite: the wider the arthroplasty gap the more important it is that the material be of sufficient bulk and substance to support the ramus adequately and to maintain its vertical height.

Temporalis muscle can be inserted between the bone ends. A strip of temporalis muscle ~2–3 cm wide is mobilized up to the superior attachment of the muscle to the temporal bone, where it is detached. The muscle strip and its overlying fascia, now based inferiorly, are further mobilized and passed inferiorly to the zygomatic arch and interposed between the bone ends, where the muscle strip is kept in place by suturing it to tissue at the margins of the glenoid fossa (Rowe 1982). The edges of the donor defect in the temporalis muscle are hard to approximate but success in doing so will reduce the eventual muscle defect and the associated aesthetic blemish. The results of this procedure are variable. Re-exploration has on occasion shown a mass of fibrous tissue, indicating that the muscle has degenerated: what was an initial good result from the point of view of a space occupier may with time give rise to recurrence of the facial deformity if not loss of joint movement. Certainly, if a considerable amount of mandible has to be removed, muscle interposition will not maintain the mandibular height (Fig. 21.61).

To obviate this, insertion of a bone graft or alloplastic material may be used. In children, a costochondral graft has theoretical advantages (Munro et al 1986, Crawley et al 1993). Not only is the height preserved, but in the

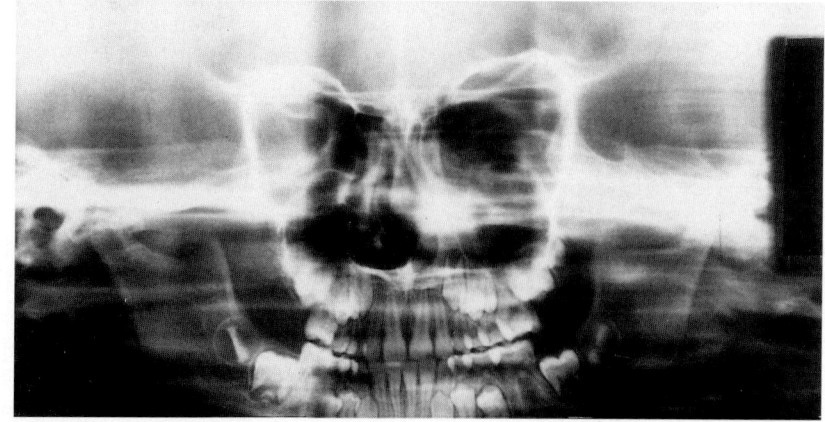

Fig. 21.61 Temporomandibular joint ankylosis. This patient suffered an intracapsular disruption of his temporomandibular joint in early childhood which, in spite of early mobilisation, developed ankylosis and marked overgrowth of bone. A continuous mass of bone fused the condyle, coronoid process, zygomatic arch, and base of skull. **A** Disruption of the joint as the ankylosis is developing.

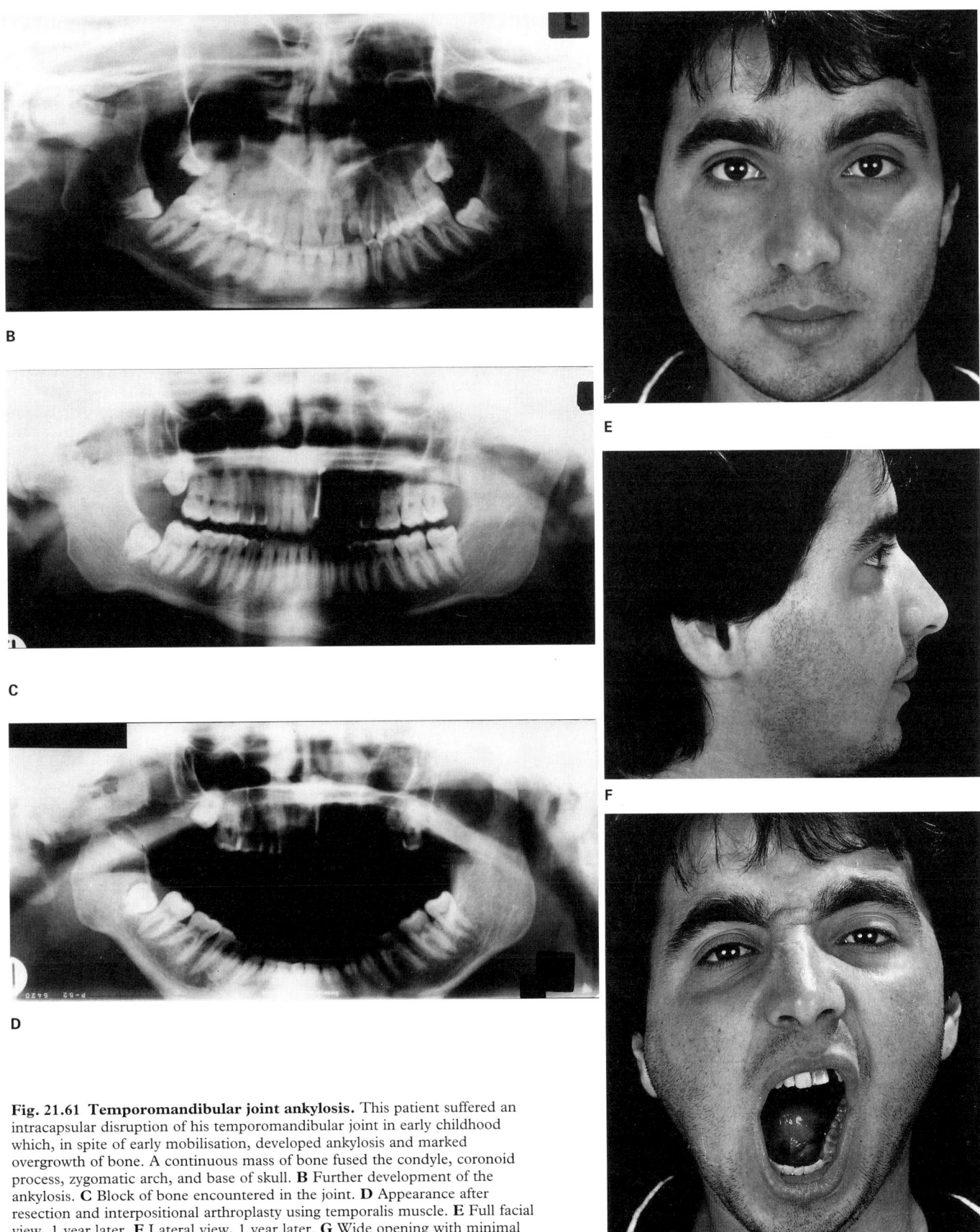

Fig. 21.61 Temporomandibular joint ankylosis. This patient suffered an intracapsular disruption of his temporomandibular joint in early childhood which, in spite of early mobilisation, developed ankylosis and marked overgrowth of bone. A continuous mass of bone fused the condyle, coronoid process, zygomatic arch, and base of skull. **B** Further development of the ankylosis. **C** Block of bone encountered in the joint. **D** Appearance after resection and interpositional arthroplasty using temporalis muscle. **E** Full facial view, 1 year later. **F** Lateral view, 1 year later. **G** Wide opening with minimal jaw deformity; however, there is some deviation of the mandible to the right.

growing individual one can hope that the grafted bone and cartilage will provide a new growing unit within the existing functional matrix (p. 77; Murray et al 1984). This thesis has been postulated for cases of hemifacial microsomia and the results are as uncertain in those cases as in post-traumatic ankylosis.

Orthodontic management

When this procedure, whether unilateral or bilateral, is proposed in the growing child, it must be planned with a view to future orthodontic control and manipulation of facial growth. After creation of the gap and mobilization of the mandible, the jaw will be positioned by an acrylic occlusal wafer and wherever possible this is made before operation. Sometimes it has not been possible to make the wafer before operation, because of lack of jaw opening; impressions of the occlusion cannot be taken if the mouth will not admit impression trays. The appropriate positioning must be then determined at the time of operation and the device made postoperatively (Fig. 21.62).

The wafer serves as a splint and often has to be supplemented by vertical elastic bands. Oral hygiene is often a problem when this appliance is installed; the parents should remove it daily and replace it after cleaning the teeth and also the surface of the appliance as any residual food may cause enamel decalcification. The orthodontist

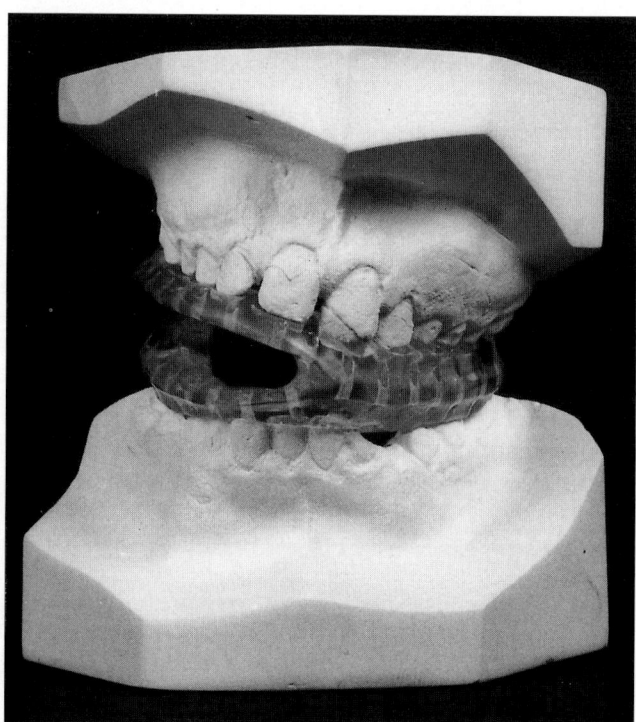

Fig. 21.62 Appliance designed to facilitate the gradual eruption of the maxillary teeth. The acrylic is shaved progressively as eruption occurs.

can instruct the patient on how to remove the appliance from the mouth; the parents are given the necessary instruments for dental hygiene. The wire ligatures securing the acrylic wafer to the maxillary teeth must be readily accessible so that the patient and parents can carry out the necessary hygiene. The wafer should be worn for at least 6 months after operation, and the longer it is worn the better: 18 months is the ideal.

Arthroplasty with costochondral graft

The contralateral chest is used for harvesting the sixth or seventh rib. More than 1 cm of costal cartilage needs to be attached to the rib, care being taken to preserve the periosteum and the perichondrium at the junction. The cartilaginous end is shaped nicely and seated into the glenoid fossa using a strong nylon stitch passed through a burrhole in the bone of the costochondral graft which is then sutured into the tissues of the temporal fossa. We have used a free piece of perichondrium from the rib to line the glenoid fossa on a number of occasions, or sometimes a small Silastic® disk, but because easy displacement has been noted, we have ceased to use this technique. Crawley et al (1993) use a vascularized segment of temporoparietal fascia. The ramus of the mandible must be shaped to receive the graft which is secured with three titanium screws, preferably placed in a triangle to give better fixation. Once the seating and fixation of the costochondral graft are achieved, occlusion should be released and checked. In the adult the costochondral graft can also be used, but like all autogenous implants it may undergo resorption, with or without re-ankylosis. This is not common and the costochondral graft has become our preferred implant in the treatment of severe cases. What is more controversial, however, is the combination of this form of reconstruction with other osteotomies of the facial bones at the same operation as advocated by Munro et al (1986). While we have done this to good effect, there is no place for hard and fast rules in this field of reconstruction. The view expressed by Lello (1990) is that when further growth retardation and skeletal deformity have been prevented by successful release of the ankylosis, secondary osteotomies for the correction of facial deformity can be undertaken later, with perhaps more precise planning. This consideration is only relevant in the period of growth; adult cases can be treated in one or two stages at the preference of the treating team (Fig. 21.63).

Postoperative care

After the insertion of a costochondral graft, it is often difficult to decide whether to re-establish the intermaxillary fixation for a short period of time. There is a delicate

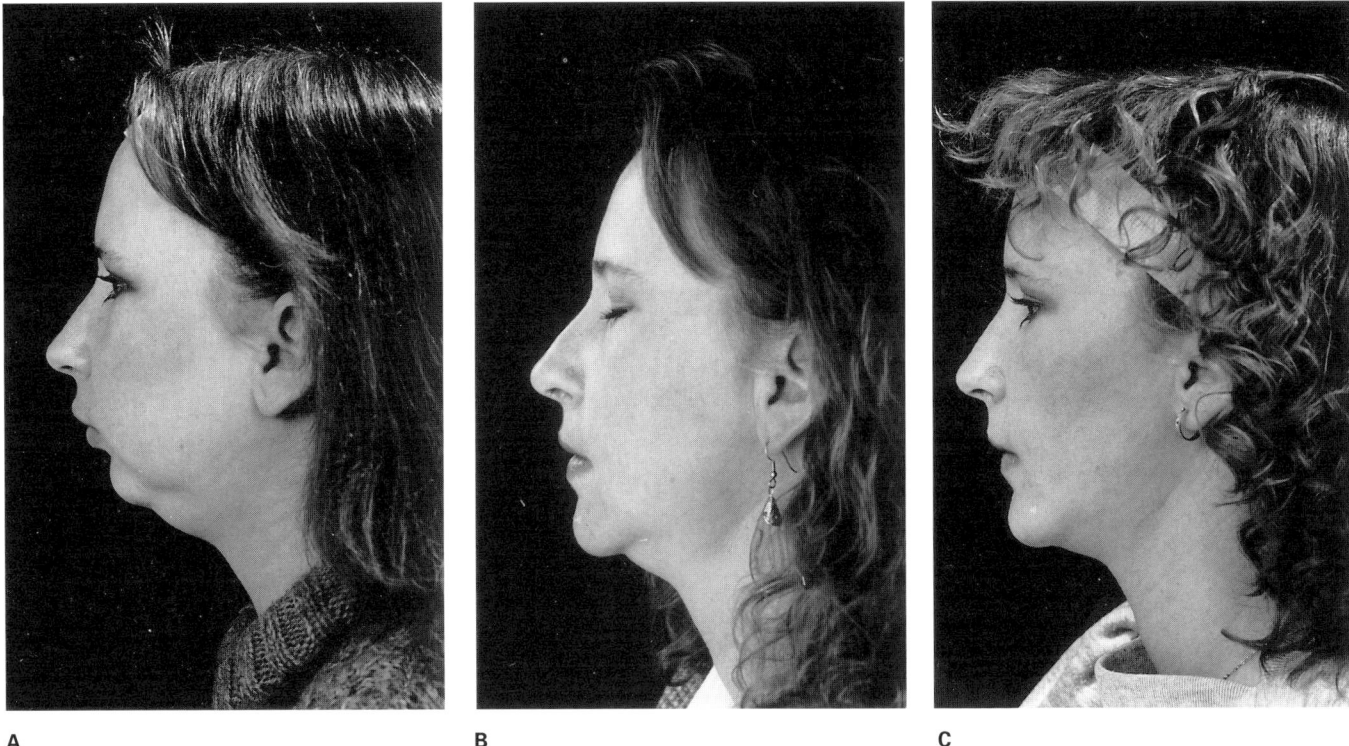

Fig. 21.63 Costochondral joint reconstruction. Case 1: ankylosis in early life. A girl presented with mandibular hypoplasia and trismus as a result of a fracture sustained when she was 3 years of age. Multiple surgical interventions had been made to overcome her trismus. She had release of the left ankylosis, costochondral grafting, bilateral sagittal split osteotomies for advancement, and genioplasty. Osteotomies and costochondral grafting were done at the same time, an extensive but quite practical solution to such difficult problems. **A** Profile seen at presentation with mandibular hypoplasia. **B** Appearance 1 year after costochondral grafting plus sagittal split advancement and genioplasty. **C** The profile after 10 years. Slight relapse is noted but the profile is still acceptable.

balance in planning the period of immobilization: immobility may promote adhesions and limit function, while early mobility may impair healing and promote graft resorption and future dysfunction. It was initially our practice to maintain maxillary fixation for at least a week, followed by controlled mobilization. However, as experience has been gained we have increasingly favoured immediate mobilization within the limits of discomfort. Munro et al (1986) advocate the early postoperative use of chewing gum as a form of immediate exercise and this is now our recommendation. The importance of postoperative oral hygiene has been emphasized.

Long-term care

This also demands judgement and resolution. Where the gap has been maintained with a costochondral graft in a young patient, the long-term supportive regimen is often very demanding. The patient is supervised by the team orthodontist and must often use the wedge-shaped occlusal splints mentioned above, which require frequent adjustments to encourage and control the eruption of the maxillary teeth to rectify the occlusal plane. It is an arduous programme for the child, the family and the treating team. Even with the best of techniques there may be collapse and shortening of the reconstructed ramus.

Complications and results

Good results have been achieved in less severe adult cases by release of the ankylosis, minimal reconstruction and the insertion of perichondrium and a thin Silastic disk to maintain the joint space, although the disk may need to be removed at a later date.

The more severe ankyloses, especially those with onset in childhood, tend to recur and the younger the ankylosis

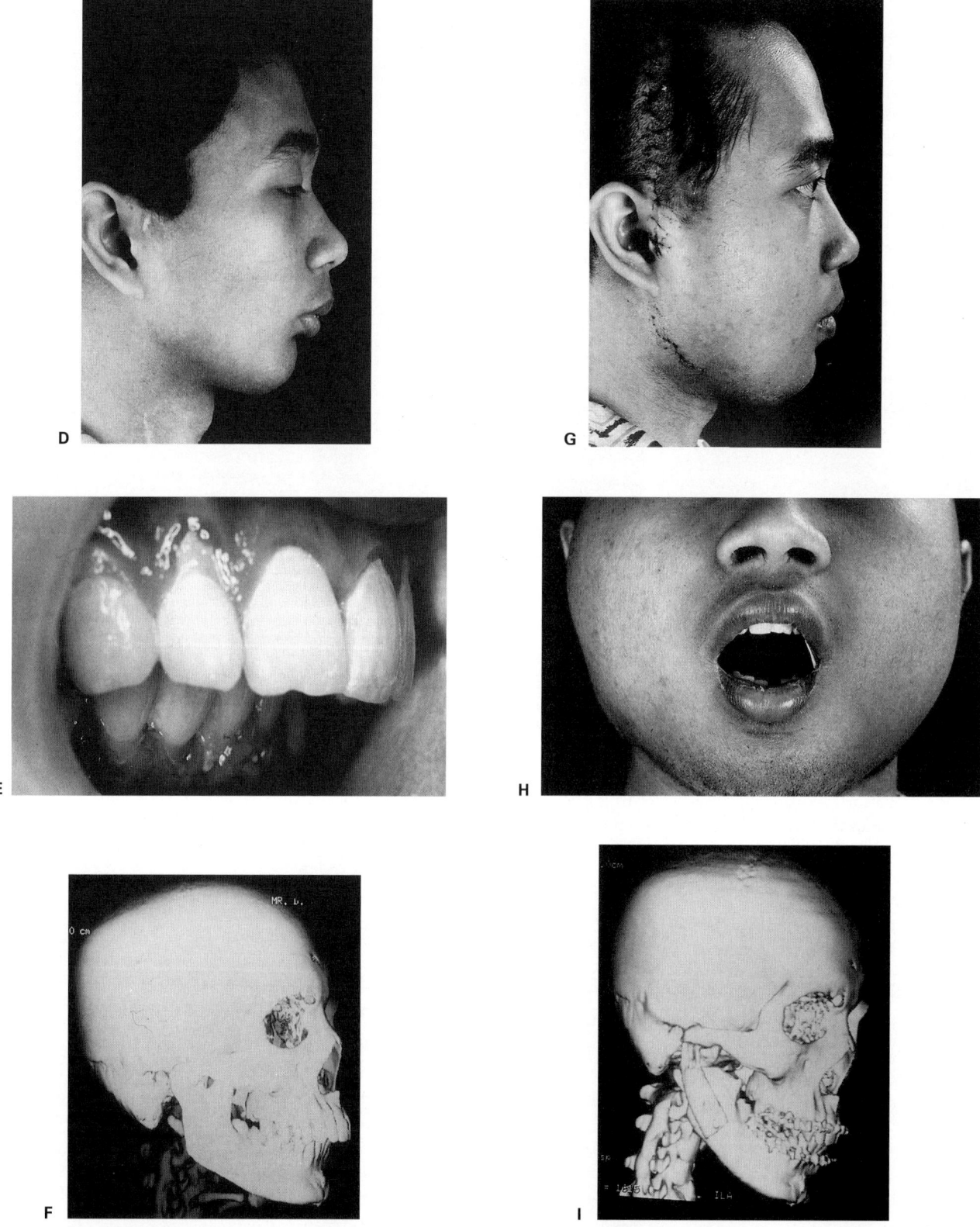

Fig. 21.63 Case 2: ankylosis in adult life. A man was injured in a vehicular accident at the age of 21 years, in another country. He suffered an impact on his chin which drove both condyles into the mandibular fossae. He had no initial treatment and the condyles fused with the skull base, producing ankylosis and retrognathia. **D** The situation at presentation 10 months after injury. **E** The occlusion with no movement of the lower jaw. **F** The lateral 3D CT scan showing the foreshortening and fusion of the jaw with the base of skull. **G** The situation after costochondral graft. **H** The degree of opening, gently controlled with a very light rubber band. **I** Postoperative 3D CT scan.

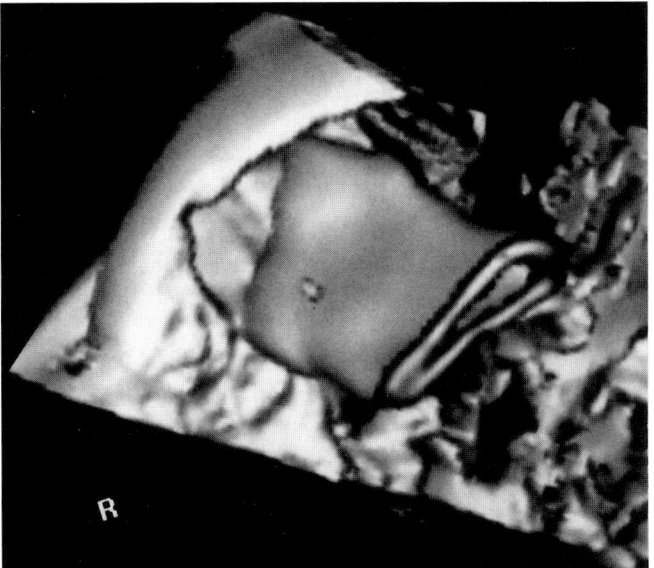

A

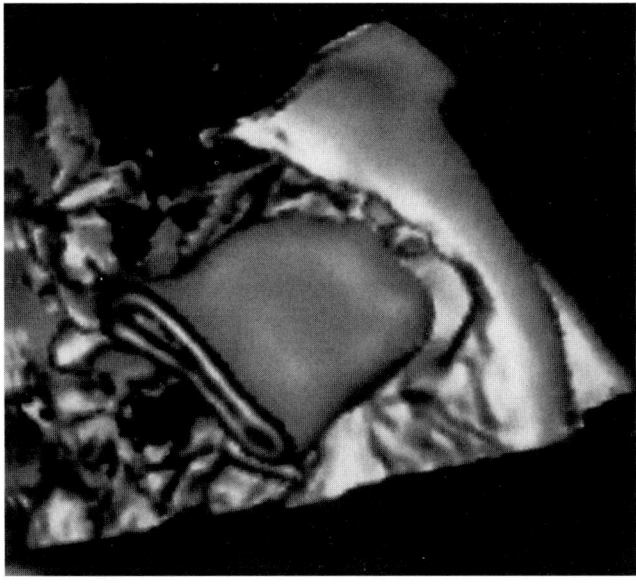

B

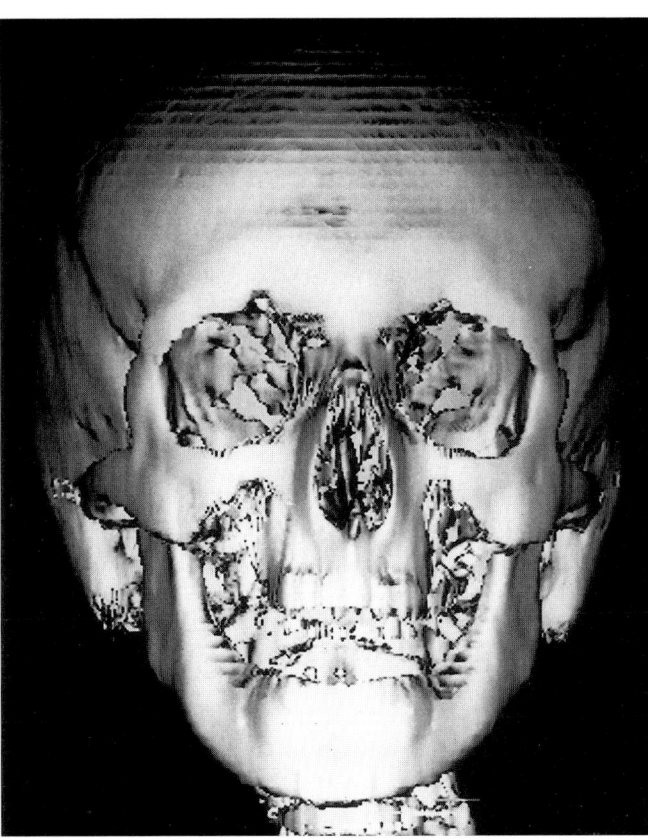

C

Fig. 21.64 Extensive surgical treatment of temporomandibular joints. Three-dimensional reconstructions of the temporomandibular joints after radical excision in a woman who had undergone numerous operations for bilateral temporomandibular joint ankylosis. This is a cautionary tale, as the problem started with supposed minor trauma and pain with some joint clicking, and proceeded to increasingly radical excision of her jaw joints. The last procedure involved replacement with carved Silastic®, which was subsequently extruded. The woman presented complaining of persistent intense pain and further restriction of movement. Under general anaesthesia, however, the jaw opened easily to 4.5 cm.
A 3D reconstruction of the right joint, seen obliquely from below where the mandible has been resected at the level of the sigmoid notch. The reconstruction has been cut away below for clarity.
B Similar view of the left side. **C** Frontal view 3D reconstruction, with the foreshortened mandible recessed beneath the zygomatic arches.

however, we have observed changes in the shape of the cartilaginous component and a diminishing of the vertical height in some cases over time. Where pain has become part of the symptom complex, it may or may not be diminished; when it is not, we are faced with the ongoing difficulties of the patient who suffers chronic pain in this region (p. 659) (Fig. 21.64).

MANDIBULAR DEFORMITIES

Surgical pathology

Residual deformities of the mandible may be extensive and grotesque, especially after gunshot wounds. Deformity may result from loss of tissue, from non-union or from malunion due to inadequate treatment — or no treatment at all. The consequences in terms of function and form depend on the extent of the malunion and on its site. The mandible supports the tongue through its extrinsic muscles, especially the genioglossus (p. 68); deformity of the mental region may affect speech and

is operated on, the more likely it is to recur. Nevertheless Ohno et al (1981) favour early operation to restore normal growth. These two views are not incompatible. The cases described in Figs 21.58–63 exemplify our management of ankylosis in childhood and the results which can reasonably be expected.

In the adult, we favour the insertion of a costochondral graft as a space-filler after wide release of the ankylosis;

swallowing while complete absence of the mandible in this region may affect the airway by allowing the tongue to fall back. The aesthetic consequences of mandibular ablation or deformity can be appalling. For a century, surgeons have been looking for a suitable material to replace the damaged or absent mandible. Metals, acrylic and bone have had their advocates, but autogenous bone is of course the material of choice in replacing mandibular defects.

If malunion occurs during the period of growth there may not only be malposition of the fragments but also deformity of the whole mandible, which is misshapen by altered growth dynamics: there is antigonial notching, deviation to the affected side and a shortened body. The chin may manifest the deformity most clearly and its shape depends on whether the mandibular lesion is unilateral or bilateral (Souyris 1990). Not only is the chin deviated to the affected side, but it is also retruded, with a secondary effect on the lower lip which may be everted. In the bilateral lesions there is typically a retruded misshapen mandible and deformed chin.

Assessment

In cases of malunion and non-union there is malocclusion, loss of chewing efficiency, pain, and perhaps stress on the TMJ. In cases with widely distracted bone ends and fibrous union, there is abnormal mobility. The symptoms relate to the malocclusion and to the malfunction of the jaw, as well as to the aesthetic deformity. On clinical inspection, the defects of the face may be obvious; palpation should confirm the abnormal mobility.

The work-up includes photography, radiology and dental assessment, which includes attention to the condition of the teeth, the taking of impressions, and the production of dental casts for study models used in multidisciplinary planning. In the preparation of a management plan, the opinion of the team prosthodontist will often be decisive.

Management

Principles of treatment

Surgical reconstruction may entail operations carried out on the alveolar process of the mandible, operations to change the shape of the body or ramus, operations to change the position and shape of the chin, and operations combining any or all of these.

Where there is loss of tissue a decision has to be taken concerning bone grafting of the mandible. If the defect is at the angle behind the tooth-bearing part of the bone, some small extent of approximation of the posterior and main fragments is permissible to close the gap. However, in the tooth-bearing part of the bone the fragments must be placed in their correct occlusion with the upper

jaw and the defect must be grafted. This situation occurs most typically after gunshot wounds causing massive tissue loss.

Mandibular deformity in edentulous patients

Special consideration must be given to secondary deformity due to malunion in the edentulous mandible. Minimal deformity may be compensated for by the prosthodontist in the manufacture of a prosthesis. More severe malunion may make it impossible for dentures to be worn and the decision to offer surgical correction may depend on the ability to construct an adequate denture. The decision should therefore be made in conjunction with the prosthodontist. Surgical problems occur especially in the elderly where the bone is atrophic: it may be very difficult to treat a deformity which requires refracturing, plating and immobilization with Gunning splints, all requiring the greatest possible respect for the poor blood supply of the ageing bone (p. 518).

Surgical correction

After the multidisciplinary work-up has been completed, three types of treatment are available:

1. Refracturing and resetting the bone with minimal bone grafting
2. Osteotomies to re-establish a suitable occlusion and/or facial shape
3. Bone grafting defects of the ramus or body of the mandible together with onlay bone grafts to recontour the misshapen bone.

Refracture and reposition

An operative plan is made after preliminary model surgery and subsequent preparation of an acrylic wafer. This wafer determines the correct relationship of the teeth and hence the new position of the jaw. The dental models are available in the operating theatre; from these models, preformed arch bars are manufactured before the operation. X-ray pictures show the position of the fracture and its relationship to the tooth roots. An appropriate surgical approach is made to the region of the fracture; this may be through either an intraoral or an external submandibular incision.

When the fracture site is exposed, the fracture is divided and the method of division depends on how solid the fracture is. If solid it may require division with a power saw; if not, mobilization by gentle insertion of an osteotome is sufficient. Callus and other interposed tissues are removed and the bone ends are freshened. Intermaxillary fixation is then established to place the jaws in predetermined position, the condyles being enlocated in the glenoid fossa. The bone fragments may then be plated. If there is still a small gap, cancellous bone from the hip is placed into the space. The plating technique employed in stabilizing osteotomies of the body and angle is usually monocortical (p. 271), using two plates in the body and one plate at the angle. In most cases, intermaxillary fixation may be removed at the end of the operation. In patients who are less likely to be compliant or who may be lost to medium- and long-term follow-up, bicortical plating system is used with a stronger plate and/or intermaxillary fixation, which is established for 1 month or as long as the patient's tolerance will permit within this time.

Osteotomies

Repositioning the body and ramus of the mandible deformed by trauma and malunion can be achieved by a variety of osteotomies. The workhorse in our unit is the sagittal split osteotomy of Trauner & Obwegeser (1957) and Dal Pont (1961). Corrections in the anteroposterior plane are well tolerated. Correction of asymmetry is less well tolerated as TMJ pain may result from angular and/or rotational stresses on the proximal fragment on the side to which the jaw is being moved. The mandible can also be rotated after a sagittal split osteotomy to correct an anterior open bite. This manoeuvre is said to be limited by the natural tendency for recurrence of the deformity from the pull of muscles opposing the correction. This tendency is recognized but has been diminished by the use of rigid screw fixation of the fragments. Side-to-side movements are well accomplished by the vertical subsigmoid osteotomy, which does not rotate or push the joint-bearing fragments laterally. More extensive lengthening of the ramus and angle region can be accomplished by the inverted 'L' osteotomy with interpositional bone grafting. This is the surgical treatment most often used in patients suffering from the 'bird face' deformity resulting from severe mandibular damage during growth.

Sagittal split osteotomy of the ramus

The technique develops the principle of the sagittal osteotomy which produces overlap of fragments. Trauner & Obwegeser (1957) applied the split to the retromolar region; Dal Pont (1961) extended the area of contact along the lateral cortical plate of the mandible (Fig. 21.65).

Like all intraoral osteotomy procedures on the jaws, the operation is very dependent upon the use of appropriate tools, adequate assistance and good lighting by a head lamp. An adrenaline-containing solution carefully injected under the periosteal plane on both sides of the mandibular ramus is very helpful in controlling bleeding and in defining the plane of dissection. The incision is small, ~3 cm in length, and runs a little lateral to the anterior line of the ramus. It extends downward over the buccal surface of the body of the mandible to the region of the second molar tooth; care is taken to keep the incision sufficiently far lateral to leave enough soft tissue for easy closure at the end of the operation. The cut is made down to the bone. The lateral aspect of the mandible is then dissected in the subperiosteal plane. The masseter muscle is lifted away to allow the introduction of a Munro–Dautrey retractor, the lip of which fits around the ramus, angle or body of the mandible depending on the area being operated upon. The posterior attachment of the muscle sling must be dissected sufficiently to allow this protective metal retractor to be fully located. However, the surgeon must be mindful not to detach more muscle than is necessary to achieve this as every bit of blood supply to the bony fragments is helpful. The medial dissection is carried out above the level of the lingula; a channel retractor protects the neurovascular bundles.

The instruments and techniques for performing the osteotomy vary. The horizontal cut is made just above the lingula through the medial cortex: we prefer a Lindemann burr on a Hall drill to facilitate this, but some operators use a sagittal saw. The lower the cut the thicker the bone but the more risk to the neurovascular bundle, so good judgement has to be used in siting this horizontal cut. As originally described the cut extends to the posterior border of the mandible; Hunsuck (1968) made the cut to just beyond the mandibular foramen before the bone starts to thin off towards the posterior border, thus producing a more robust lateral fragment. The cut is extended down the anterior border of the mandible, medial to the oblique line. Classically, this is done by a series of burrholes which are then connected. With more experience the operator can dispense with burrholes and make the cut with a series of stroking movements of a sharp side-cutting burr. The lateral cortical cut is made vertically in the region of the second molar tooth. The lower border can and must be effectively cut through and care must be taken to 'pop' through the outer cortex in the region of the neurovascular bundle and the tooth roots. Throughout the procedure, the retractor is moved by the assistant to protect the soft tissues. The original splitting technique used a thick wedge osteotome inserted into the osteotomy and with a twisting movement split the two fragments asunder; insertion of the osteotome was done with the protection of a 'ring of steel' supplied by the retractors. Dautrey (1974) introduced an elegant osteotome designed to cleave the cortices apart with the curve towards the outer cortex. With this technique, the inferior dental nerve is safer from brutal surgery, but the outer cortex may be breached if it is fragile and great care must be used to position the protecting retractors to prevent damage to the adjacent soft tissues. Unless the protection of the soft tissue is meticulous, the use of this sharp osteotome in a cleaving technique makes it possible to damage the facial nerve by plunging the osteotome into the substance of the cheek (Jones & Van Sickels 1991). After the split has been achieved the fragments are gently separated and the neurovascular

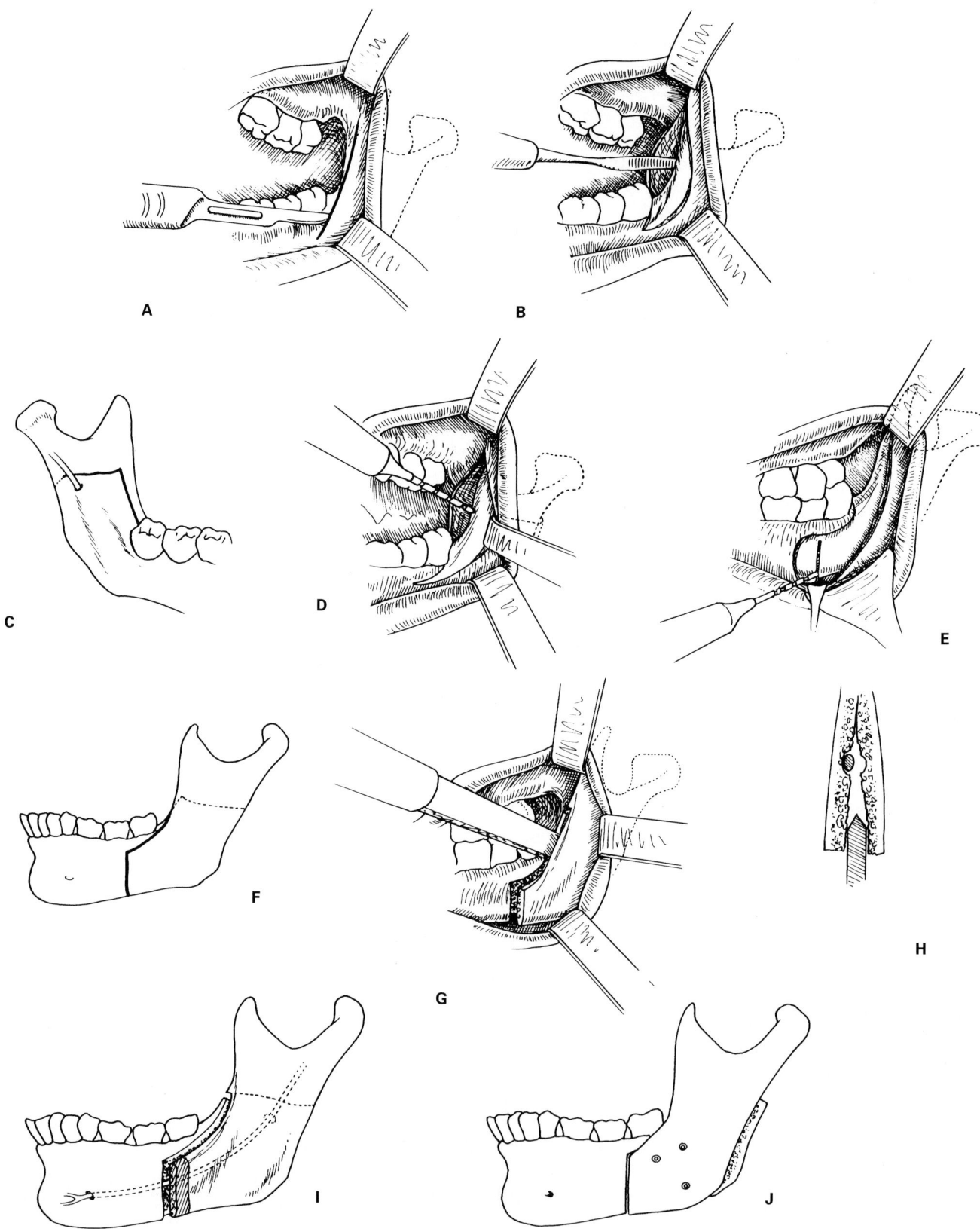

Fig. 21.65 Sagittal split osteotomy technique. A Intraoral incision just lateral to the anterior border of the mandibular ramus, extended to the bone over the external oblique ridge. **B** Elevation of the flaps medially and laterally. **C** Schematic view of the osteotomy as if seen from the medial aspect. **D** Medial cut being made with a side-cutting burr. The soft tissues are protected by the channel retractor. **E** Vertical component of the lateral cut. **F** Schematic representation of the line of the split. **G** Cleaving or splitting of the fragments. **H** Separation of the lateral fragment (proximal segment) away from the neurovascular bundle. **I** Osteotomy segments in new position. **J** Positioning of the screws for rigid fixation.

bundle is preserved and if necessary teased out of any attachments to the lateral fragment.

When the fragments have been freed on both sides, the tooth-bearing components are fixed into position with the maxilla using the preformed acrylic wafer. For fixation, it is our custom to use orthodontic bands to which are attached fine arch bars; this appliance is usually fixed earlier, thus saving time at operation. The wafer is tied to the maxilla with fine wires with the twists above the acrylic wafer for easy identification. The intermaxillary fixation is achieved with further wiring or tightly twisted rubber bands. The proximal fragment is then grasped with a long artery forcep and the condylar head properly located in the fossa. It is very important to do this lest

there be movement and relapse postoperatively. Some surgeons have devised special techniques to ensure exact placing. A miniplate may be attached to the proximal fragment of the mandible prior to the osteotomy and the other end attached to an identifiable point on the maxilla, usually a slot in the maxillary appliance. The miniplate is then removed and replaced in the same situation after the osteotomy has been made; the jaw is thus repositioned to ensure that the proximal fragment is in its original position and well seated into the condylar fossa. We have not had the necessity for this or any other similar device. With the proximal fragment held in position and the teeth in occlusion the bone fragments are secured by percutaneous insertion of three screws, two above and one below

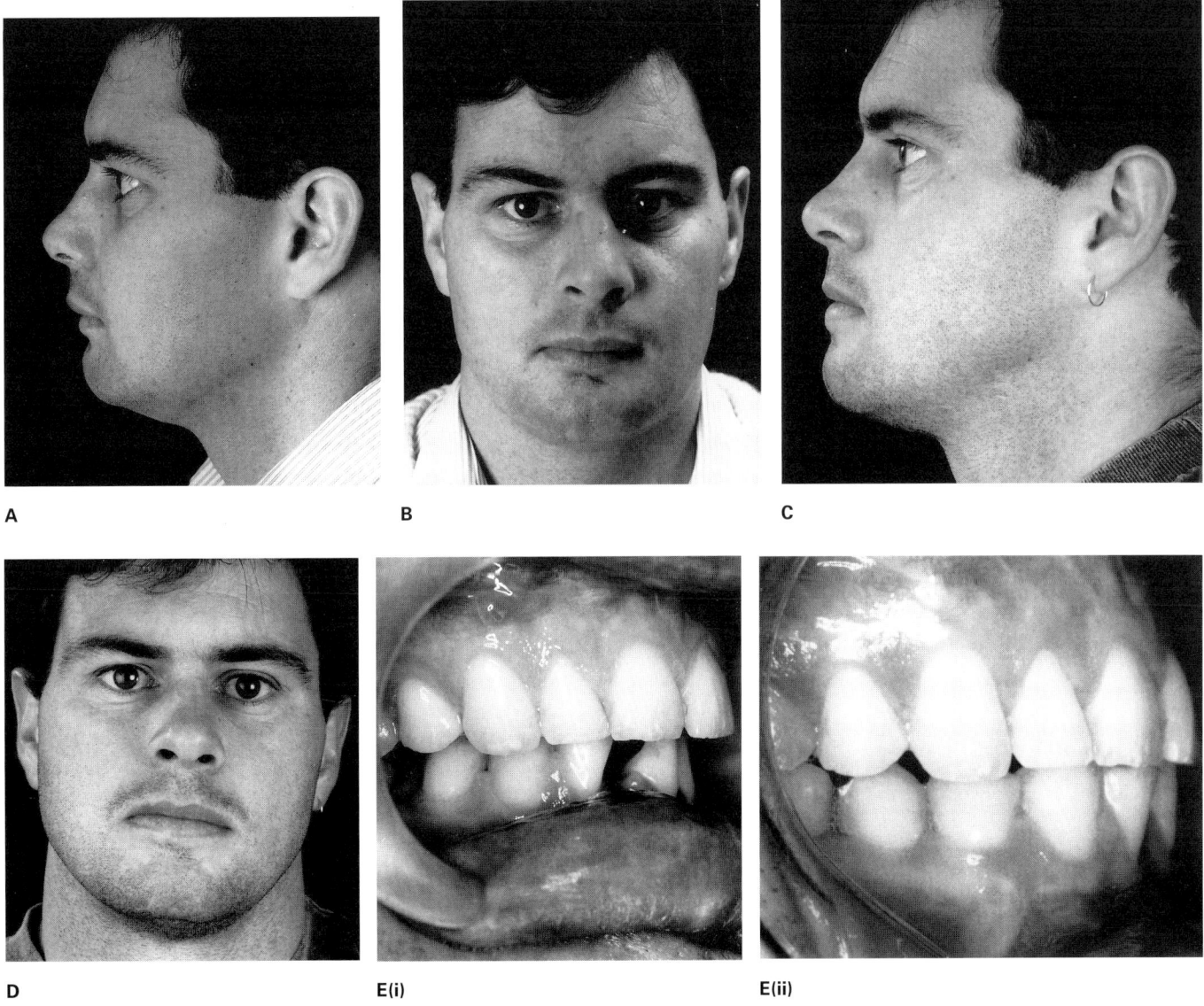

A   **B**   **C**

D   **E(i)**   **E(ii)**

Fig. 21.66 Post-traumatic retrognathia. A young man had a malposition of his mandible. He had subsequent advancement of 11 mm on one side and 7 mm on the other to centralize his facial skeleton and reconstitute the pre-injury facial appearance. **A** Retruded profile. **B** Facial asymmetry, including the nose. **C** Postoperative profile. **D** Facial symmetry improved in the final result.
E (i, ii) Occlusion before and after surgery and orthodontic treatment.

the neurovascular bundle. To achieve this the operator needs good lighting, good assistance and the appropriate use of retractors. The intermaxillary fixation is released to check the occlusion and to check that the mandible will easily come into the new position. It is a matter of judgement of the severity of the deformity as to whether the patient is left in intermaxillary fixation at this stage or not. The facial stab wounds used for percutaneous screw fixation of the mandibular fragments are closed with 6/0 nylon and the intraoral wounds with 3/0 chromic cat gut sutures. We do not dress these wounds. It is a common custom to use dexamethasone postoperatively to reduce swelling; this is not our practice. Ice-packs are used by some for the same purpose. The jaws may need to be supported with interdental rubber bands over the next few weeks and this need is monitored very carefully by the surgeon and orthodontist (Fig. 21.66).

Vertical subsigmoid ramus osteotomy (Fig. 21.67)

This osteotomy was originally used for the correction of mandibular prognathism (Caldwell & Letterman 1954) and has undergone a number of modifications. In post-traumatic cases we have used the subsigmoid ramus osteotomy when there is a tilting of the occlusal plane and where there is a necessity for significant lateral movement of the mandibular segment. Using this the condylar fragment can remain enlocated, unangulated and unrotated in the new position of the mandible.

An *intraoral approach* has become popular. The obvious advantage is the absence of an external scar, but others include simple and rapid dissection and virtual elimination of risk to the facial nerve. A 3 cm incision is made over the external oblique ridge of the mandible parallel with and just inferior to the mucogingival junction. This placement avoids formation of a scar in the buccal sulcus, which often creates an annoying 'food trap'. Blunt dissection reflects the periosteum from the entirety of the lateral surface of the ramus, which is fully visualized with Bauer retractors placed in the sigmoid and antegonial notches. To afford the greatest protection to the inferior alveolar nerve, the initial osteotomy is made with an oscillating saw 6–7 mm anterior from the posterior border of the ramus, and therefore just posterior to the antilingula if one is discernible. From this starting point the osteotomy is carried superiorly to end at the sigmoid notch and inferiorly to end just forward of the gonial angle. Various authors have advocated trimming or grooving of the proximal segment to improve positioning during the healing phase. Although there has been a trend toward shorter periods of intermaxillary fixation, several weeks at least are necessary to prevent postoperative malocclusion.

Because rigid fixation and minimal use of intermaxillary fixation have become priorities in our unit, and

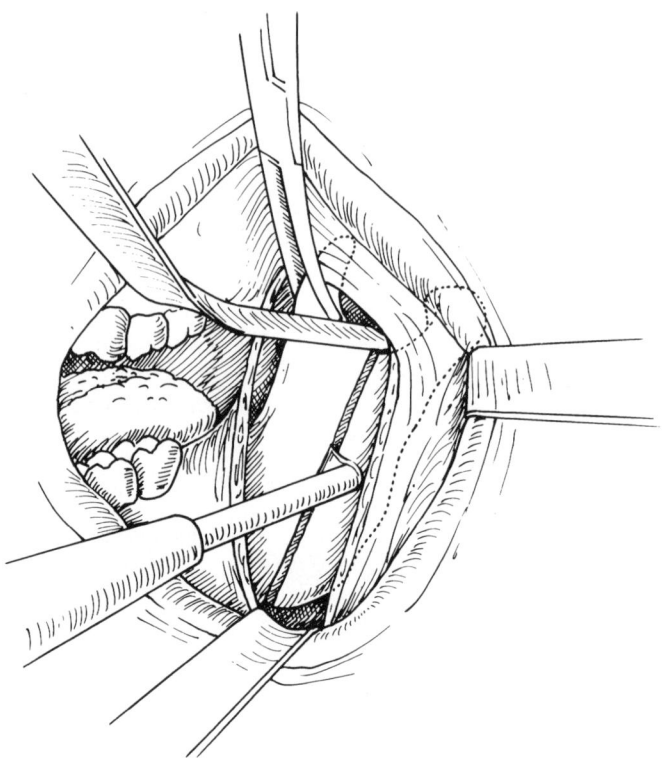

Fig. 21.67 Intraoral approach to the subsigmoid osteotomy (after Bell et al 1992). Incision is made over the external oblique ridge as for the sagittal split osteotomy, and subperiosteal dissection exposes the lateral aspect of the ramus. Retractors secured at the sigmoid and antegonial notches allow broad access, and the osteotomy is performed with an oscillating saw 6–7 mm from the posterior border of the ramus.

a satisfactory technique for achieving this from the intraoral approach has yet to be devised, we have favoured the *external approach*. The incision is 2–3 cm in length and 1 cm below the angle of the mandible. The platysma is incised at a lower level than the skin and lifted superiorly with care to avoid the mandibular branch of the facial nerve (Fig. 21.68). The lower border of the mandible is approached by blunt dissection and the muscles and periosteum are elevated from the body up to the sigmoid notch on both lateral and medial surfaces of the mandible, care being taken to dissect posterior to the lingula. A malleable retractor placed on the deep surface and an angulated retractor with a reverse lip fitting into the sigmoid notch give together good protection and exposure. The osteotomy is made with a reciprocating saw. The cut extends from the depths of the sigmoid notch to a point in front of the angle of the mandible. When the osteotomies have been completed on both sides the position of the distal segment is determined by intermaxillary fixation with an acrylic wafer. Care is taken to have the posterior segments relatively unangulated and the condyles correctly placed in the glenoid fossa. The bone fragments can then be rigidly fixed with plates and/or screws. It has

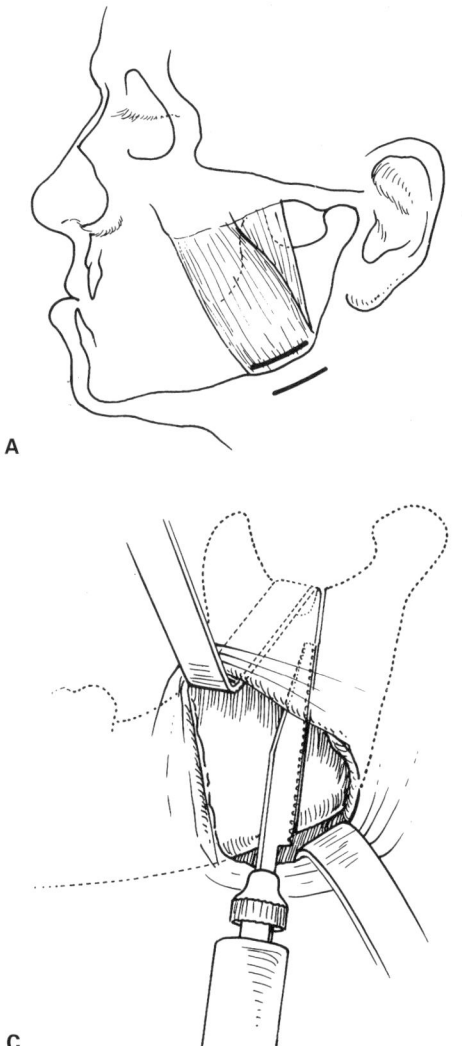

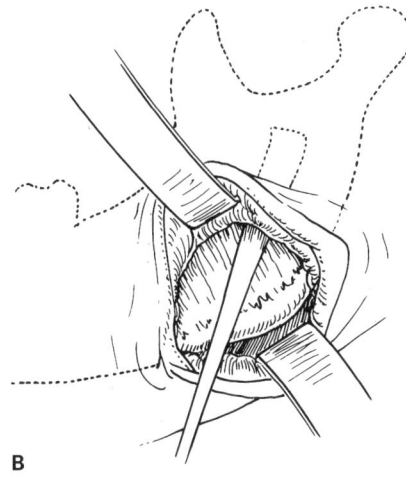

Fig. 21.68 External approach to the subsigmoid osteotomy.
A Incision is made below the angle of the mandible specifically to avoid the mandibular branch of the facial nerve. The masseter is divided from the inferior border. **B** Subperiosteal dissection on both sides of the mandible posterior to the entry of the neurovascular bundle. **C** Adequate protection with retractors allows the osteotomy to be safely performed with a reciprocating saw.

been said that rigid fixation of these fragments is not possible (McCarthy et al 1990b) but this has not been our experience. The wounds are closed in layers without drainage. The jaw is supported with intermaxillary fixation for a short period of time postoperatively; this may be achieved with rubber bands (Fig. 21.69).

Inverted L osteotomy of the ramus

This osteotomy is applicable in cases of severe mandibular hypoplasia resulting from trauma during growth (Fig. 21.70). Where significant forward projection has to be achieved and where the TMJ joint is functional or has been made to function, the L-osteotomy of the ramus is performed at the point above the entry of the neuro-vascular bundle. The TMJ, the coronoid process, and the posterior part of the ramus are left in position, and the body and angle together with the nerve and blood supply are advanced and rotated. The intervening gap may then

be bone-grafted. This approach leaves the opportunity for variation in the rotation of the tooth-bearing fragment and hence in the shape of the bone graft used to fill the gap. The bone graft is fashioned in such a way as to augment the shape of the mandible in the region of the angle. Wassmund described such an osteotomy in 1927 and Rushton (1942) also reported the osteotomy combined with bone grafting.

The ramus is exposed through the submandibular neck incision described above. The masseter and medial pterygoid muscles are elevated and the muscle sling is widely released. A horizontal osteotomy is placed above the entry of the neurovascular bundle and continued verti-cally to the lower border. After wide soft-tissue dissection, which is necessary to advance the mandible, the jaws are fixed into position with the preformed bite wafer and intermaxillary fixation. The bone graft is then inserted and fixed with miniplates. Further bone grafting may be needed to fashion the angle and enhance the stability.

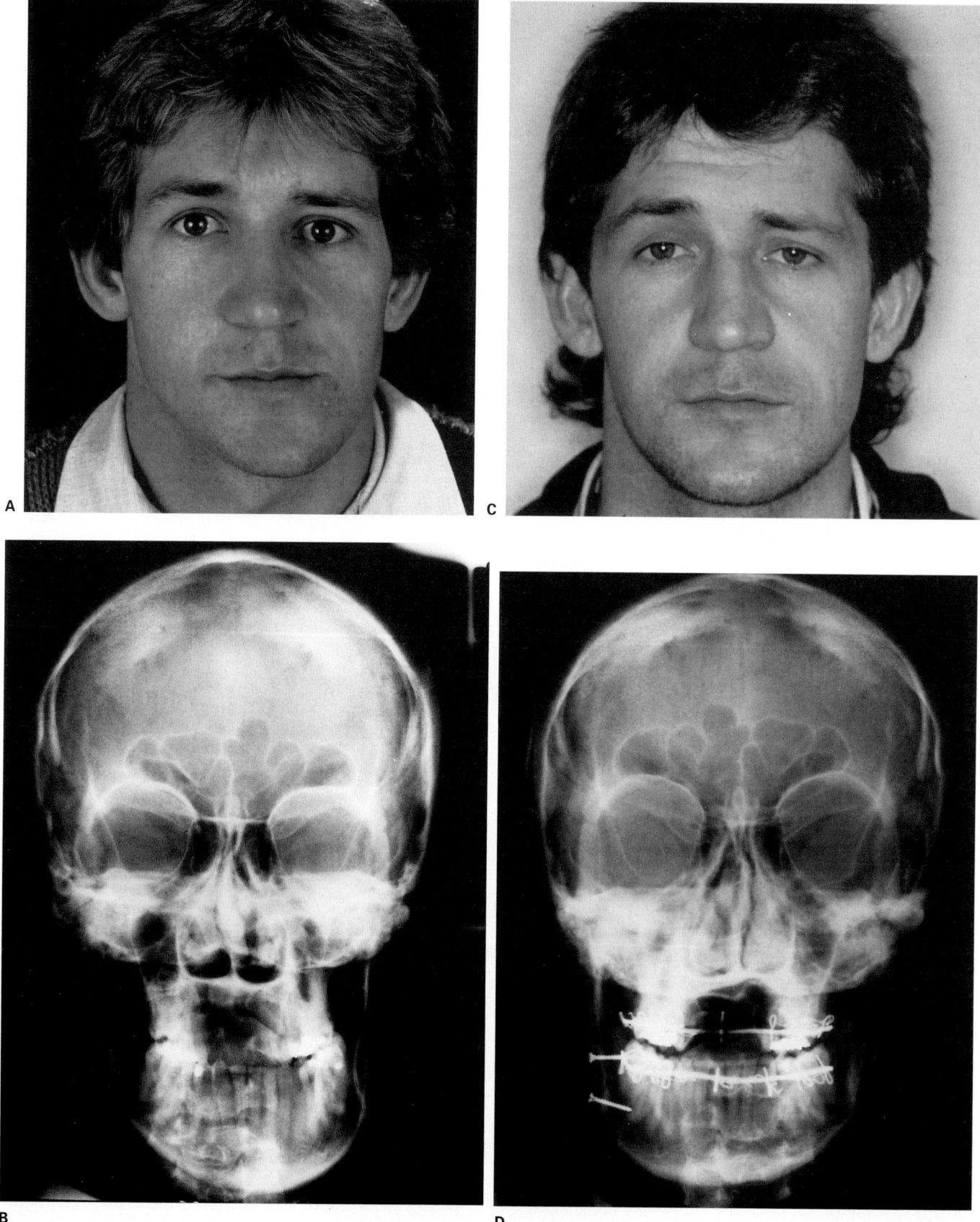

Fig. 21.69 Post-traumatic asymmetry with mandibular deviation. A childhood injury led to asymmetric facial growth. **A** Asymmetry with deviation of the chin to the left. **B** X-ray further demonstrates the defect. **C** Postoperative appearance showing the restored symmetry. **D** Vertical subsigmoid osteotomy was performed on the right side and sagittal split osteotomy on the left. Intermaxillary fixation with lag screws fixing the two overlapping fragments on the right side.

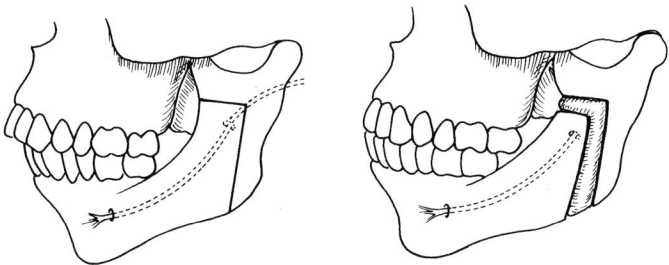

Fig. 21.70 Inverted 'L' osteotomy. The inverted 'L' ramus osteotomy is performed above the entrance of the neurovascular bundle. After freeing the muscles, the distal segment can be distracted and bone graft inserted into the gaps. Plate fixation is preferred. There may be both onlay and inlay components in the bone grafting.

Restoration of chin position and shape

In the post-traumatic setting, restructuring of the chin can best be made by osteotomies with or without bone grafting. There is an extensive literature concerning chin restoration with alloplastic materials such as silicone rubber; in our view, these techniques are best reserved for minor cosmetic deformities where there is no associated soft-tissue or bony damage (Fig. 21.71).

A horizontal osteotomy can be used to reshape the chin in three dimensions, moving the mobilized chin forwards, backwards, laterally and/or upwards, as well as downwards, when an intervening bone graft is needed. The surgical approach is made by a degloving dissection begun in the buccal sulcus. The incision is initially made through adequate soft tissue and passes obliquely down to the bone leaving some muscle on the dental side. Subperiosteal dissection leaves the soft tissue adherent to the chin point; the mental foramina are located and cleared. A reciprocating saw will easily make the osteotomy at the desired level, with wide clearance of the tooth roots. The posterior muscle attachments of the chin point can be retained for all but the 'jump' type of advancement, in which the distal segment is advanced and jumped entirely on top of the proximal segment. In all other chin reconstructions the attachments are left to ensure the

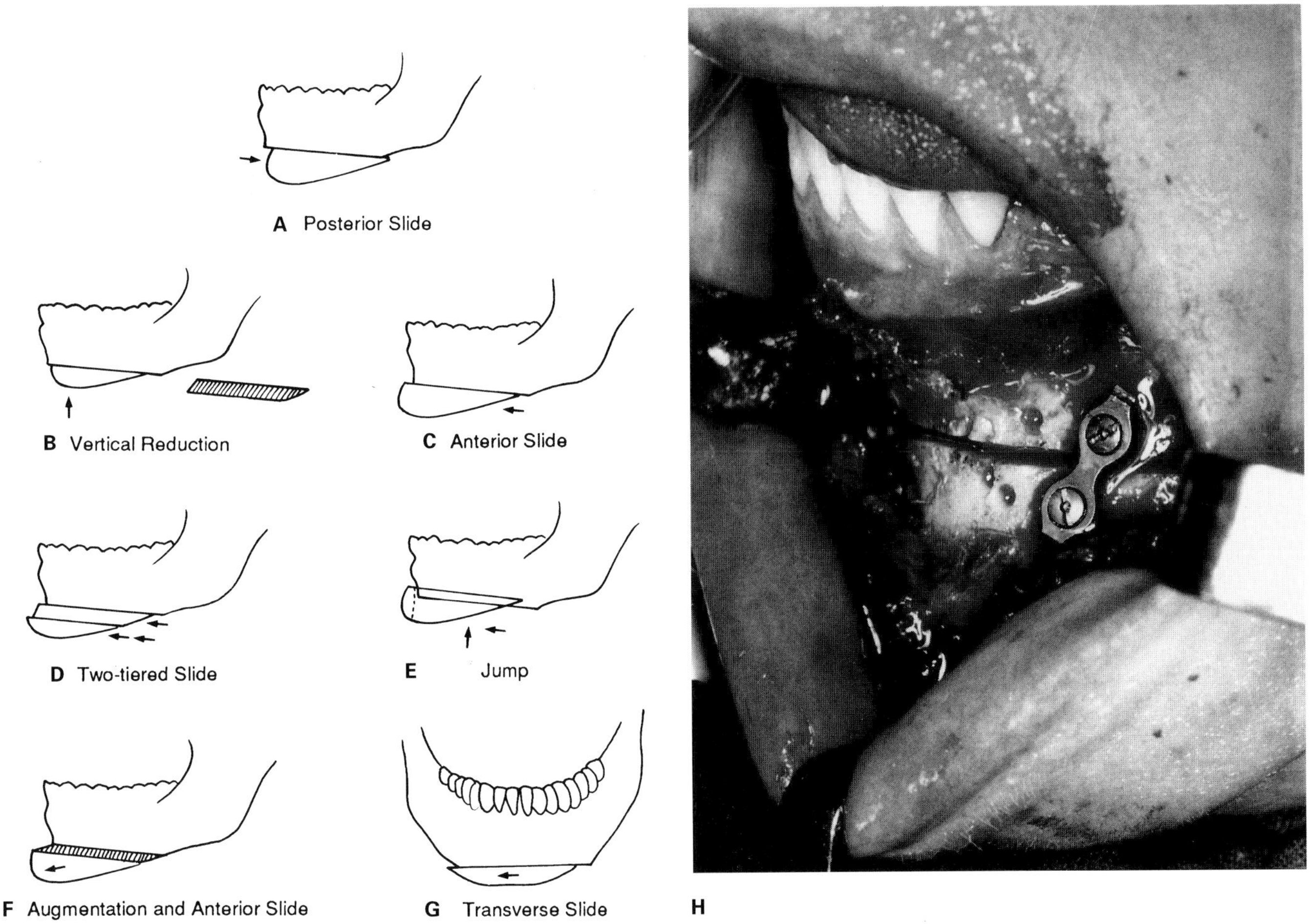

A Posterior Slide

B Vertical Reduction

C Anterior Slide

D Two-tiered Slide

E Jump

F Augmentation and Anterior Slide

G Transverse Slide

H

Fig. 21.71 Genioplasty. A–G A variety of repositioning osteotomies can be performed on the chin using similar basic technique: retrusion, vertical reduction, advancement, 'jumping,' side-to-side, and bone grafting as onlay or inlay. **H** Reduction genioplasty. The osteotomy is placed inferior to the mental foramina and the fragments are fixed with a pair of two-hole titanium plates.

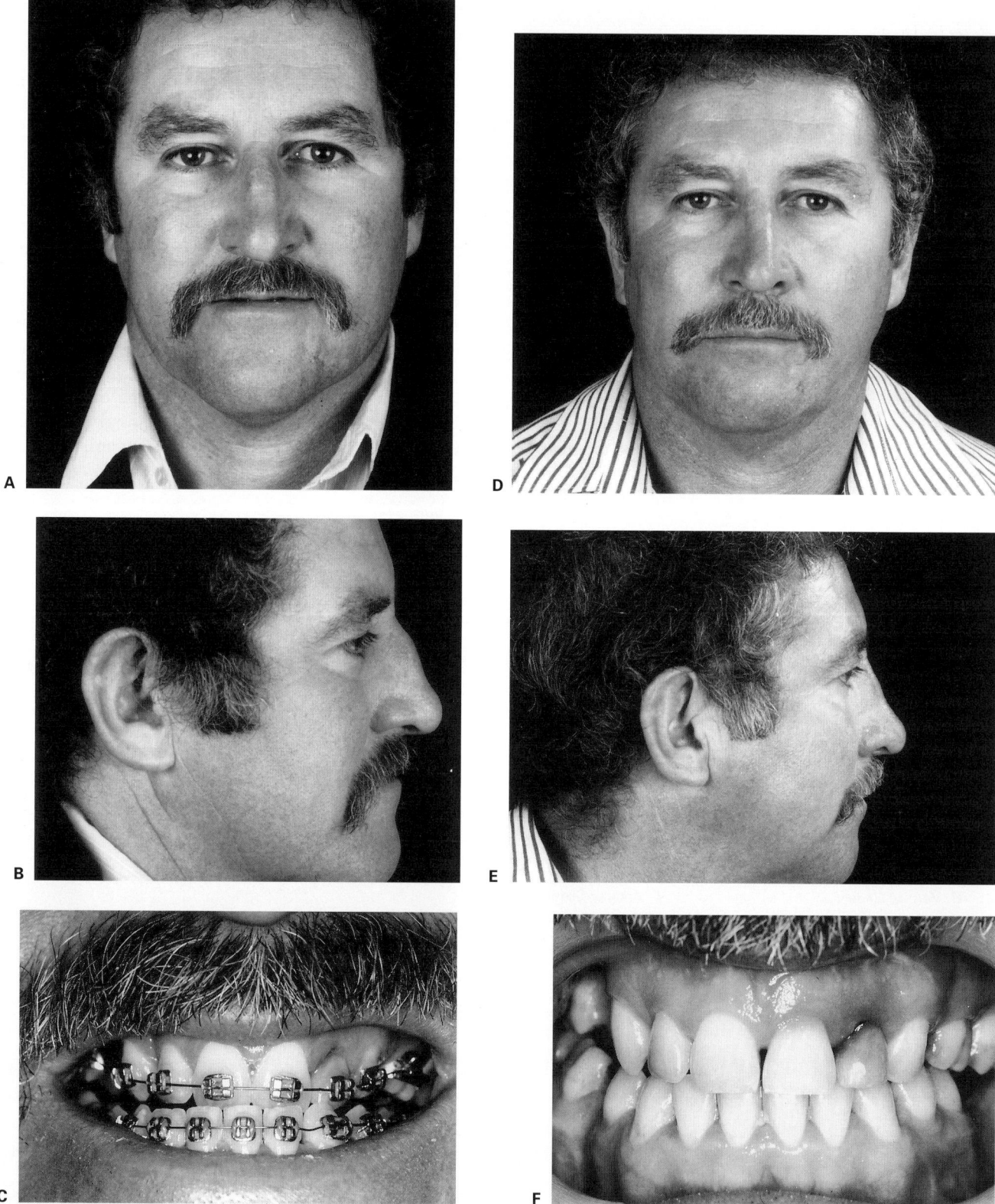

Fig. 21.72 Traumatic displacement with pre-existing skeletal deformity. 'It is an ill wind that blows no good.' A middle-aged man presented with a mandibular fracture which was accurately reduced, restoring him to his previous class III malocclusion. 2 years later he presented with a maxillary fracture and requested that his occlusion and facial shape be changed at this opportune time. **A** Anteroposterior view after the first mandibular fracture. **B** Profile view. **C** Close-up view of the occlusion with orthodontic treatment in progress. **D** Profile view. **E** Occlusion after the maxillary fracture has been repositioned anteriorly. **F** Facial appearance after the second fracture has been corrected.

blood supply to the fragment and to move the soft-tissue attachments with the bone. It is important when reducing the chin that the segment removed is taken from the body of the chin, not the chin point: if the point is resected, the soft tissue may fall away from its bony support, producing the 'witches chin' appearance (Gonzalez-Ulloa 1972). The fragment or fragments can be manipulated according to the surgical plan. Fixation is achieved by plates and/or screws. Two titanium miniplates may be used, but direct screwing is possible where there is an overlay of the apposed bones.

Contour restoration of body and ramus

It is unusual for the shape of the body of the mandible to need alteration after injury, but onlay grafts are sometimes needed to correct contour defects. Onlay bone grafting to the lower border of the mandible has been much enhanced in efficiency by the ability to secure the grafts rigidly with screws. Exposure can be via the degloving approach or externally through the submandibular incision described on p. 612.

Complications and results

In our experience, osteotomies performed on patients who have acquired a mandibular deformity from trauma complicated by non-union or malunion and whose growth is complete, do not produce different complications or different results from osteotomies performed for other reasons. However, there are two important points to make about the aesthetic outcome of these osteotomies.

First, the assessment of the patient must provide a detailed appraisal of the deficit that existed as a result of the trauma itself, and/or previous surgery, as the results of the current treatment must be seen against this background. Second, the treating team must have a clear knowledge of any preexisting congenital deformity, and clearly separate, in the minds of both the treating team and the patient, what is to be achieved by the current treating plan. The question as to whether the aim is to return the mandible to its pretraumatic state or to an ideal state must be spelled out (Fig. 21.72).

The results are less predictable when the primary deformity has occurred during growth, for example the bird face deformity; in such cases, a compromise between ideal occlusion and facial form may be necessary.

The chief complications of mandibular osteotomy are infection, recurrent deformity and nerve damage.

Infection

Prophylactic antibiotics are used during surgery and for 24 h postoperative; nevertheless, and not surprisingly, infection is an important complication in most reported series. In 236 cases of mandibular osteotomy, our infection rate is 2.2%. Onlay bone grafts of the angle of the body of the mandible have been in our experience especially prone to infection. The use of rigid fixation with titanium screws has improved the infection rate and decreased the resorption rate; however, more than half our patients treated with onlay grafts have had trouble with infection and resorption in this site. If infection does occur it generally will not settle until the underlying screw, plate or bony sequestrum is removed.

Recurrent deformity

This can be due to bad planning, bad execution of the surgery or massive infection and loss of bone.

Nerve damage

This may result from the original injury; it is therefore very important to examine the status of the fifth and seventh nerves before operation. The cervical branch of the seventh nerve may be damaged during the submandibular approach, although we have seen no occurrence of this in nearly 20 years of practice. The trunk of the facial nerve may be damaged as a result of poor technique in the sagittal split osteotomy. We have one experience where there was a temporary facial paresis. The nerve was explored and found to be intact but swollen and oedematous; spontaneous recovery took place. The inferior dental nerve is easily injured in mandibular osteotomy; in patients where this nerve was not been previously damaged almost 50% showed some sensory deficit for up to a year after definitive surgery and 15% have remained with some permanent sensory loss.

MASSIVE DEFECTS OF THE MANDIBLE AND MAXILLA

Surgical pathology

Deformities entailing massive bone and soft-tissue loss are most commonly due to missile wounds; pathology, general management and treatment strategies are discussed in Chapter 16. The size of the bone defect needing replacement and the quantity and the quality of the soft tissues in the area are the pathological factors of chief relevance in planning a reconstruction. Also important are foci of chronic infection, which may form around indriven bone chips and tooth fragments.

The mandible has received prime attention. It is not only of importance for facial appearance but is also vital functionally since it supports the tongue; it is necessary for mastication, speech and maintenance of the airway. There appears to be relatively little written on the techniques of reconstruction for major deficiencies of the maxilla: nevertheless, these deficiencies are also very deforming and may be associated with defects of jaw function and airway, as well as with damage to the eyes.

Assessment

Investigations include the radiological imaging necessary to determine the size and shape of the bone defect and if necessary the nature of any associated TMJ dysfunction. In these, 3D reconstruction from the CT scan comes into its own, as it not only gives a very good image of the bone shape to be replaced but also displays the abnormal positions and relationships of the fragments. Programs are now available which are able to model the shape and size of the defect to produce a template upon which the bone graft can be modelled. Dental models help in surgical planning to restore whatever occlusion can be salvaged, and are also useful in defining the bony and soft-tissue defects. Speech, swallowing and oral competence are necessarily affected by massive trauma of the jaws; the team speech pathologists are therefore involved in the planning, assessment and rehabilitation of these patients (Fig. 21.73).

Principles of management

The history of the repair of massive jaw injuries has until recently been intimately bound up with the history of war. Excellent historical reviews are presented by Rowe (1971) and McCarthy et al (1990b), and the theme is explored in Chapter 1.

Today, the options for jaw reconstructions are:

- Insertion of metallic spacers
- Insertion of alloplastic trays containing cancellous bone
- Replacement with heterogeneous treated bone
- Replacement with autogenous bone graft
- Insertion of a vascularized bone graft:
  (i) pedicled, or
  (ii) sustained by microvascular anastomosis.

The choice of procedure depends not only on the size of the defect in the bone but also on the quality of the soft tissue cover. A significant factor to be taken into account is the nature and the success of the primary treatment (p. 448). Unless it has an independent blood supply, a bone graft cannot survive without immobilization, excellent soft-tissue cover and a good local blood supply. The assessment of the capacity of existing soft tissue to sustain a bone graft is a vital judgement that has to be made by any team treating such deformities. If it is thought that the soft tissue cannot do this, the bone graft must have its own blood supply from a pedicle or be supported by microvascular anastomosis. Alternatively new soft-tissue cover may be provided for the bone graft.

Insertion of metallic spacers

A good example of such devices is the Bowerman Conroy kit which became popular during the 1970s (Evans et al 1985). This kit provided large malleable titanium plates, which were used to bridge mandibular defects, being bolted to the lingual side of the mandible. This technique initially held some promise but experience has shown that exposure of the plate through the soft tissues often occurs, and leads ultimately to removal of the spacer. In the post-traumatic setting spacers are at best temporary manoeuvres to separate bone ends for subsequent bone grafting; the use of long titanium plates for this purpose is discussed on p. 455. In the light of modern techniques of bone grafting and its own poor record, this form of reconstruction is probably now obsolete as definitive treatment.

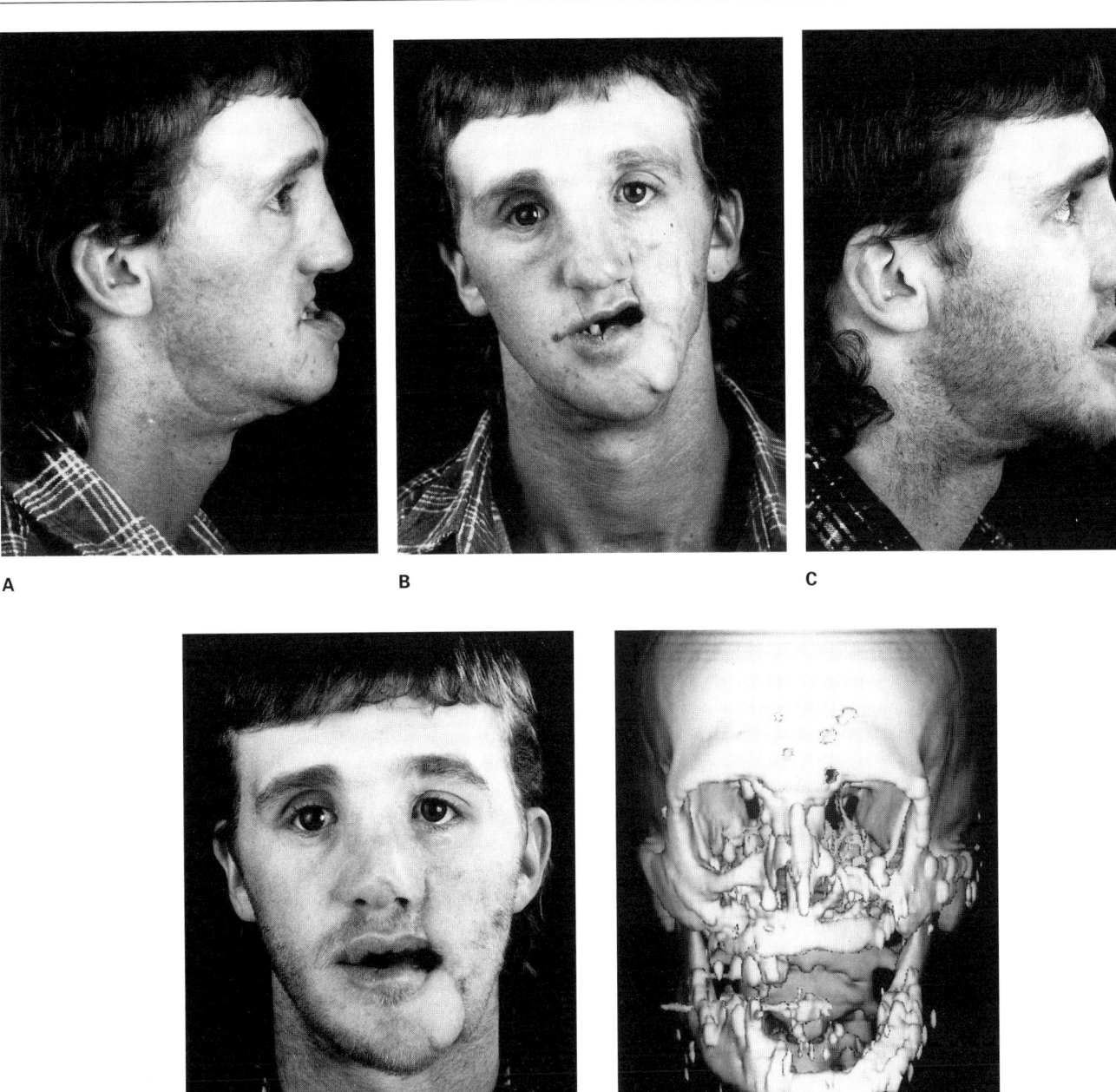

A   B   C

D   E

Fig. 21.73 Extensive trauma to the jaws. A boy suffered a gunshot wound and was originally treated in an outlying community. He lost the upper segment of the maxilla leaving only a remnant on the right side. On the left side a large portion of the body of the mandible was absent, as was soft tissue of the floor of mouth and tongue. The mandible on the left side had been partially reconstructed by a free flap which had failed to heal properly. The lip was incomplete and a deficit remained in the floor of the mouth. X-rays indicated residual fragments from the gunshot. Treatment began with microvascular lower jaw reconstruction (iliac crest based on the deep circumflex iliac artery) and upper jaw reconstruction (vascularized rib). At the second stage the soft tissue from the floor of mouth was removed in preparation for osseo-integrated implants, on which a clip-on prosthesis will rest. **A** Initial presentation, lateral view, indicating the absence of a significant amount of upper jaw. **B** Destroyed left cheek and remnant of the free flap covering the lower lip, under which was an unhealed remnant of the previous vascularized bone graft. **C** Lateral view after reconstruction of the upper jaw with vascularized rib and lower jaw with vascularized hip, and bone grafting of the nose. **D** Anteroposterior view indicating the remaining deficiency of the orbicularis muscle and soft tissue paddle on the chin. **E** 3D CT scan indicating the reconstituted mandible and maxilla, repositioned left cheek bone, and the bone graft to the dorsum of the nose.

Insertion of alloplastic trays containing cancellous bone

The principle of this technique is that the bone chips act as a receptive scaffolding for the growth of new bone and the tray acts as support and spacer to facilitate this. We have no experience of this technique and reference is therefore made to the reviews by McCarthy et al (1990b), Evans et al (1985) and Marx & Stevens (1991). Taher (1990), reporting on a series of 128 mandibular defects sustained in the Iran–Iraq war, used titanium mesh trays containing bone and hydroxylapatite granules in some 34 cases, and achieved good results with a very low incidence of complications. Tayapongsak et al (1993, 1994) have also employed titanium trays to support autogenous bone chips and marrow, held together with autologous fibrin glue (p. 380) (Fig. 21.74). Other authors have used steel trays, which have to be precast, or plastic cribs.

Heterogeneous treated bone

Bone harvested from cadavers has been used. Marx & Stevens (1991) favour the use of freeze-dried ribs, ilium or even whole mandibles, hollowed and shaped to serve as trays to contain autogenous cancellous bone chips; these authors believe that with appropriate tissue bank precautions, the risk of viral transmission is negligible. We have no experience of this technique and believe that it has been supplanted by bone flaps and microvascular methods.

Autogenous bone grafts

For a century surgeons have been looking for material to replace the damaged or absent mandible. Autogenous

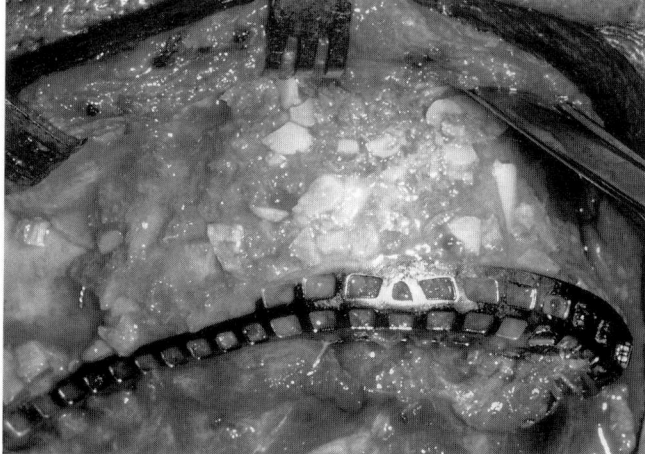

Fig. 21.74 Particulate bone and autologous fibrin polymer.
Particulate cancellous bone graft, in a matrix of autologous fibrin polymer, is used to reconstruct a large mandibular defect. A titanium crib replaces the inferior border only. (Photo courtesy of Dr Pairot Tayapongsak.)

bone is of course the material of choice in replacing a mandibular defect. Bone grafting is now the most commonly used method of reconstructing significant defects of the mandible. The bone can be harvested from the rib, hip or calvaria (p. 240). Although all of these donor sites are used from time to time, it is the hip that provides the most predictable source in terms of quality and quantity of both cortical and cancellous bone. We have found rib grafts to be less successful because they are often less robust and unpredictable in their shape and size. There is nothing more disturbing when harvesting ribs for jaw reconstruction than to find that the grafts are friable and lack substance. However, the costochondral junction is the preferred graft for TMJ reconstruction where there is a previous ankylosis (p. 604).

The general principles of bone grafting are very relevant in mandibular reconstructions. A bone graft will not 'take' unless it is placed in an adequate bed, hence the soft-tissue cover must be complete and of good vascularity. The defect to be filled must be recreated by fixing the mandibular fragments in their predetermined correct position, usually by means of intermaxillary fixation and some form of locating splint. The bone graft must be harvested carefully, shaped in all of its three dimensions, inserted into the gap and fixed rigidly (Fig. 21.75). Watertight closure is important and great care must be taken to avoid haematoma formation. Under these circumstances quite large segments of mandible can be replaced (Manchester 1965).

Defects of the angle of the mandible behind the occlusion are best dealt with by fixing the lower jaw to the upper jaw by intermaxillary fixation, in a predetermined acceptable position. The posterior fragment is then manipulated into what appears to be an acceptable position and an iliac crest graft is cut and shaped to bridge the defect. There are a number of ways to fix this graft. Fixation can be done by overlapping the graft ends and fixing each end by direct screwing with at least a triangle of screws, or by abutting the ends and using plates, or by using a single long malleable plate with screws into the mandibular fragments and the bone graft. Except in rare circumstances the soft-tissue cover of skin and muscle in this region is very conducive to healing. Calvarial bone graft can also be used; it is possible to use calvarial bone pedicled on the temporalis muscle (see below).

Where large segments of mandible are missing and there is a good soft-tissue bed remaining then large bone grafts can be used as free grafts. Since World War I, restorative procedures have often involved the use of rib grafts (Gillies 1920). Ribs, however, are often of inadequate strength and when split to facilitate curving they become weaker. Levant (1977) has used whole ribs impacted into the mandibular stumps. Iliac crest can be used and segments of mandible may be carved out of the full

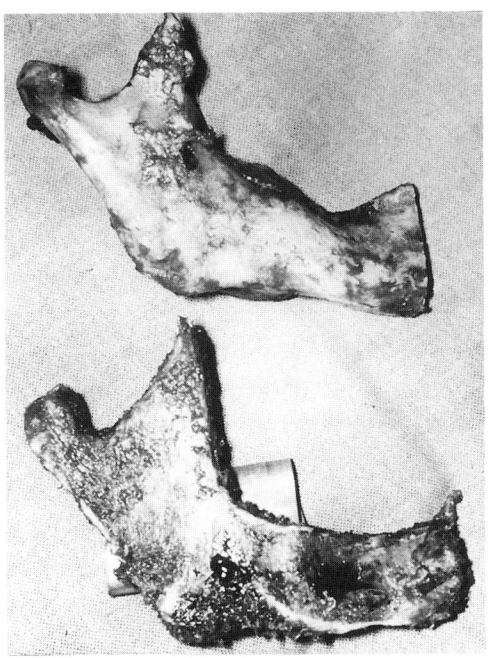
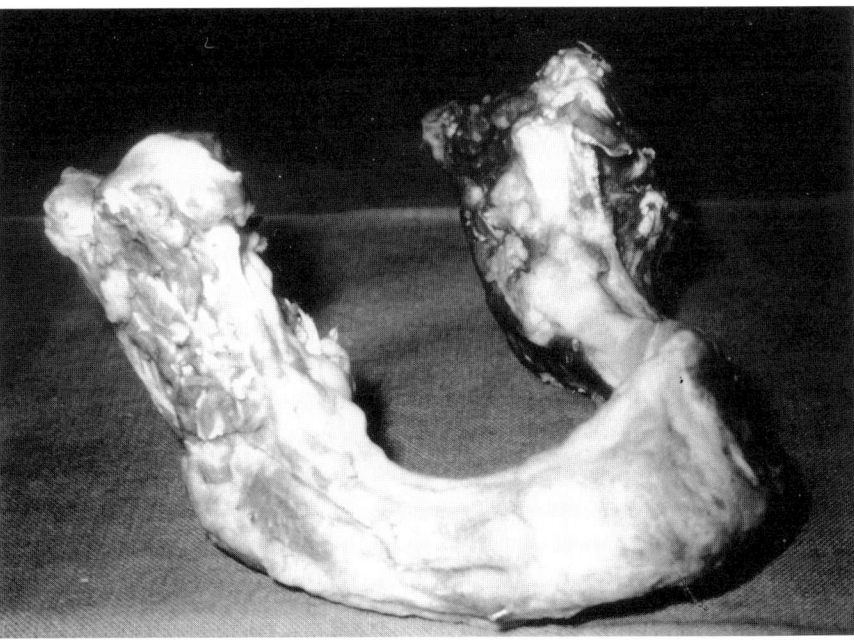

A   B

Fig. 21.75 Mandibular reconstruction with non-vascularized ilium. A The desired mandible is carefully carved from the ilium to match the resected bone. **B** A similarly reconstructed mandible removed many years later at post mortem, showing remodelling. (Photographs by courtesy of Sir William Manchester and *Plastic and Reconstructive Surgery.*)

thickness of the ilium. Various authors have suggested appropriate patterns. Dingman (1950) and Seward (1967) described U-shaped grafts to replace the anterior mandible. Manchester (1965) carved a half mandible and was able to retrieve it post-mortem many years later (Fig. 21.75). Alternatively segments of bone can be strung on a K-wire or in more modern technique united with a long titanium miniplate.

All these bone grafts depend on vascularization from the bed for survival; they require long periods of immobilization, vary in thickness and often do not become robust with time. They are subject to displacement by muscle pull and subject to the complication of infection and bone loss to an inordinate degree. Nevertheless the work of Manchester bears further consideration (Manchester 1972). His clinical studies showed that where there was an adequate soft-tissue bed and where the surgical technique was absolutely meticulous with respect to preparation of the bed, carving of the bone, fixation of the bone, immobilization and prevention of haematoma, then large segments could be replaced which would survive. Indeed, there is strong evidence from his superb clinical studies to indicate that the transferred bone itself survived and underwent healing processes; healing was evident even in fractures in the bone made at the time of reconstruction for the purpose of shaping. Manchester was careful to point out that special circumstances must exist before these grafts would succeed;

nevertheless his techniques and his subsequent theses for the success of 'bone taking' are worthy of note (p. 132). The majority of Manchester's cases came for reconstruction after excision of benign mandibular tumours and the application of his technique in the very different traumatic setting requires careful appraisal.

Vascularized bone flaps and transfers

In view of the problems that have always arisen in reconstructing large defects of the mandible with bone grafts, especially when associated with a compromised soft-tissue bed and cover, vascularized bone transfers and composite bone muscle and skin flaps have been used more and more frequently. There is now a vast experience of vascularized transfer of bone for restoration of the mandible in reconstructions carried out after tumour resections both benign and malignant. These techniques are eminently applicable to reconstruction after trauma. Vascularized flaps usually involve skin, muscle and bone, and numerous flaps of this type have been described. Initially these flaps were vascularized by pedicles dissected in continuity from parent arteries and veins.

Rib flaps

Pedicled flaps including a rib have been described by many authors, but the technique goes back to the very

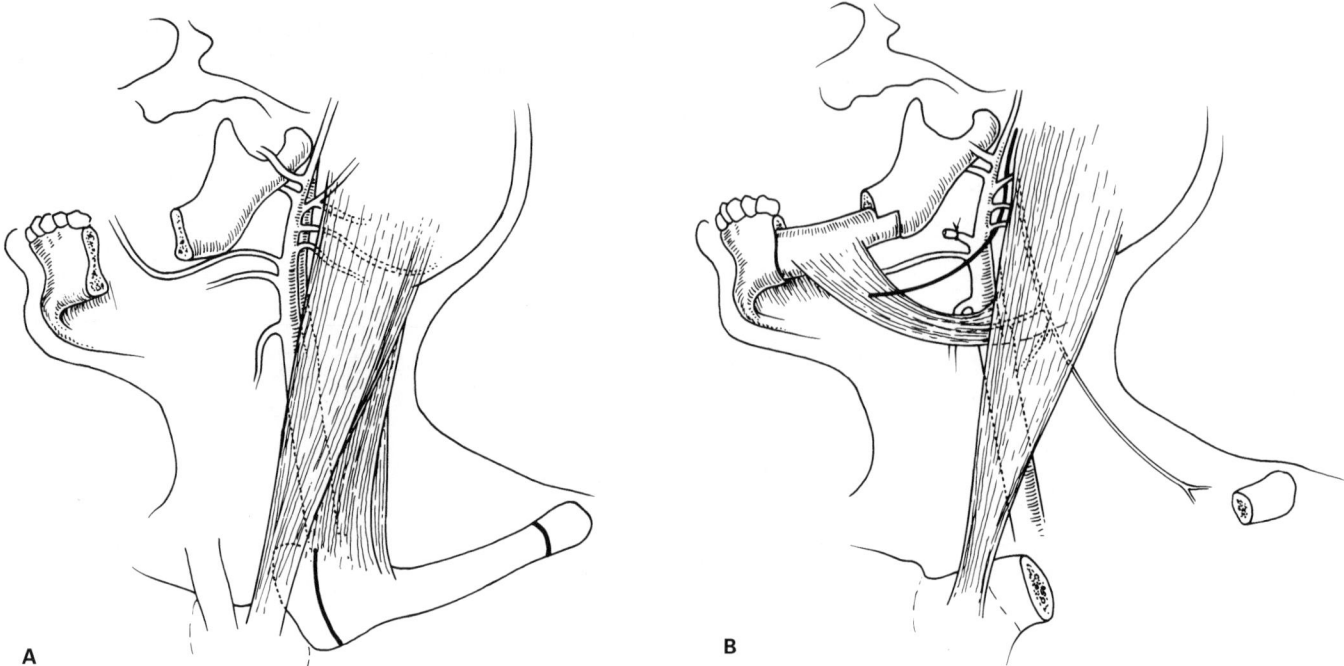

Fig. 21.76 Transfer of the clavicle on the sternocleidomastoid muscle. After Siemssen et al (1978), by courtesy of *Plastic and Reconstructive Surgery*. **A** The mandibular defect. **B** Transposition of muscle and bone.

early part of the century when Vilray Blair described the transfer of rib as part of a complex flap for mandibular reconstruction (Blair 1918). Cuono & Ariyan (1980) used a part of the fifth or sixth rib associated with a pectoralis myocutaneous flap, using the pectoral part of the muscle based on its arterial supply from the thoraco-acromial artery. The transfer of rib as an island flap based on the internal mammary vessels alone was described by Strauch et al (1971). This was done first in dogs; the seventh rib was isolated on skeletonized internal mammary vessels and the clinical application was made by Ketcham et al (1974) who repaired a mandibular defect with a portion of the seventh rib and adjacent sternum. Rib transfer using the latissimus dorsi muscle and thoracodorsal artery has been reported (Schmidt & Robson 1982, Maruyama et al 1985). Although Ariyan (1980) demonstrated that rib grafts can survive when transferred on their periosteal blood supply, this source of bone is very much second best in restoring a significant post-traumatic defect: the quality of the rib may be poor, its dimensions are inadequate for much more than a functional spacer, and it will not provide an adequate skeleton for framing a soft-tissue complex capable of fitting dentures, or stout enough to take osseo-integrated implants.

The clavicle flap

Conley (1972) described a compound flap involving the clavicle; Siemssen and his colleagues from Denmark (1978) also reported such a flap, a large segment of the whole clavicle being pedicled on the sternocleidomastoid muscle (Fig. 21.76).

The sternal flap

The lateral border of the sternum can be transferred using the pectoralis major myocutaneous flap as a carrier. Green et al (1981) described this procedure and Robertson (1986) also reported the results of using this technique.

The trapezius–scapula flap

A flap of trapezius muscle bearing the scapula spine has been described by Demergasso & Piazza (1979). The technique is also described by Panje & Cutting (1980) and Dufresne et al (1987) (Fig. 21.77).

Calvarial flap

All these flaps bearing bone to reconstruct the jaw are pedicled from below; in contrast, the calvarial full thickness or outer table graft is pedicled on temporalis muscle and rotates down from above (McCarthy & Zide 1984, Van Der Meulen et al 1984, McCarthy et al 1987). Where the bone has good diplöe and can be split, cautious dissection can leave the inner table in situ. When this is not so, the aid of a neurosurgeon must be employed and the procedure becomes much more considerable, with all the problems attendant upon opening the skull, the least

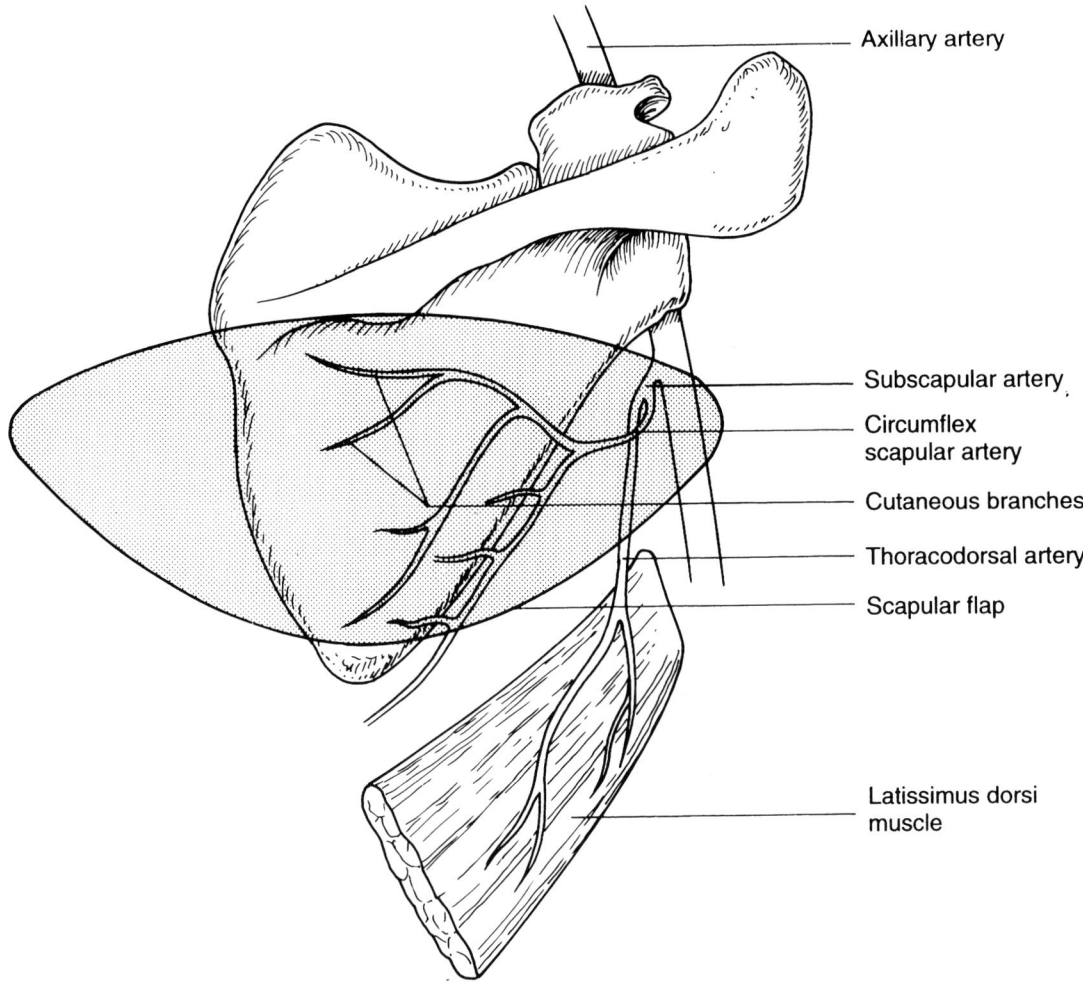

Fig. 21.77 Scapular osteocutaneous flap. After Swartz et al (1986), by courtesy of *Plastic and Reconstuctive Surgery.* Inclusion of the thoracodorsal pedicle with the scapular osteocutaneous flap allows the additional use of the latissimus dorsi muscle or myocutaneous skin paddle.

of which is the need to repair the defect with bone from elsewhere, usually split calvaria or bone from another site, hip or rib. The pedicled flap has been used to reconstruct the zygoma and orbital floor as well as the ramus of the mandible (Fig. 21.78).

Many of these techniques for pedicled bone grafting have grown out of procedures used in the reconstructions necessary after resection of the mandible for oral cancer, and have been applied to post-traumatic reconstruction. The calvarial flap had its origins in the need to reconstruct the orbit and the ramus of the mandible in Treacher Collins syndrome (Raulo & Tessier 1981). McCarthy et al (1990b) noted that bone transferred thus is best reserved for smaller segments; failures have occurred with more heroic attempts to fill large gaps. In our own practice the pedicled flaps have by and large been suplanted by more elegant and accurate reconstruction with microvascular anastomosis. They are described here because they represent a stage in the evolution of techniques of reconstruc-

tion of the bony facial skeleton, and still remain relevant where microsurgical skills and technology are not available, or where less happily microvascular techniques have failed and some salvage procedure is necessary. All these techniques have been enhanced by the availability of rigid interosseous fixation through mini- and microplating.

Osseomyocutaneous vascularized transfers

Where microvascular anastomosis provides an intact blood supply to the bone graft, there is no loss of osteogenic potential in the bone, and less risk of compromise by an inadequate environment such as that resulting from scar or irradiated tissue. The historical progress of this technique from experiment to clinical application is one of the true success stories of modern plastic and reconstructive surgery. McCullough & Fredrickson (1973) inaugurated the use of microvascularized bone flaps in experimental procedures on dogs. Ostrup and his col-

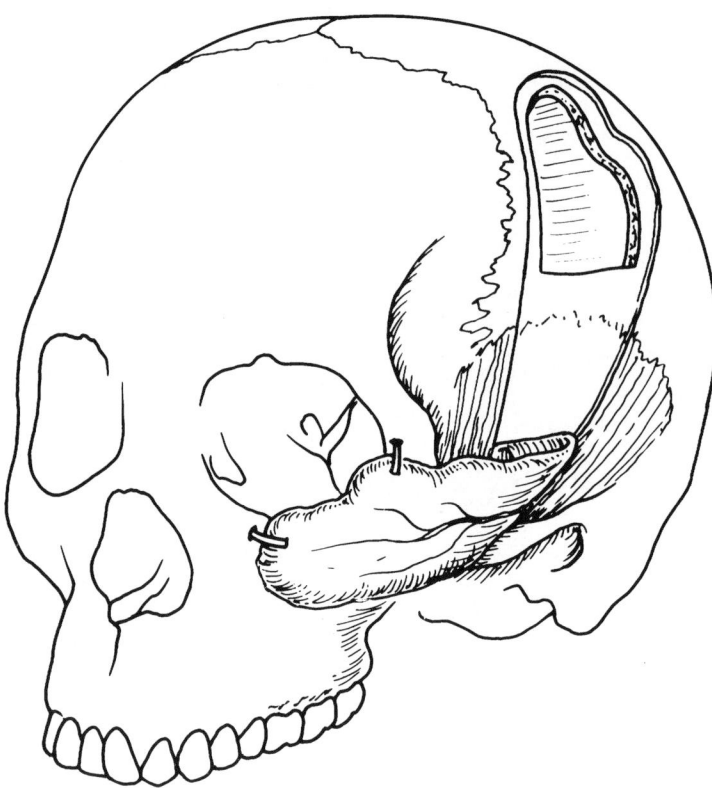

Fig. 21.78 Pedicled calvarial flap. The calvaria can be pedicled on the temporalis muscle as described by McCarthy et al (1987), yielding an extremely versatile flap for the reconstruction of congenital deformities including Treacher Collins Syndrome. If the calvaria is thick enough to be split, the outer table can be carried in this way. More frequently it is a matter of carrying the full thickness, involving the neurosurgeon to protect the underlying dura. This pedicled flap can be turned down to reconstruct the ramus of the mandible as well as the areas around the orbit.

leagues (Ostrup & Fredrickson 1974, Ostrup & Tam 1975) completed this work. In their 1974 study, angiography demonstrated that the flow of blood in the ribs was from the nutrient arterial supply. Doi et al (1977) showed that rib transferred by microvascular anastomosis to the femur of the same animal did not lose substance and rapid bone union took place. When Taylor et al (1975) successfully transferred a vascularized fibula in the human in a case of lower limb trauma, the crucial step of clinical application was put into place. Harashina et al (1978) reconstructed the mandible using a posterior rib graft. We (David & Tan 1979) reported a case performed 18 months previously of reconstruction of the hemimandible using iliac bone vascularized by the peri-

osteal vessels from the groin flap as demonstrated by Taylor (1982) (Fig. 21.79). To this day we dissect both pedicles when using bone based on the deep circumflex vessel. There has been controversy as to the relative values of the blood supply taken from nutrient vessels or from periosteal vessels, but for practical purposes this does not seem to matter. Successful transfers with good long-term follow-up have been widely reported with bone flaps supplied from the nutrient vessels, or from the periosteum or from both, and the source of the blood supply to the bone no longer seems to be of great moment. The transfers used by us in mandibular reconstruction are described below; some of them have also been used in maxillary reconstruction.

Fig. 21.79 Iliac crest free flap. A teenage girl presented with craniofacial microsomia, having had a series of operations including a metatarsal transfer and a Bowerman's prosthesis which was subsequently removed. Non-vascularized rib was used to reconstruct her zygomatic arch and joint, and the hemimandible was reconstructed from iliac crest (supplied by the superficial circumflex iliac artery) with overlying soft tissue used for contour restoration. She is seen at the time of the operation and a decade later. It is notable that after 10 years the rib has disappeared but the ilium is intact. **A** Plain radiograph showing the Bowerman's prosthesis. **B** Operative photograph showing the zygoma reconstructed from rib with a costochondral condylar fossa suspended by wire. **C** OPG showing the reconstruction. **D** 3D reconstruction made a decade later demonstrating the mandible intact but the zygoma having disappeared. **E** Initial presentation. **F** Final appearance.

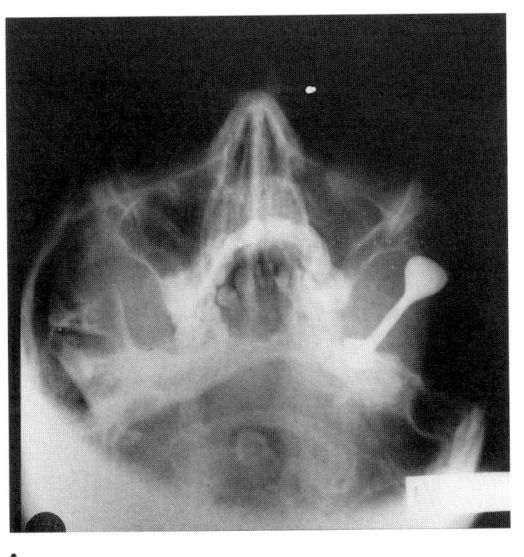

A

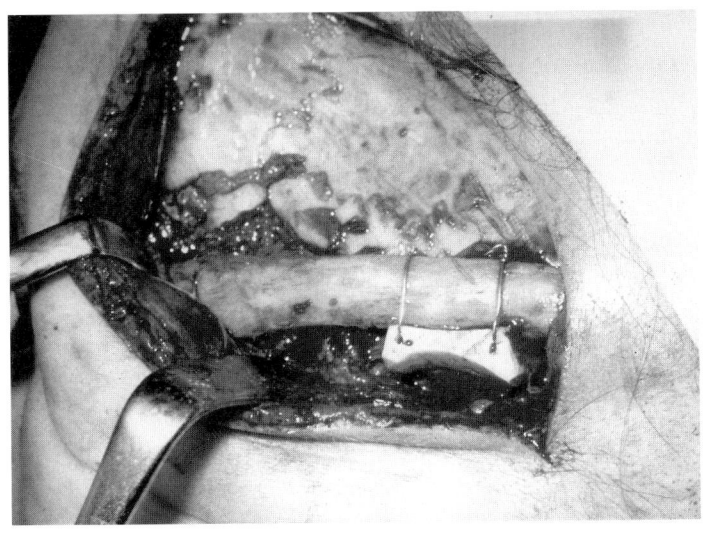

B

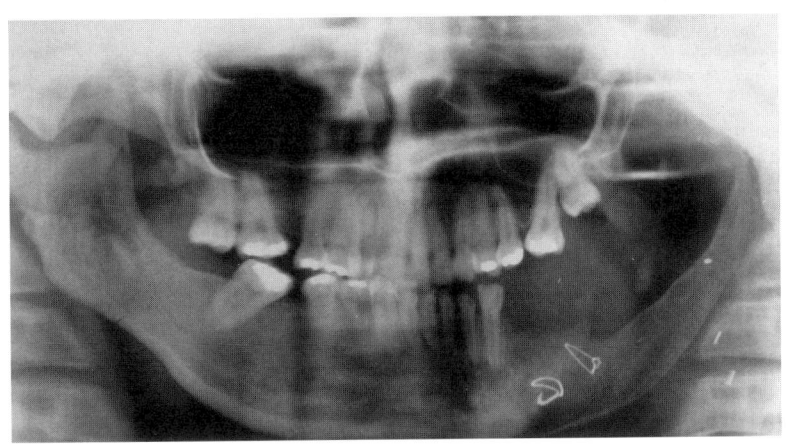

C

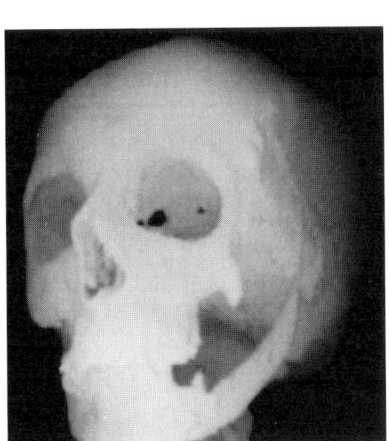

D

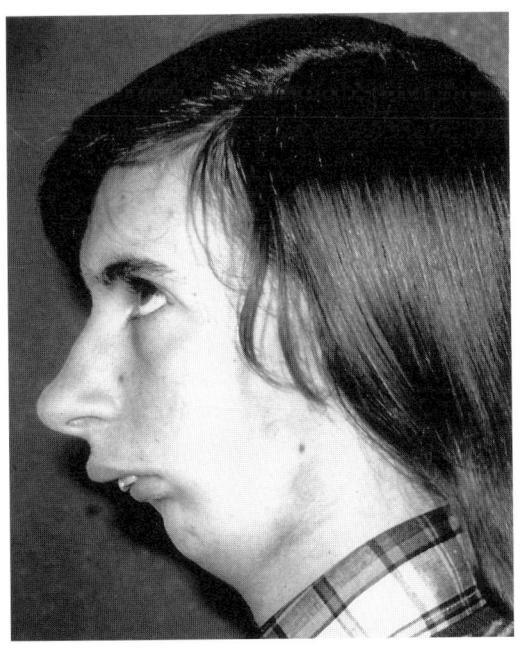

E

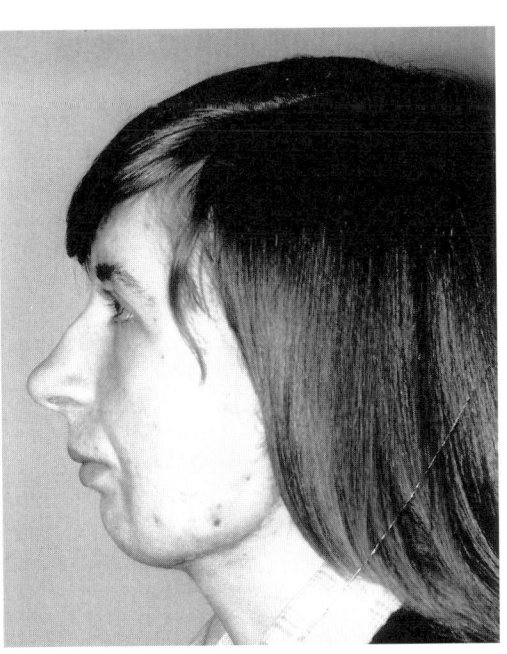

F

RECONSTRUCTION OF MANDIBULAR DEFECTS

Management

Complex mandibular reconstructions require large bone replacements and multiple osteotomies in a compromised soft-tissue environment, and constitute a prime indication for microsurgical reconstruction. These procedures can be adapted for lesser deformities, tailoring the operation to the defect to create an elegant bone and soft-tissue reconstruction. Onlay and inlay techniques can be used and combined with miniplate and lag screw fixation; the grafts have the capacity to support osseo-integrated implants, and this versatile technique has greatly expanded our capacity to reconstruct the jaws successfully. A further advance is the use of multiple free flaps in a single procedure, taking the best from each flap: thus, an iliac bone graft supported by the deep circumflex iliac artery is used for jaw reconstruction and a thin hairless forearm flap for reconstructing the oral lining (David et al 1988).

Vascularized tissue transfers

The transfers now in use offer various possibilities in reconstructing mandibular defects. We review here the chief sources of vascularized bone, and describe in detail the operative techniques which have been developed by us in mandibular reconstructions for traumatic and non-traumatic deformities.

Rib transfers

Rib flaps pedicled on the nutrient vessel have fallen into disuse because an extensive transthoracic approach is necessary to harvest the rib. Free rib transfers were described by Ariyan & Finseth (1978) and Ariyan (1980) who showed that ribs can be transferred successfully if vascularized by a periosteal blood supply from the intercostal arteries, or by a muscular attachment to a revascularized muscle. Additional supply from a nutrient artery is not necessary, and this simplifies the dissection of the free rib flap. Anterior intercostal flaps (Ariyan & Finseth 1978, McKee 1989), posterior intercostal flaps (Daniel 1978, Serafin et al 1979, 1980) and lateral intercostal flaps (Badran et al 1984) have been used for mandibular reconstruction. We prefer to take a serratus anterior free flap as a carrier to vascularize a rib graft through the muscular attachment. One or two ribs can

be raised, usually the fifth and/or sixth ribs, the length of rib being up to ~12 cm in an adult. A small skin flap can also be taken over the selected rib.

The patient is placed supine, arm abducted, with a sandbag under the shoulder. An incision is made in the posterior axillary fold, curved gently forward to include a skin ellipse if this is desired. The lateral border of latissimus dorsi is found; finger dissection opens the plane between this muscle and the lateral chest wall, and exposes the serratus anterior with its nerve and its vascular pedicle from the lateral thoracic artery. The nerve supply is segmental, and if the central slips of muscle are taken, it is possible to preserve the upper and lower slips and so to avoid winging of the scapula. The vascular pedicle can be elongated by dissecting to the thoracodorsal artery or even to the subclavian.

When the appropriate slip or slips of serratus anterior have been isolated, the rib graft is taken by incising the upper border of each rib and separating it from the pleura; the posterior periosteum is stripped. This lessens the risk of intrathoracic complications and promotes rib regeneration. The rib graft may be shaped by subperiosteal osteotomy (Fig. 21.80).

The scapula transfer

Swartz et al (1986) described a free osteocutaneous scapular flap which can provide a significant amount of bone for mandibular or maxillary reconstructions. This flap has been used for rebuilding the hard palate and anterior maxillary arch, when one or both sides of the oronasal cavity require lining tissue (Fig. 21.77). The flap may also be used in nasal or upper lip reconstruction in conjunction with repair of the anterior maxillary arch.

The lateral edge of the scapula below the glenoid fossa is thick, but the bone thins to 2–3 mm thickness in most of its body; a scapula bone graft can be up to 10 cm long. The blood supply is derived from branches of the circumflex scapular artery, especially its branch to the teres major muscle. The skin over the scapula tends to be thick, with a considerable layer of subcutaneous fat, making it a difficult flap to use except in a slim individual. The skin is supplied by a cutaneous branch of the circumflex scapular artery which emerges through the triangular space bounded by the two teres muscles and the long head of triceps. The skin flap may be taken horizontally or obliquely in line with the lateral border of the scapula;

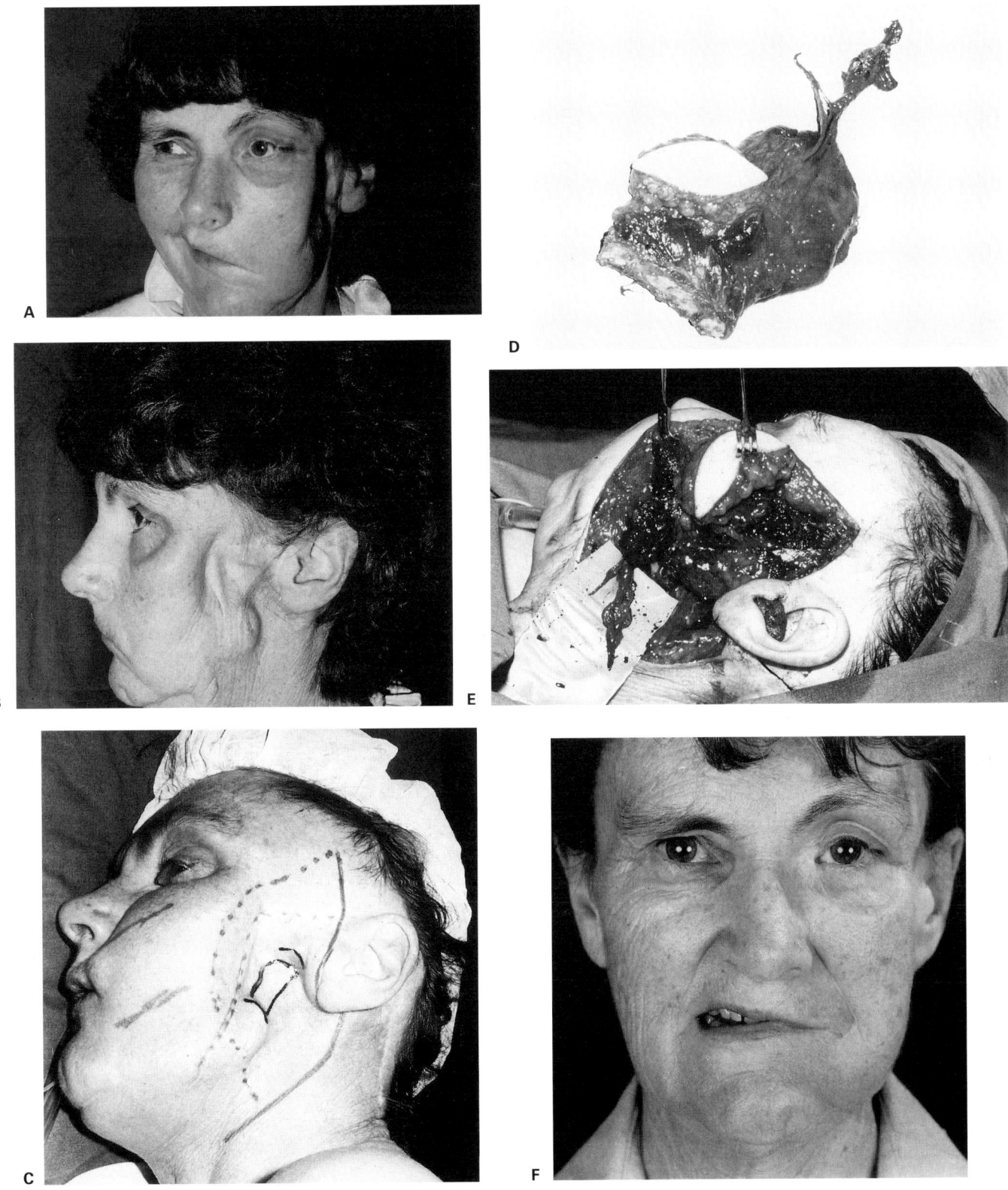

Fig. 21.80 Vascularized rib graft. A 60-year-old female underwent resection of a left parotid adenoidcystic carcinoma. Microvascular transfer of rib and innervated serratus anterior muscle was performed for reconstruction of the complex deformity in the left parotid area, including a left facial palsy. **A** Pre-operative view from the front showing the facial palsy and the contour defect. **B** Lateral view shows absence of the zygomatic arch, condyle, and condylar neck, as well as the effects of the facial palsy. **C** Design of the operation in which a composite flap of rib and serratus anterior with an overlying skin and fat paddle, together with nerve and artery, are to be placed into the defect. The muscle provides an innervated soft tissue bulk. **D** Disconnected flap. **E** Dissection at time of surgery. The flap is shown in situ prior to the anastomosis of the vessels. **F** The patient 2 years later with the capacity for facial mass movement, reasonable static tone, and good facial contour.

in marking the skin incisions, the flap should be sited over its blood supply from the triangular space.

The flap is best raised with the patient in the lateral position and the arm supported in abduction. The skin flap includes the deep fascia, and dissection usually proceeds from medial to lateral, so that the cutaneous blood supply can be identified and traced to the triangular space. Further dissection requires deep retraction to identify the circumflex scapular artery and the subscapular artery from which it arises. If necessary, the subscapular artery is exposed by an additional anterior dissection — this helps to get a longer pedicle, and is especially useful in obese patients. The area of bone to be taken is left with some attached teres muscle and soft tissue around the circumflex scapular artery because small periosteal branches, especially one descending along the lateral border of the scapula, may contribute to the supply of the graft. If a long piece of bone, rather than a plate, is taken, it may be shaped by subperiosteal osteotomy as desired.

The lateral arm osteocutaneous transfer

This flap, described by Song et al (1983) and Katsaros et al (1984), is based on the posterior radial collateral artery, a branch of the profunda brachii artery. This vessel gives several cutaneous branches to the overlying skin and muscular branches to the adjacent brachioradialis and triceps muscles, through which a periosteal blood supply goes to the humerus in the area of the lateral supracondylar ridge. In an adult, this will provide a segment of bone ~10 cm long and 1 cm wide. An osteocutaneous flap can be designed with a very small skin component based on a single cutaneous perforating artery and a small piece of bone which can be used to repair palatal or maxillary arch defects. A larger vascularized bone graft can be used in mandibular reconstruction.

The skin flap is centred over the surface marking of the lateral intermuscular septum — the lower half of a line drawn from acromion to lateral epicondyle. The flap is raised subfascially over the triceps tendon posteriorly and the brachioradialis anteriorly. As the dissection progresses proximally, the radial nerve is encountered anteriorly passing between the brachioradialis and the brachialis, together with the anterior radial collateral artery. Above this point, the pedicle can be developed by dissecting out the profunda brachii artery and its accompanying veins in the spiral groove, giving more length and larger vessels for the anatomosis.

In taking the bone graft, a 1-cm-wide cuff of muscle is preserved on each side of the supracondylar ridge. The selected piece of bone is cleaned, marked and then cut, preferably with an electric reciprocating saw, in the desired shape — usually gently curved. Further shaping may be done by subperiosteal osteotomy.

The radial forearm flap

Since its introduction by Yang (1981), this flap has found a firm place in intraoral reconstructions as a source of thin skin for lining and as an osteocutaneous flap for mandibular reconstruction. The blood supply to the bone is periosteal through the attachment of the lateral intermuscular septum. Up to 10 cm of the radius can be taken between the insertions of pronator teres and brachioradialis, but no more than half the thickness of the bone can be taken to avoid the risk of fracture. A very large skin flap can be raised if necessary, from the elbow to the wrist, or alternatively a very small flap can be designed, provided that a larger fascial component carrying a cutaneous branch is taken.

An Allen test (p. 254) is done to ensure that the hand will be viable without the radial artery. The course of the artery is marked between the palpable brachial artery and the radial pulse at the wrist. The desired skin flap is raised subfascially, leaving intact paratenon to receive a skin graft. Care is taken to preserve the lateral intermuscular septum and its attachment to the periosteum of the radius on its lateral aspect. Medially a cuff of flexor pollicis longus and pronator quadratus is left attached to the area of bone to be taken. Many large deep muscular branches of the vascular pedicle must be carefully ligated or clipped, as these may cause excessive bleeding when the flap is revascularized. The bone is then removed with an electric saw; if necessary it can be shaped by subperiosteal osteotomy in one or two places. The donor area usually requires a spilt-skin graft. A plaster splint is applied for 3 weeks to protect the weakened radius.

Ulnal and fibula transfers

Lovie et al (1984) have described a forearm free flap based on the ulnar artery (Fig. 17.17): its utility is discussed on p. 21.86. The fibula free flap has advocates, but we have not found it helpful in facial reconstruction.

The second metatarsal transfer

This was first described by O'Brien et al (1979). The authors described this composite flap apparently at the suggestion of another prominent Australian microsurgeon, D. W. Robinson of Brisbane, whose help was acknowledged. The second metatarsal gains its blood supply from the dorsalis pedis system; the venous drainage is via one of the accompanying veins which communicates with the superficial long saphenous vein. The second metatarsal is removed with its articular surfaces; remnants of the small muscles are left attached to produce soft-tissue connections to the overlying skin paddle.

In the original report, a reconstruction was undertaken to restore the mandible after a gunshot wound. The central mandibular bone was missing as well as soft tissue. Facial vessels were used for the anastomosis; interosseous wire fixation was used at one end and a plate fixation at the other. Union was reported as sound. The contour of the mandible achieved with this technique was deficient and needed further augmentation to produce an aesthetic result. Other authors have reported their experience with this technique (MacLeod & Robinson 1982, Duncan et al 1985) and it has proved possible to give adequate chin prominence. MacLeod & Robinson (1982) believe that this transfer is the technique of choice for reconstructing the anterior mandible; the pedicle is long and the vessels of large diameter.

Iliac crest transfers

In recent years, vascularized iliac grafts have been accepted as one of the methods of choice for achieving a satisfactory reconstruction of the mandible, especially when larger bone segments are required (O'Brien et al 1979, Taylor et al 1979a, b, Taylor 1982, Salibian et al 1985, David & Tan 1979, David et al 1988). In our unit, this is indeed the technique of first choice and it has been used and developed in clinical practice for the last 15 years.

In our initial experience with microvascular jaw reconstruction, segments of iliac crest based on the superficial circumflex iliac artery (SCIA) were used. This vessel anastomoses with perforating arteries emerging from the iliac crest in the line of the external oblique attachment (Fig. 21.81). When raising this composite flap, the initial dissection is the same as that used for raising a free groin skin flap (p. 454). Attachments of the skin to the fascia are preserved to retain a periosteal blood supply to an estimated 2-cm-thick segment of bone. Thigh muscle fascia and the external and internal oblique muscles are then incised to expose the desired height of the iliac

crest which is then sectioned. This composite flap is now rarely used because of the inadequacy of the bone segment that can be attached to the flap and the unpredictability of the vessel size. Retrograde blood flow to the underlying iliac crest via small vessels in the fascia may be inadequate to sustain a large segment of bone. The perforating vessels from the deep circumflex iliac artery (DCIA) are more reliable. These vessels emerge 2–3 cm medial to the iliac crest to anastomose with branches of the SCIA, and an adequate cuff of external fascia and external and internal oblique muscles must be taken if blood flow is to be possible in either direction. With the advent of the DCIA flap it became possible to provide a large amount of vascularized iliac crest for reconstruction of extensive defects (Taylor et al 1979a,b) (Fig. 21.82). Further development of the technique enabled the ilium to be split, thus improving the cosmetic result in the hip. As this procedure has become our workhorse for mandibular reconstruction, it is described in detail.

The operation is planned so that the shape and size of the mandibular bone defect can be predetermined either from study of the dental model or from 3D CT reconstruction (Fig. 21.91), which has proved very helpful in preoperative planning (Rose et al 1993). An acrylic template is made to assist in cutting out the exact shape of bone required for the graft. The appropriate intermaxillary fixation is determined in advance and a bite wafer is used to locate the mandibular fragments. Intraoperative organization is carefully planned beforehand: usually two teams are deployed, one to prepare the jaw and the other to harvest the bone.

The team dissecting the jaw prepares the ground, recreates the defect and exposes the recipient vessels. Simultaneously, the DCIA flap is harvested. The DCIA runs a course 1 cm above the inguinal ligament from the

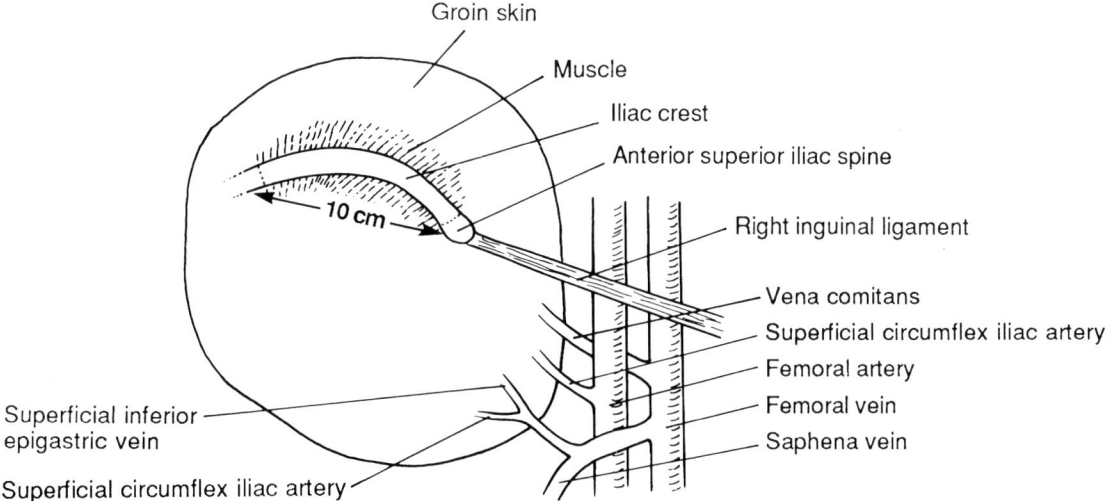

Fig. 21.81 Osteocutaneous flap from the right groin. After O'Brien et al (1979), by courtesy of *British Journal of Plastic Surgery*. Also see Fig. 21.80 for its early application.

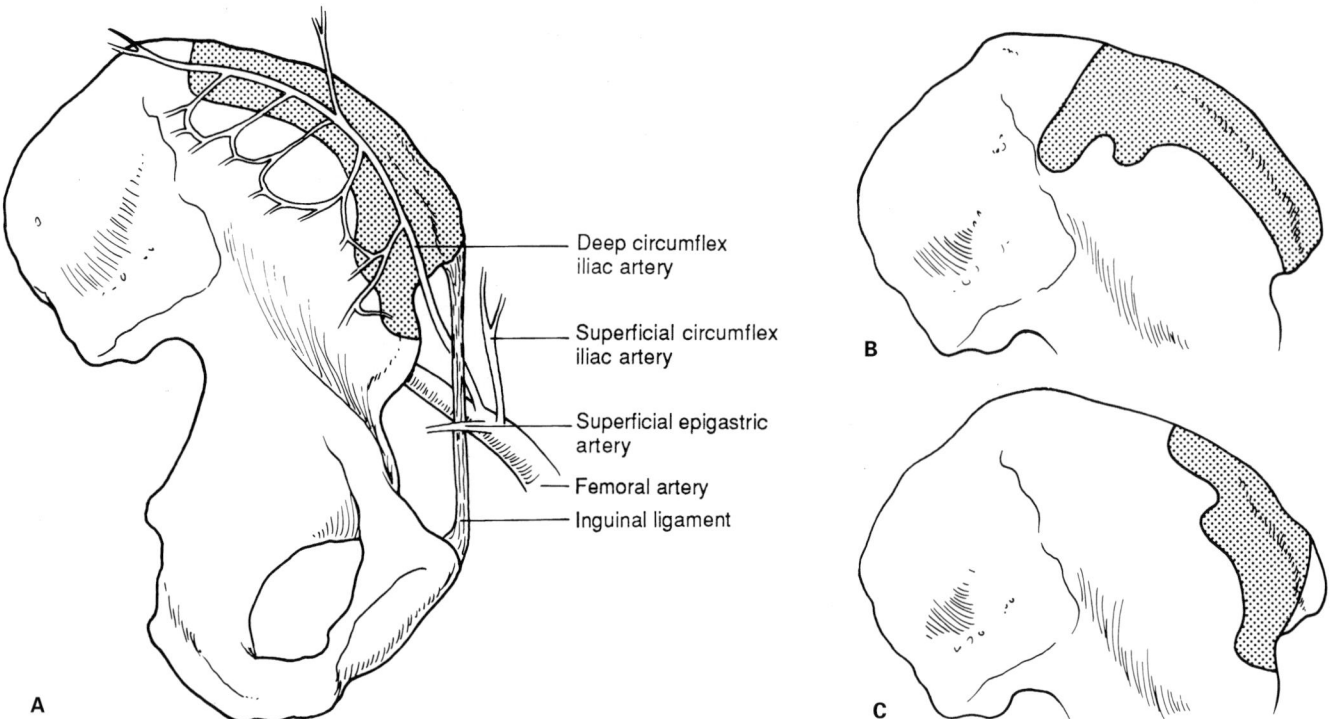

Deep circumflex
iliac artery

Superficial circumflex
iliac artery

Superficial epigastric
artery

Femoral artery

Inguinal ligament

Fig. 21.82 Fashioning the deep circumflex iliac artery (full or split thickness) flap for mandibular reconstruction from the contralateral ilium. A The bone with vessels superimposed. **B, C** Alternative methods.

external iliac artery towards the anterior superior iliac spine, deep to the transversalis fascia. The markings for a skin paddle are made over the anterior superior iliac spine and the iliac crest, usually as a lentiform shape, the medial end of which can be continued to the origin of the DCIA. The skin incision starts medially, and the external oblique aponeurosis is exposed; its fibres are split parallel to and 1 cm above the inguinal ligament. The internal oblique muscle fibres are cut transversely, and the DCIA is then identified. This is usually easy, first by palpation and then by sharp dissection through the transversalis fascia. The vessels are then followed medially to the external iliac artery and its accompanying vein, and laterally towards the anterior superior iliac spine. The ascending branch of the DCIA is encountered at a variable position in this dissection, and is divided. The main vessel lies between the iliacus and transversalis fascia, ~2 cm below the iliac crest. The skin paddle incisions are then completed and deepened to the aponeurosis of the external oblique muscle, which is divided 2–3 cm medial to the crest. Care is taken to preserve any perforating vessels appearing in the vicinity. The dissection is further deepened until the DCIA is seen on the iliacus; the iliacus is then incised and pushed away medially, leaving the periosteum of the inner table of the ilium intact. Further laterally and posteriorly, the external oblique aponeurosis becomes muscular, and a small (2 cm) cuff of the muscle is taken with the flap as more perforators often come through in this area. The line for splitting the iliac crest is marked by incising about midway along the top of the iliac crest; periosteal elevators are then used to push away the muscular and fibrous attachments from the lateral half of the iliac crest, the medial attachments being preserved. Near the anterior superior iliac spine, it is often necessary to divide the lateral cutaneous nerve of the thigh, though it is sometimes possible to identify and save this nerve when the DCIA pedicle is divided from the external iliac vessels.

The segment of the ilium is harvested according to the shape and size of the mandibular defect. Manchester's inspiration (Manchester, 1972) has influenced Taylor and others (Fig. 21.83) in the designing of the bone graft to be cut from the iliac crest. With the wide exposure obtained, the acrylic template is placed on the medial side of the iliac crest and the area to be resected is delineated with a marking pencil after the periosteum has been stripped away from the part of the ilium that will not be harvested. Often, the amount of iliac bone to be taken

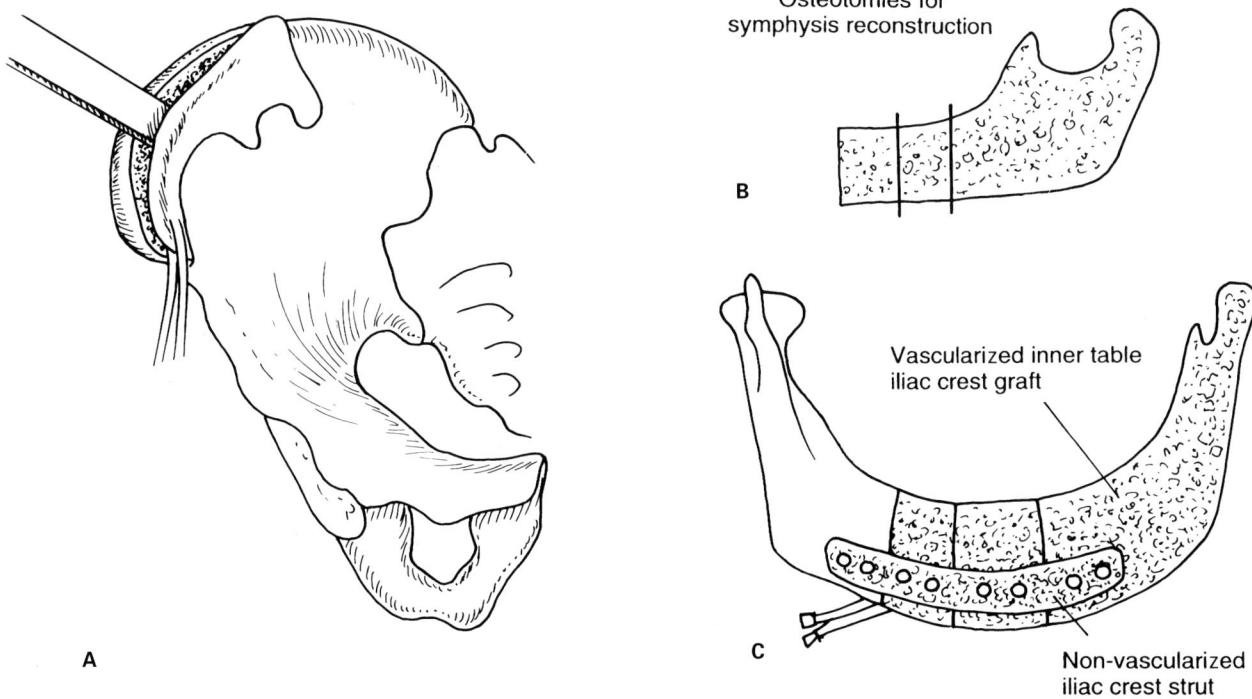

Fig. 21.83 Contouring the iliac crest graft for mandibular reconstruction. A The iliac crest is split at its rim with a reciprocating saw, and the cut is completed with an osteotome which will lever the fragment away gently with the overlying soft tissue and vessels intact. **B** Saw cuts are made through the substance of the graft subperiosteally so that the desired curvature can be produced. **C** Reconstruction of the symphysis is achieved with vertical osteotomies, preserving the periosteum on the lingual side. Non-vascularized iliac crest can be shaped and placed on the facial side to secure the segments and augment the chin prominence. If the vertical osteotomies have opened they can be filled with cancellous bone.

is estimated from measurement of the length and height of the bone defect, by now exposed by the other surgical team, taking into account possible osteotomy and reshaping. Similarly, the size and shape of the soft-tissue elements of the graft will have been determined by the need for soft-tissue, external skin and mucosal replacement.

The iliac crest is split along its rim with a reciprocating saw (Fig. 21.83), and along the outline of the graft on the inner table with either an oscillating or a reciprocal saw. The final stages of removing the bone graft are facilitated by cuts with curved or straight osteotomes. It is helpful to divide the vascular pedicle before the saws are used; at all stages of the operation this pedicle must be safeguarded. The vessels are clamped with Ligaclips® and divided between the clips. If it is intended to use the grafted bone to support osseo-integrated implants, then the harvested split iliac crest must have a minimum width of 8 mm at the projected upper border, which is usually the deeper part of the crest, so that the splitting has to be executed with care to preserve that width. In most cases, the height of the mandibular replacement is 2 cm.

Closure of the donor site is carried out with careful approximation of the internal oblique muscle to the re-

sidual fascial attachments on the outer border of the iliac crest; the external oblique aponeurosis is attached to the superior gluteal fascia and the fascia over the tensor fasciae latae with 2/0 PDS or Maxon®. Before closure, any sharp spicules of bone on the ilium are removed or smoothed by burring, as perforation of large bowel has been known to occur after this operation. This careful closure of the oblique layer should prevent herniation of large bowel through a weak point in the abdominal wall.

When the desired graft is removed, together with its vascular pedicle, it may be shaped by subperiosteal osteotomy. The use of a burr in sculpting the graft is very dangerous — one slip may avulse the pedicle in a split second! The shaping of the graft is done on a side table; the surgeon is helped by the prepared template. Osteotomies can be made in the graft; the symphysis can be built from the centre of the crest or the whole hemimandible may be shaped together with its condyle. The osteotomies performed to shape the flap leave the inner periosteum intact; the osteotomized bone is fixed with miniplates and screws. Strips of non-vascularized iliac bone can be added to secure the segments and shape the bone grafts (Fig. 21.84). Additional bone can be

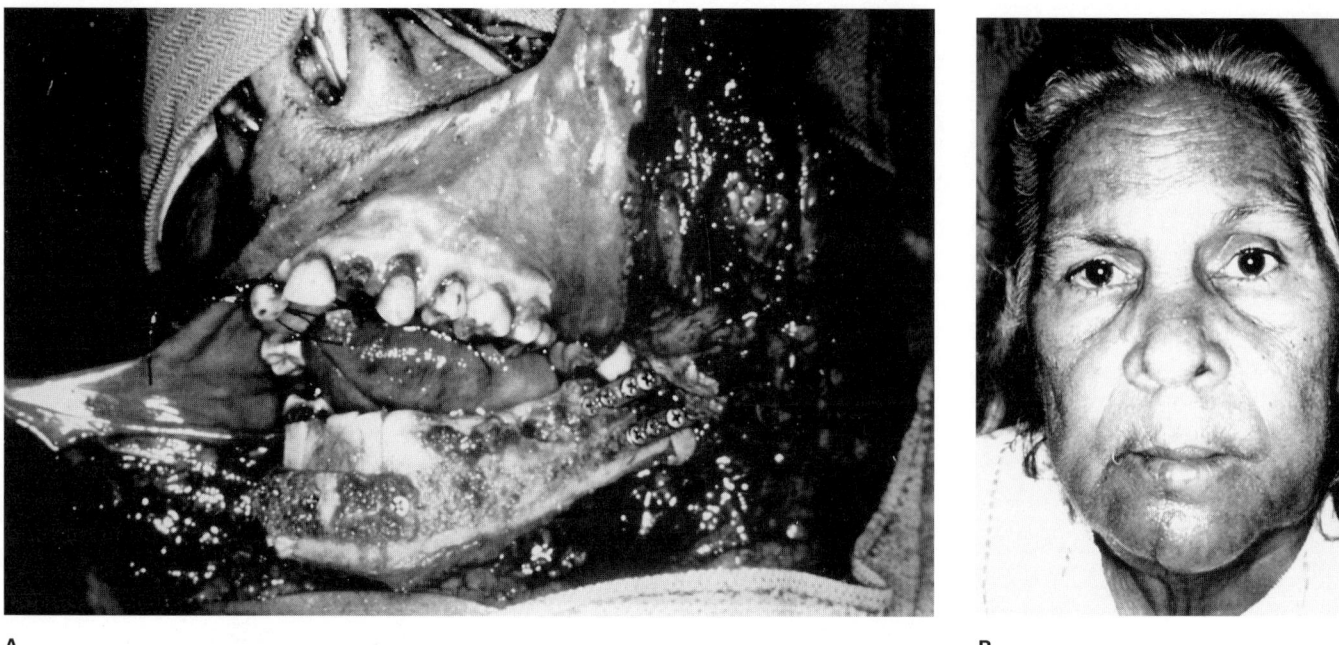

A   B

Fig. 21.84 Iliac crest graft for mandibular reconstruction. A Reconstructed mandible with strips of non-vascularized bone overlying the vascularized bone to enhance contour. **B** Post-operative appearance with a very acceptable mandibular contour.

placed on the flap or into the osteotomies as they are opened by bending; the additional grafts are fixed with long shaped titanium miniplates. The graft is so easily shaped that either step joints or end-to-end apposition can be effected, and the ends can be very strongly secured with plates and screws to obviate the need for intermaxillary fixation. In cases of anterior mandibular replacement, the graft must be made secure against downward rotation. If the infrahyoid or other upper cervical muscles still exist they can be attached to the bone graft. Where a cuff of suprahyoid musculature still exists it can be anchored to the muscle attached to the ilium to give anterior support to the tongue. If epithelial replacement is needed, the skin of the vascularized transfer can be used as oral lining or as additional skin cover. Careful planning ensures that the vascular pedicle lies in appropriate juxtaposition to the recipient vessels.

When intraoral lining is required the split iliac crest graft may be combined with a free forearm flap. The ulnar rather than the radial forearm flap is preferred as it provides more hairless skin and the donor site is less conspicuous (Lovie et al 1984). This thin flap helps to recreate the contours of the floor of the mouth, the labial sulcus and the alveolar margin; this may facilitate the fitting of dentures. It is often necessary to resect some of the soft tissue and reapply it to the underlying bone or to resect the skin from the flap and skin graft the underlying soft tissue as a secondary procedure prior to the fitting of a superstructure to support osseo-integrated implants (Fig. 21.91).

After the bone graft has been fixed with miniplates and the lining flaps stitched in place, the microvascular anastomoses are carried out. For arterial supply of the flap, the facial artery may be used, or the superior thyroid artery; for venous drainage, the anterior facial vein or the superior thyroid vein may be selected, though any sizeable venous channel in the submandibular region can be used. Rarely, we have used the superficial temporal artery and its accompanying vein. The choice of vessel depends largely on what is available, and in post-traumatic mandibular defects, the regional blood supply may have been devastated by the causative missile injury. It could be helpful to visualize the vessels by preoperative external carotid angiography; however, we have never had occasion to do this. Nor have we been prevented from performing a DCIA anastomosis because of destruction of recipient arteries, even in cases of wartime missile mutilations, though occasionally it has been necessary to use a vein graft to obtain arterial supply from a distant vessel. The microvascular anastomoses are performed with 10/0 nylon sutures on a 70 μm tapered needle. Interrupted sutures are first placed on the posterior walls of the approximated vessels, and the suture line is then brought forward around the circumference of the vessels to meet in the midline anteriorly. In the past, we began with stay sutures on each side, and completed the anastomosis by rotating the vessels in microvascular clamps, but we now prefer the sequential procedure. When the anastomoses are completed, the skin wounds are closed.

In massive defects, secondary surgery is usually necessary to trim excess soft tissue or skin. Sometimes soft tissue can be advanced into areas of contour deficiency. Excess bone is easily sculpted away. These secondary procedures are best done after 3–6 months; then, even if the vascular pedicle is inadvertently cut, the bone and soft tissues will survive the secondary surgery provided that this is not excessive or associated with too much dissection of soft tissues.

Complications and results

The success of jaw reconstruction supported by microvascular anastomosis has transformed expectations of surgical reconstruction of this area. Flap failure has been rare in our experience (David et al 1988). In more than 100 of these mandibular reconstructions performed for traumatic, neoplastic or developmental conditions, only four flaps have undergone complete necrosis; in two others, there has been partial bone necrosis and in one there was necrosis confined to the skin.

In our view, all large post-traumatic mandibular defects are best treated by the DCIA flap. In our recent experience of patients wounded in the Iran–Iraq war, we used microvascular free flaps for both upper and lower jaw defects; of special value was the capacity of the free flap to add soft-tissue cover for bone grafts and to maintain grafts without later resorption.

Although the use of DCIA microvascularized grafts seems to us the treatment of choice for massive defects of the mandible, it must be said that good results have been achieved by other methods. The work of Taher (1990), cited above, and other surgeons has shown that cancellous bone supported in titanium trays will often give a satisfactory aesthetic outcome.

RECONSTRUCTION OF MAXILLARY DEFECTS

Assessment

Nowhere is multidisciplinary planning more relevant than in this area of reconstruction. The radiological assessment, particularly sophisticated 3D imaging of the defect, allows the missing bony maxilla to be considered as part of the organ complex involving the orbit, nose and mouth. The multidisciplinary team must not only contain surgeons with maxillofacial and microvascular expertise but also dental and prosthetic experts who can argue the case for prosthetic replacement of defects. The modern technology of osseo-integrated implantation now brings these specialists closer together; surgeons can provide not only tissue for total reconstruction but also tissue into which osseo-integrated implants can be placed to give

more adequate support for whatever prosthesis may be necessary.

Prosthetic correction

Some upper jaw defects can treated by obturation of the defect with a prosthesis, constructed of silicone rubber, acrylic or a combination of such soft and hard materials; the techniques are well described by Conroy (1985). The prosthesis is designed to engage in a palatal defect or other ledge or pocket in the damaged maxilla; the prosthesis may be extended to support the anterior cheek and the orbit, sometimes by fitting in several component parts. Dentures may be fitted to the prosthesis. In mastication, the forces are considerable and the supporting tissues may suffer; surgical attention has been focused on providing a suitable lining to the defect to withstand the pressure of the prosthesis. Maxillary prostheses need to be changed with the changes in the supporting tissues which result from healing and ageing.

It is possible that the potential benefits of surgical replacement of the upper jaw have been disregarded in the past, because the defects were most often created by excision of the maxilla for cancer and there was a subsequent need to inspect the area for recurrent disease: hence the preference for prosthetic replacement. Additional problems arose from the connection of the sinus cavities, oral cavity, orbital cavity and nasal cavity once the maxilla was removed. Such complicated anatomy made this area of surgical reconstruction even more difficult than that of the mandible.

Surgical correction

Simple onlay bone grafts can be used to restore contour to a maxilla deficient in shape. But more difficult problems arise when the entire framework structure needs to be restored to support the eyeball above and the teeth and roof of mouth below. The inherent difficulty in performing this type of reconstruction from autogenous tissue has always been to provide soft-tissue cover on both sides of the grafted bone.

Smaller wounds of the alveolus and hard palate may be dealt with secondarily by mobilizing local mucoperiosteal flaps and inserting cancellous bone grafts, much as when a cleft lip and palate demands prosthetic bone grafting because the alveolus has resorbed due to loss of dentition and ageing. Operations of this type are often performed with a view to future osseo-integrated implantation of the area to support dental or orbital prostheses (see below). Obwegeser (1973) described how the hard palate and alveolar components can be reconstructed in two stages. In the first, a two-layer soft-tissue closure is provided by buccal flaps: (i) from the nasal septum above joined to flaps mobilized from the rim of the defect, and (ii) large rotation flaps from the remaining oral lining from below.

At a second stage bone is inserted between the two layers and fixed to the remnants of the bony palate. This method should be kept in mind because trauma has no respect for time, place and the availability of surgical expertise: all techniques, old and new, may need to be used at some time. However, this technique was described for a pre-planned maxillectomy and not for a traumatic case.

Losses of major segments of the midfacial skeleton are not common except as a result of high velocity missile injuries, whether military or suicidal (Moore et al 1991). This represents a vastly different scenario from that which pertains after selective dissection of the maxilla for cancer. The defect reflects the missile cavity (p. 115) and may extend from the base of the skull through the orbits, nose and both jaws (Fig. 21.85). Reconstruction of such major composite tissue loss demands the provision of adequate intraoral soft-tissue coverage together with restoration of the midfacial skeleton. Modern microvascular composite free-tissue transfers and osseomuscular flaps provide the basis of reconstitution of the missing elements with autogenous tissue. In this way, efforts to restore form and function (including aesthetic balance, speech, mastication, swallowing and occlusion) are maximized.

The strategy of repair is to reposition the existing tissues and to recreate the defect according to the fundamental principles of plastic surgery, and then to transfer vascularized autogenous tissue, if possible at one stage, to rebuild the bony structures of the orbit, alveolus, anterior maxilla together with soft tissue, lining and cover.

Timing

If one is seeing such an injury de novo then the timing of the secondary reconstruction poses an interesting question. While it is not appropriate to do this reconstruction as part of the initial surgical intervention it should be performed before really dense fibrosis has developed, as there is nothing worse for the surgeon than trying to recreate the defect from what may be a 'porridge' of scar, bone fragments and foreign material.

Surgical techniques

It may appear trite advice, but it is important to stress that the deeper reconstructions must be done first and the more superficial procedures such as scar revision of the face and reconstruction of the orbicularis oris and nasal pyramid must come later. These reconstructions used to involve many stages over a long period of time. The advent of microvascular tissue transfer has cut the stages down (Fig. 21.86). The techniques have already been described in the section on orbital and mandibular reconstruction: it is a matter of how to organize them. Cases of avulsive injury in the midface are so diverse in their anatomical deficiencies that it is impossible to give a stepwise guide to their repair: even more than in the mandibular replacements, each case is unique and requires its own operative sequence.

The orbital floors can be reconstructed from above using the temporalis muscles to support the globe on their own or with bone attached as in the pedicled calvarial flap (p. 621). Gillies (1920) described the use of the temporalis muscle for repair in this region, particularly for defects in the orbital floor. McCarthy & Zide (1984) described a calvarial bone flap pedicled on the temporalis muscle to be used to reconstruct the orbit and zygoma (Fig. 21.78).

The microvascular osseocutaneous flap has now assumed a prime role in the restoration of the upper jaw and indeed the rest of the face in massive post-traumatic deformities. The alveolar arch can be reconstructed by microvascular techniques; the buttresses between the zygoma and the palate and alveolar arch can often be rebuilt with free bone. Once this is achieved, it is possible at another stage to reshape the reconstituted tissue. All the osseomyocutaneous flaps described for reconstruction of the mandible can be used in maxillary reconstruction. Reference has already been made to Swartz et al (1986) and the use of the scapula flap. When free flaps are combined with rigid fixation, osseointegrated implants, CAD/CAM produced titanium attachments and tissue expansion, we are able to advance the reconstruction of this difficult area very significantly.

When the transferred bone is supported by microvascular anastomosis it will provide the arch for the alveolus and the supporting strut to the base of skull; if sufficient bone is not readily available from the same flap, the orbital floor can be reconstructed either by ordinary bone grafting if the soft-tissue support is still intact, or by the above-mentioned osteomuscular calvarial flap.

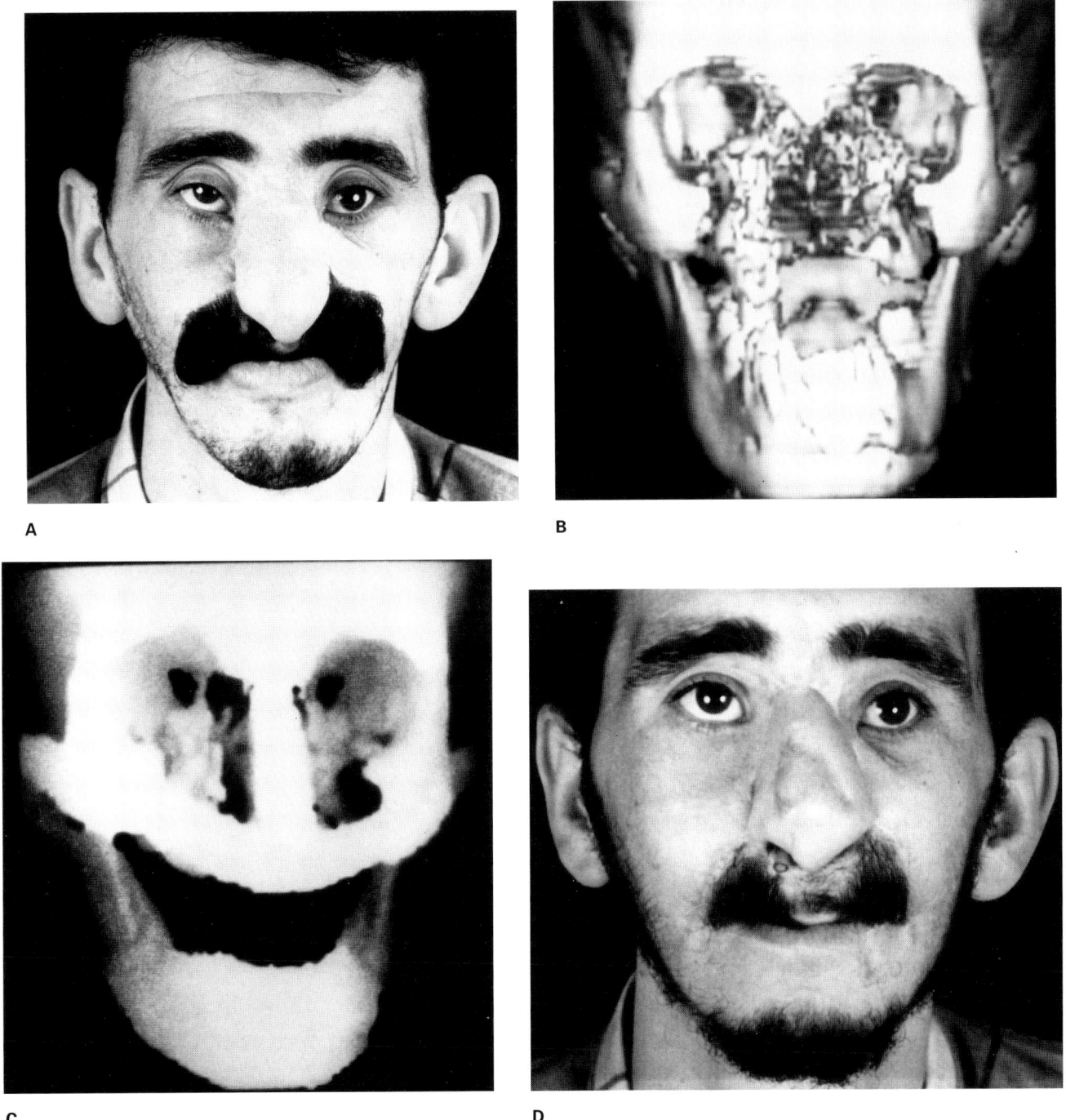

Fig. 21.85 Avulsive midfacial injuries. A soldier suffered a missile injury in the middle third of the face. **A** The nose has been reconstructed from a distant flap and the upper lip from a bipedicled scalp flap. **B** Three-dimensional reconstruction shows the massive bony defect affecting most of the maxilla to the base of skull. **C** The central buttress of the nose and the maxillary arch were reconstructed with a microvascular free flap to give support for the middle third of the face and provide a basis for further prosthetic restoration. **D** Postoperative appearance.

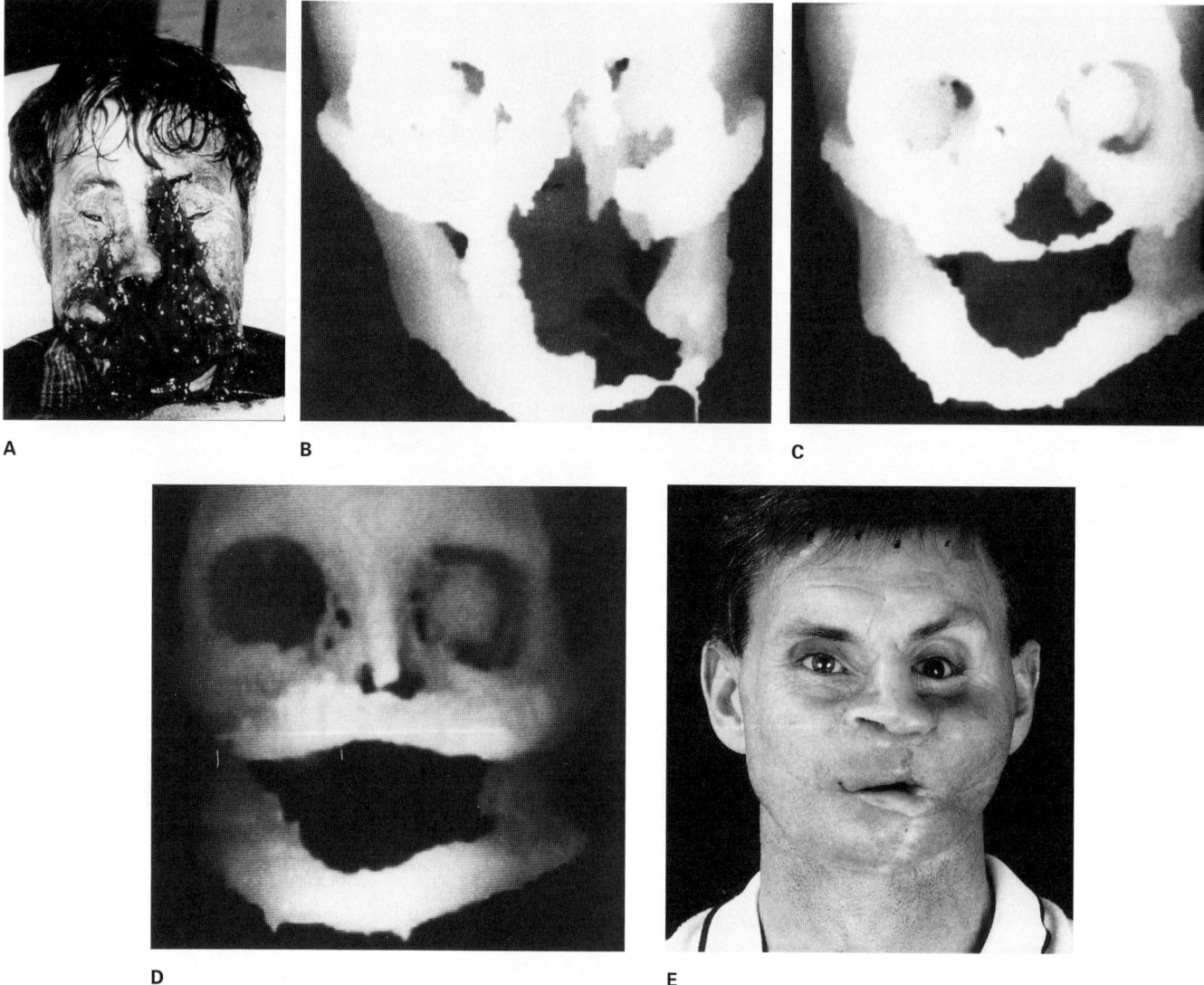

Fig. 21.86 Reconstruction of massive avulsive injuries. A young man suffered a shotgun wound which destroyed the mandible from the right of the symphysis to the left angle, carved a swathe through the upper jaw leaving a small remnant on the right and a tiny bit of buttress on the left, removed the left nasal bone, avulsed the soft tissue to the glabellar region, and destroyed the left eye. He had a retroclival subarachnoid tear and a number of pellets in the frontal intracranial region. Cardiovascular stability was gained and an urgent tracheostomy was done. A subdural catheter was inserted for intracranial pressure manometry. The mandible was stabilised with a K-wire, the wounds were debrided, and primary closure was performed where possible. Several days later his left eye was enucleated and an implant was placed into the socket. The first reconstruction of his mandible was performed using a vascularized iliac crest, with jejunum employed for restoration of the oral lining. 5 months later he underwent further reconstruction of his lower lip by cheek transfer, and rib grafting to his maxilla inserted under the mucosal lining. The first 6 months provided this man with some stability of his lower jaw, lining of the nose and mouth, and a tracheostomy. At the end of this he was able to be nourished and had an intact integument. The jejunum gave a very unsatisfactory florid lining which wept inappropriately and looked dreadful.
A Initial presentation with a massive disruption of the face. The blast has cut its way through the mandible and removed a good deal of the middle third of the face. **B** CT scan shows the situation with the temporary spacer of the mandible and the absence of the upper jaw and the defect extending into the left orbit. **C** Subsequent CT scan shows the mandible reconstructed and a rib graft supported by bowel mucosa in the upper jaw. 2 years later he had insertion of tissue expanders to both cheeks and a forehead flap to reconstruct the left side of the nose. **D** A third CT scan shows the stage of removal of the intraoral jejunal tissue and replacement of the upper jaw with superficial circumflex iliac artery flap with overlying skin. He required further fashioning of flaps and releasing of scar inside his mouth, and further widening of the nostrils. **E** His current situation is reflected with the iatrogenic scar on the left forehead from whence the nasal reconstruction was taken, a prosthetic left eye, a misshapen mouth with deficient orbicularis oris muscle on the left side, and a deficiency of tissue on the left alar base. He is capable of feeding and speaking.

OSSEO-INTEGRATED IMPLANTS IN SECONDARY RECONSTRUCTION

Osseo-integration

Titanium and hydroxyapatite can become integrated into bone, forming a solid and permanent structure into which can be inserted pegs which pass through skin or mucosa and form a basis for prosthetic superstructures which may be permanent or detachable. The biocompatibility of these substances is discussed in Chapter 5 (p. 155). However, biocompatibility is not the only factor relevant in the process of osseo-integration. The acceptance of the osseo-integrated implant depends on the viability of the bone, and this can be prejudiced by heat. Above 56°C, irreversible bone damage occurs; alkaline phosphatase and other enzymes are denatured, and bone synthesis is prevented, thus preventing the process of osseo-integration. Mechanical force effects are also important; if the implant is loaded during the process of osseo-integration, the balance between bone deposition and resorption is disturbed, new bone is not laid down, and the implant is not integrated. In the maxilla, a minimum healing time of 6 months is required, while in the mandible a period of three months may be sufficient. This variance in healing times is related to differences in bone quality.

Techniques for intraoral implantation

In post-traumatic cases, the alveolus may need to be reconstructed with bone grafts to ensure suitable depth and width of bone to receive the metal implant. Various implant designs are available, including screw implants and simple bullet-shaped implants. The implants used by us are 10, 13 and 16 mm in length and 3.75 mm in diameter. Implants may be placed into previously reconstructed jaws including jaws reconstructed with microvascularized bone grafts. A high torque, low cutting speed surgical drilling unit is required. To prevent bone damage from heat, copious irrigation is needed; in some drill systems, the longer drills embody the capacity of internal irrigation at the cutting surface.

Implants are allowed the appropriate minimum period of time to osseo-integrate. They are then uncovered and attachments are made for the superstructure. Where wider and more extensive prostheses are required and where solid bone is at a distance from the site of the necessary prosthesis, an appropriate structure can be milled in titanium from CAD/CAM planning; this is screwed into the bone, and when covered with mucoperiosteum will achieve enough osseo-integration to support a prosthesis (Figs 21.87 and 21.91).

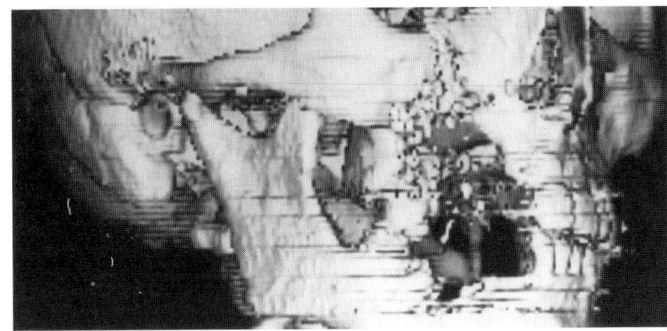

A

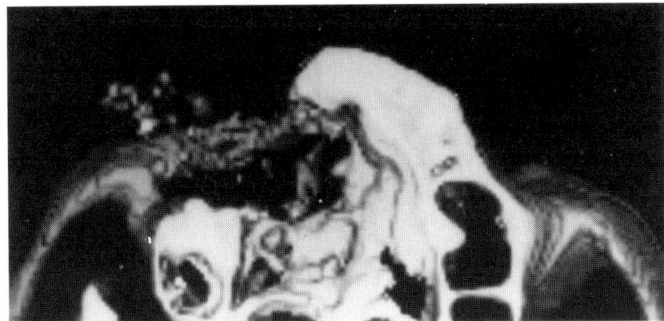

B

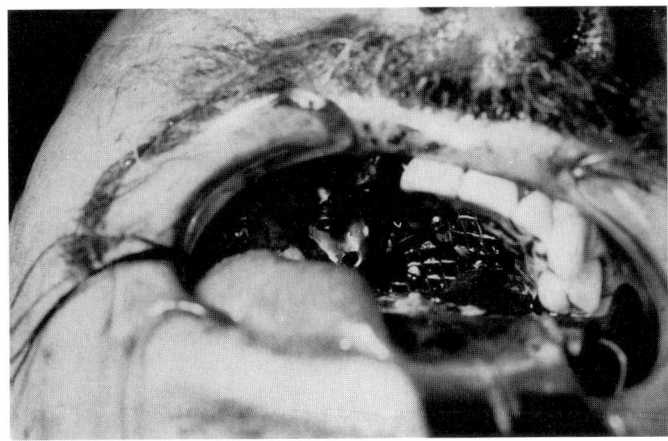

C

Fig. 21.87 Custom prosthetic fabrication from CT data. A 3D CT reconstruction of a 39-year-old male who had suffered a gunshot wound to the right side of the face. **B** Reconstruction viewed from the palate. The extensive nature of the defect is demonstrated. **C** Clinical insertion of custom made titanium prosthesis. The prosthesis was constructed from a solid model produced from the patient's CT scan.

Techniques for extraoral implantation

Extraoral implants may be established to support ocular, nasal, or auricular prostheses. In the past, such prostheses — which have a long history (Fig. 1.11) — were mounted on a spectacle frame or secured to the skin by glues or adhesive tape. These traditional methods of fixation were

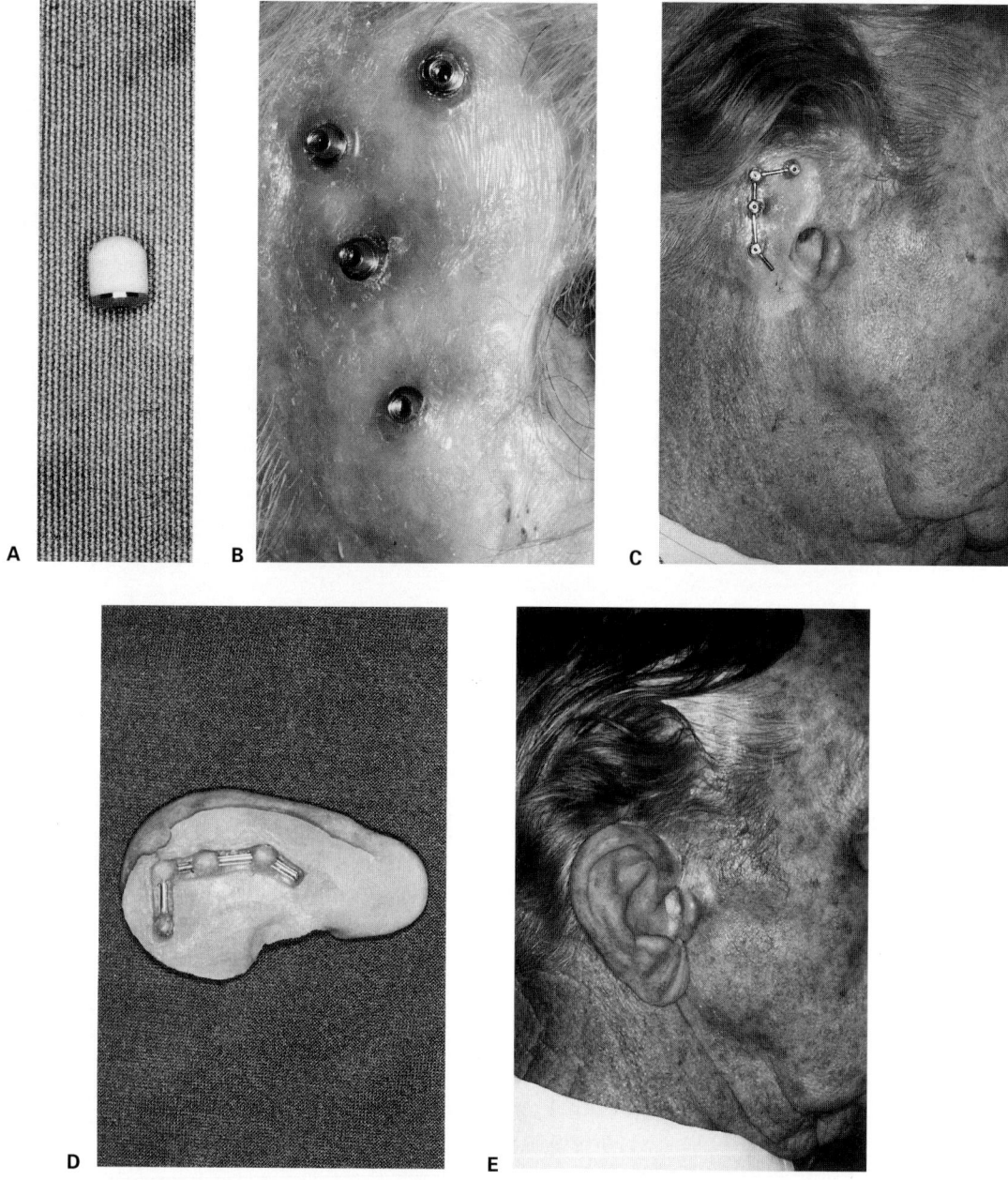

Fig. 21.88 Implant-borne auricular prosthesis. A Hydroxyapatite-coated implant. **B** Appearance after attachment of percutaneous abutments. **C** Bar clip. **D** Medial surface of auricular prosthesis. **E** Auricular prosthesis in place.

not very satisfactory; prostheses were easily dislodged and skin adhesives were associated with discoloration of the prosthesis. They have been partially superseded by the techniques of osseo-integration described by Branemark (Albrektsson et al 1987). Osseo-integrated implants provide very stable prosthetic retention with minimal inconvenience. Nevertheless, older methods of prosthetic correction of a facial defect still have roles, to give temporary aesthetic cover before a definitive procedure can be done, and where individuals or societies are unable to meet the cost of osseo-integrated implants.

Implantation is routinely performed in two stages. In the first, the implant is inserted into bone and covered with soft tissue, which may need to be thinned. The second stage comes 3–6 months later, when the implant is exposed and attached to the transcutaneous abutment to which the prosthesis is attached. The bone in the usual sites for extraoral implants (orbit, midface, temporal bone) accepts implants well and the necessary duration of the subcutaneous implantation is often reduced. This apart, the techniques of implant insertion and exposure are as for intraoral implantation. Prostheses are attached

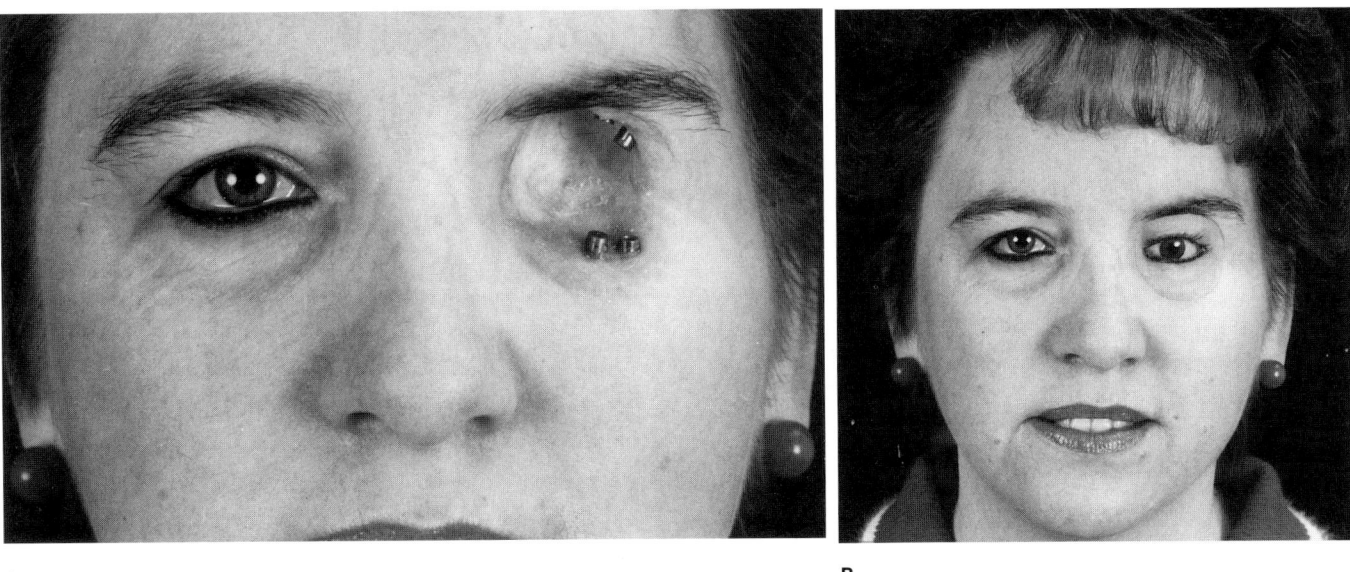

A   **B**

Fig. 21.89 Implant-borne orbital prosthesis. A Implant placement in the left orbit after exenteration. **B** Orbital prosthesis in place with magnet fixation.

by various devices, such as magnets, clips and O-rings.

The overall success rate of extraoral osseo-integration approximates to that achieved with intraoral implants. Bony integration with pure titanium and with hydroxyapatite-coated titanium implants is routinely successful, the only exception in our hands being seen when adequate soft-tissue cover was not achieved in the initial implantation (Moore & Hawker 1993). In the longer term, low grade inflammation sometimes develops around the percutaneous abutment; this is managed by regular cleaning and topical antibiotics, and has not led to loosening of the implant in the bone (McComb 1993, Moore & Hawker 1993).

Applications of this form of surgical prosthetic reconstruction are illustrated by the cases described in Figs 21.88–21.90.

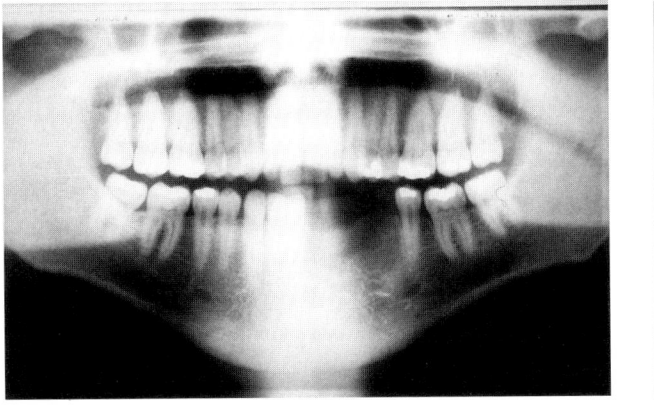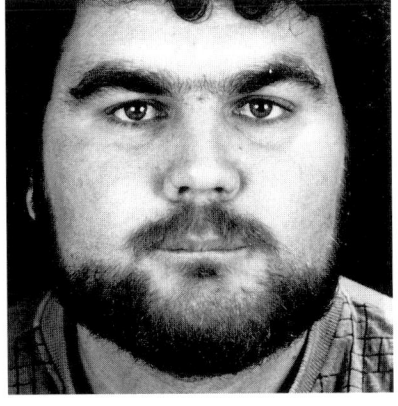

A   **B**

Fig. 21.90 Osseo-integrated implants for dental rehabilitation. A young man had the anterior part of his mandible removed for a squamous carcinoma arising in odontogenic epithelium. He had a deep circumflex iliac artery replacement which was then fitted with osseo-integrated implants. **A** The mandible before excision. **B** Appearance following the mandibular excision and DCIA reconstruction.

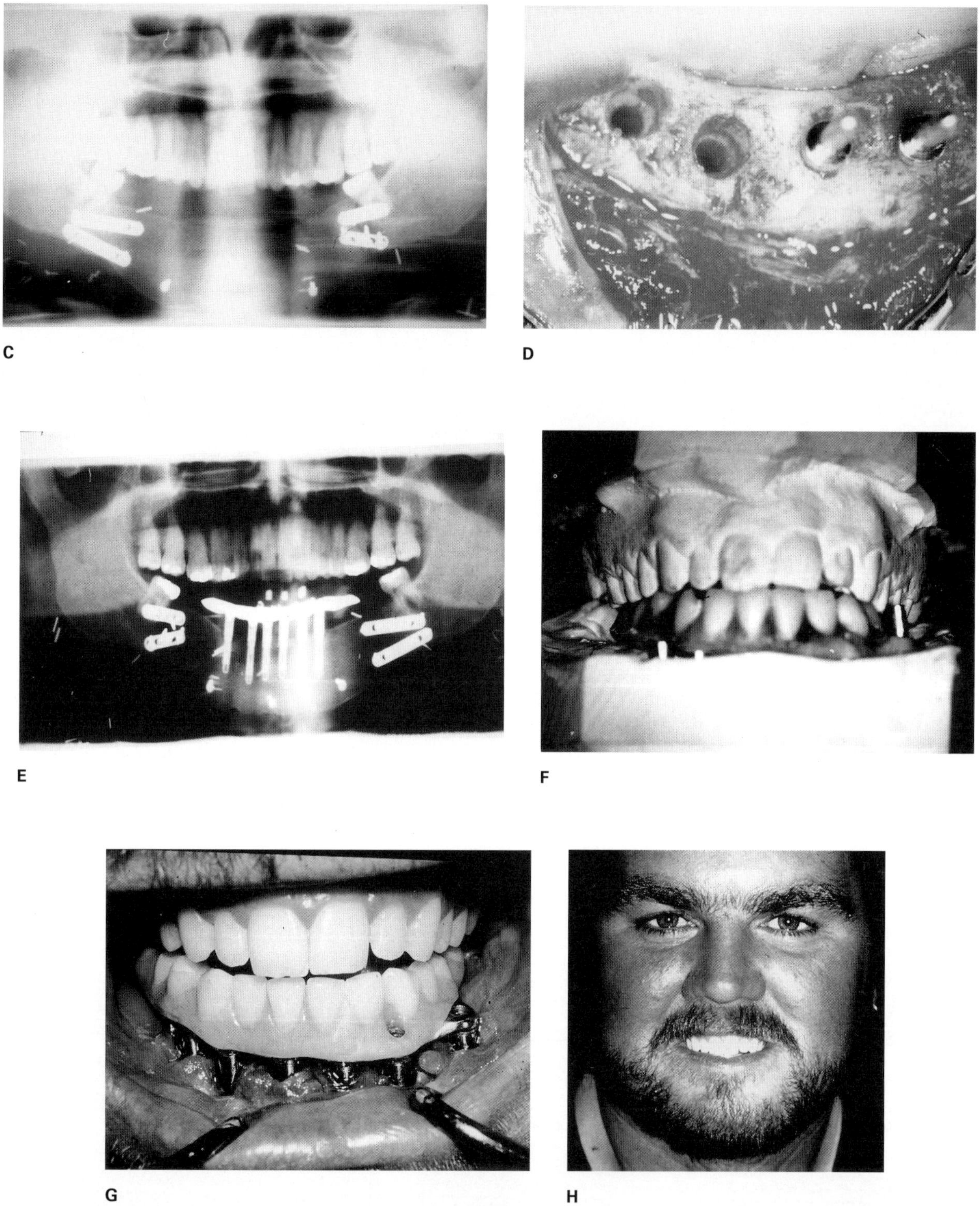

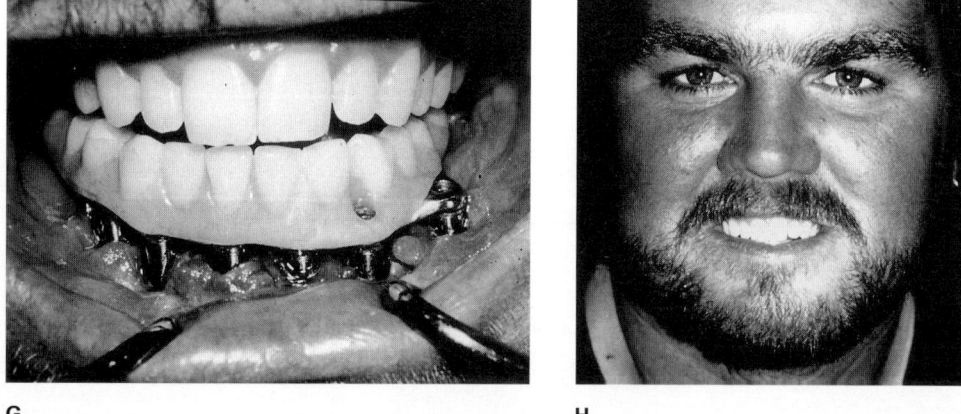

Fig. 21.90 Osseo-integrated implants for dental rehabilitation. A young man who had the anterior part of his mandible removed for a squamous carcinoma arising in odontogenic epithelium. He had a deep circumflex iliac artery replacement which was then fitted with osseo-integrated implants. **C** Orthopantomogram after reconstruction. **D** The process of osseo-integration. **E** Osseo-integrated implants with superstructure. **F** Model planning of the prosthesis. **G** Prosthesis in place. **H** The patient fully reconstructed.

THE ACQUIRED ANOPHTHALMIC SOCKET

Surgical pathology

The aesthetic and psychological problems that result from removal of the globe or destruction of orbital contents depend on the severity of the initial wound and the quality and extent of the treatment given at that time. It is not uncommon, especially in cases from remote places, for these problems to present essentially untreated many months or years after the injury.

Secondary changes occur in an anophthalmic socket, and these may lead to difficulties in fitting and retaining an ocular prosthesis and in associated problems with the motility of that prosthesis. Enophthalmos, superior sulcus deepening and lower lid laxity are several of the most common characteristics of the anophthalmic socket (Soll 1982). Studies done using monkeys as an experimental model suggest that the contributory factors most likely to cause these complications include insufficient volume replacement by using an ocular implant that is too small, mechanical alterations and contractile scar formation (Kronish et al 1990). Smit et al (1990) used high resolution CT scans to evaluate the orbits of anophthalmic patients in whom there was no ocular implant. These showed sagging and retraction of the superior muscle complex as well as downward and forward distribution of orbital fat. These findings help to explain the frequent tipping forward of the base of implants after some years. Another problem associated with the anophthalmic orbit is chronic mucous discharge from goblet cells in remnants of the conjunctiva.

Where the globe itself has been damaged and judged to be useless it may be removed by enucleation or evisceration; these operations are described in Chapter 14. This is done as soon as the indications for removal are established and accepted by the patient. A number of manoeuvres may be undertaken to ensure function of the muscles and retention of the space in which the prosthesis will be placed; increasingly, we are taking the opportunity to insert a coralline implant at the primary operation (p. 419) to mount a prosthesis. However, where there is more extensive orbital injury, with destruction of the globe and also damage or displacement of orbital contents, then there may be a significant deficiency of soft tissue within the orbit. Soft tissues are likely to be replaced by scar, which may also extend to the conjunctival sac and lids. Where there is additional damage to the bony orbit, the orbital contents may escape into the maxillary antrum, temporal fossa or into the ethmoid sinus and the orbital rim and walls may be widely displaced. Displacements affect the lids and adnexae even if these are not themselves damaged (Fig. 16.1).

Assessment

Close liaison between surgeon, ophthalmologist and prosthetist is necessary. When there has been a planned sequence from initial injury to reconstruction by the same team this is relatively easy; when the patient is referred from elsewhere with established deformity and secondary psychological problems, then a very careful multidisciplinary assessment is required. The loss of an eye from trauma can produce a lifelong psychological disability. The technical challenges of producing a satisfactory artificial eye and normal appearing eyelid structures are often not met from the patient's point of view (Perry 1991) and the initial evaluation must include a careful discussion of the patient's wishes and expectations.

Appropriate settings of the CT scan will show not only the bony orbit but also the soft-tissue remnants; from these images, the relationship between soft tissues and bone can be accurately gauged (Fig. 21.91).

Management

Where one is presented with a secondary orbital deformity of large proportions, previously untreated or inadequately treated, then the surgical requirements are:

1. To reconstruct the bony orbit, rim and walls — described in Chapter 11
2. To fill the orbit adequately to ensure projection of the artificial globe and consequently to provide sufficient projection of the lids
3. To reconstruct the conjunctival sac to contain the prosthesis
4. To reconstruct the eyelids if this is necessary.

Filling the orbit

To provide adequate forward projection of a prosthesis the orbital cavity needs to be filled and there are a number of manoeuvres to do this.

The temporalis flap. The anterior portion of the temporalis muscle can be mobilized and passed through a hole burred in the lateral orbital wall. This manoeuvre is effective in the exenterated orbit, where the flap may be covered with lid skin or skin graft, and also where the orbital contents are more or less intact, when the flap is placed behind the conjunctiva to bring the conjunctival sac forward. The technique is similar to that for mobilization of the temporalis muscle in TMJ ankylosis. The hole burred in the lateral orbital wall can be made with a large acrylic burr. The temporalis muscle is sutured to adjacent soft tissue or if necessary to the bone through

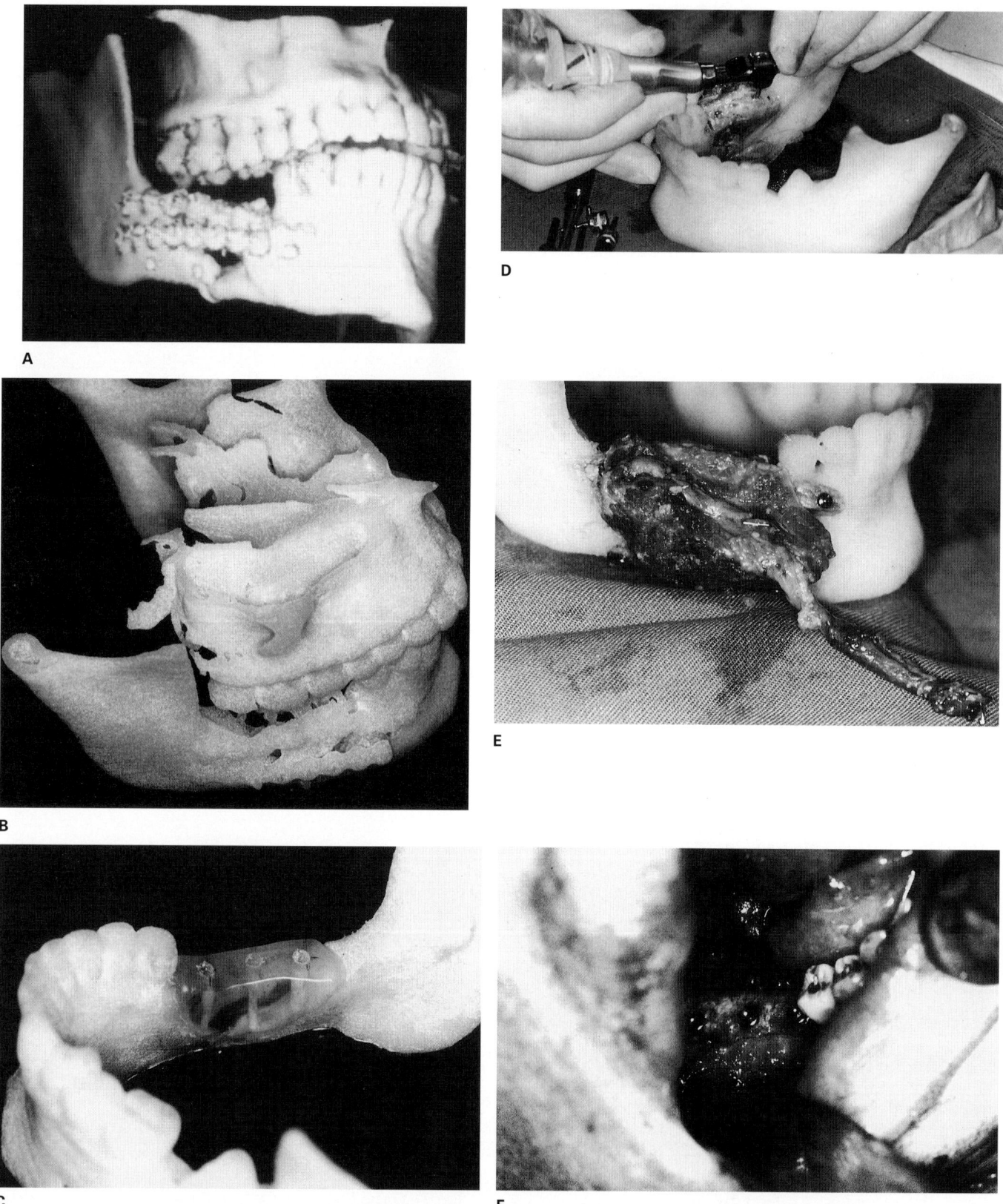

Fig. 21.91 Osseointegrated implants in a vascularized bone graft. A fracture of the body of the mandible was complicated by bone loss both from the trauma and from subsequent infection. **A** The 3D CT scan shows the bone defect on the right side. **B** A three dimensional model milled in nylon has been produced, here seen obliquely from above in articulation with the maxilla. **C** The planned bone graft is milled in acrylic and the precise sites for the osseointegrated implants are defined on this model. A titanium support has been produced for the lower border.
D Vascularised ilium is cut to the exact shape and the implants placed into position according to the template. **E** The vascularised flap on the model. **F** An intraoral view of the osseointegrated implants in their correct position prior to closure.

a few burrholes passed in the orbital rim. However, there are drawbacks in this procedure. Ultimately the flap shrinks as the muscle becomes fibrotic. Moreover, moving the flap leaves a residual temporal hollowing which may be filled secondarily but still remains something of a deformity.

Bone or cartilage grafts. These can be inserted posteriorly to achieve the same effect, particularly if the walls of the orbit have been reconstructed. Bone is subject to resorption and volume changes may occur over the next year. Cartilage from the rib may be diced and packed into the orbit posteriorly. These grafts are quite effective and less likely to resorb, but have a tendency to move.

Vascularized flap. With more extensive orbital damage, the reconstruction can be achieved with a free vascularized flap from the forearm or lateral upper arm (p. 618) (Fig. 21.93).

Filling the orbit continues to be one of the most difficult problems in this area of reconstruction, particularly where there has been previous contraction resulting from fibrosis.

Reconstructing the conjunctiva

The conjunctival sac may require expansion to form adequate fornices above and below in which an appropriate prosthesis can be placed. This is done by a combination of grafting and long-term obturation. The appropriate substances are split skin, full-thickness skin or buccal mucosa. Split skin of course takes better but is subject to further fibrosis, and long-term obturation is necessary. Full-thickness skin often does not take as well and may indeed be too thick; it may lead to problems of difficulty in cleaning. The ideal substance is buccal mucosa, which is self-cleaning; unfortunately the amount available from the cheek is limited.

The operation involves wide release of the scar under the lids, down to the orbital margins, with meticulous haemostasis. The grafts are inserted and sutured with 6–0 catgut; a preformed prosthesis is then inserted. If the prosthesis is not available then an acrylic stent can be manufactured during the operation. The lids are then closed over the prosthesis or stent with tarsorraphy-type sutures and left for as long as possible: for 3–6 months if the patient's compliance and the tarsorraphy can be maintained. When the graft has taken and the fornices are well maintained the temporary prosthesis or stent can be replaced with a permanent prosthetic eye.

Reconstructing the eyelids

The position of the lids may need to be readjusted by medial and/or lateral canthopexies. The lower lid is often too lax and sags under gravity; it may need support. This can be achieved by tightening the lid. There are several ways of doing this:

- Wedge resection of the lid
- Attachment of the lid to the lateral orbital walls (Patterson et al 1987)
- A lateral canthal sling procedure combined with a medial canthoplasty
- Insertion of ear or nasal cartilage into the lower lid to supply support.

We favour where possible the lateral sling and medial canthoplasty.

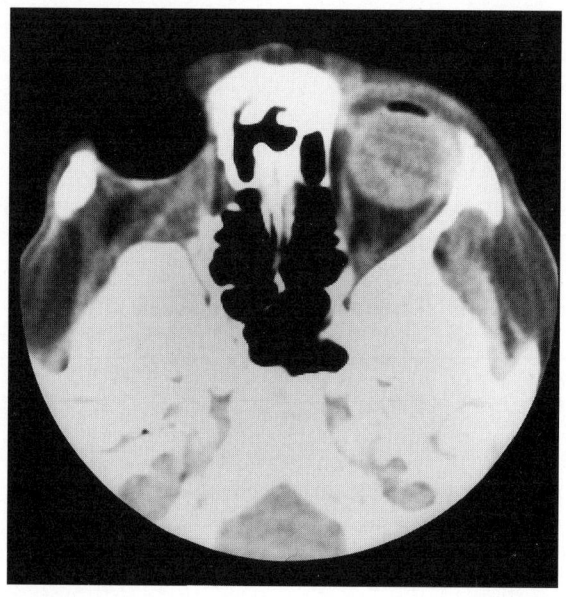
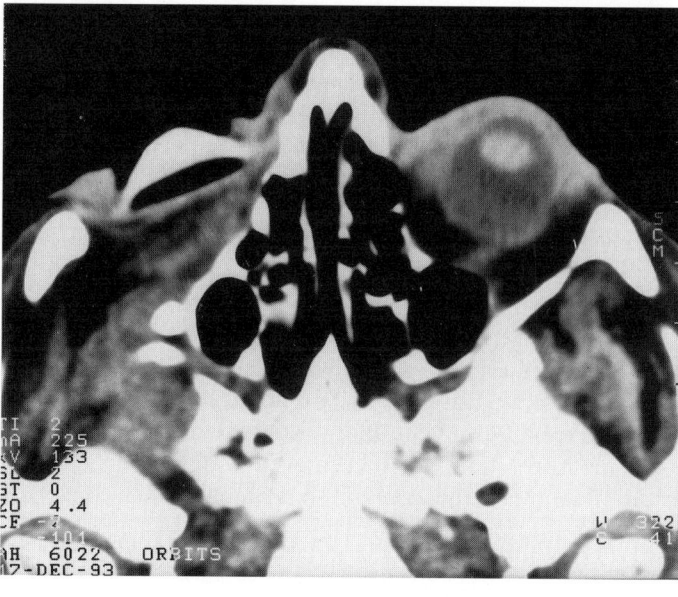

A   **B**

Fig. 21.92 CT evaluation of the orbit. A Axial CT scan of an enophthalmic orbit. The orbital rim is displaced and the residual soft-tissue contents of the orbit are shown. **B** Prosthesis in place. The deficiency in projection of the prosthetic globe is shown to be due to the relationship of the prosthesis, soft tissue, and bony wall.

Complications and results

Except in the simplest and most straightforward cases the anophthalmic orbit remains one of the most challenging areas for secondary post-traumatic reconstruction. Almost all the tissues and substances used for forward projection of the globe are subject to resorption, fibrosis or movement. The effect of gravity on the lower lid together with the ageing process may require constant readjustment to the soft tissue and to the prosthesis. Lacrimation and lid movement may be defective, and frequent cleaning may be needed to prevent the eyelashes being stuck to the prosthesis with dried mucus; for the patient, this is a continuing nuisance. The prosthetic eye is best cleaned with the fingers under running water; chemical agents and soaps should not be used as they may be absorbed by the plastic prosthesis, giving rise to chemical or allergic conjunctivitis in the socket. It is not uncommon for anophthalmic patients to abandon the use of a prosthetic eye and either to use a patch or frosted glasses.

CONCLUSION

Simple problems are rare in secondary facial reconstruction after trauma; almost always, more than one organ system is involved, and therefore more than one discipline. Even the seemingly simple deformity of a displaced zygoma causing depression of the cheek prominence will by definition involve the orbit and potentially the globe; aesthetic correction must take into account any need for orbital dissection, and the possible ophthamological complications.

This chapter has dealt with the selection of surgical and prosthetic manoeuvres necessary to correct deformities; we have attempted to explain how this is done by organized team assessment. The planned sequences of reconstruction should be worked out in advance on a rational basis. But it must be accepted that the surgical intervention itself will produce some unwanted results. Complications should not be unforeseen: any treatment plan should be considered to be a working thesis and therefore subject to falsification and the re-emergence of a stronger thesis.

The seriously damaged face will never be entirely normal in spite of the huge healing forces of nature, enhanced and manipulated by good treatment. The team and the patient will have to decide when enough surgery has been done and when surgery should give way to acceptance and rehabilitative support, at first promoted by professionals but ultimately by the patient.

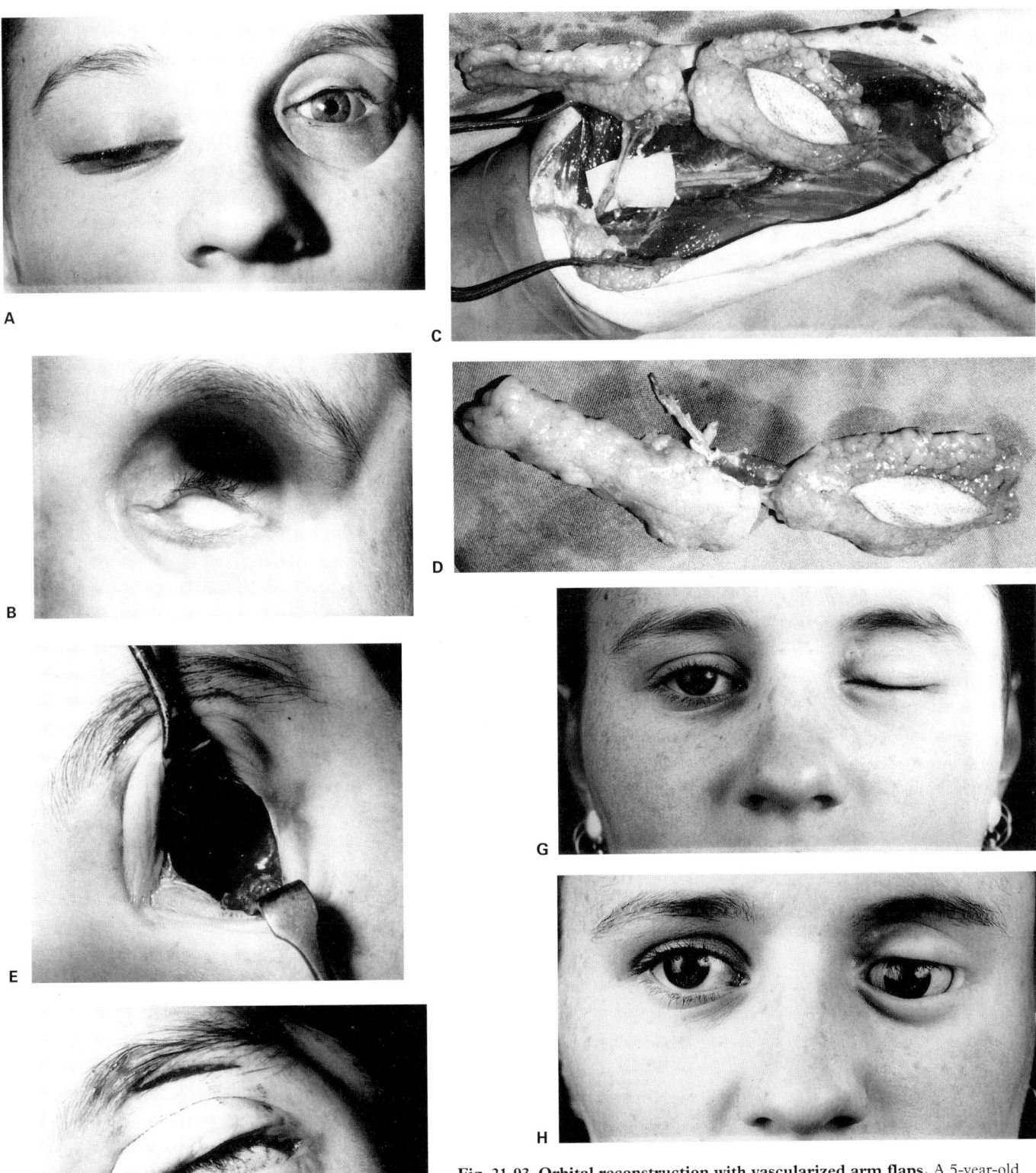

Fig. 21.93 Orbital reconstruction with vascularized arm flaps. A 5-year-old girl had a past history of retinoblastoma in the left eye at 18 months of age. She was initially treated with chemotherapy, radiotherapy, and enucleation of the left eye. **A** Prosthesis in place over the empty eye socket. **B** Contour deficit in the left temporal area. **C,D** A fascio-lipomatous lateral arm flap is raised and split. A small skin ellipse is preserved for enlarging the new eye socket and as a flap monitor. **E** Left orbit prepared to receive the flap. **F** Immediately after flap transfer and revascularization. **G,H** 2 months postoperatively, a satisfactory orbital volume has been achieved and she was able to retain a glass eye. Since this time lateral canthoplasty has also been performed, and correction of the entropion is planned.

REFERENCES

Abbott A H, Netherway D J, David D J, Brown T 1990 Application and comparison of techniques for three-dimensional analysis for craniofacial anomalies. J Craniofac Surg 1: 119–134

Albrektsson T, Branemark P-I, Jacobsson et al 1987 Present clinical applications of osseointegrated percutaneous implants. Plast Reconstr Surg 79: 721–731

Adamson J E 1988 Nasal reconstruction with the expanded forehead flap. Plast Reconstr Surg 65: 12–20

Ariyan S 1980 The viability of rib grafts transplanted with the periosteal blood supply. Plast Reconstr Surg 65: 140–151

Ariyan S, Finseth F J 1978 The anterior chest approach for obtaining free osteocutaneous rib grafts. Plast Reconstr Surg 62: 676–685

Austad E D 1987 Complications in tissue expansion. Clin Plast Surg 14: 549–550

Badran H A, El-Helaly M S, Safe I 1984 The lateral intercostal neurovascular free flap. Plast Reconstr Surg 73: 17–26

Bell W H, Yamaguchi Y, You Z 1992 Treatment of temporomandibular joint dysfunction by intraoral vertical ramus osteotomy. In: Bell W H (ed) Modern practice in orthognathic and reconstructive surgery. Saunders, Philadelphia, Ch 29

Blair G A S, Gordon D S, Simpson D A 1980 Cranioplasty in children. Child's Brain 6: 82–91

Blair V P 1918 Surgery and diseases of the mouth and jaw. Mosby, St Louis

Blake G B, MacFarlane M R, Hinton J W. 1990 Titanium in reconstructive surgery of the skull and face. Br J Plast Surg 43: 528–535

Caldwell J B, Letterman G S 1954 Vertical osteotomy in the mandibular rami for correction of prognathism. J Oral Surg 12: 185–201

Conley J 1972 Use of composite flaps containing bone for major repairs in the head and neck. Plast Reconstr Surg 49: 522–526

Conroy B 1985 Maxillofacial prosthetics and technology. In: Rowe N L, Williams J L (eds) Maxillofacial injuries. Churchill Livingstone, Edinburgh, Ch 19

Converse J M 1942 New forehead flap for nasal reconstruction. Proc R Soc Med 35: 811–812

Converse J M, Ransohoff J, Mathews E S, Smith B, Molenaar A 1970 Ocular hypertelorism and pseudohypertelorism. Advances in surgical treatment. Plast Reconstr Surg 45: 1–13

Converse J M, Smith B, Wood-Smith D 1977 Malunited fractures of the orbit. In Converse J M (ed) Reconstructive plastic surgery, 2nd edn. Saunders, Philadelphia, Ch 28

Courtemanche A D, Thompson G B 1968 Silastic cranioplasty following craniofacial injuries. Plast Reconstr Surg 41: 165–170

Crawley W A, Serletti J M, Manson P N 1993 Autogenous reconstruction of the temporomandibular joint. J Craniofac Surg 4: 28–34

Cuono C B, Ariyan S 1980 Immediate reconstruction of a composite mandibular defect with a regional osteomusculocutaneous flap. Plast Reconstr Surg 65: 477–484

Dal Pont G 1961 Retromolar osteotomy for correction of prognathism. J Oral Surg 19: 42–47

Daniel R K 1978 Mandibular reconstruction with free tissue transfers. Ann Plast Surg 1: 346–371

Dautrey J 1974 Reflexions sur le traitement des laterognathies. Orthod Fr 45: 367–371

David D J 1974 Exploration of the orbital floor through a conjunctival approach. Aust NZ J Surg 44: 25–27

David D J, Moore M H 1989 Cantilever nasal bone grafting with miniscrew fixation. Plast Reconstr Surg 83: 728–732

David D J, Tan E 1979 Microvascular surgery in maxillo-facial reconstruction. Ann Acad Med Singapore 8: 481–485

David D J, Tan E, Katsaros J, Sheen R 1988 Mandibular reconstruction with vascularised iliac crest: a ten year experience. Plast Reconstr Surg 82: 792–803

Demergasso F, Piazza M V 1979 Trapezius myocutaneous flap in reconstructive surgery for head and neck cancer. An original technique. Am J Surg 138: 533–536

Dingman R 1950 Use of iliac bone in the repair of facial and cranial defects. Plast Reconstr Surg 6: 179–195

Dingman R 1978 In: Symposium on plastic surgery in the orbital region. Mosby, St Louis, p 122

Doi K, Tominaga S, Shibata J 1977 Bone graft with microvascular anastomosis of vascular pedicles: an experimental study in dogs. J Bone Joint Surg 59A: 809–815

Dolwick M F, Aufdemorte T B 1985 Silicone induced foreign body reaction in lympadenopathy after temporomandibular joint arthroplasty. Oral Surg Oral Med Oral Pathol 59: 449–452

Dufresne C, Cutting C, Valauri F, Klein M, Colen S, McCarthy J G. 1987 Reconstruction of mandibular and floor of mouth defects using the trapezius osteomyocutaneous flap. Plast Reconstr Surg 79: 687–696

Duncan M J, Mankeltow R T, Zuker R M, Rosen I B 1985 Mandibular reconstruction of the irradiated patient. The role of osteocutaneous free tissue transfers. Plast Reconstr Surg 76: 829–840

Edwards R M 1993 Awake blind nasal intubation: letter. Anaesth Intens Care 21: 258

Evans A J, Burwell R G, Merville L et al 1985 In: Rowe N L, Williams J L (eds) Maxillofacial injuries. Churchill Livingstone, Edinburgh, Ch 18

Galicich J H, Hovind K H 1967 Stainless steel mesh–acrylic cranioplasty. J Neurosurg 27: 376–378

Gallagher D M, Wolford L M 1982 Comparison of Silastic and Proplast implants in the temporomandibular joint after condylectomy for osteoarthritis. J Oral Maxillofac Surg 40: 627–630

Georgiade N G 1977 Disturbances of the temporomandibular joint. In: Converse J M (ed) Reconstructive plastic surgery, 2nd edn. Saunders, Philadelphia, Ch 31

Gillies H D 1920 Plastic surgery of the face. Oxford University Press, London

Gillies H 1968 The diagnosis and treatment of residual traumatic deformities of the facial skeleton. In: Rowe N L, Killey H C (eds) Fractures of the facial skeleton, 2nd edn. Livingstone, Edinburgh

Gillies H, Harrison S H 1951 Operative correction by osteotomy of recessed malar maxillary compound in a case of oxycephaly. Br J Surg 3: 123–127

Gonzalez-Ulloa M 1972 Ptosis of the chin: the witches' chin. Plast Reconstr Surg 50: 54–57

Gordon D S, Blair G A S 1974 Titanium cranioplasty. Br Med J 2: 478–481

Green M F, Gibson J R, Bryson J R, Thompson E 1981 A one stage correction of mandibular defects using a split sternum pectoralis major osteomusculocutaneous transfer. Br J Plast Surg 34: 11–16

Gruss J S 1992 Rigid fixation of naso-ethmoidal fractures In: Yaremchuk M J, Gruss J S, Manson P N (eds) Rigid fixation of the craniomaxillofacial skeleton. Butterworth-Heinemann, Boston

Gruss J S, McKinnon S E, Kassel E E, Cooper P W 1985 The role of primary bone grafting in complex cranio-maxillo-facial trauma. Plast Reconstr Surg 75: 17–24

Gruss J S, Van Wyck, Phillips J H et al 1990 The importance of the zygomatic arch in complex midfacial fracture repair and correction of post traumatic orbitozygomatic deformities. Plast Reconstr Surg 85: 878–890

Harashina T, Nakajima H, Amai T 1978 Reconstruction of mandibular defects with revascularised free rib grafts. Plast Reconstr Surg 62: 514–522

Henderson D 1974 The assessment and management of bony deformities of the middle and lower face. Br J Plast Surg 27: 287–296

Henry H M, Guerrero C, Moody R A 1976 Cerebrospinal fluid fistula from fractured acrylic plate. J Neurosurg 45: 227–228

Homma K, Ohura T, Sugihara T, Yoshida T, Hasegawa T 1993 Prefabricated flaps using tissue expanders; an experimental study in rats. Plast Reconstr Surg 91: 1098–1109

Hunsuck E E 1968 A modified intraoral sagittal technique for correction of mandibular prognathism. J Oral Surg 26: 249–252

Jackson I T 1989 Advances in craniofacial tumor surgery. World J Surg 13: 440–453

Jones J K, Van Sickels J E 1991 Facial nerve injuries associated with orthognathic surgery: a review of incidence and management. J Oral Maxillofac Surg 49: 740–744

Katsaros J, Schusterman M, Beppu M, Banis J C, Acland R D 1984 The lateral upper arm flap: anantomy and clinical applications. Ann Plast Surg 6: 489–500

Kazanjian V H 1938 Ankylosis of the temporomandibular joint. Surg Gynecol Obstet 67: 333–348

Kent J N, Misiek D J, 1991 Biomaterials for cranial, facial, mandibular, and TMJ reconstruction. In: Fonseca R J, Walker R V (eds) Oral and maxillofacial trauma. Saunders, Philadelphia, Ch 29

Kent J N, Misiek D J Aikin R K et al 1983 Temporomandibular joint condylar prostheses: a ten-year report. J Oral Maxillofac Surg 41: 245–254

Ketchum L D, Masters F W, Robinson D W 1974 Mandibular reconstruction using composite island rib flap. Plast Reconstr Surg 53: 471–476

Körlof B, Nylen B, Rietz K-A 1973 Bone grafting of skull defects. A report on 55 cases. Plast Reconstr Surg 52: 378–383

Kronish J W, Gonnering R S, Dortzbach R K et al 1990 The pathophysiology of the anophthalmic socket: Part II. Analysis of orbital fat. Ophthalmic Plast Reconstr Surg 6: 88–95

Lash H, Zimmerman D, Loeffler R 1964 Silicone implantation: inlay method. Plast Reconstr Surg 34: 75–80

Laurie S W, Kaban L B, Mulliken J B et al 1984 Donor site morbidity after harvesting rib and iliac bone. Plast Reconstr Surg 73: 933–938

Lello G E 1990 Surgical correction of temporomandibular joint ankylosis. J Craniomaxillofac Surg 18: 19–26

Levant B R 1977 Total reconstruction of the mandibular body. Ann R Australas Coll Dental Surgeons 55: 90–93

Lovie M J, Duncan G M, Glasson D W 1984 The ulnar artery forearm free flap. Br J Plast Surg 37: 486–492

MacAfee K A, Quinn P D 1992 Total temporomandibular joint reconstruction with a Delrin titanium implant. J Craniofac Surg 3: 160–169

McCarthy J G, Zide B M 1984 The spectrum of calvarial bone grafting: introduction of the vascularized calvarial bone flap. Plast Reconstr Surg 74: 10–18

McCarthy J G, Cutting C B, Shaw W W 1987 Vascularized calvarial flaps. Clin Plast Surg 14: 37–47

McCarthy J G, Jelks G W, Valauri A J, Wood-Smith D, Smith B 1990a The orbit and zygoma. In: McCarthy J G (ed) Plastic surgery. Saunders, Philadelphia, Ch 33

McCarthy J G, Kawamoto H K, Grayson B H, Colen S R, Coccaro P J 1990b Surgery of the jaws. In: McCarthy J G (ed) Plastic surgery. Saunders, Philadelphia, Ch 29

McComb H 1993 Osseointegrated titanium implants for the attachment of facial prostheses. Ann Plast Surg 31: 225–232

McCullough D W, Fredrickson J M 1973 Neovascularized rib grafts to reconstructive mandibular defects. Can J Otolaryngol 2: 96–100

McKee D M 1978 Microvascular bone transplantation. Clin Plast Surg 5: 283–292

MacLeod A M, Robinson D W 1982 Reconstruction of defects involving the mandible and floor of mouth by free osteocutaneous flaps derived from the foot. Br J Plast Surg 35: 239–246

Maejima S, Tajima S, Tanaka Y 1993 Cranioplasty with ceramics (Seratite) used 3D solid model. J Japan Cran Maxillofac Surg 9: 1–6

Manchester W M 1965 Immediate reconstruction of the mandible and temporomandibular joint. Br J Plast Surg 18: 291–303

Manchester W M 1972 Some technical improvements in the reconstruction of the mandible and temporomandibular joint. Plast Reconstr Surg 50: 249–256

Manson P N, Sargent L 1992 Naso-ethmoid orbital fractures. Quoted in: Yaremchuk M J, Gruss J S, Manson P N (eds). Rigid fixation of the craniomaxillofacial skeleton. Butterworth-Heinemann, Boston

Manson P N, Crawley W A, Hoops J A 1986 Frontal cranioplasty risk factors and choice of cranial vault reconstructive material. Plast Reconstr Surg 77: 888–904

Marks M W, Argenta L C, Thornton J W 1987 Rapid expansion: experimental and clinical experience. Clin Plast Surg 14: 455–463

Maruyama Y, Urita Y, Ohnishik K 1985 Rib latissimus dorsiosteomyocutaneous flap in reconstruction of the mandibular defect. Br J Plast Surg 38: 234–237

Marx R E, Stevens M R 1991 Reconstruction of avulsive maxillofacial injuries. In Fonseca R J, Walker R V (eds) Oral and maxillofacial trauma. Saunders, Philadelphia, Vol 2, Ch 30

Merville L C, Vincent J, Thomas H 1974 Dislocations multiple de la face. Ann Chir Plast 19: 105–120

Merville L V, Derome P, Saint-Jorre G 1983 Fronto-orbito-nasal dislocations: secondary treatment of sequelae. J Maxillofac Surg 11: 71–82

Moore M H, Hawker P B 1993 Biointegrated hydroxylapatite coated implant fixation of facial prostheses. Ann Plast Surg 31: 233–237

Moore M H, Abbott J R, David D J 1991 The missing maxilla: restoring aesthetic balance with mandibular surgery. J Craniofac Surg 2: 95–100

Munro I R, Chen Y R, Park B Y 1986 Simultaneous total correction of temporomandibular ankylosis and facial asymmetry. Plast Reconstr Surg 77: 517–529

Murray J E, Swanson L T 1968 Mid-face osteotomy and advancement for craniosynostosis. Plast Reconstr Surg 41: 299–306

Murray J E, Kaban L B, Mulliken J B 1984 Analysis and treatment of hemifacial microsomia. Plast Reconstr Surg 74: 186–199

Mustardé J C 1959 The treatment of ptosis and epicanthal folds. Br J Plast Surg 12: 252–258

Neumann C 1957 The expansion of an area of skin by progressive distension of a subcutaneous balloon: use of the method for securing skin for subtotal reconstruction of the ear. Plast Reconstr Surg 19: 124–130

Nguyen P N, Sullivan P 1992 Advances in the management of orbital fractures. Clin Plast Surg 19: 87–98

Norman J E 1978 Ankylosis of the temporomandibular joint. Aust Dental J 23: 56–66

O'Brien B M, Morrison W A, MacLeod A M, Dooley B J 1979 Microvascular osteocutaneous transfer using the groin flap and iliac crest and dorsalis pedis flap and second metatarsal. Br J Plast Surg 32: 188–206

Obwegeser H L 1973 Late reconstruction of large maxillary defects after tumour resection. J Maxillofac Surg 1: 19–29

Ohno K, Michi K, Ueno T 1981 Mandibular growth following ankylosis operation in childhood. Int J Oral Surg 10: 324–238

Ostrup L T, Fredrickson J M 1974 Distant transfer of free living bone graft by microvascular anastomoses. An experimental study. Plast Reconstr Surg 54: 274–285

Ostrup L T, Tam C S 1975 Bone formation in a free, living bone graft transferred by microvascular anastomoses. A quantitative microscopic study using fluorochrome markers. Scand J Plast Reconstr Surg 9: 101–106

Otto E 1958 Posttraumatische Spätkomplikation nach Paladonplastik des Schädels. Zentralbl Neurochir 18: 162–165

Ousterhout D K 1985 Clinical experience in cranial and facial reconstruction with demineralized bone. Ann Plast Surg 15: 367–373

Ousterhout D K, Zlotolow I M 1991 Prosthetic forehead augmentation: In: Ousterhout D K (ed) Aesthetic contouring of the craniofacial skeleton. Little, Brown & Co., Boston, Ch 17

Panje W, Cutting C 1980 Trapezius osteomyocutaneous island flap for reconstruction of the anterior floor of mouth and mandible. Head Neck Surg 3: 66–71

Patterson S, Munro I R, Farkas L G 1987 Transconjunctival lateral canthopexy in Down's syndrome patients: a nonstigmatising approach. Plast Reconstr Surg 79: 714–720

Perry A C 1991 Understanding and treatment of the congenital and acquired anophthalmic socket. Curr Opin Ophthalmol 2: 607–611

Phillips J H, Gruss J S 1991 Factors affecting bone grafting especially the effects of fixation on membranous and endochondral bone. In: Ousterhout D K (ed) Aesthetic contouring of the craniofacial skeleton. Little, Brown & Co., Boston, Ch 13

Phillips J H, Rahn B 1988 Fixation effects on membranous and endochondral onlay bone graft resorption. Plast Reconstr Surg 82: 872–877

Phillips J H, Rahn B 1990 Fixation effects on membranous and endochondral onlay bone graft revascularization and bone deposition. Plast Reconstr Surg 85: 891–897

Posnick J C, Goldstein J A 1993 Surgical management of temporomandibular joint ankylosis in the paediatric population. Plast Reconstr Surg 91: 791–798

Radovan C 1982 Breast reconstruction after mastectomy using a temporary expander. Plast Reconstr Surg 69: 195–208

Radovan C 1984 Tissue expansion in soft tissue reconstruction. Plast Reconstr Surg 74: 482–492

Raulo Y, Tessier P 1981 Mandibulo-facial dysostosis analysis: principles of surgery. Scand J Plast Reconstr Surg 15: 251–256

Robertson G A 1986 A comparison between sternum and rib in osteomyocutaneous reconstruction of major mandibular defects and also plastic surgery. Ann Plast Surg 17: 421–433

Rose E H, Norris M S, Rosen J M 1993 Application of high-tech three-dimensional imaging and computer-generated models in complex facial reconstructions with vascularized bone grafts. Plast Reconst Surg 91: 252–264

Rowe N L 1971 The history of the treatment of maxillofacial trauma. Ann R Coll Surg 49: 329–349

Rowe N L 1982 Ankylosis of the temporomandibular joint. Parts 1–3. J R Coll Surg Edinb 27: 67–79, 167–173, 209–218

Rushton M A 1942 Malformations of the mandibular ramus treated by bone graft. Dental Rec 62: 272–274

Salibian A H, Rapaport I, Alison G 1985 Functional oral mandibular reconstruction with the microvascular composite groin flap. Plast Reconstr Surg 76: 819–828

Schmidt D R, Robson M C 1982 One stage composite reconstruction using the latissimus myo-osteocutaneous free flap. Am J Surg 144: 470–472

Serafin D, Villarreal-Rios A, Georgiade N G 1979 A rib-containing free flap to reconstruct mandibular defects. Br J Plast Surg 30: 263–266

Serafin D, Riefkohl R, Thomas I, Georgiade N G 1980 Vascularized rib-periosteal and osteocutaneous reconstruction of the maxilla and mandible: an assessment. Plast Reconstr Surg 66: 718–727

Seward G R 1967 Method of replacing the anterior part of the mandible by a bone graft. Br J Oral Surg 5: 99–105

Siemssen S O, Kirkby B, O'Connor T P 1978 Immediate reconstruction of resected segment of the lower jaw using a compound flap of clavicle and sternomastoid muscle. Plast Reconstr Surg 61: 724–735

Simpson D 1965 Titanium in cranioplasty. J Neurosurg 22: 292–293

Smit T J, Koornneef L, Zonneveld F W, Groet E, Otto A J 1990 Computed tomography in the assessment of the post enucleation socket syndrome. Ophthalmology 97: 1347–1351

Smith R M, Goldwasser M S, Sabol S R 1993 Erosion of a Teflon–Proplast implant into the middle cranial fossa. J Oral Maxillofac Surg 51: 1268–1271

Soll D B 1982 The anophthalmic socket. Ophthalmology 89: 407–423

Song R, Song Y, Yu Y, Song Y 1982 The upper arm free flap. Clin Plast Surg 9: 27–35

Souyris F 1990 The chin in temporomandibular joint ankylosis. In: Levignac J (ed) The chin. Churchill Livingstone, London. Ch 10

Steenfos H, Tarnow P, Blomqvist S 1993 Skin expansion. Long term follow-up of complications and costs of care. Scand J Plast Reconstr Surg Hand Surg 27: 137–141

Strauch B, Bloomberg A E, Lewin M L 1971 An experimental approach to mandibular replacement: island vascular composite rib grafts. Br J Plast Surg 24: 334–341

Swartz W M, Banis J C, Newton E D, Ramasastry S S, Jones N F, Acland R 1986 The osteocutaneous scapular flap for mandibular and maxillary reconstruction. Plast Reconstr Surg 77: 530–545

Taher A A 1990 Reconstruction of gunshot wounds of the mandible. J Craniomaxillofac Surg 18: 310–314

Tajima S, Aoyagi F, Maruyama Y 1978 Free perichondrial grafting in the treatment of temporomandibular joint ankylosis. Preliminary report. Plast Reconstr Surg 61: 676–880

Tayapongsak P, Pijut L, Scheffer R B 1993 Inferior border titanium crib in mandibular reconstruction. J Oral Maxillofac Surg 51(8) (Suppl 3): 151–153

Tayapongsak P, O'Brien D A, Monteiro C B, Arceo-Diaz L Y 1994 Autologuous fibrin adhesive in mandibular reconstruction with particulate cancellous and bone marrow. J Oral Maxillofac Surg 52: 161–166

Taylor G I 1982 Reconstruction of the mandible with free composite iliac bone grafts. Ann Plast Surg 9: 361–376

Taylor G I, Daniel R K 1975 The anatomy of several free flap donor sites. Plast Reconstr Surg 56: 243–253

Taylor G I, Miller G D, Ham F J 1975 The free vascularized bone graft. A clinical extension of microvascular techniques. Plast Reconstr Surg 55: 533–544

Taylor G I, Townsend P, Corlett R 1979a Superiority of the deep circumflex iliac vessels as the supply for free groin flaps: experimental work. Plast Reconstr Surg 64: 595–604

Taylor G I, Townsend P, Corlett R 1979b Superiority of the deep circumflex iliac vessels as the supply for free groin flaps: clinical work. Plast Reconstr Surg 64: 754–759

Tessier P 1971 The definitive plastic surgical treatment of the severe facial deformities of craniofacial dysostosis. Plast Reconstr Surg 48: 419–442

Tessier P 1973 The conjunctival approach to the orbital floor and maxilla in congenital malformation and trauma. J Maxillofac Surg 1: 3–8

Tessier P 1982 Inferior orbitotomy a new approach to the orbital floor. Clin Plast Surg 9: 569–575

Tessier P 1991 Methods and long term results of bone grafting of the nose in aesthetic contouring of the craniofacial skeleton. In: Aesthetic contouring of the craniofacial skeleton. Ousterhout D R (ed) Little, Brown & Co., Boston, Ch 21

Timmons R L 1982 Cranial defects and their repair. In: Youmans J R (ed). Neurological surgery, 2nd edn. Saunders, Philadelphia, Vol 4

Topazian R G 1964 Etiology of ankylosis of the temporomandibular joint: analysis of 44 cases. J Oral Surgery 22: 227–233

Trauner R, Obwegeser H 1957 The surgical correction of mandibular prognathism and retrognathism with consideration of genioplasty. Parts I and II. Oral Surg Oral Med Oral Pathol 10: 677–689, 787–792

Van der Meulen J C, Hauben D J, Vaandrager J M, Birgenhager-Frenkel D H. 1984 The use of a temporo osteoperiosteal flap for reconstruction of malar hypoplasia in Treacher Collins syndrome. Plast Reconstr Surg 74: 687–693

Waite P D, Morawetz R B, Zeiger H E, Pincock J L 1989 Reconstruction of calvarial defects with porous hydroxylapatite blocks. Neurosurgery 25: 214–217

Washio H 1972 Further experiences with the retroauricular temporal flap. Plast Reconstr Surg 50: 160–162

Wassmund M 1927 Frakturen und Luxationen des Gesichtsschädels unter Berucksichtigung der Komplikationen des Hirnschädels. In: Klinik und Therapie praktischen Lehrbuch. Herman Meusser, Berlin, Vol 20, p 384

Whitaker L A 1987 Aesthetic augmentation of the malar midface region. Plast Reconstr Surg 80: 337–346

Whitaker L A 1991 Aesthetic alteration of the malar-midface structures. In: Aesthetic Contouring of the Craniofacial Skeleton. Ousterhout D R (ed). Little, Brown & Co., Boston, Ch 28

Wolfe S A, Berlowitz S 1989 Plastic surgery of the facial skeleton. Little, Brown & Co., Boston, p 593

Yab K, Tajima S, Imai K (In press) Clinical application of a solid three-dimensional model for orbital wall fractures. J Craniomaxillofac Surg

Yang G F 1981 Forearm free skin flap transplantation (Chinese; no English abstract). Nat Med J China 61: 139–141

Yih W Y, Zysset N, Merrill R G 1992 Histologic study of the fate of autogenous auricular cartilage grafts in the human temporomandibular joint. J Oral Maxillofac Surg 50: 964–967

22 | Impairments and disabilities

M. Wood   M. Hammerton
Contributing authors: J. L. Crompton   M. Jay   D. Simpson
J. Abbott   T. Brown

INTRODUCTION

However well managed, injuries of the face, brain and eyes will often cause permanent impairments, and the victims will be disabled in many ways. With some injuries, the eventual disability is obvious at once. Evaluation is easy; counselling and rehabilitation can begin early. More often, however, the long-term effects are unpredictable and remain so for some time. The aesthetic effects of a mutilating facial wound cannot be assessed until reconstructive surgery has achieved the best possible result. The intellectual and behavioural disabilities resulting from frontal lobe damage cannot be evaluated until neuronal recovery and cerebral reorganization have reached a level that has to be accepted as stable — a process that may take several years. Nevertheless, despite these uncertainties, the reciprocal processes of assessment and rehabilitation should begin as soon as possible after the injury (p. 258).

All members of the multidisciplinary craniofacial team are engaged in the assessment of impairment, and many are also engaged in rehabilitation. Senior specialists in the various disciplines are responsible for counselling the victim and the family on what can be done, and on when the limits of physical recovery have been reached: it is most important that this is not delegated to someone without the necessary experience and empathy, or to a junior team member who cannot speak with convincing authority (p. 249).

A senior specialist is also usually responsible for the medicolegal evaluations that are, in most parts of the world, needed for the increasingly elaborate (and expensive) processes of litigation and compensation. In many countries, settlement of a claim for injury compensation requires a final medicolegal evaluation of the permanent disability; for such assessments, the assessor must know whether the impairment has become stable, since a premature evaluation may exaggerate the claim, or alternatively omit some serious late disability such as epilepsy.

For some impairments, specialists in rehabilitation are needed. Visual rehabilitation has for long been a separate discipline and, in many centres, this is also the case with head injury rehabilitation, where the role of the neuropsychologist has become increasingly valuable in therapy as well as in evaluation. In all kinds of post-traumatic disability, the social worker plays a vital role, in counselling and in organizing the supporting services that may be essential in helping the victim to return to an independent, self-respecting life.

FACIAL DISFIGUREMENT

Significance

An individual's face is the first source of information for social interaction and it is on the basis of the information gleaned from the face that the subsequent tenor of social contact is determined (Argyle 1983). The extent to which an individual is judged to be an attractive person is determined, at least at the initial contact, largely from the face. Faces play a very prominent role in the media, particularly magazines and newsprint where photographs are usually selected and retouched to exclude even the slightest irregularity or blemish, portraying an unrealistic ideal. There is an extensive and lucrative industry which advertises products to correct and cover up any minor 'imperfections' while accentuating features which conform to the fashionable mode for that particular era.

Research into facial characteristics has demonstrated that there are considerable advantages for those who are seen as physically attractive. Attractive individuals generally have more opportunities for social interaction and as a consequence are likely to develop sophisticated social interactive skills. They are more likely to be helped and are seen as more successful and as having more satisfying lives (Benson et al 1976, Sroufe et al 1977). In contrast, the most common complaint reported by those who have suffered facial disfigurement is impaired social interaction. Facial disfigurement is hard to conceal, even with the most advanced modern surgical techniques; within any culture, human beings are extraordinarily adept at scanning and identifying the most subtle anomalies, whether of facial expression or physiognomy. And even when the disfigurement is not apparent to the casual observer, the impact on the individual's self-image is often still incapacitating.

The victim of disfigurement from trauma often experiences anguish and resentment and may be emotionally disabled as a consequence. In addition, the direct effects of the physical trauma in disrupting function, especially cognitive function, need to be taken into account in evaluating the impact on the individual and the steps which need to be taken to achieve a reasonable quality of life.

Andreason & Norris (1972) found that a minority of severely burned adults object to the pity and curiosity that they perceive in the eyes of strangers. Females are often unwilling to go out into the community to be subjected to this scrutiny and even to adverse comment. Those who have suffered facial disfigurement often report that they find it difficult to make friends and lack opportunities for marriage. There have also been reports of horror or disgust observed in the faces of those presented with individuals who have suffered facial disfigurement. There is documented evidence that those who have suffered facial disfigurement report negative reactions from members of the public and they also complain of being rejected. While these negative reactions and feelings of rejection may be the result of misperception on the part of the facially disfigured, several studies suggest that there is substance to their perception. Experimental studies using a confederate carefully made up to show the signs of bruising and scarring from a motor-vehicle accident or with a large port-wine stain, indicate that people distance themselves physically from individuals with facial disfigurement. They also tend to move to the side of the individual away from the disfigurement, thus actively maintaining a greater personal space from the disfigurement. This supports the claims by the facially disfigured that there is discrimination against them and that this discrimination occurs solely on the basis of appearance and not as result of conduct or manner.

However, Rumsey & Bull (1986) have shown that discrimination has an interesting twist. In situations in which some degree of help is required from the general public, such as in providing donations to collectors for charity on busy shopping streets, fewer offerings are made to those who are facially disfigured, but when a donation is made the actual amounts are larger. Similarly in comparing street interviewers who were or were not facially disfigured, fewer people agree to answer the questionnaires posed by the disfigured interviewer, but when they do comply they are more helpful and answer more questions.

These authors have also looked at the interaction between level of social skill and disfigurement. The presence or absence of disfigurement was significantly less influential than the level of social skill displayed; Hill (1985) reviewed the literature on disfigurement from burns and came to similar conclusions on the importance of personality and social support rather than severity of visible disfigurement. These findings do not throw the blame for the attitudes of society on the disfigured individual, but do suggest that development of social skills in the victim of disfigurement would make an important contribution to improving the quality of life by breaking the cycle of rejection and withdrawal. There is ample evidence that once there has been some effective social interaction, the appearance or other impairment plays a far less important role as a social handicap.

The complaint of the facially disfigured that they are often avoided or rejected by other people, in settings where social interaction was possible, was also examined by Rumsey & Bull (1986) and the results confirmed to some extent the views of the facially disfigured about the general population. However, it is also evident that many people are willing to engage in positive forms of social interaction with the disfigured, but are repelled by deficits in the behaviour of the disfigured individual, such as shyness, withdrawal, and preoccupation with appearance. This reinforces the belief that social skills training has the potential to alleviate some of the social impact for the facially disfigured.

It has been argued that the severity of a deformity is inversely related to the psychological impact that it has on the victim (Lansdown et al 1991). Solely on the basis of clinical experience, MacGregor (1990) proposed that the severely deformed child copes better with teasing than the mildly deformed child. A number of potentially important factors have not been acknowledged in this argument. The period of time during which the individual had experienced the deformity may be important: when a deformity is congenital, the child may have suffered from other handicaps including cognitive or educational impairment. Children who are seen as attractive are also seen by the public as happy, clever and friendly, but children who are seen as less attractive are stared at more by others. Lansdown et al (1991) found that children with mild deformity had the lowest level of self-concept in comparison with the more severely deformed children and with children without any apparent facial deformity, though the association did not quite reach a level of statistical significance. The results of this study point to social stereotyping with regard to facial appearance. Parents and teachers in frequent contact with the children saw no differences in the behaviour of those with facial deformity and those who were undeformed, although they did report disturbed behaviour in the siblings. The conclusion drawn is that the obviously deformed child has come to terms with being stared at, but the mildly deformed may be placed in situations where the child does not know whether the deformity has been noticed or not. Where there is uncertainty about the way others may respond, anxiety is more likely to develop.

MacGregor (1990) investigated more than 500 patients who had suffered facial deformity and concluded that distress was experienced when the patients looked at themselves in a mirror. However, the behaviour of others during face-to-face interactions was far more damaging to self-esteem. These interactions tend to occur in all aspects of life including work, recreation, socializing or simply walking down the street. Most people when travelling on public transport or walking down the street can retreat into their own personal space without the intrusive continual gaze of strangers, but the facially deformed continue to be the subject of stares, whispered comments, and openly insensitive remarks and behaviour.

In the normal course of daily life there are unwritten rules governing social interaction with others, particularly on first acquaintance, such as avoiding issues which may be of a sensitive or inappropriate nature and achieving eye contact without any threat to the other person. These social rules tend to be broken for those with deformity. People often do not know how to behave with those who have suffered facial deformity and tend either to stare or to avert their gaze. There is clearly a strong case for education of the public and probably this should begin in integrated schools. But unfortunately, in the foreseeable future, the social burden will as a rule lie with those who are facially deformed.

The social setting in which the individual is functioning also has to be evaluated in assessing the extent to which the deformity has had an impact on the individual, and also the individual's personality: some people overcome adversity and cope well, whereas for others the deformity is devastating. Age and gender must also be taken into account.

Age and disfigurement

Hill-Beuf & Porter (1984) presented the results of a series of 19 in-depth interviews with children who had been treated for depigmentation of the skin (vitiligo), most noticeably on the face. They noted four types of response

to negative incidents associated with the disfigurement, ranging from mild concern to very considerable concern with evidence of depression, hostility and anger. The younger children in the age range 3–6 years appeared to be relatively unaffected, but prepubertal and pubertal children were much more affected. At 12–13 years of age, considerable changes in the child's life are taking place. The child is usually in transition from primary or junior school to high school where the issues of meeting new people as well as changes in levels of expectations about achievement become a primary focus. It is also at this stage that body image becomes of particular significance in relation to peers of both sexes. Unfortunately the study lacked control or comparison group and the numbers were small; nevertheless, the results provide some understanding of the sources of distress for different age groups. Lefebvre & Arndt (1988) point out that facially attractive children tend to be better adjusted, with higher self-esteem, and their academic performance and social competence are higher than the less attractive; they are generally regarded more highly by teaching staff at school. They also grow up to be less emotionally disturbed adults (Krebs & Adinolfi 1975). In a 15 year follow up of young patients with craniofacial deformities at the Hospital for Sick Children in Toronto, it was noted that corrective surgery resulted for most in an improvement in body image, self-esteem and social adjustment, even if no aesthetic improvement was detectable by independent observers (Arndt et al 1986). The authors stress the importance of preparation of both the parent and the child for the circumstances that will need to be faced in the immediately postoperative period.

Adolescence is a particularly important time of development. Long & DeVault (1990) provide two case reports of persons who had suffered facial disfigurement in early adolescence. Both suffered loss of self-concept and disruption of their ability to adjust to their changed circumstances. In one case there was a significant deterioration in academic achievement, which raised the question of a neuropsychological deficit which was not supported by formal psychological testing. There was no evidence that either young person ever successfully overcame the trauma of the disfigurement and both remained to some extent socially and functionally disabled.

Disfigurement may also occur in old age, but has attracted less attention. We believe that most old people come to terms with the inexorable changes imposed by the ageing process, but may still be vulnerable to the trauma and distress of sudden disfigurement; however, this belief deserves further study.

Gender and disfigurement

Kleck & Strenta (1985) explored the effects of gender differences to disfigurement in self and in others. They pointed out that cosmetic surgery is predominantly carried out on females, with the exception of corrective surgery for protruding ears. There appears to be an assumption that facial appearance is more important for females than it is for males but the evidence to date contradicts this view; it seems that disfigured males are at least equally disadvantaged as far as social and occupational advancement is concerned. Kleck & Strenta (1985) found remarkably few differences between males and females in their responses to disfigurement either of their own faces or of others; moreover, autonomic reactions measured by skin conductance were similar. Both sexes reported feelings of aversion when faced with disfigurement. However, females tended to use negative descriptors such as 'disgust, distress or fright' when describing reactions to their own disfigured image, whereas males reported that they found it 'humorous or silly'. It is possible that this single gender difference in response is culturally determined and is reflected in the lower frequency of males electing to undergo cosmetic surgery.

Bull & Brooking (1985) explored the effect of being perceived as having a facially normal marital partner on the social evaluation of a facially disfigured individual. Men who were facially disfigured, but had no partner, were seen as less attractive than when presented as having a normal partner. Women who were presented as married to a normal partner were seen as equally attractive independently of whether or not there was any facial disfigurement.

Disfigurement in the community

There is no doubt that those who have suffered some facial disfigurement are at a social disadvantage. Bull & Stevens (1981) showed that facial disfigurement was associated with a reduced likelihood of help and assistance from the public. Not only are there social costs of disfigurement, but Lees-Haley (1987) showed that there are very real economic costs also. Employers appear to follow the popular stereotyping of the disfigured and believe that other workers may object to working alongside a disfigured worker or that in some way the visible presence of a disfigured person will adversely affect the viability of the business. In view of the strength and generality of the public's attitudes towards disfigurement, there may be some validity in the employer's concerns.

Rodin et al (1989) argued that the extent to which an individual's social flaw (disfigurement) was seen as controllable by that individual would be an important determinant of the negative attitude of others. Their results confirmed that people find it easier to justify discrimination when the flaw is seen to have been in some way controllable than when it is perceived as uncontrolled. This has implications for the perception of potential employers of those who have suffered disfigurement as a result of trauma. If the cause of the disfigurement is seen to have been under the control of the individual, the employer or indeed any other person will have less compunction in acting in a discriminatory fashion.

Management

Many people with disfigurement develop their own strategies for coping and for controlling social interactions in such a way that meaningful social contact can be achieved and maintained. Much more research is needed to explore the efficacy of these strategies. Some victims adopt an assertive or even aggressive stance; others cope by avoiding situations in which they are confronted with the effects on others of their own disfigurement. Humour is a strategy adopted by some, and so is making light of the disfigurement, but the maintenance of these pretences is itself a source of considerable strain.

People are constantly attempting to draw comparisons between themselves and others in a way which will enable them to deduce a slight difference in their favour. Thus a person who has lost an ear may cope by pointing out that to have lost an eye would have been worse. Social comparisons have been shown to be a coping strategy adopted by people wherever they have suffered significant losses in their lives. Those who have suffered the loss attempt to reduce or nullify the impact by a strategy of cognitive distortion, of which the phrase 'it could have been worse if . . .' is the core component. When a disfigurement can be even partially corrected, the outcome may be very rewarding. A number of studies have shown that there is a high level of satisfaction with the results of craniofacial surgery for the correction of facial deformities by the parents and the patients themselves, despite low ratings by independent observers on the aesthetic benefits. Lefebvre & Barclay (1982) reviewed 250 patients who had undergone craniofacial surgery for congenital (178 cases) or acquired (72 cases) deformities. The authors found no difference between the two groups regarding level of improvement following surgery. At 12 month follow-up an improvement in body image was reported in 76% of cases; there was an associated improvement in emotional status, including diminished self-consciousness when meeting strangers, an increased interest in appearance and grooming and a general feeling of being more attractive to others. In 39 of the 96 patients there had also been a demonstrable improvement in the academic achievement or work performance or increased heterosexual activity. The reasons for dissatisfaction were not explored in detail although it was argued that unrealistic expectations or limited involvement in the decision-making prior to surgery were likely to have been important factors, both for the patient and for close relatives.

Despite the considerable advances which have been made in reconstructive surgery for post-traumatic craniofacial deformities there can be no guarantee that the patient will have a perfectly normal face. The appearance will often be more presentable, and it is hoped that this will help an individual who is totally withdrawn from society to achieve some degree of socialization with an attendant improvement in quality of life. But for a proportion of surgically treated cases, there is no way in which the person will blend into a crowd and appear to all intents and purposes as 'normal' in appearance, despite heroic surgical efforts and several years of treatment. In such cases, counselling aims to promote acceptance.

Acceptance of a facial prosthesis can be especially difficult. Koster & Bergsma (1990) identified major problems which confront patients who have suffered facial disfigurement from facial cancer. These problems included coming to terms with the fact that a prosthesis was necessary and that alteration or correction is never the same as the original face, though modern prostheses provide a remarkable facial likeness. The major source of concern for these patients was with the effects of their altered facial structures on social and interpersonal interactions. The treatment goal for rehabilitation is to return the individual to a life that is as normal as possible. This involves a team approach in which the skills of social workers, psychological counselling, vocational guidance, group therapy and instruction in the skilled use of cosmetics can play an important role. It is at this point that medical treatment, in the narrow sense, ceases; the growth and learning of the patient as well as those close to him or her become of primary importance. The several forms of intervention are designed to deal with anxiety and depression, self-esteem and body image. Social skills training plays an important part in facilitating the individual's return to social and work-related activities.

Counselling

This enables the patient to ventilate feelings of anger and frustration concerning the disfigurement. A common question which is central to the distress that patients undergo is to ask 'Why me?'. Anger may also be directed towards the source of the injury or towards the surgical team members, usually in cases where there were unrealistic expectations. It is important in counselling that these issues are gradually resolved and the focus turned towards realistic goals and return to former activities as much as possible, given the particular residual impairment. The issues of dealing with the outside world and particularly the comments and behaviour of other people need to be addressed. A useful process of therapy is to identify possible responses and social situations and to rehearse various strategies for dealing with them through role play. The issues need to be carefully defined and the fears of the patient uncovered and addressed. This form of therapy is well suited to providing 'homework' assignments with regular consultation and feedback. Some-

times patients will have formulated or developed their own strategies which need to be incorporated into the therapeutic process. For example, humour is one effective method which enables the individual to deal with the pain of disfigurement and to ease the burden on other people. The strategies which are eventually adopted are very individualized and need a skilled and innovative therapist to implement them. There is considerable merit in having the therapist involved in the counselling and evaluation of the patient's expectations before surgery as well as in the period of adjustment. The professional background of the therapist varies: surgeons have undertaken this role, increasingly it is being done by psychologists, but social workers, nurses and chaplains may play vital parts as counsellors in appropriate circumstances. It is important that the counsellor be an experienced member of the multidisciplinary team, or at least in full cognizance and agreement with the management plan. Despite the well-documented importance of psychological research into the functional problems of the facially disfigured individual, there is a paucity of research into the contribution of psychologically oriented therapies for those who have suffered facial trauma. Deaton & Langman (1986) outlined the role of psychologists in a large American plastic surgery unit. Approximately 10% of those who are treated in any one year are also referred to the psychologist for appraisal and/or treatment. Routinely the craniofacial patients were referred for psychological evaluation and assessment, as were the patients who had suffered burns. Most clinicians are impressed by the value of these services, yet it is hard to demonstrate this objectively.

NEUROPSYCHOLOGICAL DISABILITIES

Significance

Changes in personality are often seen after head injury, and many studies have identified frontal lobe damage (p. 53) as the usual basis for these changes. In analysing the considerable difficulties in emotional adjustment suffered by the victims of facial disfigurement, it is essential not to overlook the possibility that behavioural and emotional disorders may have a neurological basis. Damage to the frontal lobes may not result in any demonstrable impairment of attention, memory or cognitive function, but may leave the victim with a gross lack of initiative and an inability to monitor behaviour and actions. The changes in personality often seen after frontal lobe damage include disinhibition, impaired impulse control, impairment of ability to plan, poor judgement, poor organization and retention of information and inability to recognize the extent of the disability.

Disinhibition and impaired impulse control constitute a significant handicap in social interaction and employment.

The victim may behave in an inappropriate way, causing distress or social embarrassment to other people; in the employment setting, such behavioural aberrations are usually not tolerated. Weddell et al (1980) pointed out that the personality changes which follow brain injury are the most common reason for the individual's loss of friendships and the experience of such losses reinforces the feelings of isolation which the brain-injured frequently complain about. Families often cannot comprehend the change in personality which follows from brain injury and may wrongly blame the patient for lack of motivation. Families may cope well with the brain-injured individual's inability to obtain employment, but have major difficulties in coping with the marked change in personality, the inability of the individual to recover interpersonal skills and the paranoid, depressed or belligerent behaviour. It has been shown that there is often a factual basis when the facially disfigured victim of a CMF injury senses active discrimination because of the disfigurement. However, there is also evidence to show that paranoid ideation may be responsible when a victim of brain injury fails to comprehend the intentions and actions of others and becomes more suspicious and uncooperative (Prigatano 1987a). Prigatano (1987b) cites a victim of severe closed-head injury who insisted that others actively avoided her, did not talk to her and despised her. Social withdrawal is indeed a common characteristic of the patient who has suffered frontal lobe damage without facial disfigurement; it is usually progressive, as the individual withdraws further into what is perceived as a safe environment. There is some indication that the likelihood of social withdrawal is directly related to the severity of the neuropsychological deficits. Denial that there is a problem operates as a considerable social handicap as well as a significant barrier to rehabilitation. Several studies have suggested that this is a symptom most commonly arising from damage to the right hemisphere of the brain rather than the left, although at present the data are limited (Gainotti 1972, Lishman 1968, Ruckdeschel-Hibbard et al 1987). Generally patients with right hemispheric lesions tend to minimize their complaints. Although frontal impacts are especially likely to cause frontal lobe damage, patients with CMF injuries may show diffuse or multifocal cerebral damage (p. 138); temporal lobe contusions are also not unusual. This emphasizes the need for full neuropsychological and radiological investigation in such cases.

Incidence

We have found that in 44 (83%) of 48 cases who had suffered fractures of Le Fort type, there was evidence of neuropsychological deficits consistent with damage to the central nervous system (Wood et al 1990). Prolonged post-traumatic amnesia, low Glasgow Coma Scale score on admission, vault fractures and fractures of the floor of the anterior fossa were often associated with deficits indicating damage to the frontal lobes. However, some cases with subcranial facial fractures also suffered neuropsychological disabilities, suggesting that the facial skeleton does not always protect the brain from the effects of facial impacts (p. 106). In our series there was evidence of cognitive impairment and social disability in some cases with only brief loss of consciousness. It is now recognized that even mild brain trauma may produce measurable although usually transient neuropsychological deficits (Gronwall & Wrightson 1974, Binder 1986, Varney 1988) which would have been discounted in the past as resulting from 'compensation neurosis' (Miller 1961, Rutherford et al 1977). The implications are important in counselling and future management.

Neuropsychological assessment

Where CMF trauma of any magnitude has occurred, a full neuropsychological investigation is usually desirable (Fig. 22.1). If there was prolonged loss of consciousness this is mandatory, but even where loss of consciousness was brief, the surgeon should consider referral to a neuropsychologist if there are continuing symptoms. Appendix III sets out suitable psychological tests for adults and children. The results of testing provide information about premorbid as well as current levels of intellectual functioning and this may be invaluable at a later stage for vocational rehabilitation. The neurological sequelae of the injury should be documented and correlated with the neuropsychological findings.

Radiological assessment

If there is evidence of neuropsychological impairment, magnetic resonance imaging (MRI) is preferable to computed tomography (CT) as an indicator of the anatomical substrate of the impairment. Levin et al (1992) have found high signal MRI abnormalities even in mild and moderate levels of head injury. MRI will often show structural damage in the frontal or temporal lobes in the victims of CMF trauma (Figs 22.2 and 22.3), and the investigation is being increasingly used in medicolegal evaluation. But it must be emphasized that a normal MRI scan does not necessarily invalidate the findings of a neuropsychological evaluation, nor are the anatomical correlations of MRI and neuropsychological tests always in accord with expectations. Single-photon emission computed tomography (SPECT) has promise as a simple means of visualizing local impairments of blood supply in damaged cerebral tissue (Newton et al 1992).

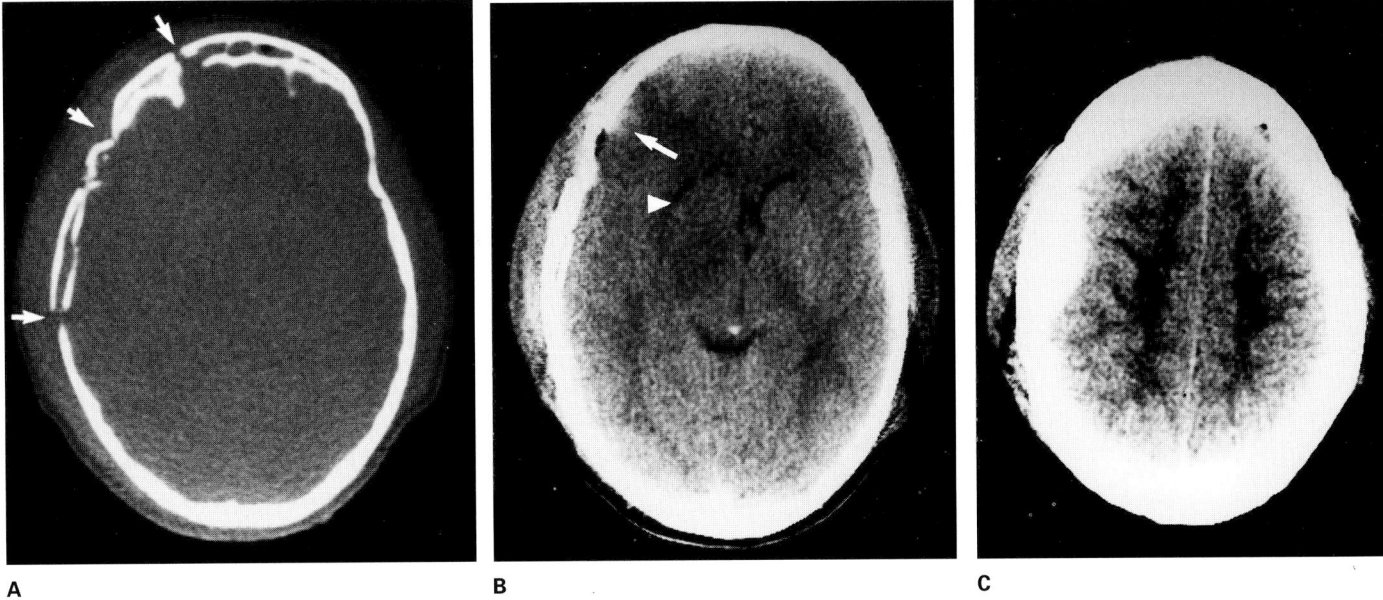

A   **B**   **C**

Fig. 22.1 Psychological evaluation of effects of frontal impact. A 12-year-old girl suffered a severe CMF injury in a road crash, with a residual left motor hemiparesis (see Fig. 22.6A) and loss of the right eye. She underwent a series of craniofacial operations to correct the facial deformity. CT scan showed: **A** multiple fractures (arrows) at site of impact in right frontotemporal region; **B** right frontal lobe cortical contusion (arrow) and probable contusion in anterior internal capsule (arrowhead) with some midline shift; **C** small right frontoparietal extradural clot.
Six years later, she complained of impaired memory and concentration. She was intolerant of criticism and had difficulty in controlling her emotions and temper. She had adapted poorly to her disfigurement and to a prosthesis for her right eye; she was socially withdrawn. Her verbal intelligence was average, but complex visual and spatial task performances were impaired. Memory for verbal information, verbal fluency, and performance on a conceptual tracking task (Trail Making Test) were all impaired.

Management

Impairments of cognition, emotional control and memory are common sequelae of neurotrauma. Their identification is very important in determining the nature and goals of a rehabilitation programme and will guide those involved in the rehabilitation to pace and structure the programme. Rehabilitation after brain injury ideally begins in the acute hospital; in more severe injuries, rehabilitation is continued in a special centre such as a head injury rehabilition unit, but as soon as possible patients should return to their normal environments, and it is there that the long-term effects of disabilities become evident. In head injury rehabilitation, the demarcation between active therapeutic intervention and social support is ill defined, and it is often difficult to determine when therapy ceases: when the disability has to be accepted as permanent. From the first, counselling is vital. The effects of brain injury on behaviour are little understood by the general public, and few relatives or friends of the patient will understand the nature and causes of the symptoms. Hence explanation of the nature of the impairments to relatives and others close to the patient can prevent much stress and misunderstanding about the patient's behaviour and conduct. Explanation must be undertaken early, before discharge from hospital, and must often be reiterated. Several authors, notably

Gronwall et al (1990), have published guides for families and lay care-givers which provide a general picture of the effects of brain damage, to be related to the problems of individual victims.

Behavioural management

There are several models which can be applied in the rehabilitation of individuals who have suffered brain impairments resulting in behavioural and social handicaps. The environmental model seeks to overcome the disability by intervening in the patient's environment rather than by attempting to focus directly on the individual. Thus, cues are given by persons who are in some way significant to the patient, or physical cues (e.g. notes or lists of tasks) are presented in well-frequented places, in the hope that a directive environment will lead the patient to modify behaviour and so reduce the social or functional disability. Another approach which may be complementary involves direct intervention. This may be used with a patient who has developed maladjusted behaviour through loss of previous competence in skilled behaviour, whether of a social nature or of self-care skills, including self-monitoring. Appropriate reinforcers of behaviour for the patient are identified and applied in the selective reinforcement of behaviour which would 'shape' and facilitate the relearning

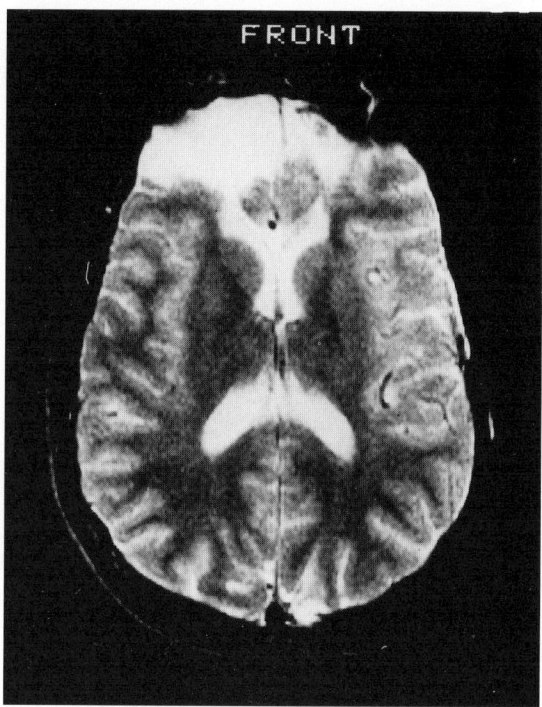

Fig. 22.2 Frontal lobe damage causing subtle intellectual impairments. A 4-year-old boy suffered a severe frontal impact in a road crash; window glass penetrated his right frontal lobe and his right eye. He later developed meningitis from a cranionasal fistula. He nevertheless made a good recovery, and at 12 years his scores in the Wechsler Intelligence Scale for Children were in the normal range. But the Halstead–Reitan Neuropsychological Test Battery suggested poor logical analysis and rigidity of thinking, and this was in accord with other evidence. MRI scan at age 15 years showed extensive atrophic changes in both frontal lobes, especially on the right side; this is well seen in T2-weighted axial sequences.

of skills agreed to be desirable by both patient and therapist. Another model also focuses the intervention on the patient. In the case of maladaptive behaviour, attempts are made to train the individual in appropriate behaviour in social settings; a system of rewards has been advocated in patients with very severe impairments (Eames & Wood 1985). An important assumption of this model is that the improvement in behaviour will generalize to other settings. Most approaches to rehabilitation involve combinations of these approaches rather than a prescriptive application of a single method; behavioural rehabilitation can also be combined with endeavours to improve cognition, insight, memory and physical disability in an integrated holistic rehabilitation programme. The first step in rehabilitation is the identification of the functional deficits likely to result in handicaps, whether in social settings or in the work place. The second step involves the establishment of goals. Goal setting in rehabilitation is a dynamic and changing rather than a static process. Initial goals are likely to be very circumscribed; with the development of basic competencies, more ambitious

goals, such as return to full independent living, are set. When the injured person has returned home, new goals may be set in collaboration with family members (see below). Goals can be used to measure outcome. Malec et al (1993) used a Goal Attainment Scale to audit the success of a holistic rehabilitation program organized from the Mayo Clinic. For this scale, goals regarded as realistic and attainable were given a zero rating, better-than-expected achievements being rated at +1 or +2 and worse-than-expected achievements at –1 or –2, depending on records of objectively stated behaviour. Goals were scaled in this way for group programmes in six fields: orientation, cognition, social awareness, communication, fitness and leisure skills. This system of goal scaling is under trial in a head injury service associated with our unit. Early discharge from hospital is always desirable, especially in paediatric rehabilitation, but often brings into prominence psychosocial problems that were not evident earlier.

Psychosocial maladjustment problems in patients who have suffered traumatic brain injury can be helped with a combination of psychotherapy and cognitive retraining. It is very important for the patient to recognize and understand the neuropsychological deficits and in particular how these affect performance in employment and in interpersonal interactions. Prigatano (1987a) has used insight-oriented psychotherapy in a group setting to help patients to come to an understanding of their failure to cope with the changes which they have suffered. However, these therapies have to be placed in the context of rehabilitation where attainable goals have been set and behaviorally oriented programmes devised to achieve these goals. Wood (1982, 1986) described examples of non-compliant and inappropriate behaviour by brain-injured patients which responded successfully to the application of a contingent management programme. The implementation of such procedures can be of assistance in facilitating the achievement of rehabilitation goals where non-compliance has interfered with treatment. Aggressive and disinhibited behaviour has also been treated by management techniques with some success, both in the ward and home settings. Finally, psychotherapeutic work with families of those who have suffered brain injury is almost always essential. Family members need to have a realistic understanding of the patient's capabilities. They also need to develop an understanding of the nature of the cognitive deficits, and their effects on behaviour, if rehabilitation is to progress in the home setting: if this is not done, gains achieved in the clinic may not be reinforced or maintained in a different environment.

Cognitive retraining

Psychosocial maladjustment in patients who have suffered damage to the frontal regions of the brain as a result of trauma has been treated successfully with a combination of cognitive retraining and psychotherapy. Deficits of attention and concentration are common sequelae of frontal lobe brain injury. The symptoms include insufficient alertness and fluctuations in attention which result in failure to attend to relevant stimuli or to exclude irrelevant and distracting stimuli. Deficits in the individual's ability to maintain sustained attention result in failures to adjust and relearn former skills. Patients are often unable to read or follow even undemanding television programmes; they may have difficulty in conversations, particularly where there is more than one contributor. As a result they often become frustrated and distressed, developing symptoms of poor self-esteem and depression. Fortunately there are techniques for overcoming these deficits which have emerged as reasonably successful (Wood 1986, Ben-Yishay et al 1987a,b). Ben-Yishay and his colleagues have developed a series of tasks which are graded for level of performance in response to demands for attention. The patients are individually trained to focus attention on the task to the exclusion of irrelevant stimuli. As the level of performance improves the complexity of the task is increased and the magnitude and variety of the distractors are also increased. The results from controlled outcome studies point to significant improvement having taken place as determined from performance on the individual training items. These changes were still evident 3 and 6 months later. Performance on several independent measures drawn from standardized neuropsychological tests also showed improvement as a result of the training. Clinical observation of patients who have undergone the programme developed by Ben-Yishay indicated that not only was there improvement on tests, but the individual patients were more alert and better oriented to their environment, with which they interacted in a more meaningful and efficient manner. There was also evidence to support the view that the individuals were better adjusted and more able to comprehend their capabilities and were more open to reason.

Medication

Psychotherapy may be helped by pharmacological therapy, aimed to stimulate lethargic patients or to control mood swings and abnormal behaviour. Zasler (1992) has reviewed the use of pharmacological agents in facilitating head injury rehabilitation; he emphasizes their many toxic or adverse effects, and in brain-injured persons, these may have a severity disproportionate to the dosage. We make very little use of such drugs. However, in occasional cases, depression may benefit from amitryptiline, or manic behaviour from lithium carbonate (Craft et al 1987). In such cases, supervision by a psychiatrist is necessary. Of all disturbed behavioural patterns, bursts of aggression are hardest to manage, and an effective psychotropic drug would be invaluable. In our experience, none of the agents now on offer have been very effective, but Tardiff (1992) has reported encouraging results from carbamazepine, propanolol and lithium.

Memory retraining

Deficits in memory and attention are common symptoms of brain damage and often disrupt the victim's quality of life and ability to function effectively. Information which is part of a continual flow of events in everyday life is never registered or is forgotten, and so are specific instructions. Memory training has focused on attempting to ensure that desired information is retained. There is unfortunately little evidence to suggest that memory, like a muscle, can be trained by constant exercising although several therapists continue to adopt this approach, which has been criticized by Schacter & Glisky (1986). On the basis that storage of verbal information is largely sited in the left hemisphere, patients with left hemisphere damage have been trained to use visual imagery (right hemisphere skill) to recall words (Patten 1972, Leftoff 1981). The results have so far been promising, although not dramatic. Visual imagery is an old technique which can result in improved recall of specific information, usually word lists, but does lend itself to retaining more useful information. The best-known technique is the 'peg method' in which an association is established between the list of items to be remembered and the 'pegs', a previously learned list of words. It is helpful to use phonetically similar or rhyming words as the pegs. The method has been used extensively in children's games or in teaching basic information. Familiar locations or objects in the home such as tables, clocks or pictures, can also be used as pegs so that an association is established between the items to be remembered and the locations or objects. Anomalies in facial features have also been used effectively to remember names (McCarty 1980). Combinations of the peg system with other mnemonic methods have proved to be much more effective in improving retention of information, compared with repeated rehearsal of the information or simple imagery. Pegs are less vulnerable to the loss of an item in a sequence (Roediger 1980, Van Der Linden & Van Der Kaa 1989). However, patients' compliance and motivation are very important. Some success has been obtained using absurd cues and it has been argued that the more ridiculous the peg stimuli the more likely that the items will be recalled. Crovitz (1979) used an 'airplane list' in which items to be recalled were associated with animals (pegs) which comprised the crew and passengers. Severely amnesic patients were able to retain significantly more verbal information using this technique. Despite the effectiveness of imagery in facilitating the recall of specific information by some amnesic patients, the practical relevance of the technique has not received as much attention as it deserves. There are certainly some situations in which there are benefits in learning associations, such as remembering the names and faces of people with whom the individual comes into frequent contact (Wilson 1987). Verbal strategies such as phonemic similarity or semantic cues are also effective in aiding recall (Baddeley 1988). Jaffe & Katz (1975) demonstrated for a severely amnesic patient that the provision of cues at both the storage and the retrieval levels is essential for the retention of new information. Without storage cues, retrieval of information was markedly impaired. The task for rehabilitation is to ensure that new information is always presented within a structure with adequate cueing both at input and retrieval levels. Although it does not appear to have received recent interest, motivation is an important component in the learning and retention of information. Dolan & Norton (1977) used positive reinforcement to facilitate the retention of visual and verbal information relevant to life on the ward in a group of amnesic patients. With reinforcement more information was recalled than without it, and training with reinforcement was more economical in staff time. Training in relaxation has also been found to improve recall when used in combination with mnemonic devices in amnesic patients (Yesavage & Jacob 1984, Yesavage et al 1988). Preliminary instruction in imagery and relaxation prior to the specific memory training also appears to improve retention (Hill et al 1988). Amnesic patients are in danger from domestic appliances in the home. O'Reilly et al (1990) developed a programme based on a combination of prompts and checklists that identified potential in-home hazards and improved the safety behaviour of the amnesic patients to an acceptable level. One month later most of the skills had been retained. A number of behavioural aids, mostly based on electronic circuitry have been developed as memory aids. The principle underlying the behavioural prosthetic is either to provide a simple cue for behaviour or to produce for the patient a complete or partial set of instructions at specified intervals of time. The simplest form of cueing is a pocket diary and instruction in diary use is given in most rehabilitation centres, but there are problems in achieving compliance once the patient is outside the structured environment. The relevant information has to be inserted in an organized manner and has to be accesssed at regular intervals. For amnesic patients both tasks may prove to be insuperable obstacles to the effective use of the diary. Despite regular cueing by ward staff or relatives, patients often fail to comply with the instruction to check their diaries. The use of an alarm of the type commonly available in digital wrist watches overcomes this problem to some extent. Kurlychek (1984) described the successful use of a wrist-watch alarm which sounded every hour and cued

the checking of a diary for information and instructions. Wood (Harris 1984) reported favourable results using an alarm chronograph which sounded every 15 min, reminding the patients to review a diary and notebook for relevant information. Digital wrist watches with alarms provide an inexpensive device to cue behaviour, provided that the patient can retain the new information over the interval which exists between checking the diary and executing the specified behaviour. Electronic notebooks and diaries can provide a means for programming more complex strings of behaviour into an 'artificial memory'. One of our patients who had suffered a severe closed head injury resulting in demonstrable amnesia was able to return to full-time employment in an office with the assistance of a 'Sharp' electronic diary. He learned to enter information using the alpha-numeric keyboard regularly during the day and received an audible cue at set times which reminded him to check the electronic diary. Although effective means are available to facilitate the retention of information which can be specified in advance, there is unfortunately no convincing evidence that they generalize to other aspects of everyday life. Memory is such a complex phenomenon that it is unreasonable to expect that a general improvement in the ability to remember information is currently possible. Yet this is what many patients and families hope for, and it is often their expectation when memory retraining is offered.

Outcome

Frontal lobe deficits are often very disabling. In our study of 48 cases of facial fractures (Wood et al 1990) assessed 7–47 (mean 17.7) months after injury, families reported difficulties in social adjustment in 66%; in 58% there were reports of uncontrolled aggression. Of those who had suffered only minor cerebral damage, about one third had failed to make adequate social adjustments. Severe frontal damage often renders the victim unemployable, though it is hard for the victim or the family to accept this because the physical impairments are often minimal. Nevertheless, with competent rehabilitation begun early, and good family support, some individuals with overt frontal lobe damage manage to return to work, though often at a lower level, and most become socially independent (Fig. 2.21). With the advent of better planned programmes for rehabilitation embodying the concepts of Ben-Yishay and Prigatano, it is hoped that satisfactory outcomes will be seen more often; to quantify the success of such programmes, objective measurements of outcome are needed and some of these measures are discussed below (p. 670).

EPILEPSY

Significance

Post-traumatic epilepsy can be very disabling, and unfortunately there is no certain way to prevent it. The seizures complicating wounds in the frontal cortex are especially detrimental, since they are typically of grand mal type with no warning aura. Temporal lobe seizures with some kind of aura are occasionally experienced after frontal impacts, perhaps from coincident contusion of the temporal lobe or from secondary kindling of a new epileptogenic focus by repeated fits. Post-traumatic epilepsy may be lethal; in long-term studies of wartime brain injuries causing epilepsy (Walker & Blumer 1989), it has been shown that there is a significant reduction in expectation of life. Status epilepticus can result in death and fits may cause fatal accidents: one of our cases of frontal lobe injury died when he fell into an acid bath in a factory. Even one post-traumatic fit may have important social consequences, as some jurisdictions regard a single fit as an absolute bar to driving a motor vehicle; in Australia, traffic authorities allow a more flexible policy and driving licences are not usually withdrawn unless there is a presumption that an epileptic tendency is established. Other adverse consequences stem from the need for anticonvulsant medication: the various drugs in common use have well-known toxic effects (Eady & Tyrer 1989), and these include subtle impairments of cognitive functions.

Incidence

Post-traumatic epilepsy is very unlikely to develop in a person who has been rendered briefly unconscious by a blunt impact on the face or elsewhere in the head. Jennett's data show a high (21%) incidence of late epilepsy when the impact is severe enough to cause a depressed frontal fracture; intracranial haemorrhage also entails a high risk, and the risk rises when both complications are present (Jennett 1975). The incidence of epilepsy after frontal missile wounds is even higher; Russell & Whitty (1952) reported an incidence of 39% in a large series of wartime brain wounds, and Salazar et al (1985) reported that 53% of 421 brain-injured veterans of the Vietnam war had experienced at least one fit in a 15 year period after injury. The seizure incidence appears to be proportional to the volume of brain destruction (p. 393). The incidence is high among cases with brain injuries severe enough to need referral to a rehabilitation unit: Armstrong et al (1990) recorded epilepsy in 87 (37%) of 238 persons referred to them after blunt head injury, and found also that their epileptic patients tended to have more severe functional disabilities.

Management

The prophylaxis and early management of post-traumatic epilepsy have been considered in Chapter 13. When a seizure occurs some time after a CMF injury, brain abscess and other treatable lesions should be excluded by CT or MRI scan, and seizure control should be established as soon as possible. For grand mal epilepsy after frontal trauma, our drug of first choice is carbamazepine, but phenytoin or sodium valproate may be preferred. Referral to a medical neurologist is advisable, and indeed mandatory if the seizures recur. Cases of medically intractable post-traumatic epilepsy should be fully investigated to assess the possible benefits of surgical ablation of an epileptogenic focus. In our experience, it is very unusual for this to be necessary in cases of epilepsy after CMF injury, and we have yet to see a case in which satisfactory indications for surgery have been found (Fig. 22.3). But increasing experience may enlarge the scope of surgical treatment; if so, it will be wrong to procrastinate too long, since uncontrolled post-traumatic epilepsy is socially devastating, and frequent epileptic discharges may kindle secondary foci elsewhere in the brain. When control of post-traumatic epilepsy has been achieved by medication, the drug(s) should be continued at least 2 years after the last fit, and withdrawn by progressive decrements over 3 months. In the UK and Australia, a driving licence may be granted if there have been no seizures for 2 years; in some USA jurisdictions, the obligatory seizure-free period is much shorter (Dickey & Morrow 1993).

Outcome

Post-traumatic epilepsy usually appears within the first 2 years after injury, though Jennett (1975) found that in 19% of his cases the first fit occurred after more than 4 years; a long latent period seems especially common in children. There is happily a tendency to eventual cessation of seizures; Caveness (1974) found this in about half of his cases of post-traumatic epilepsy complicating wartime brain injuries. Chronic post-traumatic epilepsy has medicolegal implications, especially in occupations that entail car driving or working with machinery. After a CMF injury with a high (> 20%) risk of seizures, it may be wrong to recommend a final medicolegal settlement until 4 years have elapsed; even after this period, the statistical likelihood of future fits should be stated. Jennett's data are invaluable in calculating the empiric risks in an individual case.

CHRONIC FACIAL PAIN

Significance

The face and scalp have a rich sensory innervation, chiefly from branches of the trigeminal nerve, and nerve injury is a common complication of CMF trauma. With fractures of the mandible, the inferior dental nerve is often compressed or even transected; the infraorbital nerve is likely to be injured when the zygomatic bone is displaced;

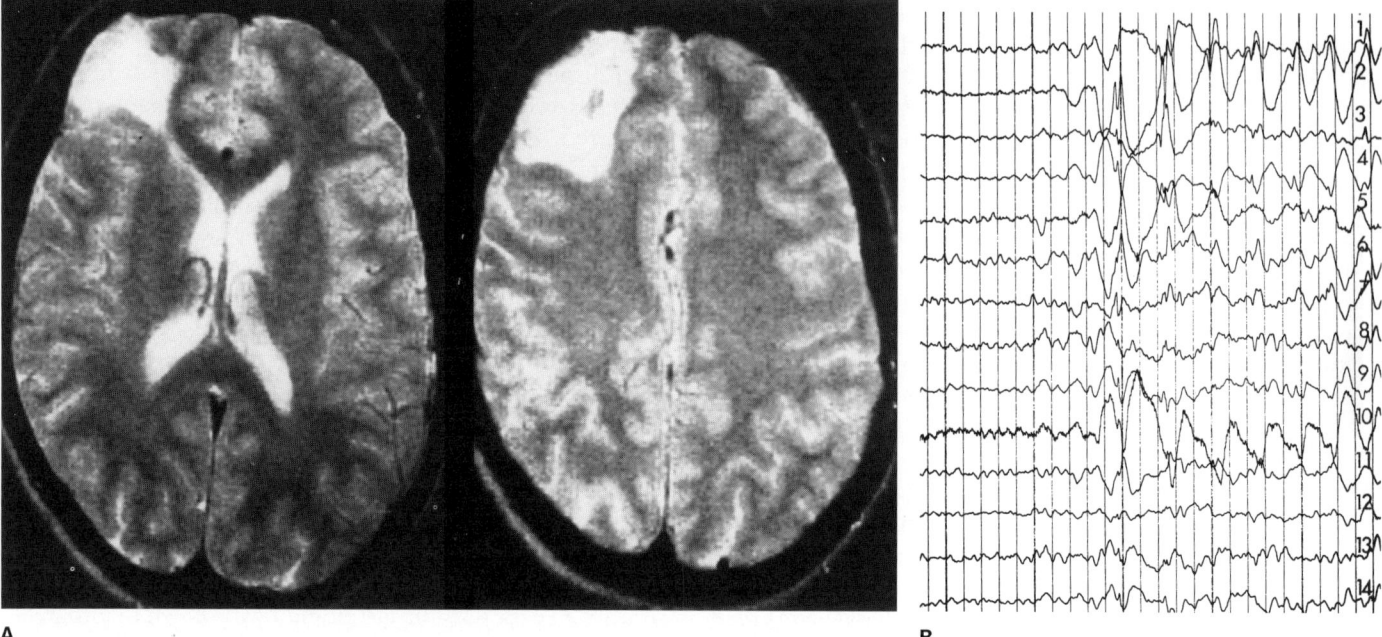

A   **B**

Fig. 22.3 Unilateral frontal lobe damage causing disabling epilepsy. A 10-year-old girl suffered a right compound frontal fracture in a road crash. Immediately after, she had several epileptic seizures, chiefly on the *right* side of the body. She made a good recovery, and was seizure-free for nearly 4 years. She then began to suffer major epileptic fits, which persisted despite medication; at the age of 21, she reported also partial seizures, initially associated with a nauseating smell and later with a strange noise and lapse of memory.
A MRI scan showed right frontal lobe damage, well seen in T2-weighted sequences. **B** Electroencephalography, including depth electrode recordings, showed seizure activity arising independently both in the right frontal and left temporal lobes; in this sequence, the picture is dominated by bifrontal seizure activity without real lateralization.
Operation was not recommended. She coped with her poorly controlled epilepsy with great courage. She recently responded well to lamotrigine.

the supraorbital nerve may be damaged in injuries of the upper third of the face. Victims of nerve injury may complain of numbness, abnormal sensation and discomfort but very few go on to complain of chronic pain. Conversely, when CMF trauma is complicated by intractable pain, there is often no objective sign of nerve damage. It seems likely that chronic post-traumatic facial or cephalic pain is often based on a sense of loss or resentment of damage to the image of the self. This interpretation seems especially plausible when there is obvious mutilation, such as the loss of an eye. Nevertheless, psychogenic interpretations have their dangers; moreover, they are often bitterly resented. The formation of a traumatic neuroma is often postulated, and in some cases this does appear to be the cause of pain.

Incidence

We have no data on the real incidence of intractable pain after injury to the facial nerves. Seddon (1972) studied 1250 war wounds of peripheral nerves of all types and sites; he recorded complaints of 'fairly severe' pain in about 10%. The incidence after injury to peripheral branches of the trigeminal nerve is probably lower, but not negligible, and every effort should be made to prevent this disabling complaint by primary nerve repair. It is even more difficult to give meaningful estimates of the inci-

dence of chronic pain attributable to injuries involving other facial structures, such as the teeth or the temporomandibular joint, or to psychogenic causes. One can only say that many patients with CMF injuries do admit to long-term discomfort in mastication, or to headache, but very few come with pain as an intractable and disabling problem.

Clinical assessment

In the investigation of chronic pain, a careful unhurried history is essential. The pain may be described as an ache, or a lancinating pain in the territory of a single nerve, or a burning sensation. There may be a trigger point or local tenderness or some form of dysaesthesia. There may be a background of previous functional illness: it has been well said that hysteria is not a disease but a way of life. It is useful to map the distribution of pain, tenderness, and sensory loss on a standard diagram of the face. Figure 22.4 records a case in which the pain was not confined to an area of well-marked sensory loss, and appeared to relate to a large number of subcutaneous foreign bodies in the middle and lower face. Such a diagram is useful as a guide to changes in the pain loci over a period of time. Examination includes a full neurological and psychological evaluation. Attention must be given to possible local causes for chronic pain, such as an im-

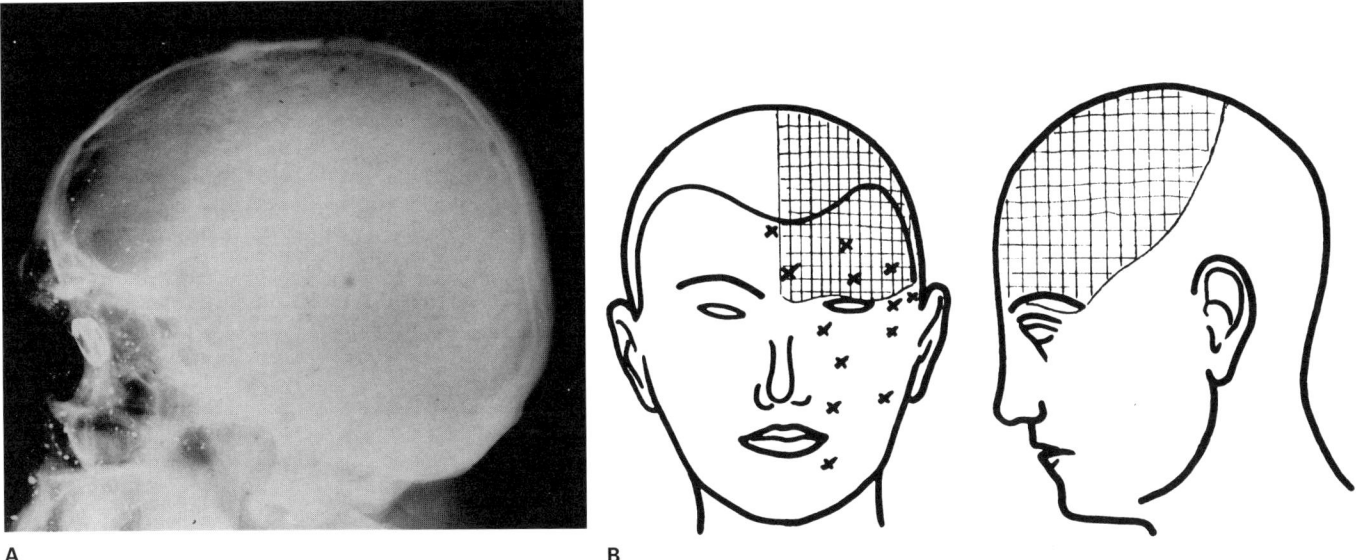

Fig. 22.4 Pain and disfigurement as a longstanding disability. A 38-year-old miner was injured in an underground explosion. Much earth and mineral material was blown into the left side of his face; his left eye was destroyed. He complained of left facial pain. **A** Lateral skull X-ray picture shows metallic density foreign bodies in the facial soft tissues, also a glass eye prosthesis. **B** Pain diagram: he complained of pain in the sites marked X; the pain was described as 'like a needle' and might last for 10–12 h. He was aware that the skin was anaesthetic, and he had anaesthesia in the shaded area. He sued the mining company, and recovered damages for loss of sight in one eye and chronic disabling pain.

planted foreign body. Implanted wood is easily missed and can be very irritative.

Management

Treatment of chronic facial pain is notoriously unsatisfactory. In some cases, reassurance and explanation may be effective after a full examination has excluded some treatable lesion or overt psychogenic problem. Where there is clinical evidence of a nerve injury, local anaesthesia may be diagnostic and even therapeutic. Where there is a persistant neurological deficit indicative of an injured nerve, decompression and neurolysis are sometimes effective, but there is no guarantee of success from such procedures. Burchiel et al (1993) reported pain relief from surgery in only 40% of 42 traumatic neuromas in various sites. Pain relief from section or alcohol injection of clinically normal nerves has often been reported. Supraorbital neurectomy has been recommended for frontal pain, and infraorbital neurectomy for cheek or alveolar pain; anterior ethmoidal neurectomy has been advocated for pain in the bridge of the nose (Golding-Wood & Brookes 1991) and section of the zygomaticotemporal nerve for malar pain. But in the absence of proof of a nerve injury, such operations are of very dubious value: success may only mean gratitude that a complaint of pain has been taken seriously. In the older literature, there are many reports of more drastic neurosurgical responses to complaints of intractable facial pain. White & Sweet (1969) reported on 29 cases of severe pain in the cephalic area, of which 18 followed accidental injuries of various

kinds. Their repertoire of operative treatment included neurectomy, trigeminal rhizotomy, and medullary trigeminal tractotomy; they achieved a remarkably high success rate. But this was not the general experience, and modern concepts of pain physiology have left little place for these major operations. Counselling on pain control and the use of drugs such as amitryptiline are less dramatic and may be ineffective, but do not cause irreversible denervation, which in itself can lead to permanent complaints of pain and unpleasant sensations.

TEMPOROMANDIBULAR ARTHRALGIA

Significance

The common disorders of the temporomandibular joint (TMJ) are derangement, arthritis and dislocation. Any of these disorders may result from trauma and may be a source of chronic post-traumatic pain; fortunately, however, relatively few patients with serious injuries in the region of the TMJ do have long-term complaints referable to the joint. On the other hand, there are patients who complain of symptoms seemingly referable to the TMJ after minor injury; in such persons, caution and very careful assessment are needed, because the results of operation are often extremely disappointing (Fig. 21.64). TMJ arthralgia is a chronic pain syndrome which is likely to result in increased emotional reactivity and a 'neurotic' presentation on personality inventories. It is characterized by pain and limitation of movement of the mandible and local tenderness over the joint: complaints may be referable to the joint itself, or to adjacent muscles, or to both origins (Proffit, 1986). Bell (1985) has identified three groups of pain-sensitive structures in the TMJ: the collateral ligaments attaching the disc to the mandibular condyle, the retrodiscal tissue lying between the disc and the posterior wall of the joint capsule, and the joint capsule itself. All these structures may be injured in fractures of the condyle and the joint itself may be secondarily affected by malocclusion. It has been claimed that derangements of the TMJ may cause a wide range of symptoms referable to remote structures, such as headache vertigo and tinnitus. But scepticism has been expressed about the causality of the relation between these symptoms and any associated joint injury. Van der Laan et al (1988) have advanced evidence to suggest that persons who complain of pain referable to the TMJ tend to have neurotic personalities, but this correlation does not necessarily imply psychogenic causation. There is some evidence to suggest that persons suffering from TMJ pain are especially susceptible to imposed mental stress, and this has been demonstrated in records of electromyographic activity in the masticatory muscles (Schumann et al 1988).

Clinical assessment

If there is any suggestion of dental or TMJ causation, an evaluation by an oral specialist is mandatory. Bell (1985) has correlated TMJ pain syndromes with specific anatomical structures:

1. Disc attachment pain is intermittent, worse on clenching the teeth in full intercuspation, and reduced by biting on a separator. There may be associated protective muscle splinting.
2. Retrodiscal pain is also worse on clenching the teeth in full intercuspation, and reduced by biting on a separator. Pain is accentuated by forced ipsilateral excursive movement of the mandible, but not by resisted protrusion.
3. Capsular pain is more or less continuous, it is not related to clenching the teeth, with or without a separator, and it is associated with local tenderness and sometimes fluctuant swelling.

In cases with an established pattern of chronic disabling pain, the multidisciplinary pain clinic is the best forum for comprehensive investigation as well as for treatment. It has been stated that ~30% of persons referred to a facial pain clinic have suffered major injuries (Clark & Solburg 1987).

Radiological assessment

The TMJ can best be visualized by MRI scan, though arthrography has also been used (p. 189); however, it is not always easy to relate the findings to the complaints.

Fibre-optic arthroscopy has been developed in Japan and elsewhere, but we have no experience of this technique.

Management

The management of chronic TMJ pain has attracted much interest, especially in view of the allegedly high prevalence of this complaint in the general community: Dworkin et al (1990) have reported an incidence of 12.1% in an adult population. In addition to the various dental, anaesthetic and even surgical measures that can be considered, psychological intervention may be helpful. Many patients with symptoms referable to the TMJ respond well to an explanation of the benign nature of the pain, reassurance and perhaps relaxation therapy and muscle biofeedback — or to the passage of time (Pogrel 1987). Prolonged use of an occlusal splint, to rest tense masticatory muscles, has been recommended (Chong-Shan & Hui-Yun 1989).

ANOSMIA AND DYSOSMIA

Significance

Both in diagnosis and as a disability, damage to the olfactory nerves (p. 57) is a very important and often neglected component of many CMF injuries. Bilateral anosmia, which entails loss of the olfactory component of taste, is a serious disability in cooking, wine-tasting and several other jobs in which perception of odours and perfumes is required. Failure to smell burning or escaping gas may be dangerous. Loss of olfaction deprives the victim of many pleasures, ranging from the glutton's delight in the approach of good food to the Proustian enjoyment of memories evoked by a forgotten smell. Yet many persons with anosmia complain very little, and some are seemingly unaware until the impairment is demonstrated. Dysosmia is a perverted perception of smell, in which all smells are the same, and all or some are unpleasant (cacosmia); this perverted perception should not be confused with olfactory hallucinations, a form of epilepsy usually associated with damage of the medial temporal lobe, in or near the olfactory cortical projection. Anosmia is often associated with damage to the orbital frontal cortex, and this may cause subtle neuropsychological impairments not related to the anosmia. Varney (1988) reported on 40 patients with total post-traumatic anosmia: almost all (93%) had serious vocational disablilities not explained by mental or physical impairments, and indeed all had been found fit to work 2 years or more before the evaluation. In some cases, the head injury had not appeared to be very serious.

Incidence

Sumner (1976) reviewed a number of large series of head injuries and concluded that the overall incidence of anosmia was ~7%. In fractures of the skull base the incidence is higher: Lewin (1954) found impaired olfaction in 78% of his cases of cerebrospinal fluid rhinorrhoea. Frontal impacts account for the majority of cases of post-traumatic anosmia, though anosmia is also a well known sequel of falls with impact in the occipital region.

Management

In all head injuries, but especially those resulting from impacts in the CMF region, the sense of smell should be tested (p. 166) as soon as the patient is cooperative enough for reliable evaluation; in cases with facial fractures one must wait for nasal patency. If anosmia is found, the patient must be told, with sympathy, the nature of the impairment, the likelihood that it will be permanent, and the associated risks and inconveniences. There is no treatment.

Outcome

In our experience, post-traumatic anosmia has almost always been permanent. Some authorities, notably Sumner (1976), have reported a significant incidence of recovery, sometimes after some years, and this should be kept in mind in making medicolegal assessments. When the anosmia follows anterior fossa repair in which avulsive damage to the olfactory nerves was seen, there can be no hesitation in giving a hopeless prognosis. When the anosmia is associated with less serious facial injury, or when there is the possibility that injury to the olfactory epithelium rather than to the nerve is responsible, then one may give a more guarded forecast.

MOTOR AND SENSORY DISABILITIES

Significance

For anatomical reasons discussed in Chapter 2, impacts in the CMF region are not especially likely to damage the sensorimotor cortex or the long tracts which govern limb movement. But some cases of CMF injury do suffer from hemiparesis, cerebellar ataxy or other limb dysfunction. This may result from diffuse axonal injury, or deep penetration by a missile wound, or some secondary complication such as intracranial haemorrhage. Impairments of limb function may increase the quantum of permanent disability.

Incidence

In our series of 238 fractures of the anterior cranial fossa, significant hemiparesis was recorded in six and spinal paraparesis in one. This incidence (2.9%) of major sensorimotor impairments may be an underestimate.

Assessment

Gross motor impairments are easily detected and can be assessed qualitatively by standard neurological methods. Until recently, these have not often been used to give quantitative measures of impaired limb function; even simple dynamometry of hand grip strength has often been omitted. Increasing attention is now being given to measures of function in stroke victims, and these can be usefully extended to cerebral disabilities in victims of head injury. The Rivermead Mobility Index, which is based on personal observation and on a 14-point questionnaire, appears particularly suitable (Collen et al 1991). Arm function has also to be quantitated as a measure of response to physiotherapy (Sunderland et al 1992). Pegboard tests have been found helpful in quantitating manual facility, and we have used the Purdue pegboard test for this purpose both in adults and in children older than 7 years. This test was devised for selecting industrial workers (Tiffin 1968); in the simplest form of the test, the subject inserts metal pegs in a row of holes in a standard board (Fig. 22.5) as rapidly as possible. A score

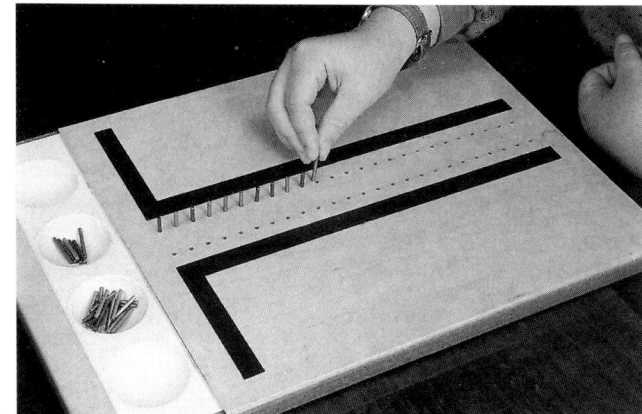

A

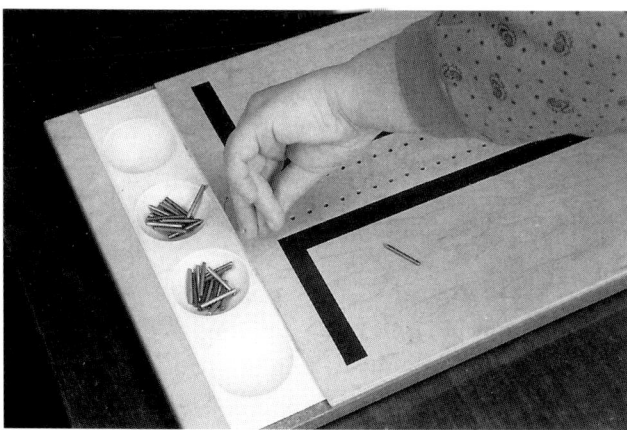

B

Fig. 22.5 Motor impairments quantified by the Purdue pegboard. A 4-year-old girl suffered a sensory hemiparesis in a road crash, with little motor weakness. Her disability remained static over the next 14-years. **A** Normal performance with right hand. **B** Grossly impaired performance with left hand.

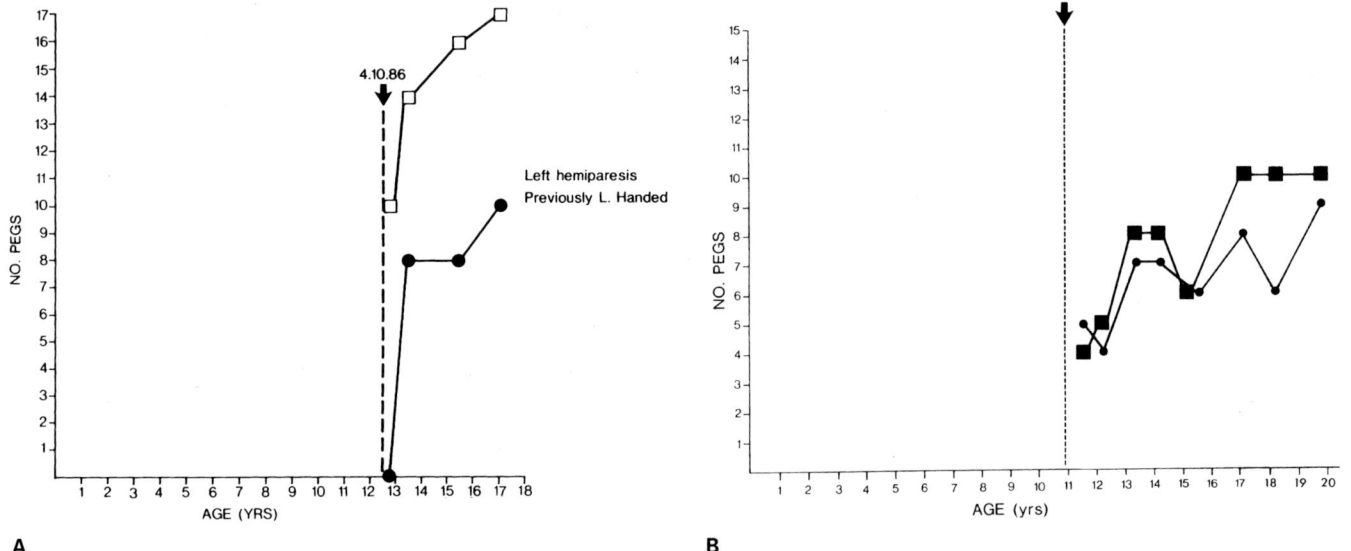

A **B**

Fig. 22.6 Motor impairments quantified over time by the Purdue Pegboard. The graphs show the number of pegs inserted in test periods of 30 s under standard conditions, the test being repeated by the same examiner at intervals of not less than six months. Care was taken to ensure that both patient and examiner were unaware of the previous score.
A A 12-year-old girl suffered a severe CMF injury in a road crash, with a residual left motor hemiparesis (Fig. 22.1 shows the CT findings in this case). There was rapid improvement over the first 6 months, but thereafter very little change over some 3 years despite intensive efforts to improve function in the previously preferred left hand.
B A 11-year-old girl suffered a severe closed head injury, complicated by bilateral motor impairments. There was slight but definite improvement, especially on the right, which continued over at least 6 years.
Key to Purdue scores: square = right hand score, circle = left hand score; black symbol = clinically affected hand, white symbol = clinically normal hand.

is obtained for each hand over a period of 30 s. Gardner & Broman (1982) have found this an excellent test of minimal brain damage.

We have followed 41 cases of brain injury, including some due to CMF impacts (Fig. 22.6), for periods of 2–19 years (mean period 8.0 years); we have been impressed by the reproducibility of the results, and by the value of the test as a guide in determining when a stable level of recovery has been attained. Other quantitative tests of hand–arm function are described by Gloss & Wardle (1982).

Management and outcome

There is evidence from animal experiments (Black et al 1975) and from studies of recovery after stroke (Sunderland et al 1992) to support the routine use of early and energetic physiotherapy in rehabilitating people with motor disabilities from head injury. Occupational therapy is also valuable in neurorehabilitation. It is not at present possible to say how long such rehabilitation should be continued, and with what intensity; economic considerations make it impossible to continue a high level of professional physiotherapy, or occupational therapy, for indefinite periods. It is generally believed that functional recovery from brain injury is greatest during the first 12 months; this was evident in the case shown in Fig. 22.6A.

However, some cases have shown worthwhile improvement after a longer period, and this is especially seen in children (Fig. 22.6B). At present, it seems appropriate to plan intensive rehabilitation for a finite period of 6 months, and then to obtain objective measures of motor function; arrangements can then be made for continued rehabilitation by the injured person and the family. A review in 6 months or more will allow repetition of the assessment, and sometimes justifies another finite course of intensive rehabilitation.

SPEECH DISABILITIES

Significance

After a CMF injury, speech may be impaired in several ways. If there was a cerebral injury, the neurological mechanisms subserving speech may be damaged. When the dominant cerebral hemisphere is injured, the cortical centres for conceptual organization of speech may be affected (p. 53), causing some kind of dysphasia or dyspraxia. Alternatively, there may be subcortical damage causing dysarthria or eating difficulty; these may also be the result of bilateral cortical damage. When the facial skeleton has been severely damaged, the muscles of articulation may be affected; the palatal muscles are especially vulnerable. Velopharyngeal incompetence may result from facial injury: this tends to give hypernasal speech, and the victim may be accused of mumbling. On the other hand, nasal obstruction may give rise to hyponasality and snoring (see below). Speech impairments may also result from post-traumatic occlusal difficulties: these often affect one phoneme only, or a single phoneme group, e.g. the sibilants. Impaired oral or labial sensation may reduce the control of saliva, which collects during speech or even at rest, causing social embarrassment.

Assessment

The team speech pathologist plays a key role in assessing the nature and treatment of impairments of speech, language and swallowing. When there is a cerebral basis, a full neurological evaluation is appropriate. Standardized tests for dysphasia, dyspraxia and dysarthria are administered, to explore both expressive and receptive language and to provide a baseline against which later progress can be evaluated. Speech recording is always undertaken, again as a baseline for future evaluations; nasendoscopy with lateral videofluoroscopy is required if velopharygeal sphincter incompetence is suspected (David & Bagnall 1990).

Management

Speech pathologists are concerned in the treatment of neurological impairments of speech as part of general neurological rehabilitation. In adults especially, dysphasic and dysarthic impairments may be quite intractable, and more so when associated with intellectual and emotional disabilities. Post-traumatic dysphasias in children have a much better prognosis, but unhappily the recovery of fluent speech is often associated with subtle learning impairments (p. 512). Speech impairments from malocclusions, such as cross-bite or lateral shift of the mandible during speech, often cause subjective concern, but usually subside with reassurance and the passage of time. Impaired control of salivation may be permanent, but can be overcome by making the victim aware of the accumulation of saliva and encouraging more frequent swallowing; self-examination with a small mirror after meals is sometimes helpful.

DENTAL DISABILITIES

Significance

In the multidisciplinary management of CMF injuries, dental treatment is often the last step in the aesthetic restoration of the disfigured person (p. 358) and may be very successful both from the functional and the psychological viewpoint. However, there are limits to what can be achieved and these limits are financial as well as technical. Throughout the world, systems of accident insurance provide financial support to persons with permanent disabilities but, in many of these, there is a financial ceiling on the provision of appliances, and for many persons with impaired dentitions, the ceiling precludes many desirable forms of prosthetic restoration. Loss of teeth or an uncorrected malocclusion may have important psychological and economic consequences. Thus, loss of maxillary anterior teeth may be disfiguring: if the accident was not compensatable, the patient may not be able to afford the costly dental implants, crown and bridgework described in Chapter 12. Instead, an acrylic partial denture may be made to replace the missing teeth. This may change lip support, interfere with speech, change taste perception and alter eating habits.

Management

Dental treatment can range from the restoration of a single tooth to the rehabilitation of the entire dentition. Single teeth that have been fractured can be restored to full function, while missing teeth can be replaced with fixed or removable prostheses that will improve comfort and masticatory ability, and may also strengthen the self-image. If extensive rehabilitation is required, the dental treatment may extend over several months and it is interesting to observe the patient's physical and mental changes during this time. There is always a potential danger that the dental disability may be viewed without regard to the overall management. Loss of teeth or a permanent malocclusion can entail a change in lifestyle, and this can influence the manner in which the patient recovers and adjusts after injury. Some patients, especially those who have suffered major trauma, will need prior psychosocial counselling, and so may their families. If an associated cerebral injury has left the patient with impaired manual dexterity and unable to clean the teeth or the denture, dental decay and soft-tissue damage will inevitably result. It is often found that the patient feels cheated because the dental restoration does not — and cannot — perfectly replace the natural dentition, either functionally or aesthetically. Whatever the legal implications of an accident may be, the injured person should bear in mind that even when there is a valid entitlement to damages, the dental contract is usually with the patient personally, and consequently it is the patient who is liable in the first instance to pay the dentist. Furthermore, the patient should know that dental restorative procedures and prostheses have a finite life-span; for a young patient, the dental work may have to be repeated three times in a lifetime. This predictable need to replace dental prostheses or to repeat restorative procedures must be taken into account when a claim for damages is formulated. Systems of accident compensation vary in different societies and change with time and political mutations; it is imperative, in all forms of rehabilitation, to know how costs will be met for the individual. This is of particular concern in the case of extensive dental implantology and associated crown and bridge work, where treatment may be very expensive; moreover, as noted above, there is often a need to repeat treatment, or to replace prostheses, at a later date.

OPHTHALMOLOGICAL DISABILITIES

Significance of eye disfigurement

Figure 22.7 illustrates the importance of the eyes as the focus of attention during social interaction. Disfigurements in this region have a significant effect on the victim's interaction with other people, resulting in all the problems discussed in relation to facial disfigurement in general. Adults record difficulty in obtaining jobs and self-consciousness during job interviews. Children are often teased at school and teenagers and adults find their social interactions stressful. Eye disfigurement may result from disturbances of the shape of the globe itself and the eyelids, disturbances in the colour of the eye, disturbances in the clarity of the eye and disturbances in the position of the eye. Each of these can be considered separately. To the lay person the shape of the eye includes the shape of the lids, eyebrow, cheek bone and lashes. Injury to the lids and the orbital bone may produce ugly scarring; in the primary repair of such injuries, attention to detail in anatomical restoration is essential to minimize this. The shape of the pupil is also cosmetically important. Penetrating injuries to the eye, or even planned surgical procedures, may leave the pupil distorted. Many techniques have been described to repair the shape of the pupil surgically; if this is impossible cosmetic contact lenses with a round pupil incorporated into the lens can be used. Blunt injury may produce a permanent traumatic mydriasis which is also cosmetically somewhat disfiguring. A severely injured eye which has poor ciliary body function may become soft and sunken, producing significant cosmetic impairment. The loss of an eye is disfiguring; a good prosthesis is an effective substitute, but lacks the mobility and fixation of a normal eye, though a better simulation of normality is given when the prosthesis is mounted on a coralline implant attached to the extraocular muscles (p. 412). Disturbances of lid function and tear function due to injury and prolonged inflammation will produce a red eye, which in social situations may be embarrassing. The clarity of the cornea may also be disturbed by scarring related to the injury or by alterations in the intraocular pressure as a secondary effect of injury. Inflammation and damage to the corneal endothelium may produce corneal swelling and lack of lustre. In common folklore, the clarity of the eye — its 'brightness' — is often associated with the clarity of the soul, mental brightness and intelligence. The dull, lustreless cornea, which indeed may become opaque and white after severe injury, is therefore cosmetically very disfiguring. Changes in the position of the eye are seen when there has been severe bony injury to the orbit with either displacement

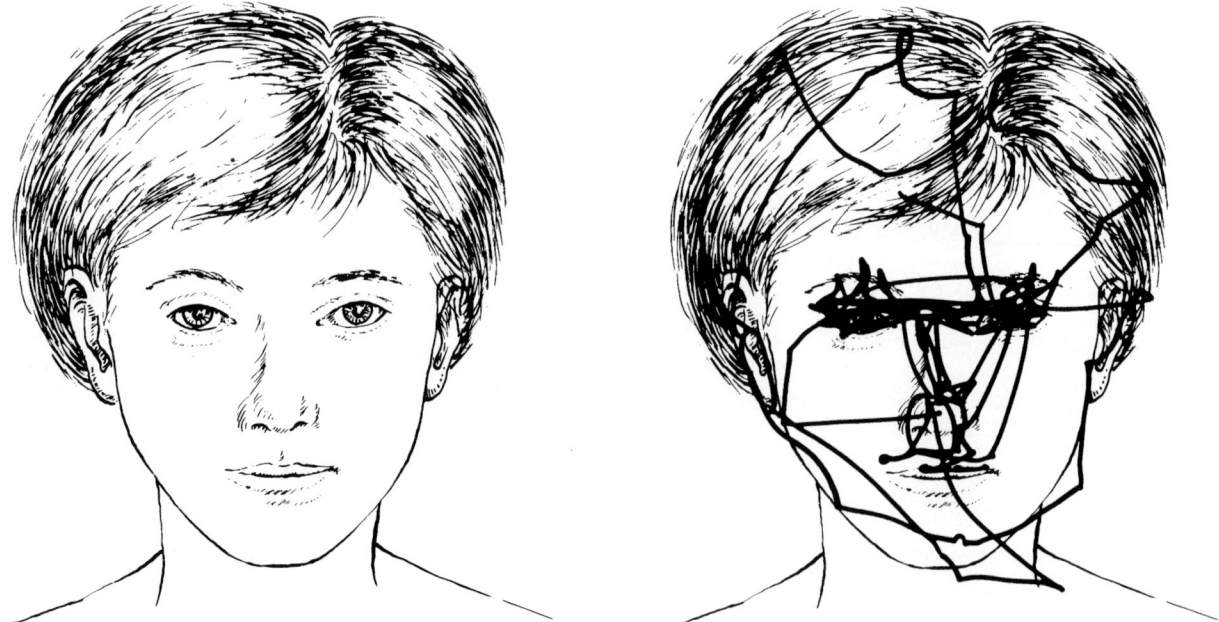

Fig. 22.7 The eyes as a focus of attention. The diagram is created from a photograph of a girl's face. Superimposed on the second picture are the recorded eye movements of a person observing the face. The movements show how much of the time an observer's eyes search the eyes of the person observed. This highlights the importance of the eyes in social interactions. After Feldon & Burde (1987).

of the bones and/or loss and atrophy of intraorbital supportive tissue. The eye may be displaced vertically or horizontally or may appear proptosed or enophthalmic. Enophthalmos is a frequent disfigurement and is very difficult to correct surgically (p. 559). Damage to the extraocular muscles or their nerve supply results in paralytic strabismus which produces further cosmetic impairment.

Significance of visual loss

This varies in degree. There may be only a partial loss of central visual acuity, or a defect of the visual field. A homonymous hemianopia may affect the victim's working capacity, by disturbing the ability to read efficiently and quickly, or by increasing the risks of driving or when using dangerous equipment. Loss of vision in one eye, to the level of no light perception, produces subtle impairments related to the reduced visual field and the loss of three-dimensional depth perception. Bilateral blindness is a rare but most important result of impact in the CMF region. The effects on the individual and on the family are devastating. The victim becomes dependent on others in everyday life, and suffers severe loss of self-esteem. Loss of vision means that car driving is impossible, and in our society this often represents for a man a sense of lost virility; for a breadwinner, it is the loss of the ability to provide for his or her dependants. It is vital to treat such patients with frankness and honesty, as well as with sympathy and empathy.

Significance of diplopia

This is an important complication of injury to the eye and orbit. Diplopia may be monocular or binocular. Monocular diplopia may be psychogenic, but it may also result from corneal scarring, cataract or pupillary damage. Monocular diplopia may often be resolved by refractive correction or by fitting contact lenses with a small pupillary aperture; cataract surgery or corneal grafting may be appropriate in some cases. Binocular diplopia may result from disorders of ocular movement, and may rectifiable by using spectacles with prisms and/or by squint surgery. These rarely give complete relief from double vision. Intractable diplopia may require the use of an eye patch or other form of occlusion. In children below the age of about 8 years, one must constantly be aware of the danger of amblyopic visual loss in such cases (p. 517).

Other visual impairments

Corneal scarring, lens opacities and disturbances of the pupil may cause sensitivity to glare and dazzle, and also photophobia. These complaints are difficult to assess objectively, but are none the less troublesome. An uneven, scarred corneal surface can benefit, both symptomatically and optically, from an appropriate contact lens. Visual impairments due to lens opacities may require lens extraction and a posterior chamber lens implant.

Abnormalities of the pupil, such as permanent mydriasis, are usually masked by the use of tinted spectacles or contact lenses; we have rarely used a coloured contact lens with an artificial pupil. Intractable pain around the eye is an occasional debilitating sequel of CMF injury; it may result from intraocular inflammatory changes, especially when secondary glaucoma has followed a retinal detachment, ischaemia and neovascularization. Chronic uveitis is a less common cause. Pain arising from the surface of a damaged eye can be diagnosed by the application of topical anaesthetic drops; relief of pain indicates a surface cause. Chronic pain from an intraocular lesion is sometimes relieved by retrobulbar injections of alcohol; when the painful eye is blind, enucleation will usually give more satisfaction in the long term. However, full assessment by a pain clinic is advisable before these procedures are recommended, especially if there is no obvious ocular cause for the pain.

Visual impairments from cortical injury

These are very unusual after CMF impacts, in which the frontal lobes commonly take the brunt, and the parietal and occipital lobes are rarely involved. However, disorders of visual and spatial perception may occasionally be seen, and these can take very complex forms. Newcombe (1987) has discussed the evaluation of these impairments, and remedial strategies are outlined by Sohlberg & Mateer (1989). Cerebral injuries may also produce intolerance of light.

Incidence

Visual impairment is often seen as a permanent disability after impacts in the upper third of the face, either as a result of direct injury of the globe or from damage to the optic nerve or chiasm (p. 422). In our series of 237 anterior fossa fractures, there were 27 (11.4%) cases with major visual impairments and six (2.5%) of these were blind.

Management

When there is significant loss of sight, visual rehabilitation starts immediately, with appropriate training in mobility and emotional and psychological support. Family members need to be counselled so that they understand the problems that the victim and the family will face; they should be given roles in the process of rehabilitation. In counselling, it is worth pointing out that very few people are totally blind to the point that they can see nothing — that they live in complete blackness. This is often a misconception in the mind of the patient and the family. It is also worth saying that children adapt very well to visual impairments, and constantly surprise us by their ability to use their remaining vision. Referral to a specialist visual rehabilitation centre should be undertaken as soon as possible.

During the immediate post-traumatic period, only the more obvious ocular and neuro-ophthalmic problems will be detected. It often happens that problems such as disorders of ocular motility, visual fusion, and field defects become apparent during the convalescent period after discharge from the acute trauma centre. Thus, for example, a fourth nerve paresis will only become apparent to the trauma victim once he is up and walking, and needing to look down to see where he is going, or to see what he is eating and reading. The management of diplopia has been discussed in Chapter 14. It has been our experience that homonymous field defects, particularly those in the superior quadrants, are only detected on routine field screening, the patient being usually unaware of the defect. Patients who have traumatic loss of central vision in one or both eyes or who have acquired homonymous visual field defects, will benefit from visual rehabilitation; and most large cities have organizations that specialize in these areas, for example Guide Dogs for the Blind. In similar fashion, referral to such agencies as schools for the visually handicapped, societies for the visually impaired and so on, will be beneficial. Patients with central scotomata resulting from loss of central vision benefit from the use of low visual aids: there is a variety of magnifiers, from simple stand-held video cameras which enlarge films on visual display screens, to binocular or monocular telescopes. Patients with tunnel vision due to loss of peripheral fields (usually due to occipital cortical damage) benefit from the use of reversed miniature telescopes wherein a greatly enlarged field of vision is obtained although it is minified. We have not found that patients with homonymous field defects benefit sufficiently from the placing of prisms over their blind hemi-fields to justify their use.

Driving

Persisting visual handicaps often lead to the loss of a driver's licence and this leads to lowering of the morale and loss of personal self-esteem, particularly in the young. In South Australia it is mandatory to notify the licencing authorities when a patient no longer fulfils the visual and medical requirements for holding a driver's licence. Once adaptation has occurred however, the authorities view such patients with sympathy and many can regain their licences once they have been rehabilitated and had driver retraining and satisfactory reassessment. Patients who are no longer able to drive a motor car are sometimes relicenced to drive low-powered motor bikes.

EAR, NOSE AND THROAT DISABILITIES

Otological disabilities after injury in the CMF region are usually due to damage to the inner ear. Common complaints include hearing loss, hearing distortion, tinnitus and vertigo or disequilibrium. Management begins with referral to an otologist at an early stage for assessment and appropriate treatment. Sometimes a remediable cause of hearing loss is found, but for post-traumatic vertigo, one can, as a rule, often give only reassurance and sympathy. Nasal disabilities include obstruction, recurrent rhinosinusitis and loss or distortion of the sense of smell (see above). Again, full investigation is warranted in the hope of finding some remediable cause. Nasal skeletal deformities causing obstruction are usually correctable, but soft-tissue injuries, especially in the vicinity of the anterior nares, are hard to rectify and often leave some degree of airway obstruction. Crusting can be persistent and annoying, especially when the delicate respiratory epithelium near the anterior nares, overlying the septum, is scarred and replaced by squamous epithelium; the loss of efficient mucociliary transport causes drying and crusting of the immobile mucus. Zinc-based ointments and the use of glycerine and bicarbonate drops may be helpful. Crusting, bleeding and whistling noises are caused by nasal septal perforations. Smaller perforations can sometimes be repaired, but often these surgical endeavours fail, when one has to resort to palliative treatment with the same ointments and drops. The insertion of nasal silastic buttons often gives good symptomatic relief. Recurrent sinus disease is usually due to traumatic deformities of the lateral wall of the nose, impairing the ventilation and drainage of the sinuses. Recurrent suppurative sinusitis can usually be eradicated by appropriate surgery.

ASSESSMENT OF IMPAIRMENT AND DISABILITY

Purposes

It is often necessary to estimate, and if possible to quantify, the long-term effects of CMF injuries. In doing so, one must distinguish if possible between objectively verified impairments resulting from structural or functional damage, and the social or vocational disabilities that result from impairments. Disabilities are sometimes less easily verified, and their severity often depends on the personality and the vocation of the injured person. Disability may be assessed holistically, as a measure of employability or ability in the activities of daily living; it is often desirable to rank disabilities in this way for social or epidemiological purposes. Reproducible estimations of both impairments and disabilities are necessary in planning rehabilitation and for vocational guidance; such estimations are also used in research, in longitudinal studies of the recovery process after injury, and in the assessment of the results of therapeutic or social interventions. Reports on impairments and the resulting disabilities may be needed for medicolegal purposes, in claims for personal injury, in connection with work-related injuries, or in insurance claims. In the USA, the American Medical Association (AMA) has published guides to the evaluation of permanent impairments of the various parts of the body: for CMF injuries, the relevant guides are those dealing with the brain and the cranial nerves, the visual system, the ear, nose and throat (including the face) and mental and behavioural disorders (American Medical Association 1990). The guides quantify impairments, which are defined as loss or derangement of a body part or its functions and expressed in percentages of impairment of 'the whole person'. Two or more impairments are combined by a simple formula in which the combined value of two percentage impairments $a\%$ and $b\%$ is given by the formula:

$$\text{Combined impairment} = A + B(1 - A)$$

where A and B are the decimal equivalents of the percentages a and b. Tables are given to facilitate this calculation, which is repeated when more than two impairments must be combined. These guides aim to measure only impairment, arguing that quantifying disability — inability to meet personal, social or occupational demands — is not a medical decision. However, some of the guides do rate impairments on estimates of disability in daily living or social intercourse. We have not used this system of assessment, except in a modified form, to evaluate visual impairments. Instead, we have preferred to evaluate specific functions by quantitative tests wherever possible, making value judgements on the total disability in the light of the objective findings and the subjective belief of the individual, and taking into account the employment and vocation before injury.

Facial disfigurement

Scars should be described and measured, and mention should be made of the victim's ability to conceal them by cosmetics, hair, a scarf or a veil. Mention should also be made of the effects of injury to the facial muscles and/ or nerves in impairing the normal expressive movements of the face; this will not be evident in a photograph. Deformities should also be described as objectively as possible. The AMA guide grades facial disfigurement in four grades (Table 22.1). This grading is arbitrary in its evaluation of impairments as percentile losses; nevertheless, it does rank facial disfigurements in a logical way. In the USA, damages are often awarded by juries; a grading of this type is no doubt useful in helping a jury

Table 22.1 Facial disfigurement quantified by the American Medical Association (1990) guide

Class 1. Impairment of the whole person: 0–5%
  The facial abnormality is limited to a disorder of cutaneous structures such as visible scars and abnormal pigmentation

Class 2. Impairment of the whole person: 5–10%
  There is loss of supporting structure of part of the face, with or without cutaneous disorder. A depressed cheek, nasal or frontal bone would constitute a class 2 impairment.

Class 3. Impairment of the whole person: 10–15%
  There is absence of a normal anatomical area of the face, e.g. loss of an eye or part of the nose, with a resulting cosmetic deformity.

Class 4. Impairment of the whole person: 15–35%
  Facial disfigurement is so severe that it precludes social acceptance. Massive distortion of normal facial anatomy constitutes a class 4 impairment

to make monetary awards in relation to other awards. In England, most Australian states and many other countries, damages are usually awarded by a judge or tribunal, guided by previous awards in more or less similar cases. One might suppose that the detached wisdom of a judge would produce more predictable awards than the warm empathy of a jury. However, Munkman (1989) says that it is impossible to make any sense or pattern of awards made by British courts in cases of disfigurement. It is of some interest that the British Criminal Injuries Compensation Board has suggested that gender should be taken into account in assessing damages for scars: for comparable injuries, females should receive 55% higher damages than males. In Australia, a judge has criticized gender discrimination of this type, apparently on ideological grounds, but his fellow judges accepted that such discrimination does exist and could affect the feelings of a disfigured woman (Luntz 1990). The findings of Kleck & Strenta (1985), summarized above (p. 652), suggest that this issue should be reconsidered in the light of changing community attitudes to gender discrimination.

Brain injury

The disabilities resulting from brain injury are infinitely diverse, and the design of quantitative measures has received much attention. Jennett & Bond (1975) devised the well-known Glasgow Outcome Scale (GOS) to assess the results of management on the basis of social capability. Among survivors, four categories are recognized:

Vegetative state: the patient is unresponsive and speechless, though showing cycles of sleep and wakefulness, and there are no psychologically meaningful responses.

Severe disability: the patient is dependent for daily existence on other persons.

Moderate disability: the patient is independent with respect to daily living, can travel by public transport, and may work in a sheltered environment, but is usually disabled from his or her former employment.

Good recovery: the patient has resumed normal life and could return to work, though there may be persisting sequelae.

This scale has been widely used in international comparative studies. It has been found that the definitions are not so precise as to avoid divergences in interpretation; nevertheless, the scale has been shown to be an effective measure within neurosurgical units using agreed criteria. In our series of 237 anterior fossa fractures, there were no cases of persistent vegetative survival, 17 (7.2%) cases of severe disabilities, 38 (16.0%) moderate disabilities, and 99 (41.8%) good recoveries; in the remainder, no grading was made, either because follow-up was inadequate, or because the case was assessed before the GOS was introduced. The scale has been used for prognosis, and its authors have found that the ratings show few changes after 6 months (Jennett & Teasdale 1981); however, in making assessments for medicolegal purposes, we believe that a final assessment of a disabling cerebral impairment should not be made until at least 2 years have passed — and in a child the period should be longer (see below). The absence of impairment can usually be asserted sooner. As variants on the GOS categories, different outcome gradings, both more and less precise, have sometimes been considered useful (Jennett & Teasdale 1981). Ben-Yishay et al (1987a) reviewed some 31 published reports on outcome after head injury and noted an absence of uniform criteria for employability. They rated employability on a rather complicated 10-point scale, in which 1 was total unemployability, 2–4 subsidized employability in rising grades of independence, and 5–10 competitive employability in increasing levels of skill. Such global evaluations of functional disability are an essential prelude to an assessment of specific cerebral impairments. In such assessments, an atomistic analysis of the various components of the disability can be undertaken; some impairments are objectively verifiable and can be measured by reproducible tests. The sequelae of a severe brain injury may include:

- Neurophysical impairments: after CMF injuries, these are chiefly in the field of motor function
- Disturbances in speech, receptive and expressive language, mastication and swallowing
- Cognitive impairments
- Impairments in memory
- Behavioural disorders, including impaired insight
- Epilepsy and other episodic disorders.

Motor impairments commonly affect hand function and mobility. Hand–arm performance can be measured; the Purdue pegboard test (see above) has been especially useful, since norms for adults and for children are available. Dynamometry is routinely used to quantify impaired hand grip, and can be used to measure other motor

actions. Impairments in mobility can be described; we have not used the Rivermead Mobility Index (see above), but it appears very practicable. For grading motor power, the British Medical Research Council 0–5 scale — well described by Seddon (1972) — is often used, but this is to be condemned in evaluations of cerebral impairment: the scale was designed for testing peripheral nerve motor function, and is often misleading when used in cases of hemiparesis.

Impaired language function can be graded in many ways, but for practical purposes it is necessary to determine whether the injured person can communicate normally with strangers, with family members only, or not at all. The AMA guide identifies four levels of speech impairment, representing whole-body percentage impairments in the range 0–95%: the criteria for these are not very well defined. We prefer to give a descriptive account, with an explanation of the neurological nature of the impairment: subcortical dysarthrias may cause less disability in communication than speech impairments of dysphasic or dyspraxic type. The disability resulting from a speech impairment has to be related to the vocation of the victim: a singer, newscaster or politician will suffer a more severe handicap than a person not reliant on vocal skills or communicative capacities.

Impairments in cognition and memory can be described and quantified by the tests described in Appendix III. These tests are repeatable over time and give percentage estimates of mental efficiency, but they must be used with great care. In some head injuries, it is possible to give a very misleading impression by quoting, for example, a normal score on the Wechsler scale; to have even limited meaning, the intelligence must be related to the estimated pretraumatic state, and this requires careful evaluation of the school and vocational history and of the social and cultural milieu. A value judgement by an experienced neuropsychologist is essential in the interpretation of quantitative tests of memory and cognition. The well known Rancho Los Amigos scale defines cognitive function in eight levels on the basis of behaviour observed during rehabilitation; it has been used especially in defining progress in recovery from severe head injury in a rehabilitation unit (Diller & Ben-Yishay 1987), but can be employed in definitive evaluations, especially in cases of severe disability.

Disorders of behaviour are often the chief disabilities after impacts in the CMF region. They are often, though not always, associated with lack of insight. In our practice, these disabilities are assessed chiefly by the neuropsychologist and the neurosurgeon, but there is often also a need for psychiatric evaluation, especially when depression is a factor, or where antisocial aspects of the pretraumatic personality have been accentuated by frontal lobe damage. Assessment depends very much on the opinions of family members and workmates, and for these to be reliable, some time must pass before the disability can be determined. It is hard to see how these aspects of a CMF disability can be quantified, though the AMA guide makes a brave attempt to do so in terms of whole-body percentages.

Epilepsy is an important cause of disability and an occasional cause of delayed death after CMF injury. In assessing the significance of post-traumatic seizures, attention should be given to the frequency after the institution of appropriate medication: in general, frequent poorly controlled seizures suggest the likelihood of a permanent epileptic tendency. The seizure severity must be described: How long is the patient incapacitated? Is hospital admission needed? Do injuries result from the fit? Are there side effects of the medication? The social and vocational impact must be described: is employment still possible? Has driving been prohibited? The emotional repercussions may also be important. The AMA guide on the evaluation of epilepsy and other episodic disturbances of neurological function quantifies seizures solely as disabilities in daily living; depending on this, the percentage impairment of the whole person is 5–15% when the interference is slight, 20–45% when moderate, 50–90% when severe and requiring care or confinement, and 95% when causing total incapacity. We have not used this somewhat arbitrary grading.

When epilepsy does occur after CMF injury, a medicolegal evaluation should be deferred until the effects of medication are known. If good control is achieved, it may be appropriate to give a reassuring opinion after two seizure-free years, and perhaps a subsequent period of freedom off medication. If the seizures do recur despite medication, it is probable that a permanent epileptic tendency has been established.

In victims of CMF injury known to be at risk of future seizures (see above), but who have not had any fits, the risk should be mentioned in an evaluation prepared for medicolegal purposes. It has been noted that the risk diminishes after 2 years, but later onset is not by any means unknown and in high-risk (> 20%) cases, a waiting period of 4 years may be appropriate if a once-and-for-all settlement is to be made. In 1982, the UK courts were empowered to make a second assessment of damages if a forecast risk of a condition such as epilepsy should declare itself at a later date (Munkman 1989); in jurisdictions where this is accepted, the responsibility of the medical assessor to advise on the percentage risk of epilepsy becomes much less burdensome. In some Australian courts, an interim award may be made when there is uncertainty over the long-term disabilities.

In assessing impaired cerebral function of any kind, one may use various special investigations to validate a clinical opinion. Brain imaging by CT or preferably MRI scan is used to show evidence of brain damage more or less appropriate to the neurological findings; it should

be emphasized that the absence of such anatomical evidence need not negate clinical findings of impaired function. Similarly, electroencephalography (EEG) may be abnormal in cases of possible post-traumatic epilepsy; however, the EEG is often normal in the presence of overt epilepsy, and a normal EEG should not be given much prognostic significance.

Visual impairments

A full ophthalmological examination is a very exact process and provides data of high scientific content. It is therefore possible to formulate convincing quantitative estimates of visual impairments. The AMA guide on visual impairment lays down a precise method of determining the whole-person impairments due to impairment of near and distant central vision, visual fields, and diplopia. In this, total loss of one eye represents 25% impairment of the visual system and 24% impairment of the whole person; bilateral blindness is — obviously — 100% loss of vision and 85% impairment of the whole person.

The Royal Australian College of Ophthalmologists has issued a simpler guide, and this is reprinted as Appendix IV. We have found it user-friendly. In this system of evaluation, the calculation of percentage disability takes into account the post-traumatic visual acuity level compared with the known or assumed level before injury, the presence or absence of visual field loss and the presence or absence of diplopia. Allowance is made for aphakia or pseudo-phakia (intraocular lens implant). Formulae are given to calculate the percentage impairment of vision, regardless of whether there are single or multiple impairments of the visual apparatus.

There are varying estimates of total blindness. For legal purposes and for pension entitlement, legal blindness may be diagnosed if:

- the visual acuity after correction with suitable lenses is less than 6/60 [20/200] by the Snellen scale, or
- the field of vision in the better eye is constricted to 10° of arc, irrespective of the corrected visual acuity, or
- there is a combination of visual defects resulting in the same degree of visual impairment as that occurring in the above situations.

Impairments of cranial nerve functions

Anosmia is difficult to quantify. Some victims seem unaware of the loss of smell and the virtual loss of taste; others find it a great sensuous deprivation (Elliott 1984); in some vocations, the inability to taste food or to smell dangerous fumes is a significant disability. The AMA guide grades total anosmia as a 3% whole-body impairment, but this arbitrary estimate may have no relation to the actual disability.

Injuries of the motor nerves of the eye and extraocular muscles are quantified as impairments of vision. Injuries of the eighth cranial nerve are usually experienced and measured as loss of hearing, though tinnitus and loss of balance may also be important complaints.

Total paralysis of both trigeminal nerves is a serious disability, but we are not aware that this has been reported as a complication of CMF injury. Unilateral trigeminal paralysis (sometimes seen in crushing head injury), and the much commoner paralyses of peripheral sensory branches, are to varying degrees unpleasant, and may affect vision if the cornea is anaesthetic.

Facial nerve paralyses may complicate skull base fractures (p. 439); if there is no spontaneous recovery after 3 months, the paralysis is likely to be permanent unless nerve repair is possible. Facial paralysis is a significant aesthetic impairment; its functional effects are less troublesome, and can to some extent be ameliorated by partial tarsorrhaphy, muscle transplants and other procedures.

Reduction in life expectancy

CMF injuries may sometimes constitute long-term threats to life, from epilepsy, meningitis or the risks of respiratory infection that may result from neurological or structural damage to the airway. However, it is hard to quantify these dangers in particular cases; in relevant parts of this book, we have set out our experiences and those of others, but it is not possible to give these as actuarial data. The call to do so comes especially when there is a severe brain injury resulting in dependency in activities of daily living, or needing institutional care. The persistent vegetative state is a clearly hazardous condition, and most persons who remain in this state for > 6 months will die, but occasional prolonged survival is known (Braakman et al 1988). The expectation of life has been determined in a large number of World War I brain injuries severe enough to require referral to a special unit, and compared with a cohort of veterans from the same war. Up to the age of 55 years, the annual mortality in the wounded men was the same as that of the control group, but between 55 and 65 years the mortality rate of the brain-injured group was 5.8% greater. It appeared that epilepsy was a significant cause of this reduced life expectancy (Caveness 1976). It is obvious that the life expectancies of men surviving missile brain injuries in the medical conditions of 1914–1918 have very limited bearing on the life expectancies of persons injured in other ways and treated very differently; however, in the absence of better data, this study may be quoted. Also relevant is the Oxford study of severe head injuries by Roberts (1979), though the follow-up period (10–24 years) in shorter.

Medicolegal reports

It is often necessary to describe the impairments listed above, and others which have not been discussed, in the form of a medicolegal report. It is advisable to do this in a standard sequence and format. We begin a report by describing its factual basis. This may be an examination made specifically for medicolegal purposes, or a retrospective review of hospital records and radiographs, or a study of reports prepared by other specialists. Sometimes all these sources of information are available, and this is very desirable, since they are complementary. The views of family members are often necessary, especially in childhood injuries, and the presence of parents, spouses or friends should be noted — unless a request not to do this is made.

The report then gives a succinct account of the accident causing injury, and the chronological course of events thereafter. The age at injury, the previous health, and the previous social status should be listed. Previous injuries should be mentioned, because injuries, especially head injuries, sometimes have a cumulative effect, and because — despite what is sometimes said to the contrary — proneness to accidents is a common phenomenon. The educational record and the job record are described, and also any relevant family history; this is important when epilepsy is a complaint.

The patient is then asked to list and describe his/her present complaints in the order of their perceived importance. Each complaint is dissected and its significance as a disability, whether in work, family life or self-care, is discussed. The patient's own ranking of the complaints is often very revealing. Aesthetic impairments and neurological disabilities that are very obvious to the examiner may have little or no prominence in the mind of the victim; conversely, the complaints may relate to multitudinous problems which are not based on objectively verifiable impairments. Time must be made available to give a sympathetic hearing to all the complaints, and after the patient's catalogue is exhausted, direct questioning should check possible omissions. Each complaint should be discussed with family members, either at the same session or in separate interviews. Spouses and parents are essential witnesses, especially in cases of neuropsychological impairment.

The enquiry is followed by an appropriate physical and/or psychological examination, along the lines set out above in relation to the various impairments. Wherever possible, quantitative estimations of impaired function are made and related to the reported disabilities. The depth and sequence of the examination varies with the examiner's specialty and the nature of the complaint. It may be a waste of time to examine a function which has been or will be assessed by a specialist better qualified in that field, but it is often wise to do so, both to reassure the patient that all complaints are being taken seriously, and because the various impairments in the CMF area often interact in surprising ways. In reporting on the findings of the examination, the sequence should parallel the patient's own sequence of complaints, and objective impairments should be related to the complaints. The findings should be described in simple terms; lawyers are often well versed in medical terminology and jargon, but medicolegal reports will usually be read by the patient, who should not be confused by professional mysteries. Great care should be taken in describing findings which are likely to be wounding to the patient.

The report should state what additional information is needed, whether from records, or from some special procedure such as an EEG or MRI scan. The need and nature of these should be explained to the patient, who is in most circumstances legally entitled to refuse any procedure that is seen as invasive; it is one of the advantages of MRI scanning that it does not entail X-irradiation.

Any need for further treatment should be discussed, and it may be appropriate to forecast the costs. This is especially important in dental impairments, when expensive prostheses with a limited period of usefulness may be needed, and in aesthetic disfigurements. The likely outcome of treatment should be stated frankly; possible complications may be cited, though it is often preferable to mention these only in broad outline and to set aside time for a later interview to explain the risks of the procedure in detail.

Finally the report should give a summary. Some lawyers provide the examiner with a written list of questions for this purpose; these should always be answered as precisely as possible. Where the questions omit some matter of relevance, it should be dealt with separately in the summary. It often happens that the examiner will be unable to answer a question with certainty; it may then be necessary to give an answer on the balance of probabilities. This useful expression does not imply scientific probability: it means 'more likely than not', and in giving such an opinion, the evidence for it should be stated.

The report will almost always have to state whether the impairment, or the consequent disability, is permanent and stable. In some impairments, such as visual loss, a definitive evaluation can often be given relatively early, perhaps even before the rehabilitation process is complete. Aesthetic impairments can be evaluated when treatment is completed and the scars have faded. The recovery from severe cerebral impairments, as has been discussed above, may be prolonged. It is often stated that 'meaningful' cerebral recovery ceases after 2 years; there are many qualifications to this dictum, and in brain-injured children, a definitive estimate of impairment and long-term disability should be deferred until the end of growth and education is in sight. We prefer to make the definitive assessment of a brain-injured child at about 14 years of age, arguing that a longer delay may be psychologically detrimental for the child who is the subject of repeated, sometimes threatening examinations; this belief is unproven but seems reasonable.

The preparation of a medicolegal report raises many ethical and professional issues beyond the scope of this book; these vary in different legal jurisdictions, and they are changing rapidly in many parts of the world. Nevertheless it is still true that the specialist who gives an expert opinion has an overriding obligation to avoid taking a partisan role in an adversarial contest; the report must present the facts, and the facts should not be selected or obscured on behalf of one or other party in the contest. It often happens that the reporting specialist does have a conscious or unconscious bias; this is especially so when it is clear that a favourable financial settlement will help to rehabilitate a disabled person, and promote reconciliation when there is resentment or anger over loss. When this is so, we advise a frank statement of the benefits in rehabilitation and adjustment to be expected from an award financially favourable to the injured person, so that the court or tribunal can take into account this aspect of the case; a surgeon is inevitably biased in favour of an injured person needing help, and if this bias is made evident, then the court will make allowance for it.

REFERENCES

American Medical Association 1990 Guides to the evaluation of permanent impairment, 3rd edn. (Revised) American Medical Association, Chicago

Andreason N J, Norris A S 1972 Long-term adjustment and adaptation mechanisms in severely burned adults. J Nerv Ment Dis 154: 352–362

Argyle M 1983 The psychology of interpersonal behaviour, 4th edn. Penguin, Harmondsworth, Middlesex

Armstrong K K, Sahgal V, Bloch R, Armstrong K J, Heinemann A 1990 Rehabilitation outcomes in patients with posttraumatic epilepsy. Arch Phys Med Rehabil 71: 156–160

Arndt E M, Travis F, Lefebvre A, Niec A, Munro I R 1986 Beauty and the eye of the beholder: social consequences and personal adjustments for facial patients. Br J Plast Surg 39: 81–84

Baddeley A 1988 Working memory. Clarendon Press, Oxford

Bell W E 1985 Orofacial pains. Classification, diagnosis, management, 3rd edn. Year Book Medical Publishers, Chicago

Benson P L, Karabenick S A, Lerner R M 1976 Pretty pleases: the effects of physical attractiveness, race and sex on receiving help. J Exp Social Psychol 12: 409–415

Ben-Yishay Y, Silver S M, Piasetsky E, Rattok J 1987a Relationship between employability and vocational outcome after intensive holistic cognitive rehabilitation. J Head Trauma Rehabil 2: 35–48

Ben-Yishay Y, Piasetsky E B, Rattok J 1987b A systematic method for ameliorating disorders in basic attention. In: Meier M J, Benton A L, Diller L (eds) Neuropsychological rehabilitation. Guilford Press, New York & London

Binder L M 1986 Persisting symptoms after mild head injury: a review of post-concussive symptoms. J Clin Exp Neuropsychol 8: 323–346

Black P, Markowitz R S, Cianci S N 1975 Recovery of motor function after lesions in motor cortex of monkey. In: Outcome of severe damage to the central nervous system. Ciba Foundation Symposium 34 (new series). Elsevier, Amsterdam

Braakman R, Jennett W B, Minderhoud J M 1988 Prognosis of the post-traumatic vegetative state. Acta Neurochir (Wien) 95: 49–52

Bull R, Brooking J 1985 Does marriage influence whether a facially disfigured person is considered physically unattractive? J Psychol 119: 163–167

Bull R, Stevens J 1981 The effects of facial disfigurement on helping behaviour. Ital J Psychol 8: 25–33

Burchiel K J, Johans T J, Ochoa J 1993 The surgical treatment of painful traumatic neuromas. J Neurosurg 78: 714–719

Caveness W F 1974 Etiologic and provocative factors: trauma. In: Vinken P J, Bruyn G W (eds) Handbook of clinical neurology, Vol 15, The epilepsies. North-Holland, Amsterdam, Ch 15

Caveness W F 1976 Sequelae of cranial injury in the armed forces. In: Vinken P J, Bruyn G W (eds) Handbook of clinical neurology, Vol 24, Injuries of the brain and skull, Part II. North-Holland, Amsterdam, Ch 25

Chong-Shan S, Hui-Yun W 1989 Postural and maximum activity in elevators during mandible pre- and post-occlusal splint treatment of temporomandibular joint disturbance syndrome. J Oral Rehabil 16: 155–161

Clark G T, Solburg W K (eds) 1987 Perspectives in temporomandibular joint disorders. Quintessence, Chicago

Collen F M, Wade D T, Robb G F, Bradshaw C M 1991 The Rivermead Mobility Index: a further development of the Rivermead Motor Assessment. Int Disabil Stud 13: 50–54

Craft M, Ismail I A, Krishnamurti D et al 1987 Lithium in the treatment of aggression in mentally handicapped patients. A double-blind trial. Br J Psychiat 150: 685–689

Crovitz H F 1979 Memory retraining in brain-damaged patients: the airplane list. Cortex 15: 131–134

David D J, Bagnall A D 1990 Velopharyngeal incompetence in plastic surgery. In: McCarthy J G (ed) Cleft lip & palate & craniofacial anomalies, Vol 4. Saunders, Philadelphia

Deaton A V, Langman M I 1986 The contribution of psychologists to the treatment of plastic surgery patients. Professional Psychol Res Pract 17: 179–184

Dickey W, Morrow J I 1993 Epilepsy and driving: attitudes and practices among patients attending a seizure clinic. J R Soc Med 86: 566–568

Diller L, Ben-Yishay Y 1987 Outcomes and evidence in neuropsychological rehabilitation after closed head injury. In: Levin H S, Grafman J, Eisenberg H M (eds) Neurobehavioural recovery from head injury. Oxford University Press, New York

Dolan M P, Norton J C 1977 A programmed training technique that uses reinforcement to facilitate acquisition and retention in brain-damaged patients. J Clin Psychol 33: 496–501

Dworkin S F, Truelove E L T, Bonica J J, Sola A 1990 Facial and head pain caused by myofascial and temporomandibular disorders. In: Bonica J J (ed) The management of pain. Lea & Febiger, Philadelphia

Eady M J, Tyrer J H 1989 Anticonvulsant therapy, 2nd edn. Churchill Livingstone, Edinburgh

Eames P, Wood R H 1985 Rehabilitation after severe brain injury: a follow-up study of a behaviour modification approach. J Neurol Neurosurg Psychiat 48: 613–619

Elliot B 1984 Lost bouquets. In: Potter J M, Briggs M (eds) The practical management of head injuries, 4th edn. Lloyd-Luke, London

Feldon S E, Burde R A 1987 The extraocular muscles. In: Moses R A, Hart W M Jr (eds) Adler's physiology of the eye, 8th edn. Mosby, St Louis, Ch 5.2, p 163

Gainotti G 1972 Emotional behaviour and hemispheric side of lesion. Cortex 8: 41–55

Gardner R A, Broman M 1982 The Purdue Pegboard Test: normative data on 1334 school children. J Clin Child Psychol 8: 156–162

Gloss D S, Wardle M G 1982 Reliability and validity of American Medical Association's guides to permanent impairment. J Am Med Assoc 248: 2292–2296

Golding-Wood D G, Brookes G B 1991 Post-traumatic external nasal neuralgia — an often missed cause of facial pain? Postgrad Med J 67: 55–56

Gronwall D, Wrightson P 1974 Delayed recovery of intellectual function after minor head injury. Lancet 2: 605–609

Gronwall D, Wrightson P, Waddell P 1990 Head injury: the facts. A guide for families and care-givers. Oxford University Press, Oxford

Harris J 1984 Methods of improving memory. In: Wilson B, Moffat N (eds) Clinical management of memory problems. Croom Helm, London

Hill C 1985 Psychosocial adjustment of adult burns patients: is it more difficult for people with visible scars? Br J Occupat Ther 48: 281–283

Hill R D, Sheikh J I, Yesavage J A 1988 Pretraining enhances mnemonic training in elderly adults. Exp Aging Res 14: 207–211

Hill-Beuf A, Porter J D 1984 Children coping with impaired appearance: social and psychologic influences. Gen Hosp Psychiat 6: 294–301

Jaffe P G, Katz A N 1975 Attenuating anterograde amnesia in Korsakoff's psychosis. J Abnorm Psychol 84: 559–562

Jennett B 1975 Epilepsy after non-missile injuries. Heinemann, London

Jennett B, Bond M 1975 Assessment of outcome after severe head injury. A practical scale. Lancet 1: 480–484

Jennett B, Teasdale G 1981 Management of head injuries. Davis, Philadelphia

Kleck R E, Strenta A C 1985 Gender and responses to disfigurement in self and others. J Soc Clin Psychol 3: 257–267

Koster M E, Bergsma J 1990 Problems and coping behaviour of facial cancer patients. Soc Sci Med 30: 569–578

Krebs D, Adinolfi A A 1975 Physical attractiveness, social relations and personality style. J Pers Soc Psychol 31: 245–253

Kurlychek R T 1984 Use of a digital alarm chronograph as a memory aid in early dementia. Clin Gerontol 1: 93–94

Lansdown R, Lloyd J, Hunter J 1991 Facial deformity in childhood: severity and psychological adjustment. Child Care Health Dev 17: 165–171

Lees-Haley P 1987 Disfigurement and economic loss: how cosmetic injuries impair earning capacity. Trial 23: 64–68

Lefebvre A M, Arndt E M 1988 Working with facially disfigured children: a challenge in prevention. Can J Psychiat 33: 453–458

Lefebvre A, Barclay S 1982 Psychosocial impact of craniofacial deformities before and after reconstructive surgery. Can J Psychiat 27: 579–584

Leftoff S 1981 Learning functions of unilaterally brain damaged patients for serially and randomly ordered stimulus material. J Clin Neuropsychol 3: 301–313

Levin H S, Williams D H, Eisenberg H M, High W M, Guinto F C 1992 Serial MRI and neurobehavioural findings after mild to moderate head injury. J Neurol Neurosurg Psychiat 55: 255–262

Lewin W 1954 Cerebrospinal fluid rhinorrhoea in closed head injuries. Br J Surg 42: 1–18

Lishman W A 1968 Brain damage in relation to psychiatric disability after head injury. Br J Psychiat 114: 373–410

Long D, DeVault S 1990 Disfigurement and adolescent development: exacerbating factors in personal injury. American College of Forensic Psychology Sixth Annual Symposium in Forensic Psychology (1990, Las Vegas, Nevada). Am J Forens Psychol 8: 3–14

Luntz H 1990 Assessment of damages for personal injury and death, 3rd edn. Butterworth, Sydney

McCarty D L 1980 Investigation of a visual imagery mnemonic device for acquiring face-name associations. J Exp Psychol (Hum Learn) 6: 145–155

MacGregor F C 1990 Facial disfigurement: problems and management of social interaction and implications for mental health. Aesthet Plast Surg 14: 249–257

Malec J F, Smigielski J S, DePompolo R W, Thompson J M 1993 Outcome evaluation and prediction in comprehensive-integrated post-acute outpatient rehabilitation programme. Brain Inj 7: 15–29

Miller H 1961 Accident neurosis. Br Med J 1: 919–925

Munkman J 1989 Damages for personal injury and death, 8th edn. Butterworths, London

Newcombe F 1987 Psychometric and behavioural evidence: scope, limitations, and ecological validity. In: Levin H S, Grafman J, Eisenberg H M (eds) Neurobehavioural recovery from head injury. Oxford University Press, New York, Ch 10

Newton M R, Greenwood R J, Britten K E et al 1992 A study comparing SPECT with CT and MRI after closed head injury. J Neurol Neurosurg Psychiat 55: 92–94

O'Reilly M F, Green G, Braunling-McMorrow D 1990 Self-administered written prompts to teach home accident prevention skills to adults with brain injuries. J Appl Behav Anal 23: 431–446

Patten B M 1972 The ancient art of memory. Usefulness in treatment. Arch Neurol 26: 25–31

Pogrel M A 1987 Letter from California — the wonders of the temporomandibular joint. Br Dent J 163: 207–208

Prigatano G P 1987a Psychiatric aspects of head injury: problem areas and suggested guidelines for research. In: Levin H S, Grafman J, Eisenberg H M (eds) Neurobehavioral recovery from head injury. Oxford University Press, New York, Ch 16

Prigatano G P 1987b In: Meier M J, Benton A L, Diller L (eds) Neuropsychological rehabilitation. Guilford Press, New York & London

Proffit W R 1986 Contemporary orthodontics. Mosby, St Louis

Roberts A H 1979 Severe accidental head injury. An assessment of long-term prognosis. Macmillan, London

Rodin M, Price J, Sanchez F, McElligot S 1989 Derogation, exclusion, and unfair treatment of persons with social flaws: controllability of stigma and the attribution of prejudice. Pers Soc Psychol Bull 15: 439–451

Roediger H L 1980 The effectiveness of four mnemonics in ordering recall. J Exp Psychol (Hum Learn) 6: 558–567

Ruckdeschel-Hibbard M, Gordon W A, Egelko S, Langer K 1987 Issues in the diagnosis and cognitive therapy of depression in brain-damaged individuals. In: Freeman A, Greenwood V B (eds) Cognitive therapy: applications in psychiatric and medical settings. Human Sciences Press, New York, pp 183–198

Rumsey N, Bull R 1986 The effects of facial disfigurement on social interaction. Hum Learn J Pract Res Applcns 5: 203–208

Russell W R, Whitty C W M 1952 Studies in traumatic epilepsy. 1. Factors influencing the incidence of epilepsy after brain wounds. J Neurol Neurosurg Psychiat 15: 93–98

Rutherford W H, Merrett J D, McDonald J R 1977 Sequelae of concussion caused by minor head injury. Lancet 1: 1–4

Salazar A M, Jabbari B, Vance S C, Grafman J, Amin D, Dillon J D 1985 Epilepsy after pentrating head injury. 1 Clinical correlates: a report of the Vietnam head injury study. Neurology 35: 1406–1414

Schacter D L, Glisky E L 1986 Restoration, alleviation and the acquisition of domain-specific knowledge. In: Uzzell B P, Gross Y (eds) Clinical neuropsychology of intervention. Martinus Nijhoff, Boston

Schumann N P, Zwiener U, Nebrich A 1988 Personality and quantified neuromuscular activity of the masticatory system in patients with temporomandibular joint dysfunction. J Oral Rehabil 15: 35–47

Seddon H 1972 Surgical disorders of the peripheral nerves, 2nd edn. Churchill Livingstone, Edinburgh

Sohlberg M M, Mateer C A 1989 Theory and remediation of visual processing disorders. In: Introduction to cognitive rehabilitation. Guilford Press, New York

Sroufe R, Chaiken A, Cook R, Freeman V 1977 The effects of physical attractiveness on honesty: a socially desirable response. Pers Soc Psychol Bull 3: 59–62

Sumner D 1976 Disturbance of the senses of smell and taste after head injuries. In: Vinken P J, Bruyn G W (eds) Handbook of clinical neurology, Vol 24, Injuries of the brain and skull, Part II. North-Holland, Amsterdam, Ch 1

Sunderland A, Tinson D J, Bradley E L, Fletcher D, Langton Hewer R, Wade D T 1992 Enhanced physical therapy improves recovery of arm function after stroke. A randomised control trial. J Neurol Neurosurg Psychiat 55: 530–535

Tardiff K 1992 The current state of psychiatry in the treatment of violent patients. Arch Gen Psychiatr 49: 493–499

Tiffin J 1968 Purdue Pegboard Examiner Manual. Science Research Associates Inc., Chicago

van der Laan G J, Duinkerke A S H, Luteijn F, van de Poel A C 1988 Role of psychologic and social variables in TMJ pain dysfunction syndrome (PDS) symptoms. Community Dent Oral Epidemiol 16: 274–277

Van der Linden M, Van der Kaa M A 1989 Reorganisation therapy for memory impairments. In: Seron X, Deloche G (eds) Cognitive approaches in neuropsychological rehabilitation. Lawrence Erlbaum, Hove

Varney N R 1988 Prognostic significance of anosmia in patients with closed-head trauma. J Clin Exp Neuropsychol 10: 250–254

Walker A E, Blumer D 1989 The fate of World War II veterans with posttraumatic seizures. Arch Neurol 46: 23–26

Weddell R, Oddy M, Jenkins D 1980 Social adjustment after rehabilitation: A two-year follow-up of patients with severe head injury. Psychol Med 10: 257–263

White J C, Sweet W H 1969 Pain and the neurosurgeon. A forty-year experience. Thomas, Springfield, IL

Wilson B 1987 Rehabilitation of memory. Guilford Press, New York

Wood M M 1982 Behavioural methods in rehabilitation of head injury. In: Dinning T A R, Connelley T J (eds) Head injuries: an integrated approach. Wiley, Brisbane

Wood M M 1986 Brain impairment. In: Remenyi A, King N J (eds) Health care: a behavioural approach. Harcourt Brace Jovanovich, Sydney

Wood M M, Reilly P, David D 1990 Neuropsychological correlates of cranio-facial surgery in trauma patients. J Craniofacial Surg 1: 163–166

Yesavage J A, Jacob R 1984 Effects of relaxation and mnemonics on memory, attention and anxiety in the elderly. Exp Aging Res 10: 211–214

Yesavage J A, Sheikh J, Tanke E D, Hill R 1988 Response to memory training and individual differences in verbal intelligence and state anxiety. Am J Psychiat 145: 636–639

Zasler N D 1992 Advances in neuropharmacological rehabilitation for brain dysfunction. Brain Inj 6: 1–14

Craniomaxillofacial injuries: the wider view

D. J. David   T. Brown

INTRODUCTION

This book sets out a system of management for injuries in the craniomaxillofacial (CMF) region. These often complex injuries have been discussed from the viewpoint of a specialist multidisciplinary craniofacial unit, but we have tried to keep in mind the very different perspective of the general surgeon who must often deal with cases of severe CMF trauma without the resources of a modern Level 1 trauma centre. If we have failed to do full justice to the problems of such surgeons, it is because in our environment the development of long range communications and air retrieval has been very successful in extending the range of the trauma centre (p. 222). We know from discussions with colleagues working elsewhere, and especially colleagues in various developing countries, that it is possible to achieve excellent results in CMF trauma management by methods that to us seem less than ideal.

The concept of the integrated regional trauma service is now generally accepted (p. 26), at least as an ideal. A craniofacial unit providing multidisciplinary treatment for CMF injuries is readily integrated in such a service. If this is done, three closely related themes demand consideration: the organizational basis of the CMF trauma unit, its roles in research, and the educational challenges inherent in the multidisciplinary management of injuries in the CMF region.

ORGANIZATION

This book has team-work as its central theme. The organization of craniofacial teams is based on certain fundamentals. These include:

- the relationship of the team to a wider trauma service

designed to provide life-saving emergency care and specialist care for extracranial injuries
- the inflow of sufficient diagnostic challenges to maintain the skills needed in multidisciplinary assessment
- the availability of all of the disciplines necessary to treat the patient in the short and long term.

The key elements are the clinical team and the clinical focus. The obvious focus for clinicians, especially surgeons, is clinical action: what can be done for the injured person. Particularly attractive are the operative aspects of management, and especially those that involve recent technical advances that can produce even better results for the patient and job satisfaction for the treating team. Conservative policies are never so appealing; the clinical team should therefore have members temperamentally inclined to argue for older techniques or for non-operative management plans when this is appropriate. Improved imaging methods such as three-dimensional computed tomography (3D CT) and magnetic resonance imaging (MRI), wide exposure of the craniofacial skeleton, power saws, titanium mini- and microplates, and microvascular tissue transfer have been discussed in more or less detail in this book. But for those people and communities looking to establish a service for the victims of CMF injuries, wider issues must be considered. How is all this expertise to be made part of a health care system?

As this book is being written (1993/4), new and old models of health care delivery are under review and revision in almost every country in the world. Devotees of the absolutes at both ends of the spectrum — the centralized socialist system at one end and the capitalist free market system at the other — are both trying to assume the best elements of the other system and moving towards the centre; most are driven by desire to control cost and increase efficiency.

Developing countries often find it hard to adopt a suitable model, especially when models evolved in the developed countries are changing so rapidly; we have seen health authorities adopting a system that has been recently rejected or greatly modified by the country in which it was first implemented. This can lead to much saddening waste of scanty resources: for example, to the purchase of complex items of equipment for use in an environment where medical and nursing skills and other support systems do not allow for their effective use. Another example is the focus by health planners on the repair of injuries from vehicular accidents in a rapidly motorizing society without putting in place proven preventive measures such as seat belt legislation or effective alcohol control (p. 89) or providing adequate primary care and transport from the accident site. These issues are well explored in relation to injuries in outback Ghana by Mock et al (1993) and in New Delhi by Colohan et al (1989).

Costs of CMF trauma

In presenting experiences that illustrate the complexity of the restoration of facial integrity after trauma, this book and other similar studies give testimony to the huge cost in human misery, the cost in loss of function and the subsequent cost to the community from permanent disability. This is most obvious in judicial awards that endeavour to cost the lifetime care needed for a child with frontal lobe damage resulting from a vehicular accident, in which payments may have to be made on the assumption of permanent dependency for the term of the child's natural life expectancy. The ongoing cost of dentofacial restoration after complex jaw fractures is also well known. Given that a structured community service is necessary to the delivery of this type of health care, how can it be provided in a cost-effective manner?

Deployment of services for CMF trauma management

The question of population ratio per special unit has always been a vexed one since Tessier (1971) argued that a craniofacial unit treating complex congenital deformities should serve approximately 20 million people. At that time, he saw trauma management as an important but secondary role for such a unit. Munro (1988) considered the appropriate workload for units treating major craniofacial trauma as well as trauma in other parts of the body, on the basis of his long experience in Canada and the USA. He suggested that a regional trauma centre could handle such cases arising from a population of

about 3 million people; the implication of this may be that such a regional team needs a case load of this magnitude to be competent and thus, in managing major trauma well, to reduce the incidence of late traumatic deformities.

The concept of centralized multidisciplinary craniofacial units for complex cases serving distinct populations with a guaranteed work load has been endorsed in principle over and over again (David 1977, Munro 1975, McCarthy 1976). But while the principle remains unchanged, and indeed is central to many health care delivery systems, it is often very hard to achieve. Moreover, a different set of numbers is applicable to units which provide primary treatment of CMF trauma as well as elective treatment of congenital and acquired deformities. The number of units and their interactions should be the subject of constant review. That organization is necessary is a truism, but how it should be achieved in a government system is more difficult.

In our community, it can be hypothesized that a metropolitan area of 2 million people should be served by two to four major hospitals with all specialist disciplines, and that one of these should house a superspecialized craniofacial unit which does the more complex secondary work and takes the lead in teaching and research. This superspecialized central unit should relate to other major hospitals; in such relationships, unifying structures are necessary and these may be:

* Agreed treatment protocols
* Agreed guidelines for transferral of patients between institutions
* Unified medical and paramedical appointments
* Joint undergraduate and postgraduate teaching programmes
* Specialist medical and surgical college or board facilitation of joint rotating training programmes and recognition of these programmes rather than appointments to individual institutions.

Such an ideal is hard enough to achieve in the Australian context, but becomes even more difficult in some emerging communities. Nevertheless, we believe that this ideal is realizable, at least in part, and we have seen impressive moves in this direction in many parts of the world.

Rehabilitation and community support

Considerations of the clinical management of CMF trauma cannot be separated from rehabilitation and its organizational basis. Rehabilitation implies long-term follow-up of patients and measurement of outcomes. The complexity and difficulties in rehabilitation of patients with frontal lobe damage, diminished or absent vision, loss of jaw and tooth function, compromised nasal airway, and changed appearance are discussed in Chapter 22. That clinical

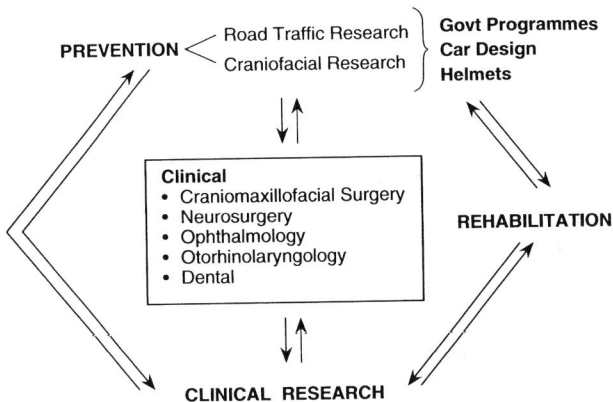

Fig. 23.1 A craniofacial unit providing multidisciplinary treatment for craniomaxillofacial injuries can deal with treatment, research and teaching and be integrated into a wider regional trauma service.

and social systems are necessary to support the long term rehabilitation and care of people thus affected may seem obvious, but the difficulties of meeting these needs are enormous, even in countries with well-established social services.

The person permanently disabled by brain damage has many needs, and the social help available varies greatly; even in affluent nations, health and welfare services may be unable to do much for the victim of traumatic brain injury or gross disfigurement. Murphy et al (1990) concluded that, in London, the vast majority of severely head-injured patients were discharged home to the care of relatives who were then left to cope alone. Family care is seen by most authorities as the ideal, but places an often intolerable burden on parents or spouses; family support groups have been formed in many communities, with variable success. Institutional state care is expensive and often of niggardly quality; it is resented and seems inappropriate except in cases of very severe brain damage. Other alternatives depend on the structure and resources of the society; community care by volunteers is being assessed in many countries.

The patient with significant jaw deformity and subsequent reconstruction may be rehabilitated by surgery, dental prosthetic restoration, and physiotherapy, only to be plunged into a new state of crisis and need for support with the onset of old age and loss of bone and teeth. It may then be that the supporting systems once available in hospital are no longer available. In some developing countries, patients may undergo sophisticated reconstructive treatment with no prospect of effective long-term treatment to accommodate for the ageing process or for changing of dental or facial prostheses: in this setting, consideration must be given to implementing other forms of primary treatment that do not require the long-term social support that will not be available. In planning a

community trauma service, rehabilitation and social support cannot be overlooked.

RESEARCH IN CMF TRAUMA

Research in a trauma unit

The clinical application of knowledge derived from basic and applied research has been an important factor in the development of CMF surgery to its present high status. Craniofacial biology, for example, is a rapidly expanding field of research covering many topics with direct relevance in the diagnosis, immediate care and postoperative evaluation of victims of CMF trauma. These include the longitudinal evaluation of the short- and long-term consequences of trauma and of its management, the investigation of craniofacial morphology and growth, the responses of soft and hard tissues to trauma, tissue responses to implant materials and the quantification of medical images in two and three dimensions. The physical and social sciences also have much to offer: important fields for collaborative research include the design and manufacture of products used in CMF surgery, the application of computer technology to the production of custom prostheses, the improvement of imaging techniques, the causes and prevention of CMF trauma and the social aspects of CMF trauma from the personal, family and community points of view.

Members of a CMF trauma unit should be aware of current research findings in the fields applicable to their work, and able to evaluate them. Ideally, some members of the unit should be involved in research either independently or as a partner in a research team, even though the time available for such activities may be limited. In some instances it may be possible for a CMF unit to engage personnel whose primary duties are in research, although the costs for staff and facilities are likely to be high.

The type of research conducted in a CMF trauma unit will be determined by the backgrounds and expertise of those involved as well as by the facilities available. In some, radiology and the computerization of medical images may form an important research thrust; this is so in our unit. Other units have been more involved in implant design, bioengineering or other aspects of the biological or behavioural sciences. The evaluation and reporting of surgical procedures and their effectiveness should always form a major area of research.

Collaboration

Trauma units usually have affiliations with institutions outside the parent hospitals; fruitful research collaboration can often be established with universities and other tertiary institutions, other local and national hospitals, government research organizations, industry and privately endowed research units. With the ever-increasing cost of research, the trend in funding is towards the successful and productive research team rather than the individual. Important and well-argued proposals may attract adequate funding for a clinical unit to employ a qualified person to pursue a particular research goal; however, research is highly dependent on the expertise of the members involved, and in a small unit the loss of a key research worker may lead to termination of a promising line of enquiry. Consequently it makes good sense to liaise with the research staff of outside bodies to establish a true multidisciplinary approach to specific research challenges. By sharing staff and facilities, this approach is likely to be cost-effective and beneficial to all concerned.

Graduate and postdoctoral programmes in medical, surgical or dental disciplines that include a research component are usually a source of effective assistance, even though the candidates may have a limited time commitment. These candidates, who work under the guidance of an experienced supervisor should be encouraged to present their research progress at regular seminars attended by all members of the CMF trauma unit.

Research staff

Research workers, whether clinical or laboratory, need to establish, refresh and maintain contacts with colleagues working in similar or related fields of interest. Regular presentation of personal research findings at local, national and international meetings, where peer comment is available, is an essential component of good research. From time to time the opportunity to visit or work in other research units, preferably in foreign countries, will arise; these opportunities are very rewarding particularly for the younger researcher. The spread of international computer communications and the widespread use of electronic mail services have simplified the task of maintaining rapid and regular contact with colleagues located in other institutions. Personal computers operated with a modem from home are now in everyday use by researchers to simplify the exchange of information and data.

Research in prevention of CMF injury

It is a truism that prevention of injury is more rewarding than trauma treatment. Road traffic research has generated legislation on traffic speed, alcohol consumption, restraining devices for front seat and rear seat occupants in vehicles, restraining devices for children, helmets for motor and pedal cyclists and the development of various forms of motor car design aimed at injury prevention or mitigation. The enactment of such legislation has been constantly driven by the results of research coupled with

public awareness campaigns, which are necessary to publicize the enactments and obtain the cooperation of the community.

In Australia and many other countries, such campaigns have been generally mounted by government-sponsored health promotion agencies, most obviously in the area of road traffic accidents, for example 'belt up' campaigns. In the USA, grass roots community feeling, exemplified in bodies such as MADD (Mothers Against Drunk Driving) has been a dynamic force, and appears to be changing social patterns in alcohol consumption (Evans 1991). Public education has also been undertaken in other areas where people may be damaged, for example 'safety in the home' campaigns, child protection campaigns, and industrial safety education. Some aspects of these endeavours to prevent injury have been reviewed in Chapter 3; here, it is sufficient to direct attention to the steady fall in the numbers and rates of road deaths in the USA, Australia and other developed countries in recent years (Fig. 3.2).

The technical research behind these advances in injury prevention is complex and beyond the expertise of most members of the multidisciplinary team. Nevertheless, there should be a close relation between clinicians who see trauma and the research workers and designers who may prevent it. Historically, surgeons have been among the leaders in accident prevention; in Chapter 1, the achievements of Hugh Cairns and Elisha Gurdjian (p. 25) were briefly discussed, and they have had many less well known successors. There has been a constant trade-off between the marketability of motor vehicles in respect to speed and design against the ability to make them safe for drivers and pedestrians; this is part of the tension between the safe and the profitable. Helmet design is another area of controversy that involves clinicians, designers and users in a complex debate that is yet to be resolved (p. 111). It is — or should be — the role of clinicians to give warning of changes in accident patterns; the rise in CMF injuries from assault exemplifies this (Levy et al 1993), and it seems likely that the sociology of crime will be an area for multidisciplinary research in the near future (p. 93).

Research and audit in clinical practice

Whatever the framework of practice, the CMF team should feed back to research workers in the following areas:

1. The measurement of outcomes, both physical and psychological
2. The development of therapeutic techniques.

In measuring and evaluating the outcomes of treatment, properly conducted audits are essential. Where possible, controlled trials should be used, though it is by no means easy to do this in testing new surgical and medical techniques for the treatment of CMF injury (Miller & Teasdale 1985). For reliable auditing, it is desirable to have one or more team members with training in research and ready to call on a statistician for advice on the design of audits and trials. Auditing the results of treatment and awareness of the outcomes have received new significance in the need for clinicians to respond to governmental demands for specific practice parameters. Throughout the world, health administrators are using case-mix systems as analytical tools in controlling costs and monitoring quality of care. The Diagnosis Related Groups (DRG) system, developed in the Yale School of Management, has been widely used for these purposes in the USA and elsewhere. Difficulties have arisen in applying the system in some surgical specialties (Sanderson et al 1989). The relevance of a case-mix costing system should be studied in the community in which it is to be applied (McKee & Petticrew 1993), and clinical audits should be used for this purpose. Habal (1993) points out the need for craniofacial surgeons to be involved in establishing proper coding systems in measuring outcomes in the multidisciplinary setting.

It is the area of applied research that has had greatest impact on the management of CMF trauma. In our own practice, this has been evident in two fields: most dramatically in the development of 3D CT, and more slowly in the evolution of titanium in facial reconstruction.

Herman & Liu (1979) first described the display of 3D information derived from CT scanning, and the method was introduced to us in the context of craniofacial deformity by David Hemmy in 1980 (Hemmy et al 1983, David et al 1991); it was soon used also in trauma. From this have come extensions in the numerical evaluation of deformity and in the production of prostheses by computer aided design/computer-aided manufacture (CAD/CAM) reconstruction, and in other technical advances described in this book.

This interplay between technological advance and clinical exploitation is also evident in our experience of titanium in CMF surgery. Titanium plates were used in cranioplasty in 1961 at the recommendation of a local industrialist, but the methods of shaping and contouring remained primitive until 1977 when the Belfast method of moulding in a high pressure chamber was adopted (Gordon & Blair 1974). In the 1980s titanium miniplates were made for fracture fixation (p. 270) and with increasing experience, more complex implants are being fabricated by casting (p. 554). These developments are enticing for the surgeon, who is offered the use of more and more beautifully crafted titanium plates and screws; there are related implantable devices for securing dentures and other prostheses both intra- and extraoral, metallurgical triumphs which are now part of the craniofacial surgeon's armamentarium. Particularly impressive

are the dimensionally accurate castings made from 3D hard models generated by computer from CT scans.

Basic research offers other possibilities; even transplant surgery may be just around the corner. Growth factors (p. 121) have great promise in the promotion of wound healing; neuroprotective drugs may have roles in promoting recovery after brain injury. But technical advances and therapeutic interventions frequently proceed well in advance of the creation of organizational systems in which they are used and before their ethical implications and cost-benefit ratios have been worked out.

Research and delivery of its benefits

Notwithstanding the exciting achievements that have been made and that will be made in the not too distant future, the exploitation of the technical possibilities remains limited by inability to deliver therapeutic applications to the people in need, and this often expresses deficiencies in organizational structures. With the best will in the world, institutions and governments still struggle with the concept of the integrated multidisciplinary delivery of this type of health care. Moreover, individualistic surgeons are often most reluctant to embrace it, let alone have it imposed on them.

Funding research and development

Research is intended to make new contributions to the body of scientific knowledge; development is the application of established knowledge to improve clinical treatment and to assess its results. Innovative and productive research in CMF trauma requires adequate funding to cover salaries, equipment, materials, publications and other costs involved. Unless privately endowed, a research unit must rely on its parent institution, usually a hospital or university, as well as on external funding bodies to support its activities.

In most countries, government departments concerned with health, education or science offer publicly funded research grants for open competition. Many forms are available: these include project grants for a specific research proposal, large-scale grants to establish and fund research centres, setting-up grants for young researchers, contract grants for a government-determined research priority and training fellowships for graduate and postdoctoral programmes. Competition for such grants is usually intense.

Privately endowed funding bodies will often be interested in proposals for research projects in CMF trauma. It is essential for the leaders of a craniofacial unit or a trauma service to know what sources are available, and how approaches should be made; even if research is not seen as a major commitment, the need to develop new technology will often call for more funding than can be met from normal departmental budgets. It is usually profitable to maintain a list of the many sources of funds available together with their terms and conditions. The art of 'grantsmanship' is a skill that the successful researcher must master, and several texts have been published to assist in reaching this goal (e.g. Margolin 1983).

Today, in the more affluent countries, trauma research receives financial support from many sources. These include:

- National institutions committed specifically to support research, such as the National Institutes of Health and Centres for Disease Control in the USA and the Medical Research Council in the UK
- Military establishments
- Health agencies: hospitals and similar institutions committed to patient care, and government departments concerned with trauma in various ways
- Universities and other tertiary educational or professional bodies with research commitments
- Commercial firms — especially the pharmaceutical industry and surgical instrument manufacturers
- Private foundations, trusts and similar endowed bodies.

National research institutions dispose of large sums; applications are usually assessed by very well qualified committees, and success in an application confers prestige that will often generate further funds from less exalted sources. It has been said that research in trauma management tends to have low priority in national health planning. In the USA, it was recently stated that the annual Federal research expenditures relating to trauma care are approximately 5% of those for cancer, heart disease or AIDS (Third National Injury Conference 1992). In the UK, the Medical Research Council (1991/ 92) allotted to trauma research in the broadest sense the large sum of £2 017 000, but this represented only about 1.0% of the annual expenditure of the Council (V. Chandy, personal communication). In Australia, the analogous body is the National Health and Medical Research Council (NH&MRC); in 1992 it funded trauma projects and a trauma research unit with substantial grants. (The epidemiological and neuropathological research reported in Chapters 3–5 was in part funded by the NH&MRC and other governmental agencies.) But as in the UK, these grants represented only about 1% of the year's budget.

Nevertheless, there is reason to believe that this attitude towards trauma research is changing. In the USA, the Centres for Disease Control are playing an important part in funding research in trauma and related fields, and other US government agencies are also active. It has to be said, however, that grants from such bodies are usually made to research workers with good track records, and laboratory studies tend to be favoured, while projects aimed at developing a new technology ordinarily receive funding only if embodied in a valid research project. It is never easy to do this, and still less easy to convince the vigilant assessors that the research is valid.

We have no experience of research funded by the armed forces, but much excellent trauma research has been funded in this way, especially with respect to missile injury. The fields of military interest are necessarily specialized, and at times may raise ethical issues. Nor have we much experience of research or development funded by commercial institutions, though again much excellent research has been done in clinical trials of new pharmaceuticals and similar collaborative projects. In the development of 3D scanning, our work has benefited very substantially from support by Silicon Graphics, General Electric and Toshiba.

Much clinical and laboratory research is done in university departments, and this is surely appropriate. This is one among many reasons which make it very desirable that the Level 1 CMF Trauma Centre should be located in a teaching hospital and closely affiliated with university medical, dental, engineering and other faculties. It is unfortunate that, in times of economic recession, university research budgets are often cut.

Finally, something must be said of the roles of private research foundations. These may have been endowed to promote research in a particular age group, or for victims of specific categories of diseases, or to support a particular hospital or clinic. There are sometimes very specific requirements regarding the age of the applicant, the proposed research and its objectives, and the time frame envisaged. Trauma research and development will often benefit when such a foundation develops a relationship with a clinical group: funds may be made available at relatively short notice, or given for a development project that is not a research project in the strictest sense. Much of our work has been fostered by two such bodies, both founded initially by surgeons concerned by the difficulties encountered in beginning research activities in a new discipline without academic affiliations. For a successful partnership between foundation and research group, the leadership of the research team must have skills in public relations, or must be able to call on such skills; it is also essential for the financial basis of the collaboration to be impeccable and for the activities of the research group to be monitored by an independent research committee responsible to the foundation, and through it to the donors. If these requisites can be provided, and if the research work attracts community support, the outcome can be rewarding both to donors and to research workers.

TRAINING AND QUALIFICATION

Career structures

It goes without saying that the specialists involved in the

management of CMF trauma should have some special training in the area. Each medical and dental discipline provides its own specialty training in which training in trauma is included and upon which further, more specialized training can be superimposed. But specialized training must have a realizable goal. Individual clinicians must always have a special interest in their area of work, but this interest can only be channelled into productive growth if there is an appropriate career path and an employment structure that offers at least adequate remuneration and sufficient job satisfaction. The craniofacial unit and the associated units in neurosurgery and other disciplines should develop such employment structures. Trauma is not an attractive surgical field, and those committed to it should be offered the prospect of a satisfying career.

The craniofacial surgeon

The craniofacial surgeon has a central role in the CMF team. The term 'craniofacial' now forms part of the description of a surgical service in many countries, and substance should be given in the description of this service and the related training programmes. Training for this role has been a controversial issue since the introduction of the craniofacial concept by Tessier in the late 1960s (Tessier 1971). In France, Tessier and his disciples grew out of the tradition of general surgery and its speciality of plastic and reconstructive surgery (p. 26). There were at that time other models for the new subspecialty that emerged from Tessier's concept. In Germany there were already maxillofacial surgeons, trained both in surgery and dentistry, and this development owed much to the leadership of Martin Wassmund (1892–1956). In some other European countries, there were stomatologists, medical specialists with dental training. In the UK, there were plastic surgeons with no formal training in dentistry who performed maxillofacial procedures, and oral surgeons some with only a dental qualification and some with both dental and medical degrees; from this situation, British maxillofacial surgery evolved into a complex surgical discipline with a strong dental background (Poswillo 1977).

In the USA, there were plastic surgeons who performed maxillofacial surgery and have latterly engaged in craniofacial surgery, and there were maxillofacial surgeons with both dental and medical degrees. Today, US craniofacial surgery exemplifies these traditions: some craniofacial work is done from a dental background, other maxillofacial surgeons proceed from a medical and dental background, and others from a purely surgical background. In all three, the scope of practice is subject to the checks and balances that prevail in countries with a lively medicolegal arena. Wolfe (1993) has given a historical view of US experience. Maxillofacial surgery began informally

in that country in 1923, when an American Association of Oral and Plastic Surgeons was formed. Both dentistry and medicine were recognized in training and in qualification. Wolfe suggested that training in craniofacial surgery should include special dental components of instruction, formally organized by dental schools. This view has long been held by many in Australasia, and would provide an excellent link between dentistry and medicine, parallel with the current provision of training in medicine for dentally based oral surgeons. In both approaches, the aim would be to bring dental and medical specialties closer together.

In the past 20 years, much time and effort has been expended in designing training courses for craniofacial surgeons and maxillofacial surgeons. These efforts continue as we write this book. The tendency to train one surgeon to do all things has been replaced by training a particular type of surgeon who works within a team of other people who do other things.

This conceptual change is very relevant in the organization of CMF trauma services. Craniofacial surgery as a plastic surgical discipline arose from the elective surgery of malformations and secondarily entered further into the field of trauma. A similar sequence took place in neurotrauma management: neurosurgery began with tumours and only secondarily and reluctantly entered trauma. There has been a different course in oral surgery which entered trauma very early and has moved on to the correction of dentofacial and craniofacial aesthetic deformities.

Each discipline has its own traditions, and these have to be taken into account in the formulation of programmes for craniofacial surgical training by colleges, certifying boards, and specialist societies. These bodies have to match their qualifications with the problems needing to be solved in an area that has expanded very rapidly.

There is an outstanding dilemma for the non-medically qualified oral surgeon who may be called upon to manage a seriously ill patient and feels that he is not armed with the necessary medical background to fill this role. In several leading countries in continental Europe, this dilemma is resolved: both dental and medical qualifications can lead through a general surgical training to a specialized maxillofacial qualification which may now be extended to encompass craniofacial surgery, although to our knowledge that specific add-on is not yet formally established. The European Union now recognizes maxillofacial surgery as a distinct surgical specialty (Wolfe 1993). In the British system (now closely resembling that of other European countries), two of the Royal Colleges have established fellowships in maxillofacial surgery for surgeons who have a dental degree; in these, the emphasis is on surgical training and in future both oral and maxillofacial surgeons will have degrees in medicine and dentistry.

An alternative training in parts of Europe, the UK and the USA is exemplified by the medically trained plastic surgeon who trains according to the guidelines of the International Society of Craniofacial Surgeons as promulgated in 1981. This career was adopted by most of the founding and subsequent members of this organization — now the International Society of Craniofacial Surgery.

At the time of writing, a number of propositions concerning the role and training of craniofacial surgeons are before the American Society of Maxillofacial Surgeons, the American Society of Craniofacial Surgeons and the International Society of Craniofacial Surgery.

It is now recommended that in future the craniofacial surgeon should be broadly competent and should experience an extra 2 years' training in craniofacial surgery on top of Board certified plastic surgical or maxillofacial training. These proposals raise contentious issues. One is the argument that entry into craniofacial surgery should be only from plastic surgery. Another is the argument that craniofacial surgery should be separated from maxillofacial surgery in higher training, on the basis that it entails transcranial procedures. Yet more contention exists on the definition of an adequate and relevant workload for a training programme.

From these fruitful debates have emerged some agreed views that we see as crucial to the role of the craniofacial surgeon in a CMF trauma service:

- additional training is necessary for a craniofacial surgeon
- the emphasis in training should be on the team approach
- the craniofacial surgeon should be trained as a potential team leader
- an adequate dental background is essential
- recognition that craniofacial surgery is intrinsically transcranial but with considerable overlap between craniofacial and maxillofacial surgery
- recognition (Tessier 1971) that trauma is an integral part of the training regimen for a craniofacial surgeon.

The problem of demarcation has bedevilled the delivery of health care since antiquity. This problem appears to have its origin in the concept of exclusivity. Throughout the world, there are today massive problems in the management of CMF trauma. If we accept the principles of team management set out in this book, then the question of who should be the deliverers and what they should know can be addressed, and what the deliverers should do and know will determine who they are. We need to develop some very broad policies that avoid named disciplines and established institutions. A tentative effort to do this is now outlined.

The craniofacial surgeon should be able to manage the facially traumatized patient. He should be able to perform the necessary major surgical procedures on the craniofacial skeleton, but within a team of skilled peers. He should be sufficiently knowledgeable and skilled to have the respect of other team members. He should have a knowledge of the scientific method, and also be aware of the need for quality assurance and quality control (Habal 1993). He should have sufficient administrative skills to be able to organize his team. Common in all this are medical skills, but the superadded expertise necessary to achieve the stated ends is not necessarily embedded in any traditional discipline, whether medical or dental. Therefore, the future craniofacial surgeon could enter the training program from many origins — from maxillofacial surgery, from plastic and reconstructive surgery, from ear, nose and throat surgery, from ophthalmology or neurosurgery — always providing that the medical background is adequate.

Poswillo's seminal paper on the relationship between oral and plastic surgery (Poswillo 1977) gave an excellent historical and philosophical analysis of this complex relationship. He spoke of the dynamism that would produce rapid change and development and in this he was prophetic: that the specialty of plastic surgical and the dental specialties have changed their grounds is now a matter of history. Poswillo quoted Claude Bernard: 'a science that is halted in a system remains stationary, and is isolated, because systematisation is really scientific encystment, and every encysted part of an organism ceases to take part in the organism's general life.' Poswillo warned against those who might attempt to prevent development by oversystematization and restriction, rather than to develop tolerance, intellectual freedom and the skills necessary to work in a team situation.

Trainee orthodontists and maxillofacial surgeons should also have the opportunity to work for a period as members of a craniofacial team and follow all procedures closely from initial examination through the unit's planning meetings to the operative procedure and the postoperative follow-up.

Fellowships in craniofacial surgery

One popular way to gain proficiency in craniofacial surgery is a fellowship, an attachment of an apprenticeship type to a unit which performs an adequate amount of craniofacial surgery. Recent efforts have been made by the International Society of Craniofacial Surgery to recognize such fellowships and it is acknowledged that they should fulfil certain standards. Fellowships range from 6 months to 2 years, the most popular being 1 year fellowships. This method of training may well be a step on the road to the formalization of training in craniofacial surgery (see above) but at the moment there is no way to measure the quality of outcome of the training offered in such programmes. It seems sensible at this stage:

- to define an entry point, namely that the candidate entering such a fellowship should have an adequate surgical background, not necessarily restricted to one discipline

- to accept that the fellowship should be for a sufficient period (we see one year as the minimum)
- to ensure that the content of the training should be identifiable and adequate
- to measure the outcome in terms of some form of assessment and possibly ultimately by examination.

CMF surgery in undergraduate and postgraduate courses

We believe that some contact with modern craniofacial surgery and trauma management should be included in the undergraduate curricula of most health sciences, and especially those of medicine and dentistry. Dental students benefit from the experience of watching members of a craniofacial team working together, particularly if the dentition or jaws are involved and there are disturbances of dental occlusion and normal oral function. Medical students benefit from seeing the work of a very broadly based multidisciplinary team, and especially from hearing the interplay of patient and clinical counsellor.

Trainee surgeons should be aware of the breadth of modern dental materials and restorative procedures and the scope of maxillofacial surgery, orthodontics and other specialties of dentistry by secondment for a period to units specializing in these fields.

A craniofacial unit should be well placed to teach at all levels of the health care curriculum — at the graduate and postgraduate levels and at the various levels of scientific education through programmes for masters and doctoral study. A craniofacial unit with international linkages may be able to design education packages to suit the particular needs of developing communities with respect to varying aspects of the managing of facial trauma. Those who argue that plastic surgery should be the only entry point for craniofacial surgery should consider the diversity of medical structures in the world today. In several developing countries known to us, craniofacial and maxillofacial trauma are major problems. In countries struggling (often with admirable success) to provide health services of all kinds, it could be very damaging if a prestigious national or international organization should demand that only plastic surgeons should enter into this field of expertise; indeed, craniofacial surgeons working in developed countries should be given every encouragement to provide training in their discipline that is appropriate to the needs and wishes of colleagues working in countries where medico-economic conditions are different. The delivery of health care in relation to CMF trauma can be very difficult in developing countries, where such injuries are only one in a wide range of demanding priorities. Specialist resources may be sparse, and training programmes should be structured to produce surgeons with the skills requisite in the real environment. Under such circumstances, we believe that entry into craniofacial surgery can well come from various specialties, given that training is adequate and that the multidisciplinary concept is kept in mind. Collaboration with colleagues in several neighbouring countries has taught us that this is not impossible.

REFERENCES

Colohan A R T, Alves W M, Gross C R et al 1989 Head injury mortality in two centers with different emergency medical services and intensive care. J Neurosurg 71: 202–207

David D J 1977 Craniofacial surgery: the team approach. Aust NZ J Surg 47: 193–198

David D J, Hemmy D C, Cooter R D 1991 Craniofacial deformities. Atlas of three-dimensional reconstruction from computed tomography. Springer, New York, Ch 1

Gordon D S, Blair G A 1974 Titanium cranioplasty. BMJ 2: 478–481

Evans L 1991 Traffic safety and the driver. Van Nostrand Reinhold, New York

Habal M B 1993 Impacts on the future practice of craniofacial surgery (editorial). J Craniofacial Surg 4: 121

Hemmy D C, David D J, Herman G T 1983 Three-dimensional reconstruction of craniofacial deformity using computed tomography. Neurosurgery 13: 534–541

Herman G T, Liu H K 1979 Three dimensional display of human organs from computed tomograms. Comput Graphics Image Processing 9: 1–21

Levy M L, Masri L S, Levy K M et al 1993 Penetrating craniocerebral injury resultant from gunshot wounds: gang-related injury in children and adolescents. Neurosurgery 33: 1018–1025

McCarthy J G 1976 The concept of a craniofacial anomalies centre. Clin Plast Surg 3: 611–620

Margolin J B 1983 The individual's guide to grants. Plenum, New York

McKee M, Petticrew M 1993 Disease Staging — a case-mix system for purchasers? J Publ Hlth Med 15: 25–36

Miller J D, Teasdale G M 1985 Clinical trials for assessing treatment for severe head injury. In: Becker D P, Povlishock J T (eds) Central nervous system trauma status report. National Institute of Neurological and Communicative Disorders and Stroke, Washington, DC, Ch 1

Mock C N, Adzotor K E, Conklin E, Denno D M, Jurkovich G J 1993 Trauma outcomes in the rural developing world: comparison with an urban level 1 trauma center. J Trauma 35: 518–523

Munro I R 1975 Orbito-cranio-facial surgery: the team approach. Plast Reconstr Surg 55: 170–176

Munro I R 1988 Craniofacial surgery: technique and philosophy. Plast Reconstr Surg 81: 970–974

Murphy L D, McMillan T M, Greenwood R J, Brooks D N, Morris J R, Dunn G 1990 Programme development. Services for severely head-injured patients in North London and environs. Brain Inj 4: 95–100

Poswillo D 1977 The relationship between oral and plastic surgery. Br J Plast Surg. 30: 74–80

Sanderson H F, Storey A, Morris D, McNay R A, Robson M P, Loeb J 1989 Evaluation of diagnosis-related groups in the National Health Service. Community Med 11: 269–278

Tessier P 1971 The scope and principles — dangers and limitations — and the need for special training in orbitocranial surgery. In: Hueston J T (ed) Trans 5th Int Cong Plast Reconstr Surg. Butterworth

Third National Injury Conference 1992 Position paper on acute care treatment. J Trauma 32: 130–132

Wolfe S A 1993 Maxillofacial surgery: past, present and future. Plast Reconstr Surg 91: 1334–1336

Standard international units commonly employed in biomechanical studies of impact injury

D. A. Simpson   A. J. McLean

Force

Usually expressed in newtons (N) or kilonewtons (kN).
1 N = force required to give an acceleration of $1 \, \text{m/s}^2$ to a mass of 1 kg.

In the USA force is sometimes expressed in pounds force (lbf).

1 lbf = gravitational effect of 1 lb avoirdupois = approximately 4.45 N.

Pressure

Usually expressed in pascals (Pa) or kilopascals (kP).

1 Pa = pressure of $1 \, \text{N/m}^2$.

In the USA and elsewhere, pressure is often expressed in pounds per square inch (psi); 1 psi = 6.9 kP.

Acceleration

Linear acceleration is usually expressed in m/s^2.

However, it is often more convenient to express acceleration (or deceleration) in terms of the gravitational acceleration (g).

$g = 9.81 \, \text{m/s}^2$.

Angular acceleration is expressed in radians per second: rads/s^2

1 radian (rad) = 57.3°.

Energy

Usually expressed in joules (J).

1 J = work done to displace 1 N by 1 m in direction of force.

In the USA, energy is often expressed in foot pounds force (ft-lbf).

Protocols for examination of craniomaxillofacial injuries by computed tomography. Parameters for the GE Hi Speed Advantage Helical Scanner

A. Abbott   B. Clark

HEAD POSITIONING AND STABILIZATION

Head immobilization

The patient's head is secured within the head holder by straps across the forehead and chin. Straps are not used when soft-tissue superficial detail is to be imaged, as they may distort the anatomy; in such imaging, Micropore® tapes are used. The ears are held in normal position, and not bent forward. A reasonable degree of patient cooperation is essential.

Head alignment

This must be symmetrical: the head must not be rotated. The Frankfort anatomical plane (line joining superior margin of external auditory meatus and infraorbital margin) must be perpendicular to the floor.

SCANNING TECHNIQUE

Axial scans are used in all cases of craniomaxillofacial (CMF) trauma; if possible, coronal scans are also performed in cases of fracture of the facial skeleton. The protocol described here is given only as a guide: in practice, the examination is modified to meet the needs of the individual patient. Four basic procedures are used:

Scanning procedure A: Orbital trauma. This procedure is appropriate in midfacial, orbital blow-out and frontal fractures.
Scanning procedure B: Trauma affecting occlusion. This procedure is appropriate in midfacial and/or mandibular fractures involving the occlusion.

Scanning procedure C: Full facial trauma. This procedure is used for panfacial fractures, and also for extensive soft tissue injuries, burns and facial gunshot wounds. Although the selective procedures A and B are in routine use, this full axial scan from chin to vertex is often performed at the request of the surgeon concerned.
Scanning procedure D: Cerebral trauma. This procedure is used when coexisting cerebral pathology is suspected, or as a baseline investigation for future comparisons.

Scanning procedure A: Orbital trauma

An axial scan using 3.0-mm-thick (3.0/3.0 mm) abutting slices is done from the maxillary teeth to above the orbital roofs. For fine detail 1.0/1.0 mm slices may be obtained. A retrospective scan may be done with 3.0/1.5 mm slices.

A direct coronal scan using 3.0/3.0 mm slices is done through the orbits, with retrospective coronal scans with 3.0/1.5 mm slices.

The parameters are set out in Table II.1; Fig. II.1 shows the extent of the scan.

Scanning procedure B: Trauma affecting occlusion

An axial scan using 3.0/3.0 mm slices is done from chin to above the orbital roofs. For fine detail 1.0/1.0 mm slices may be obtained. A retrospective scan may be done with 3.0/1.5 mm slices.

A direct coronal scan using 3.0/3.0 mm slices is done from the temporomandibular joints to the anterior nasal spine inclusive; a retrospective coronal scan with 3.0/1.5 mm slices may be done.

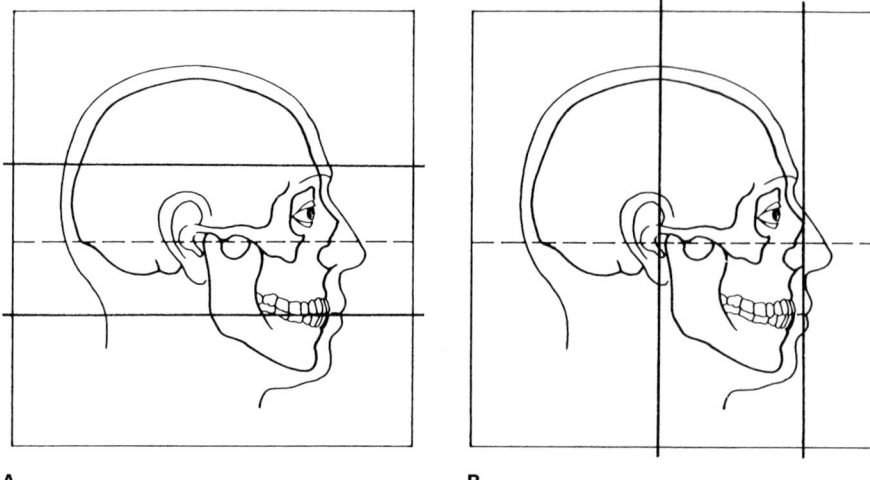

A   B

Fig. II.1 Scanning procedure A (orbital trauma). A The dotted line shows the Frankfort baseline; axial scans cover the area between the solid lines parallel to the baseline. **B** Coronal scans cover the area between the lines perpendicular to the baseline.

Table II.1 Parameters for facial trauma scanning

		Patient age		
		≤ 3 months	≥ 3 months – 16 years	Adult
kV		100	120	120
mA		140	150	170
Field		250 mm		
Slice thickness		3.0 mm (helical pitch 1:1)		
Scan spacing		3.0 mm (produce retrospective axials at 1.5 mm)		
Filter select		Standard algorithm with iterative bone option; bone retrospective if needed		
Patient transport		Chin to vertex		
Patient posture		Supine		
Viewing direction		From feet		
Reconstruction field		250 mm		
Gantry tilt		No tilt to baseline		
Film format		12 images/film		
Axial scans to be filmed		All 3.0 mm slices; 2 slices/frame		
Tissues		Bone < 1 year	Bone > 1 year	Brain (ventricles etc.): photograph every 3rd slice
Window*		1000	2000	320–400
Level*		150	450	40–90

* Hounsfield units.

The parameters are set out in Table II.1; Fig. II.2 shows the extent of the scan.

Scanning procedure C: full facial trauma

As stated above, this is done for panfacial fractures and also when a full scan of the facial soft tissues is required. An axial scan using 3.0/3.0 mm slices is done from chin to vertex; for fine detail 1.0/1.0 mm slices may be obtained. A retrospective scan may be done using 3.0/1.5 mm slices.

A direct coronal scan using 3.0/3.0 mm slices is done from the temporomandibular joints to the anterior nasal spine inclusive, as in scanning procedure B; retrospective coronal scans using 3.0/1.5 mm slices may be done.

The parameters are set out in Table II.1; Fig. II.3 shows the extent of the scan.

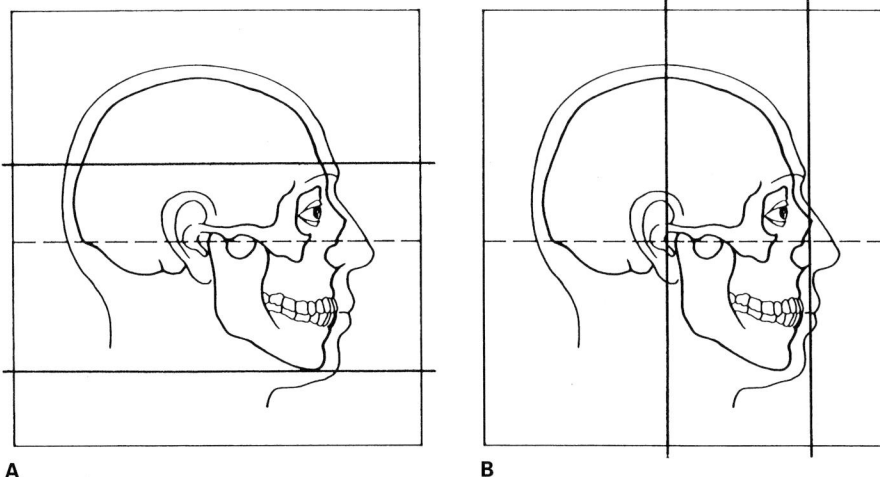

Fig. II.2 Scanning procedure B (trauma involving the occlusion). A Axial scans cover the area between the solid lines parallel to the baseline. **B** Coronal scans cover the area between the lines perpendicular to the baseline.

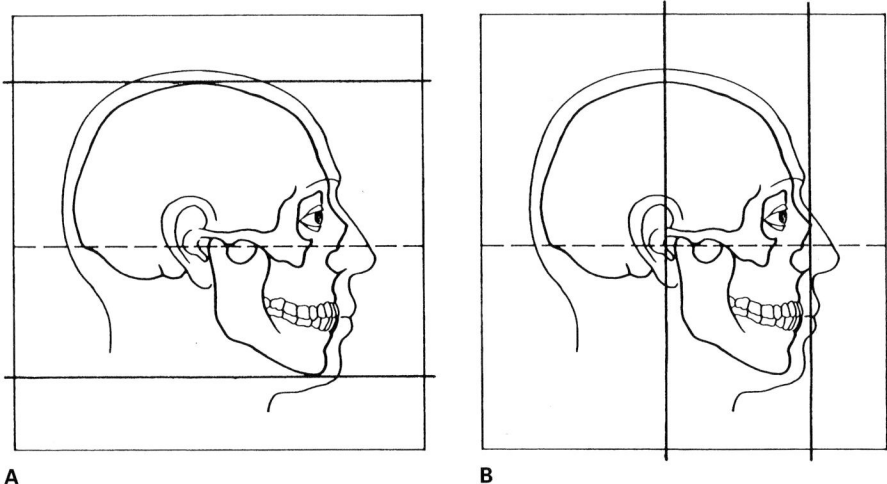

Fig. II.3 Scanning procedure C (full facial trauma). A Axial scans cover the area between the solid lines parallel to the baseline. **B** Coronal scans cover the area between the lines perpendicular to the baseline.

Table II.2 Parameters for reformatting scans

Presentation	As indicated
Pixel thickness	1.5 mm
Window*	
< 1 year	1000
> 1 year	1200
Level*	240 270

*Hounsfield units.

Table II.3 Parameters for 3D bone imaging

Threshold	Bone setting
Volume to reconstruct	Head: all slices
	Subregion: as marked
Axes of rotation	X
	Z
Number of images	12
	12

3D imaging

This may be requested in any case of CMF trauma. The parameters for bone imaging are set out in Table II.3. In addition, we now routinely utilize 3D soft-tissue images of the face and head. Six views are presented: antero-posterior, Waters 30° up, right lateral, bird's eye, Towne's 30° down, and left lateral.

Complete reconstruction

A 3D reconstruction of all slices is used to produce 12

images rotated by 30° increments about both the Z and X axes.

Subregion reconstruction

3D reconstruction of slices from mandible to the supra-orbital ridge superiorly is used routinely; the second most common option is a reconstruction from the mandible to just past the foramen magnum posteriorly. Other subregions may be selected in particular injuries.

Scanning procedure D: cerebral trauma

This is routinely done when intracranial effects of CMF trauma are suspected, or where a baseline record of the cerebral state is needed. Even when the procedure is not done, the state of the brain should always be reviewed when customized facial scans have been made.

For this procedure, the scanning parameters are those in general use for cerebral CT scans. 10 mm slices are obtained in scanning the cerebral hemispheres; 5 mm slices are used for the posterior fossa. Helical scanning is used when the patient is restless, to reduce scan time.

Reformats

These are done in all patients with CMF trauma. Fig. II.4 shows the seven standard reformat planes now in routine use.

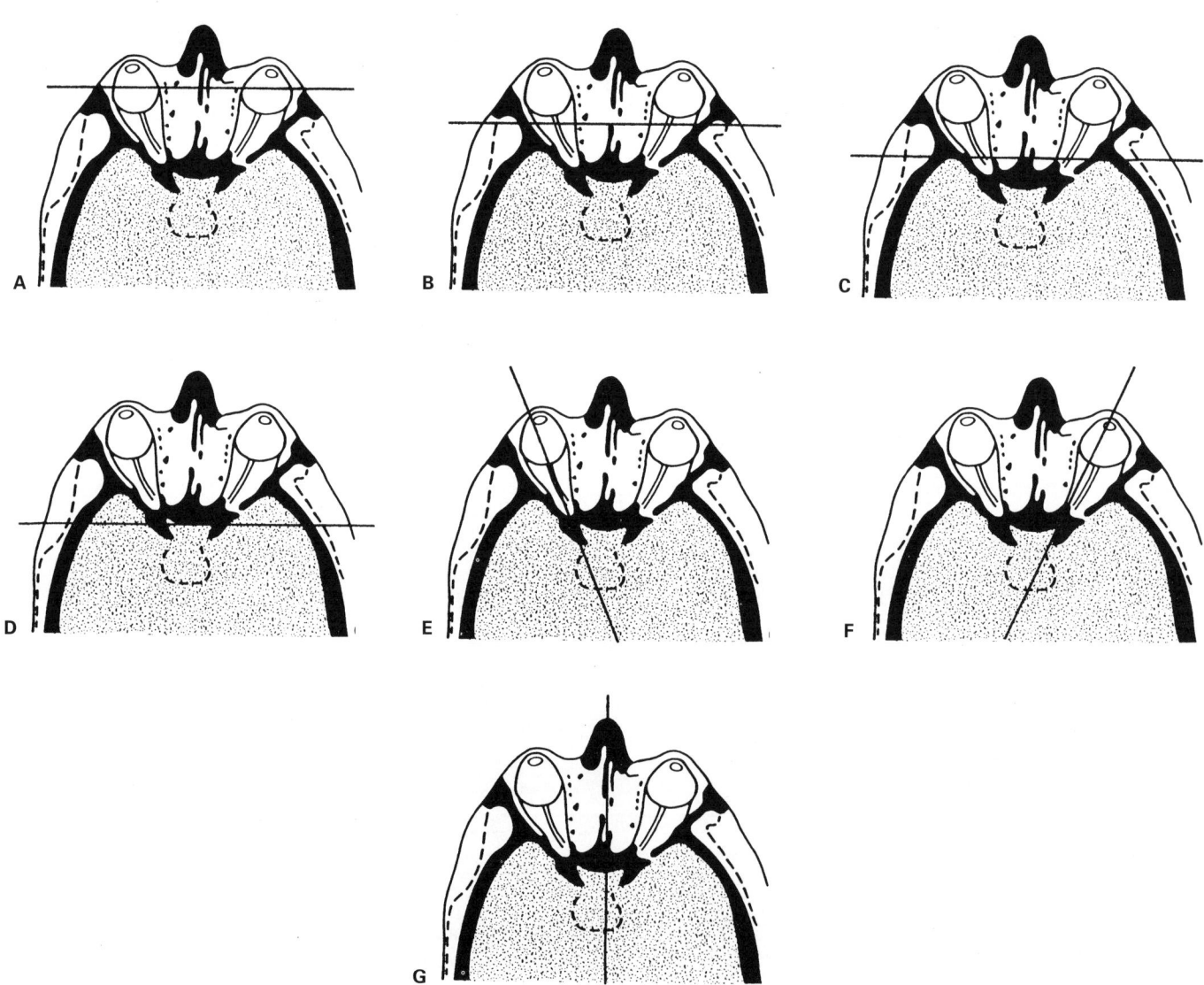

Fig. II.4 Reformatting in facial skeletal trauma. Axial scans in diagrammatic form: a standard reformat plane is indicated in each diagram. The number of reformats requested depends on whether a direct coronal scan was performed, as this may render coronal reformats superfluous. If only an axial scan was done, the following reformats are obtained: **A** through the lateral orbital rim (anterior); **B** through the lateral orbital wall (posterior); **C** through the orbital apex; **D** through the anterior clinoid process; **E** right oblique sagittal through lens and optic foramen; **F** left oblique sagittal through lens and optic foramen; **G** sagittal.

The reformat parameters for the GE Hi Speed Advantage Helical Scanner are set out in Table II.4.

Storage of CT data

In all scans of cases of CMF trauma, the scout films, the prospective axial (3.0/3.0 mm) scan data, and the retrospective axial data (i.e. all slices) are stored on optical discs and on digital data cartridges. For research purposes, selected data are stored on magneto-optical discs, which can be accessed by a remote graphic workstation (p. 187) via a fibre-optic cable.

A daily logbook is kept for all CT scans, in which patient data and related storage media reference numbers are recorded.

Neuropsychological testing

M. Wood   P. Woodroffe

INTRODUCTION

The goal of neuropsychological assessment is to evaluate systematically the cognitive performance of patients suspected of having sustained brain damage by using a series of psychological measures. In patients who have suffered craniomaxillofacial (CMF) trauma, attention must be addressed to the extent to which there has been damage to the frontal lobes of the brain and the associated subcortical structures, with the well-known attendant neuropsychological impairments. Nevertheless, depending upon the severity of the original trauma and the direction and mechanics of the forces, other structures may be affected. It is therefore important to carry out a comprehensive assessment in which the major areas of cognitive and executive functioning are evaluated.

ASSESSMENT IN ADULT LIFE

The comprehensive neuropsychological assessment must consider:

- Speech lateralization
- General intelligence
- Visuoperceptual skills
- Memory
- Spatial skills
- Somatosensory functioning
- Language functioning
- Hippocampal function
- Frontal lobe function
- Motor function
- Attention and concentration.

Premorbid functioning

The initial phase of neuropsychological assessment should focus on obtaining a family, educational and occupational history with supporting documentation where possible. An overall impression can then be gained of the intellectual ability of the individual in relation to academic and occupational achievement. Where injury has occurred in childhood, particularly early childhood, estimates of premorbid functioning are inevitably inexact and family history may then be the only source of information. Several formulae have been derived using sociodemographic data for the prediction of premorbid intellectual assessment in adults (Barona et al 1984).

The ability to define the meanings of words as demonstrated by the Vocabulary subtest from the Wechsler Adult Intelligence Scale — Revised (WAIS—R: Wechsler 1981) has been used as a measure of premorbid intellectual functioning. While this may produce a reasonable approximation, it is affected by educational opportunities and is also vulnerable to the effects of impaired memory, as the response is dependent in part on the ability to recall meanings. An alternative approach is based on the high correlation between intelligence and ability to pronounce words. The National Adult Reading Test (Nelson, 1982) has been found to be a reliable indicator of premorbid functioning, within certain constraints. Actors or those who have training in public speaking produce spuriously high scores and it is obviously inappropriate for use with those who are not native speakers of English. For the vast majority of our population, it provides a very useful measure.

Speech lateralization

Speech lateralization is usually assessed using the handedness questionnaire of Annett (1967) or obtained from asymmetries in dichotic listening (Kimura, 1967).

General intelligence

Most neuropsychological investigations commence with a measure of intelligence and the instrument of choice is usually one of the Wechsler scales. For adults the WAIS—Revised is most commonly used. Special constraints in the testing situation, particularly where there are handicaps such as a speech disorder, lead to the use of other instruments such as Raven's Progressive Matrices (Raven et al 1985), which do not require any other response than pointing by the patient, or the Peabody Picture Vocabulary Test (Revised) which again requires only limited (non-verbal) responses (Dunn & Dunn 1981).

Visuoperceptual functioning

Visual and perceptual skills are complex and can be assessed with a number of measures including the ability to copy the Complex Figure of Rey (1964) and the ability to recognize faces as determined by the test designed by Benton & Van Allen (1968).

Spatial functioning

Spatial functioning refers to the ability of the individual to orientate his or her own body in relation to space. The relevant tests include the Personal Orientation Test, which is based on the work of Semmes et al (1963) who evaluated orientation in personal and extrapersonal space by asking the patient to identify body parts in diagrams. In the version of this test used by us, the patient is asked to:

1. Touch the parts of his/her body named by the examiner
2. Name the body parts touched by the examiner
3. Touch the examiner's body parts named by the examiner
4. Touch his/her body parts in imitation of the examiner.

Right–left orientation is assessed by the Right–Left Body Parts Identification 'Show me' test (Smith 1981); this is part of the Michigan Neuropsychological Test Battery.

Somatosensory awareness

Somatosensory awareness involves a number of distinct measures for which standardization is either unnecessary or for which limited information is available. The extent to which passive movement can be detected is a standard part of the neurological examination. Single-point and two-point discrimination are often evaluated by both neurologist and neuropsychologist; other classical tests for somatosensory awareness include object recognition, identification of figures written on the hand and appreciation of weight differences. These tests can be adapted to test for interhemispheric transfer of sensory information, and thus for the integrity of the corpus callosum; Jeeves et al (1979) list tests used by us for research purposes. However, though the corpus callosum is often injured (p. 139), clinical evidence of disconnection is unusual and we have not used such tests in routine neuropsychological evaluations.

Language functioning

Speech and other forms of language are often disrupted, especially after trauma involving the left cerebral hemisphere. Because of its complex nature there is no single comprehensive measure of language function. Object naming is an important component, and easily tested; the Boston Naming Test is most frequently used (Goodglass & Kaplan 1972; Kaplan et al 1983). Spelling and reading can be assessed by standard age-related tests; the Wide-range Achievement Test (Wilkinson 1993) is applicable in adults as well as school children, and although devised in the USA, has been found useful in other English-speaking countries. The Token Test (Spreen & Benton 1969, Walsh 1978) is a very sensitive test of the disrupted linguistic processes that are at the core of aphasic disabilities. The test is easy to administer and involves a series of oral commands for which the response is either pointing to or moving coloured disks and squares. It may be used in testing residual language comprehension in patients for whom there is concern about their ability to produce a correct response, such as those who have no way of speaking or writing. However, patients in the locked-in state sometimes seen after lesions in the pontomedullary region (pp. 139 and 212) are unable to execute the simple motor reponses needed to perform this test; the locked-in state should be kept in mind in seemingly demented patients, and tests of eye movement may demonstrate considerable preservation of language comprehension.

Memory

One of the oldest and most commonly used combined measure of human memory is the Wechsler Memory Scale (Wechsler 1987), originally published in 1945. Despite numerous criticisms it was used over the ensuing decades until the revised and much improved version was published in 1987. The new version provides measures of attention and concentration and measures of verbal memory for both logically arranged information (passages of prose) and for associative learning. Memory for designs is also assessed by recognition memory, by reproduction of the information and by associative learning for visual information. The test unfortunately omits any measure of memory for faces, and the assessment of attention is for only brief intervals using digit span. No material is included to assess memory for rhythms or melodies, which is an important omission in assessing the effects of right temporal lesions. Nevertheless the test is a landmark in this field, by reason of the careful standardization achieved by the authors and the publishers.

Less often used is the Denman Memory Test, which attempts to overcome some of the limitations of the Wechsler test and does include a memory for faces test and a measure of memory for rhythm and melodies (Denman 1984). The attempt to assess remote memory using symbols and well-known information is contextually dependent on life in the USA and to date has not been adapted and standardized outside that country.

Other tests of memory which are commonly used include the Auditory Verbal Learning Test of Rey (Rey 1964), which consists of 15 unrelated words which are presented over five successive trials. The test produces useful information about learning as well as memory; a helpful adjunct is the measure of the effects of interference on retention of information obtained using a separate, but comparable, list of words.

A variation of this test is the California Verbal Learning Test, which uses a shorter list of words and has been standardized more effectively (Delis et al 1987). A further variant which is gaining increasing popularity because of its excellent construction and validation is the Selective Reminding Test, originally produced by Buschke (1973) but revised by Ruff et al (1988).

Memory for visual information is well assessed by Benton's Visual Retention Test (Benton 1974) in which 10 designs are presented individually for 10 s and then reproduced from memory. The designs increase in level of complexity although, like the visual designs in the Wechsler Memory Scale — Revised, they can be encoded verbally, raising the question of whether they are a pure measure of visual memory.

Attempts to produce pure measures of visual memory have met with varying success. The most commonly used is the Complex Figure of Rey (1964) from which an initial copy is made by the patient. Immediately after its presentation, the patient is required to produce the design from memory and a further reproduction is required at about half an hour later. Most research has found this test to be a good measure of perceptual organization (copy) and of impairment of visual memory.

For patients who are significantly impaired and for whom the above tests prove too taxing, Inglis (1959) produced a paired associate learning task using only three pairs of words. The pairs are repeated in different order, but maintaining the same pairing of words, until all three pairs can be reliably recalled. The procedure lends itself to visual stimuli as well as words and an attempt has been made to produce an equivalent tactile version.

Frontal lobe function

Frontal lobe function has been assessed by measures of attention and concentration, verbal fluency, planning and the capacity to flexibly shift concepts.

The measurement of attention and concentration must address both attention over brief periods, which is usually determined from the ability to recall lists of digits immediately after their presentation, and sustained attention which is recognized as an important deficit in patients who have sustained brain damage, particularly in the frontal regions of the brain. Well-standardized measures of immediate memory span for digits are included in a number of psychological tests including the WAIS—R, the Wechsler Intelligence Scale for Children — Revised (WISC—III; Wechsler 1992) and the Denman Memory Scale. All follow a similar format, usually providing different lists which can be useful for repeated assessments.

Tests of sustained attention are inevitably more arduous for patients. The Paced Auditory Serial Addition Test (PASAT) of Gronwall & Sampson (1974) requires the patient to add sequential pairs of digits. As each new digit is presented, it has to be added to the immediately preceding digit and this total is reported verbally. Thus for five digits there would be four totals. It is important to note that this is not an accumulative total, which would be relatively easy. The time interval between the digits is decreased from 2.8 s successively to 0.8 s, at which stage an average person would produce approximately 20% correct responses. PASAT is a well-designed test although more severely impaired patients often fail to comprehend the basic instructions. It has been used to evaluate the effects of a variety of toxic substances on human performance, including general anaesthetics, but most notably in studies of the evolution and regression of the effects of minor head injury (p. 654).

A recent test of sustained attention which is less taxing has been produced by Ruff et al (1988) and involves the cancellation of specified digits which are randomly embedded in sets of either letters or digits. Only 15 s are permitted for each set before the respondent must move on to the next one. Most patients can easily understand the task and an index of the extent to which attention can be sustained is obtained.

Verbal fluency is also susceptible to the effects of frontal lobe damage, particularly to the left hemisphere. Spoken fluency is assessed using the Controlled Word Association Test (Benton & Hamsher 1978) or in a written form by the Thurstone Test of Verbal Fluency (Milner 1975).

The Wisconsin Card Sorting Test is a widely used test of 'abstract ability' and ability to shift set (Heaton 1981). Performance on this test is particularly sensitive to the effects of frontal lobe damage. The basis for the categorization is shifted without warning after 10 successive correct responses. Some never achieve a single correct sort of the cards. Achievement of four categories is considered to be within normal limits (Berg 1948).

The maze tests were designed to assess planning and foresight, characteristics which are often impaired following frontal lobe damage. The Porteus Maze Test (Porteus 1965) is a paper and pencil test which increases in level of complexity approximating to years of education. The test is particularly sensitive to the effects of brain damage. Other maze tests are reviewed by Walsh (1978, 1985).

The Trail Making Test was originally designed as part of the Army Individual Test Battery, but has been found to provide a useful measure of difficulty in producing conceptual shifts. The task is in two parts (A and B) of which the initial part only requires simple tracking, by joining circled numbers in sequence. The second part involves double tracking, joining letters and numbers in an alternating sequence.

In practice most, but not necessarily all of the above tests are likely to be used, partly because of constraints on time and partly because of duplication of modality. It is common for most of the frontal lobe function tests to be used because of the complexity of that part of the brain.

ASSESSMENT IN CHILDREN

Psychological assessment of the child with a head injury can be of great value in determining the degree of recovery and the residual deficits in cognitive functioning and personal–social adjustment. Deficiencies noted after the child's condition has stabilized can be compared with premorbid performance, although this can usually be estimated only roughly from the developmental history or from school reports. A pattern of diffuse effects is often found in children who have suffered a head injury. Serial assessments over a substantial period of time are important because initial recovery and improvement can be followed by deterioration.

Although many tests are available, depending on the child's age and capability, members of our paediatric neurosurgical rehabilitation service have found the following standard test battery very helpful in children aged 7 years or more:

- General intelligence: the WISC — III, which is the most recent revision (Wechsler 1992).
- Scholastic attainments: the Wide Range Achievement Test (Wilkinson 1993).
- Physical co-ordination: the Stott Test of Motor Impairment (Stott et al 1984).
- Memory: the Wide Range Assessment of Memory and Learning (Sheslow & Adams 1990).
- Neuropsychological functioning: the Halstead–Reitan Neuropsychological Test Battery (Reitan & Wolfson 1985). This battery includes measures of flexibility of thinking, sustained attention, and comparison of one side of the body with the other (hence testing the two cerebral hemispheres). It also examines for aphasias, apraxias and sensory–perceptual disturbances.

Further information on the child's coping is obtainable from parent and teacher ratings of behaviour. The Conners Parent and Teacher Rating Scales (Goyette et al 1978) and the Child Behaviour Checklist (Achenbach & Edelbrock 1983, 1986) are examples of these.

REFERENCES

Achenbach T M, Edelbrock C 1983 Manual for the child behaviour checklist and revised child behaviour profile. VTL University Associates in Psychiatry, Burlington

Achenbach T M, Edelbrock C 1986 Manual for the teacher's report form and teacher's version of the Child Behaviour Profile. VTL University Associates in Psychiatry, Burlington

Annett M 1967 The binomial distribution of right, mixed and left handedness. Q J Exp Psychol 19: 327–333

Barona A, Reynolds C R, Chastain R 1984 A demographically based index of premorbid intelligence for the WAIS—R. J Consult Clin Psychol 52: 885–887

Benton A L 1974 The Revised Benton Visual Retention Test, 4th edn. Psychological Corporation, New York

Benton A L, Hamsher K deS 1978 Multilingual aphasia examination. Manual. University of Iowa, Iowa City

Benton A L, Van Allen M W 1968 Impairment in facial recognition in patients with cerebral disease. Cortex 4: 344–358

Berg E A 1948 A simple objective test for measuring flexibility in thinking. J Gen Psychol 39: 15–22

Buschke H 1973 Selective reminding for analysis of memory and learning. J Verbal Learning Verbal Behav 12: 543–550

Delis D C, Kramer J H, Kaplan E, Ober B A 1987 California Verbal Learning Test. Psychological Corporation. Harcourt Brace Jovanovich, New York

Denman S D 1984 Denman Neuropsychology Memory Scale. Sidney B. Denman, Charleston

Dunn L M, Dunn I M 1981 Peabody picture vocabulary test — revised. Manual for forms L and M. American Guidance Services, Circle Pines

Goodglass H, Kaplan E 1972 The assessment of aphasia and allied disorders. Lea & Febiger, New York

Goyette C, Conners K, Ulrich R 1978 Normative data on revised Conners Parent and Teacher Rating Scales. J Abnorm Child Psychol 6: 221–236

Gronwall D, Sampson A 1976 The psychological effects of concussion. Auckland University Press/Oxford University Press, Auckland

Heaton R K 1981 Wisconsin card sorting test manual. Psychological Assessment Resources. Odessa, Florida

Inglis J 1959 A paired-associate learning test for use with elderly psychiatric patients. J Ment Sci 105: 440–443

Jeeves M A, Simpson D A, Geffen G 1979 Functional consequences of the transcallosal removal of intraventricular tumours. J Neurol Neurosurg Psychiat 42: 134–142

Kaplan E, Goodglass H, Weintraub S 1983 The Boston Naming Test. Lea & Febiger, Philadelphia

Kimura D 1967 Functional asymmetry of the brain in dichotic listening. Cortex 3: 163–178

Milner B 1975 Psychological aspects of focal epilepsy and its neuro surgical management. In: Purpura D P, Penry J K, Walter R D (eds) Neurosurgical management of the epilepsies. Advances in neurology, Vol 8. New York, Raven Press

Nelson H 1982 National Adult Reading Test. National Foundation for Educational Research, Slough

Porteus S D 1965 Porteus Maze Test; fifty years application. Psychological Corporation, New York

Raven J C, Court J H, Raven J 1986 A manual for Raven's progressive matrices and vocabulary scales. H K Lewis, London

Reitan R M, Wolfson D 1985 The Halstead–Reitan Neuropsychological Test Battery. Theory and clinical interpretation. Neurospychology Press, Tucson

Rey A 1964 L'examen clinique en psychologie. Presses Universitaires de France, Paris

Ruff R M, Evans R W, Light R H 1986 Automatic detection vs controlled search: a paper and pencil approach. Percept Mot Skills 62: 407–416

Ruff R M, Light R H, Quayhagen M 1988 Selective reminding tests: A normative study of verbal learning in adults. J Clin Exp Neuropsychol 11: 539–550

Semmes J, Weinstein S, Ghent L, Teuber H-L 1963 Correlates of impaired orientation in personal and extrapersonal space. Brain 86: 747–772

Sheslow D, Adams W 1990 Wide range assessment of memory and learning. Jastak Assessment Systems, Delaware

Smith A 1981 Principles underlying human brain functions in neuropsychological sequelae of different neuropathological processes. In: Filskov S B, Boll T J (eds) Handbook of clinical neuropsychology. Wiley-Interscience, New York

Spreen O, Benton A L 1969 Neurosensory center comprehensive examination for aphasia. Neuropsychological Laboratory, Dept of Psychology, University of Victoria, Victoria, BC

Stott D H, Moyes F A, Henderson S E 1984 Test of motor impairment. Brook Educational Publishing, Guelph, Ontario

Walsh K W 1978 Neuropsychology. A clinical approach. Churchill Livingstone, Edinburgh, Ch 4

Walsh K W 1985 Understanding brain damage. A primer of neuro-psychological evaluation. Churchill Livingstone, Edinburgh, p 235

Wechsler D 1981 Wechsler Adult Intelligence Scale — Revised 1981 Psychological Corporation: Harcourt Brace Jovanovich, New York

Wechsler D 1987 Wechsler Memory Scale — Revised 1987 Psychological Corporation. Harcourt Brace Jovanovich, New York

Wechsler D 1992 Wechsler Intelligence Scale for Children III. Psychological Corporation. Harcourt Brace Jovanovich, New York

Wilkinson G S 1993 Wide Range Achievement Test, 3rd edn (WRAT 3). Wide Range Inc, Wilmington, Delaware

Definition of legal blindness: guidelines for the blind pension in Australia

J. L. Crompton

In 1988, Council of the Royal Australian College of Ophthalmologists endorsed the following guidelines for the Blind Pension:

1. Visual acuity on the Snellen scale after correction with suitable lenses must be less than 6/60 (20/200) in both eyes; or

2. The field of vision in the better eye is constricted to 10° or less of arc irrespective of corrected acuity; or

3. A combination of visual defects resulting in the same degree of visual impairment as that occurring in paragraph 1 or 2.

Index